DENTAL ASSISTING

A COMPREHENSIVE APPROACH

THIRD EDITION

DENTAL ASSISTING
A COMPREHENSIVE APPROACH

THIRD EDITION

Donna J. Phinney, CDA, BA, MEd
Spokane Community College

Judy H. Halstead, CDA, BA
Spokane Community College

DELMAR
CENGAGE Learning™

Australia • Brazil • Japan • Korea • Mexico • Singapore • Spain • United Kingdom • United States

Dental Assisting: A Comprehensive Approach, Third Edition
Donna J. Phinney, Judy H. Halstead

Vice President, Health Care Business Unit: William Brottmiller

Editorial Director: Matthew Kane

Acquisitions Editor: Kalen Conerly

Senior Product Manager: Darcy M. Scelsi

Editorial Assistant: Meaghan O'Brien

Marketing Director: Jennifer McAvey

Marketing Channel Manager: Christopher Manion

Marketing Coordinator: Andrea Eobstel

Technology Director: Laurie Davis

Technology Project Manager: Carolyn Fox

Production Director: Carolyn Miller

Art Director: Jack Pendleton

Content Project Manager: Kenneth McGrath

For product information and technology assistance, contact us at
Cengage Learning Customer & Sales Support, 1-800-354-9706

For permission to use material from this text or product, submit all requests online at **cengage.com/permissions**
Further permissions questions can be emailed to
permissionrequest@cengage.com

Library of Congress Control Number: 2007003672

ISBN-13: 978-1-4180-4873-0

ISBN-10: 1-4180-4873-9

Delmar
Executive Woods
5 Maxwell Drive
Clifton Park, NY 12065
USA

Cengage Learning is a leading provider of customized learning solutions with office locations around the globe, including Singapore, the United Kingdom, Australia, Mexico, Brazil, and Japan. Locate your local office at:
international.cengage.com/region

Cengage Learning products are represented in Canada by Nelson Education, Ltd.

For your lifelong learning solutions, visit **delmar.cengage.com**

Visit our corporate website at **www.cengage.com**

Notice to the Reader

Publisher does not warrant or guarantee any of the products described herein or perform any independent analysis in connection with any of the product information contained herein. Publisher does not assume, and expressly disclaims, any obligation to obtain and include information other than that provided to it by the manufacturer. The reader is expressly warned to consider and adopt all safety precautions that might be indicated by the activities described herein and to avoid all potential hazards. By following the instructions contained herein, the reader willingly assumes all risks in connection with such instructions. The publisher makes no representations or warranties of any kind, including but not limited to, the warranties of fitness for particular purpose or merchantability, nor are any such representations implied with respect to the material set forth herein, and the publisher takes no responsibility with respect to such material. The publisher shall not be liable for any special, consequential, or exemplary damages resulting, in whole or part, from the readers' use of, or reliance upon, this material.

Printed in Canada
2 3 4 5 6 7 11 10 09 08

CONTENTS

SECTION VII
DENTAL SPECIALTIES

SECTION IX
DENTAL PRACTICE MANAGEMENT

Introduction

The world of health care changes rapidly. As we enter the twenty-first century, health care professionals will encounter more challenges than ever before, but with challenge comes opportunity. Job prospects for dental assistants have never been better. The Bureau of Labor Statistics expects employment to grow much faster than average for all occupations through the year 2014. Population growth and greater retention of natural teeth will fuel demands for dental services. As the health care industry requires more work to be done by dentists, the dental assistant will be more valuable and needed than ever before.

As dental assistants, you'll be expected to take on an increasing number of clinical and administrative responsibilities to stay competitive. Now is the time to equip yourselves with the range of skills and competencies you'll need to excel in the field. Now is the time to maximize your potential, to expand your base of knowledge, and to dedicate yourself to becoming the multifaceted dental assistant required in the twenty-first century.

As a dental assisting student, this text and complete learning system, *Dental Assisting: A Comprehensive Approach,* 3rd edition, will guide you on this journey. The result of years of research, writing, and testing, this system is designed to prepare the dental assisting student for Dental Assisting National Board (DANB) certification examination and the workplace. It presents information in a unique manner, using a variety of formats that account for the many ways in which today's students learn.

To receive the full value of *Dental Assisting: A Comprehensive Approach,* 3rd edition, it's important to understand the structure of the text, chapters, and supplements and how they are all integrated into a complete learning system. Together, these materials will make your dental assisting education comprehensive and meaningful, providing you with the skills, knowledge, principles, values, and understanding to excel in your chosen profession into the twenty-first century.

The Learning System

The components of the learning system were developed with today's learner in mind. The authors and Delmar Cengage Learning recognize that students learn in different ways—they read, write, listen, watch, interact, and practice. For this reason, we've created a variety of products learners can use to fully comprehend and retain what they're taught. An instructor's manual ties the components together, making classroom integration easy and fun.

■ The Text

This text delivers comprehensive coverage of dental assisting theory and practice, supported by full-color illustrations and photographs throughout and 146 step-by-step procedures in 9 sections. Section I—*Introduction*—introduces learners to the profession, its history, communication, and legal issues. Section II—*Prevention and Nutrition*—covers general techniques to maintain health and wellness of the oral cavity and the dentition. Section III—*Basic Dental Sciences*—covers the basics of dental anatomy, embryology, histology, tooth morphology, charting, and microbiology, creating a foundation on which learners can move forward to skills training. Section IV—*Preclinical Dental Skills*—prepares students in the areas of infection control, hazardous materials management, patient care, pharmacology, and emergency management, critical elements to the profession. Section V—*Clinical Dental Procedures*—covers chairside assisting, instruments, and the management of pain and anxiety. Section VI—*Dental Radiography*—provides updated information on radiographic techniques and procedures, including the latest on digital radiography. Section VII—*Dental Specialties*—introduces learners to the specialized areas of endodontics, oral maxillofacial surgery, oral pathology, orthodontics, pediatric dentistry, periodontics, fixed prosthodontics, and removable prosthodontics. Section VIII—*Restorative and Laboratory Materials and Techniques*—covers chairside restorative materials and techniques and laboratory and impression materials and techniques. Section IX—*Dental Practice Management*—contains coverage of dental office management, dental computer software, dental insurance, employment portfolios, and legal and ethical considerations, important components for managing a dental practice properly. Advanced Chairside Functions, such as dental dam placement, coronal polishing, and retraction cord placement, have been moved to the individual chapters where that coverage would be provided in states that are teaching expanded functions.

Each textbook comes with **free practice software**. The disk contains over 1,500 exercises that use a variety of formats—multiple choice, short answer, true/false, matching, and concentration—to further reinforce content.

HANDWASHING

GLOVES

MASK AND PROTECTIVE EYEWEAR

BASIC SETUP

EXPANDED FUNCTIONS

LEGAL

SAFETY

TECHNOLOGY

GLOBAL/CULTURAL ISSUES

DANB EXAM COMPONENT

"How to Use this Text" and "How to Use the Practice Software" sections guide instructors and students through the text and software programs, enabling teaching and learning in the best way possible. Appendices and a comprehensive glossary and index are also included.

Chapters include the following pedagogical features:

- Chapter outline
- Specific Instructional Objectives
- Key terms (key terms also appear in color in the text)
- Pronunciation of difficult terms the first time they appear in the text
- Introduction
- Step-by-step procedures with icons indicating handwashing, gloves, mask and protective eyewear, basic setup, and expanded functions
- In-text icons identifying legal, safety, technology, global/cultural issues, and DANB exam components
- Boxed information containing tips and summaries
- Summary
- Case studies
- Web activity boxes
- Review questions, including critical thinking

A second **Skills CD**, optionally available packaged with the text, offers activities that simulate dental assisting skills such as dental charting, tray setup, radiograph mounting, pathology identification, and taking vital signs. These activities give learners a chance to practice and test their understanding of content in the text.

■ INSTRUCTOR'S MANUAL (ORDER #1-4180-4875-5)

The *Instructor's Manual* ties the learning system together, providing the traditional components of course objectives, outlines, answers to text and workbook questions, skills competency checklist sheets to gauge student achievement, and teaching strategies.

■ ELECTRONIC CLASSROOM MANAGER (ORDER #1-4180-4876-3)

An Electronic Classroom Manager (ECM) is available to facilitate classroom preparation, presentation, and testing. Components include a(n):

- Computerized test bank, a 2300-question bank with questions geared to text chapters and the DANB exam
- PowerPoint presentation with talking points, designed to support and facilitate classroom instruction
- Electronic version of the *Instructor's Manual*, so notes and ideas can be customized
- Electronic image library containing files of hundreds of images from the text
- Dental assisting curriculum cross referencing all of Delmar Cengage Learning's dental assisting materials to create a dynamic learning system
- Correlation guide to help make a smooth transition from the second edition to the third edition
- Conversion grids to help make the change from one of our competitor's books to our books
- Additional Handouts on Key Terms Review and additional activities such as crossword puzzles, word searches, matching, and labeling exercises
- Skill checklists to use for student evaluation.

■ STUDENT WORKBOOK (ORDER #1-4180-4874-7)

The workbook, which corresponds to the text, contains chapter objectives, summaries, exercises in a variety of formats, and skill sheets to test competencies.

■ WEB TUTORS

The self-paced Web Tutor modules include chapter objectives, PowerPoint files, quizzes, Web links, critical thinking questions, a discussion board, and video links. Both Web CT (order #1-4180-4878-X) and Blackboard (order #1-4180-4879-8) formats are available.

■ TRANSPARENCIES (ORDER #0-8273-9072-6)

Fifty-four color transparencies support the text concepts.

■ OTHER SUPPORTING MATERIALS INCLUDE:

- Delmar's Dental Assisting Exam Review (Melissa Thibodeaux-Campbell, CDA, RDA, BS)
- Dental Drug Reference (Elena Bablenis Haveles, PharmD)
- Dental Terminology, 2nd Edition (Charline Dofka)
- Dental Office Management (Ellen Dietz, CDA, AAS, BS)
- Dental Assisting Video Series

When you use all these components together, you'll discover an innovative, comprehensive system of teaching and learning that prepares students for success in the twenty-first century.

About the Authors

Donna J. Phinney is the Program Director for Spokane Community College's Dental Assisting Program. She has spent more than 20 years in the dental field as a dental assistant, a dental office consultant, an office manager, and an educator. Donna holds a bachelor of arts from Eastern Washington University, a master in education from Whitworth College, and an associate of science and certificate in dental assisting from Spokane Community College. A certified dental assistant, she is active in the Washington State Dental Assisting Association, where she served as president from 1992–1993. Donna was a consultant for the American Dental Association, Commission on Dental Accreditation for 17 years and was on the Dental Assisting Review Committee, and she was a Commissioner for the American Dental Association, appointed by the American Dental Assistants Association.

Judy H. Halstead is a dental assisting instructor at Spokane Community College. She has more than 20 years' experience teaching and more than 10 years' experience as a dental assistant. She was a program director for dental assisting in a private college and for a high school skills center. Judy holds a bachelor of arts from Eastern Washington University, is a certified dental assistant, and has an expanded functions certificate. She has been a member of local, state, and national Dental Assistants Associations for the past 25 years. She served as president of the Washington State Dental Assisting Association from 1994–1995. Judy has presented lectures and workshops at local, state, and regional dental conferences.

Acknowledgments

The authors would like to thank Delmar Cengage Learning and its staff, whose assistance and encouragement in this pursuit are greatly appreciated.

We would also like to thank the many dentists with whom we have had the opportunity to work and who made dental assisting a career to be proud of.

We would like to thank our peers across the nation, especially the Allied Health Department and staff and friends at Spokane Community College, who encouraged us throughout this endeavor. The students, who in the end make everything worthwhile, are to be thanked for their desire to learn and the ongoing challenge they present to their instructors.

We would like to thank our daughters, Heidi and Traci, who continue to love and support us and who took part in this revision.

Last, but never least, we would like to thank our husbands, Dwayne and Chuck, and our families, who supported and encouraged us throughout this project. Their understanding, patience, and love allowed us to stay on track and to complete the task at hand. Thank you!

We also want to thank the following individuals and facilities for providing valuable assistance in the development and production of this project:

- Pat Norman, CDA, who continues to give so much; we appreciate all her help in obtaining the figures for the text and the many other areas where she picked up the slack for us.

- Julie Davitt, CDA, who supported and encouraged us throughout this project.

- Peg Jacobs Bloy, CDA, RDH, MS, and Middlesex Community College, for the coordination and assistance while allowing us to photograph in their facility.

- Rita Johnson, CDA, COA, RDH, MA, and Dr. Vincent DeAngelis, who provided assistance and many pictures for the text.

- Dr. Clifton Caldwell, who continues to help us with our endeavors both in student education and now in publishing.

- Dr. Dale Ruemping, Dr. Steven Crump, Dr. Ola England, Dr. George Velis, Dr. Gary Shellerud, Dr. Dwight Damond, Dr. Earl Ness, Drs. Rodney Braun and Chris Chaffin, and Dr. Steven Gregg, who continue to help us with student education and provided pictures for the text.

- The reviewers who spent their time and energy to make this a better text.

- Anderson's dental laboratory, for continuing to help us with student education and providing pictures and models for the text.

- Dr. Joseph Konzelman, who provided many pictures for the text.

- Nici Roberts, CDA, who assisted with photos and time.

- Dr. Jay Enzler, pediatric dentist, who allowed us to take numerous photos of his entire pediatric office, including photos of his staff and patients during routine procedures.

- Dr. Charles Rigalotto general and cosmetic dentist and his assistant Judy Miner, for assisting us with numerous photos of his office, equipment, and tray-setups

- Students in the Dental Assisting Class of 2006–2007. With special thanks to Marissa Baker, Danielle Dacar, Nataliya Dubinets, Annali Furgason, Jessica Hisks, Katie Johnson, Stephanie Mueller, Laura Potts, Kristine Smasel, Hong-Van tran, and Amorette Verduin for going the extra mile.

- Dr. Dale Ruemping, pediatric dentist; Dr. Kenji Higuchi oral maxillofacial surgeon; Dr. Steven Crump general dentist, for providing pictures of various procedures and techniques.

- Troy Schmidt, sales representative for KaVo Technologies/Gendex Imaging.

Reviewers of the Third Edition

Valerie Blackenship, CDA, RDA
Program Director
Simi Valley Adult School and Career Institute
Simi Valley, California

Denis Campopiano, CDA, RDH, BS
Dental Assisting Program Director
Ogeechee Technical College
Statesboro, Georgia

Cynthia S. Cronick, CDA, AAS, BS
Dental Assisting Instructor
Southeast Community College
Lincoln, Nebraska

Heidi Denson
Instructor
Ogden Weber Applied Technology
Ogden, Utah

Sharon K. Dickinson, CDA, CDPMA, RDA
Professor
Dental Assisting Program Director
El Paso Community College
El Paso, Texas

Dennis Garcia, DMD, RDA
Curriculum Manager Health Sciences
Corinthian Colleges, Inc.

Linda Kay Hughes, RDA, NRDA
Owner/Educator
PDE/Excelle College
San Diego, California

Paulette Kehm-Yelton, CDA, EFDA, MPA
Assistant Professor
Northeast State Community College
Elizabethton, Tennessee

Vivian Koistinen, ASDA
Corporate Dental Assistant Program Manager
High Tech Institute, Inc.
Phoenix, Arizona

Krista M. Rodriguez, RDH, CDA, BA, NYCDA, FADAA
Assistant Professor
Monroe Community College
Rochester, New York

Stephanie J. Schmidt, CDA, RDAEF, CDI, CDT, BA, MS
Faculty
Pasadena City College
Pasadena, California

Le Ann Schoelne, CDA, RDA, RF, BS
Director Dental Assisting Program
Central Lakes College
Brainerd, Minnesota

Jenny Schuler, CDA, BS
Dental Assistant Instructor/Program Coordinator
Bellingham Technical College
Bellingham, Washington

Lynette Sickelbaugh, CDA
Dental Assisting Instructor
Washington Local Adult Education
Toledo, Ohio

Karen F. Sperry, CDA, RDA, BVE
Professor Emeritus Dental Assisting
College of the Redwoods
Eureka, California

Diana M. Sullivan
Director Dental Assisting Program/Instructor
Dakota County Technical College
Rosemount, Minnesota

Lynn Tyler
Director Dental Assisting Program
The American Institute of Medical-Dental Technology
Provo, Utah

Janet Wilburn, BS, CDA
Director Dental Assisting Program
Phoenix College
Phoenix, Arizona

Pamela G. Zarb, CDA, RDA, RDH, MA
Dental Assisting Program Discipline Chair
Wayne County Community College
Detroit, Michigan

Reviewers of the First and Second Editions

Robert Bennett, DMD
Texas State Technical College
Harlingen, Texas

Robin Caplan, CDA
Medsafe, Inc.
Waltham, Massachusetts

Cindy Cronick, CDA, BS
Southeast Community College
Lincoln, Nebraska

Marie Desmarais Cecil, CDA, MA
Central Community College
Hastings, Nebraska

Betty Ladley Finkbeiner, CDA, RDA, BS, MS
Washtenaw Community College
Ann Arbor, Michigan

Kathy Foust, CDA, MS
Western Wisconsin Technical College
LaCrosse, Wisconsin

Linda Kay Hughes, RDA, NRDA
Excelle College
San Diego, California

Sandra Lo, DDS
Sacramento City College
Sacramento, California

Rebecca Mattney, CDA, RDA
Vatterott College
Springfield, Missouri

Fred Rich
Gwinnett School of Dental Assisting
Lilburn, Georgia

Sheila Semler, CDA, RDH, MS, PhD
San Juan College
Farmington, New Mexico

Kelly Svanda, CDA
Southeast Community College
Lincoln, Nebraska

Susan Thaemert, CDA, RDA, BS
Hennepin Technical College
Minneapolis, Minnesota

Dental assisting is an ever-evolving profession full of opportunity and challenge. *Dental Assisting: A Comprehensive Approach,* 3rd edition, is designed to help you acquire the knowledge, skills, and values necessary to become a successful dental assistant. The text is organized into nine main sections that reflect the broad areas of dental assisting responsibility. These sections are then divided into a total of 37 chapters of related information. The text has many unique features that will make it easier for you to learn and integrate theory and practice, including:

Technology

CD icons indicate when a chapter has corresponding activities on the enclosed Practice CD or optional Skills CD.

Chapter Outline

At the beginning of each chapter is an outline listing the main headings covered in the chapter. Review these headings of topic areas before you study the chapter. They will be a roadmap to the material in the chapter.

Objectives

Learning objectives identify the key information to be gained from the chapter. Use these objectives with the review questions to test your understanding of the chapter's content.

Key Terms

All key terms are listed at the beginning of each chapter. Read the text to understand how the term is used in context; turn to the glossary for the term definition. In the text, the term is always blue boldface at its first occurrence, for easy identification.

Icons

Graphic icons pinpoint information that relates to legal, safety, technology, global or cultural issues, and certified dental assisting (CDA) competencies.

Procedures

Step-by-step procedures give detailed information on dental assisting competencies. Icons at the beginning of procedures indicate which function, instruments, and protective equipment are required for the procedure.

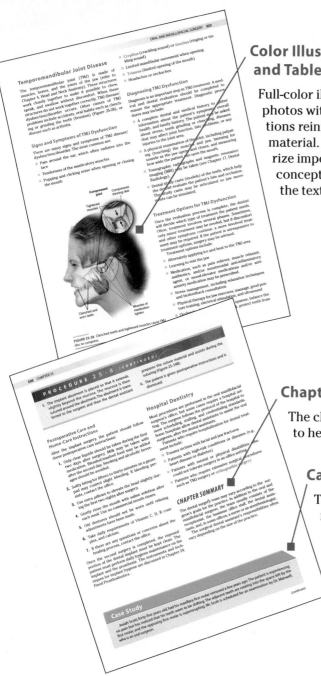

Color Illustrations, Photos, and Tables

Full-color illustrations and photos with detailed captions reinforce chapter material. Tables summarize important facts or concepts presented in the text.

Chapter Summary

The chapter summary emphasizes key concepts from the chapter to help you focus your study.

Case Studies

The case studies and review questions present real-life scenarios requiring a problem/solution approach. Use the case studies to put your knowledge into practice and to arrive at a deeper understanding of the dental assisting profession.

Review Questions

Test your comprehension of the chapter with structured multiple choice questions and open-ended critical thinking questions that require you to combine an understanding of chapter material with your personal insight and judgment.

Web Activities

Internet exercises in each chapter encourage Web searches to locate information.

StudyWARE includes learning activities, quizzes, animations, and video clips to help you study key concepts from *Dental Assisting: A Comprehensive Approach,* 3rd Edition, and to test your comprehension. By using these exercises and games, you'll challenge yourself and other students, making your study of dental assisting more effective and fun.

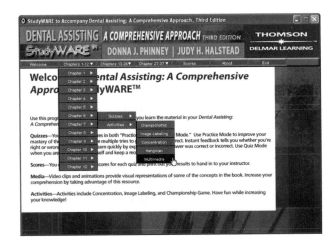

Main Menu

The main menu follows the chapter organization of the book—which makes it easy for you to find your way around. Just click on the button for the chapter you want, then click on the activity that you wish to practice.

Minimum System Requirements

- Operating System: Microsoft Windows 2000, Windows XP, Vista
- Processor: Pentium PC 500 MHz or higher (750 Mhz recommended)
- Memory: 64 MB of RAM (128 MB recommended)
- Screen Resolution: 800 x 600 pixels
- Color Depth: 16-bit color (thousands of colors)
- Macromedia Flash Player 9. The Macromedia Flash Player is free, and can be downloaded from http://www.adobe.com/products/flashplayer/

Installation Instructions

1. Insert disc into CD-ROM drive. The StudyWare™ installation program should start automatically. If it does not, go to step 2.
2. From My Computer, double-click the icon for the CD drive.
3. Double click the *setup.exe* file to start the program.

Technical Support

Telephone: 1-800-648-7450, 8:30 A.M.–5:30 P.M. Eastern Time
Fax: 1-518-881-1247
E-mail: delmar.help@cengage.com
StudyWare™ is a trademark used herein under license.
Microsoft® and Windows® are registered trademarks of the Microsoft Corporation.
Pentium® is a registered trademark of the Intel® Corporation.

Exercises and Activities

StudyWare acts as your own private tutor. For each exercise, it chooses from a bank of over 1500 questions covering all 37 chapters. Putting these exercises to work for you is simple:

- Choose either practice or test mode. You'll encounter a series of questions from the chapter. The questions are generated randomly so you can practice more than once and receive different questions each time.

- Question styles include multiple choice, fill-in-the-blank, matching, and true/false.

- Instant feedback in practice mode tells you whether you are right or wrong—and helps you learn quickly by explaining why the answer is correct or incorrect.

- Your test scores are saved and can be reviewed to determine the questions you missed.

Fun and Games

- Championship Game—a jeopardy-style quiz game that can be player solo or with a partner.

- Concentration—match terms and key concepts to their corresponding definitions or descriptions.

- Hangman—Review spelling and vocabulary by choosing the correct letters to spell dental words appropriate to the chapter.

- Media—Review video clips and animations to reinforce comprehension of the concepts discussed within the chapters.

Dental Assisting Interactive Skills and Procedures Software has been designed to help you practice essential dental assisting skills covered in *Dental Assisting: A Comprehensive Approach,* 3rd edition. In these interactive exercises you will read patient profiles and then take blood pressures, complete oral and periodontal charts, mount radiographs, and set up dental trays for many different types of procedures, such as amalgam and composite restorations, oral surgery, periodontics, endodontics, and prosthodontics.

Main Menu

From the main menu, you can select the type of skill you want to practice. You can choose Taking and Recording Vital Signs, Charting Procedures, Basic Operative Setups, Specialty Setups, Radiographs, Pathology or Instrument Identification.

Case Study Menu

Many of the exercises are based on case studies of individual patients. From the case study menu, choose a patient file and then practice the dental assisting skill for that patient's procedure. When you are finished with one case, you can choose another or go back to the main menu.

Taking and Recording Vital Signs

The Vital Signs exercises let you practice taking and recording blood pressure and TPR (temperature, pulse, and respiration). In the simulated blood pressure exercise, you can read the patient's chart, then pump up the sphygmomanometer, watch the pressure gauge, listen for the systolic and diastolic pressure, and record the patient's blood pressure on the chart.

Charting Procedures

The Charting Procedures exercises will give you practice filling in interactive oral exam and periodontal charts while listening to the dentist's dictation. You can vary the rate of the dentist's dictation, increasing your skill by beginning with very slow and progressing to normal speed dictation.

Basic Operative Setups

The Basic Operative Setups exercises will give you practice assembling anesthetic syringes, punching and assembling dental dams, and setting up dental trays for amalgam and composite restorations. In the anesthetic exercises, you will choose the correct anesthetic carpules, the correct syringe, and the correctly assembled syringe for the patient. The dental dam exercises ask you to select the correct armamentarium for the tray, correctly punch the dental dam, and choose the properly assembled dental dam for the patient.

Specialty Setups

The Specialty Setups exercises will give you practice in recognizing the appropriate tray setups for the specific procedures the patients are going to have done. You can review many different trays set up for oral surgery, periodontics, endodontics, orthodontics, and prosthodontics, and then choose the correct tray for the patient's procedure.

Radiographs

The Radiographs exercises will give you practice in mounting radiographs. In each Mounting Radiographs exercise, you are given a full set of x-rays and you identify them, rotate and position them, and place them correctly in the mount.

Pathology Identification

This exercise presents you with a series of images and you must choose the correct name of the disease/disorder represented. This will help you to learn the various pathologies that may be encountered in the dental field. It is imporant for the dental assistant to be alert to abnormal conditions and to update the patient's history and communicate any concerns to the dentist.

System Requirements for Skills Software:

Operating System: Windows 98, 2000, or XP
Processor: Pentium 400Mhz or faster
Memory: minimum memory required for Operating System.
Hard disk space: 250MB or more
CD-ROM drive: 4x or faster

Set-up Instructions for Skills Software:

Insert the *Dental Assisting Interactive Skills and Procedures* CD-ROM.
Double-Click on your My Computer icon on the desktop, then double-click on the CD-ROM drive icon.
Double-click on the *setup.exe* file to start the installation.
Follow the prompts from there.

SECTION 1

INTRODUCTION

INTRODUCTION TO THE DENTAL PROFESSION

SPECIFIC INSTRUCTIONAL OBJECTIVES

The student should strive to meet the following objectives and demonstrate an understanding of the facts and principles presented in this chapter:

1. Identify oral disease indications from the "beginning of time."

2. Identify the items on the time line of dental history.

3. Name the individuals who had a great impact on the profession of dentistry.

4. Identify the people who promoted education and organized dentistry.

5. Explain what DDS and DMD stand for.

6. Identify the nine specialties of dentistry.

7. Describe, generally, the career skills performed by dental hygienists, dental assistants, and dental laboratory technicians.

8. List the education required for, and the professional organizations that represent, each profession.

KEY TERMS

American Dental Assistants Association (ADAA) *(11)*

American Dental Association (ADA) *(9)*

American Dental Hygienists' Association *(10)*

American Dental Laboratory Technician Association (ADLTA) *(11)*

certified dental assistant (CDA) *(11)*

Black, Dr. Greene Vardiman *(6)*

de Chauliac, Guy *(5)*

Dental Assisting National Board, Inc. (DANB) *(11)*

dental public health *(9)*

endodontics *(9)*

Flagg, Josiah *(5)*

Fauchard, Pierre *(5)*

forensic dentistry *(10)*

Greenwood, John *(5)*

Harris, Chapin A. *(6)*

Hayden, Horace H. *(6)*

Hippocrates *(4)*

Kells, Dr. C. Edmund *(11)*

Morrison, James B. *(6)*

oral and maxillofacial pathology *(9)*

oral and maxillofacial radiology *(9)*

oral and maxillofacial surgery *(9)*

orthodontics and dentofacial orthopedics *(10)*

pediatric dentistry *(10)*

periodontics *(10)*

prosthodontics *(10)*

Revere, Paul *(5)*

Roentgen, Wilhelm Conrad *(5)*

Southard, Juliette *(11)*

Woofendale, Robert *(5)*

INTRODUCTION

Humans, from the very beginning of time, have been plagued with dental problems. Over the years, a number of different dental treatments were tried and perfected. Tools of various types were developed and used to repair and clean teeth.

It is important to be familiar with the historic struggles in, and contributions to, dentistry that took place to advance the profession into what it is today (Table 1-1).

History of Dentistry

Beginning in ancient times, dental work was done by physicians. Often, each physician specialized in only one area of care for one part of the body. In fact, during the fifth century B.C., a Greek historian named Herodotus wrote that medicine had become so separate that each physician was a specialist in a disease. "All the country is full of physicians, some of the eyes, some of the teeth, some of what pertains to the belly and some of the hidden diseases." One Egyptian doctor of teeth, named

TABLE 1-1 Time Line of Dental History

Era	Events
Beginning of time	Tooth decay is noted.
3000 BC	First dentist, Hesi-Re, is recorded.
460-322 BC	Written information about tooth decay is recorded by Aristotle and Hippocrates.
460-377 BC	Oath of Hippocrates (Hippocrates).
384-322 BC	Attention to oral hygiene (Diodes of Carystus).
1300-1368	Hygienic rules (Guy de Chauliac).
1452-1519	Tooth morphology identified (Leonardo da Vinci).
1678-1761	Founder of modern dentistry (Pierre Fauchard).
1760-1819	Josiah Flagg develops the dental chair.
1768-1770	Paul Revere places advertisements in a Boston newspaper offering his services as a dentist.
1790	James B. Morrison constructs the first known dental foot engine, which he adapted from his mother's spinning wheel foot treadle.
1832	James Snell invents the first reclining dental chair.
1840	Horace Hayden and Chapin Harris establish the Baltimore College of Dental Surgery.
1841	Alabama enacts the first dental practice act to regulate dentistry.
1844	Horace Wells, a Connecticut dentist, discovers that nitrous oxide can be used for dental pain relief.
1859	American Society of Dental Surgeons established.
1859	American Dental Association (ADA) created.
1866	Lucy Beaman Hobbs, the first woman to earn a dental degree, graduates from Ohio College of Dental Surgery.
1869	Dr. Robert Tanner Freeman, the first African-American to earn a dental degree, graduates from Harvard University Dental School.
1871	First commercially manufactured foot-treadle dental engine is patented by James B. Morrison.
1885	First "lady in attendance" employed by Dr. C. Edmund Kells.

(continues)

TABLE 1-1 Timeline of Dental History *(continued)*

Era	Events
1890	Ida Gray, the first African-American woman to earn a dental degree, graduates from University of Michigan School of Dentistry.
1895	X-rays discovered (Wilhelm Conrad Roentgen).
1907	"Lost wax" casting machine is invented by William Taggart.
1913	Fones School of Dental Hygiene established.
1923	American Dental Hygienists' Association (ADHA) created.
1924	American Dental Assistants Association (ADAA) established; first president was Juliette Southard.
1930	First dental specialty board is founded, the American Board of Orthodontics.
1938	First synthetic bristle (nylon) toothbrush appears on the market.
1945	Water fluoridation era begins in the cities of New York, Newburgh, and Grand Rapids, Michigan.
1947	Dental Assisting National Board, Inc. (DANB) is established.
1950	First fluoride toothpastes are marketed.
1960	Four-handed, sit-down dentistry is utilized.
1970	The Occupational Safety and Health Administration is created by U.S. Congress.
1982	Hepatitis B vaccine becomes available.
1989	Tooth whitening commercial products are marketed.
1992	Occupational Safety and Health Administration's Bloodborne Pathogen Standard becomes effective.
1997	The laser, approved by the Food and Drug Administration, is used to treat tooth decay.

Hesi-Re (the first dentist whose name was recorded), practiced in 3000 B.C.

Dentistry during these early times primarily consisted of removing teeth when pain occurred. Some evidence of drilling holes near the roots to allow infection to drain so that pressure in an abscessed tooth could be relieved has been found on human skulls. Other dental problems that date from ancient times derived from food preparation techniques. Grains were ground in stone bowls with stone pestles. During this process, particles of stone mixed with the grain. This grit in the food caused severe wear of the biting (occlusal) surfaces of the teeth and possible pulp exposure.

The father of medicine, **Hippocrates** (460–377 B.C.), attempted to explain health and disease. He suggested that four main fluids in the body, namely blood, black bile, yellow bile, and phlegm, along with heat, cold, dry air, and wet air, must remain in balance. Disruption of these four fluids and four elements would result in disease. Among Hippocrates' numerous writings is a book titled *On Affections*. In this book he wrote, "Teeth are eroded and become decayed partly by the mucus, and partly by food, when they are by nature weak and badly fixed in the mouth." Even though much of what Hippocrates thought about health and teeth was inaccurate, his writings provided much-needed information for the progress of medicine. Even today, the Oath of Hippocrates is used as a basis for the code of ethics used by the medical and dental professions in regard to the solemn obligation these professionals undertake when caring for patients.

During Aristotle's time (384–322 B.C.), some attention was given to oral hygiene and was reflected in his writings. An Athenian physician, Diocles of Carystus, stated that oral hygiene should get proper attention, and he even gave instructions to this end. During the next couple of centuries, more importance was placed on good oral hygiene. A number of cleaning powders were made from crushed bones, oyster, and egg shells. At times, these substances were mixed with honey to make a paste to clean with. Guests in the homes of the wealthy who were invited to dinner were given silver- and even gold-decorated toothpicks with which to clean their teeth after the meal. At the time, picking one's teeth was proper etiquette.

Later Progress of Dentistry

In France, a surgeon named Guy de Chauliac (1300–1368) became one of the most influential authors on surgery of the fourteenth century. He also wrote hygienic rules for oral hygiene.

Hygienic Rules for Oral Hygiene, Written by Guy de Chauliac

1. Avoid food that putrifies readily.
2. Avoid food or drink that is too hot or too cold, and especially avoid swallowing extremely cold food after extremely hot food, and vice versa.
3. Do not bite into things that are too hard.
4. Avoid foods that stick to the teeth, such as figs and confections made with honey.
5. Avoid certain foods known to be bad for the teeth (his example was leeks).
6. Clean the teeth gently with a mixture of honey and burnt salt to which some vinegar has been added.

It is now known that the information given by de Chauliac was not entirely accurate. However, because it was based on sound logic, much of it is used today. For example, it is well known that sticky, sweet foods increase dental decay. In his writings, de Chauliac noted that surgery on the teeth should be performed under the supervision of doctors but could be done by "barbers or dentatores." This notation was the first to refer to "dentatores," the specific group of practitioners caring for the oral cavity and the teeth.

During the fifteenth and sixteenth centuries, artists became more interested in human anatomy to enhance the accuracy of their artwork. Leonardo da Vinci (1452–1519) painstakingly dissected the human skull and then drew his discoveries. He was the first to make a distinction between premolars and molars. His writings further define the morphology of teeth.

Pierre Fauchard (1678–1761) organized all known information about dentistry in a book that was clearly written and had step-by-step pictures that depicted easy-to-follow procedures. He rejected the idea that a tooth-worm caused decay and noted that caries (his term for decay) were a result of a "hormonal imbalance." Fauchard wrote of his perceived causes of decay and prevention techniques and was an early advocate of treating diseased gingival tissue. Fauchard perfected a number of dental treatments that are still used in part today, almost three centuries later. Many refer to Pierre Fauchard as the founder of modern dentistry.

Wilhelm Conrad Roentgen (1845–1923), a German physicist, discovered x-rays in 1895. This discovery allowed dentists to further their knowledge of the diseases and structures of the mouth.

Progress of Dentistry in the United States

One of the first dentists to arrive in the United States from England was Robert Woofendale. Woofendale placed an advertisement in the *New York Mercury* on November 17, 1766, stating that he "performs all operations upon the teeth, sockets, gums, and palate, likewise fixes artificial teeth, so as to escape discernment." Soon after Woofendale arrived, John Baker came and started advertising in the Boston area. He spoke and wrote about fillings and artificial teeth. Baker was well known and was one of the dentists who treated George Washington. John Greenwood (1760–1819) was said to be the first president's favorite dentist. Greenwood had very little formal education but was a proficient practitioner in the eighteenth century. He thought children should care for their teeth and offered parents reduced rates for children's dental care. He also thought that tartar came from bad breath and was adamant about the regular removal of it for good oral health.

George Washington, at one time or another, was probably treated by every notable dentist of the time. A number of references in his diary note continual pain and discomfort from his teeth. At the time the picture that is currently on the one-dollar bill was taken, the president had only one tooth left, a lower left bicuspid (premolar). In fact, the artist had to pad out the cheeks and lips with cotton to give the president's sunken face a more normal appearance. Washington's last set of dentures, made by Greenwood, were comprised of ivory and gold and had two springs holding them together (Figure 1-1). A number of dentures were made for the president, but, contrary to popular belief, they were not made of wood.

Paul Revere (1735–1818), a silversmith (Figure 1-2), was involved in dentistry for several years, but his greatest contribution was making artificial teeth and surgical instruments. He may have had a part in training a notable dentist of the late 1700s, Josiah Flagg. Flagg's father was a partner to Revere. Flagg was a skilled surgeon, accomplishing corrective procedures on cleft lips, orthodontics, endodontics, and operative dentistry. However, one of his major contributions to dentistry was the construction of a dental chair. It had an extension on the arm to hold dental instruments and an adjustable head rest.

In the early 1800s, U.S. dentistry took a giant leap forward. The establishment of a popular democracy, with the chance of personal financial gain, free public school education, and population growth, prompted some of the most notable dentists in the world to relocate to America. The literature and knowledge base expanded a great deal during this time. Most large cities now had resident dentists rather than traveling barbers who extracted

FIGURE 1-1 The last dental prosthesis worn by George Washington was made for him by John Greenwood. It is made of gold and ivory and is held together with springs. *(Courtesy of the National Museum of Dentistry, Baltimore, MD)*

FIGURE 1-2 Paul Revere, shown as a silversmith. *(Courtesy of the Paul Revere Memorial Association, Gift of Miss Marion Cole. Photo: John Miller.)*

FIGURE 1-3 One of the founders of professional dentistry in the United States, Horace Hayden, helped established the world's first dental college. *(Courtesy of the National Museum of Dentistry, Baltimore, MD)*

teeth and sold tooth powders. The dentists of the time were better educated and involved in the communities they served. The profession was progressing far beyond massive tooth removals and occasional cleanings. Additionally, dental materials improved and developed as techniques did. The first dental engine with functioning handpiece, motor, and foot treadle was manufactured and patented by **James B. Morrison** in 1871. This apparatus allowed dentists to restore teeth much more quickly. Organized dentistry was rapidly approaching.

Education and Organized Dentistry

Horace H. Hayden (1769–1844) (Figure 1-3) sought dental care from John Greenwood (the dentist who cared for George Washington). Hayden was inspired and encouraged to take up dentistry as a vocation. He became very active in the dentistry profession, writing for journals and lecturing on medical and dental topics.

One of the students who studied with Hayden was **Chapin A. Harris** (1806–1860) (Figure 1-4). Harris believed in education and built an extensive library of dental literature, including his work, *The Dental Art: A Practical Treatise on Dental Surgery*. Due to the efforts of Hayden and Harris, the first dental college in the world, Baltimore College of Dental Surgery, was founded on March 6, 1840. It is now called the School of Dentistry at the University of Maryland, and is the home of the Dr. Samuel Harris National Museum of Dentistry.

Dr. Greene Vardiman Black (1836–1915), known as G.V. Black (Figure 1-5), taught in dental schools such as the University of Iowa and the Northwestern University Dental School in Chicago. As the dean, he increased the library holdings and authored more than 500 articles and several books. He invented numerous machines for

FIGURE 1-4 One of the founders of professional dentistry in America, Chapin Harris, helped establish the first dental college in the world and the first national association representing dentistry. *(Courtesy of the National Museum of Dentistry, Baltimore, MD)*

FIGURE 1-5 The "grand old man of dentistry," G.V. Black. *(Courtesy of the National Museum of Dentistry, Baltimore, MD)*

testing alloys and instruments to refine cavity preparations. Black later enlarged these instruments for demonstration to students in the classroom. Many refer to him as the "grand old man of dentistry." His son, Arthur D. Black, followed in his footsteps, becoming dean of the Northwestern University Dental School in Chicago. He developed the *Index to Dental Periodical Literature in the English Language* in 1921. This allowed not only researchers to access the literature, but also provided access to general practicing dentists who wanted to improve their knowledge and skills.

Lucy Beeman Hobbs-Taylor (Figure 1-6), the first woman to graduate from a recognized dental college, earned her dental degree in 1866. She was a teacher who became interested in medicine, and then pursued further education. She met with resistance, but after the Iowa State Dental Society amended its constitution

FIGURE 1-6 The first female graduate of a recognized dental school, Lucy Beeman Hobbs-Taylor. *(Courtesy of the Kansas State Historical Society)*

and bylaws, she was admitted into the dental college. Dr. Robert Tanner Freeman (Figure 1-7), the first African-American to earn a dental degree, graduated from Harvard University Dental School in 1869. Eleven years later in 1890, Ida Gray became the first African-American woman to earn a dental degree upon graduation from the University of Michigan School of Dentistry.

American Dental Association

At a time when education and literature were developing, it was thought that organizing dentists would promote sharing of information concerned with excellence in dentistry. Horace Hayden and Chapin Harris collaborated on endeavors such as forming the first nationwide association of dentists. In 1840, the American Society of Dental Surgeons was formed but was dissolved in 1856.

FIGURE 1-7 The first African-American to earn a DMD, Dr. Robert Tanner Freeman graduated from Harvard School of Dental Medicine in 1869. *(Courtesy of Harvard University Library)*

FIGURE 1-8 Logo for dentistry. *(Courtesy of the American Dental Association)*

Harris had long believed in the need for an informative dental periodical and was instrumental in founding it in 1839. This journal was called the *American Journal of Dental Science (AJDS)*. Later, in 1859, twenty-five delegates gathered in Niagara Falls, New York, and organized the American Dental Association (ADA) (Figure 1-8). The association was small at first, but, after grouping all local associations according to states and then all states having representation in the national organization, membership began to increase. Each state now has its own organization with bylaws approved by the ADA, and each local (regional) organization has ADA-approved bylaws that are sent to each state organization. For instance, Texas is represented by the Texas State Dental Association to the ADA, and the Texas State Dental Association comprises individual local dental associations. The official publication of the ADA is the *Journal of the American Dental Association (JADA)*. The ADA also has a Web site, http://www.ada.org, which provides a link to the ADA for dental professionals and dental consumers.

The Dental Team

Many people working together make up the dental health team. Each member of the team has specific skills, roles, and responsibilities. This team approach to dentistry improves efficiency and the overall patient experience.

Dentists

Once dentistry was established as a profession, the need for formal education became apparent. Only half the dentists practicing during the nineteenth century had formal educations. The requirements for state regulations began in Alabama in 1841, and by 1899 every state had enacted laws regulating the practice of dentistry. The requirements set forth for dentistry include an undergraduate education and graduation from a dental school approved by the ADA Commission on Dental Accreditation. Currently, three to four years of undergraduate work and four years of dental school (five at Harvard) are required to achieve a dental degree. Depending on program emphasis, a doctor of dental surgery (DDS) or a doctor of medical dentistry (DMD) degree is granted. Specialist training includes two or more additional years of postgraduate education in an approved, specialized training area. All dentists must take and pass both written and clinical examinations in the states in which they practice. All dental team members are responsible for following the regulations in their states. These regulations are defined in each state's dental practice act. The dental practice acts are defined to protect the public. The act specifies what can be performed legally by the dental professionals in that state. Dentists supervise the dental team members in their offices.

Dental Specialists. A dentist who practices all phases of dentistry is called a general dentist. General dentists may encounter cases for which treatment that goes beyond the scope of their training is required. The general dentist would refer these cases to a dental specialist. The ADA recognizes the following nine specialties:

1. **Dental public health** is the specialty concerned with the prevention of dental disease. The public health dentist works with the community to promote dental health.

2. **Endodontics** is concerned with the pathology and morphology of the dental pulp and surrounding tissues due to injury and disease. Patients referred for root canals would see an endodontist.

3. **Oral and maxillofacial pathology** is the specialty concerned with the diagnosis and nature of the diseases affecting the oral cavity. A patient who has a lesion unknown to the general dentist may be referred to the oral pathologist for further treatment and diagnosis.

4. **Oral and maxillofacial radiology** is the specialty of dentistry and the discipline of radiology concerned with the production and interpretation of images and data produced by all modalities of radiant energy that are used for the diagnosis and management of diseases, disorders, and conditions of the oral and maxillofacial region.

5. **Oral and maxillofacial surgery** is concerned with the diagnosis and surgical treatment of the oral and maxillofacial region due to injury, disease, or defects. A patient having third molars (wisdom

teeth) removed may be referred to an oral and maxillofacial surgeon.

6. **Orthodontics and dentofacial orthopedics** is concerned with the diagnosis, supervision, guidance, and correction of malocclusion in the dentofacial structures. Braces for straightening teeth are placed by the orthodontist.

7. **Pediatric dentistry** is concerned with the prevention of oral disease and the diagnosis and treatment of oral care in children, from birth through adolescence. Other patients requiring special care due to emotional, mental, or physical problems are referred to the pediatric dentist.

8. **Periodontics** is the specialty concerned with the diagnosis and treatment of the diseases of the supporting and surrounding tissues of the tooth. The periodontist is also concerned with the prevention of disease in this area. Patients who have plaque and calculus buildup and have lost some of the bone around the tooth due to periodontal disease would be referred to the periodontist for further evaluation and treatment.

9. **Prosthodontics** is concerned with the diagnosis, restoration, and maintenance of oral functions. This specialty is also concerned with the replacement of missing teeth through artificial means.

Another area that requires additional training but is not regarded as a specialty of dentistry is **forensic dentistry**. This is a relatively new area that deals with a wide range of services, such as the identification of bite marks on the body and/or the identification of an individual through tooth restorations and morphology using dental records.

The specialist works with the general dentist to provide the optimum oral health and patient care. During and once the specialty treatment is completed, the patient continues regular visits with the general dentist.

Dental Hygienists

Early in the 1900s in Bridgeport, Connecticut, several dentists, along with a leader named Dr. Alfred Civilon Fones, stated that the dentists would not be able to be surgeons and give preventive treatments. It was suggested that women be trained to clean teeth because "they have smaller and more gentle hands." At that time, it was uncommon for women to work outside the home. A dental assistant, Irene Morgan, was the first to be trained by Dr. Fones in dental hygiene. Dr. Fones established a school in 1913, and it survives today as the Fones School of Dental Hygiene, University of Bridgeport. Graduates of two- or four-year dental hygiene schools receive the title registered dental hygienist (RDH) after passing written and clinical tests in the states in which

they practice, and they are granted licenses. Dental hygienists specialize in providing dental prophylaxis, including the removal of plaque, stains, and calculus from the teeth, along with patient education. Many state practice acts allow licensed hygienists to apply tooth sealants; to expose, process, and mount dental radiographs; and to chart conditions in the oral cavity. Some of the states allow hygienists to place restorative materials and to administer local anesthetics.

American Dental Hygienists' Association. The **American Dental Hygienists' Association (ADHA)** was formed in 1923 in Cleveland in conjunction with the ADA annual meeting (Figure 1-9). In 1927, the *Journal of the American Dental Hygienists' Association* was founded and continues to be the official publication of the organization. This organization, like the ADA, has the leadership of national, state, and local societies working together to promote oral health.

Dental Laboratory Technicians

Dental laboratory technicians may not work in the dental office with the other members of the team, but they are essential team members. Some dental laboratory technicians are employed by the dentist; others work in privately owned dental laboratories.

Originally, dentists performed their own laboratory procedures; however, they eventually became too busy to complete the laboratory work and hired trained technicians to perform these tasks. The first commercial dental laboratory was opened in Boston in 1883 by Dr. William H. Stowe, a dentist, and Frank F. Eddy, a tool-

FIGURE 1-9 Logo for the American Dental Hygienists' Association. *(Courtesy of the American Dental Hygienists' Association)*

maker. By the turn of the century, dental laboratories were firmly established. Today, whether the technicians are in the dental office or in a commercial dental laboratory, they provide such extraoral services as fabricating gold and porcelain restorations and partial and full dentures.

In most states, a dental laboratory technician is not required to have formal training and may be trained on the job. Many technicians have graduated from two-year, ADA-accredited, dental laboratory technician programs. These programs require extensive knowledge of dental anatomy and dental materials and the development of detailed mechanical skills. Individuals seeking credentials must pass an examination to become certified dental technicians (CDTs). Membership in the American Dental Laboratory Technician Association (ADLTA) is also offered to dental technicians.

Dental Assistants

Before the early twentieth century, dentists hired men and boys to assist them in their dental practices. Dr. C. Edmund Kells, who practiced in New Orleans, hired a female to replace a male assistant in 1885. He wanted this "lady assistant" to be "quick, quiet, gentle, and attentive." A number of dentists were unsure about a female in the dental office, but the public accepted it quickly. This change allowed a woman to go to a dental office without being accompanied by her husband or maiden aunt. Due to the popularity of "ladies in attendance," dentists advertised the fact that they had hired female dental assistants by displaying signs in their windows.

Today, the educationally qualified dental assistant normally graduates from an institution accredited by the ADA Commission on Dental Accreditation. Training is approximately one academic year in length, and includes didactic, laboratory, and clinical content. Each state has a dental practice act that governs which duties dental assistants can perform. This varies from performing intraoral procedures, such as placing retraction cord and dental dams, to extraoral procedures, such as patient education. Dental assistants enable dentists to care for many more patients and to produce more dentistry than they could alone. Almost all dental offices employ one or more dental assistants. In the office, the person working directly with the dentist during patient procedures is the dental assistant.

Certified Dental Assistants. A 104-hour course was developed in 1947, along with a certifying board, to give credentials to assistants who passed the written and clinical examinations. The Dental Assisting National Board, Inc. (DANB) provides a means for competent, qualified dental assistants to obtain credentials. By passing a comprehensive written examination from DANB the dental assistant can use the title of certified dental

assistant (CDA). Other specialized certification can be obtained in areas such as certified dental practice management assistant (CDPMA) and certified orthodontic assistant (COA). Some state dental practice acts allow assistants to obtain the credential of registered dental assistant (RDA). Others may require registration in expanded functions (functions and skills considered to be above the normal scope of dental assisting, such as performing a coronal polish and placing a dental dam), thereby earning the title of registered dental assistant in expanded functions (EDAEF) (see Chapter 37, Employment Strategies).

Dental Receptionists/Dental Practice Management Assistants. The dental receptionist position is becoming a more specialized area of dental assisting with the use of computers and computerized insurance claims. The dental receptionist or practice management assistant attends seminars to upgrade skills in front office management, computer technology, marketing, and accounting.

American Dental Assistants Association. The American Dental Assistants Association (ADAA) was founded in 1924 by Juliette Southard, its first president (Figures 1-10 and 1-11). It was founded on four principles: education, efficiency, service, and loyalty. Membership offers a voice in national affairs regarding the career of dental assisting, opportunities in continuing education, professional liability insurance, and interaction with other professionals in the field. ADAA members can remain current in their knowledge through the ADAA publication *The Dental Assistant, Journal of the American Dental Assistants Association,* or by accessing the ADAA Web site (http://www.dentalassistant.org).

FIGURE 1-10 Logo for the American Dental Assistants Association. *(Courtesy of the American Dental Assistants Association, Chicago, IL)*

FIGURE 1-11 Juliette Southard, founder and first president of the American Dental Assistants Association. *(Courtesy of the American Dental Assistants Association, Chicago, IL)*

Creed

for Dental Assistants

" To be loyal to my employer, my calling, and myself.

To develop initiative - having the courage to assume responsibility and the imagination to create ideas and develop them.

To be prepared to visualize, take advantage of, and fulfill the opportunities of my calling.

To be a co-worker - creating a spirit of co-operation and friendliness rather than one of fault-finding and criticism.

To be enthusiastic - for therein lies the easiest way to accomplishment.

To be generous, not alone of my name but of my praise and my time.

To be tolerant with my associates, for at times I too make mistakes.

To be friendly, realizing that friendship bestows and receives happiness.

To be respectful of the other person's viewpoint and condition.

To be systematic, believing that system makes for efficiency.

To know the value of time for both my employer and myself.

To safeguard my health, for good health is necessary for the achievement of a successful career.

To be tactful - always doing the right thing at the right time.

To be courteous - for this is the badge of good breeding.

To walk on the sunny side of the street, seeing the beautiful things in life rather than fearing the shadows.

To keep smiling always."

- Juliette A. Southard

American Dental Assistants Association

FIGURE 1-12 The "Creed for Dental Assistants" by Juliette A. Southard. *(Courtesy of the American Dental Assistants Association, Chicago, IL)*

When pursuing a career in dental assisting, it is beneficial to use the "Creed for Dental Assistants" (Figure 1-12) and the "Dental Assistants Pledge" (Figure 1-13) as guidelines for professional behavior.

Other Members of the Dental Team

Additional members of the dental team are dental service technicians, dental representatives, and dental supply companies and representatives. The dental service technicians maintain dental equipment. The dental assis-

tant works with the technicians and identifies equipment problems. The technicians may be required to make service calls, or they will direct the assistant to rectify a problem. Dental representatives demonstrate how to use new materials. Normally, they are trained in the materials they represent. Dental supply companies and representatives also give information on new materials and help the dental assistant order supplies for the dental office. They normally make weekly calls to the dental office. Dental supply companies could be mail order companies through which the assistant can order office supplies.

"I solemnly pledge that,
in the practice of my profession, I will always be loyal
to the welfare of the patients who come under my care,
and to the interest of the practitioner whom I serve.

I will be just and generous to the members of my profession,
aiding them and lending them encouragement to be loyal,
to be just, to be studious.

I hereby pledge to devote my best energies to the service
of humanity in that relationship of Life to which I consecrated
myself when I elected to become a Dental Assistant."

- Dr. C.N. Johnson

Printed and Distributed through the American Dental Assistants Association

FIGURE 1-13 "The Dental Assistants Pledge" by Dr. C.N. Johnson.
(Courtesy of the American Dental Assistants Association, Chicago, IL)

CHAPTER SUMMARY

It is important to know the historic struggles in and contributions to dentistry that advanced the profession into what it is today. Organized dentistry was formed with the intent to promote the sharing of information concerned with excellence in dentistry. To provide excellence in dentistry, additional dental team members would become recognized and add contributing roles. Therefore, the dental assistant will need to be able to identify and define those who contribute to the dental profession.

Case Study

Lori Ann Smith was eighteen years old in 1880 and was seeking a position in a dental office. The opinion of the dentists was to not allow women access to the profession. Lori's career dreams were denied. Over 100 years later, her great-great-granddaughter, Traci Lynd, was seeking a position in a dental office and found a very different environment. What changes and advancements took place for dental assistants during that time frame to allow Traci to reach her goal?

Case Study Review

1. When were gender barriers eliminated for dental assistants?

2. What career changes for dental assistants took place over four generations?

3. With the current educational advancements in the profession, what credentials are available to dental assistants today?

REVIEW QUESTIONS

Multiple Choice

1. The basic code of ethics used by the medical and dental professions originated with
   a. Aristotle.
   b. Leonardo da Vinci.
   c. Pierre Fauchard.
   d. Hippocrates.

2. Who is the teacher and inventor recognized as the "grand old man" of dentistry?
   a. Chapin A. Harris
   b. C.V. Black
   c. John Greenwood
   d. Josiah Flagg

3. Which of the following is not an ADA-recognized dental specialty?
   a. Endodontics
   b. Oral and maxillofacial pathology
   c. Forensic dentistry
   d. Pediatric dentistry

4. The first president of the ADAA was
   a. Juliette Southard.
   b. Dr. Lucy Hobbs-Taylor.
   c. Dr. C. Edmund Kells.
   d. Dr. Alfred Fones.

5. Whose greatest contribution to early dentistry was the creation of artificial teeth and dental tools?
   a. George Washington
   b. Robert Woofendale
   c. Paul Revere
   d. John Greenwood

6. Who was the first African-American woman to earn a dental degree?
   a. Ida Gray Taylor
   b. Juliette Southard
   c. Lucy Beeman Hobbs
   d. Loretta Fones

7. Which dental specialty deals with the diagnosis and nature of diseases affecting the oral cavity?
   a. Endodontics
   b. Periodontics
   c. Oral and maxillofacial pathology
   d. Oral and maxillofacial surgery

8. Where was the first commercial dental laboratory opened?
   a. Boston, Massachusetts
   b. Bridgeport, Connecticut
   c. Baltimore, Maryland
   d. Chicago, Illinois

9. Which dental specialty is concerned with the replacement of missing teeth through artificial means?
   a. Periodontics
   b. Prosthodontics
   c. Pediodontics
   d. Endodontics

10. Which dental team member allows the dentist to care for more patients and increase productivity?
    a. Dental assistant
    b. Dental laboratory technician
    c. Dental practice management assistant
    d. Dental hygienist

Critical Thinking

1. If a patient fell and fractured a front tooth and it seemed to have pulpal involvement (nerve damage), what specialists could the general dentist refer the patient to?

2. Who would you contact for information about dental assisting organizations?

3. Which dental team member (nationally), besides the dentist, requires a license?

Web Activities

1. Go to http://www.dentalmuseum.org and identify which exhibits are available for viewing at the Samuel Harris Museum of Dentistry.

2. Go to http://www.ada.org and identify how many people have ADA membership.

3. Go to http://www.dentalassistant.org and download and print a membership application for the ADA.

CHAPTER 2

PSYCHOLOGY, COMMUNICATION, AND MULTICULTURAL INTERACTION

SPECIFIC INSTRUCTIONAL OBJECTIVES

The student should strive to meet the following objectives and demonstrate an understanding of the facts and principles presented in this chapter:

1. Define psychology and paradigm.
2. Describe the three steps in communication.
3. List the skills used in listening.
4. Differentiate the terms used in verbal and non-verbal communication.
5. Demonstrate the following body language used in non-verbal communication behavior: spatial, posture, facial expression, gestures, and perception.
6. Discuss how Maslow's hierarchy of needs is used and how it relates to communication in today's dental office.
7. Discuss how defense mechanisms can inhibit communication.
8. Describe some general behaviors of multicultural patient populations.

KEY TERMS

communication *(16)*

culture *(22)*

encoding *(17)*

ethnicity *(22)*

Maslow, Abraham *(20)*

Maslow's hierarchy of needs *(20)*

non-verbal communication *(19)*

paradigm *(16)*

psychology *(16)*

race *(22)*

INTRODUCTION

Communication is the foundation for dental care. The dental assistant must gain an understanding of the individuals being treated and how and why patients think and act as they do. The assistant must develop good communication skills. Communication is behind every action taken by the dental team. The message is to be transmitted to the other individual as clearly as possible, and when the patient or other staff member sends the response it is critical to listen before providing feedback. Watching for nonverbal communication is essential to obtaining the entire message. The dental assistant must develop skills in overcoming the patient's defense mechanisms and understanding how people from other cultures interact.

Psychology and Understanding Individual Paradigms

Dental team members are all responsible for communicating well and treating each patient and co-worker respectfully. Through these efforts, patients can overcome the fear of dental treatment. Employees can do many things to enhance the mental and physical comfort of patients, but those employees must have a positive attitude toward patients and their treatment. The dental assistant must understand patients and how to meet patient needs during dental treatment.

Psychology is the science of the mind and of the reasons people think and act as they do. Historically, individuals associate discomfort with dental treatment. Patients may think and react using past reasoning. Today's dentistry works diligently, striving to make treatment pain free and doing whatever is possible to make every patient comfortable. It is critical to understand the patients' attitudes toward dentistry and to listen to their views of their dental experiences. With this information, the dental assistant can better help patients overcome any fears they may have.

A person's **paradigm**, or acquired belief system, may also be a factor. Individuals have different life experiences that have contributed to their personal belief systems or paradigms. For example, people may believe that a toothbrush with hard bristles gets the teeth cleaner. They may have always used hard-bristled brushes and have no cavities. Therefore, they believe hard brushes clean the teeth better. Even though the evidence now shows that soft-bristled brushes do a better job, the dental assistant may have a difficult time changing these people's paradigm. Through good communication, the dental assistant can make an assessment. If the teeth are indeed clean in all areas and it does not appear that damage is being done to the tooth or tissue, then the dental assistant can encourage the patient. If the hard-bristled brush is damaging the tooth or gums or failing to clean the entire tooth surface, then the dental assistant will have to begin educating the patient and changing the patient's paradigm. It may be difficult for the patient to associate clean teeth with a soft-bristled brush. Good communication skills, such as listening, are essential. Listen, and then try to help patients find the right answers and understand how a hard-bristled brush may do damage. Know that the brush is going to feel different in the mouth, that the patient may try to brush harder, and that the brush may wear more quickly. Tell the patient what to expect. Continue to listen to the patient. Watch the patient's non-verbal behavior and work with the patient to understand necessary changes in behavior. The patient's behavior may not change immediately. Share with the patient that it may take a while before the change feels comfortable and that this is normal. Motivate the patient to continue the behavior.

Communication

Understanding how individuals think and feel is only part of interacting successfully with patients. A dental assistant must also have excellent communication skills. These skills, which can be learned and developed, are important in patient care. **Communication** is the act of passing along information (the message), transmitting an idea (receiving the message), or connecting with another individual (providing feedback). Transmitting thoughts, ideas, feelings, facts, and other information is done through verbal and nonverbal behavior. Every time a person communicates with another person, even if no verbal comments are taking place, information is being transmitted. In fact, people cannot avoid communicating with each other. In dental assisting, this communication is essential in establishing a relationship with the patient. This method of connecting with patients allows for patient comfort and safety so that the treatment can take place. The quality of the communication and the way the patient feels connected to the dental assistant and dentist directly relate to the patient's total experience while in the dental office. Listening is important. The adage, "You have two ears and one mouth so you can listen twice as much," is true. Often, people begin formulating their responses before they hear the entire question. In the dental office, pay special attention to what the person is saying, and then give the correct response.

In the dental office when a staff member is going over the case presentation, a patient may say something like, "I just want to fix the front teeth." This may communicate a message to the dentist or auxiliary staff that appearance is important to this individual. Other communication with the patient will help determine why she or he wants the front teeth restored. If staff members listen carefully, they may find that this individual is applying for new employment, or that she/he is going to be in a daughter's wedding and wants to look good in the pictures. Once an understanding is reached of where patients are coming from and what their desires and needs are, then the treatment plan can be established to help meet these needs.

Communication Process Components

The communication process consists of five major components: sender, message, channel through which the message is delivered, receiver, and feedback (Figure 2-1).

Sender

The sender is the individual who begins the communication process by generating a message. The senses of taste, touch, smell, or other external stimuli may inspire the individual to begin communication. Other external stimuli include, for instance, feelings of delight, hunger, fatigue, or anger; and thinking or fantasizing about a particular activity or scenario. Anything could be a source (or encoding) of the stimulus for communication. **Encoding** involves the use of specific signs, symbols, interpersonal communication, or language in sending the message.

An example of a sender is a really good teacher who everyone talks about. Most people remember that the teacher could really get the message across. A good sender engages others when sending the message, and can "transmit" the message in a manner that is clear and concise. It may be beneficial to evaluate what an admired person in your life did to enhance the message. Use those qualities to become a better sender.

Message

An individual starts with an idea, then formulates that idea and sends it through a message to another individual. The sender must shape the idea, which often starts as an image the sender visualizes, into a message by translating the image into words others can understand. This complicated process happens so routinely during the day that most people are unaware of it.

The message is the stimuli—written, verbal, or nonverbal communication—produced by the sender to which the receiver will respond. Reception of the message could occur through visual, auditory, or kinesthetic channels. The message may be received by different individuals in different manners depending on the individual's paradigm.

Channel

The channel is the communication medium through which a message is delivered. Three major communication channels are auditory, which is hearing or listening to the verbal message; visual, which is observing, perceiving, and seeing the visual message; and kinesthetic, which is the caring touch or the procedural touch. Dental assistants use each of these channels during a clinical procedure. It is critical to be a good listener. Patients may feel comfortable because of the "connection" they have with the auxiliary, and share more information than they would with the dentist. In addition, when the dentist arrives, items are placed into the mouth and it is more difficult for the patient to communicate verbally. Dental assistants also observe the patient during the procedure. Is the patient tightening his or her eyes or are the knuckles white and tightly clutching the arms of the chair? The dentist is focusing on the procedure at hand, and the assistant can view the entire situation. Many dentists count on assistants to be their eyes and to notify them if the patient is uncomfortable. Dental assistants normally possess the quality of empathy with patients and the ability to communicate through the kinesthetic channel using the procedural touch by asking the patient, "How does that feel?" The dental assistant may also use the caring touch by touching a patient's arm during the anesthesia process or any other procedure that appears to make the patient fearful or uncomfortable. This reassuring touch shows the auxiliary to be compassionate, concerned, and empathetic.

It is important to note that in the dental office, the channel can be lost due to the pressure of time. Often a dental assistant or dentist does not follow up on the channel method in which the message is being sent. The dental assistant may read the signs and ignore them due to lack of time and the fact that the next patient is waiting for treatment. Often in such a rushed atmosphere, patients may feel that it is not worth going into what is bothering them, and they hold back because they feel that they cannot share how they feel about something. The dental assistant needs to develop skills to identify

FIGURE 2-1 A communication model.

when the time should be taken to ensure that patient needs are met. These skills are developed over time after the assistant understands the entire operation of the office, when time can be made up, and when more time is needed with the patient. Understanding how communication is channeled and how to read the signs that individuals are transmitting is a lifelong learning process.

Receiver

The receiver takes the message and must make some sense of it. This process uses the feelings, intentions, and thoughts from the person's paradigm. Much of the message encoding comes from all the non-verbal clues the sender used to transmit the message. Much credence is given to the way in which the message was delivered.

Feedback

It is critical that the message is decoded correctly before providing feedback. Is the intent of the message clear? If not, state it back to the sender for correct interpretation. After making sure the message is clear, the individual formulates the response, much like the initial sender did. An idea is given shape and words are picked to mirror or express the idea to the other person. This interchange occurs until both people feel their ideas are expressed in the manner in which they wanted them to be or they continue to another area of discussion.

Listening Skills

As noted, listening is an important element of communication. We spend more time listening than doing any other type of communication. Most college students spend about 50 percent of their time listening and 35 percent reading and writing. About 15 percent is spent talking. Some of the barriers to listening are preoccupation, message overload, external noise, and effort. People are often preoccupied with concerns that are more important to them and therefore diminish their ability to listen. We experience overload because the quantity of messages we encounter each day is tremendous. Spending half our time listening, it is impossible to stay focused and listen actively. The mind wanders and listening stops. Often, there is additional external noise that distracts and makes it hard to listen. The external noise comes from others speaking, telephones ringing, music, or any number of other things. Each person identifies when to actively listen to a message of great importance.

When active listening takes place, the receiver encodes the message and responds during two-way communication. People can tell if they are listening actively, because they understand what has been said (Figure 2-2). In a dental office, it is critical to train your mind to listen to the patient so you can understand other people more often and more clearly. The dental assistant may be required

FIGURE 2-2 Good posture and position encourage positive communication with the patient. Shown here are open spatial seating, and an operator with a smile and a positive attitude.

to listen to the concerns of the patient and respond accordingly or to chart medical and dental patient history correctly. The dental assistant may need to listen to the directions of the dentist in carrying out patient treatment. Often, listening in the dental office is accompanied by analyzing and interpreting information. It may help to repeat the content back to the patient. For example, "I understand you to say that the discomfort started several days ago in the upper left side of your face, close to this tooth." The dental assistant should spend time developing and becoming more adept at active listening skills.

Telephone Listening

Listening on the telephone is especially critical. It is often said that the telephone is where the patient derives his or her first impression of the office, and that the telephone is the office's life-line. That being said, a telephone conversation is often like a conversation between two blindfolded individuals. The inflections in each person's voice along with the verbal communication dialogue give the message to the patient. Speaking in short sentences with a hard tone to the voice may not be inviting to the patient. Patients may interpret this communication to mean that the auxiliary does not want them in the office. The message could say something like, "Looking forward to seeing you in our office on May twenty-fifth," but the tone and perceived attitude may reflect a different message. The dental assistant will need to concentrate and obtain feedback from others on how the message is coming across. When listening on the telephone, sit in the correct posture and respond with the correct facial expression. These actions will have an effect on the message sent to the caller, and will relay the message that you want to listen.

FIGURE 2-3 Give the patient on the telephone your full attention, and make certain the message is sent and received correctly.

FIGURE 2-4 Body language and gestures often say more than the spoken word.

Listen with full attention to make certain that the message sent and received is correct and accurate when talking on the telephone (Figure 2-3).

Verbal and Non-Verbal Communication

It is often said that communication is less than 20 percent verbal and 80 percent non-verbal. **Non-verbal communication** is defined as communication without words. It is the way we express ourselves or by what we do and not what we say. Body language can communicate more than spoken words (Figure 2-4). Body language includes the unconscious way we move our bodies, the physical/spatial distance between individuals, posture and position, facial expressions, gestures, and perceptions.

Non-verbal communication is learned first when we are infants. The tone of a voice and the presence or absence of a smile are picked up readily by an infant through non-verbal means. The infant adapts learned behaviors that bring positive responses from the caregiver.

In the dental office, much of the communication with the patient is non-verbal. Sometimes, the patient cannot respond verbally due to the placement of the dental dam or other items in the oral cavity. The dental assistant should become aware of patient's non-verbal communication, which could be a tightening of the hands on the chair arms, a look that indicates a need the patient may have, posture or movement in the chair, or just a muffled noise the patient makes. Watch for this non-verbal communication and try to identify, with the patient's help, which feelings and emotions are being communicated non-verbally.

Territoriality or Spatial Relation

Territoriality or spatial distance indicates the amount of space an individual needs to feel comfortable with others. This distance changes with the group we are in. Intimate touching, normally within 6 inches, is usually encountered with close family members or close friends. In the classroom, students often define their space on the first day of class with textbooks and papers. In the dental office, sometimes the procedures the dental assistants are doing require the assistants to invade the patient's space. It is best that the dental assistant tells the patient of the procedure so that it will not be perceived as threatening. The patient can then feel empowered by deciding to allow the treatment to proceed. This interaction helps to build a sense of trust with the patient. After informing the patient, if possible, sit and perform invasive procedures from the side of the patient. When working straight toward a patient, the spatial distance required for comfort is much greater. Individuals are normally much more comfortable sharing the space to their side. Territoriality and personal space are handled differently by people of various cultures.

Posture and Position

Posture indicates to dental assistants how patients are responding. If the patient is tight, it may indicate that the patient is feeling threatened. The patient may be seated with the arms and legs crossed, which is a message of closure or resistance. Slumped shoulders may indicate

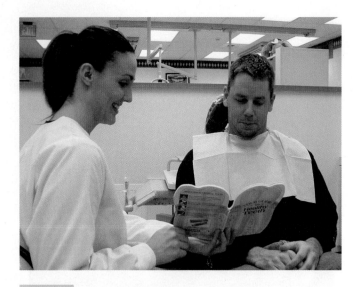

FIGURE 2-5 The operator's posture and correct positioning make patients feel more comfortable and that the dental assistant is interested in them.

the patient is depressed or discouraged. The patient who sits with legs uncrossed, hands loose on the chair arms, and a slightly laid back posture in the chair may appear to be open to suggestions. The manner in which dental assistants position themselves is also important. Standing over the patient may indicate superiority. Sitting close to the patient and leaning toward the patient express interest, warmth, acceptance, and caring (Figure 2-5). This arrangement allows the patient to feel valued, listened to, and cared for.

Facial Expression

Facial expression is considered one of the most observed and critical components of non-verbal communication. The eyes give the message receiver great insight; emotions such as happiness, sadness, and anger are reflected in the eyes. The eyebrows also indicate such non-verbal clues as puzzlement, worry, questioning, and surprise. The dental assistant should check the patient's eyes during the procedure and watch for the non-verbal communication. Practitioners, hygienists, and assistants should be mindful of facial expressions (e.g., eye expressions) behind treatment masks.

Gestures

Like facial expressions, gestures are a common form of non-verbal communication and one of the most observed. Even while in a car at a stoplight, non-verbal communication can be observed inside a car close to us. Gestures make it fairly easy to see if someone is angry, happy, or just trying to make a point to another individual. When we talk, we often use our hands to communicate. It is a form of enhancing the spoken word by emphasizing the content and holding the attention of the receiver.

Perception

It is critical that dental assistants develop good perception skills as they relate to patient communication. The dental assistant must be aware of the feelings of others and be able to sense patients' moods and their attitudes toward the dental treatment. Initially, the dental assistant can watch and observe other health care workers using good perception skills and then emulate others' examples. Soon, the dental assistant will master good perception skills.

Maslow's Hierarchy of Needs

Abraham Maslow (1908–1970), an American psychologist, is considered the founder of a movement called humanistic psychology. Maslow studied well-adjusted persons in society and identified several levels of human needs. His philosophy is that the most basic needs must be satisfied before the next levels can be fulfilled. The most basic needs are bodily drives, such as hunger, thirst, and sleep. The succeeding levels include the needs for safety, then belongingness and love. Following that is the needs of prestige and esteem. The highest need is the one for fulfillment of one's unique potential or, as Maslow termed it, self-actualization. Maslow's hierarchy of needs (Figure 2-6) aids in communication and patient treatment. When patients' most basic needs are not met, they cannot go forward and feel safe and cared for. Keeping this hierarchy in mind helps the dental assistant understand the patient's perceptions and needs, and it helps facilitate dental treatment and care.

Survival or Physiological Needs

In the context of Maslow's hierarchy of needs, an individual will seek to fulfill survival or physiological needs first. These needs include the need to breathe, regulate body temperature, quench thirst, sleep, eat, and dis-

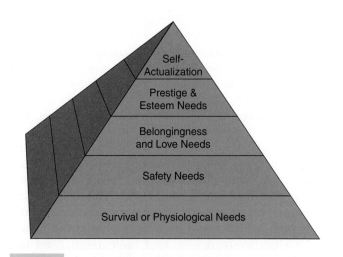

FIGURE 2-6 Maslow's hierarchy of needs.

pose of bodily waste. In the dental office, most patients would try to have their basic needs met prior to the dental appointment. However, some patients may indicate that they are having difficulty breathing through the nose if fluid in the mouth during the treatment prevents breathing through the mouth. The treatment must stop or the fluid must be removed so that the patient can swallow and breathe. Breathing through the nose may be obstructed in several other ways, such as the rubber dam covering the patient's nose or the nosepiece on the nitrous mask becoming dislodged. The dental assistant should recognize that this need must be taken care of immediately, that is, before the patient becomes too anxious and panics. The need to dispose of bodily wastes is another area that cannot wait and often in the dental office patients may need to excuse themselves to use the restroom. Survival or physiological needs cannot be ignored and they are immediate in nature. When a particular need is not being met, a person becomes entirely focused on the same, and it is all the individual can think about until it is fulfilled.

Safety Needs

After survival or physiological needs are met, the most critical is the need for safety. This need covers a variety of areas, such as safety from violence, family and health security, security in employment, and being able to pay the bills. In the dental office, this security most often comes into play under the area of insurance and the individual's need to understand the fee that will be charged for the service and what portion is paid by insurance. If patients lose a job or otherwise have to contend with lower income or higher expenses, they may contact the office to discontinue services, make arrangements to pay for services over time, or both. They would seek out ways to meet financial obligations until their employment status changes. People often do not receive necessary services due to loss of insurance or not being able to pay for the services rendered.

Dental office staff may also observe this need being met by parents who watch over their children during services to ensure their safety and security. Even auxiliaries seeking employment may prefer employment in one office over another because the former provides better insurance and thus fulfills his or her security issues. The latter may be more important to the prospective employee than other benefits or a higher salary.

Belongingness and Love Needs

After physical and safety needs are fulfilled, the focus shifts to the desire to be accepted. Individuals want others to accept them and they wish to be needed. This level of Maslow's hierarchy is focused on social needs, which encompass belonging to or having a family, feeling loved (sexually and nonsexually), and having inter-actions with friends. Patients may wish to belong to the dental office and wish to be cared for (and thus they wish to be needed as a patient in that practice). It is very important that all members of the dental team feel that they belong and are accepted as part of the team providing quality patient care. Working with individuals every day, dental assistants who feel fulfilled with the work (and that they belong in their workplace) will be more effective. The workplace will be more harmonious the greater the feeling that all individuals are part of the team and each can contribute and feel needed. Successful office teams that experience the friendships and acceptance in the workplace show greater satisfaction, and patients often notice this positive atmosphere in the office. Dental office staff often attend seminars to aid in positive interpersonal communications within the office.

Prestige and Esteem Needs

Humans have a need to gain recognition and self-esteem. This can only be realized after the previous needs have been fulfilled. At this level individuals respect others and find a level of self-respect whether it be in work or personal accomplishments. At this level, it is a balancing act of low self-esteem and feeling inferior or second rate to others and the opposite of pretentiousness, arrogance, and vanity. Ideally a person needs to have confidence, and value others' successes. Dental assistants work to feel the accomplishments of elevating their own skill level and confidence in performance without walking over other individuals in the office who seek to obtain the same. Many dentists work to provide recognition and meet employees' need for self-value within the workplace. A dental team that respects others and values each employee's accomplishments is primary to job satisfaction and enjoyment. When a dental assistant feels that she or he is not valued and has low self-esteem, it affects all office personnel; the problem is either overcome or the dental assistant eventually seeks employment in another office in search of feeling self-value.

Self-Actualization

Self-actualization is the highest level on Maslow's hierarchy of needs. This is where the individuals seek to become the best that they can be. Maslow described self-actualization as follows: "Self-actualization is the intrinsic growth of what is already in the organism, or more accurately, of what the organism is" (*Psychological Review*, 1949).

Maslow wrote that self-actualizing people are spontaneous in their ideas and actions. He stated that they are creative, interested in solving problems, feel close to others, generally appreciate life, judge others without prejudice, are spontaneous, and embrace the facts and realities of the world.

Maslow stated that the reason some individuals do not seek self-actualization is that obstacles have been placed in their way by society to hold them back. Education (i.e., lack thereof) can become such an obstacle; individuals should be taught to transcend their cultural conditioning and become world citizens, gain an understanding that life is precious, understand that controls are good, and must be taught to make good choices. In short, Maslow's message was that each individual should seek to reach his or her fullest potential.

Defense Mechanisms

Individuals often use defense mechanisms to block communication. The individual may feel ashamed, guilty, or threatened and therefore respond with defense mechanisms. It becomes difficult to go forward when the patient may be unconsciously defensive to gain control. For instance, when talking to the patient about the course of treatment to care for an area of decay, the patient may say, "The last dentist didn't find decay there!" or "You said that if I brush and floss, I won't get cavities!"

To go forward, the dental assistant must recognize common defense mechanisms and work with patients so that communication can be more effective. Denial is a common defense mechanism in health care. When patients do not brush and floss and believe they will never get decay because they have not had it in the past, they are in denial. Patients may respond with regression and move back to a former time to escape the fear, a tactic that creates temporary amnesia and the inability to cope with a situation. Often in the dental office, the patient uses rationalization to justify a situation. For instance, a patient may say, "We live in Spokane, a city that does not have fluoride in the water. Therefore, of course my children have a great deal more decay."

Understanding and recognizing patients' defense mechanisms help the dental assistant get to the truth. This in turn helps patients improve communication and get beyond their defenses to better outcomes. Dental assistants must constantly observe non-verbal behaviors and look for cues, as well as listen intently to verbal messages. Give patients your full attention so that communication has every opportunity to succeed.

Culture, Ethnicity, and Race

Understanding the concepts of culture, ethnicity, and race is necessary to gain insight into people of different backgrounds. **Culture** encompasses the beliefs, behavior, attitudes, customs, languages, symbols, ceremonies, rituals, knowledge, and practices that are distinctive to a specific group. Individuals in a particular cultural group may behave according to strictly "traditional" dictates of their culture, or their behavior may diverge from this pattern in minor to major ways. Diversity within a cultural group originates in long-term changes in the social environment (e.g., political or economic transformation and pressures) that cause cultural change, which in turn may affect group members unevenly.

Cultural traditions are transferred from one generation to the next by grandparents and parents may model behavior or through discussions within the family or group. Many families have traditions that date from previous centuries. Often traditions are shared through informal or formal activities such as mealtimes (Figure 2-7).

Defined as a subgroup's shared ancestry, history, linguistic characteristics, religion, and/or culture, **ethnicity** emerges and is made relevant through ongoing social situations and encounters, and through people's ways of coping with the demands and challenges of life. Typically, members of an ethnic group share a sense of solidarity and a desire to preserve their culture, traditions, religion, or language, or some combination of these. An ethnic group is self-conscious with a strong sense of "oneness." People usually do not become members of an ethnic group voluntarily; they are born into it. By choice or necessity, members of an ethnic group tend to marry within the group.

A **race** is a subgroup that is believed to be distinct in some way from other groups based on real or imagined *physical* differences (Figure 2-8). Racial classifications are rooted in the idea of biological classification of humans according to morphological features such as skin color or facial characteristics. Individuals are usually externally classified (meaning someone else makes the classification) into a racial group rather than choosing where they belong as part of their iden-

FIGURE 2-7 Mealtimes are often opportunities for families to share traditions and cultural customs.

tity (as occurs with ethnic identity). Conceptions of race, as well as specific racial groupings, are often controversial due to their impact on social identity and how those identities influence an individual's position in social hierarchies.

Many social scientists believe that race is a social construct, meaning that it does not have a basis in the natural world but is simply an artificial distinction created by humans. Others continue to believe that race is a valid measure when understood as genetic clusters or extended families.

In general, regardless of whether *race* is accepted as a useful descriptor, social and physical scientists agree that genetic variation *within* racial groups is much greater than genetic variation *between* them. In the face of the increasing rejection of race as a valid classification scheme, many have replaced the concept *race* with *ethnicity.*

Cultural subgroups are also based on other individual differences, such as gender, age, profession and occupation, political/ideological beliefs and attitudes, nationality, socioeconomic status, skills, education, residence, geographic location, and family structure. One or more of these (or other distinctions) may be more salient or important to an individual than ethnicity.

Multicultural Interaction

It is important that dental assistants avoid stereotyping individuals according to their cultures, customs, traditions, and beliefs. Each patient is to be treated with respect and care. Make no assumptions about the behaviors and paradigms of the multicultural patient populations you serve. According to the U.S. Census Bureau, vast numbers of immigrants have relocated to the United States and Canada in recent years; many speak English as their second language. It would benefit any dental assistant to study the geographical data, cultural beliefs, and practices that have shaped the paradigms for the patients in the region where employment is sought.

Treating everyone in the manner in which you would like to be treated may not work across cultures. Eye contact, for example, may be disrespectful in some cultures; a person may instead show respect by looking down and away. In Western culture, because doing so may be viewed as disinterest, some communication difficulties may occur. When calling a patient back for treatment, it may be appropriate in Western culture to use a patient's first name to put the patient at ease. In other cultures, it may be appropriate to use the formal name to address the patient. Right away, a person can see that mistakes can be made and therefore inappropriate messages can be inadvertently given to the patient. Speak with patients and discover how to give them the best care. Individuals may come to the dental office having used folk medicine in the past, or they may be using it currently. Find out what is working for the patient, and then inform the doctors, so they can design treatments that will achieve the best results.

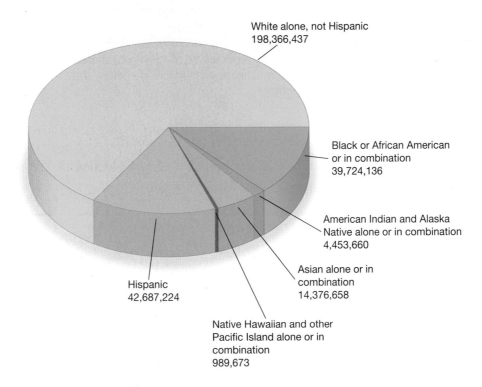

White alone, not Hispanic
198,366,437

Black or African American
or in combination
39,724,136

American Indian and Alaska
Native alone or in combination
4,453,660

Asian alone or in
combination
14,376,658

Native Hawaiian and other
Pacific Island alone or in
combination
989,673

Hispanic
42,687,224

FIGURE 2-8 U.S. population of 296,410,404 divided into racial/ethnic categories. *(From U.S. Census, July 1, 2005)*

When addressing individuals who speak English as a second language, face the patient and speak slowly, not more loudly. Try to avoid unnecessary words. Lots of information may be information overload. In Western culture, the belief is that the caregiver is to tell us everything and that the patient is included in the health care decisions. Many other cultures rely on the caregiver to make decisions without consulting the patient. Summarize information in a simple manner and obtain feedback from the patient by asking questions that require more than a "yes" or "no" answer.

Make sure that the information is accurate and unchanged in the translation. If necessary bring a translator to the dental office. When using an interpreter for your patient, make sure the interpreter understands the information. It may be appropriate to state it a couple of different ways for the interpreter to translate.

Also, always try to avoid behavior or treatment that conflicts with the patient's belief system. Some cultures find it inappropriate to have the female patient alone with the dental team. The dental team should respond to this and allow someone to accompany the patient to the office and in the treatment room during treatment. This is also true for many male dental assistants in the field today. If both doctor and dental assistant working on a female patient are male, having a female assistant in the room as well is advisable. Occasionally an instrument is placed on the patient's chest. This is not appropriate, especially with the female patient, and is even more inappropriate if a male assistant is working with a female patient. Be conscious of gender boundaries to ensure that no patient will feel uncomfortable with the treatment methods. When providing patient care, it is prudent to err on the conservative side in order to avoid conflict with the patient's cultural beliefs and preferences. Remember, do not assume that everything should be handled in one manner; listen without judgment and provide the optimal care for every patient.

CHAPTER SUMMARY

The role of the dental assistant includes making dental treatment comfortable for patients of any culture by understanding those patients' psychological backgrounds and their paradigms of dentistry. Appropriate communication is the key to successful interaction. A dental assistant should have skills in listening and verbal and non-verbal communication and know how to overcome defense mechanisms to meet patient needs.

Case Study

Maci Smith is a dental assistant in Dr. Jones's office. The office is currently working on dental teamwork and Maci cannot stay focused. In the past, Maci was involved and ready to accomplish the task at hand, but now everyone has noticed that Maci is not part of the team. What the rest of the dental team members do not know is that Maci's husband had left her and she is about to have her home repossessed. Maci has not shared this with anyone at the office. According to Maslow's hierarchy of needs, what must happen in Maci's life before she can be present in the discussions and seek to become part of team at the office?

Case Study Review

1. What levels of Maslow's hierarchy of needs are addressed in this scenario?

2. According to Maslow, is it true that the basic levels need to be met before seeking a higher level?

3. At what level in the hierarchy of needs does the dental office teamwork belong?

REVIEW QUESTIONS

Multiple Choice

1. Self-actualization is a term used by:
   a. Laurence Peter.
   b. Carol Rogers.
   c. Abraham Maslow.
   d. Harry Levinson.

2. The American psychologist that is considered the founder of a movement called humanistic psychology is called:
   a. Edmund Kells
   b. Horace Hayden
   c. Chapin Harris
   d. Abraham Maslow

3. Communication is said to be ___ % verbal and ___ % non verbal.
   a. 50   50
   b. 30   70
   c. 70   30
   d. 20   80

4. Communication without words is said to be ____.
   a. gestures
   b. expressions
   c. non-verbal communication
   d. perceptions

5. When treating individuals from other cultures it is best to treat the patient in the manner that you would like to be treated.
   a. true
   b. false

6. The science of the mind and the reasons people think and act as they do is ____.
   a. Communication
   b. Psychology
   c. Paradigms
   d. Encoding

7. A person's acquired belief system is their _____.
   a. Communication
   b. Psychology
   c. Paradigms
   d. Encoding

8. Most college students spend about ____ percent of their time listening.
   a. 25
   b. 35
   c. 50
   d. 70

9. The communication channels that are most often used are:
   a. auditory
   b. visual
   c. kinesthetic
   d. all of the above

10. Intimate spatial relationship with family members or close friends is normally within ____ inches.
   a. 3
   b. 6
   c. 10
   d. 24

Critical Thinking

1. Identify defense mechanisms that you may have used, and then identify what helped you to go forward and communicate.

2. What non-verbal communication might be seen in the dental office? What could be the intent of this behavior?

3. Define self-actualization.

4. Outline Maslow's hierarchy of needs.

Web Activities

1. Go to Cross-cultural communication in Wikipedia, the free encyclopedia. Find intercultural communication principles, improving intercultural communication, and identify the four essential principles therein. Be prepared to discuss the principles in class.

2. Go to http://www.diversityhotwire.com. Identify some common issues related to diversity in the workplace, as well as effective strategies for overcomintg diversity issues.

3. Visit words-at-work.com. Go to the articles listed on the site and read those related to diversity in the workplace and communication.

ETHICS, JURISPRUDENCE, AND THE HEALTH INFORMATION PORTABILITY AND ACCOUNTABILITY ACT

SPECIFIC INSTRUCTIONAL OBJECTIVES

The student should strive to meet the following objectives and demonstrate an understanding of the facts and principles presented in this chapter:

1. Identify the difference between civil and criminal law.

2. Define the Dental Practice Act and what it covers.

3. Identify who oversees the Dental Practice Act and how licenses for the dental field are obtained.

4. Define expanded functions.

5. Identify the components of a contract.

6. Identify due care and give examples of malpractice and torts.

7. Identify fraud and the service that can be given under the Good Samaritan Law.

8. Identify the four areas of the Americans with Disabilities Act.

9. Identify the responsibilities of the dental team in regard to dental records, implied and informed consent, subpoenas, and the statute of limitations.

10. Define ethics and give examples of the American Dental Association and American Dental Assistants Association principles of ethics.

11. State how dentistry follows ethical principles in regard to advertising, professional fees and charges, and professional responsibilities and rights.

12. State how the HIPAA law has impacted the dental office and identify the parameters of the law.

13. Identify how patient health information can be used and disclosed, as well as the rights of patients.

14. Gain an understanding of the training that the staff must follow to be compliant with the HIPAA laws.

15. Identify the CDT transactions and code sets.

KEY TERMS

abandonment *(30)*
agent *(29)*
Americans with Disabilities Act *(31)*
assault *(30)*
battery *(30)*
breach of contract *(29)*
business associates *(34)*
civil law *(27)*
common law *(27)*
contract *(29)*
covered entity *(34)*
criminal law *(27)*
Current Dental Terminology (CDT) *(33)*
day sheet *(35)*
defamation of character *(30)*
defendant *(27)*
dental jurisprudence *(27)*
Dental Practice Act *(28)*
direct providers *(34)*
doctrine of respondeat superior *(28)*
due care *(30)*
ethics *(27)*
expanded functions *(28)*
expert witness *(30)*

expressed contract *(29)*
fraud *(31)*
Good Samaritan Law *(31)*
health information (HI) *(33)*
HIPAA *(33)*
implied consent *(32)*
implied contract *(29)*
indirect providers *(34)*
informed consent *(31)*
law *(27)*
libel *(30)*
malpractice *(30)*
negligence *(30)*
noncompliant *(30)*
plaintiff *(27)*
preemption *(37)*
privacy officer *(33)*
protected health information (PHI) *(33)*
reciprocity *(28)*
res gestae *(29)*
security rule *(37)*
slander *(30)*
statute *(28)*
subpoenas *(32)*
tort *(30)*

INTRODUCTION

Each dental team member is faced with daily decisions that require judgments regarding legal and ethical principles. Maintaining professional ethical standards at all times is essential. The area of **dental jurisprudence,** the

law(s) that governs dentistry, is more clearly defined than dental **ethics,** or moral judgment(s). Ethics in dentistry covers a broad range of activities, from not taking extra toothbrushes from the dentist without the dentist being aware of this act to treating patients with high standards of conduct. People learn ethical behavior throughout life. Examples of ethics learning experiences include schoolteachers talking about cheating, parents talking about treating others the way you would like to be treated, or simply that internal moral conduct message that tells you the difference from right and wrong. Ethics encompasses the concepts of good and evil. To be ethical would be to follow the "good" pathway. Unethical behavior can be legal or follow the jurisprudence of the law, but ethical behavior cannot be illegal. At minimum, ethical behavior in the dental office must follow the letter of the law or dental jurisprudence. The consequences of not doing what should be legally done or doing what should not be done can be imposed on an individual in the form of fines or imprisonment.

The Law

The U.S. Constitution is the supreme law in the United States of America. If a question of how to read, or interpret, this law occurs, a decision is made in a court of law. The first case that relates to that particular question is referred to as the precedent. A precedent that is familiar to many is the *Roe vs. Wade* case in which the U.S. Supreme Court established that most laws prohibiting abortion violate a constitutional right to privacy. This case remains very controversial, but is currently the precedent that all similar cases are evaluated against. From that time on, all cases relating to that same situation are based on the primary decision, the principle of *stare decisis,* meaning "let the decision stand." All future cases are determined in the same manner. Following these guidelines, everyone is treated fairly under the same circumstances. These laws and rules are known as **common laws** and are to be followed by everyone.

Civil and Criminal Law

Law (jurisprudence), the set of rules established and enforced by local, state, and federal governments, can be divided into two primary classifications: **civil law** and **criminal law.** The most frequent law exercised in the dental care setting is civil law, which can be further broken into two subclassifications: contracts and torts, which are discussed later.

If a civil charge is brought against a dentist, he or she becomes the **defendant.** The **plaintiff,** the person who is bringing the charges against the defendant, must prove that a civil wrong was committed. If able to prove wrongdoing, restitution is awarded to the plaintiff in a monetary amount for any pain, suffering, and loss of wages that the dentist or dental treatment has caused.

Criminal law addresses wrongs committed against the welfare and safety of society as a whole. Criminal charges are brought against the defendant by the state to prevent any further harm to society and its members. If a case is proven against a defendant in criminal law, the defendant faces fines and/or imprisonment. A dentist would also face disciplinary action from the board of dentistry in his or her practicing state.

Dental Practice Act

In each state, statutes are enacted by each legislative body to make rules and regulations. The state board of dentistry is an administrative agency in each state that enforces these statutes and rules in regard to performance of specific functions. Each state has a Dental Practice Act that describes the legal restrictions and controls on the dentist, hygienist, and other dental assistants. The Dental Practice Act describes the dental team members as licensed or nonlicensed and lists what are allowed or disallowed duties for each, including the expanded functions (delegated functions that require increased responsibility and skill) that may be performed by each dental team member. Even if the job classification or title is unused in the state Dental Practice Act, any employee working in a dental office is covered in the law. The Dental Practice Act of each state gives guidelines for eligibility for licensing and identifies the grounds by which this license can be suspended or repealed. Dental assistants are advised to access the current Dental Practice Act when moving to another state to determine that state's guidelines for dental auxiliaries. Changing the content of the Dental Practice Act can be done by an amendment of the dental law, by an entirely new law and regulations being enacted to replace the old law, or by a combination of the two.

State Board of Dentistry

The practice act includes the name of the administrative board that supervises the dental practice act, such as the State Board of Dental Examiners or Dental Quality Assurance Board of the state. This board has the basic responsibility of enforcing adherence to the Dental Practice Act of that specific state. The members of this board are appointed by the governor of that state, normally from a list of recommendations from the state dental association. The membership usually has one lay member from the state, and the rest of the board members are normally licensed dentists. In some states a dental assistant and/or a dental hygienist are appointed to the dental board. The dental assistant and dental hygienist are normally appointed to participate and bring their profession's viewpoints into discussions, but often are nonvoting members. Another function of this board is to examine applicants for dental licenses and grant licenses if the criteria are met.

License to Practice. A license is granted to a dentist if he or she has met all the minimum requirements. The license is to protect the public from unqualified individuals providing dental treatment. Each state requires that the dental hygienist become licensed, as well. Some of the states require dental assistants to become licensed or registered in order to perform specific dental tasks.

To obtain a license, an individual must meet educational and moral requirements and pass a written theory examination and a clinical practice examination as specified by the administrative board of that state or region. The requirements may vary from state to state, so if the individual wants to practice in another state, an additional license may be required. In some states, an individual who has passed the requirements for one state may apply for a reciprocity agreement in another state and be allowed to perform dental skills without taking a written or clinical examination again. Reciprocity is an agreement between two or more states that allows an individual licensed in one state to receive, without further examination and testing, a similar license in the other state(s) identified in the reciprocity agreement. The reciprocity agreement normally takes place in states with adjoining borders and similar testing requirements.

The factors for revoking, suspending, or denying renewal of a license vary from state to state. Most states take action if the licensed person has a felony conviction and/or misdemeanors of drug addiction, moral corruption, incompetence, or mental/physical disability that may cause harm to patients under his or her dental care.

Expanded Functions. Expanded functions are specific advanced tasks that require increased skill and responsibility. These functions are delegated by the dentist according to the Dental Practice Act within the state. Some states require additional education, certification, or registration to perform these functions. Like all functions the dental assistant performs, the expanded functions fall under the doctrine of respondeat superior. Translated this means, "Let the master answer." So, if wrongdoing took place under the guidelines of employment, the dentist is liable for the negligent act. However, this does not mean that the dental assistant is not held responsible and cannot be sued. It merely means that a suit can be filed against either the employee and the dentist or both. Dental assistants who perform expanded functions are advised to carry their own malpractice/liability insurance. The dental assistant who is a current member of the American Dental Assistants Association (ADAA) has a $50,000 professional liability insurance policy that is included in ADAA dues. Other organizations and professional groups offer medical malpractice/ professional liability insurance and risk management information. The Health Providers Service Organization and many others are available to provide this coverage. Often, the dentist is sued because the plaintiff anticipates greater recovery in financial damages from the dentist. The doctrine is based on the assumption that the dentist has the right to direct and control the employees; therefore, along with the duty comes the responsibility of the consequences. In addition, if the patient is damaged, it is due to the employer exposing the patient to his or her employee. Therefore, the dentist is required to compensate the patient for any harm that was caused.

The expanded functions are most often specified in the dental practice acts according to how they are to be delegated. They may be stipulated for general supervision, which means that the procedure authorized in the dental practice act can be performed legally on a patient of record by the dental assistant under the general supervision of the dentist. If it is specified to be delegated under direct supervision, the dentist must be in the treatment facility to authorize this function and he or she must evaluate the performance of the procedure.

Certification, Licensure, and Registration. Dental assistants can become nationally certified by the Dental Assisting National Board, Inc. (DANB) (see Chapter 36, Employment Strategies). Some states require dental assistants to be certified, licensed, or registered to perform specific functions in the dental office. The first state to grant licensure to dental assistants was Minnesota. Certification from DANB is granted after education or work requirements have been met and a written test covering general chairside, radiology, and infection control has been passed. Continuing education is required to maintain current certification from DANB, and many states require continuing education to maintain registration or licensure.

The Dentist, the Dental Assistant, and the Law

The dental assistant must thoroughly understand the law in order to protect the patient, the dentist, and the profession. Dental health care continues to change, and the dental assistant must understand how these changes are impacted by the law.

Contracts

A contract is a binding agreement between two or more people. This agreement must be between two competent people, to do or not to do something lawful, in exchange for a payment ("competent" eliminates the mentally incompetent, individuals under the influence of drugs or alcohol, infants, and minors). The dentist has a legal obligation to care for a patient under the principles of contract law after a patient arrives for dental care and the dentist accepts him or her by providing dental care.

A contract can be expressed or implied. An expressed contract is written or verbally agreed upon. It describes specifically what each party in the contract will do. An implied contract is implemented by actions, not words. Most of the dentist/patient contracts are implied. If a patient comes to the dentist with a toothache and the dentist checks the area and requests that a radiograph be taken, this is an implied contract because it exists due to the circumstances. The law says that the dentist does what is necessary and what the patient would have requested had there been an expressed contract.

Dental assistants are agents of the dentist. What a dental assistant says and does can be used in a court of law against the dentist. For instance, if a dental assistant said the dentist can cure a problem but the dentist does not cure it, the dentist—not the dental assistant—is at fault. This is considered an admission by an employee and under the doctrine of respondeat superior would be the legal equivalent of the dentist saying that this can be accomplished even if it cannot be done. The dental assistant should be cautious because his or her actions and words at work may become binding on the employer, the dentist. Any statements either pro or con made spontaneously at the time of an alleged act can be admissible as evidence in a court of law. This is true because of the principle of res gestae, which translates to "part of the action," at the time of the offense and becomes admissible evidence in a case.

Termination of a Contract. A contract can be terminated when one of the parties does not meet contractual obligation. Until the contract is broken, or a breach of contract occurs, the dentist is legally bound to treat the patient. The contract can be terminated if:

- The patient discharges the dentist or fails to return to the office.
- The patient fails to follow instructions given by the dentist.
- The dentist formally withdraws from patient care.
- The patient no longer needs treatment/all requirements agreed upon have been met.

Patient Discharges the Dentist. The patient often discharges the dentist by not continuing to return to the office to complete services or continued care appointments. Legally, the dentist should send a letter to the patient to confirm and document the termination of the contract. This is normally done with a recall notification, documentation on the chart, and follow-up notification. Ideally, it should be done through certified mail, requesting a return receipt, so that a copy is in the patient's chart.

Patient Fails to Follow Instructions from the Dentist. The patient may fail to follow the instructions of the dentist in regard to the dental treatment. For instance, a patient has dental implants and is told by the dentist that ongoing cleaning appointments are necessary in order to maintain the health of the area. The patient is warned that failing to undergo ongoing cleaning may cause the implants to fail. The dental office repeatedly contacts the patient to have the prophy (cleaning) appointments, yet the patient does not return. Further, the dentist writes a letter telling the patient again that the implants may fail without the ongoing cleaning appointments and asks the patient to schedule necessary appointments. If the patient chooses not to follow the instructions from the dentist and fails to schedule the needed appointments, the contract would be broken. Any time the patient fails to respond to or follow instructions of the dentist, the contract between the dentist and the patient is broken.

Dentist Formally Withdraws from the Case. To avoid any charges of **abandonment** (desertion), the dentist should send the patient a certified letter, with return receipt requested, to formally withdraw from a dental case. This would happen if the dentist feels that he or she can no longer provide service to the patient or if the patient becomes **noncompliant** and the dentist can no longer work with the patient.

Patient No Longer Needs Treatment. The dentist is responsible for providing treatment until the patient no longer needs treatment or the dentist has formally withdrawn from the case. For example, if an oral surgeon has seen a patient to remove four wisdom teeth and this service has been completed and the patient has healed accordingly, therefore no longer needing this treatment, the contract would be terminated.

Standard of Care

The dentist and the dental team members have the responsibility and duty to perform due care in treating all patients. **Due care** is what any reasonable and prudent dental care professional in the same circumstances would do. The dental professional must provide sufficient care, within his or her scope of training, in all dental procedures, not excluding prescribing, dispensing, or administering drugs.

Malpractice

Malpractice is failure to use due care in dental treatment, which is considered negligence. **Negligence** is the failure to exercise the standard of care that a reasonable person would exercise in similar circumstances. Negligence is the primary cause of malpractice suits. Negligence comes about when an individual suffers injury because of another person's failure to live up to the normal standard of care. Malpractice is professional negligence. There are normally four elements of negligence (sometimes called the four "Ds"): duty, derelict, direct cause, and damage. Dental professionals are held to a high standard of care by virtue of their knowledge, intelligence, and skills. It is their duty to provide high performance, and they are expected not to be derelict (careless) in their skills. If they directly cause injury due to deviation from the normal standard of care and damage or harm occurs, they are negligent. At times, in a court of law, **expert witnesses** will testify in regard to the standard of care that is to be expected.

Torts

A **tort** is a wrongful act that results in injury to one person by another. For example, a dental assistant breaks the aseptic chain and causes the patient to be exposed to infection. If this infection causes the patient damage or harm, then the case may result in litigation. If the dental assistant broke the aseptic chain and the patient care resulted in no infection, damage, or harm, then a tort did not result. A tort must have a wrongful act that is a breach in due care that causes injury because of this action. Some wrongful areas of negligence may result in torts when the standard of care is not followed. Practicing good risk management protects the dentist and dental assistant from litigation.

Assault and Battery

Assault is the threat of touching a person without consent, and **battery** is the actual touching. The basis of the tort of assault and battery is the threat of or unprivileged touching of one person by another without consent. For example, an assault would be to insinuate that a desired touch is indicated. If dental personnel touch any areas other than the oral cavity or perioral region (palpation of neck, TMJ, lymph nodes, and so on), this could be considered battery. An unwanted hug without consent is battery. If a child was refusing treatment and the dental assistant threatened and restrained him or her without parental consent, assault and battery charges could be brought against the dental assistant according to the tort law.

Defamation of Character

Another tort law protects an individual(s) from causing injury to another person's reputation, name, or character. This injury, called **defamation of character**, can come from written or spoken words. Defamation of character can come from either libel or slander. **Libel** is false and malicious written comments. In the dental office, untrue comments on the patient's chart may be libel. For instance, if the dental assistant wrote on the chart that he or she suspected the patient's grinding of the teeth was a result of a bad marriage, it would be libel if someone else read the chart and took it as truth. **Slander** is false or maliciously spoken words. For example, a patient said, "Dr. Smith removes teeth even if they do not need to be removed." If the statement was overheard by another individual, it would be considered slander if untrue. A third party must hear or see it and understand what was said in order for defamation of character to exist.

Invasion of Privacy

Another kind of tort is the invasion of privacy. It includes unwanted publicity and exposure to public view and unauthorized publicity of patient information or anything in the patient's records. (See Information on HIPAA.)

> In the dental office, unwanted exposure to public view is not a problem; this occurs in the medical field where body parts are exposed for treatment.

The dental office must take great care to protect the disclosure of any patient information, spoken or written, on patient records. A dental assistant cannot use any information about the patient, medical or personal, that was obtained as a course of treatment without the person's approval or permission.

Fraud

Fraud is deliberate deception that is practiced to secure unfair or unlawful gain. The most common area of fraud in the dental office is insurance fraud. Dental personnel who send information that is incorrect to the insurance companies for payment are committing fraud.

Good Samaritan Law

The Good Samaritan Law is for individuals who do not seek payment but render medical assistance to the injured. This care is usually given because of an accident, and the law protects people or grants immunity for acts performed while providing emergency care. If this care is given without the intent to do bodily harm and without being compensated for this care, the Good Samaritan Law provides protection. Contents of the Good Samaritan Law vary from state to state, and each individual is responsible for understanding state laws.

Child Abuse and Neglect

Each of the 50 states has passed some form of a mandatory child abuse and neglect reporting law. This allows the state to qualify for funding and meet the criteria under the Child Abuse Prevention Treatment Act (CAPTA) of 1996. Every state requires certain professionals and institutions to report suspected abuse. Included are providers of medical and dental care and mental health care, teachers and other education personnel, social workers, and law enforcement personnel. In many states, individuals who work in film processing may also fall under this law. Some states require "any individual" to be responsible for reporting child abuse and neglect. Dental assistants in all states fall under this

reporting law. Failure to report suspected child abuse and neglect can result in civil or criminal liability that may be punishable by a fine. False reports are unacceptable; cases must be made according to a standard under which a "reasonable person" would believe that the report is true.

Americans with Disabilities Act

The Americans with Disabilities Act of 1990 nationally mandates that individuals will not be discriminated against because of their disabilities. The four areas noted in the act refer to:

- Employment discrimination due to disabilities.
- The disabled are provided access to public services.
- Public accommodations and access to equal goods and services are open to the disabled.
- Telecommunication services to the hearing and speech impaired are extended.

In the dental offices, ramps must be provided to allow individuals with disabilities access. The doorways and treatment rooms should allow for care to be provided for individuals with disabilities. One dental operatory needs to have access for patients confined to wheelchairs.

Dental Records

The dentist and the dental team members must be responsible to maintain accurate, up-to-date patient records. In litigation, the accuracy of the dental record directly relates to the credibility of the professionals. All actual care and charges must be reflected in the patient's dental records. Charts must be written in ink and be legible and all necessary corrections should be made by drawing a line through the initial content and then making the correction, initialing it, and dating the new data (Figure 3-1). Many offices are now utilizing software that allows for paperless charting. The dental record, radiographs, medical and dental history, and all other aspects of the chart are maintained through a computer backup system. These electronic files constitute a legal record that must be securely maintained. All HIPAA documents should be copied and scanned into the electronic record. Any prescriptions used in patient care would also be saved as part of the record, and a copy for the patient printed.

Informed Consent

 One important area of documentation is the informed consent form. Each patient has the right to know and understand any procedure that is to be performed. The patient is informed in words that can be understood. The patient should be

Chart No. ————

Patient's Name _Bradley Plummley_____

Date _____4/9/03____ #2 MOD Amal_____

_____#3 DO Amal dycal_____

_____#4 O Amal_____

_____2 anes.____ KJM_____

5/2/03_____#15 Full cold Crown prep_____

_____acrylic temp cemented w/tempbond KJM_

5/13/03_____#15 Full Gold Crown_____

_____cemented with zinc phosphate KJM__

_____R 250 mg V-cillin K ~~20 tabs~~ 10 tabs KJM_

FIGURE 3-1 When changes are made on the dental chart, a red line must be drawn through the initial content; then the correction is made with the person initiating the change notating it by initialing the chart.

told of the procedure, risks involved, expected outcome, other optional methods to treat the same problem, and the risk of denying the treatment. The health care worker must make certain that the patient understands the treatment. In today's society, a large number of patients speak English as a second language or not at all. An interpreter must be used to explain the procedure to the patient, if necessary.

If surgical procedures are to be performed, it is advisable to receive a consent form. The dental assistant may sign as a witness on the consent form. One copy is kept in the patient's chart and one is given to the patient for his or her records.

Implied Consent

Implied consent may happen in a number of subtle ways. When a dentist sits down and the patient opens his or her mouth, the patient is implying consent for the dentist to begin treatment. Patients rolling up their sleeves prior to blood pressure being taken are implying that the action for the blood pressure procedure can be taken.

Subpoenas

Subpoenas are court orders mandating that an individual show up at a specific time and date and with a specific reason to testify. Dental records can also be subpoenaed by the court and must be released to the court. Any records that provide documentation about sensitive material, such as sexually transmitted diseases including AIDS, substance abuse, and so on, may require an additional court order. Confidentiality must

be maintained, because the information the patient shares with the dentist is always held in confidence.

Statute of Limitations

The statute of limitations is different in every jurisdiction (state, county). The statute of limitations defines the period of time in which legal action can take place. Some time limits run from the beginning of treatment, some from the time the accused neglect took place, and others from the time the treatment was completed. Most timeframes run for three to six years. With the confusion about the time limits, most dentists keep their records for indefinite time periods.

Ethics

Ethics is defined in terms of what is right or wrong, or moral judgment of these two. In dentistry, it is defined by a code as the American Dental Association Principles of Ethics. Unlike the law, which rarely changes, ethics constantly changes and evolves just as personal values and morals change and evolve.

Advertising

Traditionally, dentists as professionals did not advertise. Advertising was not illegal if the advertising was truthful and not misleading, but many thought it to be unethical. Currently, it is not thought to be unethical, and there is a trend to advertise in a number of ways, such as telephone books, television, radio, media, Internet, and dental service coupons. Advertising is becoming more popular in the dental profession. Patients who are satisfied with their dental care are still the best advertising source.

Professional Fees and Charges

Professional fees are based on what is customary to the locale and should represent the difficulty of the dental procedure and the quality of the service rendered. The services documented on the patient's chart are the ones that are charged. The office can also charge the patient for insurance processing and missed appointments if the patient has been reminded of the appointment (see Chapter 36, Dental Office Management, for further information).

Professional Responsibilities and Rights

The dentist has professional responsibilities and rights when treating patients. Dentists cannot refuse to serve a patient on the basis of race, color, religion, national origin, sexual preference, or because he or she is an HIV-infected individual. If the dentist takes a dental patient for treatment, the dentist must provide the care in a timely manner unless that patient was given official written notice of possible delays.

If a dentist is HIV infected, the dentist should refrain from performing procedures that may risk transmission of the virus to the other health care providers or patients.

A dentist is not to be influenced by financial interests. For instance, if the dentist owns a large amount of stock in a company that sells specific dental medications, the dentist should not prescribe that medication only in order to enhance personal gain.

Health Insurance Portability and Accountability Act

The Health Insurance Portability and Accountability Act of 1996 (HIPAA), also known as the Kennedy-Kassebaum Act, was enacted to establish safeguards for health care transactions transmitted electronically. This does not mean that the government will develop a database of everyone's health information; it speaks only to the way health information is transacted and protected in the office. The U.S. Department of Health and Human Services (HHS) was mandated to adopt national standards for electronic administrative and financial health care transactions. The American Dental Association (ADA) was named consultant to the secretary of HHS for this legislation. The HIPAA laws are designed to protect patient rights. Every dental office that chooses to transmit transactions electronically falls under HIPAA. It is the responsibility of providers to ensure that they are up-to-date and have the correct HIPAA information. Thus, the dental office team should check with HHS and ADA for HIPAA updates.

The Law

Prior to implementation of the current HIPAA regulations, dental offices were required to be compliant with transactions and code sets by April 14, 2003. The HHS released guidance on July 6, 2001, that provided further information and explanations about the initial HIPAA Privacy Rule. In March 2002, HHS released proposed modifications to the final rule. The principal modification was elimination of the need for written patient consent for uses and disclosures of protected health information (PHI). It was noted that a dentist having a direct treatment relationship with an individual is required to make a good faith effort to obtain that person's written acknowledgment of Receipt of Notice of Privacy Practices. Form design, however, is left to the dentist, but must be written. The Centers for Medicare and Medicaid Services (CMS) is the enforcement authority for transactions, code sets, identifiers, and security. The Office for Civil Rights (OCR) is the enforcement authority for

the privacy rule. It is critical that each dental professional know the HIPAA legislation and be familiar with the HIPAA regulations and terms used in the HIPAA. It is the provider's responsibility to ensure that the office and personnel are up-to-date and have the correct HIPAA information. The HHS administrative website is http://www.hhs.gov/ocr/hipaa/finalreg.html. It is advisable that the privacy officer, the person in the office responsible for keeping all office personnel updated on HIPAA, review HIPAA updates routinely. The privacy officer should also check with the ADA repeatedly for HIPAA updates to ensure compliance. Education and training for everyone must be completed initially upon employment and ongoing thereafter. It should include all efforts to comply with HIPAA through routine office policies and procedures. It is beneficial to evaluate the "areas of concern" and then develop an implementation plan and follow up with maintenance and monitoring to ensure adherence compliance. The HHS does not intend to disrupt the flow of patient care. They proposed new regulatory language to clarify that they did not intend to prohibit the use of sign-in sheets. It was noted that it also did not mean that the practice which uses the patients' names in the waiting room when it is time for their appointments should not be able to do this under HIPAA.

Transactions and Code Sets

Vendors, payers, providers, clearinghouses, and the government came together to state their needs and reached an agreement for a standard code set. In dentistry, the 2005 code set, Current Dental Terminology (CDT), is the eleventh version of the code. The first CDT was completed in 1969. It was initially revised every five years; in response to the HIPAA Standard Code Set, it will be revised every two years. The CDT 2005 contained thirty-nine new codes, deletion of three codes, and forty-seven revisions to the standards. The codes currently have a "D" and a four-digit number attached. There are twelve categories in the code standard. The transactions and coding normally apply to most services; there are very few exceptions (see Table 3-1).

Physicians must submit their claims to the Medicare program in the standard electronic format. Normally dentists will not have Medicare claims, but if they do, they would fall under this requirement. Physician or dentist practices that consist of fewer than ten full-time employees are not subject to this standard. Medicare contractors will not accept transactions that do not meet the new standards (i.e., electronic format, since October 16, 2003).

What Does HIPAA Encompass?

The key element of HIPAA is the safeguarding of PHI. Dental personnel must understand how HIPAA defines health information (HI) as well as PHI. The privacy rule

TABLE 3-1 CDT—2005–Current Dental Terminology Standard Codes

Diagnostic	D0000–D0999
Preventive	D1000–D1999
Restorative	D2000–D2999
Endodontics	D3000–D3999
Periodontics	D4000–D4999
Prosthodontics, removable	D5000–D5899
Maxillofacial Prosthodontics	D5900–D5999
Implant Services	D6000–D6199
Prosthodontics, fixed	D6200–D6999
Oral Surgery	D7000–D7999
Orthodontics	D8000–D8999
Adjunctive Services	D9000–D9999

regulates how PHI may be used and disclosed. It also provides certain rights to patients and contains administrative requirements to protect confidentiality of PHI. The Privacy Standard covers the following:

- Protected health information
- Rights of the individual
- New policies for dental offices that cover the Privacy Standard
- Disclosures that do not require authorization
- Uses and disclosures with patient authorization
- Minimum necessary use and disclosure
- Enforcement
- Preemption

Who Must Comply with HIPAA?

The HIPAA provisions, by statute, apply to all direct and indirect providers of health care services and supplies. **Direct providers,** referred to as **covered entities,** include hospitals, clinics, nursing homes, assisted-living facilities, home health agencies, physicians, dentists, and alternative medicine. **Indirect providers,** or **business associates,** include laboratories, pharmacies, surgical centers, and any services that deal with any patient information. Health care services and supplies would include any medical and dental supplies, information systems, record and data storage and destruction, maintenance services that may have access to

patient information, and so on. The HIPAA provisions apply to any entity transmitting health information in an electronic form. Therefore, business associates that use or disclose the protected health information (or create, obtain, and use this information) to perform a function or activity on behalf of the covered entity, or dentist in this case, are covered under the HIPAA provisions. Examples of business associates would include accounting firms, consultants, legal firms, management companies, data/record copying, storage and destruction companies, and suppliers.

Business Associates. It should be noted that both the covered entities and their business associates must comply with HIPAA. The dental office must have contracts with any business associates who will be able to access individuals' PHI. These parties may even include cleaning services and any other persons with patient file access. The covered entity (dentist) should make the business associates aware of HIPAA requirements and document that the information has been provided. The business associate contract must establish the use of information and outline safeguards against inappropriate disclosure. Contracts must prohibit other uses and disclosures of the patient information, and must provide for return and destruction of protected health information at the end of the contract, if possible, or the associates are required to continue protection. Covered entities may be penalized for HIPAA infractions, and business associates may not. If the covered entity knows of a violation by a business partner and takes no action, that entity is violating the privacy standard. The dental office needs to exercise good judgment with business associates. For instance, if remodeling occurs when no office personnel are present, all PHI should be locked up. Charts for the following day should not be left out unprotected. This does not mean that dentists cannot discuss a patient's case with other dentists and fax information back and forth on the case. If the patient is made aware of how this information is to be used in his or her treatment and he or she signs a document that allows the dentists to discuss or fax information about the case with other dentists or specialists, such PHI distribution falls within the HIPAA guidelines.

Protected Health Information

Any information that identifies the individual or gives a reasonable basis toward identifying the individual is **protected health information.** PHI covers the individual's name (including nickname) telephone numbers, fax numbers, e-mail addresses, Social Security numbers, student identification numbers, photographs, oral health information, birth date, appointment date, and any geographic identifier more specific than state (e.g., zip code, county, region, or address). It also covers any individually identifiable health information such as the individual's past, present, or future physical or mental health condition; and payment for any past, present, or future physical or mental health treatment. The privacy rule excludes any health information that a covered entity maintains in its capacity as an employer.

What this means to a dental office is that all patient records must be protected. Doors must be locked when patient records are left unattended. In an office's HIPAA policy manual, an individual should be identified as the person responsible for locking the doors. Records cannot be left out for others to see; **day sheets**—sheets that show the daily schedule and patients' names with services required—cannot be left out for everyone to see in the operatories. Day sheets can be placed in a cabinet for the staff to view when necessary (Figure 3-2). Other offices have responded to this rule by taping the day sheet upside down and toward the wall (the sheet is flipped up for viewing when necessary). Screen savers could be set to come on within a few seconds of reviewing patient information and placed out of view of other patients. Charts cannot be left in potential view of other

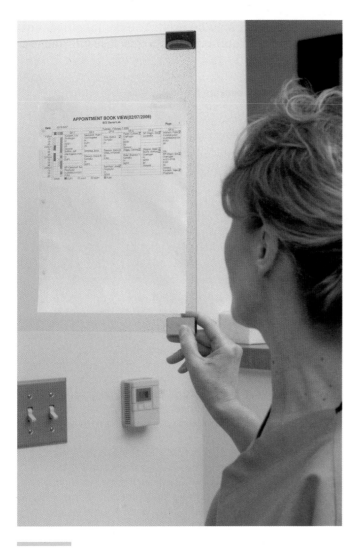

FIGURE 3-2 Due to the privacy rule, many offices are keeping the day sheets (daily schedule) with patient names on it inside a cabinet so that it is not available for viewing by other patients.

patients and individuals in the office. When the business office is confirming appointments for the following day or making an appointment for a patient, dental office employees should not repeat a patient's telephone number or any other PHI out loud if others could hear it. The last four numbers could be repeated but not the initial numbers that would identify a geographic area for the patient. If the office is located in an area where only one or a few telephone prefixes are used, then repeating out loud the last four numbers is also prohibited.

Location of the fax machine and copy machine is critical. It is important that any patient PHI that is copied or faxed is not visible or accessible to individuals passing by the machines. Spend the extra time to verify the number that any information is being sent to and remember that patient knowledge and consent for this transaction must have been obtained. If the dental office receives a facsimile that was sent in error, contact the sender and notify him or her immediately of the error.

Rights of the Individuals. Individuals have the right to access, inspect, and get copies of their dental information. They have the right to request amendments or corrections of their dental information. HIPAA requires that they receive written notice of information practices and an accounting of disclosures.

Privacy Policies and Procedure Statements. Dental offices write their own health information privacy policies and procedure statements and must present this information to patients for their acknowledgment and signature. There are a number of template formats available for adoption by dental offices. The *HIPAA Privacy Kit,* available from the ADA, contains policies and procedures for dental offices along with forms, checklists, and other helpful information (Figure 3-3).

A dental office's privacy officer (PO) may be an auxiliary, or this responsibility may be shared by two or more dental auxiliaries. The PO(s) provides information to patients about their privacy rights and how their information may be used. This information must be written so that it is easily understood by the patient. The notice of privacy practices for the patient should describe how the health information about the patient may be used and disclosed and accessed by the patient. It should also cover how a patient should proceed if he or she feels that privacy rights have been violated. It should note that retaliation against the patient will not occur if a complaint is filed. The dentist and/or privacy officer(s) are responsible for ensuring that privacy procedures are adopted and followed. Employees must be trained to ensure that they understand privacy policies. This can be accomplished by giving the employees copies of the privacy policies and having each employee read the information and sign a document that they have read the policies and understand them. It should be dated and kept as part of the office records. The office must also create and display a patient rights notice that states all rights that patients have regarding

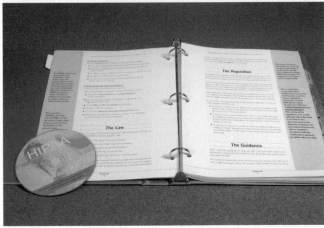

FIGURE 3-3 The American Dental Association developed the *HIPAA Privacy Kit* to aid members with HIPAA regulations.

Patients have the right to know about all instances in which their health information has been disclosed for something other than treatment, payment, or health care operations. Patients also have the right to complain about privacy violations without repercussion. Dental offices should develop a tracking system for all PHI and note each transaction so that they can ensure safety and protection for their patients.

Permitted Use and Disclosure. PHI should not be used or disclosed except as required or permitted by regulations and standards. It can be used for treatment and care coordination, to pay doctors and hospitals for health care and to help run their businesses. It can be shared with family, relatives, and friends who are identified by the patient as involved in the patient's health care or health care billing. Patient PHI can be used for public health purposes, such as in reporting flu in the locale, and to make reports to the police as required. Dental offices should minimize information release. Only "reasonably needed" information should be released from the office. Patients have the right to determine how their information may be used. The dental office must honor a patient's authorization to disclose information.

PHI. Staff training is to occur initially upon employment and annually thereafter.

HIPAA requires the following:

- Reasonable steps to protect PHI
- Identification of PO(s) by dental offices
- Employee privacy training
- Compliance with an individual's rights to notice of dental policy, access to the individual's information, and the right to ask for an amendment and accounting of how information is used
- Administrative, technical, and physical safeguards of PHI
- A policy for handling grievances
- Business associate agreements

Patient Health Information Use and Disclosure. Patients have the right to an understandable written explanation of the use and disclosure of their health information.

Consent Requirements

1. Plain language.
2. Inform the individual of the notice of information practices.
3. Refer individual to the notice of information practices.
4. Inform the individual of the right to review the notice before signing the consent.
5. State that the notice may change.
6. Inform the individual of the right to restrict use and disclosure of the information.
7. State that the individual may revoke consent.
8. Signature and date by patient.

A valid authorization must identify the nature of the information to be disclosed, must be in writing, and dated and signed by the patient. It must also identify the name, address, and institutional affiliation of the person to whom the information is being disclosed. The office may comply with this requirement by faxing a form containing all necessary information to the patient to sign and date; the patient's return fax containing signature and date is considered valid. It is a good idea to stamp any copies of PHI that leave the office so that if copies are made they can be traced to the source. Stamps for "patient copy," "insurance copy," and copied for _____ cover most areas. Stamping in red may help determine if the information has been copied again.

Remember, release only required information, and minimize information release. For instance, if patients ask for transfer of all records, what are they really asking for? Are the radiographs that were taken 20 years ago pertinent for the next provider? Dental offices can verify in the Office HIPAA Manual that office policy for transferring records states that the transfer can be limited to the past five years of information and the most recent radiographs. This would then be the standard for transferring information unless a specific request is made. The dental office does have the right to charge for copying and transferring this information for the patient. The goal is to protect the privacy and the security of PHI without hindering dental care.

Security Rule

The security rule is the ability to control access and protect information from accidental or intentional disclosure to unauthorized persons and from alteration, destruction, or loss. This rule can be understood as implementation of the privacy rules. The dental office is not required to store all PHI in a safe, nor are locks necessary on all cabinets. Instead, office staff must be responsible in preventing the inadvertent or intentional exposure of PHI to unauthorized persons.

Office Manual

An office HIPAA manual must identify the PO and a contact person to receive complaints (who may be the same person). The manual must include job descriptions for all employees. When the dental office creates a manual is a good time to evaluate how PHI is handled and what measures can be taken to ensure compliance to the HIPAA privacy standard. The manual must also include the HIPAA training plan and training dates for each employee. Training must include information about coding and electric claims submission, privacy, and security, as well as procedures and processes to be used in the office to protect the PHI. Covering relationships with business associates during the training is advisable, as well as including a copy of business associate audits and forms. The manual should contain the privacy policy statement, HIPAA forms and supporting documentation, how compliance is maintained and ongoing, method of reporting violations, confidentiality agreements, notice about contents, notice that policies may change, and employee responsibilities for following up on change notices. Document everything to maintain a record of compliance.

The dental office staff manual must include but is not limited to the following:

- PO identified
- Job descriptions for all employees
- HIPAA training plan and dates
- Business associate audits and forms
- Privacy policy statement
- HIPAA forms and supporting documentation
- Documentation of HIPAA compliance and ongoing evaluation
- Method of reporting violations
- Confidentiality agreements
- Notice that policies may change, and employee responsibilities for following up on change notices

Staff Training and Review

Dental offices should provide training for all employees in safeguarding PHI and its usage and disclosure. Training for new employees should be organized by the PO within a reasonable time from the hire date. Retraining for employees should take place when duties change or privacy policies change. If an employee appears not to follow privacy policies of the office, then discussion should occur and additional training provided. Continued violation of office privacy policies can be grounds for dismissal. Dentists should encourage incident identification by employees so that ongoing evaluation and monitoring take place. Dentists must develop a policy for disciplining employees who violate and continue to violate the office privacy policy. This policy should be part of the office HIPAA manual.

Enforcement of HIPAA

The HHS Office of Civil Rights polices HIPAA. If requested, covered entities—dentists—provide records and compliance reports. Anyone, including an employee, may file a complaint with the HHS. These complaints are covered under the whistleblower provision, and thus retaliation against the complainant is not acceptable. There are no HIPAA inspectors who will show up unannounced at the dental office to evaluate what is being done. Dental offices must self-monitor and self-evaluate HIPAA practices and be responsible for rule compliance.

Preemption. The U.S. Congress enacted several sections of the HIPAA that are known as the Administrative Simplification provisions. Congress mandated that certain standards must be followed in protecting the privacy of individually identifiable health information. Under preemption, where state laws are contrary to federal law, the federal law is to be followed. State law is therefore preempted by federal law. However, if state law provides greater privacy than the federal HIPAA, then the state law must be followed and not preempted. It should be noted that a request to make a state law provision exempt from preemption may be submitted in writing to the secretary of HHS.

Federal Civil and Criminal Penalties for Violations of Patient's Right to Privacy

Civil, or noncriminal, violations of a patient's right to privacy result in prescribed monetary penalties. Penalties for disclosures made in error with no intent of violation are $100 per incident, and up to $25,000 per year per standard or individual. Criminal penalties for "knowingly" violating the patient's right to privacy upon obtaining or disclosing PHI are up to $50,000 and 1 year of imprisonment. Other criminal penalties for "knowingly" violating a patient's right to privacy follow: up to $100,000 and 5 years of imprisonment for obtaining or disclosing PHI under "false pretenses"; and up to $250,000 and 10 years of imprisonment for obtaining PHI with the intent to sell, transfer, or use it for commercial advantage, personal gain, or malicious harm.

HIPAA Challenge

The greatest HIPAA challenge is training and monitoring office personnel. Doing so requires that everyone be responsible for protecting patients' privacy. Ongoing training is necessary as rules and regulations change. A recommended strategy for dental offices is to document, document, and document. A number of sources can be contacted for help. Many template training programs (on CD) contain sample forms that can be adapted to the dental office. Consultants are available for writing policies and procedures. Finally, many Web-based systems are available that can be adapted to the dental office.

The American Dental Assistants Association Principles of Ethics and Professional Conduct

Each individual involved in the practice of dentistry assumes the obligation of maintaining and enriching the profession. Each member shall choose to meet this obligation according to the dictates of personal conscience based on the needs of the general public the profession of dentistry is committed to serve.

The member shall refrain from performing any professional service that is prohibited by state law and has the obligation to constantly strive to upgrade and expand technical skills for the benefit of the employer and consumer public. The member should additionally seek to sustain and improve the local organization, state association, and the American Dental Assistants Association through active participation and personal commitment.

Code of Professional Conduct

As a member of the American Dental Assistants Association, I pledge to:

- Abide by the bylaws of the Association
- Maintain loyalty to the Association
- Pursue the objectives of the Association

- Hold in confidence the information entrusted to me by the Association
- Maintain respect for the members and employees of the Association
- Serve all members of the Association in an impartial manner
- Recognize and follow all laws and regulations relating to activities of the Association
- Exercise and insist on sound business principles in the conduct of the affairs of the Association
- Use legal and ethical means to influence legislation or regulation affecting members of the Association
- Issue no false or misleading statements to fellow members or to the public
- Refrain from disseminating malicious information concerning the Association or any member or employee of the Association
- Maintain high standards of personal conduct and integrity
- Not imply Association endorsement of personal opinions or positions
- Cooperate in a reasonable and proper manner with staff and members
- Accept no personal compensation from fellow members, except as approved by the Association
- Promote and maintain the highest standards of performance in service to the Association
- Assure public confidence in the integrity and service of the Association

Dental Assistants Following Ethics and Jurisprudence

The profession of dentistry will continue to advance, and dental assistants will have more decisions to make in the arena of ethics and jurisprudence. The necessity to stay abreast of the changes and to make decisions that are educated and concrete is essential. The dental assistant should always strive to stay within the law, handle patients in a professional manner, maintain a high standard of care, obtain patient consent, preserve confidentiality, maintain legible and accurate records, and avoid judging others who have belief systems that are different.

CHAPTER SUMMARY

Each dental team member is faced with daily decisions that require judgments regarding legal and ethical principles. Maintaining professional ethical standards at all times is essential. The consequences for not doing what should be legally done or doing what should not be done can include fines or imprisonment. A license is granted to protect the public from unqualified individuals providing dental treatment. Some states require dental assistants to become licensed to perform specific dental tasks. The expanded functions are most often specified in the Dental Practice Act according to how they are to be delegated. They may be stipulated for general supervision, which means that the procedure authorized in the Dental Practice Act can be legally performed on a patient of record by the dental assistant under the general supervision of the dentist, or they may be specified to be delegated under direct supervision. The dental assistant must thoroughly understand the law in order to protect the patient, the dentist, and the profession. Dental health care continues to change and the assistant must understand how the law affects these changes and stay within the law. HIPAA regulations are required to protect patient information. It is the responsibility of the dental team members to stay informed and comply with the standards.

Case Study

Two weeks ago, Dr. Greenwood treated a new patient, Deziree Jordan, for a fractured tooth. Peggy Stussi assisted Dr. Greenwood during the examination and the restoration of the tooth. Today, both Dr. Greenwood and Peggy Stussi were served with subpoenas by Deziree's attorney. Deziree is alleging that unsafe conditions took place at a local restaurant and she bit down on a rock in her hamburger. Dr. Greenwood and Peggy Stussi are called as expert witnesses in a civil hearing. Peggy is nervous about going to court and being on the witness stand. Peggy does not know what to expect.

Case Study Review

1. How will Deziree's dental record help Peggy answer questions at the hearing?

2. As an expert witness, what is Peggy expected to testify about in this case?

3. What should Peggy do to prepare for the testimony?

REVIEW QUESTIONS

Multiple Choice

1. Occasionally, a dentist is sued for negligence by a dental assistant employee, even though the dentist is not guilty of the negligent act himself or herself. This is done on the basis of the doctrine of
   a. contract law.
   b. expressed law.
   c. respondeat superior.
   d. civil law.

2. The contract that most often exists between the dentist and the patient is:
   a. civil.
   b. implied.
   c. expressed.
   d. proximate.

3. The legal restrictions and controls that governs dentistry in each state are
   a. statutes.
   b. expanded functions.
   c. Dental Practice Acts.
   d. reciprocities.

4. A binding agreement between two or more people is a(n)
   a. agent.
   b. reciprocity.
   c. contract.
   d. breach.

5. A wrongful act that results in injury to one person by another is a(n)
   a. tort.
   b. contract.
   c. assault.
   d. libel.

6. Hospitals, clinics, physicians, dentists, and alternative medicine are described as _____ according to HIPAA provisions.
   a. indirect providers
   b. direct providers
   c. covered entities
   d. b and c

7. HIPAA was enacted in
   a. 1990.
   b. 1996.
   c. 2001.
   d. 2005.

8. In dentistry, the code set Current Dental Terminology (CDT 2005) is the ____ version of the code. The first was completed in 1969.
   a. fourth
   b. eighth
   c. eleventh
   d. fourteenth

9. The office HIPAA manual must include
   a. job descriptions of all employees.
   b. PO identity.
   c. business associate audit and forms.
   d. all of the above.

10. The law that covers individuals who are not seeking payment but are rendering medical assistance to the injured is the
    a. Americans with Disabilities Act.
    b. Good Samaritan Law.
    c. ADAA Code of Ethics.
    d. HIPAA.

Critical Thinking

1. Explain the standard of care as it applies to dental assistants. Give an example.

2. What is the Good Samaritan Law? What must the dental assistant remember when giving first aid during an accident?

3. Differentiate between ethics and jurisprudence.

4. Does the HIPAA law allow patients to sign in for appointments, or is this in violation of the patient's right to privacy?

5. When calling a patient to enter the treatment room, is it allowable to use the patient's name spoken out loud in a room of other patients? Does this practice violate HIPAA guidelines?

Web Activities

1. Research the ADA site at http://www.ada.org and the U.S. Department of Health and Human Services at http://www.hhs.gov for any HIPAA updates.

2. Visit http://www.usdoj.gov and review the requirements for small businesses to aid in the treatment of individuals with disabilities.

3. Review additional information on HIPAA at http://www.hipaadvisory.com. Are there any new additions and modifications to the standard? If so, note them for class discussion.

SECTION II

PREVENTION AND NUTRITION

PRACTICE

CHAPTER 4

ORAL HEALTH AND PREVENTIVE TECHNIQUES

SPECIFIC INSTRUCTIONAL OBJECTIVES

The student should strive to meet the following objectives and demonstrate an understanding of the facts and principles presented in this chapter:

1. Describe how plaque forms and affects the tooth.
2. Identify motivation tips for oral hygiene for each age group.
3. Identify the oral hygiene aids available to all patients, including manual and automatic.
4. Demonstrate the six toothbrushing techniques.
5. Identify types of dental floss and demonstrate flossing technique.
6. Describe fluoride and its use in dentistry.
7. Define fluoridation and describe its effectiveness on tooth development and the posteruption stage.
8. List and explain the forms of fluoride. Describe how to prepare a patient and demonstrate fluoride application.

KEY TERMS

acidulated phosphate
  fluoride *(64)*
acute fluoride
  poisoning *(63)*
ameloblasts *(63)*
antibacterial
  effect *(63)*
caries *(43)*
chronic fluoride
  poisoning *(63)*
demineralization *(43)*
dentifrice *(46)*
enamel
  hypocalcification
  (63)
enamel hypoplasia *(63)*

floss holder *(49)*
floss threader *(50)*
fluoride *(61)*
fluoridation *(62)*
fluoroapatite
  crystal *(62)*
fluorosis *(62)*
gingivitis *(45)*
halitosis *(48)*
hydroxyl ion *(62)*
interproximal
  brush *(49)*
manual toothbrush *(51)*
mechanical
  toothbrush *(52)*
mottled enamel *(62)*

periodontitis *(45)*
plaque *(43)*
posteruption
  stage *(63)*
preeruption stage *(62)*
rubber dental
  stimulator *(49)*
sodium fluoride *(64)*
stannous fluoride *(64)*
systemic fluoride *(63)*
topical fluoride *(63)*
water irrigation
  device *(50)*
wooden dental
  stimulator *(49)*
xerostomia *(61)*

INTRODUCTION

Dental assistants in the dental office have an important role in preventive dentistry. Dentistry is about preventing oral disease, such as dental decay, and prevention of and caring for periodontal disease. It is important to educate the public on how to prevent disease. The dental assistant must be knowledgeable about the many products available to aid patients in maintaining their teeth and gums. The dental assistant must be a good listener and be able to evaluate the needs of patients. Dental assistants must also know how to motivate patients to be effective in their oral hygiene care. Fluoride has been proven to be effective in reducing dental caries. The dental assistant will need to have background knowledge of fluoride to educate patients in its usage and benefits. A final area of oral health and prevention is nutrition. Many patients will not be knowledgeable about the kinds of foods that will aid them in cleansing their teeth or which foods perpetuate decay. The dental assistant, after discussions with patients, can identify nutritional concerns and help patients choose foods that will benefit their oral health.

Preventive Dentistry

CDA The goal of preventive dentistry is that each individual maintains optimal oral health. Preventive concepts are woven throughout each modern dental practice. To be effective in preventive dentistry, dental assistants must first care for their own teeth properly and practice good nutrition.

- Brush and floss daily to remove plaque and bacteria.

- Disclose periodically to evaluate the effectiveness of brushing and flossing.

- Follow a fluoride program while the teeth are developing to allow them to be strong and decay resistant. The fluoride program includes office applications and home treatments.

- Follow a good nutrition and exercise program to maintain overall health. Good nutrition over a lifetime allows strong teeth and bones to develop and be maintained.

- Schedule regular dental visits for a thorough examination, cleaning, and any necessary dental treatment.

Plaque Formation

Dental **plaque** is a sticky mass that contains bacteria and grows in colonies on the teeth (Figure 4-1). Most people have missed areas while brushing their teeth and noted that a soft, white, sticky mass forms. This consists of plaque and other soft deposits. The bacteria in plaque are fed by the sugar in food. The bacteria-rich plaque converts the

FIGURE 4-1 Plaque on the gingival surface of the teeth, shown as a soft, white, sticky mass.

FIGURE 4-2 Demineralization of the tooth enamel appears as a white chalky area. *(Courtesy of Dwight H. Damon, DDS, MSD)*

sugar to acid. After a period of time, the acid attacks the tooth and eventually causes **demineralization**, in which minerals, calcium, and phosphate are lost from the enamel surface (Figure 4-2). People who have had orthodontic appliances may have demineralization on the tooth surface where the brackets were located. When the brackets are removed, demineralization appears as a whitish area on the tooth. It developed because plaque was not removed routinely around the brackets. If plaque continues to attack the tooth, it will cause decay, or **caries**. Once dental decay has begun, the area should be restored by a dentist.

> **Dental Decay (Caries) Equation**
>
> Sugar + plaque = acid + tooth = decay

Patient Motivation

Preventing dental disease is ultimately the responsibility of the patient, but dental auxiliaries spend a great deal of time educating and motivating patients to care for their teeth and oral cavities. The first aspect of patient motivation is for the dental assistant to assess oral hygiene and to listen to the patient. Listening to the patient gives insight into the patient's attitude toward oral hygiene and allows the assistant to get a better idea how to motivate and communicate with the patient. It is best to work with patients to help them recognize their dental problems, problem solve together to develop solutions, and then provide motivation and help them set oral hygiene goals.

Age Characteristics

Each patient should be treated as an individual, taking into consideration the patient's age, oral hygiene knowledge, skills, attitude, and any special considerations. Different age groups have characteristics that are normally identifiable; however, these characteristics are not absolute. A few general characteristics pertaining to each age group follow.

Infants. An infant's oral hygiene must be accomplished by the parent or caregiver. The dental assistant can show parents how to lay children back in their arms and use washcloths or infant toothbrushes to remove plaque. It should be stressed that this initial contact with oral hygiene should be positive. Making this a fun activity sets the stage as the infant develops (Figure 4-3).

Preschool Children. Preschool children have an active interest in visual aids, such as amusing toothbrushes or puppets. They lack highly developed motor skills, normally cannot read, and their attention span is less than five minutes. The child's first appointment with the dentist takes place around age three and should be a very positive contact. The dentist may not accomplish as much as desired during this appointment, but it is more

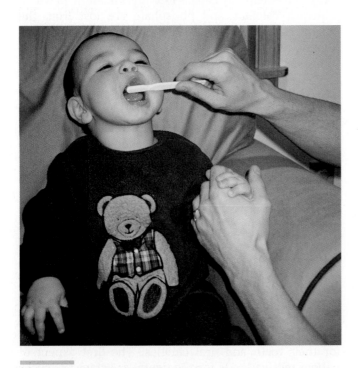

FIGURE 4-3 Parent brushing an infant's teeth.

important that it is a pleasant experience. The dental assistant can use a puppet to show oral hygiene instructions. "Mr. Air," the three-way syringe, can be used to blow "wind" on the tooth after "Mr. Water" gives the child a drink from the same syringe. Counting the "upstairs" and "downstairs" teeth for children is another fun activity to get children to open their mouths. Children can be shown how to put toothbrushes in their mouths and tickle the teeth and gum tissue. Even if a child chews on the brush, some plaque is being removed.

At home, parents can instruct children to sit down and watch television or listen to a story while brushing their teeth. If this happens on and off throughout the day, the teeth will have some care. Parents can also brush their teeth in front of the television without toothpaste to role play what the children are to do. Children of this age love to imitate their parents. Keep in mind that children like active, short procedures that give positive reinforcement. Parents must ensure that at least once (at bedtime) the child's teeth get a thorough, monitored brushing. Twice a day (morning and night) is best, especially if the parent can floss between the child's molars once daily.

Ages Five through Eight. Ages five through eight are when many changes take place in children's lives and their attention span increases to ten to fifteen minutes. Children at this age are learning to read and their vocabulary is growing. They like to please adults and enjoy learning (Figure 4-4). They love facts and require constant guidance as they strive for immediate goals with positive reinforcement. A dental assistant could teach children of this age to improve their brushing techniques and floss because the child's dexterity is getting better. Videos lasting under ten minutes with cartoons describing brushing and flossing could be used for this age group. Pictures to color, finding items in a picture, or matching a picture are also popular activities for this age group. The dental assistant can design hygiene pictures or purchase commercial ones. The ADA has videos and other aids for hygiene instruction.

Ages Nine through Twelve. Nine- through twelve-year-olds are very concerned with fitting into a group and doing what others in that group are doing. They can brush and floss proficiently and have great curiosity. They only like realistic visual aids at this age and their attention span is normally around thirty minutes. They have a mixed dentition of primary and permanent teeth that may require special directions to achieve proper hygiene in some areas. The dental assistant may provide hygiene instructions in a group of this age or may give rewards for good hygiene. One technique is to take pictures of the patients in this age group who have had success with oral hygiene. These pictures can then be posted on a bulletin board in the office. The patients love to find their friends and may strive to have their pictures among the others on the wall.

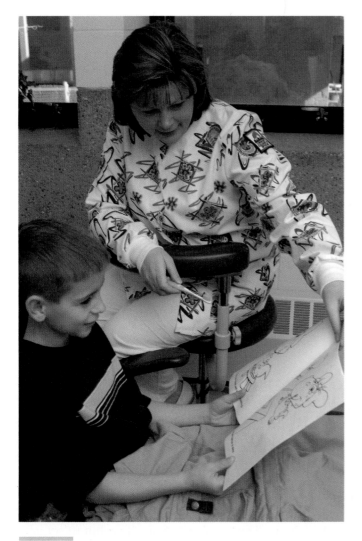

FIGURE 4-4 Seven-year-old patient is learning how to improve brushing technique.

Ages Thirteen through Fifteen. Patients in the thirteen-through fifteen-year-old group are extremely motivated by peer pressure and personal appearance. The rapid growth of individuals in this age group makes coordination a problem. Some may have to work hard at flossing and it is crucial that they do not feel silly in front of others. Another problem with adolescents is that their nutrition is often poor. Snacking is routine and, along with sporadic dental hygiene, the rate of decay rises. Motivation for this group will be individual and may change from office visit to office visit. Listen carefully to what is said at each visit and adapt the instruction to meet the current needs of the patient. Sincere positive reinforcement will be necessary to motivate this group of adolescents.

Ages Sixteen through Nineteen. Sixteen- through nineteen-year-olds are still very aware of peer pressure and experience increased concern about health and personal appearance. This group seems to question authority, so approach them as friends, allowing them to accept responsibility for their own oral hygiene. Nutritional habits are still in decline at this age, and time management is a problem. Suggestions by the dental assistant as to when oral hygiene can fit into the patient's schedule may be helpful. One area that will help motivate individuals of this age group is the desire to avoid bad breath. Talk to the individuals in this age group about the disadvantages of using a breath aid that has sugar in it. The dental assistant can give education about the process of plaque formation and tooth decay. Also, show them how to brush and floss to maintain good hygiene and fresh breath. Growth has leveled off, and coordination should be improved. Share with the patients of this age group how a good smile will help them secure employment.

Ages Nineteen through Sixty. Patients in the nineteen through sixty age group have specific needs and concerns that originate from their diverse backgrounds. One of the main concerns with this age group for the dental assistant is to help patients to unlearn habits that are not beneficial to their dental care. Help these individuals identify the problem and solve it. The patient must be involved and motivated in the action plan or no change will be made.

Patients in this age group may develop gingivitis or periodontal disease. **Gingivitis** is the inflammation of the gingival tissues. It appears as red, swollen, and/or bleeding gums. If people in this age group do not care for their teeth and plaque builds up, this condition may develop. Often when people see bleeding in their mouth, they try to stay away from that area; however, they should instead focus on that area. They should make sure to brush and floss more in that area and remove all plaque; this treatment will allow the tissues to heal and the bleeding to disappear. This oral health condition, if not cared for, may become worse, leading to **periodontitis**. In this disease process, the margins of gingival and periodontal fibers recede and the supporting bone becomes inflamed and destroyed. The patient develops periodontal pockets. The dental assistant will be instrumental in educating and motivating these adults in caring for their oral cavity.

Sixty Plus. Sixty-plus years allow patients to think about the necessity of keeping their teeth for a lifetime. Patients of this age should be made aware that tooth loss is not a part of aging. They would like to keep their teeth and be able to chew their food properly. Their dental restorations and appliances may have been placed many years ago and may need to be repaired or replaced. Routine dental appointments will assist in identifying concerns. Talk with the patients in this age group to help problem solve the life changes affecting their oral health. For example, arthritis may hamper adequate toothbrushing and flossing. The dental assistant may suggest to a patient with arthritis a larger, more pliable, handled toothbrush and a floss holder to ensure that a proper grasp can be accomplished.

Many of the patients in this group may be taking medications and need to understand what happens to their oral health when taking medications. The drug may cause the mouth to be dry, and saliva is an aid in fighting the acidity of plaque. Patients may choose to suck on hard candy to overcome dry mouth. The patient may not think of the effect on the teeth, and decay may develop rapidly between check-ups.

Home Care

Patients are ultimately responsible for caring for their oral health at home. The dental assistant can suggest ideas that will make this task simpler while still having every section of every tooth cleaned every day. The dental assistant's goals should closely resemble the ideas that stimulated the patient's desire to meet these goals. These ideas, of course, will differ for each patient. If what patients have been doing is working and they are not developing periodontal disease or dental decay, then acknowledge that they are doing a good job and encourage them to keep it up.

Patients should be made aware that the gingival tissue may be sore and may bleed when they first start a vigorous oral hygiene program. This means that the tissues are not healthy but will improve over time. It is much like the rest of the body. For instance, if a body is out of shape and an exercise program including sit-ups is started, the abdominal area will be sore for a week or so until the area is in shape. The same is true for gingival tissue. In about a week, the tissue will firm up and become healthier if the patient maintains the program. Patients should be told to expect soreness and bleeding for the first few days and not to stop because of it. They should be encouraged to continue the daily routine to maintain healthy gingival tissues and prevent decay.

Oral Hygiene Aids

A number of oral hygiene aids are on the market today for patient use. It is important to keep in mind that the simpler the task, the more chance of getting it accomplished. Adding a large number of steps will make it more difficult to accomplish the task daily. Suggestions for the proper aid and its correct usage will come from dental team members. The dental assistant should stay abreast of the aids on the market and know how they can help specific patients.

Disclosing Agents

Most individuals are visual in their approach to life. Being able to see plaque makes it easier for the dental assistant to show what it is and how and when it should be removed. Disclosing agents are used as a motivating factor in oral hygiene (Procedure 4-1). The agent is a temporary coloration (normally red) that makes plaque

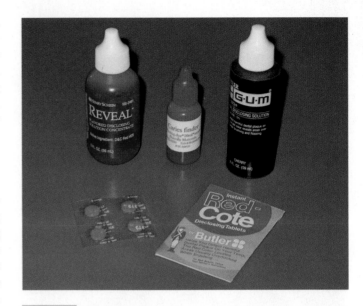

FIGURE 4-5 Examples of disclosing solutions (tablets and liquids).

visible. The disclosing agent comes in a tablet that can be chewed, a solution the dental assistant can paint on the teeth, or a drop that can be placed on the tongue (Figure 4-5). The color adheres to the plaque. Disclosing agents can be used in the dental office or at home to identify plaque. The patient should be warned that the oral cavity will change color due to the use of the disclosing agent. Before use, it is advisable to place petroleum jelly on the lips to prevent the color from sticking to the tissue. The color will go away within thirty minutes, but patients may not want it noticeable when they leave the office.

Dentifrice

Dentifrice (DEN-ti-fris) is the toothpaste used with brushing and flossing for patient oral hygiene self-care. As with all products used in oral hygiene, use those that have been tested and approved by the ADA. The ADA Seal of Acceptance will be on the packaging if the ADA Council on Dental Therapeutics has examined the product and classified it as such. The ADA classifies products as accepted, provisionally accepted, or not accepted. The accepted classification is awarded to products the ADA has found to be safe and effective for self-care. The provisionally accepted classification means that the ADA has found a product to be safe but clear evidence of dental usefulness is not available. The unaccepted classification is for products that present questionable safety and no evidence of dental usefulness. These classifications expire after three years.

Toothpaste is used by most individuals for dental care. Many toothpastes are available to patients, with numerous different flavors and consistencies (Figure 4-7). It should be chosen carefully based on the abrasives as

PROCEDURE 4 - 1

Applying Disclosing Agent for Plaque Identification

The procedure is performed by the dental assistant or dental hygienist. During the hygiene appointment, disclosing would be done to identify plaque and its location for the patient and operator. In some offices, a record of plaque location is charted and referred to during future appointments. Means of removing the plaque are then discussed and demonstrated.

EQUIPMENT AND SUPPLIES

▪ Basic setup: mouth mirror, explorer, and cotton pliers

▪ Saliva ejector, evacuator tip (HVE), and air-water syringe tip

▪ Cotton rolls, cotton-tip applicator, and gauze sponges

▪ Petroleum jelly (lubricant)

▪ Disclosing agent (liquid or tablet) and dappen dish

▪ Plaque chart and red pencil or software program

PROCEDURE STEPS

1. While seating the patient, the operator reviews the medical and dental history with the patient.

2. After washing hands and donning personal protective equipment (PPEs), such as mask, gloves, and glasses, the operator examines the oral cavity.

3. The operator applies the petroleum jelly (lubricant) to the patient's lips (some dentists may want petroleum jelly applied on any tooth-colored restorations to prevent staining).

4. The operator applies the liquid using the dappen dish and cotton-tip applicator. All accessible surfaces of the teeth should be covered with the disclosing solution.

5. If using the tablet, the patient chews and swishes for fifteen seconds.

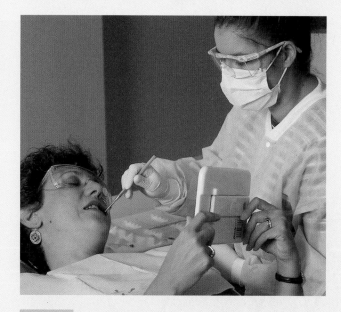

FIGURE 4-6 Dental assistant working with a patient to identify dental plaque. Disclosing agent on the patient's teeth identifies plaque.

6. The remaining solution is rinsed and evacuated from the area.

7. The patient uses a hand mirror to see the plaque, and the operator uses a mouth mirror and an air-water syringe to identify the plaque (Figure 4-6).

8. Overgloves are placed over treatment gloves to record the plaque in the chart or on the computer.

9. The operator removes the overgloves (treatment gloves remain in place), and then demonstrates for the patient methods of brushing and flossing for plaque removal.

well as caries control. The dentifrice (toothpaste) most often recommended is one that contains fluoride, especially for children and adults who are prone to caries. A small, pea-sized amount should be expelled onto the toothbrush for use. Toothpaste should not be ingested (because of the possibility of excessive intake of fluoride), and the excess should be expectorated (spit) into the sink. A toothpaste with low abrasives is also rec-

ommended because extremely high abrasives can permanently damage the patient's teeth with repeated use (they actually abrade the tooth structure). If a patient is prone to calculus (hard deposits mineralized on the teeth), there are toothpastes on the market with active ingredients that inhibit the growth of supragingival calculus. Other specialized toothpaste products whiten teeth or reduce gingival sensitivity when used routinely.

FIGURE 4-7 Examples of toothpaste used with brushing.

FIGURE 4-8 Antimicrobial mouth rinses.

Mouth Rinses

Mouth rinses are used for cosmetic or therapeutic reasons. Advertisements may lead patients to believe that mouthwashes do more than is possible. Vigorous rinsing with mouthwashes may loosen debris and give the patient a pleasant taste and feel, and temporarily eliminate **halitosis** (bad breath). They can also reduce the total number of microorganisms in the mouth, but mouth rinses (Figure 4-8) should not be used to replace brushing and flossing. The ADA has approved oral rinses that contain fluoride, which helps reduce dental decay and supragingival plaque. Individuals using these rinses must follow manufacturer's directions.

Rinses with fluoride are often prescribed for patients that have a high incidence of decay. Rinses that can be purchased at the pharmacy or the grocery store generally contain 0.05 sodium fluoride and are for daily use. The fluoride that is prescribed generally contains 0.2% sodium fluoride or 0.63% stannous fluoride. The stannous fluoride can also be used for decreasing the sensitivity of the tooth to hot and/or cold, dental hypersensitivity. The fluoride rinses are used for anti-plaque properties. When using the fluoride rinse it is best to brush and floss thoroughly and then dispense about 10 ml. of solution and swish in the mouth for 1 minute and then spit it out. Adults should not swallow the solution and children should be monitored so they do not swallow the rinse. It is not advisable to ingest excessive fluoride. After rinsing with the solution the patient should not eat or drink for 30 minutes. This allows the rinse to have time to be effective. Other fluoride rinses contain antimicrobial properties that can be used for the prevention and control of periodontal disease.

FIGURE 4-9 Xylitol containing chewing gum used to prevent tooth decay.

FIGURE 4-10 Interproximal brush.

Chewing Gum

Chewing gum designed specifically for oral hygiene purposes is a fairly new aid on the market (Figure 4-9). It is recommended for use after the intake of carbohydrates. Gum chewing stimulates saliva that buffers the plaque acid and is said to have carious inhibition properties. The chewing action also helps dislodge particles from the teeth.

Interdental Aids

Interdental aids are used to aid in cleaning the area between the teeth and to stimulate the gingival tissue in that area. In ancient oriental cultures, women would put spices between the teeth to have good breath. These women did not develop periodontal disease at the same rate as other individuals, and it was found that the spices being placed and removed routinely cleaned the plaque in that area, therefore eliminating periodontal disease. In other early cultures, it was said that a "chew stick" was used to clean the interproximal areas of the teeth. It resembled the toothpick and, after the end was chewed, the small fibers spread out slightly. As it was inserted into the area between the teeth, it cleaned the opposing surfaces. Some individuals today use the toothpick in this manner and it is quite effective at removing plaque between the teeth. A number of other products are on the market for use today.

The **interproximal brush** is a small hand-held brush with soft nylon bristles twisted in wire and adapted into a handle (Figure 4-10). It comes in different shapes and sizes and can be disposable. The brush is placed in the interproximal area and rotated back and forth using light pressure. Patients who have open contact areas or a substantial amount of bone loss due to periodontal disease would benefit from the interproximal brush. This brush is also useful to individuals who

have open bifurcation or trifurcation areas (where the roots of the teeth come together). It is also handy to use around orthodontic brackets to clean the difficult-to-access areas.

Rubber and wooden dental stimulators are placed in the interproximal area, angling them toward the occlusal (biting) surface and rotating them in a circular pattern. This action stimulates the soft tissues and removes plaque in this area. Many toothbrushes have a rubber stimulator at one end that can be used for this purpose (Figure 4-11). Wooden stimulators often come in a pack, much like a book of matches. These elongated, soft-wood wedges are first moistened before use. The wood, normally balsam, has a little give as it stimulates the tissue. Another type of wooden dental stimulator has a plastic handle device that holds a moistened toothpick tip to be used in the same manner as the rubber and wooden stimulators.

The **floss holder** is a Y-shaped device with a handle used by some individuals to hold the floss tightly as it is

FIGURE 4-11 Rubber tip stimulator on the end of a toothbrush.

FIGURE 4-12 Floss holders.

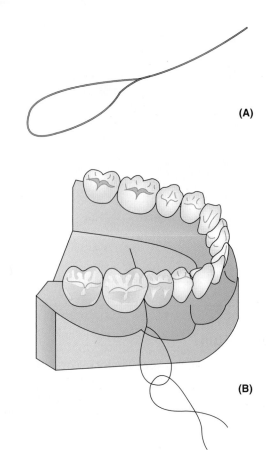

FIGURE 4-13 (A) Floss threader. (B) Floss threader threaded under the pontic area of a three-unit bridge.

placed into the interproximal area of the teeth and then around the posterior of the last tooth in each quadrant (Figure 4-12). The floss holder makes flossing easier for individuals who have arthritis, poor manual dexterity, or hands that seem too large to allow access to the posterior teeth. The patient starts in one area and cleans the side of each tooth while rotating the floss holder around the arch and then in the same manner on the opposing arch. The floss holder is placed into each area and moved up and down on the sides of the tooth and into the sulcus area (the space between the tooth and the gingival tissue) to remove plaque and clean the area.

The **floss threader** is used to remove plaque and debris from under fixed bridges, orthodontic wires, and retainers (Figure 4-13). The floss threader, which comes in a variety of shapes and is made from stiff plastic, is designed like a needle with a large eye. The floss is threaded through the eye of the threader and the needle (stiff end) portion is then threaded through the intended area by the patient. When the floss reaches the opposite side, the floss threader can be removed, leaving the floss to clean this difficult-to-reach area. This allows the patient to direct the floss under the appliance and to clean away plaque and debris. After the entire area is cleaned, the floss can be removed. The area should be flossed daily using the threader to maintain proper oral hygiene.

A **water irrigation device** is used to flush away debris from orthodontic brackets and other prosthetic devices. It does not remove plaque and should not replace brushing and flossing. The pulsating water flow allows food debris to be removed easily; some patients place mouthwash in the fluid-holding container to gain fresh breath in the process. The patients should be instructed to use the water irrigation device carefully, because it can cause tissue damage when turned on high and directed toward the gingival sulcus (it could force debris into the tissue and damage the periodontium). It should be used at low speed and in a direction that forces debris to be pushed away from the gingival area.

Toothbrushes and Techniques

Most patients use toothbrushes, but many have never been shown proper techniques and the methods recommended today. Patients should be shown that the toothbrush only cleans three of the five tooth surfaces. The proximal (between-the-teeth) tooth surfaces normally are not accessible with a toothbrush.

Patients have a variety of toothbrushes to select from today. Dental assistants must stay informed of these choices so they can answer patients' questions appropriately. Miscellaneous styles and designs of both manual and mechanical toothbrushes are on the market today. **Manual toothbrushes** are powered by the human hand. **Mechanical toothbrushes** are powered by electricity or batteries—the toothbrush moves while merely held by the individual. Automatic toothbrushes normally come with recharging units.

Correctly designed toothbrushes are sized and shaped to allow for efficient cleaning and easy management. The toothbrush should be durable and inexpensive and have bristles that are flexible and soft (normally polished on the end), allowing for repeated use. The handle must be firm and strong as well as lightweight. The choosing of a toothbrush is individual according to needs. Some adult patients use children's toothbrushes to gain access to the teeth in the most posterior areas of their mouths.

Manual Toothbrushes

The parts of a manual toothbrush are the head, shank, and handle (Figure 4-14). The bristles are placed on the head of the brush and can be multitufted or spaced and in a number of patterns. Normally, the handle, shank, and head are in a relatively straight plane. Nylon bristles are recommended because they maintain their shape longer than natural bristles and they dry quickly. The ends of the nylon bristles are often run over a flame to cause rounded ends that will not abrade the tooth. Soft bristles are recommended over medium and hard because they do not abrade the tooth or the gingival surface.

(A)

(B)

FIGURE 4-14 Manual toothbrush parts identified. A. Spaced. B. Multi-tufted.

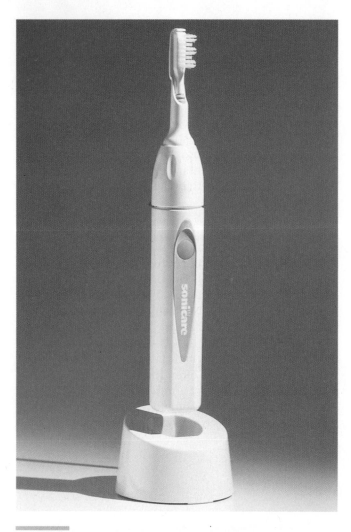

FIGURE 4-15 Mechanical toothbrush. *(Courtesy of Philips Oral Healthcare)*

Motion	Illustration
Reciprocating motion—moves back and forth in a line	
Orbital motion—moves in a circle	
Vibratory motion—vibrates quickly back and forth	
Semicircular motion—moves in an arc	
Elliptical motion—moves in an oval	

FIGURE 4-16 Motions of mechanical toothbrushes.

Mechanical Toothbrushes

Many patients use mechanical toothbrushes (Figure 4-15). Like manual toothbrushes, there are many models of mechanical toothbrushes on the market today. They have larger handles and chargers (the handles have to be larger to hold the rechargeable battery and circuit board). The heads of the mechanical toothbrush can move in several different directions. Dental assistants must be familiar with each motion to be able to recommend the appropriate toothbrushing method for each motion. The motions can be reciprocating, orbital, vibratory, arched, elliptical, or a combination of two or more of these motions (Figure 4-16). Newer models also incorporate sonic action that seems to be particularly effective in removing plaque and extrinsic stains. Some of the automatic units have built-in timing devices that allow thirty seconds for each of the four quadrants and stop when the two minutes have elapsed. An automatic toothbrush can be used in place of a manual toothbrush.

Care should be taken to apply light pressure and to let the action of the bristles clean the teeth and gums.

Brushing Techniques for the Manual Toothbrush

Several toothbrushing techniques can be used to obtain proper oral hygiene. Any technique should allow for all the surfaces of all the teeth to be cleaned. Brushing will not clean the interproximal areas. Some patients will be successful in noting the amount of time spent on brushing by using a timer. Normally, two to three minutes is recommended to clean the facial, lingual, occlusal, and incisal surfaces of all the teeth. A pattern should be developed by the patient to ensure that no area is missed. Some patients like the counting system in which five to ten strokes are made in each area. Starting at the same point each time when brushing is a good idea. The area could be the maxillary (upper) right facial surface (cheek and lip side), and then continue around the entire surface to the maxillary left. From that position, the lingual side (tongue side) of the arch can be cleaned from the left to the right. The mandibular (lower) teeth can be cleaned in the same manner starting from the right, continuing to the left, and then cleaning the lingual side from the left to the right. It does not matter what the pattern is; it only matters that no teeth are left uncleaned. The heel or the toe of the toothbrush can be used effectively on the narrower anterior areas. There are six commonly used brushing techniques: Bass or modified Bass, Charters, modified Stillman, rolling stroke, Fones, and modified scrub. The Bass or modified Bass is the most popular in the dental community.

Bass or Modified Bass Brushing Technique. The Bass technique is named for Dr. C. Bass, a dentist who was an early advocate of preventive dentistry. The Bass brushing technique is used to remove plaque next to and directly beneath the gingival margin (Procedure 4-2).

Charters Brushing Technique. This brushing technique is used to loosen plaque and debris and to stimulate the gingiva, both marginal and interdental (Procedure 4-3). The primary difference from the Bass technique is the angle of toothbrush placement.

Modified Stillman Brushing Technique. The modified Stillman technique is designed to do a good overall cleaning, remove plaque, and stimulate and massage the gingiva (Procedure 4-4). Again, bristle placement distinguishes this technique from the Bass and Charters techniques. They are positioned so that the bristles point apically (toward the root of the tooth), with the toothbrush handle level with the biting surface of the tooth.

PROCEDURE 4 - 2

Bass or Modified Bass Brushing Technique

This procedure is explained to an individual to teach a toothbrushing technique.

EQUIPMENT AND SUPPLIES

- Toothbrush

PROCEDURE STEPS

Bass

1. Grasp the brush and place it so that the bristles are at a 45-degree angle, with the tips of the bristles directed straight into the gingival sulcus (Figure 4-17).

2. Using the tips of the bristles, vibrate back and forth with short, light strokes for a count of 10, allowing the tips of the bristle to enter the sulcus and cover the gingival margin.

3. Lift the brush and continue into the next area or group of teeth until all areas have been cleaned.

4. The toe bristles of the brush can be used to clean the lingual (tongue) anterior area in the arch.

Modified Bass

1. Follow all the steps of the Bass technique.

2. After the vibratory motion has been completed in each area, sweep the bristles over the crown of the tooth, toward the biting surface of the tooth.

Maxillary

FIGURE 4-17 Initial position of the toothbrush when using the Bass technique.

PROCEDURE 4 - 3

Charters Brushing Technique

This procedure is explained to an individual to teach a toothbrushing technique.

EQUIPMENT AND SUPPLIES

- Toothbrush

PROCEDURE STEPS

1. Grasp the brush and place it so that the back of the head is directed apically (toward the end of the root), with the bristles placed downward on the maxillary and upward on the mandibular (Figure 4-18).

2. The bristles should be placed over the gingival, where the tooth and gingiva meet.

3. Press the bristles into the space between the teeth.

4. Vibrate gently back and forth while maintaining position. Count to ten.

5. Reposition and repeat the technique for each subsequent area.

6. For anterior areas, hold the brush parallel to the teeth and use the sides of the toe bristles to clean the area. Count to 10.

Maxillary

FIGURE 4-18 Initial position of the toothbrush when using Charters technique.

PROCEDURE 4 - 4

Modified Stillman Brushing Technique

This procedure is explained to an individual to teach a toothbrushing technique.

EQUIPMENT AND SUPPLIES

- Toothbrush

PROCEDURE STEPS

1. Place the toothbrush so that the bristles are pointing apically and the handle of the brush is level with the biting surface of the tooth (Figure 4-19).

Maxillary

FIGURE 4-19 Initial position of the toothbrush when using the modified Stillman technique.

(continues)

PROCEDURE 4 - 4 *(CONTINUED)*

2. Rotate the bristles downward and vibrate back and forth until the brush has rotated over the entire surface of the tooth (Figure 4-20). Do this motion slowly and count to ten.

3. Repeat this motion over the same area at least five times.

4. Continue until each area and every tooth have been cleaned in this manner.

Maxillary

FIGURE 4-20 Brush stroke used with the modified Stillman technique.

Rolling Stroke Brushing Technique. The rolling stroke is a method used to remove food debris and plaque from teeth and to stimulate the gingival tissue (Procedure 4-5). The brush is placed parallel to the tooth with the bristles pointed apically.

Fones Technique. The Fones technique is used as an initial brushing method to achieve a good overall cleaning. Most individuals can easily learn to make the small circles over the teeth as they are in the closed position. It is very easy to do on the outside surface of the teeth (see Procedure 4-6).

Modified Scrub. The modified scrub brushing technique uses a scrubbing motion to remove plaque and to stimulate the gingival tissue (Procedure 4-7).

PROCEDURE 4 - 5

Rolling Stroke Brushing Technique

This procedure is explained to an individual in order to teach a toothbrushing technique.

EQUIPMENT AND SUPPLIES

■ Toothbrush

PROCEDURE STEPS

1. Grasp the brush and place it parallel to the tooth so that the bristles are pointing apically, upward for the maxillary arch and downward for the mandibular arch, as in the modified Stillman method (Figure 4-21).

2. Firmly but gently press the bristles against the gingiva and roll them slowly over the tissue and the teeth, toward the biting surface (Figure 4-22).

3. Repeat this rolling stroke over the same surface a total of five times.

4. Move the brush to the next area and repeat the five rolling strokes.

5. Use the heel or the toe of the toothbrush to clean the lingual surfaces of the anterior teeth. The bristles will still need to be pressed gently into the area and rolled toward the biting surface.

Maxillary

FIGURE 4-21 Initial position of the toothbrush when using the rolling stroke technique.

Maxillary

FIGURE 4-22 Brush stroke used with the rolling stroke technique.

PROCEDURE 4-6

Fones Brushing Technique

This procedure is explained to an individual in order to teach a toothbrushing technique.

EQUIPMENT AND SUPPLIES

- Toothbrush

PROCEDURE STEPS

1. Close the jaws and place the brush against the cheek. Starting with the posterior teeth, the brush is placed over the maxillary and mandibular teeth (Figure 4-23).

2. The brush proceeds over the teeth in a circular motion as it progresses toward the anterior in a sweeping motion.

3. The anterior teeth are placed in the biting position and the brush is used in a circular motion sweeping from right to left.

Maxillary

FIGURE 4-23 Brush stroke used with the Fones technique.

PROCEDURE 4-7

Modified Scrub Brushing Technique

This procedure is explained to an individual to teach a toothbrushing technique.

EQUIPMENT AND SUPPLIES

- Toothbrush

PROCEDURE STEPS

1. Grasp the brush and place the bristles at a right angle to the tooth surface (Figure 4-24).

2. Use gentle but firm pressure and place the bristles over the area where the tooth and gingiva come together.

3. Activate the brush with back-and-forth scrubbing strokes.

4. Repeat this action throughout the mouth until all areas have been cleaned.

Maxillary

FIGURE 4-24 Initial position of the toothbrush when using the modified scrub technique.

Tongue Brushing

For centuries, individuals have known that it is important to clean the surface of the tongue. Bacteria can collect in the irregular dorsal (top) surface of the tongue. The daily ritual of oral hygiene historically included the scraping of the tongue with a tongue scraper (Figures 4-25 and 4-26). Several different tongue cleaners are on the market today.

FIGURE 4-25 Automatic tongue scraper. *(Courtesy of Oralgiene USA, Inc.)*

FIGURE 4-26 Toothbrush with tongue scraper on backside of the head.

A conventional toothbrush is most often used to ensure cleaning of the tongue surface. The size of the toothbrush head may limit access to the posterior area of the tongue because it may initiate gagging. To clean the tongue, the toothbrush should be placed as far back as is comfortable and then be drawn forward to the tip, allowing the bristles to clean the debris that has accumulated. Repeat this process until the entire tongue has been cleaned.

Dental Flossing

Dental flossing (Procedure 4-8), the second essential element of a good oral hygiene program, should be done daily. Dental floss has been shown to be the most effective way to remove bacterial plaque and other debris from otherwise inaccessible areas, the interproximal surfaces of the teeth.

Types of Floss

Dental floss is available in several forms. Floss should be chosen according to patients' manual skills, dental restorations, and preferences. Following the office philosophy, the dental assistant can make suggestions to the patient that will meet the patient's dental needs. Historically, patients have been advised to use unwaxed dental floss with small, individual filaments that aid in plaque removal as the floss is moved over the surface of each tooth. Some patients become frustrated while using unwaxed floss because it is thinner and more likely to shred or to catch on old dental restorations, making it difficult to remove from the interproximal areas. These patients should be encouraged to use waxed, lightly waxed, or nonshredding dental floss. Waxed floss will slide over the surface with greater ease for patients who have tight contacts and roughened surfaces.

Dental floss also can be purchased in extra fine, larger flat tape, or even a tufted texture that when tightened changes sizes. Some patients will be attracted to the different colors and flavors of floss available on the market today. Colored and flavored floss does not perform better than plain floss, but it may motivate patients to use it routinely. Daily flossing is more important than the type of floss that is used.

Hygienic Care of Prosthetic Devices

An individual may have prosthetic devices that require special oral hygiene care to obtain the desired plaque-free result each day. Professional knowledge and guidance will aid patients in the care of their prosthetic devices, such as fixed bridges, implants, orthodontic brackets, and full and partial dentures.

Fixed Bridges. A fixed bridge that is anchored on both sides with a pontic in the middle will not allow for normal flossing. The patient will need special instructions

PROCEDURE 4-8

Dental Flossing Technique

This procedure is explained to an individual to teach a dental flossing technique.

EQUIPMENT AND SUPPLIES

- Dental floss

PROCEDURE STEPS

1. Obtain the appropriate dental floss and dispense 18 inches of it.

2. Wrap the ends of the floss around the middle or ring finger as anchors (Figure 4-27).

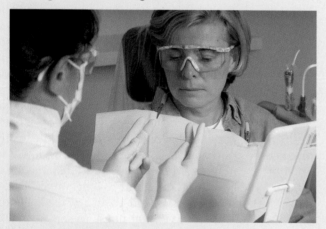

FIGURE 4-27 Adapting floss to the fingers for use.

3. Grasp the floss between the thumb and index finger of each hand, allowing $1/2$ to 1 inch to remain between the two hands (Figure 4-28).

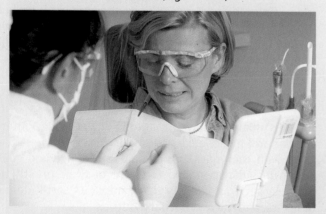

FIGURE 4-28 Floss adapted between fingers, prepared for use.

(A)

(B)

FIGURE 4-29 (A) Finger position on the floss for the maxillary arch. (B) Finger and thumb position on the floss for the mandibular arch.

4. For the maxillary teeth, pass the floss over the two thumbs or a thumb and finger, and direct the floss upward (Figure 4-29A). For the mandibular teeth, pass the floss over the two index fingers and guide it downward (Figure 4-29B).

5. Direct the floss to pass gently between the teeth, using a sawing motion. Try to avoid snapping the floss through the contacts because it may damage the interdental papilla (gingival point between teeth).

6. Curve the floss into a C-shape to wrap it around the tooth and allow access to the sulcus area (Figure 4-30). Resistance indicates that the bottom of the gingival sulcus has been reached.

7. Move the floss gently up and down the surface of the tooth to remove the plaque.

(continues)

PROCEDURE 4-8 *(CONTINUED)*

8. Lift slightly and wrap the floss in the opposite direction in a C-shape over the adjacent tooth.

9. Move the floss gently up and down the surface of this tooth before removing it from the area.

10. Rotate the floss on the fingers to allow for a fresh section to be used each time, and continue to clean between every tooth. It does not matter where an

individual begins with floss, but it is best to proceed systematically to ensure that no area is missed.

11. Use the dental floss around the distal surface of the most posterior tooth by wrapping it into a tight C-shape and moving it gently up and down with a firm pressure (Figure 4-31). Do the most posterior teeth in all four quadrants in the same manner.

FIGURE 4-30 Placing the dental floss around the tooth, wrapped into the sulcus.

FIGURE 4-31 Patient placing the dental floss around the last molar.

on how to use a floss threader (see information on the floss threader and Figure 4-13) to remove plaque and debris from under the bridge. The patient may also need special brushing instructions to clean the gingival area more carefully.

Implants. Many patients have dental implants to replace their missing teeth. The implants are a great advancement in dental care. The long-term success of implants is deter-

mined partially by the patients and how well they maintain the areas. Patients can use yarn in place of floss or a disposable elastomeric cleaning appliance and interproximal brushes to clean around the implants (Figure 4-32). A plastic scaler is used in the dental office to thoroughly clean and remove any calculus.

Full and Partial Dentures. All removable dentures and appliances should be carefully cleaned daily

(A)

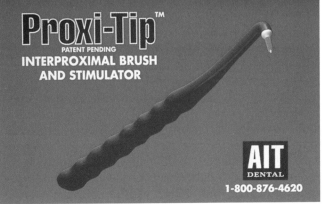

(B)

FIGURE 4-32 Dental hygiene aids for implants. (A) Proxi-Floss. (B) Proxi-Pic. *(Courtesy ATI Dental, Inc.)*

FIGURE 4-33 Denture and denture toothbrush.

FIGURE 4-34 Orthodontic oral hygiene aids.

and rinsed following a meal or as needed. A denture brush is used to brush the appliance (Figure 4-33). It is a larger brush that can be used with toothpaste or a mild soap. A soft brush should be used on the tissue under the appliance to clean and to stimulate circulation in that area.

Commercial cleaning agents can be used daily on a denture. These chemical agents remove stains and help freshen breath. The dentures normally are immersed in solutions according to the manufacturer's directions and rinsed after the specified time has elapsed. The soaking solutions can be made at home with the following ingredients:

- Warm water (1 cup)
- Bleach (1 tsp.) (*Note:* The bleach should not be used with a partial denture as it may corrode the metal.)
- An anticorrosive agent (2 tsp.)

When calculus is heavy, a solution of 1 cup of warm water with a teaspoon of vinegar can be used. These home solutions should be used only once a week.

Orthodontic Appliances. As stated earlier in this chapter, special oral hygiene techniques must be practiced to maintain orthodontic appliances. The appliances must be kept plaque free. When care is improper, the tooth structure around the brackets may decay and the gingival tissue will become irritated and virtually grow over the appliances. Special orthodontic toothbrushes and aids can be used (Figure 4-34). The bristles of the brush are designed to allow contact with the surface of the tooth. In special cases, an interproximal brush can be used to gain access to difficult areas. In addition to removing food and debris with a toothbrush and flossing, a water irrigation device can be used for overall cleaning.

Oral Hygiene for Patients with Special Needs

Dental assistants may be called on to be creative to meet the oral hygiene needs of patients with special needs (Figure 4-35). Patients who are mentally or physically compromised are often fed soft foods that lack the cleaning effects of normal foods. Devices can be developed to clean these patients' teeth. The dental assistants may need to show caregivers how to clean the patient's teeth routinely. For example, putty or a rubber ball can be wrapped over the handle of a toothbrush to allow the patient to grasp it more easily, or handles may be extended with tongue depressors or rulers so that patients can reach their oral cavities. Keep the focus on

FIGURE 4-35 Aids for patients who have difficulty brushing and flossing.

the desired outcomes and establish methods to meet those goals. A moist washcloth can be used to wipe the surfaces of the teeth, if necessary. Be creative in meeting the needs of patients with special needs.

Pregnant Patients

Pregnant patients may require special dental hygiene techniques due to the nausea that often accompanies pregnancy. Regurgitation will bring acid from the stomach repeatedly over the surface of the teeth (this will also be a concern for patients with bulimia). Patients should be educated as to the possible destruction of the teeth from this acid repeatedly contacting the teeth. In addition, placing a toothbrush into the mouth may cause the patient to gag. Problem solve with the patient and find a way to meet the goal of proper oral hygiene. Normally, eliminating toothpaste and identifying specific times of the day when the pregnant patient is less nauseated allows toothbrushing and flossing to be made more comfortable during pregnancy. The dental assistant should tell the obstetrical patient that increased gingival bleeding is normal and that routine prophylaxis (cleaning) is recommended during pregnancy. Any dental treatment should be approved by the patient's physician.

Patients with Cancer

Patients with cancer may have a number of oral manifestations due to the cancer and the therapy. Loss of muscle function, gingival bleeding, rampant caries, and xerostomia (zee-roh-STOH-me-ah) may compromise skills of good oral hygiene. Xerostomia is abnormal dryness of the mouth and may be due to radiation or chemotherapy treatments. The patient may have a number of problems to overcome, such as root caries. Home topical fluoride treatments are often suggested to help eliminate these problems. Listen and problem solve with the patient. It will be important that infection does not perpetuate in the oral cavity and compound the patient's condition. The dental assistant may suggest that an extra-soft toothbrush or a moistened foam toothbrush be used on the tender tissues with a non-abrasive fluoride toothpaste. Maintaining the teeth and tissues will allow the patient to eat properly and regain a healthier state. Use empathy, encouragement, and sincerity to motivate the patient.

Patients with Heart Disease

Patients with heart disease may express a number of the same problems that cancer patients have due to medication usage. Many have xerostomia, gingival bleeding, and rampant caries. Patients with congestive heart disease will be uncomfortable in the chair if the chair is reclined (this brings increased fluid around the heart and patients feel as if they are suffocating). Be aware of the patient's health status, address the problems that are identified, and aid the patient through education and understanding to seek a method to accomplish good oral hygiene.

Older Patients

For many older patients with arthritis, holding floss and a toothbrush is difficult. There are toothbrushes with large, soft handles that help these patients. A floss holder can be used to secure the floss tightly as it is placed between the teeth. Listen to these patients and keep in mind that they want to save their teeth to be able to eat properly. Many are afraid of having dentures. The wonderful thing about older patients is that often they have time to listen carefully to oral hygiene directions and to ask questions to clarify what is required of them to meet their oral hygiene goals.

Additional Preventive Procedures Performed in the Dental Office

Other procedures that are performed in the dental office to aid patients in good oral hygiene are topical fluoride treatments and pit and fissure sealants.

Fluoride

The use of fluoride in dentistry is based on the knowledge that when the fluoride content of the teeth is increased to the "optimum level," there is significant reduction in dental caries. Once, fluoride was thought to be beneficial only during tooth development years, but through further research fluoride has been proven to be beneficial throughout the life span.

Fluoride is a natural mineral nutrient. It is derived from fluorine, which comes from fluospar, the thirteenth most abundant chemical element in the earth's crust. Fluoride is essential to the formation of healthy bones and teeth, just as calcium and phosphorous are. These minerals are obtained from water and certain foods.

Fluoride Content in the Bones and Teeth

- Normal bone contains 0.01 to 0.3 percent fluoride.
- Dental enamel contains 0.01 to 0.02 percent fluoride.
- Carious teeth contain as little as 0.0069 percent fluoride.

History of Fluoride in Dentistry

Early in the 1900s, Dr. G.V. Black and Dr. F. McKay of Colorado first revealed the fact that people with mottled enamel (discolorations) did not have as much dental decay. In the l930s, a chemist found a definite relationship between fluoride and mottled enamel. Eventually, an "optimum" level of fluoride was found. This level prevents dental caries without mottling the teeth. The optimum level was found to be 1 part per million (1 ppm). In some climates, this level may be adjusted slightly. For example, in hot climates where people are likely to drink more water, the level may be reduced.

Fluoridation

Fluoridation is the process of adding fluoride to the water supply. The first city to test the benefits of fluoride through fluoridation was Grand Rapids, Michigan. In 1945, 1 ppm fluoride was added to the water supply. Several other cities also fluoridated their water supplies when it was proven that dental caries in Michigan were reduced by approximately 60 percent. Since then, numerous cities have added fluoride to their water supplies.

Adding fluoride to community water supplies is a very controversial issue in many areas. It has been proven that adjusting the amount of fluoride to the optimum level does reduce dental caries, but some people oppose fluoridation. Much has been written about the fluoride controversy, and dental assistants need to stay up-to-date on what is going on in their communities. Knowing whether the water is fluoridated, the benefits of fluoridation, and the effects of too much fluoride will better prepare the assistant to answer patients' questions.

Effects of Fluoride

Fluoride is a natural substance needed for the development of healthy teeth and bones. It is absorbed almost entirely through the bloodstream from the gastrointestinal tract. Fluorides also are absorbed through the lungs, as in industrial settings where people have occupational exposure to fluorine.

Once fluoride is absorbed by the body and deposited in the bones and teeth, the remaining fluoride is excreted. The developing child requires more fluoride than a forty-year-old person and so the body adjusts the amount absorbed and excretes the excess fluoride.

Tooth Development

When the fluoride reaches the tooth, it replaces part of the tooth structure called the hydroxyl ion. The hydroxyl ion is on the surface of the apatite crystal in the enamel. The new tooth structure that is formed is called a fluoroapatite crystal.

Fluoride affects the tooth both before and after the tooth has erupted into the oral cavity. During the pre-eruption stage, the fluoride ion replaces the hydroxyl ion when the teeth are calcifying. Fluoride is supplied from drinking water, some foods, and fluoride tablets or drops. During this stage, excessive amounts of fluoride may disturb the normal pattern of development. This condition is known as fluorosis, or mottled enamel (Figure 4-36).

Children who are given prescribed doses of fluoride at birth and continue receiving fluoride during the development of both the deciduous and permanent teeth benefit the most in reducing the number of dental caries.

(A)　　　　　　　　　　　　　　　　　　　　　　　　　　　　　　　　(B)

FIGURE 4-36 (A) Dental fluorosis and shade guide. *(Courtesy of Dr. Ola J. England, DDS, PS, Spokane, WA)* (B) Mild dental fluorosis.

During the posteruption stage, the absorption rate of fluoride is the highest just after the tooth has erupted; then, it tapers off as the enamel matures. Absorption is also affected by the amount of fluoride exposure. Once the teeth have erupted, they receive fluoride through the bloodstream and also through exposure in the oral cavity to fluoride in toothpastes, tablets, gels, and rinses.

Fluoride in Dental Plaque

Fluoride in dental plaque has been found to have a favorable effect. The amount of fluoride in plaque is relative to the amount of fluoride exposure. Fluoride in plaque is bound within bacteria. This condition causes an antibacterial effect that inhibits the production of acids responsible for dental decay.

Fluoride Toxicity

Fluoride, like many other substances, can be toxic when absorbed in excessive amounts. Today, fluorides are regulated carefully by occupational health legislation and governmental agencies. Over the years, it has been found that the toxicity of fluoride depends on the duration and dosage of ingestion. Fluoride used in dentistry presents little or no risk for acute toxicity. However, the dental assistant should be aware of the possibilities of fluoride poisoning and when and where it has occurred, because patients may have questions.

Dangers Associated with Fluoride Ingestion. Acute fluoride poisoning is extremely rare. It occurs when large amounts of fluoride are ingested, inhaled, or absorbed into the body at one time. The lethal dose varies from 2.5 to 10 grams in adults to as low as 0.25 grams in infants. A medical doctor should be contacted any time excessive amounts of fluoride are ingested at one time. When there is suspected toxicity, the patient should drink milk, and then seek medical treatment immediately. Milk acts as a demulcent, a medicine that soothes irritated mucous membranes. It also helps with mild nausea the patient may have.

Chronic fluoride poisoning is ingestion of high fluoride levels in the water or combinations of several fluoride sources over a period of time. Two effects of chronic fluoride overdose are crippling fluorosis (skeletal hypermineralization of ligaments) and mottled enamel. With today's health and safety controls in industry, crippling fluorosis can be avoided. Mottled enamel is caused by excess exposure to fluoride during the time of tooth development. When the fluoride level is from 1.8 to 2.0 ppm, the enamel shows varying degrees of white areas, brown lines, or enamel hypoplasia. Because high levels of fluoride occur naturally in some areas, mottled enamel would be more common unless the amount of fluoride in the water supply is adjusted to the optimum level.

Mottled enamel is pitted because of a deficiency in the number of ameloblasts (enamel-forming cells) and chalky because of a lack of mineral deposits. See Table 4-1 for the appearance of teeth with varying degrees of mottled enamel.

Benefits of Fluoride

The dental health benefits of fluoride have been shown in numerous studies. The benefits are in proportion to the length of time an individual received fluoride and the amount of fluoride given. The primary benefit is the reduction of dental caries in both primary and permanent dentition, but there are also long-term effects with the reduction of need for extensive dental care and the time and cost of such care. Through the use of fluoride, primary teeth are not lost prematurely to decay. This results in less malocclusion in permanent dentition; therefore, the need for orthodontic treatment is reduced. There is also less permanent tooth loss at early ages. Thus, adults require fewer bridges, partials, or dentures. Improved bone density can affect bone resorption and resistance to local factors. With stronger alveolar bone and less decay, the periodontal tissues stay healthier.

Forms of Fluoride

Fluorides are available for dental health care needs in two forms: systemic fluoride and topical fluoride.

TABLE 4-1 Appearance of Teeth with Exposure to Different Levels of Fluoride

Amount of Fluoride Exposure	Appearance of the Teeth
Exposure between 0.7 and 1.2 ppm—the optimum level depending on average temperature of the area	Teeth are white, opaque, and shiny without blemishes.
Exposure up to 1.8 ppm	The structure of the enamel is not affected, but chalky bands or flecks can be seen on the surface.
Exposure over 1.8 ppm	Chalky bands or flecks appear on the surface and the enamel structure is affected; this is known as enamel hypocalcification. The chalky bands and flecks discolor with time. With increased exposure to fluoride, the enamel may become cracked and pitted.

The fluoride compounds used in dentistry are sodium fluoride, stannous fluoride, and acidulated phosphate fluoride.

Systemic Fluoride. Systemic fluoride is ingested and then circulated through the body to the developing teeth. Sources of systemic fluoride include fluoridated water, foods with fluoride, fluoride tablets, and drops.

- Fluoride may be added to the community or school water supply. The level of natural fluoride is evaluated to adjust water supplies to the optimum level prescribed for dental health.

- Sodium fluoride is used in the community water supply.

- Foods such as meat, vegetables, cereals, and citrus fruits naturally contain small amounts of fluoride. Tea and fish have slightly higher amounts of fluoride.

- Tablets and drops require a prescription from a dentist or physician. They are prescribed from birth until the second permanent molar erupts. Vitamins with fluoride are also available.

- The ADA's Council on Dental Therapeutics recommends that specific amounts of fluoride be prescribed according to the child's age and weight.

- Studies have shown a 50 to 65 percent reduction in caries for patients who have received the optimum prescribed amount of fluoride during tooth development.

- Not all bottled water contains fluoride. Be sure to check the label if you want fluoride benefits and you rely on bottled water for your water supply.

The amount of natural fluoride in a water supply can be determined by tests done by private laboratories and state and county agencies. In rural areas and cities without fluoridated water, children should receive topical fluoride. The dentist will assist the parents in determining the best methods and amount of fluoride the child should receive for maximum benefit. It is important that the fluoride supplement be taken continuously during tooth development to be most effective.

Topical Fluoride

Topical fluoride is another method to make the tooth more resistant to demineralization and also to assist in the remineralization of decalcified areas. Because topical fluoride only penetrates the outer layer of the enamel, it is most effective if the tooth is cleaned before application. The cleaning can be accomplished by toothbrushing or a rubber-cup polish.

Topical fluoride is available for direct application in a variety of forms, such as gels, rinses, foams, and liquids. Polishing paste and dentifrice that are applied to the teeth also contain fluoride.

Dual Benefit of Chewing Fluoride Tablets

If fluoride tablets are chewed before being swallowed, the teeth benefit both from topical and systemic fluoride applications.

Topical Fluoride Application in the Dental Office. For a child to achieve the optimal benefit, topical fluoride is applied to clean teeth once or twice a year in the dental office. Using this method, caries can be reduced by 40 to 50 percent.

In the dental office, fluoride gels, foams, and rinses are commonly applied (Procedure 4-9). The gels and foam solutions are convenient to use and remain in the fluoride tray. Fluorides come in many flavors and usually the dental office will have several for the patients to choose from. The dental assistant should read and follow the directions for the type of fluoride being applied to determine the length of application and helpful hints. The most common agents are 2 percent sodium fluoride, 8 percent stannous fluoride, and 1.23 percent acidulated phosphofluoride.

Advantages and Disadvantages of Fluoride Preparations. *Neutral–2 Percent Sodium Fluoride* Sodium fluoride solutions are relatively stable, have an agreeable taste, are nonirritating to soft tissue, and do not discolor the teeth or restorative materials. The disadvantage is that they must be used at one-week intervals for four weeks. Sodium fluoride solutions are applied after an initial prophylaxis of the crowns. The teeth are isolated and air dried and fluoride is applied for three minutes. The complete series is performed at ages three, seven, eleven, and thirteen.

8 Percent Stannous Fluoride The aqueous solution of 8 percent stannous fluoride is not stable and must be made up immediately before application. The 8 percent solution has a disagreeable taste, is astringent, causes gingival blanching, and causes discoloration of the teeth. This discoloration is due to the tin, not the fluoride.

1.23 Percent Acidulated Phosphate Fluoride (APF) APF solutions and gels are commonly preferred because of patient acceptability and greater uptake of the fluoride by the surface enamel of the tooth. They are not irritating to soft tissue, do not discolor teeth or restorative material, and are slightly astringent. They are stored in plastic containers because they become more acidic when stored in glass. The application procedure involves prophylaxis, isolation, and drying of teeth, then application of solution, gel, or foam for one or four minutes (both solutions are available). The single appli-

PROCEDURE 4 - 9

Fluoride Application

This procedure is performed by the dental assistant after the rubber-cup polish has been completed. In some states, the application of fluoride may be an expanded function.

EQUIPMENT AND SUPPLIES

- Basic setup: mouth mirror, explorer, and cotton pliers
- Saliva ejector, evacuator tip (HVE), air-water syringe tip
- Cotton rolls, gauze sponges
- Fluoride solution
- Appropriately sized trays
- Timer (for one or four minutes)

PROCEDURE STEPS *(Follow aseptic procedures)*

1. Seat the patient in an upright position, review health history, and confirm that he or she has not had allergic reactions to fluorides.

2. Explain the procedure to the patient. Inform the patient to try not to swallow the fluoride.

3. Explain that for the fluoride to be most effective, he or she should not eat, drink, or rinse for thirty minutes after the fluoride treatment.

4. Place glasses and mask, wash hands, and don treatment gloves.

5. Select the trays and try them in the patient's mouth to ensure coverage of all the exposed teeth.

6. Place the fluoride gel or foam in the tray. The tray should be about one-third full. Show the patient how to use the saliva ejector.

7. Dry all the teeth with the air syringe. To keep the teeth dry while reaching for the tray, keep your finger in the patient's mouth and tell him or her to keep it open.

8. Place the tray over the dried teeth. The maxillary and mandibular arches can be done at the same time or individually (Figure 4-37).

9. Move the trays up and down to dispense the fluoride solution around the teeth.

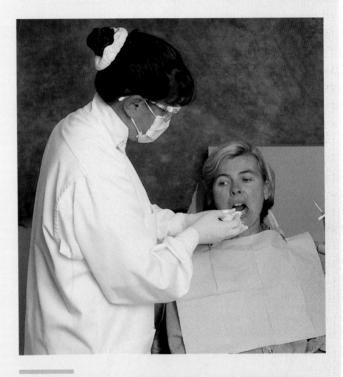

FIGURE 4-37 Dental assistant placing a loaded fluoride tray into the patient's mouth.

10. Place the saliva ejector between the arches and have the patient close gently.

11. Set the timer for the designated amount of time.

12. When the timer goes off, remove the saliva ejector and the trays from the patient's mouth.

13. Quickly evacuate the mouth with the saliva ejector or the evacuator (HVE) to completely remove any excess fluoride.

14. Remind the patient not to eat, drink, or rinse for thirty minutes.

15. Place on overgloves and make the chart entry, including the date, the fluoride solution applied, and any reactions.

cation is repeated at six- or twelve-month intervals. The choice of solution is up to the practitioner, but foams appear to be more popular at this time.

The trays used with fluoride gels and foams come in a variety of materials and sizes (Figure 4-38). It is important to select a tray that covers all the erupted teeth and does not extend beyond the most posterior tooth. Some trays come with the maxillary and mandibular arches connected so they are placed at the same time. Others are individual for each arch, with the maxillary arch slightly larger. Often, the trays are color coded for different sizes.

Contraindications. Note that fluoride should not be applied before placement of orthodontic bands, before placement of sealants, or before seating of cosmetic dentistry because it may inhibit adhesion.

Fluoride Rinses

Fluoride rinses are available as a means of fluoride treatment. The fluoride comes in a liquid that is a higher concentration and, because it is easy to swallow, the patient must be reminded not to swallow after rinsing.

After the patient's teeth have been cleaned with a toothbrush or a rubber-cup polish, apply the fluoride rinse. Follow the instructions for the individual rinse. Usually, the patient is directed to take half the dosage and then swish for a specific time (one minute). The patient then empties this amount and repeats with the second portion for the same amount of time.

Because of the taste of the fluoride, patients do not always look forward to fluoride treatments. The dental assistant can be the motivating factor and set the stage for the patient's attitude. Children under six years of age should not use fluoride rinses or mouthwashes because they may accidentally swallow them.

FIGURE 4-38 Various fluoride trays.

CHAPTER SUMMARY

To be effective in preventive dentistry, dental assistants must first care for their teeth properly. Becoming knowledgeable about the oral disease process will aid the dental assistant in educating the public on how to prevent it. The dental assistant must have the knowledge to problem solve oral hygiene concerns, know what preventive aids are available, and then aid patients in maintaining their teeth and gums.

Case Study

Heidi Ann Jones, a seventeen-year-old, came to the dental office concerned with the discoloration of her teeth. After a thorough examination by the dentist, the findings showed that she had no caries, one restoration, and marginal gingivitis. What further information would be important to ask Heidi? What preventive techniques would benefit Heidi?

Case Study Review

1. Was Heidi given fluoride drops or pills during the development of her permanent teeth?

2. Was she raised in an area that had fluoridated water?

3. What oral hygiene aids and habits were used by Heidi in her daily routine?

4. Because Heidi is seeking information about her discolored teeth and not about her gingivitis, the operator must first make sure that Heidi also wants help with the gingivitis before proceeding with home care instruction.

5. Home care instructions should include toothbrushing and flossing appropriate for a seventeen-year-old.

REVIEW QUESTIONS

Multiple Choice

1. The most widely used brushing technique is the
   a. Stillman technique.
   b. Charters technique.
   c. Bass technique.
   d. Rolling stroke technique.

2. What is the most effective way to remove bacterial plaque from the proximal surfaces of the teeth?
   a. Use of a toothbrush
   b. Use of a tongue cleaner
   c. Use of an interproximal brush
   d. Use of dental floss

3. What is the optimal level of water fluoridation?
   a. 1 ppm
   b. 5 ppm
   c. 10 ppm
   d. 25 ppm

4. When dispensing dental floss, an appropriate length is about ____ inches.
   a. 4
   b. 10
   c. 18
   d. 25

5. The condition that causes an abnormally dry mouth is called
   a. fluorosis.
   b. demineralization.
   c. caries.
   d. xerostomia.

6. A sticky mass that contains bacteria and grows in colonies on the teeth is called
   a. caries.
   b. demineralization.
   c. plaque.
   d. acid.

7. The age group in which children are very concerned with fitting into a group and doing what others in that group are doing is
   a. five through eight.
   b. nine through twelve.
   c. thirteen through fifteen.
   d. sixteen through nineteen.

8. Dentifrice refers to
   a. toothpaste.
   b. disclosing agents.
   c. mouth rinses.
   d. dental floss.

9. A condition where the enamel shows varying degrees of white areas or brown lines could be
   a. demineralization.
   b. enamel hypoplasia.
   c. caries.
   d. xerostomia.

10. Which foods naturally contain small amounts of fluoride?
    a. Vegetables
    b. Cereals
    c. Citrus fruits
    d. All of the above

Critical Thinking

1. If you have a choice of hard candy or a candy bar, which is more damaging to the teeth? Why?

2. Can dental fluorosis occur on a permanent tooth after eruption into the mouth?

3. Is it important to use one particular type of toothbrushing technique? Why?

Web Activities

1. Go to http://www.ada.org, read the article about the ADA Seal of Acceptance, and print the article.

2. Go to http://www.sonicare.com and identify the types of replacement brush heads available for the Sonicare toothbrush.

3. Go to www.crest.com, find *For Professionals,* and then go to *What's New.* See if there are any samples available for trial usage. Fill out information to obtain the free sample.

CHAPTER **5**

NUTRITION

SPECIFIC INSTRUCTIONAL OBJECTIVES

The student should strive to meet the following objectives and demonstrate an understanding of the facts and principles presented in this chapter:

1. Describe how an understanding of nutrition is used in the profession of dental assisting.

2. Define nutrients found in foods, including carbohydrates, fiber, fats, proteins, and amino acids. Explain how they affect oral hygiene.

3. Define a calorie and basal metabolic rate.

4. Identify and explain the function of vitamins, major minerals, and water.

5. Explain how to interpret food labeling.

6. Discuss the implication of eating disorders.

7. Identify the food sources, functions, and deficiencies with fat-soluble vitamins, water-soluble vitamins, and the seven major minerals.

KEY TERMS

amenorrhea *(78)*

anorexia nervosa *(77)*

basal metabolic rate (BMR) *(76)*

binging *(77)*

biotin *(72)*

bulimia *(77)*

calcium *(74)*

Calories *(76)*

carbohydrates *(69)*

cariogenic foods *(69)*

carotene *(71)*

cheilosis *(72)*

chlorine *(74)*

chromium *(74)*

cobalt *(74)*

copper *(74)*

diet *(69)*

diuretics *(75)*

electrolytes *(74)*

emaciation *(78)*

essential amino acids *(71)*

fats *(70)*

fluorine *(74)*

folic acid *(72)*

glossitis *(72)*

iodine *(74)*

iron *(74)*

lanugo *(78)*

magnesium *(74)*

malnutrition *(69)*

manganese *(74)*

metabolism *(69)*

metabolism rate *(76)*

molybdenum *(74)*

niacin *(72)*

nursing bottle syndrome (NBS) *(70)*

nutrients *(69)*

nutrition *(69)*

organic *(76)*

pantothenic acid *(72)*

phosphorus *(74)*

potassium *(74)*

preservatives *(76)*

prothrombin *(71)*

purging *(77)*

regurgitation *(77)*

retinol *(71)*

riboflavin *(72)*

selenium *(74)*

sodium *(74)*

sulfur *(74)*

thiamin *(72)*

triglycerides *(70)*

INTRODUCTION

Nutrition affects the entire body as well as the oral cavity. It directly impacts on how an individual feels and functions throughout the day. Poor nutrition can affect the dental assistant in his or her career. It is critical that dental assistants maintain good health through proper food choices. This chapter covers an overall basic understanding of nutrients, including fats and lipids, proteins, vitamins, minerals, and water. Information on how to interpret food labeling is provided. Content on implications of eating disorders is covered in this chapter. Knowledge of nutrition provides the individual with the information to make sound decisions. The old saying "You are what you eat" is true.

Nutrition

To remain healthy, dental assistants must first be knowledgeable about **nutrition**, the manner in which foods are used to meet the body's needs. Dental assistants also need to be able to help patients with diet, the food the individual eats. Many patients may have the meaning of the word diet confused with weight loss. Everything that is taken into the mouth is the **diet**. An *adequate diet* meets all the individual's nutritional needs. People can eat large amounts of food and still be **undernourished**, or lacking the correct nutrients for the body. A disorder resulting from being undernourished is **malnutrition**. This is often seen in alcoholics who may experience malnutrition due to the intake of alcohol (they feel full and do not eat the food necessary for an adequate diet).

The U.S. Department of Agriculture (USDA) first developed a guide to a balanced diet in 1992, which was later revised in 1996. This guide was presented in the shape of a pyramid with the items at the top to be used sparingly and the items at the bottom to be consumed in larger amounts (Figure 5-1). In 2005 the USDA replaced the pyramid and developed *MyPyramid*, which allows for individual assessment of food intake and physical activity (Figure 5-2). The aim of this dietary guideline is to help each individual choose the foods and amounts that are right for her or him. The individual enters age, gender, and activity level, and the *MyPyramid* will help get the most nutrition out of the calories ingested (www.mypyramid.gov). The USDA Web site helps each user find a balance between food and physical activity, and will track food intake and physical activity level.

More than 60 percent of Americans are overnourished, leading to obesity and the diseases related to obesity. Americans are eating an abundance of fast foods that are high in fat content. Along with lack of exercise, the overall population gains a minimum of a half pound a year.

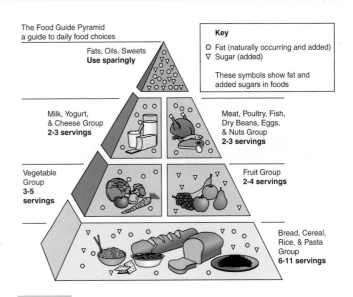

FIGURE 5-1 Food guide pyramid. *(Courtesy of USDA and HHS, 1992, "The Food Guide Pyramid: A Guide to Daily Food Choices." Leaflet No. 572. Washington, DC)*

Nutrients

Nutrients are defined as any chemical substance in food that provides the body tissues and structures with the elements necessary for growth, maintenance, and repair. Forty-plus essential nutrients are required by the human body. These can be obtained from a diet comprised of foods from all the food groups. Having a variety of foods daily helps ensure that essential nutrients are obtained and the body's **metabolism** is maintained. There are six broad classifications of nutrients: carbohydrates, fats, proteins, vitamins, minerals, and water.

Carbohydrates

Carbohydrates primarily come from fruits, grains, legumes (peas, beans, and lentils), and some vegetable roots. This group encompasses sugars, starches, and fibers, and provides quick energy. People in athletic events normally take in carbohydrates before events to increase their energy levels.

Dental assistants will need to advise patients on carbohydrates because they are potentially cariogenic. **Cariogenic foods** break down into simple sugars in the mouth and can be used by the bacteria to cause dental caries. Most patients will be aware that carbohydrates already broken down into simple sugars, such as candies, soft drinks, and sweet desserts, will cause decay. It will be the other carbohydrates that patients are

MyPyramid.gov
STEPS TO A HEALTHIER YOU

Grains: Make Half Your Grains Whole
- Eat at least 3 ounces of whole grain bread cereal, crackers, rice, or pasta every day.
- Look for "whole" before the grain name in the list of ingredients.

Veggies: Vary Your Veggies
- Eat more dark green veggies
- Eat more orange veggies
- Eat more dry beans and peas

Fruit: Focus On Fruits
- Eat a variety of fruits
- Choose fresh, frozen, canned, or dried fruit
- Go easy on fruit juices

Oils:
- Make most of your fat sources from fish, nuts, and vegetable oils
- Limit solid fats like butter, stick margarine, shortening, and lard

Milk: Get Your Calcium-Rich Foods
- Go low-fat or fat-free
- If you don't or can't consume milk, choose lactose free products or other calcium sources

Meat and Beans: Go Lean With Protein
- Choose low-fat or lean meats and poultry
- Bake it, broil it, or, grill it
- Vary your choices – with more fish, beans, peas, nuts, and seeds

Physical Activity:
- Be physically active for at least 30 minutes most days of the week
- Children and teenagers should be physically active for 60 minutes every day, or most days

FIGURE 5-2 The new food pyramid. *(Courtesy of USDA and HHS, Center for Nutrition and Policy Promotion)* .

unaware of that may cause decay, such as raisins, crackers, fruits, and a few vegetables. The intake of fruits and vegetables normally is not a problem because fruits and vegetables do not stick to the teeth and are not converted to simple sugars until they reach the stomach.

Evaluating cariogenic foods in patients' diets is accomplished by having the patients record their diets over several days. The dental assistant can review the diet and identify cariogenic foods with the patient. The assistant can discuss the texture of the foods and if they are retentive sugars, such as caramels, that remain in a concentrated sugar form on the tooth. Evaluation of each food in the patient's diet provides a better understanding of which types of foods are cariogenic.

Other pertinent information that the dental assistant can discuss with the patient is the number of times

cariogenic foods are being eaten, if they are eaten with other foods, and at what time of day they are eaten.

One other factor in the equation of decay is that the more often the teeth are exposed to cariogenic food, the greater the probability of decay. For instance, the person who drinks a soft drink very slowly and allows the sugar to soak on the teeth over and over will have a greater chance of decay.

Eating cariogenic foods with other foods may offer some neutralization of the acid that feeds the bacteria. Eating cariogenic foods at bedtime, when the flow of saliva decreases, increases the chance of decay. Saliva is a buffer to the acid and, if the flow rate of the saliva is inadequate, the washing away of cariogenic substances may not be accomplished.

Infants who have erupted teeth and are given bottles of milk, fruit juice, or sweet substances for long periods may develop **nursing bottle syndrome (NBS)** or baby bottle tooth decay (BBTD). This extensive decay of newly formed teeth is due to the sweetened liquid frequently bathing the teeth, often at bedtime. Parents should be informed and advised of the possibility of NBS so they can take preventive measures.

Suggest to patients that they choose carbohydrates that will not remain on the teeth for long periods. Caution patients about medicines and mouth fresheners that have sugars in them because they dissolve in the mouth, bathing the teeth with sugar for a long period. These may cause a large number of caries if used over time.

Fiber. Fiber is obtained from fruits, vegetables, and grain food groups. It is suggested that 20 to 30 grams of fiber be eaten daily. Currently, an average of 15 grams or fewer are taken in by most Americans. Recent evidence has shown that consuming greater amounts of fiber can reduce the occurrence of colon cancer and reduce blood cholesterol levels. Increasing the levels of fiber should be done gradually to prevent unnecessary gastrointestinal problems, such as constipation.

Fats and Lipids

Fats and lipids share one commonality: They are insoluble in water. Fats are derived from a solid, and lipids are the oils from a liquid. Fat provides an alternate source of energy to carbohydrates. It is often called a backup source of energy. Fat also insulates the body from heat loss, protects vital organs, and aids in the transportation of fat-soluble vitamins: A, D, E, and K.

The fats in normal diets derive from plant and animal foods, and are identified as **triglycerides** or neutral fats. Everyone needs fat in their diet but there is widespread concern that Americans are consuming too much fat. The American Heart Association suggests that the diet contain 30 percent fat content, but currently most Americans' diets are 40 to 45 percent fat. The excess fat has a direct correlation to cholesterol and heart disease, which is the number one cause of death of Americans over the age of forty.

Even though people know fat consumption is a problem, they are drawn to foods that have fat in them. Food manufacturers are aware that fat enhances the taste and smell of food. People need to read food labels and reduce the intake of fast-food products to reduce the fat in their diets. Choosing fat-containing foods is often difficult unless the individual has an understanding of comparative claims. For instance, if the label states *reduced fat,* it normally is reduced about 25% from the original, and if it states that it is *light* it is typically about 50% less than the original.

Proteins

Found naturally in plants and animals, protein is essential for the growth and repair of body tissue. Protein molecules are composed of a combination of twenty amino acids. The quality of a protein is determined by the distribution and kinds of amino acids in its structure. They are classified as "complete" if they have all ten essential amino acids, and "incomplete" if they do not have all ten. Most animal proteins such as eggs, milk, and meat are complete, and vegetable or grain proteins are incomplete. Incomplete proteins can be combined to make complete proteins if complementary foods are eaten at the same meal. For example, corn, an incomplete protein, can be eaten with beans, another incomplete protein, to make a complete protein. Macaroni with cheese, as well as cereal with milk, form complementary proteins.

Amino Acids. There are ten **essential amino acids** that the body cannot synthesize or produce in the needed amounts, so they must come from the individual's diet (Table 5-1). Nonessential amino acids can be produced or synthesized by the body.

Vitamins

Vitamins are a class of nutrients that do not provide the body with energy. Instead, they perform other necessary functions. *Vita* comes from the Latin word meaning life. The first vitamins were discovered by a group of scientists in 1913. They named the first vitamin A and the second vitamin B, the third C, and so on. Later, they found that Vitamin B was not a single vitamin but several, so they added numbers to the letter B (e.g., Vitamin B_1, B_2, B_3). Some of the other vitamins were given names, rather than letters or numbers. In the 1940s, a committee of scientists named the vitamins A, B, C, D, E, and K with number subscripts where applicable. All vitamins fall in one of two groups: fat soluble or water soluble.

Fat-Soluble Vitamins. The fat-soluble vitamins are Vitamins A, D, E, and K. These vitamins are stored in the fatty cells, especially the liver, and are not easily carried in the bloodstream.

TABLE 5-1   Essential and Nonessential Amino Acids

Essential Amino Acids	Nonessential Amino Acids
Arginine	Alanine
Histidine	Asparagine
Isoleucine	Aspartate
Leucine	Cysteine
Lysine	Glutamate
Methionine	Glutamine
Phenylalanine	Glycine
Threonine	Proline
Tryptophan	Serine
Valine	Tyrosine

Vitamin A. Vitamin A has two forms: the plant form **carotene** and the animal form **retinol**. Vitamin A is essential for healthy skin and maintenance of mucous membranes and gives strength to epithelial tissue (Table 5-2). It aids in the continual reshaping of bone but is best known for its contribution to vision.

Vitamin D. Vitamin D can be manufactured by the body if exposed to ultraviolet rays (Table 5-2). Dark-skinned people require additional sun exposure to manufacture the same amount of Vitamin D. Individuals need Vitamin D to ensure healthy bones and tooth development. Most milk is fortified with Vitamins A and D.

Vitamin E. Vitamin E has been related to childbearing and aging. It protects nutrients from destruction by oxidation. Scientific proof relating Vitamin E to slowing the aging process has not been demonstrated, but many feel the vitamin is effective in conditioning the skin.

Vitamin K. The last fat-soluble vitamin is Vitamin K. It promotes the formation of **prothrombin**. Prothrombin is responsible for blood clotting and coagulation. A small amount of Vitamin K is stored in the liver.

Water-Soluble Vitamins. Vitamin C, probably the most famous of all, and the B complex vitamins fall into the group of water-soluble vitamins. The body maintains the balance of water-soluble vitamins through the kidney; any excess is excreted through urine. Vitamin B_6 or niacin can become toxic when intake is excessive because the kidneys cannot easily eliminate the surplus.

Vitamin C, Ascorbic Acid. A large number of people take Vitamin C for everything from toothaches to cancer (Table 5-3). Tragic stories of individuals who developed scurvy (a disease resulting from Vitamin C deficiency)

TABLE 5-2 Fat-Soluble Vitamins

Fat-Soluble Vitamins	Food Sources	Functions	Deficiency/Toxicity
Vitamin A (carotene or retinol)	Animal 　Liver 　Whole milk 　Butter 　Cream 　Cod liver oil Plants 　Dark green leafy vegetables 　Deep yellow or orange fruit 　Fortified margarine	Dim light vision Maintenance of mucous membranes Growth and development of bones Healthy skin	Deficiency 　Night blindness 　Xerophthalmia 　Respiratory infections 　Bone growth ceases Toxicity 　Cessation of menstruation 　Joint pain 　Stunted growth 　Enlargement of liver
Vitamin D (cholecalciferol)	Animal 　Eggs 　Liver 　Fortified milk Plants 　None	Bone growth Healty tooth development	Deficiency 　Rickets 　Osteomalacia 　Poorly developed teeth 　Muscle spasms Toxicity 　Kidney stones 　Calcification of soft tissues
Vitamin E (alphatocopherol)	Animal 　None Plant 　Margarines 　Salad dressing	Antioxidant Skin conditioning	Deficiency 　Destruction of red blood cells Toxicity 　Hypertension
Vitamin K	Animal 　Egg yolk 　Liver 　Milk Plant 　Green leafy vegetables 　Cabbage	Blood clotting	Deficiency 　Prolonged blood clotting Toxicity 　Hemolytic anemia 　Jaundice

during long sea voyages, wars, and famines are widely known. Vitamin C acts to hold cells together and is a component of connective tissue. Oral manifestations of Vitamin C deficiency include improper tooth development, ulcerated gums, and slow healing processes. It was discovered that citrus products prevented and treated this deficiency. Fruits and vegetables contain Vitamin C, especially citrus fruits and tomatoes.

Vitamin B Complex. Even though all vitamins in the B classification are grouped, each has distinct functions (Table 5-3). Vitamin B$_1$ (**thiamin**), Vitamin B$_2$ (**riboflavin**), and **niacin** work together in the production of energy, but they also have separate functions. For example, thiamine prevents cardiovascular changes and a disease called beriberi, riboflavin helps produce proteins and is essential in growth, and niacin prevents gastrointestinal and nervous system disorders. Oral manifesta-

tions of Vitamin B deficiency include angular **cheilosis** (kee-**LOH**-sis), where the lips become red and fissures develop in the corners of the mouth, and **glossitis** (glos-**EYE**-tis), which is inflammation of the tongue, and pellagra, where muc ous membranes atrophy and ulcers develop (Figure 5-3).

Vitamin B$_6$ is essential in the synthesis and metabolism of protein, carbohydrates, and fat. **Folic acid** and **Vitamin B$_{12}$** are important for the functioning of red blood cells and DNA. **Pantothenic acid** and **biotin** aid in energy metabolism.

Minerals

Major Minerals. Minerals are classified as major or trace. A "major" classification indicates that the human body requires larger amounts. Minerals differ from vita-

TABLE 5-3   Water-Soluble Vitamins

Water-Soluble Vitamins	Food Sources	Functions	Deficiency/Toxicity
Vitamin C (ascorbic acid)	Fruits 　All citrus Plants 　Broccoli 　Tomatoes 　Brussels sprouts 　Potatoes	Prevention of scurvy Formation of collagen Healing of wounds Release of stress hormones Absorption of iron	Deficiency 　Scurvy 　Muscle cramps 　Ulcerated gums Toxicity 　Raise uric acid level 　Hemolytic anemia 　Kidney stones 　Rebound scurvy
Thiamin (Vitamin B_1)	Animal 　Liver 　Eggs 　Fish 　Pork 　Beef Plants 　Whole and enriched grains 　Legumes	Coenzyme in oxidation of glucose Prevention of beriberi	Deficiency 　Gastrointestinal tract, nervous and cardiovascular system problems Toxicity 　None
Riboflavin (Vitamin B_2)	Animal 　Milk Plants 　Green vegetables 　Cereals 　Enriched bread	Aids release of energy from food Help produce proteins Aids in growth	Deficiency 　Angular cheilosis 　Glossitis 　Photophobia Toxicity 　None
Pyridoxine (Vitamin B_6)	Animal 　Pork 　Milk 　Eggs Plants 　Whole-grain cereals 　Legumes	Synthesis of nonessential amino acids Conversion of tryptophan to niacin Antibody production	Deficiency 　Angular cheilosis 　Glossitis Toxicity 　Liver disease
Vitamin B_{12}	Animal 　Seafood 　Meat 　Eggs 　Milk Plants 　None	Synthesis of red blood cells Maintenance of myelin sheaths (muscles)	Deficiency 　Degeneration of myelin sheaths 　Pernicious anemia Toxicity 　None
Niacin (nicotinic acid)	Animal 　Milk 　Eggs 　Fish 　Poultry	Transfers hydrogen atoms for synthesis of ATP Prevents gastrointestinal problems Prevents nervous system problems	Deficiency 　Pellagra Toxicity 　Vasodilation of blood vessels
Folacin (folic acid)	Animal 　None Plants 　Spinach 　Asparagus 　Broccoli 　Kidney beans	Synthesis of red blood cells	Deficiency 　Glossitis 　Macrocytic anemia Toxicity 　None

(continues)

TABLE 5-3 Water-Soluble Vitamins *(continued)*

Water-Soluble Vitamins	Food Sources	Functions	Deficiency/Toxicity
Biotin	Animal 　Milk 　Liver Plants 　Legumes 　Mushrooms	Coenzyme in carbohydrate 　and amino acid metabolism Niacin synthesis from 　tryptophan Energy metabolism	Deficiency 　None Toxicity 　None
Pantothenic acid	Animal 　Eggs 　Liver 　Salmon 　Yeast Plants 　Mushrooms 　Cauliflower 　Peanuts	Metabolism of carbohydrates, 　lipids, and proteins Synthesis of acetylcholine Energy metabolism	Deficiency 　None Toxicity 　None

FIGURE 5-3 (A) Cheilosis. (B) Glossitis. *(Courtesy of the Centers for Disease Control and Prevention Public Health Image Library)*

mins in that they are elements rather than complex molecules. Some of the minerals that are positive or negatively charged are called **electrolytes**. When a person is healthy, the electrolytes are in balance.

Seven major minerals are in the body (see Table 5-4). **Calcium** (Ca) makes up the largest quantity and is found in bones and teeth. It also functions in muscle contraction, the nervous system, and the blood. **Phosphorus** (P) is found in bones and teeth and is involved in energy metabolism and maintenance of proper pH balance in the blood. **Sodium** (Na) and **potassium** (K) work together to regulate the electrolyte balance. Sodium maintains fluid balance in the blood; potassium helps release energy and synthesize protein. **Sulfur** (S) is found in protein and is involved in energy metabolism. The last two major minerals are **magnesium** (Mg), which is involved in energy metabolism and stabilizing components of bones and teeth once they are formed, and **chlorine** (Cl), which maintains the correct pH balance in the blood.

Trace Minerals. In smaller quantities, yet as important as the major minerals, are the trace minerals. **Copper, chromium, molybdenum, selenium,** and **manganese** are important to our bodies in the process of metabolism. **Iodine,** found in the thyroid gland, regulates metabolism of the body as well.

Iron primarily functions to carry oxygen through the blood to the cells. People who are deficient in iron become anemic, which reduces their energy levels. Women tend to be more prone to this condition. **Zinc** aids in tissue growth and maintenance of the immune system. **Cobalt** helps in the functioning of red blood cells. **Fluorine** helps strengthen teeth, and research also

TABLE 5-4 The Seven Major Minerals and Their Food Sources

Name	Food Sources	Function	Deficiency/Toxicity

Calcium (Ca)	Milk exchanges
	  Milk, cheese
	Meat exchanges
	  Sardines
	  Salmon
	Vegetable exchanges
	  Green vegetables
		Development of bones and teeth
		Permeability of cell membranes
		Transmission of nerve impulses
		Blood clotting
		Muscle contraction
			Deficiency
			  Osteoporosis
			  Osteomalacia
			Rickets

Phosphorus (P)	Milk exchanges
	  Milk, cheese
	Meat exchanges
	  Lean meat
		Development of bones and teeth
		Transfer of energy
		Component of phospholipids
		Maintain pH balance in the blood
			Same as calcium

Potassium (K)	Fruit exchanges
	  Oranges, bananas
	  Dried fruits
		Contraction of muscles
		Maintaining water balance
		Transmission of nerve impulses
		Carbohydrate and protein metabolism
			Deficiency
			  Hypokalemia
			Toxicity
			  Hyperkalemia

Sodium (Na)	Table salt
	Meat exchanges
	  Beef, eggs
	Milk exchanges
	  Milk, cheese
		Maintaining fluid balance in blood
		Transmission of nerve impulses
		Works with potassium to regulate fluid
		  balance in the blood
			Toxicity
			  Increase in blood pressure

Chlorine (Cl)	Table salt
	Meat exchanges
	  Fish, pork
		Gastric acidity
		Regulation of osmotic pressure
		Activation of salivary amylase
		Energy metabolism
			Deficiency
			  Imbalance in gastric acidity
			  Imbalance in blood pH

Magnesium (Mg)	Vegetable exchanges
	  Green vegetables
	Bread exchanges
	  Whole grains
		Energy metabolism
		Transmission of nerve impulses
		Activator of metabolic enzymes
		Relaxation of skeletal muscles	

Sulfur (S)	Meat exchanges Eggs, poultry, fish	Maintaining protein structure Formation of high-energy compounds	

indicates that it helps prevent osteoporosis (osteoporosis is a condition in which calcium deficiency makes the bones weak and brittle).

Water

Water, by far, is the most abundant nutrient in the body. Water makes up 60 to 70 percent of total body weight. A turnover of 5 percent of total water each day is experienced by the average human adult. A person can go far longer without food than without water. In excessive heat, the body requires additional intake of water to prevent dehydration.

Water is used by the body in several ways, but the primary function is as a solvent for biochemical reactions. For instance, a large part of the blood is composed of water, and this allows for transport and necessary reactions to occur. This solvent action also serves to remove toxic waste from the body. Water acts as a lubricant, especially in the digestive system and the joints. It also helps control body temperature, releasing excessive heat through perspiration, and dispersing heat evenly throughout the body.

The body does not store water and it must be replenished daily. It is lost primarily through perspiration, urination, and fecal output. Some water is obtained from foods, but an additional eight glasses of water per day are recommended. Note that coffee and alcohol cannot be counted as water intake; in fact, they act as **diuretics** and cause the body to lose water through increased urine output.

Balancing Energy

Ideally, people should take in enough nutrition to equal the amount of energy used daily. The amount of energy a substance can supply is measured in the form of Calories. One thousand kilo calories make up one Calorie. (When referring to a Calorie, always capitalize it or abbreviate it by using a capital C or Cal.) Carbohydrate and protein grams yield 4 Calories per gram, in contrast to 1 gram of fat, which yields 9 Calories. For example:

- 5 grams of carbohydrates × 4 Calories = 20 Calories of carbohydrates
- 5 grams of proteins × 4 Calories = 20 Calories of protein
- 5 grams of fat × 9 Calories = 45 Calories of fat

The total of all three categories would be 85 Calories. Fats are more energy rich than carbohydrates or proteins.

Calories are taken into the body to use as energy for everything from running to breathing. The body uses what it needs and the rest is stored as fat. The physical and chemical changes that take place in relationship to the usage of energy are called the metabolism rate. If the rate of metabolism is less than the consumed Calories, then the person will store fat; if the rate of metabolism is greater, the stored fat will be used.

The energy that is used when a person is at rest is called the basal metabolic rate (BMR). The BMR will be higher for pregnant women, children, and leaner individuals because it takes more energy to fuel muscle than it does to store fat in the body. Optimum energy balance would include the same amount of Calories taken into the body as are used. Ideally, most Calories would come from carbohydrates. Fats and proteins should make up less than half the Calories taken in.

Nutrition Labels

For dental assistants to make good choices and be able to advise patients to do the same, they must be knowledgeable about nutrition labels on food products (Figure 5-4). Information is provided on labels according to government standards. Manufacturers of food products know that people are attracted to words described on the products like "lite" or "healthy." These terms may or may not describe the product, so it is important to read the details on the nutrition label. Information such as preservatives (the chemicals added to food to keep it fresh for a longer period) and artificial flavors and colors is also found on the food label.

Listed Items on Labels. Standard information is listed on nutrition labels. The government requires that the labels be easy for the consumer to read, so nutritional information is most often listed in a standard format. The 1990 Nutritional Labeling and Education Act was passed by Congress and enacted in 1994. This requires manufacturers to list all ingredients in the product. Individuals who have special dietary needs can readily identify ingredients, and all consumers can make comparisons from

Nutrition Facts

Serving Size: 1/2 Cup
Servings Per Container: 4

Amount Per Serving

Calories 100 Calories from Fat 30

	% Daily Value*
Total Fat 3g	5%
Saturated Fat 0g	0%
Cholesterol 0mg	0%
Sodium 340mg	14%
Total Carbohydrate 15g	5%
Dietary Fiber 1g	4%
Sugars 0g	
Protein 2g	

Vitamin A 0% • Vitamin C 0%
Calcium 0% • Iron 2%

*Percent Daily Values are based on a 2,000 calorie diet. Your daily values may be higher or lower depending on your calorie needs:

		Calories	2,000	2,500
Total Fat	Less than		65g	80g
Sat Fat	Less than		20g	25g
Cholesterol	Less than		300mg	300mg
Sodium	Less than		2,400mg	2,400mg
Total Carbohydrate			300g	375g
Dietary Fiber			25g	30g

Calories per gram:
Fat 9 ∞ Carbohydrate 4 ∞ Protein 4

Ingredients: Flour, Water, Yeast Vegetable Oil, Salt, Artificial Flavor and Color.

FIGURE 5-4 Food label. *(Courtesy of the FDA)*

one product to another. The labels provide the serving size, percent of daily nutritional value, Calories, fat and cholesterol, sodium, carbohydrate, and other pertinent information on each label.

If the product packaging indicates that it is organic or organically grown, it must have been grown without the use of herbicides, chemical pesticides, or fertilizers. In addition, to qualify as organically grown, plant seeds must not have been prepared with the use of hormones or any other enhancement.

The *serving size* is listed on the label in a measurement or number of the product, for instance, ½ cup or 2 cookies on a cookie package. It also gives the total number of servings per package. The rest of the information pertains to a single serving size.

The *ingredients* and *percent of daily value* are also listed. The daily value percent is based on a diet of 2,000 Calories per day for one adult. So, if the amount listed for total carbohydrate is 15 grams, this indicates that it is 5 percent of the daily value required according to calculations for the carbohydrate group.

Total *Calories* per serving are noted along with specific Calories derived from fat. The Calories from fat should total less than 30 percent of total Calories. Remember that this is the Calories in one serving and not the entire package.

Fat and *cholesterol* notations are valuable to the consumer because of various health concerns, including heart disease and weight control. The listing on the sample label in Figure 5-4 breaks out total fat as well as saturated fat. Saturated fat primarily comes from animal sources, while unsaturated fat primarily comes from vegetable sources. The total cholesterol content for one serving is also noted on the label.

Patients with heart disease or other diseases on sodium-restricted diets will want to watch the levels of *sodium* in foods. The total amount of sodium for one serving is listed on the nutritional label.

The total amount of *carbohydrate* is also listed, which may be broken down into dietary fiber (complex carbohydrates) or sugar (simple carbohydrates).

The nutritional labels show other information, such as the protein, vitamins, and minerals in the product.

Eating Disorders

It seems as if everyone is either overeating or doing everything possible to stay thin. The media and the fashion industry have brought forth the idea that thin is what all individuals aspire to be. Advertisers repeatedly assert that taking this or that pill will allow for significant weight loss within a very short time. Eating disorders such as chronic dieting syndrome, compulsive overeating, bulimia, and anorexia nervosa are widespread, and can be very serious and even life-threatening. They can have psychological, physical, and medical implications. The population most affected is females (at a ratio of 10 females to 1 male), aged twelve to thirty, and often from white, affluent families.

Chronic dieting syndrome causes the individual to experience continuous weight loss and gain, and compulsive overeating can cause a number of psychological, physical, and medical implications that increase risk factors for diabetes and other disease. Bulimia and anorexia can become life-threatening.

Chronic Dieting Syndrome

Chronic dieting syndrome is commonplace. A large percentage of people are ingesting pharmaceuticals and/or diet supplements to control their weight. This is important to dental assistants because the drugs may cause problems in dental treatment. The dieting may cause the heart to race or other chemical imbalances. Adding the anxiety of dental treatment may be enough to cause problems for the patient. Paying special attention to

patients' medical and dental histories will be extremely beneficial.

Bulimia

Bulimia, also called bulimia nervosa, is a disorder that is characterized by secretive bouts of gross overeating followed by methods of weight control such as self-induced vomiting (purging), laxative abuse, excessive exercise, and overuse of diuretics (drugs that increase urine output). Bulimia is attempted when other weight loss attempts do not work. Once tried, it quickly becomes obsessive, resulting in an out-of-control cycle of overeating and purging. An estimated 3 to 5% of women in the United States have been affected by bulimia at some time in their lives. Far fewer men are affected with this disorder. Bulimia and anorexia nervosa behaviors are very secretive and therefore difficult to diagnose. Individuals with bulimia may experience weight gains and losses, but normally do not show extreme weight loss such as in anorexia nervosa. The overeating (binging) is not caused by the desire for food but is a response to stress or depression. Eating brings about overwhelming happiness or a euphoric feeling that is quickly followed by the feeling of self-hatred and depression because of the binging. The individual experiences loss of control and then begins the purging or other behaviors that allow them to feel that they have regained control. Individuals may take laxatives, participate in excessive exercise, take diuretics, or use other weight loss methods to rid the body of the weight gained during the overeating.

There are a number of systemic complications that can result from bulimia. The vomiting can erode the tooth enamel, especially on the lingual surface of the teeth (Figure 5-5). Vomit is highly acidic. When the enamel has thinned or completely eroded, the teeth are more susceptible to decay and are more sensitive to hot or cold. The recurring regurgitation (vomiting) can cause the parotid glands and the saliva glands to become tender and swell, which can be very uncomfortable.

Anorexia Nervosa

Anorexia nervosa (Table 5-5) is an eating disorder characterized by severe weight loss, an extreme aversion to food, and an extreme fear of being fat. Individuals with this disorder have a distorted body image, and see themselves as fat even though they may be overly thin. This psychological disorder centers on control, and behavioral symptoms focus on the fear of putting on weight or eating foods that contain fat or carbohydrates. Individuals with anorexia nervosa may have psychological, physical, and behavioral symptoms such as flaky skin, brittle nails, thinning of hair on the

FIGURE 5-5 Eroded tooth structure shown on the facial, lingual and buccal surfaces of the teeth due to bulimia. *(Courtesy of University of Washington, School of Dentistry)*

head, **amenorrhea** (absence of monthly periods), heart complications, kidney function issues, gastrointestinal complications, impaired organ function, **lanugo** (baby-like hair) on the body, food obsession, extreme use of laxatives, depression, social withdrawal, and obsessive exercising. The individual often feels intensely hungry but will deny fulfillment of this need. Individuals with anorexia nervosa are obsessed with food and thinking of food. They may find it difficult to go out to eat with others. They usually have eating rituals and may cut their food into small pieces and arrange and rearrange it on their plate; typically anorexics know every calorie in each bite consumed. Individuals suffering from this disorder may fix others calorie-laden foods but would feel extreme distress if they had to eat it themselves. The disorder is not focused on the weight loss or food intake but on control and/or other fears relating to the body.

Treating this disease is difficult. It is much easier to diagnose in the later stages because of **emaciation**, or extreme thinness. It is more complicated to diagnose in the early stages due to secrecy and attempts to hide the disorder from others. There are numerous types of therapies that can be helpful to people with anorexia nervosa, including psychological therapy, group therapy, family therapy, cognitive behavior therapy, and drug therapy, along with numerous hospital treatments that focus on correcting the malnutrition. Intravenous feeding may be recommended to treat the malnutrition. Working with a nutritionist during any of these therapies may enhance the outcome. The individual may require day treatment or longer inpatient care. Even if the treatment is successful, relapses can easily occur because the slightest stress triggers the disorder again. Of the individuals who have been hospitalized for anorexia nervosa, an estimated 8 to 10% later die from suicide or starvation. This condition is on the rise in the United States; an estimated one in every hundred adolescent females has anorexic symptoms.

The individuals that come to the dental office with this disorder have numerous physical problems, so special attention to the medical and dental history is crucial. They may also be very uncomfortable lying back in the dental chair if the dental treatment continues for any length of time. The oral cavity may show signs of the disorder, such as sore tissues resulting from poor periodontal health. The binging and purging may be reflected in the state of the teeth as noted in the section on bulimia. Calcium intake may be limited; therefore, the teeth may not be as strong as normal and decay may progress more rapidly.

Diet and Culture

 Dental assistants will come into contact with patients who come from a variety of cultural backgrounds. As stated in Chapter 1, each patient must be treated as an individual and stereotyping must be avoided.

Patients may eat foods that are unfamiliar to the dental assistant. Dental assistants should be informed of patients' diet choices so they can make suggestions that will aid them in achieving and maintaining oral health.

TABLE 5-5   Stacia's Story

Stacia's parents have shared this story and the pictures in the hopes that they will help someone else identify and overcome this disorder. They tried everything that they were aware of to help Stacia, but were unable to turn this eating disorder around. People with this disorder become quite skillful in their methods of weight loss and control.

Stacia was an outgoing well-liked child. She was born into a family who cared about their children, and was loved and supported throughout her life. She was not pressured to be perfect but was allowed to seek her own desires. When she was twelve years old, an incident occurred that her parents did not know about. Other things occurred that seemed to perpetuate this disorder. This is a picture of Stacia at around sixteen years old. She was a great athlete and gave it her all. She had been purging for four years at this time. Her parents were just becoming aware of what she was doing.

Stacia spent part of her senior year in treatment facilities, and missed the senior picture opportunity. In this picture, she is about twenty-one. She is five foot-6 inches tall. In this picture she weighs about one hundred pounds.

Stacia weighs about eighty-five pounds in this picture, and the disorder has progressed. She now is taking many laxatives a day, and she focuses on food. In this photo she is about twenty-two.

(continues)

TABLE 5-5 Stacia's Story *(continued)*

Stacia continues to lose weight. She now is down to eighty-two pounds, and lacks the energy to work full-time. She is about twenty-four.

The disorder becomes more apparent to everyone she comes in contact with. Stacia has a distorted view of her appearance. She does not see herself as thin and is still obsessed with controlling her food intake. Her weight has now dropped to about seventy-eight pounds.

This is one of the last pictures of Stacia. Her weight declined to around sixty-two pounds around the time that she passed away at age twenty-seven. At the time of her death, she was taking over one hundred laxatives a day.

CHAPTER SUMMARY

Dental assistants need to have a background in nutrition to maintain good overall health as well as aid patients in decision making. Having a background in eating disorders may prove beneficial in the work environment with other co-workers and patients. Everyone can benefit from knowledge on reading nutrition labels and what it means when a product is organic or organically grown.

Case Study

Maci Smith was a beautiful seventeen-year-old who had been involved in chronic dieting to keep her weight down. Recently when she came into the dental office, staff members noticed that she had lost an extreme amount of weight. Signs of erosion on the lingual surface of her teeth were also noted. She told the dentist that her teeth were sensitive to heat and cold.

Case Study Review

1. What should the dental assistant do if he/she observes this condition?

2. What diagnosis may be indicated with these symptoms?

3. Should the dentist discuss with her the possibility that she has been purging?

4. What other areas in the oral cavity could be examined?

REVIEW QUESTIONS

Multiple Choice

1. Water-soluble vitamins include
   a. B_1, B_2, D, and niacin.
   b. D, E, K, and C.
   c. D, E, B, and K.
   d. B_1, B_2, C, and niacin.

2. The major minerals are calcium, phosphorus, potassium, sodium, chlorine, magnesium, and
   a. copper.
   b. sulfur.
   c. chromium.
   d. manganese.

3. _____ primarily derive from fruits, grains, legumes, and some vegetable roots.
   a. Proteins
   b. Cariogenic foods
   c. Fats and lipids
   d. Carbohydrates

4. Fats in normal diets occur in plant and animal foods and are identified as
   a. amino acids.
   b. proteins.
   c. triglycerides.
   d. thiamin.

5. The "vita" in vitamin came from the Latin word
   a. calories.
   b. life.
   c. health.
   d. energy.

6. The fat-soluble vitamin that aids in the continual reshaping of bone, but is best known to help with vision is
   a. Vitamin A.
   b. Vitamin B.
   c. Vitamin C.
   d. Vitamin D.

7. The fat-soluble vitamin that has been related to childbearing and aging is
   a. Vitamin A.
   b. Vitamin E.
   c. Vitamin C.
   d. Vitamin D.

8. Water makes up _____ percent of total body weight.
   a. 40–50
   b. 50–60
   c. 60–70
   d. 70–80

9. The babylike hair on the body that occurs with anorexia nervosa is called
   a. amenorrhea.
   b. lanugo.
   c. emaciation.
   d. regurgitation.

10. The eating disorder that is characterized by secretive bouts of gross overeating followed by purging is called
    a. anorexia nervosa.
    b. bulimia.
    c. chronic dieting syndrome.
    d. compulsive overeating.

Critical Thinking

1. How can knowledge of nutrition benefit the dental assistant?

2. If the dental assistant learns that a patient is bulimic, what should the dental assistant do? Should this information be disclosed to the dentist? What information should be offered to the patient about effects on the oral cavity?

3. How should food labels be interpreted? What information is most helpful to the consumer? What should the dental assistant suggest that patients look at on food labels?

Web Activities

1. Go to http://www.nutrition.gov and find the Food and Drug Administration (FDA) page on food labels. Identify which foods are required to have FDA food labeling. Identify which foods require voluntary food labeling.

2. Go to www.usda.gov/wps/portal/usdahome and find food and nutrition. Proceed to good labeling and packaging. From there go to food security and emergency preparedness and learn what is new in this area.

3. Go to www.usda.gov/wps/portal/usdahome and find food and nutrition. From this point, go to *MyPyramid* and develop a customized food guide plan. This individual plan allows for tracking. Track food intake and physical activity for the following week.

SECTION III

BASIC DENTAL SCIENCES

PRACTICE

CHAPTER 6

GENERAL ANATOMY AND PHYSIOLOGY

SPECIFIC INSTRUCTIONAL OBJECTIVES

The student should strive to meet the following objectives and demonstrate an understanding of the facts and principles presented in this chapter:

1. List the body systems, body planes and directions, and cavities of the body, and describe the structure and function of the cell.

2. Explain the functions and divisions of the skeletal system, list the composition of the bone, and identify the types of joints.

3. List the functions and parts of the muscular system.

4. List the functions and the structure of the nervous system.

5. List the functions and the parts of the endocrine system.

6. Explain dental concerns related to the reproductive system.

7. Explain the functions of the circulatory system and list and identify the parts.

8. Explain the functions and parts of the digestive system.

9. List the functions and parts of the respiratory system.

10. List the functions and parts of the lymphatic system and the immune system.

KEY TERMS

abdominal cavity *(87)*
absorption process *(100)*
accessory organ *(101)*
alimentary canal *(101)*
allergy *(106)*
alveolar sac *(103)*
alveoli *(103)*
anatomy *(86)*
antagonistic pair *(94)*
aorta *(99)*
aortic valve *(99)*
aponeurosis *(93)*
appendicular skeleton *(88)*
arteriole *(99)*

artery *(99)*
articulation *(89)*
associate neuron *(94)*
asthma *(104)*
atria *(99)*
atrophy *(94)*
auricle *(99)*
autonomic nervous system (ANS) *(94)*
axial skeleton *(88)*
axon *(94)*
bacterial endocarditis *(100)*
Bell's palsy *(96)*
bicuspid valve *(99)*
bile *(102)*

blood *(99)*
bronchi *(103)*
bronchiole *(103)*
bulimia *(103)*
cancellous bone *(89)*
capillary *(99)*
cardiac muscle *(92)*
cartilage *(89)*
cell *(87)*
cell membrane *(87)*
central nervous system (CNS) *(94)*
chromosome *(88)*
chyme *(102)*
cleft palate *(90)*
compact bone *(89)*

(continues)

OUTLINE (continued)

KEY TERMS (continued)

contract *(92)*

corpuscle *(100)*

cramp *(94)*

cranial cavity *(87)*

cytoplasm *(88)*

deglutition *(102)*

dendrite *(94)*

diabetes mellitus *(98)*

digestion *(100)*

dorsal cavity *(87)*

duodenum *(102)*

elimination *(101)*

endocardium *(99)*

epiglottis *(101)*

erythrocyte *(100)*

esophagus *(102)*

eustachian tube *(103)*

excitability *(92)*

exhalation *(103)*

extensibility *(92)*

fascia *(92)*

fibromyalgia *(94)*

fracture *(90)*

frontal plane *(87)*

gallbladder *(102)*

glycogen *(94)*

heart valve *(99)*

heart *(99)*

hemoglobin *(100)*

hemophilia *(100)*

hemostasis *(100)*

hepatitis *(103)*

Hodgkin's disease *(106)*

homeostasis *(88)*

horizontal plane *(87)*

hormone *(98)*

hyperthyroidism *(98)*

hypothyroidism *(98)*

immune deficiency disease *(106)*

inflamed *(94)*

inhalation *(103)*

irritability *(92)*

isometric contraction *(93)*

isotonic contraction *(93)*

insertion point *(93)*

interneuron *(94)*

joint *(89)*

lactic acid *(94)*

large intestine *(102)*

laryngopharynx *(103)*

larynx *(103)*

leukemia *(100)*

leukocyte *(100)*

ligament *(93)*

lingual tonsil *(105)*

liver *(102)*

lung *(103)*

lung cancer *(105)*

lymph *(105)*

lymph node *(105)*

lymphatic capillary *(105)*

mid-sagittal plane *(87)*

mitral valve *(99)*

motor neuron *(94)*

mouth *(101)*

multiple sclerosis (MS) *(96)*

muscle tone *(92)*

muscular dystrophy (MD) *(94)*

myasthenia gravis *(94)*

myelin sheath *(94)*

myocardium *(99)*

nasal cavity *(103)*

nasal mucosa *(103)*

nasal septum *(103)*

nasopharynx *(103)*

nerve cell *(94)*

neuritis *(96)*

neuron *(94)*

nonspecific immunity *(105)*

nose *(103)*

nucleus *(88)*

olfactory receptor *(103)*

oral cavity *(101)*

organ *(88)*

origin *(93)*

oropharynx *(103)*

osseous tissue *(89)*

osteoblast *(89)*

osteoclast *(89)*

osteomyelitis *(90)*

osteoporosis *(90)*

palatine tonsil *(105)*

pancreas *(103)*

Parkinson's disease *(96)*

pelvic cavity *(87)*

pericardium *(99)*

periodontal disease *(103)*

periosteum *(89)*

peripheral nervous system (PNS) *(94)*

peristalsis *(102)*

pharyngeal tonsil *(105)*

pharynx *(101)*

physiology *(86)*

plasma *(100)*

pleura *(103)*

pregnancy *(98)*

pulmonary circulation *(98)*

pulmonary valve *(99)*

red bone marrow *(89)*

reflex arc *(94)*

relax *(92)*

respiration *(103)*

Rh factor *(100)*

sagittal plane *(87)*

salivary gland *(102)*

sensory neuron *(94)*

small intestine *(102)*

smooth muscle *(92)*

spasm *(94)*

specific immunity *(105)*

spinal canal *(87)*

spleen *(105)*

sprain *(94)*

stomach *(102)*

(continues)

KEY TERMS (continued)

strain *(94)*

striated muscle *(91)*

synapse *(94)*

system *(88)*

systemic circulation *(98)*

tongue *(102)*

teeth *(102)*

temporomandibular joint
disease (TMJ) *(90)*

tendon *(93)*

thoracic cavity *(87)*

thrombocyte *(100)*

thymus *(105)*

tissue *(88)*

tissue fluid *(105)*

tonsils *(105)*

tonsillitis *(106)*

tooth decay *(103)*

trabeculae *(89)*

trachea *(103)*

transverse plane *(87)*

tricuspid valve *(99)*

tuberculosis *(105)*

villi *(102)*

vein *(99)*

vena cava *(99)*

ventral cavity *(87)*

ventricle *(99)*

vocal cord *(103)*

yellow bone marrow *(89)*

INTRODUCTION

To give the quality of care each patient deserves, the dental assistant needs to be familiar with the terminology of body systems and how each system functions. **Anatomy** is the study of the body structure and **physiology** is the study of how the body functions. The anatomy and physiology of each body system will be briefly discussed.

Specific terms are used to establish a means for the health professional to communicate more effectively. Depending on the information and understanding needed, the human body can be studied on many different levels. The body is divided into systems, planes, cavities, and basic units. This chapter provides common references and terms for studying and communicating information about the human body.

Body Systems

The human body is comprised of many body systems. Each body system consists of specific organs and serves a specific purpose. Some of the body systems to be discussed relative to dentistry include: skeletal, muscular, nervous, endocrine, reproductive, circulatory, digestive, respiratory, lymphatic, and immune. Information about each system is presented according to its relationship with dentistry. Refer to Table 6-1 for a list of the systems and their major functions.

Refer to Table 6-2 for terms commonly used to describe areas of the body. The dental assistant will use these terms in many circumstances. For example, when discussing radiographic images, an abscess that shows on the radiograph may be mesial and superior to the root, or an abnormal lesion may be found on the dorsal surface of the tongue.

TABLE 6-1 Body Systems

System	Function
Skeletal	Provides the basic framework of the body; protects, shapes, and gives support to the body; source of attachment for muscles; stores minerals and manufactures blood cells.
Muscular	Muscles contract and relax to allow external body movement and production of the body's heat; internal muscles work to move food along the digestive track and keep the heart beating.
Nervous	Provides a communication system for the body; response to both internal and external stimuli.
Endocrine	Controls growth; stimulates sexual development; regulates use of calcium; aids in regulating the body's water balance; produces insulin.
Reproductive	Produces new life.
Circulatory	Carries life-sustaining substances, such as nutrients and oxygen, throughout the body; carries away waste materials; maintains a balance between intracellular and extracellular fluids.
Digestive	Takes food in, breaks it down, and converts it to substances the body needs to sustain life; provides a means for the body to eliminate solid wastes.
Respiratory	Brings oxygen into the body, which is transported to all cells; the waste product, carbon dioxide, is picked up and exhaled.
Lymphatic	Provides nutrients; drains body fluids and absorbs fats.
Immune	Protects the body from disease and harmful substances

TABLE 6-2   Terms to Describe Areas of the Body

Term	Definition	Example
Anterior	In front of; in the front of the body or body section.	The eye is anterior to the ear.
Ventral	On the front.	The belly or abdominal area of the body is on the ventral side of the body.
Posterior	In back or behind; in the back of the body or body section.	The ear is posterior to the nose.
Dorsal	On the back.	The dorsal surface is on the back of the body or organ.
Medial	Toward the middle of the body; the medial is closest to the midline.	The midline or median line divides the body into left and right halves.
Mesial	Toward the midline of the body (primarily used in dentistry).	The surface of a tooth that faces the median line is the mesial surface.
Lateral	Toward the outside or away from the midline that divides the body.	The ear is on the lateral surface of the head.
Distal	Away from the midline of the body or body section.	The hand is the distal portion of the arm. In dentistry, the surface of a tooth that faces away from the median line is the distal surface.
Proximal	Refers to the part of the body closest to the point of attachment.	The thigh is the proximal surface of the leg.
Inferior	Below or under.	The mouth is inferior to the nose.
Superior	Above or higher.	The eyes are superior to the mouth.

Body Planes and Directions

The body is divided into three primary planes (Figure 6-1). The **sagittal plane** divides the body into left and right halves. If the sagittal plane divided the body into equal left and right halves, it would be referred to as the **mid-sagittal plane**. The plane that divides the body into upper and lower sections is known as the **transverse plane**, sometimes called the **horizontal plane**. The **frontal plane** divides the body into front and back sections. This vertical division divides the body into a front section, called the ventral or anterior, and a back section, referred to as the dorsal or posterior.

Body Cavities

Body cavities are spaces or areas in the body where various structures and organs are found. The body cavities are divided into two sections: the dorsal and the ventral.

The **dorsal cavity** is in the posterior portion of the body and contains two parts: the **spinal canal**, which contains the spinal cord, and the **cranial cavity**, which contains the brain. These two occupy one continuous space.

The **ventral cavity** is in the anterior portion of the body and contains three main parts: the **thoracic cavity**, **abdominal cavity**, and **pelvic cavity**. These cavities contain organs that maintain the basic life processes. The thoracic cavity or chest cavity contains the lungs, the heart, and all accessory parts needed for their functioning. The abdominal cavity is divided into upper and lower sections. The upper cavity is called the abdominal and includes most of the digestive tract and supporting organs needed for the process of digestion. The lower portion is called the pelvic cavity and contains the urinary bladder, the rectum, and the reproductive system (Figure 6-2).

Basic Structure and Functions of the Cell

The **cell** is the basic unit of all systems and the smallest functioning unit of the body (Figure 6-3). The basic components of a cell include the cell membrane, nucleus, cytoplasm, and chromosomes. The **cell membrane** is the outer wall of the cell. This thin wall is composed of proteins, lipids, and carbohydrates. This membrane controls the exchange of materials coming into and out

FIGURE 6-1 Body planes and directions.

of the cell. The **nucleus**, the controlling body of the cell, contains genetic codes. **Cytoplasm** comprises all the substance of a cell except the nucleus. **Chromosomes** are in the nucleus and contain DNA, which transmits genetic information.

Cells differ in appearance, function, and structure according to what they do. Specialized groups of cells form **tissues** and tissues group together to form **organs**. Tissues and organs unite to form **systems**. These cells, tissues, organs, and systems all function together to maintain harmony in the body, which is called **homeostasis** (hoh-me-o-**STAY**-sis).

Skeletal System

Functions of the Skeletal System

The functions of the skeletal system include support for the body's framework and overall body shape. The skeleton provides a surface for muscles to attach to and

protects the fragile organs of the body. Also, the skeletal system manufactures blood cells and stores minerals for use when they are needed. An example is calcium.

Divisions of the Skeletal System

The skeleton is divided into two main divisions: the axial skeleton and the appendicular skeleton. The **axial skeleton** includes bones of the cranium, face, spinal column, ribs, and sternum. It is the framework of the head and the trunk of the body. The spinal column is divided into five sections including: cervical vertebrae, thoracic vertebrae, lumbar vertebrae, sacrum, and coccyx. Knowledge of the areas of the spinal cord are useful when learning the correct ergonomic positioning for the dental assistant. The **appendicular skeleton** is composed of the bones from the upper and lower extremities and includes the arms, hands, legs, feet, shoulders, and hips. Together, the two divisions total 206 bones in an adult skeleton (Figures 6-4B).

FIGURE 6-2 Body cavities.

FIGURE 6-3 Basic cell structures.

Bone Composition

The bone or **osseous tissue** is composed of connective tissue. This connective tissue is rendered hard by the deposits of mineral salts. The bone tissue is 20 percent water; of the remaining 80 percent, two-thirds is minerals and inorganic matter and one-third is organic matter, including blood cells, lymphatic vessels, and nerves.

There are two types of bone tissue: cancellous or spongy bone and compact or dense bone. The **cancellous bone** consists of a meshwork of interconnecting bone called **trabeculae** (trah-**BEK**-you-lay). The pattern of the trabeculae gives the bone a sponge-like appearance and strength without adding weight. Cancel-

lous bone is found in the ends of long bones and in the middles of other bones. The **compact bone** is the strong and hard section of the bone. Compact bone is dense and forms the main shaft of long bones and the outer layer of other bones. **Osteoclast** cells are found in the compact bone. When bone is damaged or stressed, the osteoclasts dissolve and reabsorb the calcium salts of the bone matrix. The compact bone is covered with a layer of tough, fibrous tissue called the **periosteum**. The periosteum contains blood and lymph vessels, bone-building cells called **osteoblasts**, and nerve tissue.

Inside the spaces of the cancellous bone is **red bone marrow**. Red marrow is filled with blood vessels and small amounts of connective tissue. Red bone marrow manufactures red and white blood cells and platelets. It is found in the ends of long bones and the middles of other bones. **Yellow bone marrow** contains mainly fat cells and is found in the center shafts of long bones. As the body ages, the active red bone marrow is slowly replaced with yellow bone marrow (Figure 6-5).

Cartilage is found where bones join and forms part of such structures as the nose and ears. It is a tough, nonvascular, resilient connective tissue.

Types of Joints

Joints or **articulations** are areas where two or more bones meet or form a junction. A joint is usually composed of fibrous connective tissue and cartilage. Table 6-3 illustrates the three types of joints, explains how they are divided, and gives an example of each.

Synovial joints make movement possible and comprise most of the joints in the body (Figure 6-6).

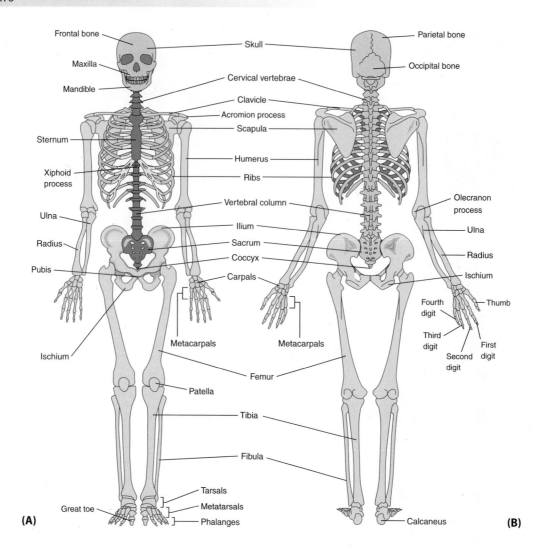

FIGURE 6-4 Axial (highlighted in blue) and appendicular (highlighted in grey) skeleton.

Importance to the Dental Assistant

The skeletal system contains the cranium and facial bones, including the maxilla and the mandible. These bones support the teeth and surrounding tissues and are the primary focus of dentistry. Conditions of the skeletal system may alter patient treatment. Knowledge of this system aids dental assistants in correct patient positioning and movement at the dental unit, as well as sound ergonomic principles for themselves.

Common Diseases and Conditions of the Skeletal System

Diseases of the bone include:

■ **Osteomyelitis** (oss-tee-oh-my-eh-**LYE**-tis)—an infection of the bone-forming tissue. There is inflammation, edema, and circulatory congestion in the bone marrow. Pus may form and inflammatory pressure may cause small pieces of bone to fracture.

■ **Osteoporosis**—the loss of bony material, thus leaving the bones brittle and soft.

■ **Cleft palate**—the failure of the palate to form and join correctly.

■ **Fractures**—breaks of the bone or cartilage.

■ **Temporomandibular joint disorder (TMJ)**—degeneration or disease of the joint where the mandible articulates with the temporal bone.

Muscular System

Functions of the Muscular System

The muscular system makes up 30 to 40 percent of total body weight. The muscles contract and relax to provide for all movements of the body, both internally and externally. Internal muscles move food along the digestive track and keep the heart beating. External muscles allow the body to walk, run, stand straight, and communicate. Muscles also produce body heat.

FIGURE 6-5 (A) Anatomic features of the bone. (B) Dental radiograph showing compact and spongy bone.

TABLE 6-3 Joints

Name of Joint	Description of Joint	Type of Movement	Example
Fibrous joint	Fibrous connective tissue	Immovable or fixed	Sutures found between the bones of the cranium.
Cartilaginous joint	Connective tissue, cartilage	Slightly movable	Joints found between bones of the vertebrae.
Synovial joint	Fluid within the joint (synovial fluid)	Considerable or free movement	There are six types of synovial joints: ball and socket, hinge, pivot, gliding, saddle, and condyloid. The temporomandibular joint is a synovial joint.

Types of Muscles

There are three types of muscle tissue: striated, cardiac, and smooth. Figure 6-7 shows these muscle tissues, locations, appearances, and functions.

Striated Muscles. **Striated muscles** are made of long, thin cells that have stripes or bands across them. Because these muscles are in bunches of fibers that attach to the skeleton, they are sometimes called skeletal muscles. This type has the largest amount of muscle tissue of the three types and its function is to provide for external body movement, from facial expression to bike riding. The skeletal muscles are under voluntary control. They are the only group of muscles an individual has conscious control over and are sometimes called voluntary muscles.

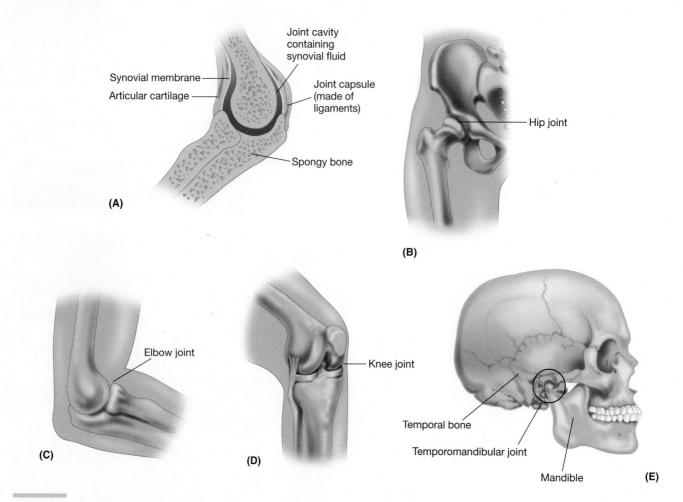

FIGURE 6-6 Skeletal joints: (A) Structures of a synovial joint and several examples of synovial joints. (B) Ball and socket joint of the hip. (C) Hinge joint of the elbow. (D) Hinge joint of the knee. (E) Temporomandibular joint.

Cardiac Muscles. Cardiac muscles have the same striated or striped appearance as the skeletal muscles but are involuntary in action. Cardiac muscles are found only in the heart, where they receive approximately seventy-five stimuli per minute. These muscle cells are specially designed in a chain-like arrangement and are able to receive an impulse, respond, and relax very rapidly, thereby keeping the heart beating in an even rhythm.

Smooth Muscles. Smooth muscles are nonstriated tissue. The smooth muscles are also involuntary, which means they are controlled by the autonomic nervous system and are not consciously controlled. These muscles are found in internal organs (except the heart), blood vessels, skin, and ducts from glands.

Muscle Characteristics

Each muscle is made of cells in various shapes and sizes depending on muscle function. Groups of muscle cells are often called fibers. Each fiber is about the size of a human hair and can support 1,000 times its own weight. Humans have over a trillion fibers in over 600 muscles in their bodies. Each fiber has nerves and a blood supply; it also has a fibrous sheet of connective tissue that covers, supports, and separates the muscle fibers. This sheet is called the fascia.

Muscle tissue has the capacity to respond to stimuli, called excitability or irritability. This response puts the muscle into motion or activity. Extensibility is the ability of the muscle to stretch or spread in order to perform tasks. Muscle tone is the tension of the muscular system. The brain and spinal cord continually send stimuli to the muscles on a subconscious level. The increase or decrease of the constant stimuli from the nervous system affects muscle tone. When the muscles are used, they stay toned and ready in a healthy state, while muscles that are not used become flabby and begin to deteriorate.

Muscles work by contracting and relaxing. When muscles contract, they become shorter and thicker.

(A) Striated Muscle Tissue

(B) Cardiac Muscle Tissue

(C) Smooth Muscle Tissue

FIGURE 6-7 (A) Striated muscle. (B) Cardiac muscle. (C) Smooth muscle.

When relaxed, they release and return to their normal form. There are two types of contractions: isometric and isotonic. **Isometric contraction** occurs when there is no change in the length of the muscle but the muscle tension is increased. Pushing against a solid object is an example of isometric contraction. Lifting weights is an example of **isotonic contractions**—the muscle tension remains the same but the muscles shorten.

Muscle Attachments

Skeletal muscles attach to the bone in various ways. They may attach directly to the periosteum of the bone or they may attach through specialized connective tissue that extends beyond the muscle. When this extension is in the form of a cord, it is called a **tendon**. Tendons attach muscle to bone (Figure 6-8). Certain muscles require a broad, flattened extension called an **aponeurosis** (ap-oh-new-**ROH**-sis). The aponeurosis attaches muscle to bone and binds muscle to muscle. **Ligaments** are composed of bands or sheets

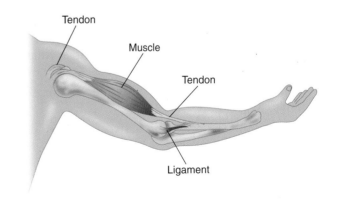

Tendon

Muscle

Tendon

Ligament

FIGURE 6-8 Muscle tissues and attachments of the arm.

of fibrous tissue and act to connect or support two or more bones.

The **origin** of the muscle is where the muscle attaches to the more stationary bone. The **insertion point** of the muscle is where the bone is moveable.

How Muscles Function

Muscles contract and relax to provide movement. Most skeletal muscles function in antagonistic pairs. This means that while one set of muscle contracts, another corresponding set relaxes. The body moves and functions through these coordinated efforts.

It takes energy for muscles to function. Energy is received in the form of oxygen and glucose. Oxygen comes to the muscle through the circulating blood and glucose is stored as a substance called glycogen. Muscles go through chemical changes to provide energy for body functions. Sometimes, when the activity is too rapid, there is not enough oxygen and an incomplete breakdown of glycogen occurs, resulting in a waste product called lactic acid. When the activity stops, the normal metabolic process readjusts and sufficient oxygen is restored.

Importance to the Dental Assistant

The muscular system is important to the dental assistant both personally and professionally. To be an effective dental assistant, it is advantageous to keep in shape and stay healthy. Muscles of the lower back and neck are used when the dental assistant assists the dentist or works directly on patients. These muscles need to be strengthened so that correct positioning can be accomplished. Professionally, the dental assistant will work with patients who have problems with their muscular systems. Understanding the muscular system can help the assistant make patients' dental visits more comfortable. Chewing, swallowing, facial expressions, and talking are all specific muscular activities that make this system pertinent to dentistry.

Common Conditions and Diseases of the Muscular System

Conditions and diseases of the muscular system are numerous and varied. Following are a few examples:

- The muscle tissue can be strained, sprained, cramped, or inflamed.

- Sometimes the muscles go into spasm, which is a sudden, involuntary muscle contraction.

- If muscles are not used, they begin to deteriorate, known as atrophy.

- Fibromyalgia (figh-broh-my-**AL**-jee-ah) is chronic pain in the muscles and soft tissues surrounding the joints.

- Muscular dystrophy is a congenital disorder characterized by progressive degeneration of the skeletal muscles. It usually strikes in early childhood.

- Myasthenia gravis (my-as-**THEE**-nee-ah **GRAH**-vis) is an autoimmune disorder that leaves the muscles weak and fatigued. One of the first symptoms is weakness in the facial or swallowing muscles.

Nervous System

Functions of the Nervous System

The nervous system transmits stimuli from outside and inside the body; it is the body's communication system. It has the ability to respond and transmit stimuli to maintain the body's unity and harmony.

Structure of the Nervous System

The nervous system consists of three sections: brain, spinal cord, and nerve cells. The brain and the spinal cord make up the central nervous system (CNS). All the nerves outside the CNS make up the peripheral nervous system (PNS). There is also a specialized group of peripheral nerves that function mainly automatically; this group is called the autonomic nervous system (ANS).

The basic structural unit of the nervous system is a neuron or nerve cell. The neuron structure includes a nucleus surrounded by a cell membrane with thread-like projections called nerve fibers. The nerve fibers that conduct impulses toward the cell body are called dendrites. Axons are nerve fibers that conduct impulses away from the cell body. Some dendrites and axons can be up to two feet long. Nerve fibers move impulses from one cell body to another through a synapse. This is a junction where chemicals are released from the ends of axons to allow the stimuli to jump to the next dendrite. Some nerves in the PNS are covered with layers of Schwann cells. These layers insulate and protect nerves, and are known as the myelin sheath (Figure 6-9).

Sensory neurons work together to carry messages from all over the body to the spinal cord and the brain. Neurons that carry a message away from the spinal cord and brain are motor neurons. Motor neurons carry messages that direct the body to act. A third type of neuron, interneurons or associate neurons, transmits impulses from sensory neurons to motor neurons in the CNS.

The Spinal Cord and Spinal Nerves

The spinal cord is a major part of the nervous system. The activity of the spinal cord is twofold. First, it is a center for reflex or involuntary responses. Reflex arc occurs when a stimulus is sent through the sensory neurons into the spinal cord and a response is automatically processed and sent back through motor neurons for an action (Figure 6-10).

Second, the spinal cord transmits stimuli from the body to the brain, where the message is interpreted and then a response is sent back to an organ or a muscle.

Thirty-one pairs of spinal nerves originate in the spinal cord. The nerves are named and numbered according to the closest vertebrae.

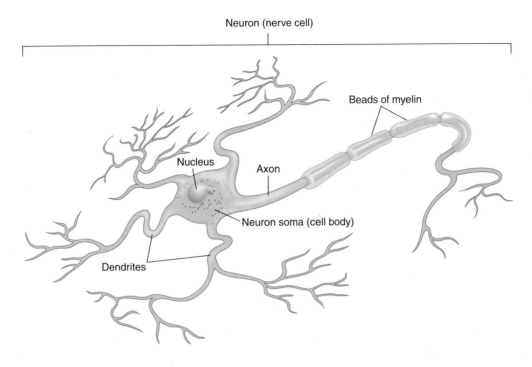

FIGURE 6-9 Structure of a neuron.

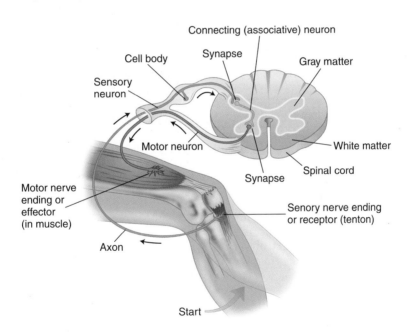

FIGURE 6-10 Simple reflex arc.

The Brain and Cranial Nerves

The brain consists of many interlinked parts. The brain receives incoming stimuli and interprets and processes the information. Stimuli are directed to various parts of the brain, depending on which area of the body the stimuli is coming from.

Twelve pairs of cranial nerves mainly involve the head. They are numbered with Roman numerals beginning in the front of the brain and moving toward the back (Table 6-4).

Importance to the Dental Assistant

Understanding its structure and how the nervous system works will help the dental assistant work with the dentist and the patient. Patients often fear going to the dentist because they assume it will be a physically painful experience. Anesthesia blocks patients' pain and makes dental procedures possible. Dental assistants must know the nerves in the face and oral cavity to effectively assist the dentist dur-

TABLE 6-4   Cranial Nerves and Their Functions

I.	**Olfactory nerves** conduct impulses from receptors in the nose to the brain and are sensory in function.
II.	**Optic nerves** conduct impulses from receptors in the eyes to the brain and are sensory in function.
III.	**Oculomotor nerves** send motor impulses to four of the external eye muscles, as well as to certain internal eye muscles.
IV.	**Trochlear nerves** send motor impulses to one external eye muscle of each eye.
V.	**Trigeminal nerves** each divide into three branches: **Ophthalmic branches** go to the eyes and forehead. **Maxillary branches** go to the upper jaw. **Mandibular branches** go to the lower jaw.
VI.	**Abducens nerves** innervate the muscles that turn the eye to the side.
VII.	**Facial nerves** innervate the facial muscles, salivary glands, lacrimal glands, and the sensation of taste on the anterior two-thirds of the tongue.
VIII.	**Acoustic nerves** each divide into two branches: **Cochlear branches** are concerned with the sense of hearing. **Vestibular branches** are concerned with the sense of balance.
IX.	**Glossopharyngeal nerves** innervate the parotid glands, the sense of taste on the posterior third of the tongue, and part of the pharynx.
X.	**Vagus nerves** innervate part of the pharynx, larynx, and vocal cords, and parts of the thoracic and abdominal viscera.
XI.	**Spinal accessory nerves** innervate the shoulder muscles. Some of the fibers of these nerves arise from the spinal cord.
XII.	**Hypoglossal nerves** primarily innervate the muscles concerned with movements of the tongue.

ing the administration of anesthetic, as well as during many types of surgical procedures. Dental team members sometimes experience physical problems themselves, especially with the sciatic nerve located in the lower back and traveling down the back of the thigh. This is due to the positions they must hold for long periods of time.

Common Diseases of the Nervous System

- **Neuritis** is the inflammation of nerves. It may be the result of a fall or blow and can affect one or more nerves in the body. The term neuritis is also used when describing nerve tissue degeneration.

- **Multiple sclerosis (MS)** is a disease that usually appears in people aged twenty to forty. This disease destroys the myelin sheath of neurons in the CNS. When this happens, impulses cannot be transmitted to their destinations.

- **Parkinson's disease** is a chronic nervous disease characterized by slowly spreading tremors, muscular weakness, and a peculiar gait.

- **Bell's palsy** is a sudden onset of facial paralysis.

Endocrine System and Reproductive System

Functions of the Endocrine System

The endocrine system, like the nervous system, is a control and communication system. The nervous system acts rapidly to transmit stimuli, whereas the endocrine system is much slower and the results are longer lasting. The nervous system and the endocrine system are connected because the nervous system controls the pituitary gland and this gland controls the other glands. The endocrine system generally controls the body's growth, protects the body in stressful situations, controls development of sex characteristics, regulates utilization of calcium, aids in regulating the body's water balance, and produces insulin, which aids in the transport of glucose into cells (Table 6-5).

Parts of the Endocrine System

The endocrine system is made of glands spread throughout the body (Figure 6-11). They are grouped according to structures and interrelated functions. These glands produce secretions and are ductless—there is no tube

TABLE 6-5   Major Glands of the Endocrine System

Gland	Main Function(s)	Examples of Hormones Produced
Pituitary	Master gland that releases hormones which affect the workings of other glands.	Growth hormone and thyroid stimulation hormone
Thyroid	Increases metabolic rate, which affects both mental and physical activities. Needed for normal growth.	Thyroxin
Parathyroid	Increases the level of calcium in the blood. Regulates the calcium between bone and blood.	Parathyroid hormone
Adrenal	Releases the fight or flight hormone, which increases heart rate and blood pressure and aids in the metabolism of carbohydrates, proteins, and fats during stress.	Cortisol and adrenalin
Pancreas (islets of Langerhans)	Produces hormones, including insulin and glucagon.	Insulin
Testes	Responsible for the development of male sex characteristics.	Testosterone
Ovaries	Responsible for the development of female sex characteristics.	Estrogen and progesterone

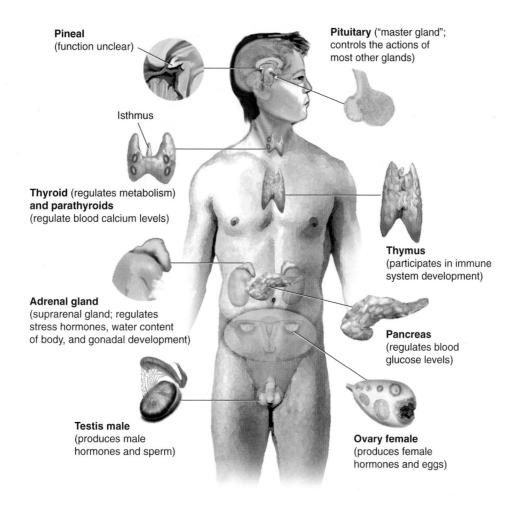

FIGURE 6-11   Structures of the endocrine system.

for secretions from the glands to pass through, so the secretions empty directly into the bloodstream and circulate throughout the body. These secretions are called hormones. Hormones are released from the endocrine glands. Hormones control the internal environment of the body from the cellular to the organ level. They are analogous to the furnaces and thermostats in our homes. We set the thermostat to a particular temperature, and when the temperature falls below that temperature, the thermostat causes the furnace to turn on. Once the temperature reaches the set temperature on the thermostat the furnace turns off. The hormonal system functions in a similar manner. When the concentration of a particular hormone reaches a certain level in the body, the endocrine gland that secretes that hormone is inhibited and secretion of the hormone ceases or decreases. Later when the concentration of that gland's hormone falls below normal levels, the inhibition of the gland stops and it begins to produce and secrete the hormone once again.

Reproductive System

The reproductive system includes male and female reproductive organs. The male and female reproductive system's main function is the creation of life. In both sexes, primary and accessory organs must be protected in certain procedures used in dentistry. Two examples of procedures requiring protection are using a lead apron when exposing radiographs and providing adequate ventilation during nitrous oxide sedation. Safety guidelines are routinely followed in the dental office to protect the patient and the dental staff.

Importance to the Dental Assistant

There are diseases and conditions of the endocrine system, such as diabetes, that affect patients and how they respond to dental treatment. The dental assistant can prepare for possible emergencies with an understanding of the patient's needs. With young patients going through puberty and older patients going through menopause, better communication and understanding will be enhanced by knowledge of this system. The dental assistant is responsible for knowing and following all precautions and standards regarding radiation and use of nitrous oxide in the dental examination room.

Common Diseases and Conditions of the Endocrine and Reproductive Systems

- **Diabetes mellitus** is a disease that occurs when the pancreas produces an insufficient amount of insulin.
- During **pregnancy**, dental treatments may need to be altered depending on the stage of pregnancy.
- **Hypothyroidism** is an underactive thyroid gland.
- **Hyperthyroidism** is an overactive thyroid gland with excessive secretion of hormones.

Circulatory System

Functions of the Circulatory System

The circulatory system is the body's means of transporting a continuous supply of oxygen, nutrients, hormones, and antibodies throughout the body while carbon dioxide and other cellular wastes are being removed from the body. This system maintains a balance between intracellular and extracellular fluids.

Parts of the Circulatory System

Circulation is divided into two pathways. The first pathway circulates blood through the heart to the lungs and back to the heart. This is **pulmonary circulation**. The second pathway, **systemic circulation**, carries the blood from the aorta to the smallest blood vessels and back to the heart (Figure 6-12). Main components of the circula-

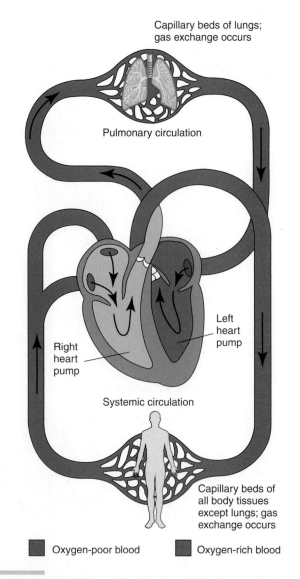

FIGURE 6-12 Systemic and pulmonary circulation.

tory system include the heart, blood vessels (arteries, veins, and capillaries), and blood.

Heart. The **heart** is a pump that circulates the blood throughout the body. It is a triangular-shaped muscular organ that is approximately the size of a closed fist (Figure 6-13). The heart is covered with three layers: the **pericardium**, the outer layer that is composed of a double-walled sac; the **myocardium**, a tough, muscular wall; and the **endocardium**, a thin lining on the inside of the heart. A wall divides the heart into right and left halves. Each half is divided again into upper chambers called the **atria** or **auricles** and lower chambers called **ventricles**. Four **heart valves** regulate the flow of blood in one direction. The blood comes into the heart through large vessels called the **vena cava**. From the superior and inferior vena cava, blood enters the right atrium, and then is pumped through the **tricuspid valve** into the right ventricle. It then goes through the **pulmonary valve** into the pulmonary artery, which carries the blood to the lungs to get rid of waste and gases, and picks up fresh oxygen. From the lungs, the blood is carried by the pulmonary vein to the left atrium, and then through the **mitral (bicuspid) valve** into the left ventricle and then through the **aortic valve** into the aorta to be distributed to all parts of the body (Figure 6-13).

Blood Vessels, Arteries, Veins, and Capillaries. The **arteries** carry oxygenated blood from the heart to the capillaries of the tissues. The walls of the arteries are tough and composed of three layers to withstand the pressure. The largest artery is the **aorta**, which receives blood directly from the heart; the **arterioles** are the smallest arteries.

The **veins** carry blood that has drained from the capillaries back to the heart. The walls of the veins are composed of three layers like the arteries, but they are much thinner and less muscular. Within the inner layer are folds that form valves that keep the blood flowing toward the heart.

The **capillaries** are the connection between the arteries and the veins. The exchange between the blood and body cells occurs in the capillaries. Here, oxygen and nutrients are delivered to the cells and carbon dioxide and wastes are removed. The walls of the capillaries are comprised of a single thin layer, which is an extension of the lining in arteries and veins. There are thousands of miles of connecting capillaries in the body.

Blood. The **blood** has three main functions: transportation of nutrients, gases, waste products, and hormones; regulation of the amount of body fluids, pH balance, and body temperature; and protection

FIGURE 6-13 Structures of the heart.

against pathogens and blood loss after injury through the clotting mechanism. Blood is a thick fluid that varies in color from bright red to a darker, brownish red. The average adult has four to six quarts of blood. The liquid portion of the blood, **plasma**, is 91 percent water and carries nutrients, hormones, and wastes. The cells or solid portion of the blood are called **corpuscles**. There are three types of corpuscles: erythrocytes, leukocytes, and platelets.

- **Erythrocytes**, or red blood cells, contain the protein **hemoglobin**, which gives the erythrocytes the ability to carry oxygen.

- **Leukocytes**, or white blood cells, protect the body from infection and disease. There are five types of leukocytes, all with specific tasks to defend the body against viruses, bacteria, and other foreign substances.

- **Thrombocytes**, or platelets, are fragments or pieces of cells that are necessary for blood clotting (coagulate). The process by which the body controls bleeding is called **hemostasis**.

Blood Groups. There are five main blood type categories: A, AB, B, O, and the ABO system. The ABO system is primarily used for blood transfusions. Refer to Table 6-6 for blood types, donors, and recipients. If patients were to receive blood that is not compatible with their blood type, the result could be fatal. Additionally, the **Rh factor** should be considered when treating patients who may require blood transfusions from a donor. Serious transfusion reactions could occur if the Rh factor is not matched. The Rh factor is also an important consideration during pregnancy; if the child is Rh positive and the mother is Rh negative, incompatibility between the mother and the fetus may result. People with the Rh antigen are Rh positive and those without are Rh negative. The mother may become sensitized by the blood of the Rh-positive fetus. To prevent problems in future pregnancies, if the fetus is Rh positive, during the second trimester of the first pregnancy the mother is given RhoGAM, an immunoglobulin.

> **Importance to the Dental Assistant**
>
> The circulatory system is important to the dental assistant as our population is aging and geriatric dentistry is growing. Understanding heart disease and frequently prescribed medications helps the assistant to be alert for possible complications. Heart disease is the leading cause of death for both men and women; therefore another consideration is to be prepared for an emergency—dental treatment can present a stressful situation to an already compromised patient.

Common Diseases and Conditions of the Circulatory System

- **Bacterial endocarditis** is an inflammation of the lining of the heart. Patients who have a history of rheumatic fever, congenital heart disease, open-heart surgery, joint replacement, organ transplants, or dental implants should always be treated with antibiotics before dental treatment.

- A disorder called **hemophilia** is the failure of the blood to clot.

- **Leukemia** is a malignant, progressive disease of the blood-forming organs that is marked by unrestrained growth of abnormal leukocytes. Leukemia cells infiltrate the bone marrow and lymph tissue. These cells then advance to the bloodstream and various body organs.

Digestive System

Functions of the Digestive System

The digestive system provides a means for consumed food to be prepared for use by the body, circulated to all cells, and eliminating wastes. This is done by **digestion**, breaking down food into small nutrient molecules the cells can use. After food has gone through digestion, it is transferred into the bloodstream; this is the **absorption**

TABLE 6-6   Blood Types, Donors, and Recipients

Blood Group/ Type	Percent of Population	Antigen/ Agglutinogen on Red Blood Cells	Antibody/ Agglutinin in Plasma	Can Receive	Can Donate to
A	41	A	Anti-B	A or O only	A or AB only
B	12	B	Anti-A	B or O only	B or AB only
AB	3	A and B	None	A, B, AB, O Universal recipient	AB only
O	44	None	Anti-A and Anti-B	O only	A, B, AB, O Universal donor

process. Here, the small nutrient molecules are circulated by the bloodstream to all cells of the body. Another function of the digestive system is the process of **elimination**, which provides a means for the body to eliminate solid wastes.

Parts of the Digestive System

The digestive system is divided into two groups: the **alimentary canal** and **accessory organs**. The alimentary canal forms a canal or tube from the mouth to the anus. The canal includes the mouth (oral cavity), **pharynx**, esophagus, stomach, small intestine, and large intestine. Accessory organs aid in the process of digestion.

Included are the teeth, tongue, salivary glands and ducts, liver, gallbladder, and pancreas (Figure 6-14 and Table 6-7).

Alimentary Canal. The **mouth (oral cavity)** receives food and begins breaking the food down. The teeth, tongue, lips, cheeks, and salivary glands all work together to mechanically break food into small pieces and then move the food to the throat area.

The **pharynx** connects the oral cavity to the esophagus, which is where food is swallowed. The pharynx also functions as part of the respiratory system. Therefore, sometimes during swallowing, food may go into the larynx instead of the esophagus. To prevent this from occurring, the **epiglottis** (a small, leaf-shaped

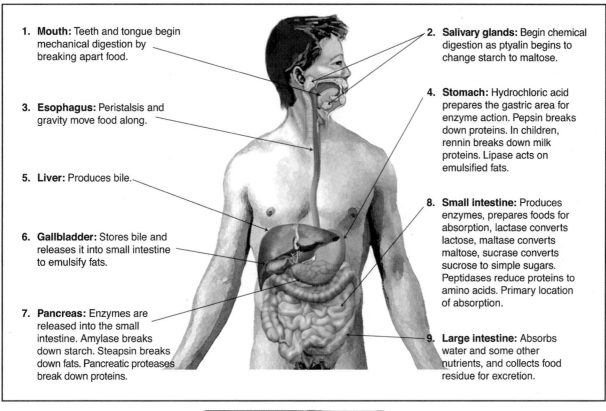

1. **Mouth:** Teeth and tongue begin mechanical digestion by breaking apart food.

3. **Esophagus:** Peristalsis and gravity move food along.

5. **Liver:** Produces bile.

6. **Gallbladder:** Stores bile and releases it into small intestine to emulsify fats.

7. **Pancreas:** Enzymes are released into the small intestine. Amylase breaks down starch. Steapsin breaks down fats. Pancreatic proteases break down proteins.

2. **Salivary glands:** Begin chemical digestion as ptyalin begins to change starch to maltose.

4. **Stomach:** Hydrochloric acid prepares the gastric area for enzyme action. Pepsin breaks down proteins. In children, rennin breaks down milk proteins. Lipase acts on emulsified fats.

8. **Small intestine:** Produces enzymes, prepares foods for absorption, lactase converts lactose, maltase converts maltose, sucrase converts sucrose to simple sugars. Peptidases reduce proteins to amino acids. Primary location of absorption.

9. **Large intestine:** Absorbs water and some other nutrients, and collects food residue for excretion.

Parotid gland
Parotid duct
Masseter muscle
Submandibular gland
Buccinator muscle
Sublingual gland

FIGURE 6-14 Structures of the digestive system.

TABLE 6-7 Mechanism of Digestion

Organ	Process	Description of Process
Oral cavity (mouth, teeth, tongue, and saliva)	Taste Mastication Swallowing or deglutition	Receives the food, tastes Mechanical breakdown of food Saliva glands produce enzymes to start chemical digestion
Pharynx	Deglutition	Movement of food as a result of swallowing Passageway for food and air
Esophagus	Deglutition Peristalsis	Mucus is secreted as food is transported in waves toward the stomach
Stomach	Churning Peristalsis	Chemical breakdown continues as stomach enzymes are released and mechanical movements churn the contents
Small intestine	Absorption Peristalsis	Absorption of digested food Move contents along intestinal track
Large intestine	Peristalsis Defecation	Mechanical movements occur Emptying of the rectum

cartilage) covers the larynx. Swallowing is a complex, multi-stepped process that is controlled by the medulla part of the brain. Swallowing or **deglutition** provides movement for the food to proceed from the mouth to the stomach.

The **esophagus** extends from the pharynx to the stomach. Muscles help to keep food moving toward the stomach, even when the body is reclined. The lower esophageal sphincter (**SFINK**-ter) muscle, at the end of the esophagus, relaxes to allow food into the stomach, and then contracts to prevent it from flowing backward.

The **stomach** is an organ that extends from the esophagus to the small intestine. It is located in the upper left area of the abdominal cavity, and can expand to hold a half gallon of food. The stomach acts as a storage area and a churn to mix the food with gastric juices. Two components of gastric juices are hydrochloric acid and pepsin. These gastric juices are secreted by glands in the stomach lining. Then, the muscular movement of the walls called **peristalsis** mixes food with gastric juices and breaks it down to a mixture called **chyme**. After about three hours, chyme leaves the stomach in spurts and enters the small intestine.

The **small intestine** connects the stomach to the large intestine. It is approximately twenty feet long and one inch in diameter. The first section of the small intestine is called the **duodenum**. Here, other digestive juices enter and the breakdown process continues. In the walls of the small intestine are finger-like projections called **villi**. Here, the digested food is absorbed into the bloodstream.

The **large intestine** extends from the small intestine to the rectum. The large intestine is shorter, approximately five feet long, and 0.5 to 2.5 inches in diameter. The large intestine stores and excretes the waste products of digestion.

Accessory Organs. The accessory organs have specific functions, but each organ relies on the functions of the others in order to complete the digestive process.

- The **teeth** begin the digestive process by biting, tearing, and grinding the food.

- The **tongue** moves food from the anterior teeth to the posterior teeth and gathers the food before it is swallowed.

- The **salivary glands** produce saliva to dissolve food, facilitate the process of chewing (mastication), and coat food for ease in swallowing. The salivary glands excrete mucus to lubricate the food; amylase, an enzyme to begin the digestive process of starches; sodium bicarbonate to increase pH, which accelerates amylase function; and water to dilute and facilitate food mixing. Three salivary glands surround the mouth. This includes the parotid gland on the cheek, which empties into the mouth through Stenson's duct; the submandibular gland in the posterior area of the mouth between the mandible and the tongue, which empties into the mouth through Wharton's duct; and the sublingual gland on the floor of the mouth, which empties directly into the mouth. More information on the salivary glands is found in Chapter 7, Head and Neck Anatomy.

- The **liver**, the largest of the glandular organs, is on the right side of the body, just below the diaphragm. The liver has many functions that aid in the digestion process, but the main function is the production of **bile**. Bile contains salts that emulsify fats.

- The **gallbladder** is a muscular sac that stores bile from the liver. It is on the right side on the inferior surface of the liver.

■ The **pancreas** produces juices that are emptied into the duodenum to aid digestion and produce insulin.

Even before food is ingested, the sight, smell, and thought of food stimulates the saliva glands to produce saliva and stomach secretions begin to flow. Then the process of digestion begins as outlined in Table 6-7.

> **Importance to the Dental Assistant**
>
> The digestive system begins with the oral cavity, which is the focus in dentistry. Knowing the components of this system and how each contributes to the processing of food enables the dental assistant to detect disease and communicate with the patient.

Common Diseases and Conditions of the Digestive System

Many diseases and conditions of the digestive system directly relate to dentistry.

■ **Tooth decay** is destruction of the tooth surface.

■ **Periodontal disease** is inflammation and deterioration of the periodontal tissues.

■ **Bulimia** is a disease in which individuals "purge" or vomit after eating large quantities of food. With time, the hydrochloric acid from the stomach, left in the oral cavity after vomiting, can cause serious dental problems for bulimic patients. The acid eventually dissolves tooth structure.

■ **Hepatitis** is inflammation of the liver caused by several viruses. There are three main hepatitis viruses: hepatitis A, hepatitis B, and hepatitis C. Hepatitis B is contracted by exposure to body fluids of infected individuals, and is of the most concern because of its serious prognosis. For more information, see Chapter 10, Microbiology.

Respiratory System

Functions of the Respiratory System

Breathing is the main function of the respiratory system. Air is inhaled through the nose into the lungs, where it is absorbed into the bloodstream and carried to all body cells. Once the oxygen reaches the cells, it is exchanged for the waste product carbon dioxide. Carbon dioxide is then transported by the blood back to the lungs and exhaled.

Parts of the Respiratory System

The respiratory system consists of the nose, pharynx, larynx, trachea, bronchi, and lungs (Figure 6-15).

The **nose** is the passage for outside air to enter the body. The nose contains two **nasal cavities**, which are divided by the **nasal septum**. The inner surface of the nose is lined with **nasal mucosa**, which warms and humidifies the air as it passes through. The nose also contains the **olfactory receptors**, which facilitate the sense of smell.

The pharynx, or throat, serves as a passageway for two systems: respiratory and digestive. Air and food pass through the pharynx as they move downward. This tube is about five inches long and is divided into three sections. The first is the **nasopharynx**, the upper section behind the **nasal cavity**. The **eustachian** (you-**STAY**-shun) (auditory) **tubes** open into the pharynx. The **oropharynx** (o-ro-**FAIR**-inks), the middle section, is the portion behind the mouth. It is lined with the same mucosa as found in the oral cavity. The lower section, the **laryngopharynx** (lah-ring-goh-**FARE**-inks), divides and has an opening in the front to the larynx and in the back to the esophagus.

The **larynx**, or voice box, connects the pharynx and the trachea. The larynx is made up of cartilage and is supported by muscles. At the upper end of the larynx is the leaf-shaped epiglottis. Its function is to close off the larynx during swallowing to prevent food from entering. The thyroid cartilage, or Adam's apple, lies anterior to the larynx. In the interior of the larynx, the **vocal cords** stretch across the width of the larynx to produce sound.

The **trachea**, or windpipe, the next section for air passage, is four to five inches long and extends to the lungs. The trachea consists of C-shaped cartilage that allows for expansion of the esophagus during the process of swallowing. The trachea can become blocked by the inhalation of an object or from swelling.

The **bronchi** are the two branches that form at the end of the trachea and enter the lungs. The bronchi branches divide into smaller tubes called **bronchioles**. At the end of the bronchioles are **alveolar sacs**, which resemble clusters of grapes. These alveolar sacs consist of individual **alveoli**. Gaseous exchange takes place here in the alveoli. The thin walls of the alveoli make for easy passage of air entering and leaving the blood capillaries.

The **lungs** are two cone-shaped organs inside the rib cage. Each lung consists of a spongy mass that is pink at birth and then darkens to blue-gray or black, depending on air quality and personal habits. Each lung is surrounded by a sac called the **pleura**.

Respiration is the process of breathing and exchanging gases (oxygen and carbon dioxide) between the body and its environment. There are two phases to this process: inhalation and exhalation. During **inhalation**, muscles contract, the chest enlarges, and air flows into the lungs. **Exhalation** occurs when the muscles relax and the air is moved out of the lungs.

> **Importance to the Dental Assistant**
>
> The dental assistant should watch the patient for signs of discomfort or problems with breathing. The use of nitrous oxide may be contraindicated when a patient has

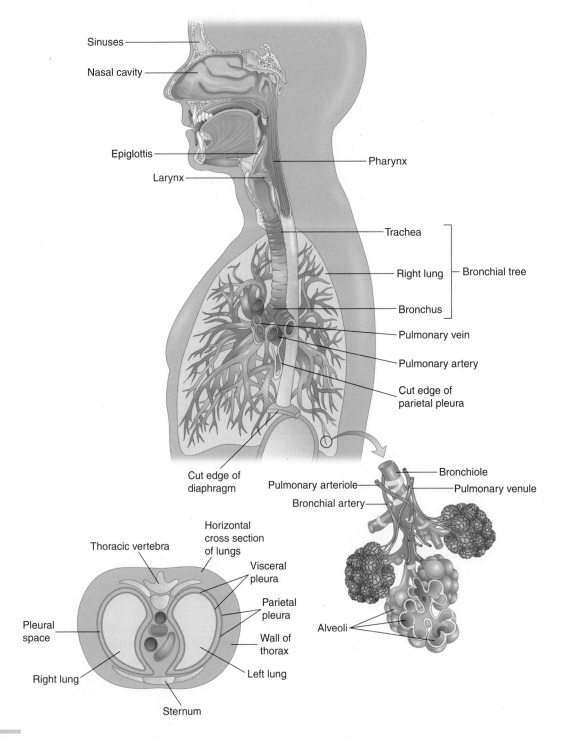

FIGURE 6-15 Structures of the respiratory system.

respiratory disease. Allergic reactions can and do occur in the dental office. A patient could choke on materials that fall to the back of the throat, and respiratory diseases or conditions can make treatment difficult. Understanding the respiratory system could save a patient's life.

Common Diseases of the Respiratory System

- **Asthma** is the muscular spasm of the walls of the bronchi. The air passages are constricted so the person cannot easily exhale.

- **Tuberculosis** is a highly contagious disease of the respiratory system. Tuberculosis is transmitted by breathing or swallowing droplets contaminated by the TB bacillus.

- **Lung cancer** is a malignancy of the lung tissue. It is a very common form of cancer and is often caused by cigarette smoking.

- Other conditions include the common cold, pneumonia, and bronchitis. Following standard precautions protects the office staff and the patient when treatment is required during times of infection.

Lymphatic System and Immune System

Functions of the Lymphatic System

The lymphatic system is a network of vessels that drains and filters the tissue fluid surrounding cells.

Parts of the Lymphatic System

The parts of the lymphatic system include the lymph, lymph vessels, lymph nodes, spleen, and thymus gland.

Lymph, also called **tissue fluid**, is a clear liquid formed in tissue spaces. The lymph enters the lymphatic capillary system and drains away excess fluid and carries proteins back to the bloodstream.

Lymph is transported through a specialized network of vessels called **lymphatic capillaries**. These capillaries are very thin-walled and only allow lymph to travel in one direction on the way back to the general circulation system.

Lymph nodes are found in groups along the lymphatic vessels. They are small, round masses that vary in size and location. The lymph nodes most commonly known are the ones in the armpit, neck, and groin. The purpose of the lymph nodes is to filter the lymph as it journeys back to the bloodstream and to manufacture antibodies and other active materials of the immunity process.

The **spleen**, located behind the stomach, is protected by the rib cage. It is the largest lymphoid organ in the body and contains a very rich blood supply. If the spleen is damaged, it may have to be removed to stop blood loss. As the blood moves through the spleen, it removes bacteria and other foreign materials, filters out old red blood cells, produces red blood cells before birth, and acts as a storage area for blood in case of hemorrhage. Humans can live without the spleen because other lymphoid tissues take over its functions. However, without the spleen, the person may be more susceptible to certain bacterial infections.

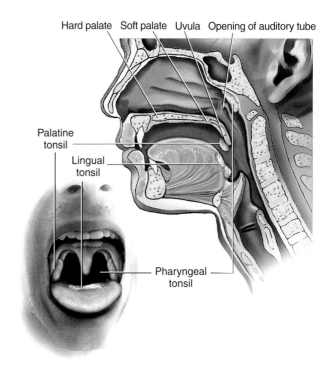

Hard palate Soft palate Uvula Opening of auditory tube

Palatine tonsil

Lingual tonsil

Pharyngeal tonsil

FIGURE 6-16 Tonsils.

The **thymus** is under the sternum, just below the thyroid. It is large and active from before birth through puberty, but then shrinks and almost disappears in adults. The thymus gland is important to immune system development.

Tonsils form a protective circle around the inside of the oral cavity. They consist of masses of lymphoid tissue that guard against bacteria that may enter the body through the digestive and respiratory systems. There are three groups of tonsils: the **palatine tonsils**, on each side of the throat; the **lingual tonsils**, on the base of the tongue; and the **pharyngeal tonsils** (adenoids), on the posterior wall of the nasopharynx area (Figure 6-16).

Functions of the Immune System

The immune system is part of the body's defense against harmful organisms. It protects the body from pathogens, foreign materials, debris, and damaged cells by removing these elements. The immune system is composed of specialized cells (phagocytes and lymphocytes) and molecules (antibodies and antigens). The system is organized into nonspecific and specific defenses. **Nonspecific immunity** is the body's defense against any harmful agents, while **specific immunity** acts against selected agents. The immune system involves organs or vessels from several other systems (Figure 6-17).

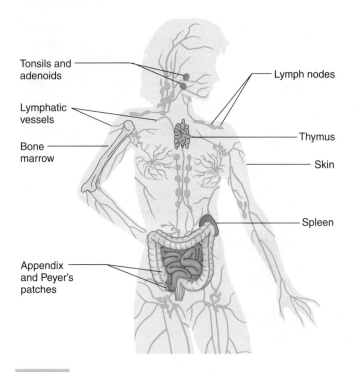

Tonsils and adenoids

Lymphatic vessels

Bone marrow

Appendix and Peyer's patches

Lymph nodes

Thymus

Skin

Spleen

FIGURE 6-17 Organs and vessels from other body systems involved in the immune system.

Importance to the Dental Assistant

The dental assistant is constantly exposed to disease and infection. A major responsibility of each dental team member is to maintain a safe environment. Continuing education on prevention of and protection from health risks is necessary for all dental professionals.

Common Diseases and Conditions of the Lymphatic and Immune Systems

- **Tonsillitis** is a chronic infection of the tonsil tissue.
- **Hodgkin's disease** is a malignant disorder that causes enlargement of the lymph nodes.
- **Allergies** are a hypersensitivity to certain substances. These are often common substances such as pollen, pet dander, or cigarette smoke, which are referred to as allergens. The reaction to allergens can cause an inflammatory response or a severe allergic reaction.
- **Immune deficiency disease** is a failure in some part of the immune system.

Bacterial and viral infections, fungi, parasites, cancer cells, and foreign tissue implants are all conditions that the immune system protects and fights against.

CHAPTER SUMMARY

Specific terms are used to establish a means for health professionals to communicate more effectively. The body is divided into systems, planes, cavities, and basic units that provide common references and terms for studying and communicating information about the body.

The dental assistant needs to be familiar with the terminology of body systems and how each system functions to provide the quality of care that each patient deserves. Both the anatomy and physiology of all body systems will need to be understood.

Case Study

Charlie T. Smith is a twenty-three-year-old patient with a history of diabetes. The patient is reclined in the dental chair. The dental assistant is placing a rubber dam clamp on a tooth when the clamp pops off and drops to the back of the patient's mouth. The patient swallows the clamp.

Case Study Review

1. List the body systems affected.

2. List the specific structures of the primary system that could become involved.

3. Would the patient's age or medical condition impact the situation? If so, how?

REVIEW QUESTIONS

Multiple Choice

1. Which of the following divides the body into left and right halves?
   a. Horizontal plane
   b. Transverse plane
   c. Sagittal plane
   d. Frontal plane

2. The skeletal muscles are comprised of what type of muscle tissue?
   a. Striated muscle
   b. Cardiac muscle
   c. Smooth muscle
   d. None of the above

3. The neurons that carry messages away from the spinal cord and brain are
   a. sensory neurons.
   b. motor neurons.
   c. associate neurons.
   d. interneurons.

4. All of the following are layers of the heart except the
   a. endocardium.
   b. myocardium.
   c. pericardium.
   d. intracardium.

5. The body system that drains and filters the fluid around cells is the
   a. respiratory.
   b. lymphatic.
   c. circulatory.
   d. immune.

6. The alimentary canal is part of what system?
   a. Circulatory
   b. Digestive
   c. Reproductive
   d. Skeletal

7. The _____ serves as a passage for the respiratory and digestive systems.
   a. larynx
   b. stomach
   c. pharynx
   d. small intestine

8. All of the following are true statements, *except:*
   a. Blood is a clear liquid formed in tissue spaces.
   b. Blood transports nutrients, gases, waste products and hormones.
   c. Blood is a thick fluid that varies in color from bright red to a darker, brownish red.
   d. Blood regulates body temperature.

9. The skeletal system is divided into two main divisions:
   a. the axial skeleton and articulations.
   b. the appendicular skeleton and articulations.
   c. the axial skeleton and the appendicular skeleton.
   d. the pulmonary system and the systemic system.

10. This system is part of the body's defense against harmful organisms.
    a. Digestive
    b. Immune
    c. Circulatory
    d. Nervous

Critical Thinking

1. Name the synovial joint that has significance to the dental assistant.

2. Explain why the pulmonary arteries are called arteries even though they carry deoxygenated blood, and the pulmonary veins are called veins even though they carry oxygenated blood.

3. Why it is harder to replace lost blood in elderly patients?

Web Activities

1. Go to: http://www.americanheart.org and look for the warning signs of a heart attack, stroke, and cardiac arrest.

2. Go to: http://www.lungusa.org and learn how to help your patients stop smoking.

3. Go to http://www.ada.org and search on topics related to the common disorders discussed in this chapter such as bulimia. What is the significance of these disorders to dental health?

PRACTICE

CHAPTER 7

HEAD AND NECK ANATOMY

SPECIFIC INSTRUCTIONAL OBJECTIVES

The student should strive to meet the following objectives and demonstrate an understanding of the facts and principles presented in this chapter:

1. List and identify the landmarks of the face and the oral cavity.

2. Identify the bones of the cranium and the face and identify the landmarks on the maxilla and the mandible.

3. Identify the parts of the temporomandibular joint (TMJ) and describe how the joint works.

4. List and identify the muscles of mastication, facial expression, the floor of the mouth, the tongue, the throat, the neck, and the shoulders. Explain their functions.

5. List and identify the nerves of the maxilla and the mandible.

6. Identify the arteries and veins of the head and the neck.

KEY TERMS

ala of the nose *(110)*

alveolar mucosa *(111)*

alveolar process *(115)*

angle of the mandible *(117)*

anterior alveolar nerve *(125)*

anterior superior alveolar artery *(128)*

anterior tonsillar pillars *(111)*

articular disc *(117)*

buccal nerve branch *(125)*

buccal mucosa *(111)*

buccinator *(119)*

circumvallate papilla *(111)*

common carotid *(125)*

condyle *(117)*

condyloid process *(117)*

coronoid process *(117)*

deep facial vein *(128)*

dental arteries *(127)*

digastric *(121)*

ducts of Bartholin *(113)*

ducts of Rivinus *(113)*

ethmoid bone *(114)*

ethmoid sinuses *(114)*

external auditory meatus *(114)*

external carotid artery *(125)*

external jugular vein *(129)*

external oblique ridge *(117)*

external pterygoid muscles *(119)*

extrinsic muscle *(119)*

facial nerve *(122)*

facial artery *(127)*

facial vein *(128)*

fauces *(111)*

filiform papilla *(111)*

fimbriated folds *(113)*

foliate papillae *(111)*

Fordyce's spots *(111)*

frena *(111)*

frontal bone *(114)*

fungiform papilla *(111)*

genial tubercles *(117)*

genioglossus *(119)*

geniohyoid *(121)*

gingiva *(111)*

glenoid fossa *(114)*

glossopharyngeal *(122)*

greater palatine artery *(128)*

(continues)

KEY TERMS (continued)

greater palatine
    foramen (116)

greater palatine
    nerve (122)

hyoglossus (119)

hyoid bone (121)

hypoglossal (122)

incisive arteries (127)

incisive nerve branch (125)

incisive papilla (111)

inferior alveolar artery (127)

inferior alveolar
    branch (125)

inferior nasal
    conchae (115)

infraorbital artery (128)

infraorbital foramen (116)

infraorbital nerve (122)

internal carotid artery (125)

internal jugular vein (129)

internal oblique ridge (117)

internal pterygoid
    muscles (119)

intrinsic muscles (119)

labial commissures (110)

labial mucosa (111)

labio-mental groove (110)

lacrimal bones (115)

lesser palatine
    foramen (116)

lesser palatine nerve (122)

linea alba (111)

lingual branch (125)

lingual foramen (117)

lingual frenum (112)

lingual vein (112)

mandibular artery (127)

mandible (116)

mandibular foramen (117)

mandibular notch (117)

mandibular nerve
    branch (125)

masseter muscles (119)

mastication (113)

mastoid process (114)

maxilla (115)

maxillary artery (127)

maxillary nerve branch (122)

maxillary sinus (116)

maxillary tuberosity (116)

maxillary vein (129)

median sulcus (111)

median suture (115)

mental artery (127)

mental foramen (117)

mental nerve branch (125)

mental protuberance (117)

mentalis (119)

middle superior alveolar
    artery (128)

middle superior alveolar
    nerve (125)

mucosa (111)

mylohyoid (121)

mylohyoid artery (127)

mylohyoid nerve
    branch (125)

mylohyoid ridge (117)

nasal bones (115)

naso-labial groove (110)

nasopalatine nerve (122)

occipital bone (114)

oral vestibule (111)

orbicularis oris (119)

palate (111)

palatine bones (116)

palatine raphe (111)

palatine rugae (111)

palatine suture (116)

palatine tonsils (111)

palatoglossal arches (111)

palatoglossus (121)

palatopharyngeal (122)

palatopharyngeal
    arches (111)

papilla (111)

parietal bone (114)

parotid duct (113)

parotid glands (113)

parotid papilla (111)

philtrum (110)

platysma (122)

posterior superior alveolar
    artery (128)

posterior superior alveolar
    nerve (122)

posterior tonsillar
    pillars (111)

pterygoid (114)

pterygoid artery (128)

pterygoid plexus of
    veins (129)

pterygopalatine nerve
    branch (122)

rami (117)

retromandibular
    vein (128)

retromolar area (117)

saliva (113)

sphenoid bone (114)

sphenoid sinuses (114)

Stensen's duct (111)

sternocleidomastoid (122)

styloglossus (119)

stylohyoid (121)

styloid process (114)

sublingual caruncles (113)

sublingual folds (113)

sublingual glands (113)

sublingual sulcus (113)

submandibular
    glands (113)

symphysis (117)

synovial fluid (117)

taste buds (113)

temporal bone (114)

temporal muscles (119)

temporomandibular joint
    (TMJ) (117)

tongue (111)

torus (111)

torus mandibularis (113)

trapezius (122)

trigeminal (122)

tubercle of the lip (110)

uvula (111)

vermilion border (110)

vermilion zone (110)

vestibule fornix (111)

vomer bone (115)

Wharton's duct (113)

xerostomia (113)

zygomatic nerve (122)

zygomatic bones (115)

zygomatic major (119)

INTRODUCTION

This chapter provides information on the anatomy of the head and neck. The dental assistant must be able to describe this anatomy, including the locations of structures and their functions. Identifying the anatomy of the head, face, and neck in normal, healthy tissues enables the dental assistant to recognize the abnormal.

Landmarks of the Face and Oral Cavity

Landmarks of the anatomy are usually skeletal or soft tissue structures that are easily recognizable. They are used as reference points in describing the locations of anatomical structures or for taking measurements. It is important for the dental assistant to be familiar with the landmarks that make up the face and oral cavity.

Landmarks of the Face

The face has the following landmarks: ala of the nose, naso-labial groove, philtrum, vermilion border, vermilion zone, the tubercle of the lip, labial commissures, and the labio-mental grooves (Figure 7-1).

The **ala of the nose** is the wing of the nose or outer edge of the nostril. From the ala of the nose to the corners of the mouth is a groove called the **naso-labial groove**, or sulcus. Between the bottom of the nose and the middle of the upper lip is a shallow, V-shaped depression known as the **philtrum**. All these landmarks are covered with skin consistent with the skin in other parts of the face. These are areas to look at for scarring from accidents, surgeries, or physical conditions, such as cleft lip.

The lips are covered externally with skin and internally with mucous membrane. The reddish portion of the lips is called the **vermilion zone**. The vermilion zone is highly vascular and covered with a thin layer of epithelium. The **vermilion border** is where the skin meets the vermilion zone and forms a line around the lips. In the middle of the upper lip is a small projection that sometimes enlarges or thickens. It is called the **tubercle of the lip**. The corners of the mouth, where the upper lip meets the lower lip, are known as **labial commissures**. The commissures should be observed for cracks, color changes, and variations in form. Just below the lower lip is the **labio-mental groove**, which runs horizontally and separates the lip from the chin.

Importance to the Dental Assistant

The dental assistant may notice scars or sores around the nose, mouth, and chin areas. By knowing the normal landmarks of the face the dental assistant can use correct terminology to describe any deviation and record information on the health history. Sometimes facial scars can indicate the person has been in an accident and may have had many x-rays taken and possible surgery. He or she may have had seizures or have had a cleft palate or lip. Knowing this information may assist in the details of the health history and treatment plan.

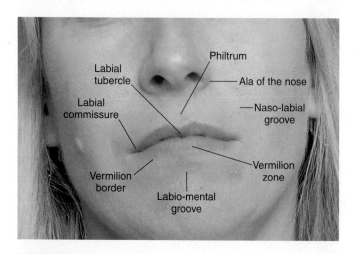

FIGURE 7-1 Landmarks of the face.

Landmarks of the Oral Cavity

Understanding the landmarks of the oral cavity aids the dental assistant when taking radiographs, placing topical anesthetic, recognizing healthy tissue, and recording information or medical history on a patient's chart.

The landmarks of the oral cavity include the following: vestibule, vestibule fornix, labial mucosa, buccal mucosa, parotid papilla, Stensen's duct, linea alba, Fordyce's spots, alveolar mucosa, gingiva, labial frenum, and buccal frenum (Figure 7-2).

(A)

(B)

FIGURE 7-2 Structures of oral cavity.

Inside the mouth, a pocket is formed by the soft tissue of the cheeks and the gingiva. This is the oral vestibule (mucobuccal fold). The deepest point of the vestibule is called the **vestibule fornix**. The fornix forms a U-shaped pocket that is continuous throughout the anterior and posterior areas. The tissue that lines the inner surface of the lips and cheeks is called **mucosa**. The mucosa is named according to location. The inner surface of the lips is called the **labial mucosa**, and the inner surface of the cheeks is the **buccal mucosa**. On the labial mucosa are small, yellowish glands near the commissures called **Fordyce's spots**, which become larger and more visible with age. On the buccal mucosa, opposite the maxillary second molar, is a flap of tissue called the **parotid papilla**, which is where the opening of the **Stensen's duct** is located. On the buccal mucosa is a raised white line that runs parallel to where the teeth meet, called the **linea alba** (Figure 7-3). Mucosa also covers the alveolar bone that supports the teeth. It is called the **alveolar mucosa**. The alveolar mucosa is loosely attached and is highly vascular, giving the mucosa a reddish color. Moving from the alveolar mucosa toward the teeth is the **gingiva**. The gingiva is firmly attached and usually pale pink or brownish pink, depending on pigmentation. This dense, fibrous tissue covered with mucous membrane can withstand pressure during chewing. The portion of the gingiva that meets the tooth is called the free gingiva or marginal gingiva.

When the lips are pulled out, frena become visible. Frena (plural form of **frenum**) are raised lines of mucosal tissue that extend from the alveolar mucosa through the vestibule to the labial and buccal mucosa. On the labial, the main frena are between the maxillary central incisors and the mandibular central incisors, with minor frena along the vestibule of both arches in the labial and buccal areas.

Palate Area of the Oral Cavity

On the inside of the maxillary teeth is the **palate**, or "roof of the mouth." The palate is divided into hard and soft sections. The hard palate, the anterior portion, is a bony plate covered with pink to brownish pink keratinized tissue. The soft palate, the posterior portion, covers muscle tissue and is darker pink or yellowish. On the hard palate is the **incisive papilla**, which is a raised area of tissue lying behind the maxillary central incisors (Figure 7-4). Extending from the back of the incisive papilla is a slightly raised line that extends down the middle of the hard palate, known as the **palatine raphe**. The ridges that run horizontally across the hard palate behind the incisive papilla are the **palatine rugae**. Occasionally, in the middle of the palate a lump or prominence of bone (exostosis) may be found. This excess bone is called a **torus** (plural is tori), or a torus palatinus, specifically.

The following landmarks are on the soft palate and in the oropharynx areas: the uvula, anterior tonsillar pillars, posterior tonsillar pillars, palatine tonsils, and

FIGURE 7-3 The oral vestibule with the linea alba on the buccal mucosa.

the fauces (Figure 7-4). The **uvula** is a projection that extends off the back of the soft palate. Extending horizontally from the uvula to the base of the tongue are folds of tissue called **anterior tonsillar pillars** or **palatoglossal arches**. Another set of arches is found farther back in the throat. This set is the **posterior tonsillar pillars** or **palatopharyngeal arches**. Between the two sets of pillars is a depressed area where the palatine tonsils are situated. The **palatine tonsils** are often marked with deep grooves and are red and inflamed due to infection. The space in the back of the oral cavity where food passes into the pharynx is the **fauces**.

Tongue

The **tongue** is a significant region of the oval cavity with the following landmarks: sulcus terminalis, circumvallate papilla, filiform papillae, fungiform papillae, foliate papilla, and median sulcus on the dorsal or top surface of the tongue. On the ventral or underside of the tongue are the lingual frenum, the lingual veins, and the fimbriated folds. When the tongue is extended, a shallow, V-shaped groove is apparent on the posterior portion. This is the sulcus terminalis. This groove separates the anterior two-thirds, or body of the tongue, from the base of the tongue. Anterior to the sulcus, covering the dorsal side of the tongue (Figure 7-5A), are small, raised projections called **papilla**, where taste buds are located. The largest papilla, mushroom shaped, are anterior to the sulcus terminalis in a row of eight to ten and are called **circumvallate papillae**. Anterior to the circumvallate papillae and covering the dorsal side of the tongue are hair-like projections called **filiform papillae**. Papillae that give the tongue the "strawberry effect" are the **fungiform papillae**. On the lateral border of the tongue near the base are the **foliate papillae**, which are slightly raised, vertical folds of tissue. The tongue is divided in half by the **median sulcus**, which runs from the base to the tip of the tongue. The median sulcus is a groove that varies in depth from person to person.

Posterior tonsilar pillar

Anterior tonsilar pillar

Uvula

Palatine tonsils

Fauces

(A)

Incisive papilla

Palatine rugae

Palatine raphe

(B)

FIGURE 7-4 Landmarks of the palate and oral pharynx area.

Foliate papilla

Filiform papilla

Median sulcus

Circumvate papilla

Foramen cecum

Fungiform papilla

(A)

Fimbrinted fold

Lingual vein

Sublingual folds

Sublingual caruncles

Lingual frenum

(B)

FIGURE 7-5 (A) Dorsal surface of the tongue. (B) Ventral surface of the tongue.

In the middle of the ventral side of the tongue, a line of tissue extends from the tongue to the floor of the mouth, called the **lingual frenum** (Figure 7-5B). On either side of the lingual frenum are the **lingual veins**. They are bluish and run the length of the tongue.

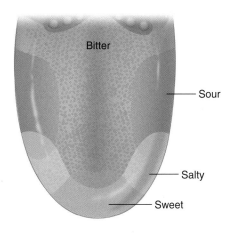

Bitter

Sour

Salty

Sweet

FIGURE 7-6 The location of the basic taste buds of the tongue.

Lateral to the lingual veins are folds of tissue called **fimbriated folds**. Sometimes, under the tongue on the alveolar bone are excess bone formations called **torus mandibularis**.

Sensation of Taste. The **taste buds**, also known as taste receptors, are oval structures that are located on the dorsal surface of the tongue. When stimulated with different chemicals these receptors carry taste impulses to the brain. To stimulate the sense of taste substances (food) must be mixed with liquid to form a solution. The solution stimulates these receptors to generate one or a combination of the four fundamental taste sensations. The four fundamental taste senses include: sweet, salty, sour, and bitter. These basic taste buds are located on different but overlapping areas of the tongue (Figure 7-6). Sweet tastes are located on the tip of the tongue, salty tastes are on the anterior sides of the tongue, sour tastes are on the posterior sides of the tongue, and the bitter tastes are located in the center posterior section of the tongue.

Importance to the Dental Assistant

The dental assistant should be aware that certain drugs cause patients to lose their sense of taste. Taste bud cells are continually being renewed because they have an average life span of only 10 to 10½ days. If a patient is receiving certain toxic agents, such as a cytotoxic agent used to treat cancer, the taste buds may be destroyed and the patient's sense of taste will take a minimum of 10 days, usually longer, to return.

Floor of the Mouth

The floor of the mouth includes the sublingual caruncles, sublingual folds, and sublingual sulcus (Figure 7-5B). Where the lingual frenum attaches to the floor of the mouth are two small, raised folds of tissue, one

on either side of the frenum. These are **sublingual caruncles**. On top of these folds of tissue lie the ducts of two salivary glands. The **sublingual folds** begin at the caruncles on either side of the frenum and run backward to the base of the tongue. Lateral to the sublingual fold is a horseshoe-shaped groove that follows the curve of the dental arch, called the **sublingual sulcus**. This sulcus marks the end of the alveolar ridge and the beginning of the floor of the mouth.

Salivary Glands

Three major pairs of salivary glands supply the oral cavity: parotid, submandibular, and sublingual (Figure 7-7). These glands secrete saliva to assist in the process of digestion. The largest of the salivary glands are the **parotid glands**, which lie just below and in front of the ear. The parotid glands empty into the mouth through the **parotid duct** (also known as Stensen's duct). The duct empties into the mouth through the parotid papilla, which is just opposite the maxillary second molar. The **submandibular glands** are about the size of a walnut and lie on the inside of the mandible in the posterior area. They empty saliva into the mouth through the **Wharton's duct**, which ends in the sublingual caruncles. The third set of glands and smallest are the **sublingual glands**, located on the floor of the mouth. These glands either empty directly into the mouth through the **ducts of Rivinus** or through the sublingual caruncles by means of the **ducts of Bartholin**. The ducts of the sublingual glands are similar in function to a "soaker hose."

There are also smaller minor salivary glands that are in the buccal, labial and lingual mucosa, the floor of the mouth, the posterior portion of the dorsal surface of the tongue, the soft palate, and the lateral (side) portions of the hard palate. The saliva from these glands is a mucous saliva.

Saliva. **Saliva** is a clear fluid secreted by the salivary and mucous glands throughout the mouth. This fluid varies in viscosity depending on an individual's chemical makeup, diet, and medications. Saliva contains water, mucin, organic salts, and the digestive enzyme ptyalin. It is normally odorless, tasteless, and slightly alkaline. Approximately 1,500 ml of saliva is produced daily.

The function of the saliva is to moisten and lubricate the oral cavity and to moisten food, aiding in the **mastication** (chewing) and swallowing of food. Saliva also initiates the digestion of starches and helps regulate water balance. Excess dryness of the mouth is called **xerostomia** (refer to Chapter 4). Dry mouth is caused by an abnormal reduction in the amount of saliva secretion. It can be related to certain diseases, such as diabetes, or result from radiation or chemotherapy. There are a number of products on the market to assist the patient with dry mouth symptoms.

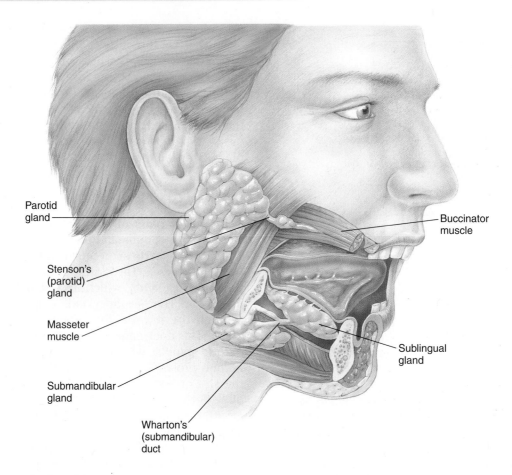

FIGURE 7-7 Salivary glands and ducts.

Salivary Gland Diseases and Problems

The mumps are a viral infection affecting the parotid glands. Characterized by swelling and tenderness, mumps often affect children between ages five and fifteen. Sometimes, the salivary glands develop crystallizations or stones. When these stones try to leave the glands, they block the ducts. Swelling immediately occurs and the stones must be surgically removed.

Bones of the Head

The skull is divided into two sections: the cranium and the face. The cranium covers and protects the brain and is composed of eight bones. The face consists of fourteen bones, including the maxilla and the mandible.

Bones of the Cranium

The **frontal bone** forms the forehead, the main portion of the roof of the eye socket (orbit), and part of the nasal cavity. On the skull just behind the frontal bone are the two parietal bones, right and left halves joining at the midline. The **parietal bones** form most of the roof of the skull and the upper half of the sides. Below each parietal bone, forming the lower sides and the base of the skull, are the **temporal bones**. Each temporal bone contains the following landmarks: external auditory meatus, mastoid process, glenoid fossa, and styloid process. The **external auditory meatus** is the opening for the ear. The **mastoid process** is the bony projection found on the bottom border of the temporal bone. A pit or depression found anterior to the mastoid process is the **glenoid fossa**, the location where the mandible articulates with the skull. The **styloid process** is a sharp projection on the under-surface of the temporal bone between the glenoid fossa and the mastoid process. The **occipital bone** forms the back and base of the skull. The occipital bone contains a large opening, the foramen magnum, through which the spinal cord passes. The **sphenoid bone** is a wedge-shaped bone that goes across the skull anterior to the temporal bones. It is a single continuous bone, shaped like a bat with its wings spread. The wings of the sphenoid bone are called the **pterygoid** process. The sphenoid bone forms the anterior base of the skull behind the orbit and contains the **sphenoid sinuses**. The **ethmoid bone** forms part of the nose, orbits, and floor of the cranium. This bone is thin and spongy or honeycombed in appearance. It contains the **ethmoid sinuses** (Figure 7-8 and Table 7-1).

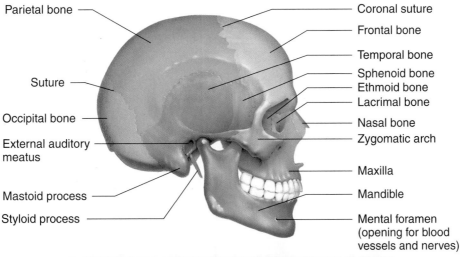

Parietal bone

Suture

Occipital bone

External auditory meatus

Mastoid process

Styloid process

Coronal suture

Frontal bone

Temporal bone

Sphenoid bone

Ethmoid bone

Lacrimal bone

Nasal bone

Zygomatic arch

Maxilla

Mandible

Mental foramen (opening for blood vessels and nerves)

FIGURE 7-8 Lateral aspect of the cranium. *(Photography by Dr. David Fankhauser, University of Cincinnati).*

Bones of the Face

The **nasal bones** form the bridge of the nose. The **vomer bone** is a single bone on the inside of the nasal cavity. It forms the posterior and the bottom of the nasal septum (the nasal septum is a cartilage structure that divides the nasal cavities). On the outside of the nasal cavities are scroll-like bones called **inferior nasal conchae**. Each concha consists of thin, cancellous bone. The **lacrimal bones** are small and very delicate. They are anterior to

the ethmoid bone, comprising part of the orbit (the corner of the eye). The tear ducts pass through the lacrimal bones. The **zygomatic bones** form the cheeks (Figures 7-8 and 7-9 and Table 7-2).

Maxilla. The **maxilla** is the largest of the facial bones and is composed of two sections of bone joined at the **median suture**. The maxilla extends from the floor of each orbit and the floor and exterior walls of the nasal cavity to

TABLE 7-1 Bones of the Cranium

Name of Cranial Bone	Number
Frontal	One (1)
Parietal	Paired (2)
Temporal	Paired (2)
Occipital	One (1)
Sphenoid	One (1)
Ethmoid	One (1)

TABLE 7-2 Bones of the Face

Name of Facial Bone	Number
Nasal	Two (2)
Vomer	One (1)
Inferior nasal conchae	Two (2)
Lacrimal	Two (2)
Maxillae	Two (2)
Zygomatic	Two (2)
Palatine	Two (2)
Mandible	One (1)

form the roof of the mouth. The maxilla is formed by four processes (outgrowths of bone). The frontal and zygomatic processes meet the frontal and zygomatic bones. The **alveolar process** forms the bone that supports the maxillary and mandibular teeth, and the palatine process is the main portion of the hard palate.

The **infraorbital foramen** (foramen means an opening) is just below the orbit on the maxillary bone and the **maxillary sinus** forms a large cavity above the roots of the maxillary molars. Just beyond the last posterior maxillary tooth is a rounded area known as the **maxillary tuberosity**.

Palatine Bones. The **palatine bones** are joined at the midline, often referred to as the median **palatine suture**

(Figure 7-10). Just behind the maxillary central incisors is the incisive (nasopalatine) foramen, which is an opening for the nasopalatine nerve. In the posterior region of the hard palate are three other openings on each side. The first of these three, the largest, is the **greater palatine foramen**. Behind the greater foramen are two smaller or **lesser palatine foramen**.

Mandible. The **mandible** is the only movable bone of the face (Figure 7-11A). The mandible consists of a horseshoe-shaped body that is horizontal, with two vertical exten-

FIGURE 7-9 Bones of the face. *(Photograph by Dr. David Fankhauser, University of Cincinnati).*

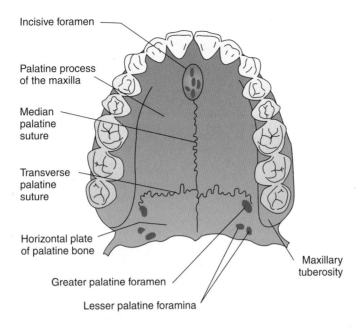

Incisive foramen

Palatine process
of the maxilla

Median
palatine
suture

Transverse
palatine
suture

Horizontal plate
of palatine bone

Greater palatine foramen

Lesser palatine foramina

Maxillary
tuberosity

FIGURE 7-10 Landmarks of the palate.

sions called **rami** (plural form of ramus). At the top of the rami are two projections. The posterior projection is the **condyle** or **condyloid process**, and the anterior projection is the **coronoid process**. The condyle articulates with the temporal bone to form the **temporomandibular joint (TMJ)**. Between the two processes is a depression known as the **mandibular notch** (also referred to as the sigmoid or coronoid notch). From the top of the rami moving downward is the body of each ramus. On the inside of the body of the ramus is the **mandibular foramen**, which is the beginning of the **internal oblique ridge** (Figure 7-11B). The internal oblique ridge, also known as the **mylohyoid ridge**, follows the inside of the ramus and the body of the mandible. Where the ramus meets the body of the mandible on the outside border is the **angle of the mandible**. On the body of the mandible near the apex of the premolars is the **mental foramen**. Extending from the mental foramen, the **external oblique ridge** follows the length of the body of the mandible past the last tooth and up to the ramus. Behind the last molar is a triangular area known as the **retromolar area**. In the center of the mandible on the external surface is a concave area where two bones of the mandible are fused. This area is known as the **symphysis**. The tip of the chin is called the **mental protuberance**. On the internal surface at the center of the mandible is the **lingual foramen**, which is surrounded by small, bony projections called **genial tubercles**. The mandibular teeth are supported in the alveolar process.

Importance of the Bones of Head and Face

Dental assistants should learn the bones of the head and the face thoroughly. This knowledge will assist them throughout their program but also in their career working in the dental profession. Two examples as to when they might use this information include understanding the landmarks seen on dental radiographs and identifying anatomy while assisting during surgical procedures.

Temporomandibular Joint

Once the bones of the cranium and the face have been identified, it is easy to locate the temporomandibular joint (TMJ). The joint is named for the two bones that form the union: the temporal and the mandible bones. The TMJ is composed of three parts:

1. Glenoid fossa of the temporal bone

2. Articular eminence of the temporal bone

3. Condyloid process of the mandible

These bones are covered with thick cartilage and are surrounded by several ligaments. There are no blood vessels or nerves in this connective tissue, but **synovial fluid** bathes these bone structures, providing nourishment and lubrication that enable the bones to glide over each other without friction. (Synovial means a thick, sticky fluid found in the joints of bones.)

The TMJ is formed by the condyle of the mandible articulating with the glenoid fossa and the articular eminence of the temporal bone (Figure 7-12). The condyle rests closer to the glenoid fossa, and then moves forward to the articular eminence when the mouth opens.

Between the condyle and temporal bone is the **articular disc** (meniscus). This disc is a dense, fibrous connective tissue that is thicker at the ends. The articular disc is attached to the condyle, so when the condyle glides forward and backward, the disc moves with it.

Condyle

Mandibular (sigmoid) notch

Ramus

Mandibular angle

External oblique ridge

Border of the mandible

Mental foramen

Mental protuberance

Coronoid process

Mandibular foramen

Retromolar area

Internal oblique ridge (Mylohyoid line)

Submandibular fossa

(A)

Coronoid process

Internal oblique ridge

Mandibular foramen

Sublingual fossa

Condyle

Mylohyoid groove

Submandibular fossa

Lingual foramen

Genial tubercles

Lingual view

(B)

FIGURE 7-11 (A) Lateral view of the external surface of the mandible. (B) Internal (lingual) view of the mandible. (C) Frontal view of the external surface of the mandible. *(Photography by Dr. David Fankhauser, University of Cincinnati).*

Surrounding the articular disc is a dense, fibrous *capsule* that encloses the entire joint. The capsule is divided into upper and lower cavities by the disc; these cavities are filled with synovial fluid.

The TMJ is supported by ligaments, and the muscles of mastication control the movements. The left and right TMJs function in unison and move in two ways: hinge (swinging) motion and gliding movement.

The *hinge motion* occurs in the lower joint cavity when the mouth opens. The condyles and the discs begin this hinge motion by rotating anteriorly. As this motion continues and the mouth opens wider, there is

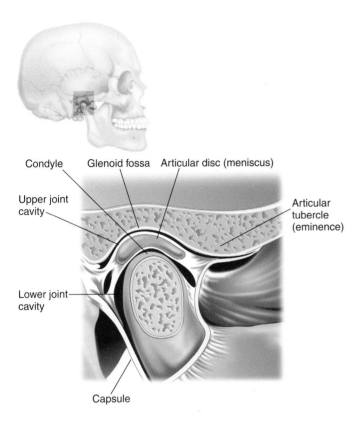

FIGURE 7-12 Temporomandibular joint (TMJ).

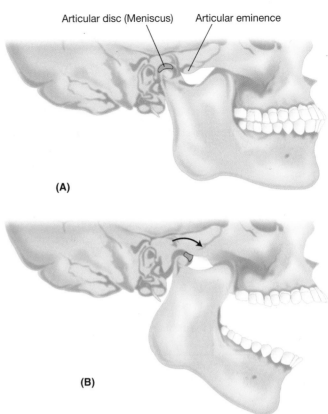

FIGURE 7-13 Movement of the TMJ. (A) Hinge joint. (B) Gliding joint movement.

an anterior *gliding movement* as well. This gliding movement involves both the upper and lower cavities. The gliding continues along the articular disc during protrusion and lateral movements of the mandible during mastication (Figure 7-13).

Some problems with the TMJ occur when the disc becomes stuck or displaced. Popping and clicking sounds may result if the disc does not stay interposed between the condyle and the temporal bone. More severe problems may occur as the condition advances. For more information on TMJ disease (dysfunction), refer to Chapter 25, Oral and Maxillofacial Surgery.

Muscles of the Head and Neck

Muscles expand and contract to make movement possible. Each muscle has an origin (fixed point) and insertion (movable point). Muscles of the head and neck include muscles of mastication, muscles of facial expression, muscles of the floor of the mouth, muscles of the tongue, muscles of the soft palate, the pharynx, and muscles of the neck.

Muscles of Mastication

There are four pairs of muscles of mastication: **temporal muscles, masseter muscles, internal pterygoid muscles,** and **external pterygoid muscles.** These muscles

provide movement for the mandible as they protrude, retract, elevate, and provide lateral movements (Figure 7-14). Nerves to the muscles of mastication originate from the mandibular division of the trigeminal labor. The origins, insertions, and functions (distributions of nerves) of the muscles of mastication are listed in Table 7-3.

Muscles of Facial Expression

The major muscles of facial expression include the **orbicularis oris, buccinator, mentalis,** and **zygomatic major**. These muscles allow for a wide variety of facial expressions, including smiling and whistling. The muscles of the face are innervated by the facial nerve, which is the seventh cranial nerve (Figure 7-15). The muscles of facial expression are described in Table 7-4.

Muscles of the Tongue

The muscles of the tongue are divided into intrinsic and extrinsic groups. The **intrinsic muscles** are all within the tongue and are responsible for shaping the tongue during speech, mastication, and swallowing. There are four **extrinsic muscles** to assist in the movement and functioning of the tongue: **genioglossus, hyoglossus, styloglossus,**

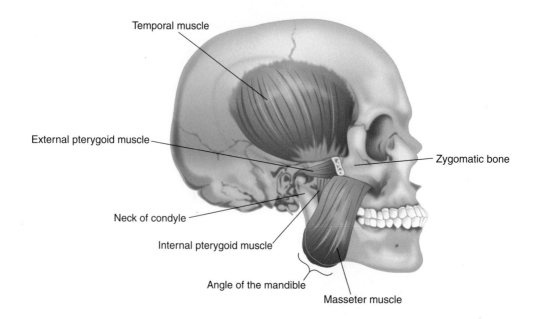

FIGURE 7-14 Muscles of mastication. Lateral view of the internal pterygoid muscle and the external pterygoid muscle. The temporal muscle and the masseter muscle.

TABLE 7-3   Muscles of Mastication

Muscle	Origin	Insertion	Function
Temporal	Fan shaped across the temporal fossa of the temporal bone.	Inserts into the coronoid process of the mandible and down the anterior border of the ramus.	Elevates the mandible—closing the jaw. Contraction of the posterior fibers retracts the mandible.
Masseter	Two portions: superficial portion (strong, tendinous fibers from the zygomatic process of the maxilla and from the anterior two-thirds of the lower border of the zygomatic arch) and deep portion (muscular and smaller from the medial aspect and inferior border of the posterior one-third of the zygomatic arch).	The superficial portion inserts into the angle and lower border of the mandible; the deep portion is inserted into the upper section of the ramus and the lateral surface of the coronoid process.	Strong elevator of the jaw. This muscle is easily seen when the teeth are clenched.
Medial (internal) pterygoids	Medial surface of the lateral pterygoid plate of the sphenoid bone, the lateral portion of the palatine bone, and the maxillary tuberosity.	The medial pterygoids insert into the interior surface of the angle of the mandible (opposite the insertion of the masseter muscle).	Elevates the mandible.
Lateral (external) pterygoids	Superior portion from the lateral surface of the greater wing of the sphenoid bone; inferior portion from the lateral surface of the lateral pterygoid plate.	Superior portion inserts into the articular capsule of the temporal mandibular joint; inferior portion inserts into the neck of the condyle of the mandible.	Opens jaw by depressing the mandible. If both lateral pterygoid muscles contract, the jaw protrudes; if only one contracts, the mandible shifts laterally.

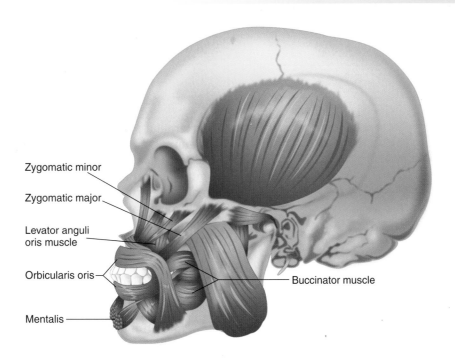

Zygomatic minor

Zygomatic major

Levator anguli
oris muscle

Orbicularis oris

Mentalis

Buccinator muscle

FIGURE 7-15 Muscles of facial expression.

TABLE 7-4 Muscles of Facial Expression

Muscle	Origin	Insertion	Function
Orbicularis oris	Complex origin—There is no skeletal attachment. The origin is from muscle fibers that surround the mouth.	Insertion is into itself and the surrounding skin.	Closing the lips or protruding them.
Buccinator	Alveolar processes of the maxilla and the mandible and the pterygomandibular raphe.	Inserts into the corners of the mouth, becoming part of the muscles that surround the mouth.	Compresses the cheeks against the teeth to assist during mastication. Assists in blowing air out of the mouth.
Mentalis	Incisive fossa of the mandible.	Inserts into the skin of the chin.	Wrinkles the skin of the chin and protrudes the lower lip.
Zygomatic major	Zygomatic bone.	Insertion into the corners of the mouth.	Lifts the corners of the mouth upward and backward, as in smiling.

and **palatoglossus** (Figure 7-16). (The palatoglossus is discussed with the palate.) All the muscles of the tongue are innervated by the hypoglossal nerve except the palatoglossus muscle. See Table 7-5 for the origin, insertion, and function of each extrinsic muscle of the tongue.

Hyoid Bone. There is also a horseshoe-shaped bone lying at the base of the tongue called the **hyoid bone**.

Muscles of the tongue and the floor of the mouth attach to this bone for support (Figure 7-17).

Muscles of the Floor of the Mouth

The muscles that form the floor of the mouth are the **digastric, mylohyoid, stylohyoid,** and **geniohyoid.** These four muscles are located between the mandible

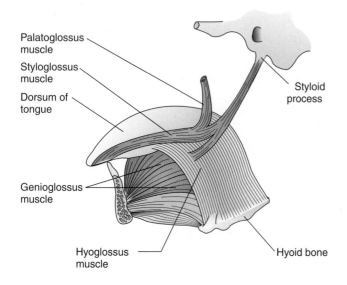

Palatoglossus muscle
Styloglossus muscle
Dorsum of tongue
Genioglossus muscle
Hyoglossus muscle
Styloid process
Hyoid bone

FIGURE 7-16 Extrinsic muscles of the tongue.

and the hyoid bone. Unlike some other muscle groups, the muscles of the floor of the mouth are innervated by distinct nerve branches (Table 7-6 and Figure 7-17).

Muscles of the Soft Palate

There are two muscles of the soft palate, called the **palatoglossus** and **palatopharyngeal** (Table 7-7). These muscles raise the soft palate during the swallowing process (deglutition) and are both innervated by the pharyngeal plexus (Figure 7-18).

Muscles of the Neck

The three muscles of the neck are the **platysma, trapezius**, and **sternocleidomastoid** (Figure 7-19). Knowing the muscles of the neck helps the dental assistant per-

form chairside functions in positions that are not tiring and will not cause injury (Table 7-8).

Nerves of the Head and Neck

Four cranial nerves innervate the face and oral cavity: **trigeminal, facial, glossopharyngeal**, and **hypoglossal**. The largest cranial nerve and the most important to dental auxiliaries is the trigeminal nerve, because this cranial nerve innervates the maxilla and the mandible. The trigeminal nerve divides at the semi-lunar (gasserian) ganglion into three branches: the ophthalmic nerve, maxillary nerve, and mandibular nerve.

Maxillary Branch of the Trigeminal Nerve

The **maxillary nerve branch** is a sensory nerve that innervates the nose, cheeks, palate, gingiva, maxillary teeth, maxillary sinus, tonsils, nasopharynx, and other facial structures. The maxillary nerve branch is divided into four branches: **zygomatic, infraorbital, posterior superior alveolar**, and **pterygopalatine** (Figure 7-20A).

Pterygopalatine Nerve Branch. After the maxillary nerve leaves the semi-lunar ganglion, one branch becomes the pterygopalatine nerve branch. This branch divides into the **greater palatine nerve**, the **lesser palatine nerve**, and the **nasopalatine nerve** (Figure 7-20B). The greater palatine nerve extends downward from the pterygopalatine nerve and reaches the palate through the greater palatine foramen. This nerve serves the soft palate, hard palate, medial gingiva, and mucous membrane as far forward as the anterior teeth. The lesser palatine nerve is a smaller branch that innervates the soft palate, uvula, and tonsils. The nasopalatine nerve extends anteriorly from the pterygopalatine nerve and exits through the incisive foramen. This nerve innervates the anterior hard palate, gingiva, mucous membrane, and the anterior teeth from the cuspids forward.

TABLE 7-5 Extrinsic Muscles of the Tongue

Muscle	Origin	Insertion	Function
Genioglossus	Genial tubercle in the center of the lingual of the mandible.	Fans out to insert in the inferior surface of the tongue and to the hyoid bone.	Most of the work of the tongue. Protrudes the tongue and retracts or depresses the tongue.
Hyoglossus	Hyoid bone.	Runs vertically to insert in the inferior sides of the tongue.	Mainly depresses the tongue.
Styloglossus	Anterior surface of the styloid process of the temporal bone.	Part of the styloglossus inserts into the sides of the tongue while the rest of the muscle continues forward to the tip of the tongue.	Retracts the tongue and raises the tip of the tongue.

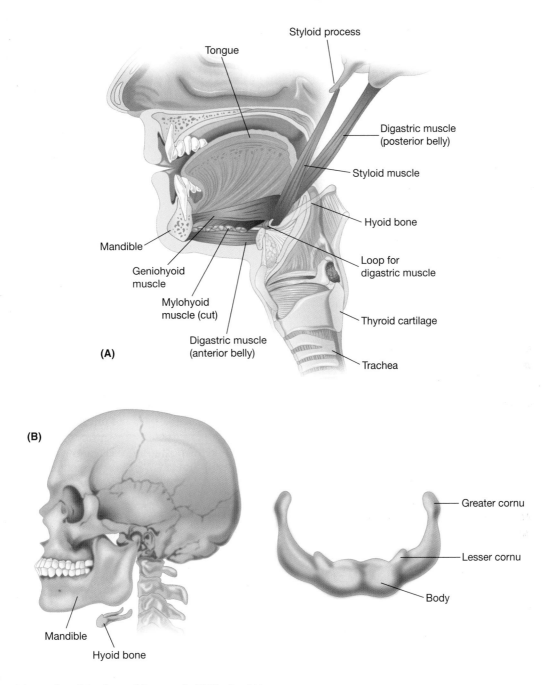

FIGURE 7-17 (A) Muscles of the floor of the mouth. (B) The hyoid bone.

TABLE 7-6   Muscles of the Floor of the Mouth

Muscle	Origin	Insertion	Function
Digastric	There are two portions, called bellies. Posterior belly originates from the mastoid process of the temporal bone; anterior belly begins on the lingual surface of the mandible at the midline.	Both the posterior belly and the anterior belly insert into the intermediate tendon on the hyoid bone.	Together the digastric muscles lift the hyoid bone and assist in opening the mouth; separately, the posterior belly draws the hyoid bone posteriorly and the anterior belly pulls the hyoid bone anteriorly.
Mylohyoid	This muscle is composed of left and right halves that join at the midline of the mandible. From the midline, each half attaches in a fan shape to the last molar area, thus following the mylohyoid line.	Inserts into the body of the hyoid bone.	Forms the floor of the mouth and assists in depressing the mandible and elevating the tongue.
Stylohyoid	The styloid process of the temporal bone.	Inserts into the body of the hyoid bone.	Draws the hyoid bone superiorly and posteriorly and stabilizes it.
Geniohyoid	Above the mylohyoid muscle the geniohyoid originates from the genial tubercle of the mandible.	Inserts into the anterior portion of the hyoid bone.	Pulls the hyoid bone and the tongue anteriorly.

TABLE 7-7   Muscles of the Soft Palate

Muscle	Origin	Insertion	Function
Palatoglossus	This muscle forms the anterior arch on each side of the throat and arises from the soft palate.	Inserts along the posterior side of the tongue.	Elevates the posterior portion of the tongue and narrows the fauces.
Palatopharyngeal	This muscle forms the posterior arch on each side of the throat and also arises from the soft palate.	Inserts into the thyroid cartilage and the wall of the pharynx.	Constricts the nasopharyngeal passage and elevates the larynx.

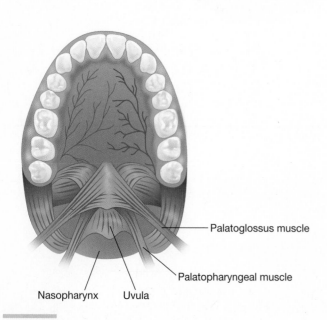

FIGURE 7-18 Muscles of the soft palate.

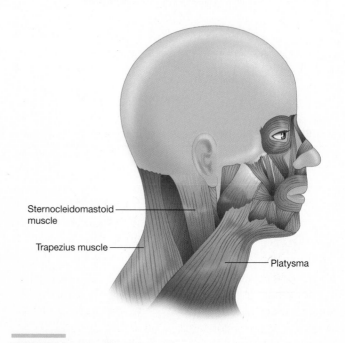

FIGURE 7-19 Muscles of the neck.

TABLE 7-8   Muscles of the Neck

Muscle	Origin	Insertion	Function
Platysma	Clavicle and the shoulder.	Inserts into the inferior border of the mandible.	This sheet of muscle draws down the mandible as well as the corners of the mouth and the lower lip.
Trapezius	Protuberance on the occipital bone.	Inserts into the clavicle and shoulders.	This large muscle moves the head backward and laterally.
Sternocleidomastoid	The top of the sternum and the clavicle.	Inserts into the mastoid process and the anterior of the occipital bone.	One on each side of the neck assists in elevating the chin.

Infraorbital Nerve. The infraorbital nerve is another branch of the maxillary nerve. Two nerves come from the infraorbital nerve before it exits through the infraorbital foramen. These are the middle superior alveolar nerve and the anterior alveolar nerve.

The middle superior alveolar nerve supplies the lateral wall of the maxillary sinus, gingiva, mesial buccal root of the first molar, and all the roots of the bicuspids (premolars). The anterior superior alveolar nerve is the next nerve to come from the infraorbital nerve. It innervates the anterior maxillary sinus, gingiva, cuspids, laterals, and central incisors.

Posterior Superior Alveolar Nerve. The posterior superior alveolar nerve branches downward from the maxillary nerve. It supplies the gingiva, maxillary sinus, cheeks, and maxillary molars with the exception of the mesial buccal root of the first molar, which is innervated by the middle superior alveolar nerve.

Zygomatic Nerve The zygomatic nerve innervates the orbicularis oculi, the area around the eye and the area around and behind the zygomatic arch.

Mandibular Branch of the Trigeminal Nerve

The mandibular nerve branch is composed of both sensory and motor neurons and is the largest division of the trigeminal nerve. There are three branches of the mandibular nerve: buccal, lingual, and inferior alveolar (Figure 7-21).

Buccal Nerve Branch. The buccal nerve branch passes through the buccinator muscle to the cheek, where it innervates the buccal mucosa and buccal gingiva, as well as the buccal of the mandibular molars.

Lingual Nerve Branch. The lingual nerve branch descends from the mandibular nerve to the underside of the tongue and extends from the posterior to the anterior of the mouth. This nerve innervates the floor of the mouth, the ventral side of the tongue, taste buds on the anterior two-thirds of the tongue, and the lingual gingiva.

Inferior Alveolar Nerve Branch. The inferior alveolar nerve branch descends from the mandibular nerve and runs parallel to the lingual nerve. The first branch is the mylohyoid nerve branch, which supplies the mylohyoid muscle and the anterior belly of the digastric muscle. The inferior alveolar nerve then enters through the mandibular foramen and runs through the mandibular canal. Within the canal, the inferior alveolar nerve supplies the mandibular teeth (specifically the molars and the premolars), the gingiva, and the mucosa. It then subdivides into the mental nerve branch and the incisive nerve branch. The mental nerve branch supplies the chin and the lower lip area, and the incisive nerve branch innervates the anterior teeth and labial gingiva.

Although learning the nerves of the head and neck can be difficult to learn, this knowledge will be very helpful to the dental assistant when studying the injection sites discussed in Chapter 20. Knowledge of the location of nerves and foramen on the bones will assist the dental assistant in determining where to place topical anesthetic before a local injection is given to the patient.

Circulation of the Head and Neck

The arteries and veins of the face and oral cavity are near each other. They supply blood and nutrients to the area and drain unoxygenated blood and waste products from the area.

Arteries of the Face and Oral Cavity

The common carotid supplies blood to most of the head and neck. As the common carotid ascends up the neck, it divides into the internal and external carotid arteries. The internal carotid artery supplies blood to the brain and eyes, while the external carotid artery

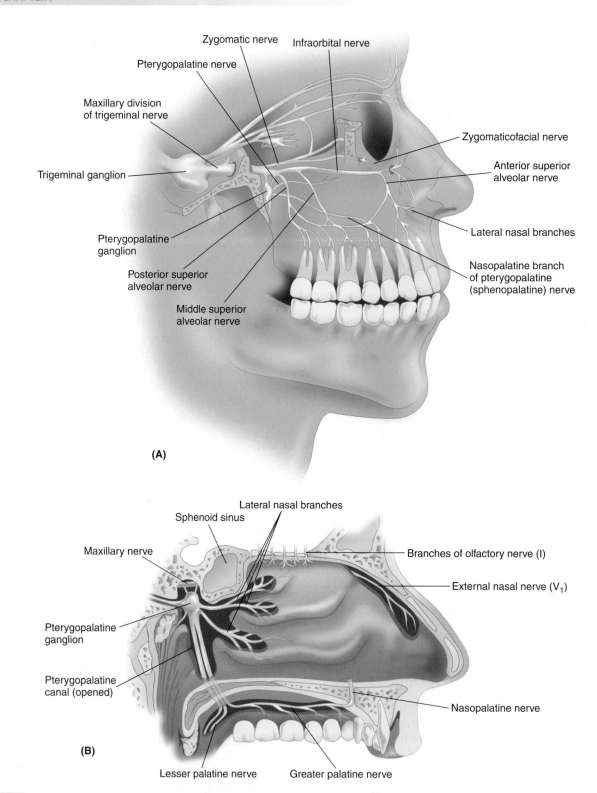

FIGURE 7-20 (A) Nerves of the maxillary arch. (B) Medial view to show branches of the pterygopalatine nerve.

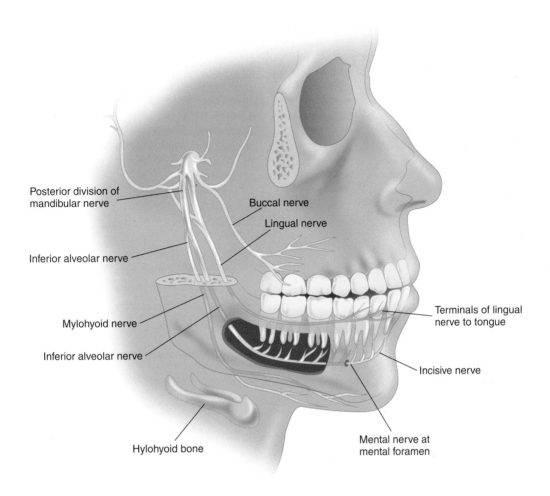

FIGURE 7-21 Mandibular nerves.

Labels in figure:
- Posterior division of mandibular nerve
- Buccal nerve
- Lingual nerve
- Inferior alveolar nerve
- Mylohyoid nerve
- Inferior alveolar nerve
- Terminals of lingual nerve to tongue
- Incisive nerve
- Hylohyoid bone
- Mental nerve at mental foramen

supplies blood to the face and oral cavity and has many branches (Figure 7-22). (Information presented is limited to the arteries that supply the teeth, tongue, and surrounding tissues.)

External Carotid Artery

The external carotid artery branches go to the throat, tongue, face, and ears and to the wall of the cranium. Branches are named according to the areas they supply and are nearer the surface (more superficial).

Lingual Artery. The lingual branch is about even with the hyoid bone and has several branches that supply the entire tongue, floor of the mouth, lingual gingiva, a portion of the soft palate, and the tonsils.

Facial Artery. The facial artery is above the lingual artery, near the angle of the mandible. It branches across the mandible to the corners of the mouth and then upward toward the eye. The facial artery has six branches that supply the pharynx muscles, soft palate, tonsils, posterior of the tongue, submandibular gland, muscles of the face, nasal septum, nose, and eyelids.

Maxillary Artery. The maxillary artery is the largest of the branches of the external carotid artery. It moves anteriorly across the ramus of the mandible, near the condyle, and supplies facial structures. The maxillary artery divides into three sections: mandibular, pterygoid, and pterygopalatine.

Mandibular Artery. The mandibular artery is behind the ramus of the mandible and branches into five arteries. The inferior alveolar artery descends into the ramus, enters the mandibular foramen, and bifurcates around the first premolar tooth to form the incisive and the mental arteries. The mylohyoid artery and the dental arteries are additional branches. The mylohyoid artery branches off the inferior alveolar artery before entering the mandibular canal. It supplies the mylohyoid muscle. As the inferior alveolar artery travels through the mandibular canal, the dental arteries supply the roots and periodontal ligaments of the molars and premolars. The incisive arteries continue anteriorly to supply blood to the roots and periodontal ligaments of the anterior teeth. The mental artery branches off the inferior alveolar artery, and then

FIGURE 7-22 Arteries of the face and oral cavity.

Labels (top to bottom, right side):
- Superficial temporal artery
- Posterior superior alveolar artery
- Infraorbital artery
- Middle superior alveolar artery
- Anterior superior alveolar artery
- Descending palatine artery
- Maxillary artery
- Facial artery
- Inferior alveolar artery
- Lingual artery
- External carotid artery
- Internal carotid artery
- Thyroid cartilage
- Common carotid artery
- Vertebral artery
- Brachiocephalic trunk
- Clavicle
- Subclavian artery

exits the mandibular canal at the mental foramen and supplies the chin and lower lip.

Pterygoid Artery. The pterygoid artery supplies blood to the temporal muscle, masseter muscle, pterygoid muscles, and buccinator muscles. The pterygopalatine artery divides into branches: posterior superior alveolar artery, infraorbital artery, middle superior alveolar artery, anterior superior alveolar artery, and greater palatine artery. The posterior superior alveolar artery branches from the maxillary artery and descends along the maxillary tuberosity, where it enters the posterior superior alveolar foramen. This artery supplies the maxillary sinus, maxillary molar teeth, and surrounding gingiva with blood. The infraorbital artery ascends from the maxillary artery and travels anteriorly to the infraorbital foramen, where it supplies the face with blood. From the infraorbital artery, the middle superior alveolar artery branches to the maxillary premolar teeth, and the anterior superior alveolar artery branches to supply the anterior teeth. The greater palatine artery travels through the greater palatine foramen to supply the hard palate and the maxillary lingual gingiva.

Veins of the Face and Oral Cavity

Some of the veins of the face and oral cavity are located with corresponding arteries and have similar names. There are many variations of venous drainage, but ultimately the blood from the face and oral cavity drains into either the external jugular vein or internal jugular vein and then into the brachiocephalic vein, which flows into the superior vena cava. The veins are divided into the superficial veins and the deep veins. Only the primary veins of importance to the dental assistant are discussed (Figure 7-23).

Superficial Veins. The facial vein drains the facial structures, beginning near the eye and descending toward the mandible. One of the tributaries is the deep facial vein, which connects the facial vein to the pterygoid plexus of veins. Near the border of the mandible, the facial vein heads posteriorly to the angle of the mandible, where it joins with the retromandibular vein. The retromandibular vein is frequently formed within the parotid gland. This vein drains the maxillary artery and the superficial temporal arteries. Below the facial vein is the lingual vein, which drains the floor of the mouth. The tongue empties into the internal jugular vein.

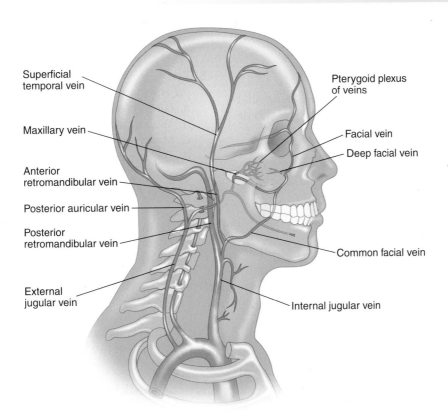

FIGURE 7-23 Veins of the face and oral cavity.

Deep Veins. The **maxillary vein** drains the pterygoid plexus of veins. It is a short vein that follows the maxillary artery. The **pterygoid plexus of veins** is a junction or center of veins that directly or indirectly drain a vast area, including the nasal cavity, eye, paranasal sinuses, muscles of mastication, buccinator muscle, palate, and teeth. The pterygoid plexus of veins is between the temporal and pterygoid muscles.

Jugular Vein. The **external jugular vein** drains the superficial veins of the face and neck into the subclavian vein. The **internal jugular vein** receives blood from the cranium, face, and neck, and drains into the brachiocephalic vein, and then into the superior vena cava, which drains into the heart.

CHAPTER SUMMARY

As a vital team member, the dental assistant needs to be able to recognize factors that may influence the general physical health of the patient. Understanding landmarks of the oral cavity, as well as being able to describe head and neck anatomy as it relates to location of structure and function, enables the dental assistant to recognize the abnormal. For this reason, accuracy is especially important when completing the patient's dental chart. This information provides a point of comparison for future visits.

Case Study

Pat Boyer is a thirty-five-year-old patient at Dr. Olson's office. Pat has had a series of headaches and pain during mastication (chewing). She also experiences clicking and popping when opening her mouth. These symptoms have continued for six months and seem to be worsening.

Case Study Review

1. List the components of the head and neck affected, identifying the specific anatomy.

2. Identify the possible conditions.

3. How might the dental assistant be involved in this patient's care?

REVIEW QUESTIONS

Multiple Choice

1. What are the raised lines of mucosal tissue that extend from the alveolar mucosa to the vestibule called?
   a. Gingiva
   b. Alveolar mucosa
   c. Frenum
   d. Papilla

2. The vertical part of the mandible that articulates with the temporal bone is called the
   a. oblique ridge.
   b. ramus.
   c. maxilla.
   d. palatal.

3. Which of the following are muscles of mastication?
   a. Temporals, masseters, buccinators, and internal pterygoids
   b. Temporal, masseters, internal pterygoids, and external pterygoids
   c. Masseters, mentalis, buccinators, and external pterygoids
   d. Orbicularis oris, buccinators, zygomatic major, and mentalis

4. Which division of the common carotid artery supplies the face and the oral cavity?
   a. External carotid artery
   b. Internal carotid artery
   c. Facial artery
   d. Maxillary artery

5. All of the following are correct statements about the veins that supply the face and the oral cavity *except:*
   a. The veins correspond to the arteries and often have similar names.
   b. The veins drain into the external or internal jugular vein.
   c. The veins are classified as deep or superficial veins.
   d. The lingual vein drains the muscles of mastication, the sinuses, and the palate.

6. The parotid gland empties into the mouth through:
   a. Wharton's duct
   b. Sublingual duct
   c. Duct of Rivinus
   d. Parotid duct also known as the Stensen's duct

7. The temporomandibular joint is composed of all of the following *except:*
   a. Glenoid fossa of the temporal bone
   b. Greater wing of the zygomatic bone
   c. Articular eminence of the temporal bone
   d. Condyloid process of the mandible

8. The _____ muscle opens the jaw by depressing the mandible.
   a. Lateral (external) pterygoid
   b. Medial (internal pterygoid)
   c. Masseter
   d. Temporal

9. The mental foramen, genial tubercles, and lingual foramen are all found on the _____.
   a. The maxilla
   b. the mandible
   c. The temporal bone
   d. the nasal bone

10. The common carotid:
    a. Drains the blood from most of the head and neck
    b. Is divided into three arteries
    c. Supplies blood to most of the head and neck
    d. Is a vein of the face and oral cavity

Critical Thinking

1. Which maxillary nerve is involved if a patient has a toothache on tooth #4?

2. Between the bottom of the nose and the middle of the upper lip is a shallow, V-shaped depression. Identify this landmark and any developmental disturbances that occur in this area.

3. Prominence of excess bone is sometimes found in the bones of the arches. What are these prominences called, and where are they located?

Web Activities

1. Go to http://www.tmjoints.org, click on What is TMJ?, and find out how a patient can avoid TMJ surgery. Which month has been proclaimed JAW-JOINTS-TMJ AWARENESS MONTH? Check http://www.tmj.org.

2. Go to http://www.bellspalsy.com and learn about facial paralysis and its causes.

3. Go to http://www.visiblehuman.org and view the video and animations related to mastication and facial expression.

CHAPTER 8

EMBRYOLOGY AND HISTOLOGY

SPECIFIC INSTRUCTIONAL OBJECTIVES

The student should strive to meet the following objectives and demonstrate an understanding of the facts and principles presented in this chapter:

1. Identify the terms and times of the three prenatal phases of pregnancy.

2. Describe how the human face develops and changes during the zygote and embryo phases.

3. Describe the life cycle of a tooth and identify the stages.

4. Identify the four primary structures of the tooth and the location and function of each.

5. Identify the substances of enamel, dentin, cementum, and pulp and their identifying marks.

6. Identify the components of the periodontium and the considerations of the alveolar bone.

7. Describe the structures of the gingiva and the mucosa.

KEY TERMS

alveolar crest *(148)*

alveolar crest fiber groups *(149)*

alveolar mucosa *(150)*

alveolar process *(148)*

alveolodental ligament fiber group *(149)*

alveologingival fiber groups *(150)*

alveolus *(148)*

ameloblasts *(144)*

apical fiber groups *(149)*

apposition *(144)*

attached gingiva *(151)*

attrition *(144)*

bilaterial cleft lip *(136)*

bud stage *(136)*

calcification *(144)*

cap stage *(143)*

cemental spurs *(148)*

cementoblasts *(144)*

cementum *(144)*

circular ligament fiber groups *(150)*

circumpulpal dentin *(146)*

cleft lip *(136)*

cleft palate *(136)*

cleft uvula *(136)*

contour lines of Owen *(146)*

cortical bone *(148)*

cytodifferentiation *(132)*

dental lamina *(137)*

dental sac *(143)*

dentin *(144)*

dentinal fluid *(146)*

dentinal hypersensitivity *(146)*

dentinal tubules *(146)*

dentogingival fiber groups *(150)*

dentoperiosteal fiber groups *(150)*

ectoderm *(132)*

embryology *(132)*

enamel *(144)*

enamel dysplasia *(146)*

enamel lamellae *(145)*

enamel matrix *(145)*

enamel spindles *(145)*

enamel tufts *(145)*

endoderm *(132)*

epithelial attachment *(151)*

KEY TERMS *(continued)*

eruption *(144)*

evanesce *(144)*

fibroblasts *(146)*

free gingiva *(151)*

gestational period *(135)*

gingiva *(150)*

gingival fiber groups *(149)*

gingival groove *(151)*

gingival hyperplasia *(151)*

gingival sulcus *(151)*

gums *(150)*

histodifferentiation *(132)*

histology *(136)*

horizontal fiber groups *(149)*

hypercementosis *(148)*

imbrication lines *(145)*

imbrication lines of Von Ebner *(146)*

initiation *(137)*

intercellular substances *(146)*

interdental gingiva *(151)*

interdental ligament groups *(149)*

interdental septum *(148)*

interprismatic substance *(145)*

interradicular fiber groups *(149)*

interradicular septum *(148)*

intertubular dentin *(146)*

labial commissures *(134)*

lamina dura *(147)*

lamina propria *(149)*

lanugo *(139)*

lines of Retzius *(145)*

mantle dentin *(146)*

mesenchyme tissue *(143)*

mesoderm *(132)*

morphodifferent- iation *(132)*

mucogingival junction *(151)*

Nasmyth's membrane *(146)*

nasolacrimal groove *(134)*

neonatal line *(145)*

oblique fiber groups *(149)*

odontoblasts *(144)*

odontogenesis *(136)*

osteoblasts *(148)*

osteoclasts *(144)*

perikymata *(145)*

periodontal fiber groups *(148)*

periodontal ligament *(148)*

periodontium *(147)*

peritubular dentin *(146)*

philtrum *(133)*

primary dentin *(146)*

primary palate *(134)*

proliferate *(132)*

proliferation *(143)*

pulp *(144)*

pulp canal *(145)*

pulp chamber *(145)*

pulp horns *(145)*

pulp stones *(147)*

pulpitis *(146)*

rod core *(145)*

secondary dentin *(146)*

secondary palate *(134)*

Sharpey's fibers *(147)*

stippled *(150)*

stomedeum *(133)*

tertiary dentin *(146)*

Tome's process *(145)*

unilateral cleft lip *(136)*

zygote *(132)*

INTRODUCTION

Dental assistants should be familiar with general embryological development of the face and the oral cavity, and general histology to understand the composition, formation, and eruption of the teeth. In addition to embryology and histology, this chapter covers the components of the periodontium and describes the strucures of the gingiva.

Embryology

The study of prenatal growth and the developing process of an individual is called **embryology**. Oral embryology refers to the study of the development of the oral cavity. The following information provides the dental assistant with a basic understanding of embryology.

Human pregnancy is approximately nine months (thirty-eight weeks [often counted forty weeks from the first day of the pregnant woman's last menstrual period]) in duration. This period starts with conception, when the ovum is fertilized by the sperm. The following terms and times identify the three prenatal phases of the pregnancy:

1. Conception through the first two weeks—zygote

2. Two weeks through the eighth week—embryo

3. Nine weeks through birth—fetus

The **zygote** phase is when cells rapidly increase in number, or **proliferate**. During the embryonic phase, many critical changes are taking place. The cells are differentiating (developing individual characteristics) and integrating to form cell layers that develop into a human being. There are three stages of differentiation:

1. **Cytodifferentiation**—the development of different cells

2. **Histodifferentiation**—the development of different tissues

3. **Morphodifferentiation**—the development of different forms

Three primary embryonic layers are formed early in the embryo phase. The **ectoderm** layer differentiates into skin, hair, nails, brain, nervous system, lining of the oral cavity, and enamel of the teeth. The second layer, the **mesoderm**, differentiates into the lining of the abdominal cavity, bones, muscles, circulatory system, reproductive system, internal organs, dentin, cementum, and pulp of the teeth. The **endoderm**, the third layer, gives rise to the epithelial linings of the respiratory system, some glandular organs, and the digestive tract. To remember the layers, recall that *derm* refers to tissue and *ecto* refers to outside, *meso* refers to middle, and *endo* refers to inside (Figure 8-1). The first sign of a developing tooth is noted during the embryonic phase, in the area that will eventually become the lower mandibular anterior region (Figure 8-2).

Primitive Facial Development

The face begins to form during the fourth week of prenatal development (Figure 8-3A). This embryonic phase involves all three embryonic layers. At this time, the

Figure 8-1

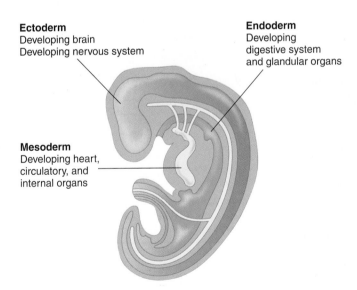

Ectoderm (outer)
Skin, brain, nervous system, hair, nails, enamel of teeth, lining of the oral cavity

Endoderm (inner)
Epithelial linings, glandular organs, digestive system

Mesoderm (middle)
Bones, muscles, circulatory system, internal organs, reproductive system, lining of the abdominal cavity, dentin, cementum, pulp of the teeth

FIGURE 8-1 The three primary embryonic layers—ectoderm (outer), mesoderm (middle), endoderm (inner)—and associated tissues.

Ectoderm
Developing brain
Developing nervous system

Endoderm
Developing digestive system and glandular organs

Mesoderm
Developing heart, circulatory, and internal organs

FIGURE 8-2 Developing embryo with primary embryonic layers identified.

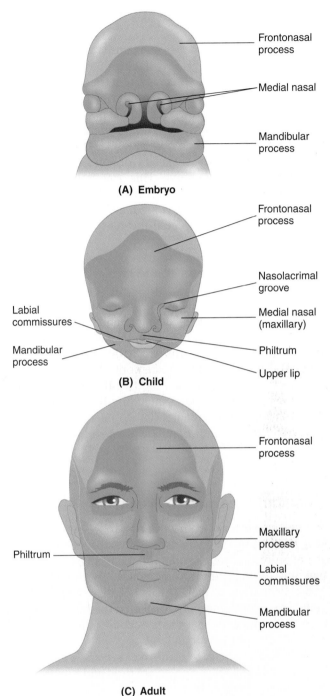

(A) Embryo
- Frontonasal process
- Medial nasal
- Mandibular process

(B) Child
- Frontonasal process
- Nasolacrimal groove
- Medial nasal (maxillary)
- Philtrum
- Upper lip
- Labial commissures
- Mandibular process

(C) Adult
- Frontonasal process
- Maxillary process
- Labial commissures
- Mandibular process
- Philtrum

FIGURE 8-3 Embryonic facial processes shown on (A) embryo, (B) child, and (C) adult.

future face appears to be squeezed between the bulging brain and the large heart, with the eyes and nose spread out toward the sides. The face further develops from the three embryonic layers (Figures 8-3B and C). The first area, the frontonasal process, forms the upper portion of the face, the forehead, eyes, nose, and the **philtrum** (vertical groove on the midline of the upper lip). The second area forms the middle of the face, called the maxillary (medial nasal) process. This area consists of the cheeks, sides of the upper lip, midface, secondary palate, zygomatic bones, portion of the temporal bones, and the maxilla embryonic surface. The third area, called the mandibular process, forms the two mandibular arches (first branchial arches) and makes up the lower lip, lower face, temporal area, and the mandible. The **stomedeum** (stoh-mah-DE-um), or primitive mouth, appears between the maxillary and mandibular processes. It initially appears as a shallow depression in the embryonic surface.

The face continues developing until the twelfth week, changing shape considerably during this time. The eyes move forward, the nose comes together, and the face appears much more narrow than during the first formation. The maxillary processes on each side of the face fuse at the **labial commissures**, or corners of the mouth, with the mandibular arch (Figure 8-3B). The frontonasal process fuses with the maxillary process along the line of the **nasolacrimal groove**. This groove extends from the medial corner of the eye to the nasal cavity along the maxillary process to the medial nasal process. This fusion normally is completed during the sixth week of prenatal development.

Inside the oral cavity, the **primary** (primitive) **palate** is developing. It appears as a triangular mass and contains the four maxillary incisor teeth. It serves to separate the developing oral cavities from the nasal cavities. The two palatal shelves develop and move medially toward each other, fusing to form the **secondary palate**, which will become two-thirds of the hard palate (Figure 8-4). The secondary palate contains the remaining teeth and forms the remaining two-thirds of the hard palate and the soft palate, including the uvula. During the twelfth week of prenatal development, the primary palate and the secondary palate meet and fuse, forming the final palate. Thus, the oral cavity and the nasal cavity are completely separated.

Stages and Features of Pregnancy

The first trimester is from week zero to week twelve. The first sign of pregnancy is usually the absence of a menstrual period, although some women have breakthrough bleeding during their normal cycles. The breasts swell and may become tender. This is because the mammary glands develop to prepare for breast-feeding. The veins over the surface of the breasts become more prominent and the nipples begin to enlarge.

During the first six to eight weeks, nausea and vomiting are common. Most women are tired and require more rest. Some women notice cravings for certain foods and may have a metallic taste in the mouth. After the vomiting decreases, weight begins to increase. All major organs in the embryo/fetus begin developing (Figure 8-5A).

The second trimester is from week thirteen to week twenty-eight. The woman begins to look noticeably pregnant. Her weight increases, as does her appetite. The nausea is less and the woman may feel better and more energetic than during the first trimester. The woman's breasts and abdomen enlarge. The woman feels the baby moving between the eighteenth and the twentieth weeks. The fetus, now with recognizable features, grows rapidly throughout the second trimester. The pregnant woman's heart rate increases, increasing blood pumped to the fetus, which helps the fetus develop correctly (Figure 8-5B).

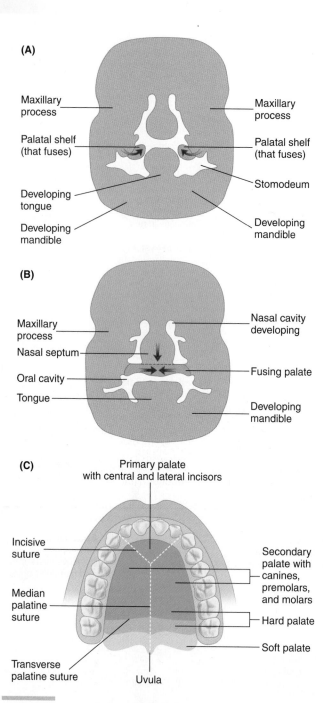

FIGURE 8-4 Development of the palate. (A) Palate forming from three sections. (B) Frontal view. (C) Palatal view of the three sections and where the secondary and primary palates fuse.

During the second trimester, the woman has a routine ultrasound. This test estimates time of birth and detects multiple fetuses or fetal malformations. The ultrasound also shows the anatomy of the normal child (Figure 8-6), often indicating the sex of the child. An ultrasound machine uses sound waves instead of radiation to create an image of a baby in the womb. The sound waves bounce off the fetus and that information is sent to a computer, which produces a three-dimensional (3D) "still" image. This technology, called sonography, is much safer than radiation and provides much of the same information.

(A) First trimester
(0 to 12 weeks)

(B) Second trimester
(13 to 28 weeks)

(C) Third trimester
(29 to 40 weeks)

FIGURE 8-5 (A) In the first trimester of pregnancy, all major organ structures are developing. (B) In the second trimester, the fetus—now with features—grows rapidly. (C) As the fetus prepares for life outside the uterus, the head drops low in the pelvis.

FIGURE 8-6 Sonogram taken in the second trimester of pregnancy. *(Courtesy of Nici Peterson)*

A four-dimensional (4D) sonograph produces an image as well as movement of the fetus (Figure 8-7A and B). Both the 3D and the 4D tests can be considered safe as long as trained medical professionals are performing them. The number of nonmedical people offering ultrasound exams has recently increased. These individuals may not be trained, and could give parents inaccurate information. The Food and Drug Administration (FDA) and professional medical organizations discourage the use of these nonmedical ultrasound examinations.

The third and final trimester is from week twenty-nine to week forty. During the **gestational period** (the time span in the womb until offspring are born), the fetus can grow to a length (height) of forty-eight to fifty-two centimeters (nineteen to twenty-one inches) (Figure 8-8). The woman may experience stretch marks on the breasts, abdomen, and thighs due to the expansion and stretching of the skin. The woman may also experience hot flashes and perspire easily. The fetus matures and prepares for birth. During week thirty-six to thirty-seven the baby's head drops low into the pelvis (Figure 8-5C). This relieves pressure in the woman's chest and aids in breathing, but puts additional pressure on the bladder and hip region. Often, women feel tired because they cannot find a comfortable position in which to rest. The woman's feet and legs may swell due to water retention and it becomes more difficult to get around. The average weight increase during a pregnancy is twenty-eight pounds; 70 percent of this weight gain occurs in the last twenty weeks. Table 8-1 summarizes the stages of fetal development.

Developmental Disturbances

Disturbances during periods of prenatal development most often occur during the embryonic period but may occur at any time. Genetic and environmental factors such as drugs and infections can initiate malformations in the unborn child. Women should avoid using alcohol and drugs immediately after suspicion of pregnancy. Infants born to women who have persisted taking alcohol during pregnancy may exhibit fetal alcohol syndrome (FAS). Symptoms of FAS include, but are not limited to, small head circumference, low nasal bridge, indistinct philtrum, thin upper lip, and a small mandible.

Specific infections contracted by pregnant women may cause malformations and developmental dis-

FIGURE 8-7 (A) 4D ultrasound at 37 weeks. (B) 4D ultrasound at 20 weeks. *(Courtesy of Kenneth and Tory McGrath)*

turbances in the unborn child. For example, German measles may cause heart, eye, or hearing defects in the unborn child. Syphilis, another infection, can cause paralysis, blindness, deafness, and defects in the incisors and molars.

Varying degrees of disfigurement may be caused by the failure of the tissues to fuse. Children born with disabilities of this kind should be seen by medical and dental specialists. Initially, the infant may face problems that limit nursing and feeding. Decisions need to be made to allow proper nutritional care for the child. Developmental disturbances that deal with the failure of tissues to fuse normally require long-term attention. If the palate has not fused, the teeth may not erupt in

the proper positions, if at all. The dentist follows the case to ensure that all needed procedures are done at the proper time. Reconstructive surgery and speech and hearing therapy may be recommended.

Disturbance in the fusion may be caused by a number of factors. It is important that the pregnant mother be healthy and enjoy good nutrition. Drugs (alcohol included) taken during pregnancy may cause birth defects. Hereditary factors may also play a role in birth defects.

Cleft Lip. When the maxillary processes fail to fuse with the medial nasal process, **cleft lip** results. Cleft lip occurs in about one in 1,000 live births. These cleft lips can occur on one side or both sides of the upper lip. One side is called **unilateral cleft lip** (Figure 8-9A); both sides are called a **bilateral cleft lip**. Cleft lips are more common in boys and more frequently unilateral on the left side. They are also more severe in boys than girls. Clefts can be as small as a notch in the lip to more severe cases that extend into the floor of the nostril.

Cleft Palate. A **cleft palate**, the failure of the palatal shelves to fuse with the primary palate or with each other, may occur with or without a cleft lip. Cleft palate occurs in one of every 2,500 births. Cleft palate occurring alone is more common in girls than boys. A **cleft uvula** is the mildest form of a cleft palate because it does not hamper eating or speaking to the same degree that the cleft palate or the cleft lip does. With a cleft uvula, only the uvula is separated slightly (Figure 8-10A). The clefts may be bilateral in only the posterior palate or complete unilateral cleft lip and alveolar process with unilateral cleft of the primary palates (Figures 8-10B and C). The clefts may also be complete bilateral cleft lip and alveolar process with bilateral cleft of the primary palatal portions (Figure 8-10D). The most complex is the complete bilateral cleft lip and maxillary alveolar process with bilateral cleft of the primary and secondary palates (Figure 8-10E).

Histology and the Life Cycle of the Tooth

Histology is the study of the microscopic structure and function of tissues. Oral histology is the study of the tissues of the teeth and the structures of the oral cavity that surround the teeth.

Each tooth goes through a number of successive periods of development during its life cycle. These periods are grouped into stages according to the shape and development of the organ.

Bud Stage

The first stage of **odontogenesis** (origin of the tooth) is called the **bud stage** (Table 8-2). During this stage, initia-

50.0 cm

36.0 cm

30.0 cm

Size (crown-to-rump length)

27.0 cm

23.0 cm

16.0 cm
14.0 cm

8.7 cm

5.0 cm

11 14   18   22 26   30   34   38   40

Gestational age in weeks

FIGURE 8-8 Fetal size by gestational age.

tion takes place. **Initiation** is when the tooth begins formation from the **dental lamina**. The dental lamina is a growth from the oral epithelium that gives rise to the tooth buds. Therefore, on a deciduous dentition, ten growths on each arch are apparent or ten buds later become the primary teeth. The first sign of a developing tooth is noted during the embryonic phase in the area that will eventually be the lower mandibular anterior region of the child's oral cavity. The permanent teeth develop in a similar manner. Each arch has sixteen buds developing into one tooth each. The last three molars in each quadrant develop behind the primary dentition. The six-year molar begins developing at birth, the twelve-year molar starts developing when the baby is about six months old, and the third molars (wisdom teeth) start when the child is approximately five years old.

TABLE 8-1 Stages of Fetal Development

Stage	Fetal Development
First Trimester **Embryonic or Germinal Stage**	
Weeks 1 and 2	Rapid cell division and differentiation.
Embryonic Stage	
Week 3	Primitive nervous system, eyes, and ears present. Heart begins to beat on day 21.
Week 4 Wt 0.4 g L 4–6 mm (crown–rump, C–R)	Half the size of a pea. Brain differentiates. GI tract begins to form. Limb buds appear. Primitive face develops. Stomedeum appears.
Week 5 L 6–8 mm (C–R)	Cranial nerves present. Muscles innervated.
Week 6 L 10–14 mm (C–R)	Fetal circulation established. Central autonomic nervous system forms. Primitive kidneys form. Lung buds present. Cartilage forms. Primitive skeleton forms. Muscles differentiate.
Week 7 L 22–28 mm (C–R)	Eyelids form. Palate and tongue form. Stomach formed. Diaphragm formed. Arms and legs move.
Week 8 Wt 2 g L 3 cm (1.2 in) (C–R)	Resembles human being. Eyes moved to face front. Heart development complete. Hands and feet well formed. Bone cells begin replacing cartilage. All body organs have begun forming.
Fetal Stage	
Week 9	Finger- and toenails form. Eyelids fuse shut.
Week 10 Wt 14 g ($\frac{1}{2}$ oz) L 5–6 cm (2 in) crown–heel (C–H)	Head growth slows. Bone marrow forms. Bladder sac forms. Kidneys make urine.
Week 11	Tooth buds appear. Liver secretes bile. Urinary system functions. Insulin forms in pancreas.

(continues)

TABLE 8-1   Stages of Fetal Development *(continued)*

	Stage	Fetal Development
	Week 12 Wt 45 g (1.5 oz) L 9 cm (3.5 in) (C–R) 11.5 cm (4.5 in) (C–H)	Oral cavity and nasal cavity are separated. Lungs take shape. Palate fuses. Heartbeat heard with Doppler ultrasound. Primary palate developing. Swallowing reflex present. External genitalia. Male or female distinguished. Eyes move forward. Nose comes together. Face narrows. Maxillary processes fuse at labial commissures. Frontonasal process fuses with maxillary process.
	Second Trimester Week 16 Wt 200 g (7 oz) L 13.5 cm (5.5 in) (C–R) 15 cm (6 in) (C–H)	Scalp hair appears. Frequent fetal movement. Skin thin. Sensitive to light.
	Week 20 Wt 435 g (15 oz) L 19 cm (7.5 in) (C–R) 25 cm (10 in) (C–H)	Lanugo (a covering of soft downy hairs) covers body. Sucks and swallows amniotic fluid. Heartbeat with fetoscope. Hands can grasp. Regular schedule of sucking, kicking, and sleeping.
	Week 24 Wt 780 g (1 lb, 12 oz) L 23 cm (9 in) (C–R) 28 cm (11 in) (C–H)	Alveoli present in lungs. Eyes completely formed. Eyelashes and eyebrows appear. Many reflexes appear. Chance of survival if born now.

(continues)

TABLE 8-1 Stages of Fetal Development *(continued)*

	Stage	Fetal Development
	Third Trimester Week 28 Wt 1,200 g (2 lb, 10 oz) L 28 cm (11 in) (C–R) 35 cm (14 in) (C–H)	Subcutaneous fat deposits begin. Lanugo begins to disappear. Nails appear. Eyelids open and close. Testes begin to descend.
	Week 32 Wt 2,000 g (4 lb, 6.5 oz) L 31 cm (12 in) (C–R) 41 cm (16 in) (C–H)	More reflexes present. Begins storing iron, calcium, and phosphorus. Central nervous system directs breathing movements and partially controls body temperature.
	Week 36 Wt 2,500–2,750 g (5 lb, 8 oz) L 35 cm (14 in) (C–R) 48 cm (19 in) (C–H)	A few creases on soles of feet. Skin less wrinkled. Fingernails reach fingertips. Sleep–wake cycle fairly definite. Transfer of maternal antibodies.
	Week 38	L/S ratio 2:1
	Week 40 Wt 3,000–3,600 g (6 lb, 10 oz–7 lb, 15 oz) L 50 cm (20 in) (C–H)	Lanugo only on shoulders and upper back. Creases cover soles. Ear cartilage firm. Less active, limited space. Ready to be born.

Adapted from Littleton, L. and Engelbreson, J. (2002). *Maternal, Neonatal, and Women's Health Nursing.* Clifton Park, NY: Thomson Delmar Learning.

FIGURE 8-9 (A) Cleft lip. (B) Cleft palate. *(Courtesy of Joseph L. Konzelman, Jr., DDS)*

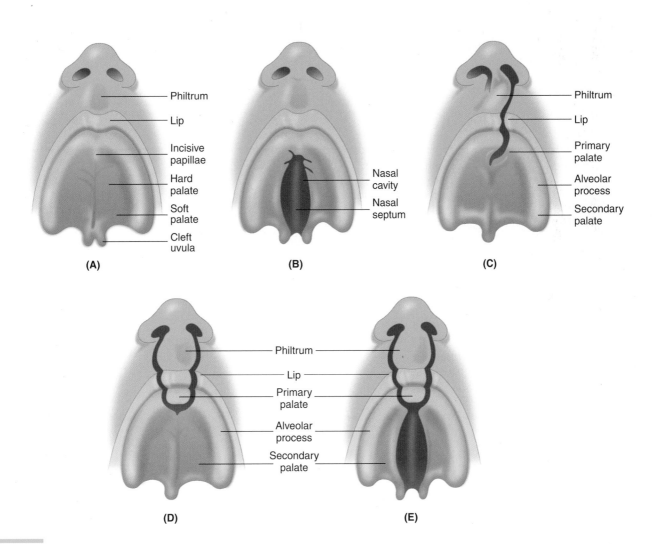

FIGURE 8-10 (A) Cleft uvula. (B) Bilateral cleft of the secondary palate. (C) Unilateral cleft lip, primary palate, and alveolar process. (D) Bilateral cleft of the lip, alveolar process, and primary palate. (E) Bilateral cleft of the lip, alveolar process, and primary and secondary palates.

TABLE 8-2   Life Cycle of the Tooth

Processes Involved	Description	Approximate Prenatal Time Span	Appearance as the Tooth Develops
Initiation	Odontogenesis (origin of the tooth) begins. The tooth begins formation from the dental lamina which is a growth from the oral epithelium that gives rise to the tooth buds.	6–7 weeks	Initiation (bud stage)
Proliferation	Cap stage (begins proliferation, histodifferentiation, and morphodifferentiation) where the primary embryonic ectoderm layer matures into the enamel of the developing tooth.	8–9 weeks	Proliferation (cap stage)
Histodifferentiation	Bell stage where the cells develop into different tissues and begin the future shape of the developing organ. Mesoderm layer develops into connective tissue called mesenchyme tissue.	9–11 weeks	Histodifferentiation (bell stage)
Morphodifferentiation	The forming organ takes shape and further resembles a bell shape.	11–12 weeks	Morphodifferentiation

(continues)

TABLE 8-2 Life Cycle of the Tooth *(continued)*

Processes Involved	Description	Approximate Prenatal Time Span	Appearance as the Tooth Develops
Apposition	The calcium salts and other minerals are deposited in the formed tooth. The tissues or enamel, dentin, and cementum are formed in layers.	Varies according to the tooth	Apposition (maturation stage)
Calcification	The layers of the tooth tissue become calcified.	Varies according to the tooth	Calcification
Eruption	The tooth emerges from the gum tissue and becomes visible.	Varies according to the tooth. See eruption schedule for teeth in appendix.	Eruption

(continues)

Cap Stage

The bud of the tooth grows and changes shape during the cap stage. The organ is indented on the lower side and appears much like a cap, therefore the name **cap stage** (Table 8-2). The primary embryonic ectoderm layer that has developed into the oral epithelium matures into the enamel of the developing tooth. The processes of **proliferation**, when the cells multiply, and histodifferentiation, when the cells develop into different tissues, take place along with early morphodifferentiation, when the cells begin to outline the future shape of the developing organ. During this process, the primary embryonic mesoderm layer develops into connective tissue that is called the **mesenchyme tissue**. This connective tissue forms an enclosed area, called a **dental sac**, and further matures into the dentin, cementum, and the pulp of the tooth. A portion of

TABLE 8-2 Life Cycle of the Tooth *(continued)*

Processes Involved	Description	Approximate Prenatal Time Span	Appearance as the Tooth Develops
Attrition	The tooth wears away the incisal or occlusal surfaces during normal function and use.	Varies according to dentition, occlusion, stress, and lifestyle	Attrition

the mesenchyme surrounds the outside of the enamel organ, the cementum, and the periodontal ligament of the tooth.

Bell Stage

Further specialization of the cells, or histodifferentiation, takes place in the bell stage (Table 8-2). The inner epithelium of the enamel organ becomes **ameloblasts**, enamel-forming cells. The peripheral cells of the dental papilla become **odontoblasts**, cells that form dentin. The **cementoblasts**, cementum-forming cells, form from the dental sac. Continued morphodifferentiation takes place, forming the organ into a shape that resembles a bell (Table 8-2).

Maturation Stage

The odontogenesis reaches completion in these final stages. The tissues of enamel, dentin, and cementum are formed in layers and fused in the appropriate manner. The process of depositing calcium salts and other minerals in the formed tooth takes place during the **apposition** stage (Table 8-2). This process, called **calcification**, is the last developmental stage before **eruption** of the tooth when the growing tooth emerges from the gum. (Table 8-2). The final stage of the life cycle of the tooth is **attrition**, or the wearing away of the incisal or occlusal surfaces of the tooth during normal function (Table 8-2 and Figure 8-11).

The root of the tooth does not develop fully before eruption. Eruption is the phase when the tooth passes through the bone and the oral mucosa and into its place in the oral cavity. An eruption schedule for the primary

and permanent teeth appears in Chapter 9, Tooth Morphology. Twenty of the permanent teeth are below and distal to the primary teeth. As the permanent teeth erupt, they apply pressure to the apices of the roots of the primary teeth. During this force, **osteoclasts**, bone resorption cells, **evanesce** (ev-a-**NES**) (dissolve) the root of the primary tooth. This resorption first takes place at the apex and continues up toward the crown of the tooth. When very little of the root structure of the primary tooth is left, the tooth loosens due to lack of support. Children often assist in the final stages of loosening the tooth by moving it back and forth until they break the attaching fibers.

The primary teeth occupy and maintain space in the dental arches for the permanent teeth and act as guides during the eruption process. If the primary teeth are removed early, the spaces may be diminished, causing crowding when the permanent teeth erupt.

Tooth Structure

Each tooth is comprised of four primary structures (Figure 8-12). The **enamel** is the structure that covers the outside of the crown of the tooth. It is the hardest living tissue in the body. Enamel can be very brittle if not supported by dentin and a vital pulp. **Dentin** makes up the bulk of the tooth structure but is not normally visible. It surrounds the pulp cavity and lies under the enamel, within the anatomical crown and under the cementum within the root. The **cementum** is the third structure and is located around the root. It covers the dentin on the root portion of the tooth. At the center of the tooth, within the **pulp** cavity, is the pulp tissue. It is made of

FIGURE 8-11 Attrition of the primary dentition. *(Courtesy of Dr. Steve Gregg)*

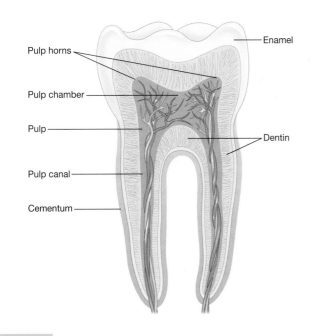

FIGURE 8-12 Tissues of the tooth.

the nerves and blood vessels that provide nutrients to the tooth. The pulp cavity is made of a pulp chamber with pulp horns and pulp canal(s). The **pulp canal**(s) is (are) in the root(s) of the teeth. The **pulp chamber** is a large portion of the pulp, which is in the crown of the tooth. The **pulp horns**, pointed elongations of the pulp, extend toward the incisal or occlusal portion of the tooth. The pulpal portion of the tooth is often larger in primary teeth and newly formed permanent teeth. As a person ages, the pulpal portion may decrease in size. For example, adults over seventy years of age may have small pulp chambers or the pulpal portion may be totally calcified.

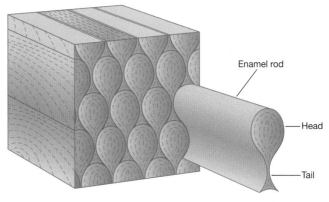

FIGURE 8-13 Drawing representing the enamel rods.

Enamel

Enamel is thicker on the biting surfaces, occlusal cusps, and the incisal edge than in other areas. Ameloblasts aid in developing enamel rods. These rods, which are not visible to the naked eye, are four micrometers in diameter, variable lengths, and shaped in the pattern of a fish (Figure 8-13). Their location in the enamel is such that the head is surrounded by the tails of two other enamel rods. The substance surrounding the inner portion, the **rod core**, of each enamel rod is the **interprismatic substance**. Of these substances, the enamel rods are hardest and the interprismatic substance is the weakest.

The enamel matrix is produced by the ameloblast cells. **Tome's process**, a secretory surface of the ameloblast, is responsible for laying down the enamel matrix. Tome's process guides the **enamel matrix** into place. As the second layer is laid down, the first becomes more mineralized and this process follows until the last layer is placed.

Enamel rods under a microscope show several developmental identification marks. The **lines of Retzius** (**RET**-zee-us) appear as incremental lines or bands around the layers, much like the growth rings on a tree. Very few lines are indicated prenatally, but one, known as the **neonatal line**, an accentuated incremental line, indicates the trauma of birth. It is found in all the primary teeth and several of the permanent teeth. Along with the lines of Retzius are the **imbrication lines**, slight ridges on the cervical third of certain teeth that extend mesiodistally, and the **perikymata** (pear-ee-**KIGH**-mah-tah), small grooves noted on some teeth.

Enamel spindles represent short, dentinal tubules that seem to have crossed over into the enamel and were trapped there during the process of enamel mineralization. Noted with bases near the dentinoenamel junction are the **enamel tufts**. They appear as small, dark brushes. Narrower and longer enamel tufts are called **enamel lamellae**. These thin structures extend from the dentinoenamel junction to the enamel surface.

Clinical Considerations Regarding Enamel

▪ Primary teeth may erupt with a covering over the enamel that is left over from the epithelium and the ameloblasts, called the Nasmyth's membrane. Nasmyth's membrane may absorb stain easily. This membrane is easily removed by a thorough polishing. No lasting effects on the condition of the enamel are observed following removal of the membrane.

▪ Certain developmental disturbances can occur during the apposition stage. A loss of nutritional support may result in the surface of the teeth becoming grooved and pitted, called enamel dysplasia. The patient may be concerned with the appearance of the tooth, and the weakened surface is more susceptible to decay. With today's dental materials, the surface of the tooth can be restored.

▪ Fluoride can aid in strengthening the enamel to prevent demineralization. Fluoride can be ingested or applied topically.

▪ Dentists prepare the teeth for the placement of restorations in a manner in which isolated enamel rods are protected from fracture.

Dentin

Mature dentin is softer than enamel but harder than cementum and bone. If the dentin is exposed, it appears yellowish white. It is what gives the translucent enamel its underlying yellow hue. The cuspid is a bulky tooth with a greater amount of dentin; therefore, it appears more yellow than the teeth surrounding it. Dentin is less dense and appears rougher in surface texture than enamel. The odontoblasts form dentin, beginning at the dentinoenamel junction and continuing toward the pulp chamber. **Dentinal tubules** pass through the entire surface of the dentin. These long tubes contain the **dentinal fluid**, which is presumably tissue fluid surrounding the cell membrane of the odontoblast.

As with enamel, developmental marks are apparent in the dentin. **Imbrication lines of Von Ebner** are the stained growth rings or incremental lines in dentin. Contour lines that demonstrate a disturbance in the body metabolism are called **contour lines of Owen**. Again, the most pronounced stained contour line is the neonatal line that occurs due to the trauma of birth.

Types of Dentin. Dentin differs from area to area and is not uniform throughout. **Peritubular dentin** is the dentin that creates the wall of the dentinal tubule. Dentin found between the tubules is called **intertubular dentin**. The first predentin that is formed and matures within the tooth is called **mantle dentin**. The layer of dentin that surrounds the pulp is called **circumpulpal dentin**. Forming the bulk of the tooth is **primary dentin**, which is formed before the completion of the apical foramen (opening of the root's pulp canal). **Secondary dentin** forms after the completion of the apical foramen and slowly throughout the life of the tooth. Due to continued growth, the pulp chamber narrows and may become calcified later in life. **Tertiary dentin** repairs and is reactive to irritations. It forms quickly in response to localized injury. Injury may be caused by dental caries, cavity preparation, recession, attrition, or erosion. Tertiary dentin may be more irregular than primary or secondary dentin.

Clinical Considerations Regarding Dentin

▪ If the antibiotic tetracycline is taken during the formation of dentin, it binds chemically to the dentin and causes permanent yellow staining.

▪ Cavities that appear small on the outside of the tooth extend more rapidly through the dentin because its density is lower than enamel.

▪ Patients may experience dentinal hypersensitivity if the dentin is exposed. This may be very painful for the patient. In some individuals, the enamel and cementum do not come together at the cementoenamel junction (CEJ), leaving exposed dentin. Using the air-water syringe in an area that is not anesthetized causes discomfort.

Pulp

The pulp of the tooth evolves from cells similar to the dentin. Its function is to provide nourishment, support, and maintenance for the dentin. Also, when the dentin or pulp is injured, sensory nerves send the messages to the brain for interpretation. The pulp identifies the temperature and chemical changes, vibrations, and bacterial invasion of the tooth and transmits this information to the brain. It is a warning system that works as a defense system for the tooth.

The pulp is made partially from **fibroblasts** (cells from which connective tissue evolve), which synthesize protein fibers and **intercellular substances** (substances between the cells) to form pulp tissue. The pulp is fed continually through the opening at the apex of the root, the apical foramen.

Clinical Considerations Regarding Pulp

▪ If the pulp is damaged due to an injury, the tissue may become inflamed, causing pulpitis. The pressure increases and cannot escape. The structures of the tooth form a hard encasement and, when the tooth becomes inflamed, cause a great deal of pressure and discomfort. The patient may need to have root canal therapy, which opens the pulp and releases the pressure.

▪ If endodontic treatment (root canal therapy) is performed on a tooth, the pulp tissue is removed and the tooth becomes nonvital.

▪ The use of water-cooled handpieces prevents overheating of the pulp during dental treatment.

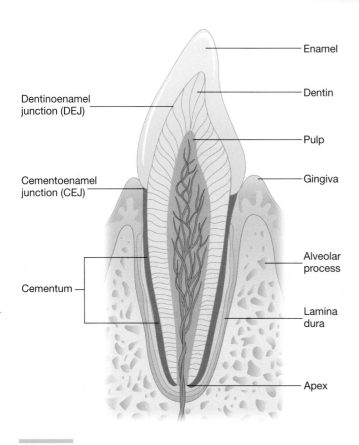

FIGURE 8-14 The tooth and surrounding tissues.

▪ **Pulp stones,** calcified masses of dentin, are sometimes found in the pulp tissue. They can be attached or unattached to the pulpal wall. They are quite common and normally cause a problem only if root canal therapy is necessary.

Components of the Periodontium

The **periodontium** consists of portions of the tooth structure that support hard and soft dental tissues and the alveolar bone. The cementum is part of the periodontium as well as the last tooth structure.

Cementum

Surrounding the root of the tooth, attaching it to the alveolar bone by anchoring the periodontal ligaments, is the cementum (Figure 8-14). It is a dull light yellow, lighter than dentin and darker than enamel. It is softer than both dentin and enamel and has a grainy feel. Cementum continues to develop throughout life, similar to dentin and pulp. Cementum is formed by cementoblasts and is thicker at the apex than elsewhere. Cementum does not resorb and regenerate like bone, which allows orthodontic treatment to move the teeth through the bone and not destroy the cementum. Within the outer part of the cementum are collagen fibers from the periodontal ligament, called **Sharpey's fibers** (Figure 8-15). They act as anchors between the alveolar bone and the tooth.

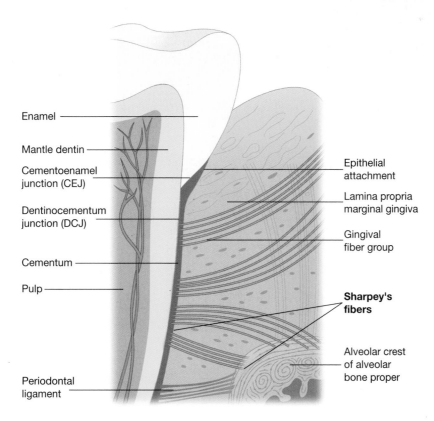

FIGURE 8-15 Section of tooth identifying Sharpey's fibers and cementum.

Clinical Concerns Regarding Cementum

■ In the case of gingival recession, the cementum may become exposed. The cementum is very thin at the cementoenamel junction (CEJ) and can quickly wear away. This exposes the dentin and causes pain.

■ Cemental spurs are found near the CEJ. During dental cleaning (scaling and curettage), the operator may find it difficult to differentiate cemental spurs from calculus. One difference is that the calculus is much easier to remove.

■ If the tooth is traumatized due to force from the occlusal or incisal surface, a condition known as hypercementosis may take place. This causes a thickening of cementum around the apex, which may show on the x-ray as a mass at the apex.

Alveolar Bone

The bones of the mandible and maxilla are formed by **osteoblasts**, bone-forming cells. The cells that remodel and resorb bone are called osteoclasts. The extended areas of bone in each arch that are tooth bearing are called the **alveolar process**. The compact bone plates on the facial and lingual surfaces are called the **cortical bone**. The bone that surrounds the root of the tooth, the socket, is the **alveolus**. On a dental radiograph, the **lamina dura**, or radiopaque line, represents the thin, compact alveolus bone lining the socket. This alveolus does not actually contact the root because the periodontal ligament suspends it in place. The two cortical bone plates come together between each tooth. This is called the **alveolar crest** and should be slightly below the CEJ

in a healthy mouth (Figure 8-16). If the tooth has multiple roots, the bone that separates the roots is identified as the **interradicular septum**. Each socket is separated by a bony projection called the **interdental septum**.

Clinical Concerns Regarding the Alveolar Bone

■ Periodontal disease can cause bone loss. The bone does not regenerate and the diseased tissue must be removed.

■ The bone is stimulated from mastication and speech. If the teeth are removed, this stimulation is lost and the bone can resorb. The bone supports the teeth and the teeth support the bone.

■ Modern implants placed in the bone are more successful if proper dental hygiene of the area is maintained. The implant has no movement in the bone; unlike teeth, it remains stable.

Periodontal Ligament

The **periodontal ligament**, like all connective tissue, is formed by the fibroblast cells and secures the tooth in the socket by a number of organized fiber groups. The Sharpey's fiber is attached in the cementum and to the alveolar bone. The periodontal ligament has two types of nerves: one sensory and one to regulate the blood vessels. This ligament is wider at the cervix (CEJ) and at the apex and narrow between these points.

Periodontal Fiber Groups. Most of the fibers in the **periodontal fiber groups** are principal fibers, meaning they are organized into bundles or groups dependent on

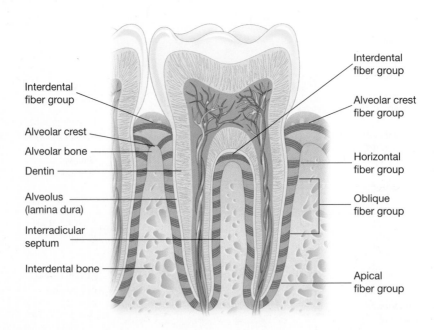

Interdental fiber group

Interdental fiber group

Alveolar crest fiber group

Alveolar crest

Alveolar bone

Dentin

Horizontal fiber group

Alveolus (lamina dura)

Oblique fiber group

Interradicular septum

Interdental bone

Apical fiber group

FIGURE 8-16 Section of a mandibular molar showing periodontal ligaments, and alveolar crest, horizontal, oblique, apical, interradicular, and interdental group fibers.

their functions. These fibers allow for some flexibility during mastication, speech, and other forces that would be exerted on the teeth. Six principal fiber groups consist of the five **alveolodental** (al-vee-oh-loh-**DENT**-al) **ligament fiber groups** and one interdental or transseptal ligament group (Figure 8-16).

The alveolodental dental ligaments include the following:

- **Alveolar crest fiber groups** function to resist rotational forces and tilting. They originate in the alveolar crest of the alveolar bone and then insert into the cervical cementum at various angles.

- **Horizontal fiber groups** function in much the same manner as the alveolar crest fiber group. They are, however, in a different area. They originate in the alveolar bone, apical to the alveolar crest, and then insert into the cementum horizontally.

- **Oblique fiber groups** constitute the most abundant of the fiber groups. Their function is to resist intrusive forces that try to push the tooth inward. The oblique fiber group covers two-thirds of the root, attaching in the alveolar bone and extending in an oblique (diagonal) manner into the cementum.

- **Apical fiber groups** function to resist forces that try to pull the tooth outward, as well as rotational forces. They attach at the apex of the tooth and radiate outward to attach in the surrounding alveolar bone.

- **Interradicular fiber groups** are found only in multirooted teeth. Their function is to resist rotational forces and to hold the teeth in interproximal contact. They run from the cementum of one root to the cementum of the other root(s), over the interradicular septum.

- **Interdental (or transseptal) ligament groups** function to resist rotational forces and hold teeth in interproximal contact. They run above the crest of the alveolar bone interdentally, from the cervical cementum of one tooth to the cervical cementum of another tooth.

Clinical Considerations Regarding the Periodontal Ligaments

- Occlusal trauma does not cause periodontal disease but can accelerate an existing disease.

- Chronic periodontal disease causes the fiber groups to become disorganized and lose attachment due to resorption.

- The fiber group that is retained the longest during periodontal disease is the interdental ligament. As the disease progresses, this ligament reattaches itself in a more apical manner.

Gingival Fiber Groups. The **gingival fiber groups** are found in the **lamina propria**, the connective tissue of the marginal gingiva (Figure 8-17). They support the mar-

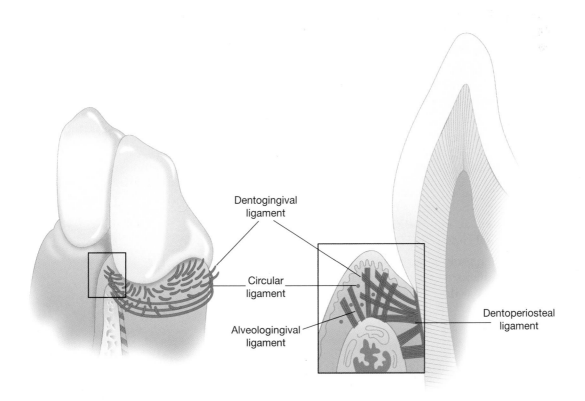

FIGURE 8-17 Gingival fiber groups: dentogingival, circular, alveologingival, and dentoperiosteal.

Dentogingival ligament

Circular ligament

Alveologingival ligament

Dentoperiosteal ligament

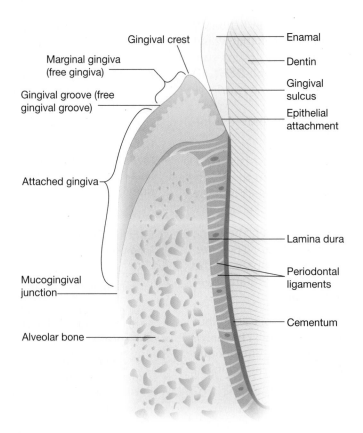

Gingival crest
Marginal gingiva (free gingiva)
Gingival groove (free gingival groove)
Attached gingiva
Mucogingival junction
Alveolar bone

Enamal
Dentin
Gingival sulcus
Epithelial attachment
Lamina dura
Periodontal ligaments
Cementum

FIGURE 8-18 Periodontium.

ginal gingival tissues in relationship to the tooth. They lie above the alveolar bone crest and below the epithelium.

- **Dentogingival fiber groups** act to maintain the gingival integrity of the marginal gingiva. They are attached to the cementum and extend into the lamina propria of the marginal gingiva.

- **Circular ligament fiber groups** circle and tighten the gingival margin around the neck of the tooth. This fiber group is in the lamina propria of the marginal gingival.

- **Alveologingival fiber groups** aid in attaching the gingiva to the alveolar bone. They extend from the alveolar bone and diffuse into the overlying lamina propria of the marginal gingiva.

- **Dentoperiosteal fiber groups** are supportive fibers that anchor the tooth to the bone. They originate from the cementum, near the CEJ, and extend across the alveolar crest.

Gingiva

The **gingiva**, composed of a mucosa that surrounds the necks of the teeth and covers the alveolar processes, is commonly called the **gums**. It can be attached to the underlying bone or unattached (free) (Figures 8-18 and 8-19). (The plural of gingiva is gingivae.) The gingival tis-

sue surrounds the teeth and, in a healthy state, is firm and tightly adapted to the tooth. The texture appears similar to the outside of an orange—**stippled**. The color of the gingiva may differ according to the pigmentation of the person.

Alveolar Mucosa. The **alveolar mucosa** appears thin and loosely attached, covering the alveolar bone.

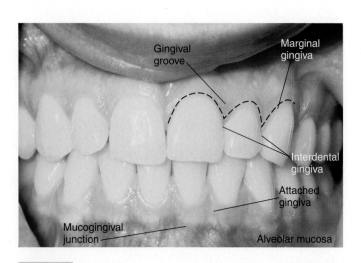

Gingival groove
Marginal gingiva
Interdental gingiva
Attached gingiva
Mucogingival junction
Alveolar mucosa

FIGURE 8-19 Periodontium identified in patient's mouth.

It flows into the tissue of the cheeks and lips and the inside floor of the mandible. It is found immediately apical to the mucogingival junction.

Mucogingival Junction. The mucogingival junction is the line of demarcation between the attached gingiva and the alveolar mucosa.

Attached Gingiva. The attached gingiva extends from the mucogingival junction to the gingival groove. The tissue is stippled and attached tightly to the alveolar bone.

Gingival Groove. The gingival groove, or free gingival groove, is the line of demarcation between the attached gingiva and the marginal gingiva.

Marginal Gingiva. The marginal gingiva, commonly called free gingiva, surrounds the teeth. This tissue, attached only at the gingival groove, appears lighter in color (if healthy) and is about one millimeter wide.

Interdental Gingiva. The interdental gingiva is an extension of unattached gingiva between adjacent teeth. It is also called interdental papilla.

Gingival Sulcus. The gingival sulcus is the space between the unattached gingiva and the tooth. In a healthy mouth, this space would not exceed two to three millimeters in depth.

Epithelial Attachment. The epithelial attachment is the gingiva in the floor of the gingival sulcus that attaches to the enamel surface of the teeth just above the CEJ of the teeth.

> **Clinical Considerations Regarding Gingival Tissue**
>
> ▪ Certain drugs can affect the gingiva and cause gingival hyperplasia, which is an overgrowth of the tissue. An example would be the drug Dilantin (trade name for phenytoin sodium), which is prescribed to treat epilepsy. These drugs cause the fibroblasts to increase output.
>
> ▪ The gingival tissue, rich in blood and fluid, can become inflamed to fight infection. It appears swollen and red, bleeds easily, and loses its stippled look. Correct hygiene measures can usually alleviate this condition.

CHAPTER SUMMARY

It is vital for the entire dental team to be able to communicate about the structure and function of the oral cavity. Therefore, it is important for the dental assistant to understand the structure/function of tissue, the prenatal growth/development process of oral embryology, and the oral cavity that surrounds the teeth.

Case Study

Joseph Tanner is a new patient at the Community Dental Clinic. He is a six-year-old with a loose primary tooth in the anterior region of the mandible. He stated that the tooth has been "wiggling" for two months. He has tried to get it out but has been unsuccessful. The dentist examines the area and documents his findings.

Case Study Review

1. Describe the process of resorption of the root of the primary tooth.

2. Identify the periodontal fibers that may remain attached around the loose tooth at this stage.

3. If the primary tooth is removed early, what possible complications may occur?

REVIEW QUESTIONS

Multiple Choice

1. The term used to identify the third prenatal phase of pregnancy from nine weeks through birth is
   a. fetus.
   b. embryo.
   c. zygote.
   d. ovum.

2. The embryonic layer that differentiates into enamel and the lining of the oral cavity is the
   a. ectoderm.
   b. mesoderm.
   c. endoderm.
   d. stomedeum.

3. Enamel-forming cells are called
   a. ameloblasts.
   b. odontoblasts.
   c. cementoblasts.
   d. fibroblasts.

4. An incremental line in the enamel indicating the trauma of birth, found in all primary teeth and several permanent teeth, is the
   a. line of Retzius.
   b. imbrication line.
   c. Tome's process.
   d. neonatal line.

5. The softest tooth structure is the
   a. alveolar bone.
   b. cementum.
   c. dentin.
   d. enamel.

6. The development of different tissues is
   a. cytodifferentiation.
   b. histodifferentiation.
   c. morphodifferentiation.
   d. proliferation.

7. The vertical groove on the midline of the upper lip is called the
   a. stomedeum.
   b. labial commissure.
   c. nasolacrimal groove.
   d. philtrum.

8. A tooth emerging from the gum is called
   a. eruption.
   b. attrition.
   c. apposition.
   d. proliferation.

9. The structure of the tooth that covers the outside of the crown is called the
   a. pulp.
   b. dentin.
   c. cementum.
   d. enamel.

10. Name the connective tissue that is formed by the fibroblast cells and secures the tooth into the socket by a number of organized fiber groups.
    a. Lamina dura
    b. Periodontal ligaments
    c. Gingiva
    d. Epithelial attachment

Critical Thinking

1. While in the hospital maternity ward, a dental assistant sees a newborn child with a severe unilateral cleft lip. Based on what the dental assistant knows about the probability of a child having this condition, what assumption would be made regarding the child's sex?

2. If a child has enamel dysplasia, a dental assistant would assume that a disturbance took place during which cycle of tooth development? Which stage?

3. If a calcified mass of dentin material is in the pulp chamber, what procedures can it inhibit? What are such masses called?

Web Activities

1. Go to http://www.operationsmile.org and read how many babies in the United States are born with cleft lips.

2. Search the Web to identify the dental specialty that would treat a child born with a cleft lip. Be prepared to discuss this in class.

3. Go to http://www.babycenter.com and compare fetal development at 4 weeks, 8 weeks, and 12 weeks.

TOOTH MORPHOLOGY

SPECIFIC INSTRUCTIONAL OBJECTIVES

The student should strive to meet the following objectives and demonstrate an understanding of the facts and principles presented in this chapter:

1. Identify the dental arches and quadrants using the correct terminology.

2. List the primary and permanent teeth by name and location.

3. Explain the eruption schedule for the primary and permanent teeth.

4. Identify the different divisions of the tooth, including clinical and anatomical divisions.

5. Identify the surfaces of each tooth and their locations.

6. List the anatomical structures and their definitions.

7. Describe each permanent tooth according to location, anatomical features, morphology, function, position, and other identifying factors.

8. Describe each deciduous (primary) tooth according to its location, anatomical features, morphology, function, position, and other identifying factors.

KEY TERMS

adjacent *(155)*

agenesis *(167)*

anatomical crown *(158)*

anatomical root *(158)*

anomaly *(167)*

apex *(162)*

apical foramen *(162)*

apical third *(160)*

bicuspid *(156)*

bifurcated *(162)*

buccal *(159)*

buccal groove *(162)*

canine *(156)*

central incisor *(156)*

cervical line *(158)*

cervical third *(160)*

cingulum *(163)*

clinical crown *(158)*

clinical root *(158)*

concave *(159)*

contact area *(160)*

convex *(159)*

crown *(158)*

cusp of Carabelli *(163)*

cusps *(156)*

deciduous *(155)*

dentition *(154)*

developmental groove *(163)*

distal *(158)*

embrasure *(160)*

exfoliated *(156)*

facial *(159)*

fissure *(164)*

fossa *(164)*

furcation *(164)*

imbrication lines *(166)*

incisal edge *(156)*

incisal third *(160)*

labial *(159)*

lateral incisor *(156)*

lingual *(159)*

lobes *(164)*

mamelons *(165)*

mandibular arch *(154)*

marginal ridges *(165)*

maxillary arch *(154)*

mesial *(158)*

midline *(155)*

mixed dentition *(156)*

molar *(156)*

(continues)

KEY TERMS *(continued)*

oblique ridge *(165)*	**ridge** *(165)*
occlusal *(159)*	**root** *(158)*
occlusal third *(160)*	**succedaneous** *(156)*
peg lateral *(167)*	**supplemental groove** *(166)*
pit *(165)*	**tooth morphology** *(154)*
posterior *(156)*	**transverse ridge** *(166)*
premolar *(156)*	**triangular ridge** *(166)*
quadrant *(155)*	**trifurcated** *(166)*

INTRODUCTION

Tooth morphology is the study of the structure and form of teeth. In this chapter, the morphology of the teeth is discussed, along with the location, eruption schedule, and function of each tooth in the primary and permanent dentition. The terms in this chapter are the building blocks of dental terminology used in the dental office.

Dental Arches

The **dentition** (natural teeth in position) are arranged in two arches. The upper arch is the **maxillary arch**, because the teeth are set in the maxilla bone. The lower teeth are located in the mandible bone, and therefore are located in the **mandibular arch** (Figure 9-1). The maxillary arch is fixed to the skull and the mandibular arch is movable, bringing the biting force toward the maxillary arch. Each arch has an identical number of teeth, and the teeth are designed so that proper function and positioning can be maintained. The teeth in the maxillary arch slightly overlap the mandibular teeth when in proper alignment. The teeth in each arch touch the

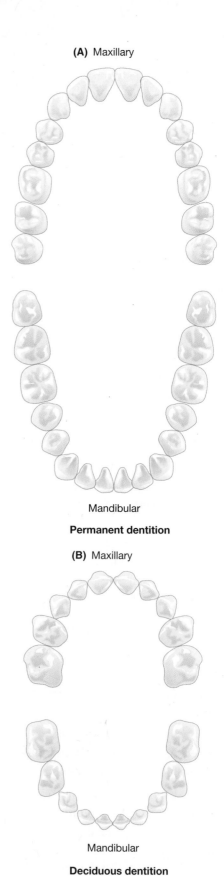

(A) Maxillary

Mandibular

Permanent dentition

(B) Maxillary

Mandibular

Deciduous dentition

FIGURE 9-1 (A) Maxillary and mandibular dentition of an adult (permanent dentition). (B) Maxillary and mandibular dentition of a child (deciduous dentition).

teeth **adjacent** (next) to them, except for the last tooth in each arch. The teeth from the maxillary arch contact the teeth from the mandibular arch each time the mouth is closed. Each tooth supports the teeth beside it and the teeth in the opposing arch so that displacement does not occur.

Dental Quadrants

Each of the dental arches is divided in two halves by an imaginary line called the **midline** (median line), which creates two sections called **quadrants** (one-fourth of the dental arches). Thus, there are four quadrants, containing eight permanent teeth each, found in the dentition. The arrangement of the teeth is identical in each quadrant, and each quadrant is named according to its location in the dentition (Figure 9-2).

The quadrants are labeled according to the patient's right or left. Looking into the oral cavity from the front of the patient makes the directions of right and left reversed to the dental assistant.

The dentition can also be divided into sextants, or sixths. There are two posterior sextants and one anterior sextant in each arch. The anterior sextant is comprised of the six front teeth (Figure 9-3).

Types of Teeth and Their Functions

Humans grow two sets of teeth: primary and permanent. The primary teeth erupt first and are replaced by permanent teeth between the ages of six to seventeen.

Primary Teeth

The primary (**deciduous** [di-**SI**-jeh-wus]) teeth in each quadrant are named similar to the permanent teeth. The deciduous (i.e., first) dentition consists of twenty teeth: ten in each arch and five in each quadrant. The follow-

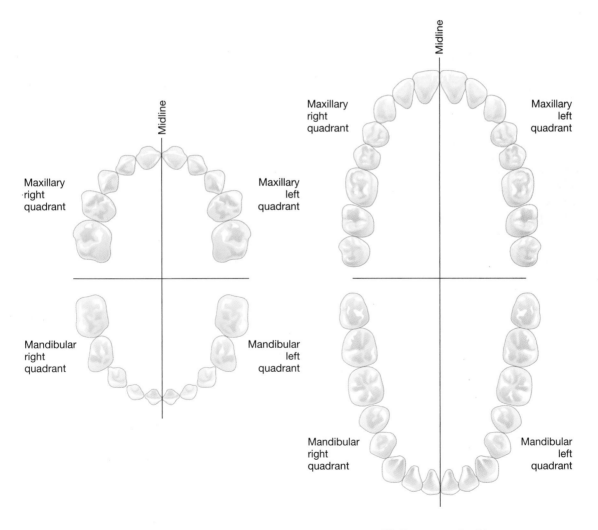

(A) Primary dentition

(B) Permanent dentition

FIGURE 9-2 Dental arches of (A) primary (deciduous) dentition and (B) permanent dentition divided into quadrants with the midline identified.

Anterior sextant

Right posterior sextant

Left posterior sextant

Maxillary

Right posterior sextant

Left posterior sextant

Mandibular

Anterior sextant

FIGURE 9-3 Permanent dentition divided into sextants. The maxillary and mandibular arches each have two posterior sextants and one anterior sextant.

ing teeth are found in each quadrant. Starting from the midline, the first tooth is called the **central incisor** and is used to cut or bite the food that is ingested. The second tooth from the midline, the **lateral incisor**, is also used for cutting. The third tooth from the midline is the **canine** (cuspid). This tooth is slightly more bulky in size and aids in tearing food. The next two teeth are molars and are named the first molar, which is the one closest to the midline, and the second molar. **Molars** are used to chew food.

> Both the first and the second primary teeth from the midline are incisors; to incise something is to cut it.

When compared to the permanent, the deciduous dentition contains an identical number of central incisors, lateral incisors, and canines, but has no premolars and one less molar per quadrant (Figure 9-4).

Permanent Teeth

Permanent teeth are arranged similarly to the deciduous teeth. Adults have thirty-two permanent teeth: sixteen in each arch and eight in each quadrant. Each quadrant has the permanent central incisor, the lateral incisor, and the canine (cuspid), as did the deciduous quadrant. Directly after the canine (cuspid) in the permanent dentition are the first and second **premolars**.

The premolars are often called **bicuspids** because they usually have two (bi) **cusps** (pointed or rounded mounds on the crown of the tooth). However, two of the eight bicuspids may have three cusps; therefore, the term is not technically correct. However, it is important to be aware of the names commonly used for the same teeth (for example, canines or cuspids and premolars or bicuspids).

The premolars are used to pulverize food. In other words, the premolars break the food down into smaller sizes to ready them for the chewing process, which is done by the molars.

After the premolars, the permanent dentition has the first, second, and third molars. The first molars are closest to the midline and the third molars, farthest from the midline, are commonly termed the "wisdom teeth."

The teeth in either arch that are toward the front of the mouth from cuspid to cuspid are the anterior teeth. The central incisors, lateral incisors, and canines (cuspids) are termed anterior teeth for both the deciduous and permanent dentition. Anterior teeth have single roots and a cutting or tearing edge called the **incisal edge**.

The teeth in either arch that are located in the back of the mouth are termed **posterior** teeth. The molars are posterior teeth in the deciduous dentition, and the premolars (bicuspids) and molars are posterior teeth in the permanent dentition. Posterior teeth normally have more than one root and multiple cusps for pulverizing and chewing.

Eruption Schedule

The primary dentition (deciduous teeth) begins eruption (emerges into the oral cavity) around six months of age. All twenty teeth are normally erupted by the age of three years (Table 9-1). The period when both primary teeth and permanent teeth are in the dentition is called the **mixed dentition** period (Figure 9-5). This period lasts from approximately six to twelve years of age. After the age of twelve, most of the primary teeth have **exfoliated** (shed from the oral cavity). The permanent dentition begins to erupt from about six years of age until around seventeen to twenty-one years of age (Table 9-2).

The permanent teeth that replace the primary teeth are called **succedaneous** teeth (Figure 9-6). The term refers to succeeding the deciduous teeth. Therefore, because there are twenty primary teeth, there are also

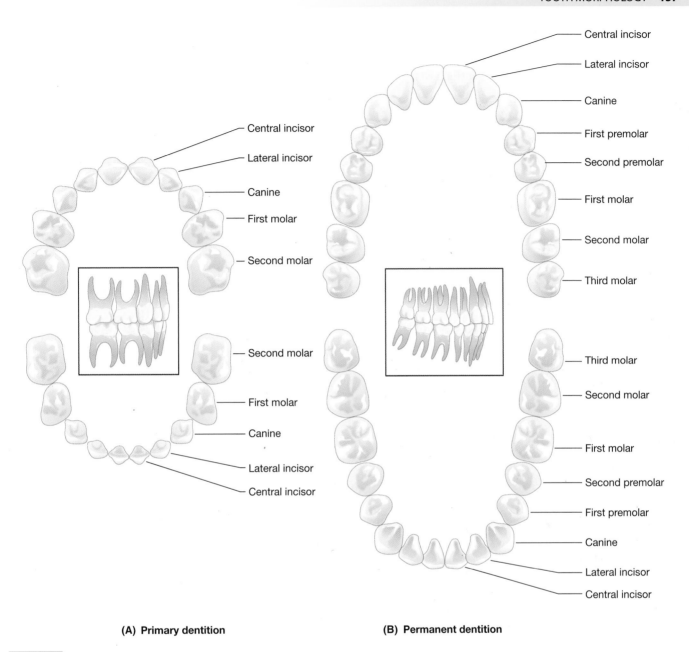

(A) Primary dentition   **(B) Permanent dentition**

FIGURE 9-4 (A) Deciduous dentition, identifying each tooth by name. (B) Permanent dentition, identifying each tooth by name.

TABLE 9-1   Eruption and Exfoliation Dates for Primary Teeth

Tooth	Eruption Date (Months)	Exfoliation Date (Years)	Maxillary Order
Central incisor	6–10	6–7	#1
Lateral incisor	9–12	7–8	#2
Canine	16–22	10–12	#4
First molar	12–18	9–11	#3
Second molar	24–32	10–12	#5

(continues)

TABLE 9-1 Eruption and Exfoliation Dates for Primary Teeth *(continued)*

Tooth	Eruption Date (Months)	Exfoliation Date (Years)	Mandibular Order
Central incisor	6–10	6–7	#1
Lateral incisor	7–10	7–8	#2
Canine	16–22	9–12	#4
First molar	12–18	9–11	#3
Second molar	20–32	10–12	#5

FIGURE 9-5 Mixed dentition of a seven- or eight-year-old.

FIGURE 9-6 Dentition of a five-year-old. Unerupted succedaneous teeth are shaded.

twenty succedaneous teeth. The only permanent teeth that are not succedaneous are the molars, because the premolars replace the primary molars.

Divisions of the Tooth

Each tooth has two basic parts: the **crown** and the **root**. The crown of the tooth is described as either anatomical or clinical (Figure 9-7). The **anatomical crown** is the portion of the tooth that is covered with enamel. The **clinical crown** is the portion of the crown that is visible in the mouth. The clinical crown may be smaller than the anatomical crown if the gingiva covers a portion of the crown (for example, during tooth eruption). The root of the tooth is also divided into anatomical and clinical portions. The **anatomical root** is the portion covered with cementum, and the **clinical root** is the portion

of the root seen in the oral cavity (for example, where the gingiva has receded). The **cervical line** divides the crown and the root; the anatomical crown and the root join together here as well. (Cervical comes from the word *cervix,* meaning "the neck of.") The cervical line is also termed the cementoenamel junction (CEJ).

Surfaces of the Teeth

All teeth have five surfaces on the crown portion. Each surface, or side, has a specific name (Figure 9-8).

Anterior Teeth

- **Mesial**—Surface toward the midline
- **Distal**—Surface away from the midline

TABLE 9-2 Eruption Dates for the Maxillary and Mandibular Permanent Teeth

Tooth	Eruption Date (Years)	Order of Eruption (Maxillary)
Central incisor	7–8	#2
Lateral incisor	8–9	#3
Canine	11–12	#6
First premolar	10–11	#4
Second premolar	11–12	#5
First molar	6–7	#1
Second molar	12–13	#7
Third molar	17–21	#8

Tooth	Eruption Date (Years)	Order of Eruption (Mandibular)
Central incisor	6–7	#2
Lateral incisor	7–8	#3
Cuspid	9–10	#4
First premolar	10–11	#5
Second premolar	11–12	#6
First molar	6–7	#1
Second molar	11–13	#7
Third molar	17–21	#8

- **Labial**—"Outside" surface, which is toward the lips
- **Lingual**—"Inside" surface, which is toward the tongue. On the maxillary arch, the lingual side may be referred to as the palatal surface
- **Incisal edge**—The biting or cutting edge

Facial Surface

The term facial may be used for either the labial surface of the anterior teeth or the buccal surface of the posterior teeth.

Posterior Teeth

- **Mesial**—Surface toward the midline
- **Distal**—Surface away from the midline

- **Lingual**—"Inside" surface, which is toward the tongue
- **Buccal**—"Outside" surface, which is toward the cheek
- **Occlusal**—Pulverizing or chewing surface

All of the above tooth surfaces are flat, convex, or concave (Figure 9-9). **Convex** means to bulge or curve outward, and **concave** means recessed or indented. (A memory cue is to think of a "cave" in concave; a cave is hollow and not bulging outward.)

Teeth surfaces are further identified by dividing them into approximate thirds. This practice helps dental staff in identifying specific areas on each surface. Also identified are the space between the teeth and where the teeth are touching.

The crown of the tooth and the root of the tooth are divided in approximate thirds (Figure 9-10). The area on

FIGURE 9-7 Clinical crown.

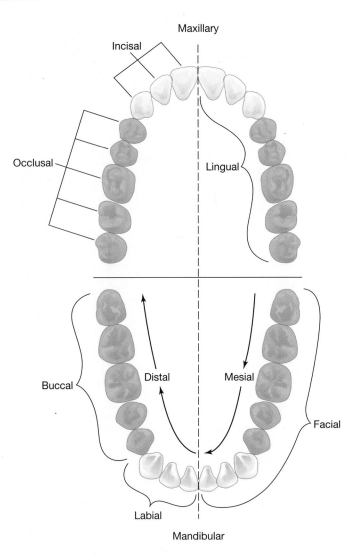

Permanent dentition

FIGURE 9-8 Surfaces of the teeth identified on the dental arches. Posterior teeth colored in blue.

the crown of the tooth that is nearest the incisal edge on the anterior tooth is called the **incisal third** of the tooth, and the occlusal surface of the posterior tooth is called the **occlusal third** of the tooth. The area on the crown of the tooth that is closest to the cervical area (or to the gingiva) is called the cervical third of the tooth. The area between the incisal third and the **cervical third** is called the middle third. The root is also divided into imaginary thirds with the area nearest the apex as the **apical third** and the area nearest the crown of the tooth as the cervical third of the root. The area between the apical third of the root and the cervical third of the root is called the middle third of the root.

Identifying these areas allows the dentist to give clearer information about a tooth. For instance, if the dentist is describing the shade of the tooth to the dental laboratory technician, the dentist can say that the incisal third is a lighter shade and the cervical third is a darker shade. This information enables better color matching, thereby preventing creation of a single-color tooth. Another example is when the dentist describes a lesion on the root of the tooth, noting that it is on the apical third of the root. These terms also facilitate better diagnosis through greater specificity in identifying location on the root. All such terms are used frequently in the dental office to identify a specific area of the tooth.

Contact

Identifying the **contact area** (Figure 9-11) on the tooth refers to where the proximal sides of two teeth come together and touch. This is normally the mesial of one tooth, and the distal of another tooth, except where the two central incisors come together in each arch. This area is generally in the middle third of the tooth, and also the area that dental floss tends to snap through. Such contact holds teeth in place so that they do not drift and shift around. It should also be noted that food impaction is common in places where teeth do not contact. Good contact areas protect the gingiva from trauma during mastication (chewing food).

Embrasure

The **embrasure** (im-*bray*-zhur) (Figure 9-11) is the triangular space in the gingival direction when two adjacent teeth are in contact. When discussing flossing with

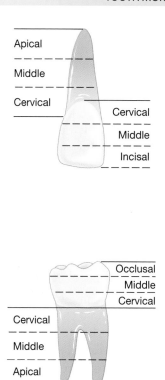

FIGURE 9-9 Concave and convex surfaces of the mandibular incisor.

FIGURE 9-10 Crown and root of tooth divided into approximate thirds.

FIGURE 9-11 Contact area and embrasure shown on two adjoining teeth.

patients, the dental assistant will show the patient how to hold the floss and guide it through the contact area and make a half circle and wrap the floss tightly around the tooth as it goes down the embrasure toward the gingival sulcus of the tooth. The floss is then wrapped around the proximal tooth on the other side of the embrasure, and this area is cleaned with the dental floss as well. The embrasure allows the dental papilla to remain healthy.

Anatomical Structures

It is important to be able to identify landmarks on each individual tooth. Each area's name should be used when identifying the anatomical structures.

- **Apex**—At or near the end of the root (Figure 9-12).
- **Apical foramen**—Opening in the end of the tooth through which nerve and blood vessels enter (Figure 9-12). There may be more than one opening at the end of the root.
- **Bifurcated**—When there are two roots on one tooth, they are said to be bifurcated, or branched in two (*bi* means two and *furca* means fork) (Figure 9-13).
- **Buccal groove**—Linear depression forming a groove that extends from the middle of the buccal surface to the occlusal surface of the tooth (Figure 9-14).

Bifurcated roots

FIGURE 9-13 Mandibular molar showing bifurcated roots.

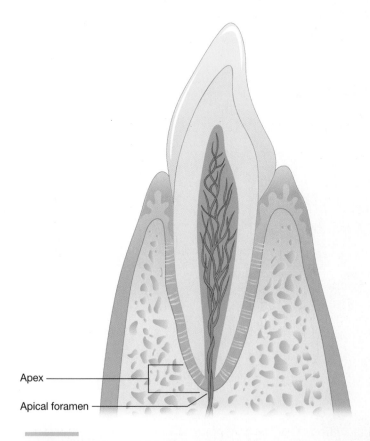

Apex

Apical foramen

FIGURE 9-12 Apex and apical foramen of a tooth.

Buccal groove

Mesial

Distal

FIGURE 9-14 Mandibular molar with buccal groove identified.

■ **Cingulum**—Convex area on the lingual surface of the anterior teeth, near the gingiva (Figure 9-15).

■ **Cusp**—Pointed or rounded mound on the crown of the tooth (Figure 9-16).

■ **Cusp of Carabelli**—Fifth cusp located on the mesial lingual surface of most maxillary first molars (Fig-

ure 9-17). (The name comes from the man who first described it.)

■ **Developmental groove**—Groove formed by the uniting of lobes during development of the crown of the tooth (Figure 9-18).

FIGURE 9-15 Lingual surface of a central incisor with the cingulum shaded.

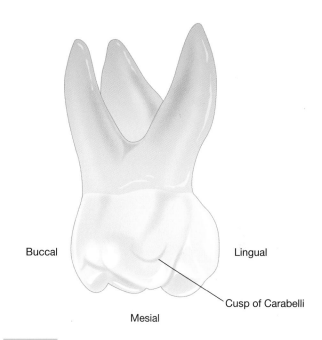

FIGURE 9-17 Maxillary first molar showing the mesial lingual side with the cusp of Carabelli identified.

FIGURE 9-16 Maxillary second premolar with the cusps identified.

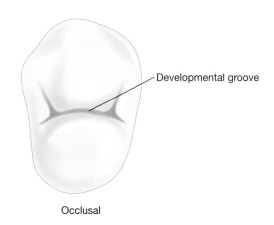

FIGURE 9-18 Developmental groove on the occlusal surface of the maxillary first premolar where lobes were united.

■ **Fissure**—Developmental groove resulting from an imperfect union where the lobes come together (Figure 9-19). Decay often initiates in the fissure.

■ **Fossa**—A shallow rounded or angular depression (Figure 9-20).

■ **Furcation**—Dividing point of a multirooted tooth (Figure 9-21).

■ **Lobes**—Separate parts that come together to form a tooth (Figure 9-22). In the molars, the lobes often become cusps.

Fissure

FIGURE 9-19 Mandibular second premolar showing the imperfect union or fissure on the occlusal surface.

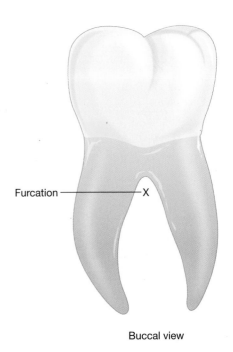

Furcation —————X

Buccal view

FIGURE 9-21 Mandibular first molar from the buccal side showing the furcation or dividing area where the roots fork off.

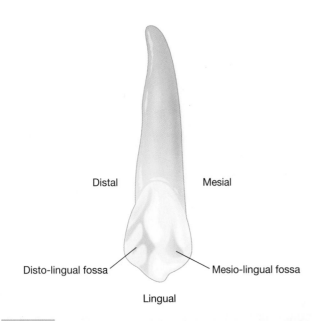

Distal   Mesial

Disto-lingual fossa   Mesio-lingual fossa

Lingual

FIGURE 9-20 Lingual view of a maxillary canine with the mesio lingual fossa and disto lingual fossa shaded.

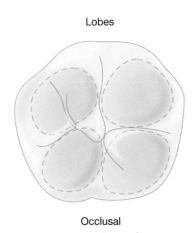

Lobes

Occlusal

FIGURE 9-22 Occlusal view of the maxillary first molar showing the lobes and how they come together.

- **Mamelons**—Three bulges on the incisal edge of the newly erupted central incisor (Figure 9-23). Mamelons normally disappear from normal wear.

- **Marginal ridges**—Elevated area of enamel that forms the mesial and distal borders of the lingual surface of the anterior teeth and the mesial and distal borders of the occlusal surface of the posterior teeth (Figure 9-24).

- **Oblique ridge**—Elevated area of enamel that extends obliquely across the occlusal of the tooth (Figure 9-25). On the maxillary first molars, the oblique ridge extends from the disto-buccal cusp to the mesio-lingual cusp.

- **Pit**—Place where the grooves come together or the fissures cross (Figure 9-26). Decay often begins in the pit.

- **Ridge**—Linear elevation of enamel found on the tooth (Figure 9-27).

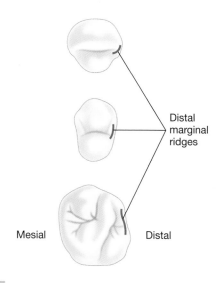

FIGURE 9-24 Marginal ridges of the maxillary central, premolar, and molar.

FIGURE 9-25 Maxillary first molar with the oblique ridge identified.

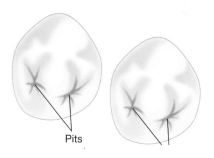

FIGURE 9-26 Permanent mandibular first premolar showing the occlusal view with pits identified.

FIGURE 9-23 (A) Newly erupted maxillary incisor showing the three bulges on the incisal edge, called mamelons. (B) Mamelons shown on the anterior of the maxillary dentition.

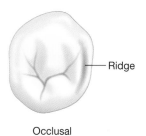

FIGURE 9-27 Ridge identified on the occlusal surface of the mandibular second premolar.

- **Supplemental groove**—Shallow, linear groove that radiates from the developmental groove (Figure 9-28). It often gives the tooth surface a wrinkled look. These grooves do not denote major divisions of the tooth.

- **Transverse ridge**—Union of two triangular ridges that produces a single ridge of elevation across the occlusal surface of a posterior tooth (Figure 9-29).

- **Triangular ridge**—Ridge or an elevation that descends from the cusp and widens as it runs down to the middle area of the occlusal surface (Figure 9-30).

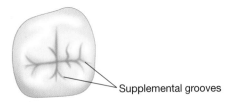

Supplemental grooves

FIGURE 9-28 Occlusal surface of the mandibular second molar showing shallow linear grooves, which are called supplemental grooves.

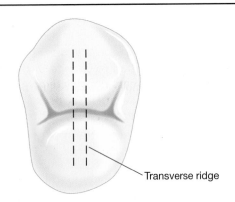

Transverse ridge

FIGURE 9-29 Maxillary right first premolar occlusal view showing transverse ridge.

Buccal

Lingual

FIGURE 9-30 Triangular ridge identified on occlusal surface of a maxillary second premolar.

Trifurcated roots

FIGURE 9-31 Maxillary first molar, buccal surface, showing the roots as trifurcated (three roots forked off from the main trunk).

- **Trifurcated**—Three roots (*tri* means three) coming from the main trunk of the tooth (Figure 9-31).

Permanent Teeth

Each type of tooth in the permanent dentition serves a specific function, and the size and shape of the tooth are related to that function. A working knowledge of each type of tooth is useful for the dental assistant.

Maxillary Central Incisor

The maxillary central incisor is the first tooth closest to the midline (Figure 9-32). These teeth, along with the lateral incisors, play an important part in a person's appearance. Their shape, color, size, and placement directly relate to how a person looks. The position of the teeth dictates the shape of a person's profile. Normal placement will provide for correct support of the face and lips. The incisors also play an important role in speech. To execute specific sounds, such as *S*s and *T*s, these teeth are necessary. Additionally, the incisors have a unique incisal edge that differs greatly from the other teeth in the mouth, which all have cusps. The ridge allows for cutting food into smaller particles.

The maxillary central incisor erupts with three bumps on the incisal edge, called mamelons (Figure 9-23). They derive from the three developing lobes coming together. The mamelons become flattened due to attrition (wear), and the incisal edge becomes a flattened surface as well. At the gingival area of the crown on the labial surface, small curved lines run parallel to the CEJ. These are called **imbrication lines** (Figure 9-33). Most central incisors have imbrication lines.

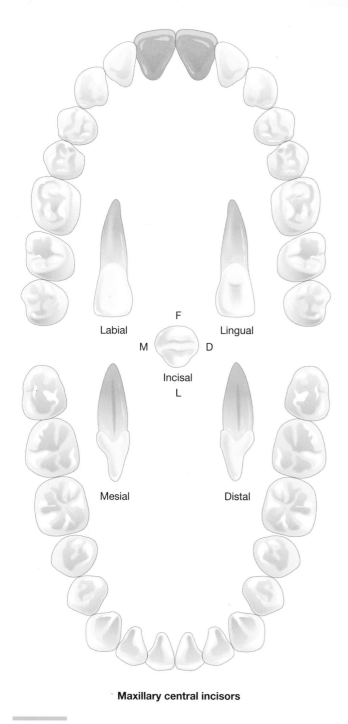

Labial   Lingual

F

M   D

L

Incisal

Mesial   Distal

Maxillary central incisors

FIGURE 9-32 Permanent dentition with the maxillary central incisors identified and maxillary central incisor viewed from the five surfaces.

The crown of the maxillary central incisor is the longest of any of the maxillary teeth. The labial surface is convex, both mesial to distal and gingival to incisal. The lingual surface is concave, except the gingival one-third where the cingulum is present. The cingulum spreads toward the mesial and distal in an arch pattern, forming the mesial and distal marginal ridges. The mesial surface is slightly longer than the distal surface. The mesial-incisal angle is rather acute, at about a ninety-degree

Imbrication lines

Developmental depression

Mamelons

FIGURE 9-33 Labial surface of the maxillary right central incisor with the mamelons, developmental depressions, and imbrication lines identified.

angle, and the distal-incisal angle is more rounded. The root is about one and a half to two times the length of the crown. The root appears constricted at the CEJ and then swells in the body, tapering suddenly at the apical portion. Therefore, it ends in a rather blunt apex. The root tends to incline slightly distally.

Maxillary Lateral Incisor

The maxillary lateral incisor is the second tooth from the midline and the smallest in the maxillary arch (Figure 9-34). It initially contacts the central incisor on the mesial and the primary canine (cuspid) on the distal. It resembles the maxillary central in most ways. The difference is primarily its size, the crown being about three-tenths smaller in all directions. The root also is smaller in all directions; however, the length has been known to be similar to that of the maxillary central. The crown of the lateral incisor appears narrower than the central, especially in females. The distal-incisal angle is more rounded than that of the central incisor, making the distal length much shorter than the mesial length.

Except for the third molars, the maxillary lateral is the tooth with the most **anomalies** (extreme variations from the norm). The most frequent is the **peg lateral**. This is a diminutive, peg-shaped crown with a smooth surface lacking contact on the mesial and distal surfaces. Maxillary laterals are sometimes congenitally missing. **Agenesis** occurs when the tooth buds do not form. Roots that are curved in unusual ways and distorted crowns may appear. Many of these deviations appear generation after generation.

Maxillary lateral incisors

FIGURE 9-34 Permanent dentition with maxillary lateral incisors identified and maxillary lateral incisor viewed from the five surfaces.

Maxillary canines (cuspids)

FIGURE 9-35 Permanent dentition with maxillary canines (cuspids) identified and maxillary canine viewed from the five surfaces.

Maxillary Canine (Cuspid)

The canine is often called the "cornerstone of the mouth" due to its placement, which is between the incisors and the bicuspids (Figure 9-35). It is the one tooth that turns the corner for the arch. The canine's purpose is to tear the food, which is much different from the incisors, which bite or cut the food, and the premolars and molars, which chew or grind it.

The canine (cuspid) is one of the most important teeth for animals, because it tears the food. This term, derived from the Latin term for dog, has carried over to humans.

The canine (cuspid) is the third tooth from the midline. Because of its placement and size, it is extremely important in supporting the muscles of the face. Therefore, the canine contributes to a person's appearance.

The root is the longest in the maxillary arch and therefore the most stable. The crown of the canine is convex on the facial surface, with a ridge running vertically. The incisal edge is fairly pointed and is off center, slightly toward the mesial (the name *cuspid* is derived from the long cusp that ends in a point on the incisal edge). The mesial surface of the canine (cuspid) is longer than the distal surface, and as they both turn toward the incisal edge, the angle is more rounded than that of the incisors. The lingual surface has two concave fossas, one toward the mesial and the other toward the distal, with a lingual ridge dividing them in the middle. On the outer sides of the fossa is a distal marginal ridge and a mesial marginal ridge. On the lingual side of the tooth, toward the gingiva, is a cingulum. The canine appears darker than the incisors because of the bulk of dentin.

Premolar (Bicuspid)

There are eight premolars: four in each arch, two in each quadrant. They are named first and second premolars because of their positions from the midline. The first premolars, closest to the midline, line up in the fourth position. The second premolars line up in the fifth position from the midline. They are transitional teeth, placed between the cuspids and the molars. They look like the canines (cuspids) from the facial side; in fact, the buccal cusp functions much like a cuspid in tearing food, but the transitional teeth have an additional cusp on the lingual side (hence "bicuspids," meaning two). The additional cusp aids in further breaking down the food or pulverizing it for the molars to chew. These posterior teeth are not as critical in personal appearance because of their placement. They do not always show when smiling or talking.

Maxillary First Premolar (Bicuspid)

The facial cusp of the maxillary first premolar is much larger than the lingual cusp (Figure 9-36). It is longer and wider and appears much like the cuspid from the facial. The cusps come together on the occlusal surface in a central groove. This central groove extends to the mesial and distal grooves. The mesial groove is bordered by the mesial marginal ridges, and the distal groove is bordered by the distal marginal ridge. The maxillary first premolar has a bifurcated root (two roots, one buccal and one lingual) that is slightly separated. Some first premolars have roots that are fused together; thus, one root has two canals. The roots have a depression on the mesial and distal sides running from the CEJ to the root bifurcation. The roots are shorter and resemble the roots of the molars in this aspect more than they do the roots of the cuspid.

This premolar is often considered for removal if the patient's teeth are overcrowded and orthodontic treatment is needed. The position allows for movement from both anterior and posterior teeth. The orthodontist closes the space and the patient's facial appearance

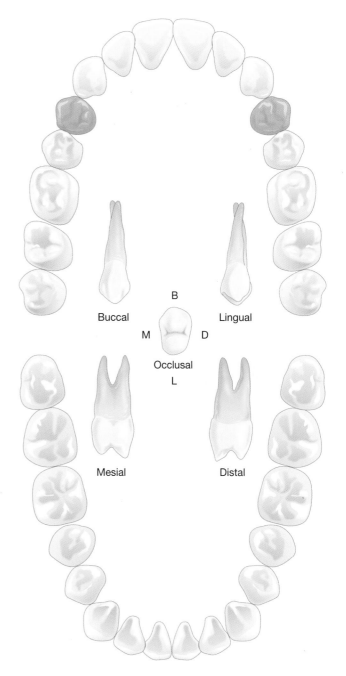

Maxillary first premolars (bicuspids)

FIGURE 9-36 Permanent dentition with maxillary first premolars (bicuspids) identified and maxillary first premolar viewed from the five surfaces.

is not changed by the removal of this tooth. Also, the depression in the root structure makes it more susceptible to periodontal disease; therefore, it is a better choice for removal than the second premolar.

Maxillary Second Premolar (Bicuspid)

The maxillary second premolar resembles the first in all but the following variations (Figure 9-37). The cusps, one on the buccal and one on the lingual, are more

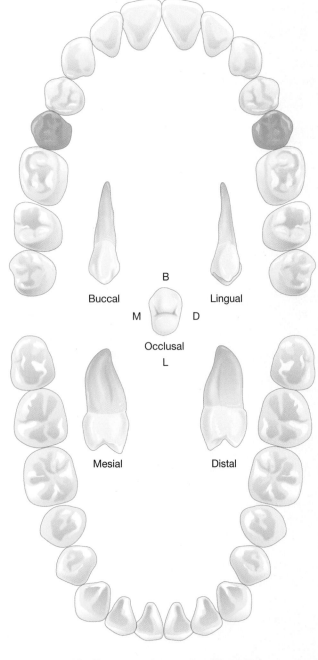

Buccal

B

M   D

Lingual

Occlusal

L

Mesial

Distal

Maxillary second premolars (bicuspids)

FIGURE 9-37 Permanent dentition with maxillary second premolars (bicuspids) identified and maxillary second premolar viewed from the five surfaces.

equal in length. The lingual cusp is slightly shorter but not as short as the cusp on the maxillary first bicuspid. The mesial buccal cusp slope is shorter than the distal buccal cusp slope. There is only one root and therefore only one root canal. There is a slight depression on the mesial root, but it is very shallow. The crowns of both the first and second bicuspids are wider bucco-lingually than mesio-distally. The second bicuspid is slightly more narrow mesial-distally than the first premolar.

Maxillary Molar

The word molar is derived from the Latin word *molaris,* referring to a millstone. This seems like an appropriate term for the teeth that chew, grind, or break down the food into tiny particles for swallowing. When normal eruption occurs, the molars are the first and last permanent teeth in the mouth. There are twelve molars in the oral cavity: six in each arch and three in each quadrant. They are called the first, second, and third molars because of their placement from the midline. The first molar is the closest to the midline. The molars are the strongest teeth in the arch due to the size of their crowns and the shape and size of their roots. The first molar is the largest and the strongest; this decreases toward the posterior, leaving the third molar the weakest and smallest of the molars. Just as the cuspids are considered the cornerstones of the anterior teeth, the first molars are considered the cornerstones of the developing occlusion in the posterior teeth. The molars do not replace any primary teeth and therefore are not succedaneous teeth. They erupt posterior to the deciduous dentition.

Maxillary First Molar

The maxillary first molar is often referred to as the "six-year molar" because of its eruption time (Figure 9-38). Often, parents do not realize that this is a permanent tooth because of its early eruption. The crown of the maxillary first molar appears square in shape with four primary cusps present: mesio-buccal, disto-buccal, mesio-lingual, and disto-lingual. There is a fifth cusp, the cusp of Carabelli, located on the largest cusp, the meso-lingual. This cusp is located about one-third the way down from the occlusal surface and appears as a "mini" cusp. The prominence of this cusp varies from tooth to tooth.

The mesio-buccal and the disto-buccal cusps are divided by a buccal groove that extends about half the length of the crown and ends in a depression often called the buccal pit. The lingual cusps are slightly longer than the buccal cusps. The mesio-lingual cusp and the disto-lingual cusp are also divided by a lingual groove that travels about halfway down the crown on the lingual side, ending in a shallow depression called the lingual pit.

The root of the maxillary first molar is trifurcated. The first two roots, a meso-buccal root and a distal-buccal root, are placed on the buccal side. These buccal roots curve slightly toward each other. The third root is the largest and longest and is located on the lingual side. These three roots are spread out from each other and normally have one canal each.

On the occlusal surface of the maxillary first molars, the four primary cusps come together in a central fossa. There is an oblique (diagonal) ridge running across the occlusal surface that unites the distal cusp ridge of the mesio-lingual cusp and the

Maxillary Second Molar

The second molar is called the "twelve-year molar" because of the time of eruption (Figure 9-39). It is similar to the first molar in many ways; however, it is smaller both in size of the crown and size of the root. The crown of the maxillary second molar has four cusps (no cusp of Carabelli). The cusps are located mesio-buccal, disto-buccal, mesio-lingual, and disto-lingual. The surface of

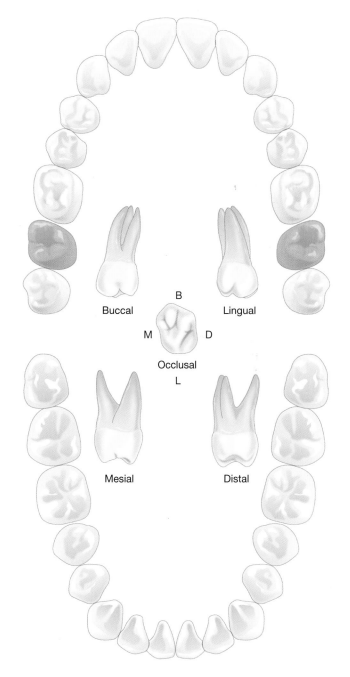

Maxillary second molars

FIGURE 9-39 Permanent dentition with maxillary second molars identified and maxillary second molar viewed from the five surfaces.

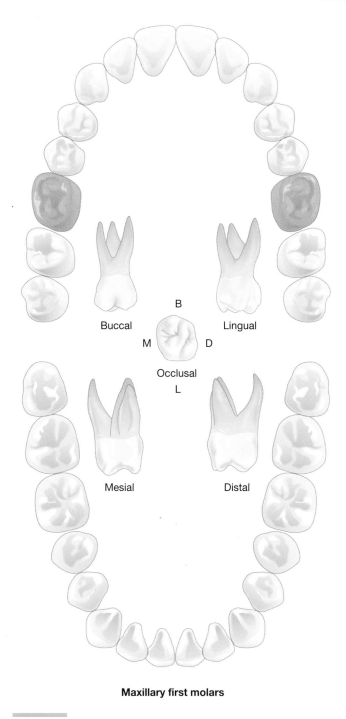

Maxillary first molars

FIGURE 9-38 Permanent dentition with maxillary first molars identified and maxillary first molars viewed from the five surfaces.

lingual cusp ridge of the disto-buccal cusp. Another ridge, a transverse ridge, runs from the buccal cusp of the mesio-lingual cusp to the lingual cusp ridge of the mesio-buccal cusp. The occlusal surface also has a mesial ridge on the mesial of the occlusal surface and a distal ridge on the distal occlusal surface. This creates a surface with additional grooves and ridges to properly grind food.

the mesial of the tooth is greater across than the distal surface. The occlusal surface of the molars tapers down in size from the first molar toward the third molar.

The occlusal surface, although smaller, is much like that of the first molar. It has more supplementary grooves than the first molar, making it more wrinkled in appearance. The roots are the same in number but smaller in size and not as spread apart as the roots of the first molar. Each root has one canal, as in the maxillary first molar.

Maxillary Third Molar

Developmental variations make it impossible to describe exactly what the third molar looks like. The maxillary third molar is called the "wisdom tooth" because it was thought that by the time these teeth erupted into the oral cavity a person would have obtained maturity or wisdom (Figure 9-40). Many people do not develop third molars. If third molars do develop, they may not erupt into the oral cavity because of lack of space in the posterior of the arches. This is the one tooth that, after careful diagnosis, the dentist may recommend be removed.

When the tooth erupts normally, it resembles the second molar, only slightly smaller. It exhibits a more wrinkled appearance on the occlusal surface because many more supplemental grooves are usually present. The roots are normally fused together and vary in number.

Mandibular Central Incisor

The mandibular central incisor is the least variable tooth in the mouth (Figure 9-41). It is also the smallest tooth in the dentition. It is smaller than the mandibular lateral, which is not the case in the maxillary arch. The maxillary central incisor is larger than the maxillary lateral incisor.

When the mandibular central incisor erupts, it has three mamelons on the incisal edge. These wear off, leaving a fairly straight incisal edge for cutting. The crown of the mandibular incisor has a labial surface that is convex but does not appear to have the developmental depressions and imbrication lines of the maxillary central. The crown is narrow and the incisal angle makes a sharp ninety-degree angle as it extends down the mesial and distal surfaces. The lingual is concave and has a cingulum near the gingiva. It is relatively smooth, and the structures are not as prominent as in maxillary centrals. The root is straight and ends abruptly at the apex.

This tooth is the first from the midline; therefore, the mesial surface of each central incisor contacts its counterpart. The distal surface contacts the lateral in its prospective quadrant.

Mandibular Lateral Incisor

The anatomy of the mandibular lateral incisor so closely resembles that of the central incisor that a detailed

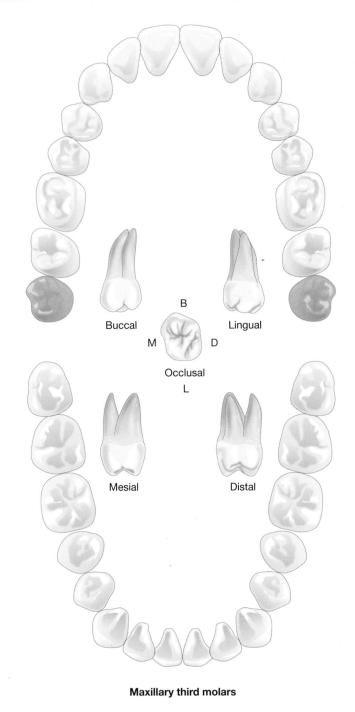

Buccal   B   **Lingual**

M   D

Occlusal

L

Mesial   **Distal**

Maxillary third molars

FIGURE 9-40 Permanent dentition with maxillary third molars identified and maxillary third molars viewed from the five surfaces.

description is unnecessary (Figure 9-42). The mandibular incisor is slightly larger. The root is also larger and slightly longer. Concavities may be present on the mesial and distal of the root. If these occur, the mesial concavity is shallower.

The crown of the lateral incisor is shaped the same as the central incisor except that the distal surface is not as long. The incisal distal angle is more rounded to accommodate this change in length. This tooth does

Mandibular central incisors

Mandibular lateral incisors

FIGURE 9-41 Permanent dentition with mandibular central incisors identified and mandibular central incisor viewed from the five surfaces.

FIGURE 9-42 Permanent dentition with mandibular lateral incisors identified and mandibular lateral incisor viewed from the five surfaces.

not have the developmental abnormalities of the maxillary lateral.

Mandibular Canine (Cuspid)

The mandibular canine is the third tooth from the midline (Figure 9-43). It resembles the maxillary canine but is not as well developed. The crown of the tooth is approximately the same length as the maxillary canine,

but the root is generally shorter (the root is still longer than the mandibular central and lateral roots). The cusp of the mandibular canine is not as well developed as the maxillary and not as sharp on the tip. The function, however, is the same: Both are designed to tear food.

The distal cusp slope is longer than the mesial cusp slope. The cingulum and marginal ridges are not as pronounced as on the maxillary canine, and the pronounced buccal ridge helps give shape to the face.

Mandibular canines (cuspids)

FIGURE 9-43 Permanent dentition with mandibular canines (cuspids) identified and mandibular canine viewed from the five surfaces.

Mandibular first premolars (bicuspids)

FIGURE 9-44 Permanent dentition with mandibular first premolars (bicuspids) identified and mandibular first premolar viewed from the five surfaces.

The canine is the longest tooth in the mandibular arch. The single root provides for stability; it is the cornerstone of the mandibular arch. The root, with one canal, has deep depressions on both the mesial and distal surfaces.

Mandibular First Premolar (Bicuspid)

The mandibular first premolar is much more of a transitional tooth than the maxillary first premolar (Figure 9-44). It does not resemble the mandibular second pre-

molar as much as the maxillary first premolar resembles the maxillary second premolar. It looks much more like the mandibular canine: It has two cusps, one buccal and one lingual. The lingual cusp is often nonfunctioning; therefore, the shape is much like the canine. The buccal cusp is larger in all directions and its convex surface is more pronounced. The mesial cusp slope is shorter than the distal cusp slope.

The occlusal surface has both the mesial and distal ridges and, as the buccal and lingual cusps incline toward the occlusal groove, a transverse ridge crosses the tooth.

The single straight root of the mandibular first premolar is slightly shorter than the mandibular second premolar and a great deal shorter than the root of the mandibular canine. It sometimes bifurcates slightly at the apex.

Mandibular Second Premolar (Bicuspid)

The buccal surface of the mandibular second premolar resembles the mandibular first premolar except it is not as long and it is wider (Figure 9-45). The lingual cusps are much more developed. Instead of one lingual cusp, it has two or possibly three functioning cusps. This tooth helps with the transition from cutting and tearing to chewing. The occlusal surface of the mandibular second premolar resembles the molars, while the first mandibular premolar resembles the canine.

The cusps of the lingual surface are shorter than the buccal cusps and are divided by a lingual groove. The mesio-lingual cusp is slightly larger than the disto-lingual cusp but more equal in size than the cusps of the mandibular first bicuspid.

Three grooves divide the occlusal surface. The disto-buccal groove and the mesio-buccal groove come together with the lingual groove to form a Y shape on the occlusal surface. All the cusps slope into these grooves in the middle of the tooth. The mesial and distal ridges outline the sides of the occlusal surface.

The root is shorter than the maxillary cuspid root but longer than the mandibular first bicuspid root. The root has a single canal and inclines slightly toward the distal.

Mandibular Molars

The mandibular molars are the largest and strongest of the mandibular teeth.

Mandibular First Molar

The mandibular first molar is referred to as the "six-year-molar" (Figure 9-46). It normally erupts slightly before the maxillary first molar and is thought to be the keystone of the dental arch. It has the widest crown of any tooth in the dentition and is the largest mandibular tooth.

There are normally five functioning cusps on the occlusal surface of this tooth. The mesio-buccal cusp is the bulkiest and the longest of the three buccal cusps; however, it is shorter than the lingual cusps. The disto-buccal cusp is a rounded cusp, found between the larger mesio-buccal cusp and the smaller distal cusp. The mesio-lingual cusp and the disto-lingual cusp are the longest and the sharpest of the five cusps. The mesio-lingual cusp may be slightly smaller than the disto-lingual cusp. All these cusps come together on the occlusal surface in the central fossa and are divided

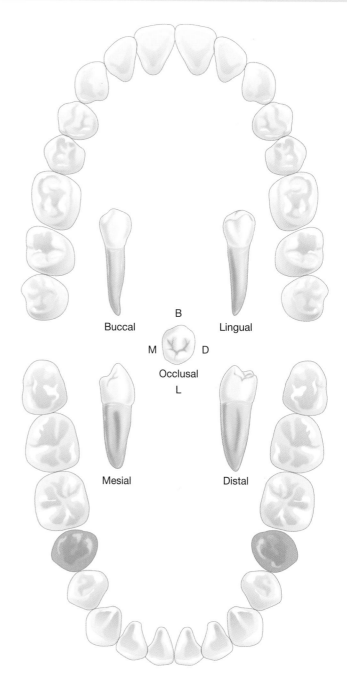

Mandibular second premolars (bicuspids)

FIGURE 9-45 Permanent dentition with mandibular second premolars (bicuspids) identified and mandibular second premolar viewed from the five surfaces.

by a groove extending between one cusp and the next. For instance, the buccal groove coming from the central fossa extends between the mesio-buccal cusp and the disto-buccal cusp and ends halfway down the buccal surface of the crown of the tooth in a buccal pit. These divisions make the occlusal surface appear as though five lobes come together. The mesial surface of the tooth is slightly concave, and the distal side is fairly straight.

The mandibular first molar has two roots: mesial and distal. The mesial root is the wider and the stron-

Buccal B Lingual

M D

Occlusal
L

Mesial Distal

Mandibular first molars

FIGURE 9-46 Permanent dentition with mandibular first molars identified and mandibular first molar viewed from the five surfaces.

Buccal B Lingual

M D

Occlusal
L

Mesial Distal

Mandibular second molars

FIGURE 9-47 Permanent dentition with mandibular second molars identified and mandibular second molar viewed from the five surfaces.

ger of the two. It normally has two pulp canals, which is unusual because most of the teeth have one canal per root. The root is fairly flat in shape from the buccal to the lingual and tends to incline first toward the mesial of the tooth and then curve back toward the distal. The distal root is the smaller and weaker of the two. It is usually straight but occasionally will curve toward the mesial or the distal. It usually has a wider canal, and the outer surface of the root is more convex on the distal portion.

Mandibular Second Molar

The mandibular second molar is similar to the first molar but smaller (Figure 9-47). It has four cusps: mesio-buccal, disto-buccal, mesio-lingual, and disto-lingual. They are nearly the same size, but the mesio-buccal cusp is normally the largest and the disto-lingual cusp is normally the smallest. They are divided by the buccal groove on the buccal surface and the lingual groove on the lingual surface. Both these grooves travel down the outside portion of the crown, about one-half of the surface, and end in pits or shallow depressions. The occlusal surface exhibits more supplemental grooves than the first molar.

The roots of the second molar are normally shorter than the first molar, but they do have more variations. The two bifurcated roots generally are closer together and may even be fused. They normally angle more toward the distal than the roots of the first mandibular molar. The mesial root is wider than the distal root and may have one or two canals (the distal root has one canal). They are shaped similar to the first molar, but the mesial root is flatter and the distal root is rounder.

Mandibular Third Molar

The mandibular third molar has many variations in shape and size (Figure 9-48). If it does develop properly and erupt, this molar resembles the second molar but is smaller. The mandibular third molar has a wrinkled surface and the roots are often fused together. The roots tend to angle toward the distal in almost a horizontal position and may be four or more in number and fused together. These teeth, like the maxillary third molars, are referred to as "wisdom teeth" and may not develop or erupt. The dentist must determine if it is to the patient's advantage to keep these teeth. If they do erupt, they normally are difficult to keep plaque free because of their location and additional grooves.

Deciduous (Primary) Teeth Descriptions

There are twenty deciduous teeth in the primary dentition: ten in each arch, five in each quadrant (Figure 9-49). There is a central incisor, lateral incisor, cuspid, first molar, and second molar (there are no bicuspids in the deciduous dentition). The primary teeth are referred to as the baby teeth, milk teeth, first teeth, or primary teeth, but the correct clinical term is deciduous teeth. They begin to erupt when the child is six months of age and finish erupting when the child is approximately two to three years of age.

It seems that less importance has been placed on the deciduous teeth because they are only temporary. Some patients prefer not to restore deciduous teeth and choose to have them removed, knowing that a permanent tooth will replace them. However, the deciduous teeth play a very important role in maintaining space for the permanent teeth, and they also aid the child in mastication and phonetics. Additionally, the appearance of the deciduous teeth plays an important role in establishing a child's positive self-image. Even though the deciduous teeth begin exfoliation by age six, they are still an important part of facial development.

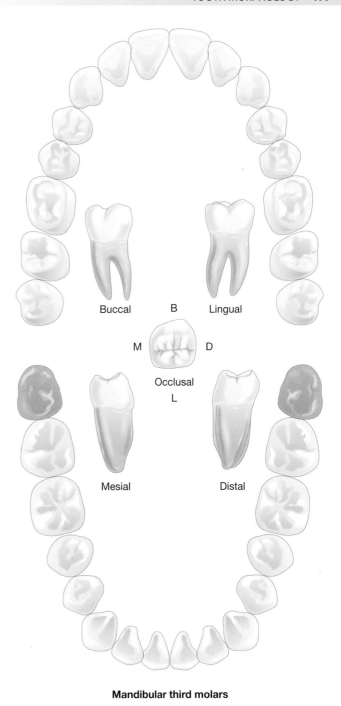

Buccal **B** **Lingual**

M **D**

Occlusal
L

Mesial **Distal**

Mandibular third molars

FIGURE 9-48 Permanent dentition with mandibular third molars identified and mandibular third molar viewed from the five surfaces.

The deciduous teeth are normally smaller than the permanent teeth that replace them. The crown portion is quite short in comparison to the root, and the cervical ridge is much more pronounced. The crowns of the deciduous teeth appear more white or light bluish in color, as compared to the yellow-gray color of the permanent teeth. This is because the enamel and dentin are much thinner and the pulp chamber is much larger. The deciduous molars have especially large mesial pulp

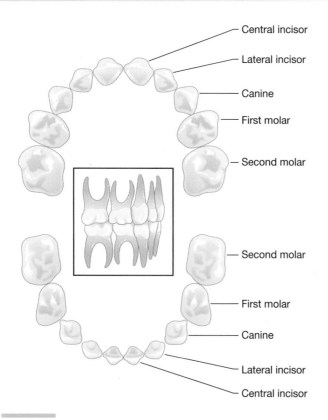

FIGURE 9-49 Deciduous dentition with tooth identification.

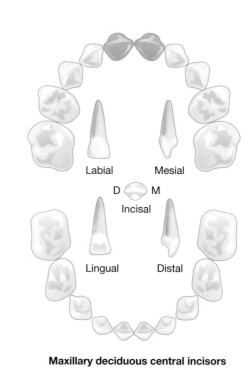

Maxillary deciduous central incisors

FIGURE 9-50 Deciduous dentition with maxillary central incisors identified.

horns. Knowing that the pulp is larger and closer to the surface of the deciduous tooth, a dental assistant should take great care during the coronal polish not to overheat the tooth and injure the pulp.

Maxillary Deciduous Central Incisor

The maxillary deciduous central incisor resembles the permanent maxillary central in shape (Figure 9-50). It is much smaller in size than the permanent maxillary central and has a more pronounced cervical line. The crown is the only anterior tooth in either dentition to have a shorter inciso-cervical height than the mesiodistal width. This tooth erupts with no mamelons, and the labial surface is convex and smooth.

Maxillary Deciduous Lateral Incisor

The maxillary deciduous lateral incisor is similar to the central incisor except it is smaller (Figure 9-51). Another difference is that it is longer than it is wide. The incisal edge of the deciduous maxillary lateral incisor is more rounded on the mesial and distal sides than the straight incisal edge of the central incisor.

Maxillary Deciduous Canine (Cuspid)

The maxillary deciduous canine appears to be wider than it is long; however, with the pointed incisal edge, it is slightly longer than it is wide (Figure 9-52). It is more

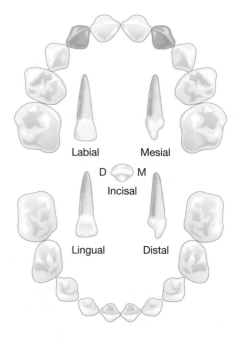

Maxillary deciduous lateral incisors

FIGURE 9-51 Deciduous dentition with maxillary lateral incisors identified.

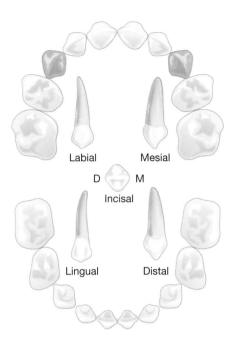

Maxillary deciduous canines (cuspids)

FIGURE 9-52 Deciduous dentition with maxillary canines (cuspids) identified.

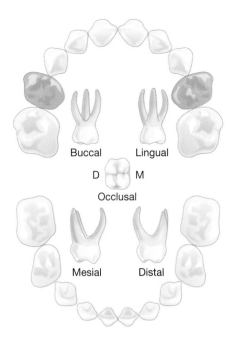

Maxillary deciduous first molars

FIGURE 9-53 Deciduous dentition with maxillary first molars identified.

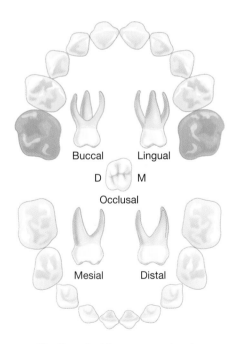

Maxillary deciduous second molars

FIGURE 9-54 Deciduous dentition with maxillary second molars identified.

convex than the permanent maxillary canine and constricts more at the cervix of the tooth. The mesio-incisal slope has a pronounced cingulum and mesial and distal marginal ridges. The root is similar to the incisors but is longer (but nothing like the permanent canine).

Maxillary Deciduous First Molar

The maxillary deciduous first molar resembles the permanent bicuspid in many respects (Figure 9-53). It has four cusps; the mesio-buccal and the mesio-lingual are the most prominent. The mesio-lingual is the longest and the largest. The disto-lingual is the smallest or may even be absent. The tooth has transverse and oblique ridges like the permanent maxillary first molar, but they are not as prominent. The roots, like those of all deciduous molars, spread out rapidly from the crown of the tooth and are widely spaced. The maxillary deciduous first molar has three roots, like its permanent counterparts.

Maxillary Deciduous Second Molar

The maxillary deciduous second molar (Figure 9-54) resembles the maxillary first permanent molar because it has four primary cusps and may even have a cusp that resembles the cusp of Carabelli. It has three roots that are widely spaced.

Mandibular Deciduous Central Incisor

The mandibular deciduous central incisor (Figure 9-55) more closely resembles the permanent mandibular lat-

eral incisor than its central incisor counterpart. The crown of the tooth is slightly wider than the permanent lateral incisor. The shape and form of the incisal edge is almost exactly the same as that of the permanent lateral. The root is slender and rather long. Mesial and distal sur-

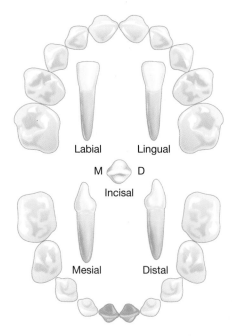

Mandibular deciduous central incisors

FIGURE 9-55 Deciduous dentition with mandibular deciduous central incisors identified.

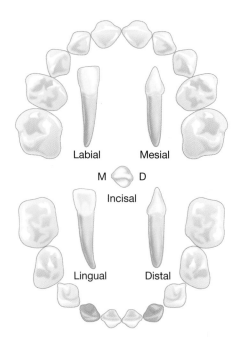

Mandibular deciduous lateral incisors

FIGURE 9-56 Deciduous dentition with mandibular deciduous lateral incisors identified.

faces of the root are flat, while lingual and labial surfaces are convex.

Mandibular Deciduous Lateral Incisor

The mandibular deciduous lateral incisor resembles the mandibular deciduous central incisor except that it is slightly longer and wider (Figure 9-56). The cingulum and the mesial and distal marginal ridges are more pronounced and the fossa is not as shallow. The root curves toward the distal at the apex.

Mandibular Deciduous Canine (Cuspid)

The mandibular deciduous canine is much more delicate in form than that of the maxillary deciduous cuspid—even the root is not as large or long (Figure 9-57). The cingulum and the mesial and distal marginal ridges are less pronounced than those of the maxillary counterpart. The mesio-incisal slope is not as long as the disto-incisal slope; the maxillary incisal slopes are more nearly equal in length.

Mandibular Deciduous First Molar

The mandibular deciduous first molar (Figure 9-58) resembles no other permanent or deciduous tooth. It has four cusps, with the mesio-buccal the largest and the mesio-lingual next in size. The disto-buccal and the disto-lingual are much smaller. The buccal surface is longer than that of the lingual and has a very prominent

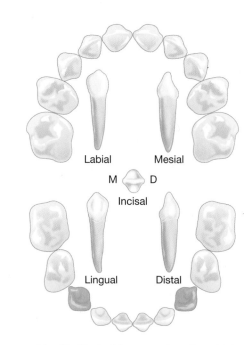

Mandibular deciduous canines (cuspids)

FIGURE 9-57 Deciduous dentition with mandibular deciduous canines (cuspids) identified.

cervical ridge across the gingival area, directly above where the tooth constricts at the cervix. The tooth has two roots, including a mesial root, which is much longer and wider, and a distal root. The apex of the mesial root is flattened or squared off.

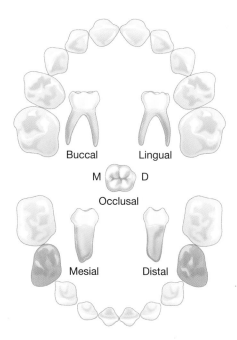

Mandibular deciduous first molars

FIGURE 9-58 Deciduous dentition with mandibular first molars identified.

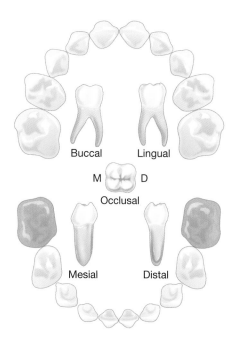

Mandibular deciduous second molars

FIGURE 9-59 Deciduous dentition with mandibular second molars identified.

Mandibular Deciduous Second Molar

The mandibular deciduous second molar closely resembles the permanent mandibular first molar (Figure 9-59). It is smaller in all dimensions, and the mesio-buccal and the disto-buccal cusps are nearly equal in size, unlike the permanent mandibular first molar. The distal root is smaller, while the mesial root is longer and wider. The permanent mandibular first molar has roots approximately the same length as this tooth.

CHAPTER SUMMARY

Understanding tooth morphology will prepare the assistant to record accurately for the dentist or hygienist and is a vital contribution to those team members to make a more accurate diagnosis. Therefore, the dental assistant will need to be able to identify each tooth form from its anatomical form.

Case Study

Travis Charles, age twelve, complains of discomfort in the back of the mouth on both sides. The patient says it feels like the skin is broken open behind his teeth.

Case Study Review

1. What probable condition is present?

2. Is the discomfort constant? Should Travis be concerned?

3. Does any one thing bring on the discomfort? Should Travis expect primary tooth loss in these areas?

REVIEW QUESTIONS

Multiple Choice

1. How many teeth are in the deciduous dentition?
   a. 32
   b. 16
   c. 20
   d. 24

2. The surface of the tooth that is away from the midline is the
   a. mesial surface.
   b. distal surface.
   c. labial surface.
   d. lingual surface.

3. Three bulges on the incisal edge of the newly erupted central incisor are
   a. marginal ridges.
   b. cingulums.
   c. mamelons.
   d. fissures.

4. Except for the third molar, the maxillary tooth that has the most anomalies is the
   a. central incisor.
   b. lateral incisor.
   c. first premolar (bicuspid).
   d. second molar.

5. The cusp on the mandibular second molar that is normally the smallest is the
   a. mesio-buccal.
   b. disto-buccal.
   c. mesio-lingual.
   d. disto-lingual.

6. The cusp on the mesial lingual surface of the permanent maxillary first molar is the
   a. oblique cusp.
   b. cusp of Carabelli.
   c. cusp of succedaneous.
   d. transverse cusp.

7. The permanent teeth that replace the primary teeth are called _____ teeth.
   a. deciduous
   b. milk teeth
   c. succedaneous
   d. mamelon

8. The number of molars in a permanent dentition is
   a. 12.
   b. 8.
   c. 16.
   d. 4.

9. When there are two roots on a single tooth, they are said to be
   a. divided.
   b. trifurcated.
   c. fused.
   d. bifurcated.

10. A convex area on the lingual surface of the anterior teeth, near the gingiva is called the
    a. cusp.
    b. fossa.
    c. cingulum.
    d. lobe.

Critical Thinking

1. If a patient has not formed a permanent mandibular first bicuspid on the left side, which deciduous tooth is retained in its place?

2. Which teeth in the maxillary arch are bifurcated?

3. Which surface of the anterior teeth is convex?

Web Activities

1. Go to http://www.Dentistry2000.com and find the listings for continuing education resources online. Review the resources and see if any articles relate to tooth morphology. Read the articles and plan to report your findings to the class.

2. Go to http://www.openchannelfoundation.org and find the tooth morphology online class. Review the sample screens and identify how many modules are necessary to complete the course.

3. Go to http://www.delmarhealthcare.com and find the listings of any tooth morphology textbooks. Are any of these textbooks being used in your classroom?

SECTION IV

PRECLINICAL DENTAL SKILLS

PRACTICE

MICROBIOLOGY

SPECIFIC INSTRUCTIONAL OBJECTIVES

The student should strive to meet the following objectives and demonstrate an understanding of the facts and principles presented in this chapter:

1. Identify Anton Van Leeuwenhoek, Ferdinand Cohn, Louis Pasteur, Robert Koch, and Richard Petri according to their contributions to microbiology.

2. Explain the groups of microorganisms and staining procedures used to identify them.

3. Identify characteristics pertaining to bacteria.

4. List the characteristics of protozoa.

5. Identify the characteristics of *Rickettsia*.

6. Explain the characteristics of yeasts and molds.

7. List the characteristics of viruses.

8. Describe the diseases of major concern to the dental assistant and explain why they cause concern.

9. Identify how the body fights disease. Explain types of immunity and routes of microorganism infection.

KEY TERMS

acquired immunity *(196)*

acquired immunodeficiency syndrome (AIDS) *(196)*

active acquired immunity *(197)*

aerobic bacteria *(187)*

allergen *(197)*

anaerobic bacteria *(187)*

anaphylactic shock *(197)*

antibodies *(196)*

antigens *(196)*

antitoxin *(196)*

aphthous ulcer *(193)*

artificial acquired immunity *(197)*

bacteria *(186)*

candidiasis *(191)*

chickenpox *(193)*

cold sore *(193)*

conjunctivitis *(194)*

corneal ulcer *(194)*

diphtheria *(187)*

diplococci *(187)*

endospore *(187)*

etiologic agent *(185)*

facultative anaerobic bacteria *(187)*

flagella *(190)*

gram negative *(187)*

gram positive *(187)*

Gram stain *(186)*

hepatitis A *(194)*

hepatitis B *(194)*

hepatitis C *(194)*

hepatitis D *(194)*

hepatitis E *(195)*

herpes simplex *(193)*

herpes simplex virus type I *(193)*

(continues)

KEY TERMS *(continued)*

INTRODUCTION

CDA The study of microorganisms is called **micro-biology**. Most microorganisms benefit humans and are often used in making vitamins, antibiotics, and food products. However, some microorganisms are harmful to humans, and these are called **pathogens** (**PATH**-oh-jens) (disease-producing microorganisms). In this chapter, five groups of pathogenic microorganisms are covered (bacteria, protozoa, rickettsiae, yeasts and molds, and viruses), along with the diseases they cause and the ways in which the body defends against them. Methods and instruments used to study microorganisms include the microscope, growing colonies in a culture medium, color or staining, and injection into an animal to observe the outcome.

Important People in Microbiology

There are several key individuals who made significant discoveries in the field of microbiology. It is helpful to know and understand the contributions of these individuals to the field of microbiology and the impact of these discoveries on the approach to the identification and treatment of diseases.

Anton Van Leeuwenhoek

Born in 1632 in Holland, Anton Van Leeuwenhoek (laye-vuhn-hook) (1632–1723) ground lenses to magnify and view things more closely. He looked at a rain-drop through these lenses and found small things that moved; he saw microorganisms for the first time. Later, he scraped his teeth and viewed the scrapings through the ground lenses and found a great number of moving microorganisms; these single–celled organisms he referred to as "animalcules." He created over four hundred different types of microscopes, several which are still used today. They were made of hand-ground lenses in metal frames made from silver or copper.

Ferdinand Julius Cohn

Ferdinand Julius Cohn (1828–1898) was a biologist from Germany who was the first person to classify bacteria as plants. He later divided bacteria into four groups: desmobacteria, microbacteria, sphaerobacteria, and spirobacteria. His studies of the life cycle of *Bacillus* showed that it will change into an endospore from its vegetative state when it is exposed to high heat or some adverse or unfavorable environment. He understood that bacteria could go into this endospore state when being boiled and therefore the bacteria would not be killed. This has become very critical information in today's sterilization procedure. In the dental office, tests must be done to ensure that the endospores have been killed during the sterilization process.

Louis Pasteur

Louis Pasteur (1822–1895), a French microbiologist and chemist (Figure 10-1), experimented with fermentation. By isolating the causative bacteria in other diseases, some affecting humans, he proved that bacteria caused disease. Pasteur found that bacteria, along with resistant spores, could be destroyed by heat. He showed that broth, when heated and kept in an airtight container, did not spoil. Pasteur suggested that food be processed by steam under pressure in an airtight container. His work led to the food-canning process used today. The sterilizers used in dental offices are based on his original premise that heat kills pathogens. Pasteur's name is noted in the pasteurization of milk, whereby the pathogens in milk are destroyed by heat. Pasteur's later work was in the area of creating vaccines. He discovered a method of using an artificially generated weak form of the disease to fight the disease or prevent its occurrence. His work has been the foundation for many of the vaccines now produced. His work helped lead to eradicating polio and typhus as health threats. He was noted as the "Father of Microbiology." It should be noted that Anton Van Leeuwenhoek was given this title earlier as well. He was awarded the Leeuwenhoek metal in 1895, microbiology's highest honor.

Robert Koch

Robert Koch (1843–1910), a German biologist (Figure 10-2), proved that a specific type of bacteria causes a specific disease, termed the **etiologic** (**EE**-tee-ol-**OH**-gic)

FIGURE 10-1 Louis Pasteur *(From* The Evolution of Preventive Medicine in the United States Army, 1607-1939. *Office of the Surgeon General Department of the Army: Washington, DC, 1968)*

agent (causative agent) of the disease. He was able to determine the etiologic agent for tuberculosis. Koch is remembered for the "Koch postulates," a procedure he developed to prove that a particular bacterium was the cause of a disease.

Koch's Postulates

1. The organism must be present in all cases of the disease.
2. The organism must be isolated in pure culture.
3. The organism must be able to produce the disease in another person or animal.
4. The organism must be recovered again in pure culture.

Richard Julius Petri

Richard Julius Petri (1852–1921) was born in Germany and as a young adult he enrolled in training as a military physician and then received a doctorate in medicine. He worked in a research facility and was the laboratory assistant to Robert Koch. As an assistant he realized the need for a method to easily culture bacteria for research. He devised the cylindrical shallow dish with

R. Koch.

FIGURE 10-2 Robert Koch *(Courtesy of the National Library of Medicine)*

the clear cover that is still being used in microbiology laboratories today, the **Petri dish** or the Petri plate. This dish is used with a medium of molten agar to grow or culture bacteria. The lid is easily removed. He further developed the technique that is used today for dispensing the bacteria onto the medium (Figure 10-3). The dish bears his name and continues to allow the growth of bacteria under sterile conditions to be accomplished for study and research.

Groups of Microorganisms

The two principal groups of microorganisms important to dentistry are **bacteria** and **viruses**. When looking through a microscope, types of bacteria are identified based on characteristics, shapes, and sizes.

Often, bacteria cells are stained to further identify the groups. Dr. Christian Gram developed a staining procedure, called the **Gram stain**, to differentiate cells into two specific groups. To aid in viewing the cells, special dyes are used. The cells are placed on a slide and dried,

FIGURE 10-3 Microorganism being grown in a medium in a Petri dish.

and then stained with an alkaline solution of violet dye. The slide is rinsed with iodine and left untouched for two minutes. Then, the slide is gently rinsed with water and next rinsed with acetone alcohol. If the cell wall keeps the color, the cells are classified as **gram positive** and appear dark purple under the microscope. If they lose the color during the procedure, they are classified as **gram negative** and appear colorless under the microscope.

Bacteria

Bacteria (back-**TEER**-ee-uh) are tiny, simple, single-celled plants that contain no chlorophyll. If an individual has 2,000 bacteria lying side by side in a line, they are about the width of the period at the end of this sentence. Bacteria divide by simple fission: They elongate and divide into two separate cells, then continuously repeat this cycle. In ideal conditions (warm, dark, nutrient-rich, and moist), they divide about every twenty minutes. Bacteria are often incorrectly called "germs." Some bacteria are **sporulating**. One example is bacilli. These **spores** become enclosed in several protein coats that resist drying, heat, and most chemicals (**endospores**). They also withstand boiling. Sporulating is a means of survival for bacteria, and bacteria have been known to survive for years in this state. Later, they may land on a surface that is moist and nutrient rich, and reactivate. The process is much like a seed that floats and then lands on rich soil and begins growing.

Bacteria's Need for Oxygen

- **Aerobic bacteria** must have oxygen to grow and live. Most bacteria are aerobic.

- **Anaerobic bacteria** are destroyed in the presence of oxygen and live only without oxygen.

- **Facultative anaerobic bacteria** grow with or without oxygen.

Bacteria Morphology

The shape of bacteria (morphology) is unique to this group of microorganisms (Figure 10-4). Under a microscope, the types of microorganisms are bacilli (rod shaped), cocci (round or bead shaped), spirilla (S shaped), and vibrios (curved like a comma).

When the bacteria are grown in colonies, or masses, they appear differently (Figure 10-5). The prefix diplo, as in **diplococci**, identifies pairs of bacteria; **staphylococci** grow in clusters, much like grapes; and **streptococci** identifies chains of bacteria.

Disease Examples Caused by Bacteria

Tuberculosis. **Tuberculosis** (to-bur-kol-**O**-sis) is caused by *Mycobacterium tuberculosis* and is most often found in the lungs. Several months may pass before signs of the disease appear. Symptoms include fatigue, low-grade fever, night sweats, loss of weight, and, finally, a persistent cough. This disease is spread to others by airborne particles released through coughing, saliva contact, and, if cross-contamination occurs, dental treatment. Dental personnel must wear masks during dental procedures to protect from the handpiece spray that may contain infectious particles if the patient has tuberculosis. The disease can be detected by a skin test and/or chest x-ray. Treatment for this disease includes antibiotics and other drugs.

Diphtheria, Pertussis, and Tetanus. **Diphtheria**, **pertussis**, and **tetanus** are diseases caused by bacteria. Diphtheria, caused by the bacillus *Corynebacterium diphtheriae*, appears as a severe throat infection and fever. At one time, diphtheria took the lives of thousands. Pertussis (whooping cough) is caused by the *Bordetella pertussis*. Pertussis is a disease of the respiratory system, and it mainly affects infants and young children. Tetanus is caused by spores of *Clostridium tetani*. The most common sign of tetanus is a stiffness of the jaw, commonly called lockjaw. All three of these diseases are prevented with a combined vaccination. The DPT immunization is given to children at two, four, and six months of age, and then a booster is given at five years of age. After age five, tetanus boosters are given every ten years.

Strep Throat. **Strep throat**, one of the most common bacterial diseases in humans, is a streptococcal infection. Symptoms are sore throat, fever, and general malaise. In some cases, toxins released by the bacterium can cause a rash to develop and become a condition known as scarlet fever. *Streptococcus mutans*, a species of streptococcus, has been implicated in dental caries and endocarditis. This same group of bacteria can give rise to pneumonia or rheumatic fever. These infections can be prevented by the prompt use of antibiot-

FIGURE 10-4 The unique shapes of bacteria. (A) Bacilli: rod shaped. (B) Cocci: round. (C) Spirilla: S-shaped. (D) Vibrios: curved. (Courtesy of the Centers for Disease Control and Prevention).

ics. The ADA recommends that a prophylactic regimen be followed for any dental procedures that may cause endocarditis. A dose of amoxicillin one hour before the anticipated procedure is recommended.

Staphylococcal Infections. Staphylococcal infections derive from bacteria that grow in clusters. Some diseases caused by these pathogens include the staph infection, gangrene, toxic shock syndrome, venereal

diseases, and some forms of pneumonia. Antibiotics are the first line of treatment.

Bacillus anthracis. *Bacillus anthracis*, which causes anthrax in grazing animals, including goats, sheep, and cattle, is a gram-positive bacillus that causes a lethal disease. Humans can get the disease through cuts in the skin (cutaneous anthrax) or by eating infected meat. If treatment is not administered before symptoms manifest,

FIGURE 10-5 The pair, cluster, and chain bacterial colonies *(Courtesy of the Centers for Disease Control and Prevention)*

the disease is normally fatal. There are 100 million lethal doses in each gram of anthrax, making it 100,000 times more deadly than any other chemical. In powder form, this chemical can be made and disseminated easily at low cost, making it a very deadly chemical weapon. Infected individuals experience symptoms within one to six days, which will start as a low-grade fever, weakness, and a dry, hacking cough. The symptoms will improve slightly before severe respiratory distress, shock, and normally

death. The disease can be prevented by a vaccination or an antibiotic treatment before symptoms manifest.

Chlamydiae. Different strains of *Chlamydia trachomatis* are responsible for various genital, eye, and lymph node infections. This microorganism is the most common sexually transmitted disease (STD) in the United States. Treatment is with antibiotics, such as tetracycline and erythromycin, and is usually quickly successful.

Protozoa

Protozoa (proh-tah-**ZOH**-ah) are about 100 microns in size, just below visibility of the naked eye (Figure 10-6). Often called amoeba, they live in fluids in the bloodstream, mouth, and intestinal tract and survive in polluted water in pools and ponds. Protozoa are single-celled animal life, and some are sporulating. They engulf their food as they change in shape to achieve mobility. Many have a long, threadlike appendage called a flagella. Flagella whip around and cause additional movement for the protozoa. Some protozoa contain chlorophyll, and most are aerobic.

Disease Examples Caused by Protozoa

Amebic Dysentery. Amebic dysentery is an infection caused by the microorganism *Entamoeba histolytica*. Symptoms include severe diarrhea and, in extreme cases, abscesses in the liver. This disease is prevalent in countries where drinking water is contaminated and overall poor hygiene conditions prevail. Drug treatment is necessary to effectively kill the parasite.

Periodontal Disease. Periodontal disease is caused by protozoa and bacteria. Both microorganisms are found in the inflamed tissue around the tooth. Protozoa are in the plaque in the periodontal pockets around the tooth. Treatment includes a thorough cleaning around the area to remove any plaque and diseased tissue and then impeccable oral hygiene maintenance.

Malaria. Malaria and sleeping sickness are two other diseases caused by protozoa. Both are prevalent throughout the tropics and have symptoms during the first two weeks, such as fever and soreness at the point of entry. Malaria is spread via mosquito bites, and sleeping sickness is spread by the tsetse fly. Both require drug therapy to kill the parasites in the bites.

Rickettsiae

Rickettsiae are parasitic bacteria. Lice, fleas, ticks, and mites are often hosts to rickettsiae. They multiply only by invading the cells of another life form. The hosts then transmit the disease to humans.

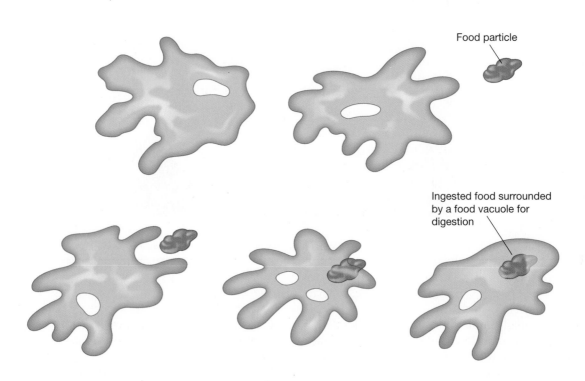

FIGURE 10-6 The protozoan changing shape as it travels to and engulfs its food.

FIGURE 10-7 Greatly magnified head lice.

FIGURE 10-8 Patient presenting with thrush. *(Courtesy of Joseph L. Konzelman, Jr., DDS).*

Disease Examples Caused by Rickettsiae

Rocky Mountain Spotted Fever. Symptoms of Rocky Mountain spotted fever occur about a week to ten days after transmission from the host and are much like those of the flu. Two to six days after the symptoms have occurred, small pink spots appear on the ankles and wrists. The body is soon covered with these spots. Treatment with antibiotics normally cures the disease, which is rare.

Typhus. Typhus is another fairly rare disease, similar to Rocky Mountain spotted fever. The microorganism is spread by a host, and symptoms appear rapidly. A severe headache, back and limb pain, constipation, and high fever develop suddenly. A rash similar to measles appears, the heart beats weakly, and confusion is common. Typhus fever is treated with antibiotic drug therapy.

Head Lice. Pediculosis is the state of being infected with head lice. Head lice (Figure 10-7) is a common occurrence for children in schools. If one child is identified as having head lice, others should be checked carefully to stop recurrence. Lice are tiny, bloodsucking, wingless parasites that are transmitted through direct contact. Mature lice produce about six eggs every day. These eggs (nits), attached to hair shafts, are visible. Treatment consists of applying medicinal shampoo and combing to loosen the nits. Bedding, towels, brushes, combs, and clothes must also be washed with very hot water and soap. Multiple shampoo treatments may be required.

Yeasts and Molds

Yeasts and molds (fungi) are smaller than protozoa and larger than bacteria. This group of microorganisms includes bread yeast, mushrooms, and bread molds. Some are sporulating, and they reproduce by budding. They cannot be killed by the antibiotics that kill bacteria (penicillin is made from mold but does not act upon fungi, from which it is made).

Disease Examples Caused by Yeasts and Molds

Candidiasis. Candidiasis (kan-dih-**DYE**-ah-sis) is an infection by the fungus *Candida albicans,* often on areas covered with mucous membrane, such as inside of the mouth or the vaginal area. It is commonly called thrush, or moniliasis (Figure 10-8). It is kept at bay with normal flora, that is, normal bacteria in these areas. If antibiotics destroy too many of the "normal" bacteria, or if the body's immune system is impaired, such as is the case with acquired immunodeficiency syndrome (AIDS), then the fungi multiply and overgrow. The disease causes thick white or creamy yellow ("cottage cheese") raised patches. These patches may become irritated and cause discomfort. Treatment for candidiasis is antifungal drug therapy.

Tinea. Tinea includes any group of common fungal infections. They are acquired from an infected person, animal, or inanimate object, such as a shower stall. Tinea pedis, commonly called athlete's foot, causes itching and cracking between the toes and on the foot. Tinea corporis, commonly called ringworm, usually appears as red circles with a raised edge on the body. Tinea unguium is characterized as white patches on the toe or fingernail (Figure 10-9). The location makes it difficult to treat because the fungus is under the nail. The nail may thicken, overgrow, become brittle or entirely destroyed. For most types of tinea, a treatment of antifungal drugs in the form of skin creams, ointments, or lotions is prescribed. Oral antifungal drugs may be necessary in persistent strains of the fungus.

FIGURE 10-9 Tinea unguium.

Prions

Proteinaceous infectious particles called prions (pree-on) is a fairly newly identified microorganism that is an infectious agent made only of protein. All mammals have prions in the nerve cells that are normal. Prions are actually the host protein that convert normal protein molecules into abnormal structures that are responsible for a group of diseases classified as transmissible spongiform encephalopathies (TSEs). The TSEs are rare, untreatable, and deadly due to the fact that they affect the brain tissue. There is some research that identifies the prions in some fungi, but much is yet to be known about prions. The prions are associated with the diseases in animals like mad cow disease (bovine spongiform encephalopathy) and in human diseases like Creutzfeldt-Jakob disease as well as others.

Mad Cow Disease

The mad cow disease or bovine spongiform encephalopathy (BSE) is a progressive disorder of the brain seen in cattle. The first time that cows were noted to have this disease was in the early 1970s. In the United States only one or two cases have been identified and they have been immediately contained. The fear is that a human will ingest the meat from an animal infected with BSE and that this will cause the diseased prions to react on the human's protein molecules, affecting the nerve cells which may lead to loss of brain function. Great precautions are being taken by the Centers for Disease Control and Prevention and the United States Department of Agriculture to monitor the beef industry.

Creutzfeldt-Jakob Disease

Two German neurologists, Hans Gerhard Creutzfeldt and Alfons Maria Jakob, were the first to describe the disease of Creutzfeldt-Jakob disease. The disease is rare with only one per million in the world and only about 200 cases in the United States each year. It belongs to the TSE group of diseases. Individuals that are affected typically are around the age of sixty years of age and they present with rapidly progressing dementia, memory loss, speech impairment, involuntary jerky movements, weakness, blindness, and then coma. The disease progresses rapidly and is fatal due to the neurological deterioration. The cause of the disease is currently unknown. It is believed that this disease is related to the prion proteins, but some think that it is a slowly growing virus that is latent, suppressed or dormant for a period of time. There are several variants of the disease that affect individuals earlier in life.

Viruses

Viruses are the smallest microorganisms known to date. They are tiny particles, one one-hundredth the size of bacteria. An electron microscope must be used to observe viruses (Figure 10-10). Like rickettsiae, they are able to reproduce only inside host cells. Viruses are difficult to grow in a culture, and their morphology is varied, like bacteria. Most are easy to kill by disinfecting or exposure to air, but the hepatitis B virus is

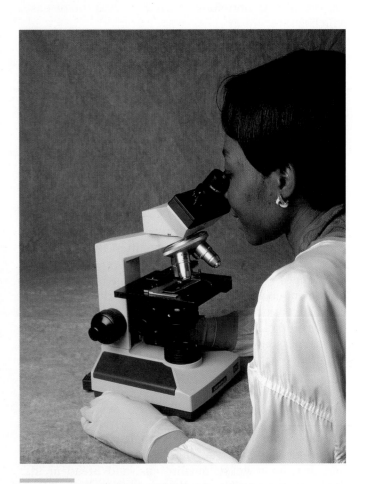

FIGURE 10-10 Pathologist looking through microscope.

very resistant. It can live on a dry surface for up to two weeks. Antibiotics will not kill any true virus. Outbreaks of viruses, such as herpes simplex, can last from ten days to two weeks, whether treated or not. Treatment is primarily aimed at the symptoms in order to make the patient more comfortable.

Disease Examples Caused by Viruses

Measles, Mumps, and Rubella. Measles, mumps, and rubella are childhood illnesses caused by viruses. Measles cause a rash and a fever, and is spread by airborne droplets of nasal secretions. An incubation period of nine to eleven days takes place before symptoms appear. The main symptom of mumps is the swelling of the parotid (salivary) glands on one side or both sides. Mumps is spread by airborne droplets. Rubella, also known as German measles, appears as a rash on the face and may spread to the trunk and limbs. This disease is serious only if it affects women in the early stages of pregnancy, because of possible birth defects. The incubation period for both mumps and measles is two to three weeks. The MMR (measles, mumps, and rubella) vaccine is highly effective in providing long-lasting immunity and is given to all children at about fifteen months of age. Treatment aims at reducing discomfort only. An analgesic such as aspirin is given for fevers, and lotion is applied to relieve itching.

Poliomyelitis. Poliomyelitis (poh-lee-oh-my-eh-**LYE**-tis), commonly called polio, attacks the central nervous system and may lead to extensive paralysis. Since the development of vaccines in the late 1950s, very few cases have been identified in the United States. The virus IPV (inactivated, or dead, polio vaccine) is given by injection; the IPV, however, is not used as much as OPV (oral poliovirus vaccine), which contains live but harmless virus and is given orally at the ages of two, four, and eighteen months. A booster dose at five years of age is also given.

Chickenpox. Chickenpox is a childhood disease caused by the varicella-zoster virus. It is characterized by a rash and slight fever. The virus remains dormant in the nerve tissue after the attack and may cause herpes zoster (shingles) later in life. Patients are contagious from about two days before the fever to five days after. The disease is spread through airborne droplets. The patient is treated for the fever but will heal within ten days. A varicella virus vaccine is recommended for this disease, but the period of immunity is unknown. Adult symptoms are quite severe, and include pneumonia.

Common Cold and Influenza. The common cold and influenza are caused by viruses. Treatment is focused on relieving fever, upset stomach, headache, and body ache. Anti-influenza vaccines are available and are highly recommended for the elderly and medically com-

promised. The vaccines are successful in about 60% of cases. Patients are contagious from twelve to seventy-two hours after the symptoms appear. Colds are spread through airborne droplets, contact with contaminated objects, or hand-to-hand contact. Flu is spread through airborne droplets.

Diseases of Major Concern to the Dental Assistant

The dental assistant is at risk of exposure to a variety of infectious diseases and disorders. Some diseases pose mild risks and recovery from exposure is quick while others may have a great risk for causing chronic illness or may even threaten the dental assistant's life. The most critical conditions to be alert to are herpes simplex, viral hepatitis, HIV, and AIDS.

Herpes Simplex

Herpes (**HER**-peez) simplex is a common and troublesome viral disease (Figure 10-11). Herpes simplex virus type 1 (HSV1) is usually associated with infections of the lips, mouth, and face, and herpes simplex virus type II (HSV2) is normally associated with the genital area. Type II, however, can appear in the oral cavity. Both viruses are extremely contagious and spread by direct contact with a fluid-filled lesion, called a vesicle, or the fluid from such a lesion.

Most adults have been infected by herpes simplex virus type I. Initially, the infection may cause flu-like symptoms and a blister or sore in the mouth. It remains in the nerve cells within that area for life. HSV1 reactions often result from fever, prolonged exposure to the sun, stress, or ingestion of certain high-acid foods. These herpes simplex viruses (cold sores or aphthous ulcers) can reactivate and appear in the same general areas. The virus may infect the fingers if open sores are present, but this virus on the finger (herpetic whitlow) is rare, and was a greater concern to dental personnel

FIGURE 10-11 Herpetic labialis lesion. *(Courtesy of Joseph L. Konzelman, Jr., DDS)*

prior to the usage of treatment gloves. The virus can be transferred to the eye and cause **conjunctivitis** or a **corneal ulcer**, which could result in blindness.

Treatment of HSV1 depends on type, site, and severity. Dental teams may suggest rescheduling the patient if the sores are apparent. This is primarily for the comfort of the patient, but it also may be office policy not to provide treatment when vesicles are present in the oral cavity. A number of topical treatments are available for patient comfort. Some people take L-Lysen, an amino acid, when they feel the symptoms coming on. Antiviral drugs such as acyclovir, generic for Zovirax, are sometimes helpful.

HSV2 is sexually transmitted genital herpes. It displays the same vesicles, erupting on the sex organs, and may erupt orally as well. As with type 1, type 2 can recur.

Bloodborne Diseases. Bloodborne diseases of concern to the dental assistant are viral hepatitis (HBV) and human immunodeficiency virus (HIV), which later develops into acquired immunodeficiency syndrome (AIDS). These diseases are transmitted directly through contaminated blood and other body fluids.

High-Risk Behavior for Acquiring Hepatitis B, HIV, and AIDS

- Injuries or sticks with sharp objects contaminated with blood or body fluid

- Multiple sexual partners, unprotected sex (homosexual, bisexual, or heterosexual)

- Sharing contaminated needles

- Exposure to non-intact skin or open wound with contaminated blood or body fluid

---

Viral Hepatitis

Viral hepatitis has five different types (Table 10-1). Hepatitis A and E are transmitted by person-to-person contact or by ingestion of contaminated water or food. The symptoms, which appear from fifteen to forty days after contact, range from flu-like symptoms to acute liver damage.

Hepatitis A Hepatitis A (often called infectious hepatitis) is in the news when a food provider has a number of customers become ill and the virus is identified. No long-term immunization has been available until recently. People who have possible contact with contaminated food or water are given an injection of gamma globulin within fourteen days of exposure, which provides short-term immunization. In 1995, a vaccine called *Havrix* was licensed by the U.S. Food and Drug Administration (FDA). A recent paper by the Centers for Disease Control and Prevention (CDC) stated the benefits of *Havrix* and, in 1997, *Havrix* was awarded the pediatric vaccine contract. Children in areas with a high rate of hepatitis A will be given the initial and booster dose of *Havrix* between the ages of two and eighteen years.

Hepatitis B Hepatitis B is of major concern to dental personnel. This disease (commonly called serum hepatitis) has been recognized only since the early 1950s. Primarily transmitted through contaminated needles and syringes, the incubation period is from fifty to 180 days. Only one-third of infected people have symptoms that can be easily identified, one-third have slight symptoms, and one-third have no symptoms at all. The symptoms include loss of appetite, digestive upset, upper abdominal pain and tenderness, fever, weakness, muscle pain, and jaundice (yellowing of the skin). According to the CDC, about 300,000 people are infected each year; of that number, 300 will die from the disease, 10,000 will be hospitalized, and 20,000 will become chronic carriers. The CDC estimates that there are over a million carriers in the United States today. The FDA approved Hepsera (adefovir dipivoxil) tablets in 2002 for treatment of chronic hepatitis B in adults. Hepsera slows the progression of chronic hepatitis B.

In 1982, a plasma-derived Heptavax-B vaccine was introduced in the United States. Since that time, Recombivax HB and Energix B have been licensed for use in the United States and are shown to be effective against the hepatitis B virus. Both these vaccines are administered in a series of three injections. The schedule is initially, then a month later, then three months from the first vaccine administration. The vaccine is administered in the form of an injection to the deltoid muscle in the arm. It has been found that administration in the buttocks did not yield the same **seroconversion** rate (vaccine causes the development of immunity).

It should be noted that, according to OSHA standards, the employer is responsible for offering the HBV 3 series vaccination to new employees in Categories I and II within ten days of employment at no cost to the employee. The employee can refuse the vaccine by signing an informed refusal form that is to be kept in the employee file. (See Chapter 12).

After completing the three series of HBV vaccines, a blood test is performed to ensure that immunity has developed. The employer is not responsible for the blood test, because it is not noted in the OSHA standard, but it is an important step for the dental assistant to take to ensure prevention of hepatitis B. If the dental assistant tests negative for seroconversion, the physician must make a determination about additional dosages of the HBV vaccine.

A booster dosage is not recommended by the CDC unless an exposure incident has occurred or a physician recommends it after testing negative for seroconversion.

Hepatitis C Hepatitis C, often called non-A and non-B, reacts somewhat like hepatitis B, but there is no vaccine available currently. About 50 percent of the people infected become chronic carriers.

Hepatitis D Hepatitis D, also known as the delta agent, cannot replicate on its own and requires the presence of hepatitis B. The vaccination for hepatitis B should also prevent hepatitis D.

TABLE 10-1 Types of Viral Hepatitis

Disease & Cause	Transmission	Symptoms	Prevention	Long Term Effects
Viral Hepatitis A HAV	Human feces of persons with HAV being transmitted to oral cavity of other person. Example: Not washing hands after bathroom and then preparing food.	fatigue, loss of appetite, fever, nausea, diarrhea, and jaundice	• Hepatitis A vaccine recommended for people 12 months and older • Wash hands • Immune globulin can be taken within two weeks of contact	• No chronic infection • Have it only once
Viral Hepatitis B HBV	• Blood from infected person enters a person who is not infected • Spread through contaminated needles, or other sharps • Sex • Infected mother to baby during birth	fatigue, loss of appetite, fever, nausea, vomiting, joint and abdominal pain and jaundice. Approximately 1/3 have no symptoms	• Hepatitis B vaccine • Use of latex condom during sexual activity • Don't shoot drugs and share needles • Don't share items that may have blood on them	• 15–25% will die from chronic liver disease • High rate of chronic liver disease in infants born to infected mothers
Viral Hepatitis C HCB	• Blood from infected person enters a person who is not infected • Spread through contaminated needles, or other sharps • From infected mother to baby during birth • It can be spread through sexual activity but that is rare	fatigue, loss of appetite, nausea, abdominal pain dark urine and jaundice	• No vaccine • Don't shoot drugs and share needles • Don't share items that may have blood on them • Wash hands	• Chronic infection in 55–85% of infected individuals • 1–5% may die • Leading indication for liver transplant • Uncommon in the United States
Viral Hepatitis D HDV	Same as viral hepatitis B: • Blood from infected person enters a person who is not infected • Spread through contaminated needles, or other sharps • Sex • Infected mother to baby during birth	fatigue, loss of appetite, nausea, vomiting, joint and abdominal pain, jaundice and dark urine	• Hepatitis B vaccine • Education to reduce risk behaviors	If co-infection with HBV the individual may have more severe symptoms and is more likely to have chronic liver disease
Viral Hepatitis E HEV	Same as HAV: Human feces of persons with HAV being transmitted to oral cavity of other person Example: Not washing hands after bathroom and then preparing food.	fatigue, loss of appetite, nausea, vomiting, dark urine, and jaundice	• No vaccine • Wash hands	• No long-term infection • More severe in pregnant women in their third trimester

This information was taken from the Centers for Disease Control web site fact sheets for Viral Hepatitis A-E.

Hepatitis E Hepatitis E is found in the feces of people and animals and is therefore spread through contaminated water and food. The symptoms are loss of appetite, dark urine, fatigue, and nausea. To prevent this disease an individual should wash hands carefully when preparing food and when traveling take special care in avoiding contaminated water.

Human Immunodeficiency Virus

Human immunodeficiency virus (HIV) belongs to the class of retroviruses and is the cause of acquired immunodeficiency syndrome (AIDS). It gains access to the bloodstream via sexual intercourse, transfusions, and sticks with infected needles that break the skin. Also, a fetus can be infected by its mother. HIV attacks

T-lymphocytes, part of the immune system, and multiplies. People in this stage pose no threat to the health care worker if standard precautions are followed. People who have HIV but are unaware that they carry it are called asymptomatic carriers. Some have vague complaints, such as fever, weight loss, or unexplained diarrhea. These individuals are referred to as having AIDS-related complex (ARC).

In most cases, the disease progresses and the infected individual develops some brain damage in the form of dementia. If the individual is in this state for a long period of time, more severe brain damage may occur; normally, the infected individual most likely succumbs to AIDS before this happens.

Current treatment focuses on symptoms and not the disease itself. A great deal of research is being done currently to develop a vaccine to fight this retrovirus.

Acquired Immunodeficiency Syndrome

Acquired immunodeficiency syndrome (AIDS) results from infection with HIV, but not all individuals infected with HIV develop AIDS. A syndrome is a group of symptoms that characterize a disease. In the United States, 100,000 cases of HIV were diagnosed in the 1980s. The first few cases were reported in 1981. The CDC was notified of a rare and unusual lung infection in young homosexual men. Also, a slow-growing skin tumor found in aging men, called Kaposi's sarcoma, was found to be growing aggressively in this same group of men. Individuals with these two symptoms reported with a number of opportunistic infections, such as pneumonia.

After much research, the virus was found to be transmitted via the semen and blood of infected individuals. "Casual" spreading of the disease does not seem to happen. For example, kissing does not spread the disease. A person with full-blown AIDS exhibits cancers, infections, diarrhea, or a number of other viral diseases. The prognosis is often fatal, but life may be sustained for a number of years with appropriate diet and health measures. Through December 2001, the cumulative number of AIDS cases reported to the CDC was 816,149. Total deaths of this same group were 467,910. The majority of these diagnosed cases are in the thirty to forty age group.

There is no cure for AIDS. The complications are treated accordingly. Several antiviral drugs are used, such as zidovudine (AZT) and acyclovir. AZT has a number of side effects but has been shown to slow progression of the disease. Research continues in an effort to find a vaccine for HIV, with several drugs showing promise.

How the Body Resists Diseases

The body fights disease in a number of ways, such as fever or chills or localized inflammation. Before these symptoms occur, however, the pathogens must pass through other lines of defense.

Our bodies repel thousands of infections that come our way every day. Intact skin makes it impossible for a number of bacteria to enter body cells. If dust or some pathogen-laden particles get into the nose, a person sneezes. If something enters the throat, a person coughs. If spoiled food is swallowed, a person normally vomits or expels it through diarrhea.

If the pathogen gains access to the body, the second line of defense, the circulatory system, begins fighting the pathogen. The area becomes inflamed and swollen. Swelling and redness are due to the engorgement of the capillaries with blood. White cells in great numbers migrate to the area and engulf large numbers of bacteria. Many of these cells die and produce enzymes that digest the dead tissues. These mobile phagocytes or leukocytes engulf the invading pathogens and destroy them. The result of this process is **purulence** (pus). While this is going on, the body is building a dam around the infected area, called the **pyogenic membrane**. This membrane is a wall that contains the infection and does not allow it to spread to other parts of the body. If the infection can be controlled, this area fills in with connective tissue and is healed.

If the pathogens overcome the body's first and second lines of defense, the infection spreads to adjoining tissues and finally to the entire body. When this happens, the body utilizes its final defenses: **antibodies**. Antibodies produce immunity against any foreign substance or pathogen. Pathogens that stimulate the production of antibodies are called **antigens**.

There are a number of antibody groups that perform different functions in response to antigens. For instance, an **antitoxin** neutralizes the toxins given off by certain bacteria.

Infection

Another way the body fights off infection or pathogens is with fever and inflammation. Few bacteria can survive a fever of 102 to 104 degrees for long. Inflammation, an increase in blood flow in the injured area, is characterized by four signs: erythema (redness), heat, edema (swelling), and pain. An increase in blood supply in the area causes the redness and heat and the walls to enlarge, allowing antibodies into the area. The swelling causes pain and pressure on nerve endings.

Immunity

The ability to resist pathogens is called immunity. People differ in their abilities to resist disease, and this resistance is stronger at various times in a person's life than at others. Two general types of immunity are natural and acquired. Humans are born with **natural immunity**. Local inflammation and blood phagocytes are part of the natural immune system.

If immunity is developed as a result of exposure to a pathogen, it is called **acquired immunity**. This also can be a borrowed immunity, called **passive acquired immunity**. This occurs when antibodies from another animal or person are injected into an individual, giving protection to the individual from a specific disease. This immediate immunity normally only lasts up to six weeks. A fetus obtains temporary passive immunity from the mother through the placenta. While breastfeeding, the mother's milk also provides some passive immunity to the baby.

Lasting longer and preferred over passive acquired immunity is **active acquired immunity**. The two types of active acquired immunity are natural acquired immunity and artificial acquired immunity. **Natural acquired immunity** occurs when an individual has had a disease, the body has manufactured antibodies to the disease, and the person has recovered from the disease. Normally, the individual is then immune to the disease and does not contract the disease again. The second type of active acquired immunity, **artificial acquired immunity**, occurs when the individual is vaccinated (inoculated) with a specific antigen. An antigen is a substance injected into the individual in order to stimulate production of specific antibodies. This antigen is often

an expired or a weakened state of the pathogen. The process is used to increase an individual's resistance to a particular disease or to provide **immunization**.

The body itself may overreact to an antigen. If the antigen causes an allergic response, it is called an **allergen**. Individuals who are generally more sensitive to certain allergens than most people are called **hypersensitive**. In severe cases, a person's antigen-antibody response stimulates a massive secretion of histamine. This severe reaction, called **anaphylactic shock** (anaphylaxis), is sometimes fatal. It is important to take a thorough health history in order to identify individuals who are hypersensitive to one or more substances.

CHAPTER SUMMARY

To safeguard against microorganism exposure in a dental office, one must understand how these pathogens pass from an infected person to a susceptible person. Therefore, within this chapter you have been given information about pathogenic microorganisms along with the diseases they cause and how the body can defend against them.

Case Study

Darin Scott came down with a low-grade fever, night sweats, and weight loss. He exhibited fatigue and finally a persistent cough.

Case Study Review

1. What is one disease you would consider?

2. Is this disease common?

3. What treatment will most likely be prescribed?

4. What microorganism caused this disease?

REVIEW QUESTIONS

Multiple Choice

1. Who developed the theory of the etiologic agent?
   a. Anton Van Leeuwenhoek
   b. Louis Pasteur
   c. Robert Koch
   d. Joseph Lister

2. Most bacteria is said to require air and is therefore called
   a. aerobic.
   b. anaerobic.
   c. facultative bacteria.
   d. gram positive.

3. Which bacteria has been implicated in dental caries?
   a. Staphylococcal
   b. *Mycobacterium tuberculosis*
   c. Bacillus *Corynebacterium diphtheria*
   d. *Streptococcus mutans*

4. The herpes simplex virus that infects the finger and was a concern before the usage of treatment gloves is called
   a. corneal ulcer
   b. herpetic whitlow
   c. tinea
   d. candidiasis

5. The name of the slow-growing skin tumor that develops from HIV is called
   a. Kaposi's sarcoma.
   b. pyogenic membrane.
   c. allergen.
   d. herpes zoster.

6. The individual credited with the creation of vaccines and the eradication of polio is
   a. Anton Van Leeuwenhoek.
   b. Louis Pasteur.
   c. Robert Koch.
   d. Joseph Lister.

7. The shape of bacteria that is rod shaped is:
   a. cocci.
   b. bacilli.
   c. spirilla.
   d. vibrios.

8. The bacteria that can grow with or without oxygen are termed _____.
   a. aerobic bacteria
   b. anaerobic bacteria
   c. facultative anaerobic bacteria
   d. all of the above

9. The individual who was instrumental in using heat to destroy bacteria and resistant spores is:
   a. Anton Van Leeuwenhoek.
   b. Louis Pasteur.
   c. Robert Koch.
   d. Joseph Lister.

10. The childhood disease that is caused by the varicella-zoster virus is _____.
   a. measles
   b. mumps
   c. chickenpox
   d. poliomyelitis

Critical Thinking

1. If two individuals kiss on the lips and neither has open sores around the mouth but one of the two has AIDS, is the probability high for the other individual to acquire AIDS because of this kiss?

2. Which two of the five microorganisms are present during periodontal disease?

3. Which of the hepatitis viruses is of greatest concern to the dental assistant and why?

Web Activities

1. Go to www.cdc.gov and find the current statistics for HIV/AIDS mortality.

2. Go to www.cdc.gov and find current statistics for tuberculosis. Has the number of reported cases increased or decreased in the past two years? In which year was the incidence of tuberculosis the highest?

3. Go to www.cdc.gov and research the most recent information on HBV. Be prepared to discuss it in class.

INFECTION CONTROL

SPECIFIC INSTRUCTIONAL OBJECTIVES

The student should strive to meet the following objectives and demonstrate an understanding of the facts and principles presented in this chapter:

1. Identify the rationale, regulations, recommendations, and training that govern infection control in the dental office.

2. Describe how pathogens travel from person to person in the dental office.

3. List the three primary routes of microbial transmission and the associated dental procedures that affect the dental assistant.

4. Demonstrate the principles of infection control, including medical history, handwashing, personal protective equipment, barriers, chemical disinfectants, ultrasonic cleaners, sterilizers, and instrument storage.

5. List various disinfectants and their applications as used in dentistry.

6. Identify and demonstrate the usage of different types of sterilizers.

7. Demonstrate the usage of several types of sterilization monitors, such as biological and process indicators.

8. Identify and show the proper usage of preprocedure mouth rinses, high-volume evacuation, dental dams, and disposable items.

9. Identify and demonstrate the correct protocol for disinfecting, cleaning, and sterilizing prior to seating the patient, as well as at the end of the dental treatment, in the dental radiography area, and in the dental laboratory.

KEY TERMS

aerosol *(206)*

agent *(204)*

airborne
  transmission *(205)*

American Dental
  Association
  (ADA) *(201)*

antimicrobial *(207)*

antisepsis *(207)*

asepsis *(200)*

aseptic technique *(200)*

asymptomatic *(207)*

autoclavable utility
  gloves *(212)*

biofilms *(224)*

**Bloodborne Pathogens
  Standard** *(201)*

**body substance
  isolation (BSI)** *(201)*

cavitation *(218)*

**Centers for Disease
  Control and
  Prevention
  (CDC)** *(201)*

chain of asepsis *(200)*

cleaning *(215)*

compromised
  host *(205)*

contact dermatitis *(210)*

contact
  transmission *(205)*

direct contact *(206)*

disinfection *(215)*

**Environmental
  Protection Agency
  (EPA)** *(202)*

fomite *(204)*

**Food and Drug
  Administration
  (FDA)** *(202)*

glutaraldehyde *(216)*

(continues)

INTRODUCTION

The dentist is responsible for ensuring that the process of **infection control** is adequate. Compliance with all regulations must be accomplished on a continuing basis; staff must be trained at the time of initial employment or when job tasks change (before the employee is placed in a position where occupational exposure may occur) and annually thereafter. Records must be maintained for the duration of employment plus thirty years, in accordance with regulations. Even though the dentist is ultimately responsible, often an employee (full-time) is designated as the infection control and hazardous waste coordinator. This person ensures that the office is in compliance with all regulations, reads updated information on infection control and hazardous waste, and presents the information to the dental team for review. The infection control and hazardous waste coordinator schedules staff training, oversees the entire process of infection control, and makes sure that procedures ensure complete **asepsis**. Asepsis means the creation of an environment free of **pathogens** (disease-causing microorganisms). It also includes the steps, or **aseptic technique**, to provide this environment. Aseptic technique is needed for all procedures in which there is a danger of introducing infection or disease into a human's body.

Rationales and Regulations of Infection Control

All efforts are made to stop infectious diseases from spreading and routine practices eliminate mistakes. **Universal precautions** mean that all patients are treated as if they are infectious. **Standard precautions** (universal precautions and body substance isolation techniques) are practiced prior to, during, and after each procedure in the dental office. Therefore, every precaution is taken to ensure that the **chain of asepsis** (aseptic procedures ensuring that no cross-contamination occurs) is not broken and that contamination does not occur.

Regulations and Recommendations for Infection Control in the Dental Office

A number of agencies have established guidelines for infection control in the dental office. These minimal standards change from time to time as the knowledge base on prevention expands. **Regulations** are made by government agencies (see below) and licensing boards that have the authority to enforce compliance. If compliance is not met, dentists may be fined, lose their licenses to practice dentistry, or face imprisonment. **Recommendations** can be made by anyone, and no authority for enforcement is mandated. When regulations are introduced, the profession has a specific timeframe in which to comply. During this time, consultants, the dental association, and other groups make recommendations on the best means for compliance. See Appendix A for addresses and phone numbers for regulating and recommending agencies.

American Dental Association (ADA). The **American Dental Association (ADA)**, the parent organization for dentistry in the United States, makes recommendations through its councils (see Chapter 1, Introduction to the Dental Profession) in the form of literature, videotapes, news broadcasts, manuals, brochures, the *Journal of the American Dental Association (JADA), ADA News,* and an Internet site (www.ada.org). The American Dental Assistants Association (ADAA), the American Dental Hygienists' Association (ADHA), and the American Dental Laboratory Association (ADLA) also provide information to their members through support services and journals.

Centers for Disease Control and Prevention. The **Centers for Disease Control and Prevention (CDC)** provides the basis for many of the regulations. This agency, part of the Public Health Service, a division of the U.S. Department of Health and Human Services, has developed a number of recommendations that were made by federal, state, and local agencies into regulations.

In 1996, the CDC issued standard precautions that augmented and synthesized universal precautions and **body substance isolation (BSI)** techniques. BSI is a system requiring **personal protective equipment (PPE)** to be worn to protect against contact with all body fluids, whether or not blood is visible. Standard precautions, adopted by numerous health care industries, protect providers, patients, and others from infectious diseases.

Occupational Safety and Health Administration. The **Occupational Safety and Health Administration (OSHA)** is a regulating body that enforces requirements that employers must protect their employees from exposure to blood and **other potentially infectious materials (OPIM)** during the time when employees are at work. This agency is part of the U.S. Department of Labor. Its overall mission is to protect workers in the United States from physical, chemical, or infectious hazards while in the workplace. The OSHA **Bloodborne Pathogens Standard** became effective in 1992. This standard applies to any facility where employees can or have the potential to be exposed to body fluids, such as in hospitals, funeral homes, emergency medical services, medical and dental offices, and research laboratories.

Other Potentially Infectious Materials

OSHA and the CDC define the following human fluids as blood and OPIM according to the standard:

- Blood and anything that is visually contaminated with blood
- Saliva in dental procedures
- Cerebrospinal fluid (brain and spinal fluid)
- Amniotic fluid (fluid around the fetus)
- **Synovial** fluid (joint and tendon fluid)
- **Pleural** (lung fluid)/**peritoneal** fluid (abdominal fluid)/**pericardial** fluid (heart fluid)
- Semen and vaginal secretions
- Unfixed tissue or organ (other than intact skin) from a human (living or dead)
- HIV-containing cell or tissue cultures, organ cultures, and HIV- or HBV-containing culture medium or other solutions
- Blood, organs, or other tissues from experimental animals infected with HIV or HBV

Compliance with these standards is monitored through investigations of the facilities by OSHA inspectors. If the facility fails to come into compliance, a citation resulting in a possible fine is given. If the facility continues to refuse to comply, the fine increases and additional steps are taken to ensure that noncompliant conditions are corrected.

When Dental Offices Are Investigated for Compliance

- After an employee or a patient complaint is made
- In any office having eleven or more employees, randomly
- By invitation of the office requesting an inspection

All states are regulated by the OSHA standard. Twenty-four states are regulated through state agency standards that run parallel to or are more demanding than the federal standard; the other states are administered through regional branches of the federal OSHA.

Overview of the 1991 OSHA Bloodborne Pathogens Standard

Every facility must:

- Review the Bloodborne Pathogens Standard

- Prepare a written exposure control plan and means to protect and train employees

- Train all employees in a timely manner (initially, after a job task change, and annually)

- Provide employees with everything needed in order to meet standard regulations

- Provide personal protective equipment (PPE)

- Maintain and dispose of necessary PPE

- Establish standard operating procedures (SOPs) in infection control

- Offer the hepatitis B vaccination series to all employees

- Establish a postexposure plan, including medical evaluation and follow-up procedures (for example, occupational exposure needlestick)

- Provide communication on biohazards

- Establish standards for handling and disposing of hazardous waste

- Maintain records of training, hepatitis B vaccinations, and exposure incidents

Exposure Determination To evaluate an employee's chances of occupational exposure to bloodborne pathogens, an exposure determination is made. An **occupational exposure** is any reasonably anticipated eye, mucosa, skin, **parenteral** (cut, needlestick, puncture, abrasions, and so on), or any contact with blood or saliva that may be a result of employment tasks. The determination is made based on three categories:

- **Category 1** includes all tasks that involve exposure to blood, body fluids such as saliva, and body tissues. (This group includes dentist, dental assistant, dental hygienist, and dental laboratory technician.)

- **Category 2** includes all tasks that involve no exposure to blood, body fluids such as saliva, or body tissues, but occasionally may involve unplanned tasks from Category 1. (This group includes the receptionist, coordinating assistant, and so on.)

- **Category 3** includes all tasks that involve no exposure to blood, body fluids such as saliva, or body tissues. (This group includes the accountant, insurance assistant, and so on.)

Written Exposure Plan This plan documents the specific exposure determination for each employee and identifies a schedule of implementation (how and when provisions of the standard will be implemented). This document must list how situations surrounding an exposure will be evaluated and what measures will be taken to correct the situation (if necessary).

Step 1. All employees list tasks they perform in each job classification, and then identify which category they fall under. Any employee who may have any occupational exposure at any time is covered under the standard.

Step 2. The office must have a schedule for implementation. This schedule must designate how and when each provision of the standard will be implemented.

- How and when are the hepatitis B vaccinations being offered to employees?

- How and when is communication of hazards to employees covered?

- How and when are the postexposure evaluation and office follow-up procedures accomplished?

- How and when is the recordkeeping accomplished and updated?

Step 3. A manual and procedure plan must be written to cover methods of compliance for office PPE and safety issues. For instance, the office must have written information covering all aspects of the following:

- Personal protective equipment

- Engineering controls

- Housekeeping controls

- Work practice controls

Step 4. A written policy on how exposure incidents are evaluated is required. Included in this area are the circumstances that surround the incident and how they can be corrected. What type of evaluation will be done by the office if an exposure incident occurs?

The Food and Drug Administration. The **Food and Drug Administration (FDA)**, which is a division of the U.S. Department of Health and Human Services, regulates the manufacturing and labeling of medical devices and solutions. The FDA requires that certain performance standards be met prior to use by the public. It requires that general controls be used with the devices and solutions and that labeling give the appropriate information to the consumer. It holds manufacturers responsible for problems that develop, unless the medical device or solution is misused by the consumer. In that instance, the liability lies with the user.

Items in the dental office regulated by the FDA are sterilizers; chemical and biologic indicators; cleaning solutions such as ultrasonic solution and cold chemicals; PPE such as gloves, masks, glasses, and disposable clothing; sterilizing solutions; and disinfectants.

Environmental Protection Agency. The **Environmental Protection Agency (EPA)** is a federal regulatory agency involved in the safety and effectiveness of disinfecting and sterilizing solutions. It also regulates the disposal of hazardous waste after it leaves the dental office. All disinfecting and sterilizing solutions must be submitted by the manufacturer to the EPA for registration. If a solution meets all claims listed and safety concerns are noted on the container, after undertaking and passing specific testing requirements the EPA assigns an EPA number that must appear on its label.

Organization for Safety and Asepsis Procedures (OSAP). The membership of the Organization for Safety and Asepsis Procedures (OSAP), a national organization, encompasses dental health care workers, distributors of dental equipment and materials, health care instructors, dentists, and others in the field of dentistry. OSAP has regional and annual meetings that cover topics of infection control and hazard communication for dental team members. Written documentation is available from OSAP to help infection control in the dental office.

OSHA-Mandated Training for Dental Office Employees

All employers must ensure that employees (full-time, part-time, and temporary) who fall into Category 1 and/or 2, where tasks involve exposure to blood, body fluids such as saliva, and/or body tissues, have training. This training must be provided at no cost to the employee. The training must be given before placement in a position where bloodborne pathogens are a factor, to all new employees, and to all employees reclassifying into new positions.

OSHA-Mandated Training for Dental Employees

The following must be available to all dental employees:

- A copy of the Bloodborne Pathogens Standard and specific information regarding the meaning of the standard
- Information about bloodborne pathogens, both the epidemiology and symptoms of the diseases
- Information about the cross-contamination pathways of bloodborne pathogens
- A written copy or means for employees to obtain the employer's/office's written exposure control plan
- Information on the tasks, category placement of employee classifications, and how each is identified in relation to bloodborne pathogens and other potentially infectious materials (OPIM)
- Information regarding the hepatitis B vaccine
- Information about exposure reduction, including PPE; work practices; standard precautions, including universal precautions; and engineering practices
- Information about the selection, placement, use, removal, disinfection, sterilization, and disposal of PPE
- Information about what to do and whom to contact if an emergency involving blood or OPIM arises
- Information about the procedure to follow if an incident of blood exposure occurs, how to report the incident, and what type of medical follow-up is available at no cost to the employee
- Information about the postexposure evaluation and follow-up the employer provides
- A copy of the OSHA Hazard Communication Standard
- Material safety data sheets (MSDSs) and information about labeling and hazardous waste
- Opportunity for employees to ask questions of the individual giving the information

---

The training cannot be accomplished by videos or interactive computer training programs alone. The training must be accomplished by an individual who has the background necessary to answer questions and to supplement the training with in-office (on-site), specific information. The information must be given in a manner for all to understand. If an employee cannot understand the content due to a language barrier or a disability, the employer must provide an interpreter or convey this information in a manner for the employee to understand completely.

A record of the date of the training session, employees present, and qualifications of the trainer must be maintained.

Cross-Contamination Pathways

Pathogens can travel from patients to dentists, dental assistants, dental hygienists, dental laboratory technicians, and other patients. Pathogens can also travel from dental personnel to patients. The transfer then can go to the families and friends of the dental personnel.

Chain of Infection

The chain of infection describes the elements of an infectious process. It is an interactive process that involves the agent, host, and environment. This process must include several essential elements or "links in the chain" for the transmission of microorganisms to occur. Figure 11-1 identifies the six essential links. Without the transmission of microorganisms, the infectious process cannot occur. Knowledge about the chain of infection facilitates control or prevention of disease by breaking the links in the chain. This is achieved by altering one or more of the interactive processes of agent, host, or environment.

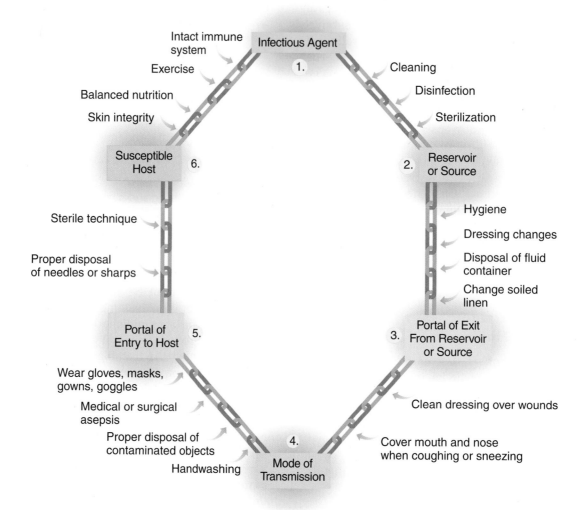

FIGURE 11-1 Chain of infection: Preventive measures follow each link.

Agent

An **agent** is an entity that is capable of causing disease. Agents that may cause disease follow:

- *Biological agents*—living organisms that invade the host, such as bacteria, virus, fungi, protozoa, and rickettsiae
- *Chemical agents*—substances that can interact with the body such as pesticides, food additives, medications, and industrial chemicals
- *Physical agents*—factors in the environment such as heat, light, noise, and radiation

In the chain of infection, the main concern is biological (infectious) agents and their effect on the host.

Reservoir

The **reservoir** is a place where the agent can survive. Colonization and reproduction take place while the

agent is in the reservoir. A reservoir that promotes growth of pathogens must contain the proper nutrients (such as oxygen and organic matter), maintain proper temperature, contain moisture, maintain a compatible pH level, and maintain the proper amount of light exposure. The most common reservoirs are humans, animals, environment, and **fomites**. Fomites are objects contaminated with an infectious agent such as instruments or dressings.

Humans and animals can have symptoms of the infectious agents or can be strictly carriers of the agent. Carriers have the infectious agent but are symptom free. The agent can be spread to others in both instances.

Portal of Exit

The **portal of exit** is the route by which an infectious agent leaves the reservoir to be transferred to a susceptible host. The agent leaves the reservoir through body secretions, such as sputum, semen, vaginal secretions, urine, saliva, feces, blood, and draining wounds.

Mode of Transmission

The mode of transmission is the process that bridges the gap between the portal of exit of the infectious agent from the reservoir and the portal of entry of the susceptible "new" host. Most infectious agents have a usual mode of transmission; however, some microorganisms may be transmitted by more than one mode (Table 11-1).

- **Contact transmission** involves the physical transfer of an agent from an infected person to an uninfected person through direct contact with the infected person. Contact with the infected person through contaminated secretions is called indirect contact. Examples of direct contact are sexually transmitted diseases, colds, and flu.

- **Airborne transmission** occurs when a susceptible person is exposed to contaminated droplets or dust particles that are suspended in the air. The longer the particle is suspended, the greater the chance it will find an available port of entry in the human host. An example of an organism that relies on airborne transmission is measles. Spores of anthrax are also transmitted in an airborne powder form. The dental handpiece, while in use, creates airborne droplets that can be transmitted.

- **Vehicle transmission** occurs when the agent is transferred to a susceptible host by contaminated inanimate objects such as dental instruments, water, food, meat, drugs, and blood. An example is salmonellosis transmitted through contaminated food.

- **Vectorborne transmission** occurs when an agent is transferred to a susceptible person host by animate means such as mosquitoes, fleas, ticks, lice, and other animals. Lyme disease is an example.

Portal of Entry

A portal of entry is the route by which an infectious agent enters the host. Portals of entry include the following:

- Integumentary system—a break in the skin or mucous membrane
- Respiratory tract—inhaling contaminated droplets
- Genitourinary tract—contamination with infected vaginal secretions or semen
- Gastrointestinal tract—ingesting contaminated food or water
- Circulatory system—bite of insects or rodents
- Transplacental—transfer of a microorganism from mother to fetus via the placenta and umbilical cord

Host

A host is a simple or complex organism that can be affected by an agent. As the term is used here, a host is an individual who is at risk of contracting an infectious disease. A susceptible host is a person who lacks resistance to an agent and is vulnerable to a disease. A compromised host is a person whose normal defense mechanisms are impaired and who is therefore more susceptible to infection.

The following characteristics of the host influence the susceptibility to and severity of infections.

- Age—as a person ages, immunity declines
- Concurrent disease—the existence of other diseases indicates susceptibility
- Stress—a person experiencing a compromised emotional state has lower defense mechanisms
- Immunization/vaccination status—certain people are not fully immunized
- Lifestyle—practices such as having multiple sex partners, sharing needles, or tobacco/drug use can alter defenses

TABLE 11-1 Modes of Transmission

Mode	Examples
Contact	Direct contact of health care provider with patient: • Touching • Secretions from client Indirect contact with fomites: • Clothing • Health care equipment • Instruments used in treatments • Personal belongings • Personal care equipment • Diagnostic equipment
Airborne	Inhaling microorganisms carried by moisture or dust particles in air: • Coughing • Talking • Sneezing • Dental handpiece
Vehicle	Contact with contaminated inanimate objects: • Water • Blood • Drugs • Food • Urine
Vectorborne	Contact with contaminated animate hosts: • Animals • Insects

- Occupation—forms of employment that involve increased exposure to pathogenic sources such as needles or chemical agents
- Nutritional status—people who maintain targeted weight for height and body frame are less prone to illness
- Heredity—some people are naturally more susceptible to infections than others

Breaking the Chain of Infection

Dental assistants focus on breaking the chain of infection by applying proper infection control practices to interfere with the spread of microorganisms. Specific strategies can be directed at breaking or blocking the transmission of infection from one link in the chain to the next. Discussion regarding each of the six links follows.

Between Agent and Reservoir

The keys to eliminating infection between agent and reservoir in the chain are cleansing, disinfection, and sterilization. These tactics serve to prevent the formation of a reservoir and environment within which infectious agents can live and multiply.

If the reservoir is an already infected individual, that individual may need to be isolated. The individual's infectious condition needs to be vigorously treated to reduce the reservoir of infectious material or eliminate the agent.

Between Reservoir and Portal of Exit

Promoting proper hygiene, maintaining clean dental operatories, and ensuring the use of clean equipment in patient care can break the chain between the reservoir and the portal of exit. The aim is to eliminate the reservoir for the microorganism before the pathogen can escape to a susceptible host.

Between Portal of Exit and Mode of Transmission

The goal in breaking the chain here is to block the exit of the infectious agent. The dental assistant must maintain clean dressings on all injuries or wounds. People should be encouraged to cover the mouth and nose when sneezing or coughing, and the dental assistant must do so as well. Gloves must be worn when caring for a person who may have infectious secretions and care must be taken to properly dispose of contaminated articles.

Between Mode of Transmission and Portal of Entry

The goal is to break the chain of infection between the mode of transmission and portal of entry. Dental assistants must always wash their hands between cases that may involve contact with contaminated items. Barrier protection must be worn when care involves contact with body secretions. Gloves, masks, gowns, and goggles are all forms of barrier protection.

Between Portal of Entry and Host

Maintaining skin integrity and using sterile techniques for patient contacts are methods of breaking the chain between portal of entry and host. The goal is to prevent the transmission of infection to an uninfected person including the dental assistant.

Between Host and Agent

To break the chain between host and agent means eliminating infection before it begins. Proper nutrition, exercise, and immunization allow an individual to maintain an intact immune system, thus preventing infection.

Routes of Microbial Transmission in the Dental Office

In dentistry, three primary routes transmit most microorganisms: direct contact, indirect contact, and inhalation/aerosol. Microorganisms may be missed because they appear as a mist or dry clear on exposed surfaces. They are overlooked if careful, consistent aseptic procedures are not followed. The dental assistant is the primary caretaker of infection control practices. Using the correct barriers, PPE, treating all patients as if they are infectious, using proper disinfection, and sterilization break the chain of infection and eliminate cross-contamination (see also Chapter 10, Microbiology).

Routes of microbial transmission are as follows:

1. **Direct contact:** An individual has direct contact with a lesion or microorganism while performing intra-oral dental procedures.
2. **Indirect contact:** An individual contacts the microorganism through another means, such as contaminated instruments, supplies, or equipment.
3. **Inhalation/aerosol:** An individual contacts the microorganism through inhalation. This normally happens when the high-speed handpiece or the ultrasonic cavitron is used in the dental office.

Infection Control in the Dental Office

A number of steps must be followed to accomplish the goal of **infection control**, or asepsis. The first step is for the dental assistant to maintain good health standards. Eating and sleeping properly aid in staying healthy.

Proper exercise, along with maintaining a positive mental attitude, provides the energy to attain individual goals for good overall health.

Immunizations

The dental assistant should have the immunizations necessary to fight off pathogens that are encountered due to close proximity to patients during dental treatment. If the dental assistant has not had the hepatitis B series, the employer must provide information about immunizations and the available vaccine during initial training and is required to pay for the series. Review the employee training information regarding the hepatitis B vaccine earlier in this chapter (see also Chapter 10, Microbiology, for additional information regarding immunizations).

Medical History

Taking the patient's medical history and updating it at each appointment is a good way to gather information but may not identify infectious diseases patients have. It is important to update this information both verbally and in writing. Patients are sometimes more willing to disclose information during conversation. Most individuals infected with HBV and HIV are asymptomatic, meaning they have no symptoms. Therefore, the medical history may give information to the health care workers, but it cannot be used alone to identify patients who place dental personnel at high risk. Standard precautions incorporating universal precautions and practicing infection control standards with each and every patient are essential in infection control.

Handwashing

One of the most important ways to prevent the transfer of microorganisms from one person or object to another person is handwashing. Handwashing is the vigorous rubbing together of well-lathered soapy hands (ensuring friction on all surfaces), concluding with a thorough rinsing under a stream of water and proper drying. Handwashing is both a mechanical cleaning and chemical antisepsis (inhibiting the growth of causative microorganisms).

Hands contain resident and transient microflora (visible by use of microscope). The mechanical process of scrubbing removes transient microorganisms and some resident microorganisms. Transient microorganisms are fresh contaminants of brief duration. Transient microorganisms are of primary concern to the dental profession because they constitute the pathogen group that includes hepatitis. Resident microorganisms survive and multiply for a longer period primarily in the top layers of the skin but can be in deeper layers of the skin. The chemical antisepsis is accomplished through the use of an antimicrobial soap. Applying the proper technique and using antimicrobial (microorganism growth

inhibitor) handwashing products can add additional protection to ensure that microorganisms are removed each time the hands are washed.

Currently, antimicrobial handwashing agents that are the most beneficial include chlorhexidine digluconate, triclosan, and para-chlorometaxylenol. These handwashing agents exhibit prolonged antimicrobial effects.

At the beginning of each day, every member of the dental team should complete *two consecutive fifteen-second handwashes*. It is important to use plenty of antimicrobial soap and water while rubbing all areas of the hands (Figure 11-2). Getting between the fingers, rubbing each finger and thumb, and cleaning beneath the fingernails is essential. Some offices provide brushes that aid in scrubbing. These brushes (often made of foam rubber pad and plastic bristles) must not be so hard that they abrade the tissue, allowing microorganisms access to the body. The brushes must be disposable or autoclavable. Remember, the skin is a barrier to microorganisms, and care should be taken to prevent cuts and lesions. A final rinse with cool water is used to close the pores in the skin. Dry the hands completely with paper towels, and use the paper towels to turn off the hand-controlled sink faucets and wipe the area clean. The brushes are sterilized or disposed of after each use.

A minimal fifteen-second handwashing should be completed before and after patient care, donning and removing gloves, breaks, ending each day, and at any other time the hands become contaminated. Due to constant handwashing, the hands may show effects of skin irritation. Hand lotions help to prevent hands from chapping. Procedure 11-1 presents an overview of proper handwashing technique.

FIGURE 11-2 Dental assistant hand washing with antimicrobial soap and scrub brush/sponge.

PROCEDURE 11-1

Handwashing

The procedure is performed by all dental team members.

EQUIPMENT AND SUPPLIES

- Liquid antimicrobial handwashing agent
- Soft, sterile brush or sponge (optional)
- Sink with hot and cold running water
- Paper towels

PROCEDURE STEPS

At the beginning of each day (two consecutive 15-second handwashes)

1. Remove jewelry (rings and watch).

2. Adjust water flow and wet hands thoroughly.

3. Apply about one teaspoon of antimicrobial handwashing agent with water; bring to a lather.

4. Scrub hands together or with a sterile brush or sponge, making sure to get between each finger, the surface of the palms and wrists, and under the fingernails.

5. Rinse and repeat Steps 3 and 4.

6. Final rinse with cool to lukewarm water for ten seconds to close the pores.

7. Dry with paper towels, the hands first and then the wrist area.

8. Use paper towels to turn off the hand-controlled faucets.

Routine Handwashing: Fifteen-second handwash before and after patients, donning gloves, and taking breaks. Routine handwashing must be completed at the end of each day and any other time the hands become contaminated.

1. Complete handwashing steps for the beginning of each day, except Step 5.

- Artificial fingernails are not recommended for health professionals. Artificial fingernails have been found to exhibit high microbe counts under the nail, even after thorough handwashing.

- Wearing fingernail polish can harbor microorganisms. Wearing red fingernail polish or within that color range can also alarm the patient if he or she sees the nails pass within his or her sight. Seeing the red from the patient's point of view may appear as blood and cause the patient undue stress during treatment. It is advisable not to wear fingernail polish.

The soap containers and the sink area become contaminated and should be disinfected routinely. Foot-operated soap dispensers prevent unnecessary hand contamination. The water controls should be foot or light sensor operated to cut down on contamination. Do not use reusable towels to dry hands; instead, use air or disposable towels.

Dental teams involved in oral surgery should perform a surgical scrub (see Chapter 25, Oral and Maxillofacial Surgery, for directions in performing a surgical scrub).

Personal Protective Equipment

The dental assistant is constantly exposed to saliva and blood during intraoral/invasive dental procedures. Even with the maintenance of good health and immunizations, it is essential for dental team members to ensure better protection from microorganisms through constant use of personal protective equipment (PPE). Employers must provide this equipment according to OSHA regulations. Barriers are used to prevent potential pathogens encountered during patient care from gaining access to dental personnel. Barriers such as protective eyewear, face masks, disposable gloves, and appropriate uniforms should be used routinely to minimize exposure.

Protective Eyewear. Dental team members must wear protective eyewear during specific phases of dental treatment. The splatter of blood and saliva can transfer infectious diseases, such as hepatitis and herpes simplex viruses, to the mucous membranes of the eye. Aerosol droplets that contain microorganisms can cause an eye infection known as pink eye (conjunctivitis). Also, during some dental procedures, particles of gold, amalgam, and tooth fragments can be hurled into the eye, causing damage. Dental offices provide protective eyewear for patients to wear during dental treatment. These glasses, like the ones worn by the dental personnel, can be disposable or disinfected or sterilized after use.

Protective eyewear should provide front, top, and side protection; several choices are available. The American National Standards Institute developed a standard for the design and characteristics of occupational glasses. Dental team members who wear corrective lenses may choose to wear goggles that fit over their glasses or side shields that fit on their own eyewear (Figures 11-3A and B). Others wear glasses designed for dental personnel that incorporate top and side shields (Figure 11-3C). In addition, a face shield can be worn that covers the entire face (Figure 11-3D). A mask must still be worn with a face shield.

Eyewear is also used to protect the eyes from high-intensity lights used for curing dental materials. These glasses or shields are normally colored orange for protection.

At times, the eyewear becomes fogged due to warm breath coming from under the dental mask. Several antifog products are available to minimize fogging. Fog spray can be used, or the eyewear can be placed under warm water to reduce the fog problem.

Gloves. Gloves are used as a barrier to microorganisms. Any time a dental team member anticipates contact with saliva or blood, gloves should be worn. This includes saliva- or blood-contaminated surfaces, instruments, or mucous membranes. Numerous gloves are on the market that meet FDA regulations. The FDA regulates the gloves specific for the health care industry. Five primary types of gloves are used in the dental office (FDA regulated*):

1. Latex gloves (nonsterile and sterile)*

2. Vinyl gloves (nonsterile and sterile)*

3. Overgloves (nonsterile)

4. Utility gloves (nonsterile)

5. Polynitrile, nitrile (autoclavable)

Choose gloves according to comfort, tactile sensitivity required, and the procedure being completed. Obtaining the best quality for the greatest value is another factor in choosing gloves.

Both latex and vinyl gloves are ambidextrous, used interchangeably for the right or left hand (Figures 11-4A, B, and C). They are supplied in a variety of sizes to provide the proper fit for most individuals. Many individuals feel that latex gloves provide a better fit. Latex-sensitive individuals use vinyl gloves as an alternative to latex. The vinyl gloves, however, are more rigid, tearing more easily and lacking tactile sensitivity. Due to increased use, however, vinyl gloves are being improved. The gloves (latex and vinyl) can be ordered with powder

FIGURE 11-3 (A) Goggles. (B) Eyewear with protective side shields. (C) Dental protective eyewear with side shields. (D) Dental face shield.

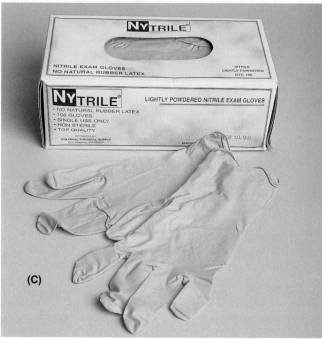

FIGURE 11-4 (A) Vinyl and (B) latex examination gloves. (C) lightly powdered colored latex examination gloves.

on the inside to aid in donning (placing the gloves on). Both types of gloves are supplied as nonsterile, referred to as examination gloves, and sterile, referred to as sterile surgical gloves. Most procedures in the dental office require only the use of the nonsterile gloves. They provide the minimal barrier protection needed for the dental personnel. Sterile surgical gloves are only used in specific surgical procedures requiring a sterile environment, such as oral, periodontal, and implant surgery.

Both the latex and the vinyl gloves need to be changed with each new patient. If, during the procedure, they become torn or punctured, they should be removed, the hands washed, and the gloves replaced with new gloves to complete the procedure. *Gloves should never be washed and reused.*

Latex Allergies

Latex is used in many of the products that are available today. In the dental office and other medical clinics, latex gloves are used routinely for patient care. This increase in latex usage has increased the number of individuals who present with latex hypersensitivity. Latex is a natural rubber that comes from a rubber tree, *Hevea brasiliensis.* It is a milky fluid that is taken from the tree much like maple is collected for syrup and then it is manufactured. The product from this tree if not treated properly releases proteins that can cause allergic reactions. An allergic reaction may develop after a person has had a large amount of exposure or a slight exposure to latex. It is unknown how an individual will react. It is known that increased exposure to latex does increase the risk of developing symptoms of an allergy. Initially the person normally has mild symptoms and does not develop life-threatening responses. However, the dental assistant should be ready to aid in treating the patient who presents with allergic symptoms. The Centers for Disease Control and Prevention (CDC) sets forth guidelines for contact dermatitis and latex hypersensitivity. It says that each patient should be screened for latex allergy during the process of taking the medical and dental history. If latex allergy is suspected, the patient should be referred to the physician for further medical consultation. All dental personnel should be educated to the signs and symptoms of latex allergy and how constant handwashing and use of latex gloves increase the possibility of contact dermatitis and latex hypersensitivity. The dental office should provide a latex-safe environment for patients and dental personnel and an emergency kit with latex free treatment available.

Latex allergies are commonly presented in three primary types of reactions. The first one is contact dermatitis and involves only irritation to the top layers of the skin, the second one is Type IV and it is the most common. Type IV allergic reaction is primarily limited to the areas that contacted the latex. The third allergic reaction to latex is Type I allergic reaction and it can be very serious. Anyone can develop a latex allergy, but it is a small group that really do. It is normally the individuals who are sensitive to allergies or individuals who are in constant contact with latex products or people in the rubber industry.

Contact Dermatitis

Contact dermatitis is an inflammation of the skin due to a chemical irritation. Contact dermatitis occurs immediately or very soon after contact. It is characterized by hands that become itchy, and sometimes cracked. Dental assistants are especially prone to have contact dermatitis due to the wearing of the gloves and the constant washing of hands. Things that increase this condition are the usage of antimicrobial agents and washing the hands so often. If the assistant uses any type of rough sponge or brush it will increase the abrasion and exaggerate the condition. If the hands are not rinsed thoroughly and dried completely the chance for contact dermatitis will increase and if the condition is present it will intensify the symptoms. When wearing the treatment gloves oftentimes the hands will perspire and this will lead to the condition as well as the contact to the cornstarch or powder in the gloves. The cornstarch in the powder does not have allergenic chemicals in it but can aid in transferring the proteins and allergenic chemicals from the latex glove to the source. It also allows the particles to become airborne when the gloves are changed. These airborne particles can be inhaled and then contact body membranes. The dental assistant can use special care to wash, rinse, and dry the hands and then choose gloves that decrease sensitivity and change them often and apply lotion to hands as necessary to inhibit this condition.

Type IV Allergic Reaction

Type IV allergic reaction to latex is also referred to as allergic contact dermatitis, delayed hypersensitivity, and chemical sensitivity dermatitis. Type IV allergic reaction is a great deal more common than type I allergic reaction. It is a result of exposure to the chemicals added to latex during harvesting, processing, and/or manufacturing. A type IV allergic reaction to latex is much like an allergic reaction to poison ivy. The skin rash usually begins 24 to 48 hours after the contact. It may even show up 72 hours after the contact. It shows up like red itching areas and may present with oozing blisters. It normally shows up in the areas of contact but may spread away from the initial site. It is an immune system response and therefore very different from contact dermatitis. If an employee shows with the symptoms of type IV allergic reaction, all employees should take care and not use powdered gloves and other latex equipment. The affected employee must be provided with hypoallergenic gloves (reduced protein, powder-free gloves), latex gloves, or non-latex gloves and/or glove liners. The employer should evaluate current prevention strategies and take steps to limit the exposure in the workplace. There are a number of items that contain latex in the office and in the home.

A few of the products that contain latex:

Office

- Treatment gloves
- Blood pressure cuffs
- Stethoscopes
- Syringe carpule stoppers
- Some goggles
- Rubber bands
- Erasers
- Dental dams
- Elastic waistbands

Home

- Hot water bottles
- Balloons
- Baby bottle nipples
- Baby bottle pacifiers
- Automobile tires
- Carpeting
- Shoe soles
- Elastic waistbands
- Many rubber devices

Type I Allergic Reaction

Type I allergic reaction can occur minutes after exposure to latex proteins and can result in death if the patient has an anaphylaxis reaction. This severe allergic reaction is the most serious of allergic reactions to latex. It causes the airway to close due to swelling. Type I allergic reaction to latex is not common in the dental office but the dental assistant should always be prepared for an emergency. The patient may show signs of coughing, wheezing, respiratory distress, runny eyes and nose and becomes unable to breath. Emergency medical treatment should be summoned immediately.

Type I allergic reaction is not due to the chemical additives as in type IV but is in response to the proteins in the latex. The proteins can be released during contact or they can adhere to the cornstarch or powder in the gloves and become released when the gloves are donned or removed during normal treatment. These released proteins that are attached to the powder then become airborne and are suspended in the air. Sensitized individuals can breathe in these proteins and a reaction may occur. Individuals who have extreme sensitivity should be treated in latex-free environments. It may be that these patients will have to seek treatment in places that latex has not been used and will not be in the air system. This is life and death and should be treated as such. Individuals who have latex allergies should practice prevention and not place themselves in areas of latex usage. There is no cure available. Testing can be done to confirm that an individual is sensitive or has an allergy to latex. If a patient is sensitive to latex, non-latex gloves (vinyl) can be used as well as other non-latex products such as rubber dam material.

Gloves in the Dental Office

- Use new gloves for each patient.
- Never wash gloves.
- If gloves become penetrated during treatment, remove gloves, wash and dry hands, and place new gloves on hands.

Overgloves, also known as food handlers' gloves, are placed over the latex or vinyl gloves during a procedure to prevent cross-contamination if the dental assistant has to reach inside a drawer, write on a chart, or touch an area that is not contaminated (Figure 11-5). Overgloves are big, loose gloves that do not have the tac-

FIGURE 11-5 Overgloves used to open a drawer or write on a chart. *(Courtesy of Biotrol International 1-800-822-8550)*

FIGURE 11-6 Utility gloves.

tile touch that the latex and vinyl gloves have, but they quickly fit over the gloves so that the user can obtain something in a sterile area. They are not to be used as examination gloves. Overgloves can be placed on rapidly to accomplish a secondary task, such as opening a container. They should be discarded after each use.

Thick **utility gloves** are used during disinfection and cleanup procedures (Figure 11-6). These gloves are used for "dishwashing" and like overgloves, are not regulated by the FDA. An assistant carries the tray to the sterilization area, removes the latex or vinyl gloves, washes his or her hands, and dons the utility gloves to complete the cleanup. The utility gloves can be washed and reused. If they do become cracked or punctured, they should be discarded and replaced.

Autoclavable utility gloves have an added benefit in that they can be sterilized in the autoclave after use. Each dental team member involved in cleanup and instrument recycling must have his or her own set of polynitrile gloves.

Donning and Removal of Gloves. The donning (placement) of gloves is done after carefully washing and drying the hands. The dental assistant should not place petroleum-based hand lotion on prior to placement of gloves because it may cause the integrity of the gloves to break down, therefore weakening them.

When removing the gloves, tuck the fingers of one glove into the cuff of the first glove, coming from the glove side and not from the skin side. Lift it off, taking care not to touch the tissue with the gloves. It can be inverted as it is removed and remains in the palm of the gloved hand. After the first glove is removed, use the thumb of the freed hand inside the cuff (skin side) of the remaining glove and pull it down and off the hand and invert over the first glove. Carefully dispose of the gloves into a biohazard waste receptacle (Figure 11-7A–C).

Masks. Masks are worn at any time that splatter or aerosol of saliva or blood can occur (Figure 11-8). The dental assistant must wear a mask to protect the mucous membranes of the nose and mouth. The aerosol mist that remains suspended in the air may come from the use of the dental handpiece, the ultrasonic scaler, or the air-water syringe. At times, due to the use of the air-water syringe, splatter occurs where a concentrated amount of saliva or blood projects from the oral cavity to the dental health worker. Proper placement of the high volume evacuator and the air-water syringe (Chapter 17, Introduction to the Dental Office and Basic Chairside Assisting) aids in the reduction of splatter; however, it can still occur. Wearing a mask that covers the nose and mouth protects dental personnel in such cases.

The dental mask also protects the patient and the dental assistant from communicable diseases. The mask should be placed along with the eyewear before washing hands and donning gloves (Figure 11-9). It is important that the mask be placed properly so that it fits snugly against the face and stays in place during the procedure. Normally, the face mask has an outside and an inside (next to the face); place it according to the manufacturer's directions. Often, a color is on the outside surface for quick identification. Masks are also available in a variety of designs for a positive practice image. For example, cartoon images are available for a pediatric practice.

The mask is secured with elastic that goes around the head or over the ears, or with ties that are fastened behind the head. Some masks can be pinched above the nose to fit better and not allow the breath to fog the protective eyewear. Always adjust the mask to proper position prior to the procedure. Masks should be removed

(A)

(B)

(C)

FIGURE 11-7 (A) Grasp the outside of the cuff of the first glove. (B) Invert as removing, and then keep the removed glove in the palm of the gloved hand. (C) Insert the thumb of the freed hand inside the cuff of the second glove. Pull outward and over the hand while inverting the glove over the glove inside the palm and off the second hand.

after the procedure by grasping the ties or attachments. Never reuse a mask; replace after every patient or during the procedure if the mask becomes moist. Never slip the mask down on the neck area or let it dangle from the ear after treatment is over. Remove the mask and dispose of it.

FIGURE 11-8 Face masks used in dentistry.

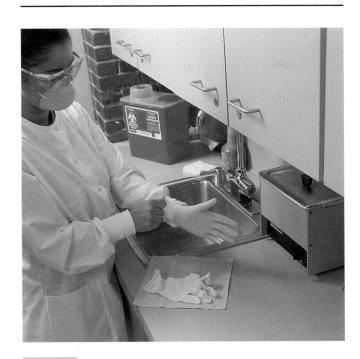

FIGURE 11-9 Dental assistant is putting on PPE before performing dental procedures.

Masks During Dental Treatment

- Use a new mask for each patient.
- Replace the mask if it becomes moist or wet.
- Never let the mask dangle around the neck or from the ear; remove and discard after use.

Protective Clothing. Special protective clothing worn only in the dental office is regulated by OSHA. Protective clothing includes uniforms, laboratory coats, gowns, and clinic jackets. According to OSHA, the dentist must provide protective clothing that is worn in the office and laundered in the office or by a commercial laundering service. One uniform for each staff member each day is appropriate. Dental personnel enter the office and change into uniforms or other PPE overgarments (Figure 11-10). The employer is required to clean, launder, and dispose of PPE at no cost to the employee. The uniforms or other PPE overgarments, such as laboratory coats, should be removed if the dental assistant is going out to lunch or going into the staff lounge for lunch.

Long isolation gowns are worn by the dental team members who fall in Category 1 or 2 (Figure 11-11). Gowns and uniforms cover the arms and fit closely around the neck and the wrists and provide the greatest protection if impermeable to fluids. During the time the gloves are on, the gloves fit over the cuffs of the uniform.

Protective clothing should be changed daily or immediately if splattered with body fluids. Special attention to the design of the protective clothing should be taken. Any buttons, zippers, and ornamental design should be kept to a minimum, because they can harbor pathogens. Disposable outer gowns are an option for dental personnel. The specific types of uniforms or gowns worn during patient care are dictated by office policy.

When removing protective clothing, care must be taken to keep the side of the clothing that has been possibly contaminated with pathogens folded inward. The assistant should remove one arm first, then fold the clothing inward, then slowly remove the rest of the lab coat, all the while taking special care to fold the clothing together as it is removed. OSHA notes that special care is to be taken with items that are considered potentially infectious.

Protective Clothing in the Dental Office

- Worn only in dental office (not in staff lounges or lunch rooms)
- Must close tightly at neck and around cuff area
- During a high-risk procedure, must be knee length when sitting
- Must be removed at the end of the day, prior to going home
- Must be laundered in the office or sent to a laundry service

---

Barriers

Barriers are used in all aspects of the dental office where possible. In the operatory, the patient dental chair, light (handles and operating switch), hand-

FIGURE 11-10 Dental assistant in uniform.

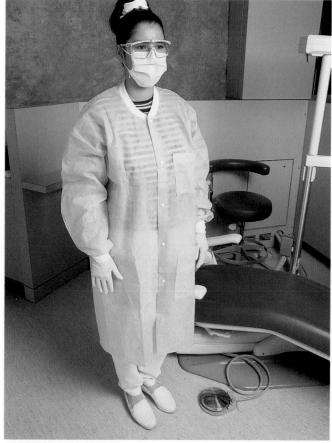

FIGURE 11-11 Dental assistant in treatment gown.

pieces, air-water syringe, high-volume evacuator, saliva ejector, tubing, writing utensils, and surfaces are covered with barriers (Figure 11-12). Any area that can be covered where contamination is possible during dental treatment should be covered. Barriers have been made specifically for areas that have been hard to disinfect or sterilize in the past, such as tubing and hoses for the handpieces. The patient should wear protective eyewear and a patient napkin or bib for protection from splatter and debris.

> ▪ Using disposable shower caps to cover the light and handles provides a barrier to the entire light. It allows light to pass through it but can be disposed of quickly.
>
> ▪ The dental chair can be covered with plastic dry-cleaning bags to shield them from contaminants. The dry-cleaning bags are fairly inexpensive and can be purchased on a roll. After the procedure is completed, the bag is turned inside out (contamination inside), and all disposable supplies are placed in the bag for easy cleanup.

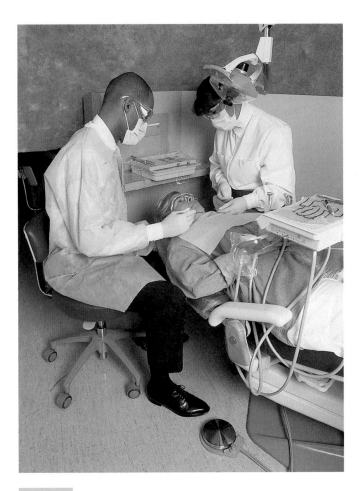

FIGURE 11-12 Barriers in place in a dental treatment room. Doctor, patient, and assistant with PPE.

Disinfection

Areas that do not lend themselves to the use of barriers in the dental office need to be disinfected if they cannot be sterilized. Some dental offices use barriers and also disinfect. As long as all surfaces are disinfected and/or protected by a barrier, the requirement of asepsis is met.

> Using paper mixing pads makes proper disinfection difficult. However, the plastic ends in the dental x-ray film boxes can be used to mix some cements. These ends can be cleaned and placed in a submersion sterilization solution and reused.

Cleaning the Area

All areas where dental procedures are performed must be cleaned prior to disinfection and sterilization. **Cleaning** is the physical removal of organic matter, such as blood, tissue, and debris. The process of cleaning decreases the number of microorganisms in the area and removes substances that may hinder the processes of disinfection and sterilization. This process is much like washing off dishes before placing them in the dishwasher. If the substances stay on the instruments, they cannot be disinfected or sterilized properly.

If something is **sanitized**, the process is much like cleaning. Sanitization means that the area has been decontaminated, but it does not mean that all microorganisms in the area have been destroyed.

Environmental Protection Agency Approval

The EPA registers disinfection and sterilization solutions only after the products have undergone careful testing. The disinfecting and sterilization solutions must have EPA approval on their labels. Each product registered with the EPA must have determination as to whether a solution sterilizes or disinfects and what types of microorganisms it will destroy. **Sterilization** means that all forms of microorganisms are destroyed and **disinfection** occurs when *some* microorganisms are destroyed. The contact time needed for each product is also defined on the label. Some products disinfect after ten minutes but need to have ten hours of submersion to sterilize. The disinfection levels according to the EPA are rated as high, intermediate, and low.

▪ *High-level disinfection* is a tuberculocidal that kills most but not all bacterial spores. If it is extremely strong and can kill all the bacterial spores, it is noted as a sporicidal on the label.

▪ *Intermediate-level disinfection* is a tuberculocidal that normally does not kill bacterial spores.

■ *Low-level disinfection* kills some viruses and fungi and most of the bacteria microorganisms. It does not kill tuberculosis or bacterial spores.

When choosing the products for disinfection and sterilization for the dental office, be aware that no one product meets all the needs. Each product has advantages and disadvantages for use with specific materials. Staining and corrosiveness to instruments and equipment, along with the toxicity of the material, should be considered when choosing solutions. Read labels carefully to gain information needed about product effectiveness. Reading the information recommended by the dental organizations or asking the dental supply representative assists dental personnel in choosing the proper solutions for the dental office.

Chemical Disinfectants

There are many solutions that can be used for disinfection. The dental assistant should be familiar with the solutions used in the dental practice. This includes becoming familiar with the properties of the solutions, the proper uses of the solutions, the time required for the solutions to be effective when used, and proper storage and disposal of the solutions. The dental office should maintain MSDS forms for each solution used in the practice.

Chlorine Dioxide. Chlorine dioxide (EPA registered) is a high-level disinfectant that should be used only on items not subject to corrosion. Any materials made of or having parts made of stainless steel, carbide steel, copper, or brass will corrode if chlorine dioxide is used. The solution should be stored only in glass or plastic containers. Follow the manufacturer's directions for dilution and contact time. Normally, disinfection is rapid, but sterilization takes six to ten hours. Proper ventilation is necessary when using this product.

Glutaraldehyde. Glutaraldehyde (EPA registered) is used for high-level disinfection and sterilization. Some of the solutions are corrosive to metals. Read the manufacturer's directions regarding the dilution and contact time for disinfection and sterilization. Time for disinfection is normally ten to ninety minutes and sterilization is normally six to ten hours. Whenever additional instruments are added to the solution, the time countdown must be started over. Therefore, most sterilization done with glutaraldehyde must be done overnight and is more efficiently done in a steam or an autoclave sterilizer. Some glutaraldehydes, after activation, are only effective for twenty-eight days. Fumes from glutaraldehyde are toxic and can irritate the skin and eyes, so proper ventilation is essential.

Sodium Hypochlorite. Sodium hypochlorite can be obtained in a number of different concentrations. The concentration referred to here is the same as "household bleach," which is 5.25% sodium hypochlorite.

The desired concentrations for use in the dental office is 1:10 dilution. This is obtained by placing one cup of household bleach in one gallon of water. The mixed solution is ready for use. It is highly effective for an intermediate-level disinfection and is effective against a broad spectrum of microorganisms. A 1:100 dilution of 1/4 cup bleach to one gallon of water is used for general-purpose disinfection. Sodium hypochlorite works rapidly (within ten minutes) on surfaces. The solution is extremely unstable and has to be mixed daily. It is also extremely corrosive to metals. Sodium hypochlorite is irritating to the eyes and skin and can harm clothing. PPE should be worn while using all cleaning and disinfection solutions. Good ventilation is essential when using sodium hypochlorite, and caution should be used when mixing it with other cleaning agents because it can become extremely toxic.

Iodophor. Iodophor is used as an intermediate-level disinfectant. Care should be used when diluting the solution to procure the correct concentration. One of the active ingredients in iodophor is iodine. The iodine in this solution can stain white countertops and light-colored vinyl with repeated use. Iodophor works rapidly, taking five to twenty-five minutes of surface contact to be effective. It is corrosive to some metals and has a short life span. Solutions should be changed every three days minimum to remain active. Iodophor can be irritating to skin; thus, utility gloves should be worn while disinfecting surfaces.

Phenolics. Phenolics are used for intermediate-level disinfection. They are irritating to the skin and eyes. Follow manufacturer's directions when diluting the solution. The surface contact time is normally ten minutes. Many phenolics come premixed in spray or pump containers. They are destructive to plastic surfaces but are effective overall surface disinfectants.

Alcohol. Isopropyl alcohol was used routinely for disinfection prior to the 1980s. Essentially, it cleaned the areas and had some disinfecting qualities, but it provides limited properties. *Alcohol is no longer recommended for disinfection in the dental office.* Alcohol evaporates so quickly that it is difficult to have surface contact for the length of time necessary to be effective.

Table 11-2 compares the commonly used disinfectants in the dental office.

Disinfection Technique

A universally accepted technique for cleaning and disinfecting surfaces is the spray-wipe-spray-wipe technique. First, the surface is sprayed, then wiped to eliminate debris and to accomplish initial surface cleaning. The second spray, which must be a surface disinfectant, is left on the item and/or surfaces for the specific time indicated by the manufacturer (normally ten minutes) and then items and surfaces are wiped and items are put away.

TABLE 11-2   Disinfectant Comparisons

Disinfectant	Level	Advantages	Disadvantages	Time Required for Effectiveness
Chlorine dioxide	High	Rapid disinfection	Corrosive to metals Requires ventilation Irritating to eyes and skin	5–10 minutes
Glutaraldehyde	High	Used to disinfect some impressions Instrument can be submerged Many have a twenty-eight–day useful life	Some are corrosive to metal Requires ventilation Irritating to eyes and skin	10–90 minutes
Iodophor	Intermediate	Used as holding solution for impressions	May discolor white or pastel vinyls Surface disinfectant or holding solution Irritating to eyes and skin	10 minutes on surfaces
Sodium hypochlorite	Intermediate	Rapid disinfection	Corrosive to metals Irritating to skin and eyes Diluted solution is unstable, must be mixed daily	5–10 minutes
Phenolics	Intermediate	Available as sprays or liquids	Skin and mucous membrane irritation Cannot be used on plastics	10 minutes
Alcohol	Cleaner only	NA	NA	NA

Ultrasonic Cleaning

If the dental assistant is not able to recycle the instruments immediately after the procedure, the instruments may be submerged in a holding bath (precleaning), a solution that loosens hardened debris from the instruments prior to cleaning and sterilizing. It also prevents contamination from airborne bacteria and begins the process of disinfection. The instruments remain in the holding bath until the dental assistant is ready to proceed with the processing.

After dental assistants have removed the treatment tray from the operatory and disinfected the area and/or placed the instruments in a holding bath, they return to the sterilizing area to process the instruments. The utility gloves remain on during this procedure as the dental assistant takes the instruments from the tray or holding bath and places them in an ultrasonic cleaner. Metal or plastic containers sometimes are used to hold instruments as they pass from the tray to the different solutions for processing and then on to storage (Figure 11-13). In the past, the dental assistant hand scrubbed the instruments with soap, rinsed, and placed the instruments in containers for ultrasonic cleaning or in the sterilizer for processing. The chance of being punctured with a contaminated instrument was much greater than it is today, because the manual scrub was done without gloves or use of an ultrasonic unit. The use of the utility

FIGURE 11-13 Dental assistant using plastic instrument cassettes for ultrasonic cleaning procedure.

gloves, along with the containers and ultrasonic cleaning instead of hand cleaning, significantly reduces the high risk to the dental assistant. The ultrasonic cleaning device uses sound waves that travel through glass and metal using a special solution to clean the debris from the instruments (Figure 11-14). This **cavitation** process (whereby bubbles are formed) takes three to ten minutes to complete. During that time, the bubbles implode (burst inward) and produce a cleaning effect on anything within the solution. When ultrasonic cleaning is complete, the instruments are rinsed thoroughly and dried. All instruments, both loose and remaining in containers, are rinsed and dried prior to sterilization. They may be placed in an alcohol bath to aid the drying process. It does not matter which method is used to prepare the instruments for sterilization. What is important is that all the debris, blood, saliva, and tissue are removed from the instruments to ensure that the sterilization can be completed on all surfaces. The ultrasonic cleaner should be drained each night, rinsed out with water, and refilled with new ultrasonic solution each morning. It should be emptied and refilled any time the ultrasonic cleaning solution becomes exhausted, which varies depending on individual offices.

> To determine whether the ultrasonic cleaner is working properly, take a small piece of aluminum foil and submerge it in the solution vertically and run the ultrasonic for thirty seconds. Remove the foil from the ultrasonic solution, and hold it up to the light for examination. It should have no area larger than a half square inch

FIGURE 11-14 Dental assistant using the ultrasonic cleaning unit.

> without holes in it. This indicates whether the cleaner is operating properly. If the ultrasonic unit is not operating properly, the assistant should have it tested and repaired.

Sterilization

All forms of microorganisms are destroyed in the process of sterilization. The dental assistant most often is the person who ensures that all items used in intraoral procedures are sterile. Any items that touch the skin or mucosa or are involved in invasive procedures must be sterilized. Several choices are available for sterilization (Table 11-3).

Liquid Chemical Disinfectant/Sterilization

Many of the disinfecting solutions can be used for immersion sterilization. The items are placed in the liquid for six to ten hours to ensure that all microorganisms are destroyed. The instruments are then rinsed off thoroughly, dried, and stored. Some of the items used in the dental office cannot endure heat sterilization and must be placed in a cold sterile solution. This is the primary reason for using cold sterilizing. The disadvantages to this type of sterilization is the time involved and the limited shelf life of the solution. Cold sterilizing is difficult to monitor for effectiveness and the solution may be toxic to skin and inhalation, therefore requiring proper ventilation. Another disadvantage is that when the sterilizing procedure is complete, the instruments are rinsed with water that is not sterile and left unwrapped for storage; therefore, they are not maintained in a sterile state.

Ethylene Oxide Sterilization

Sterilization in the dental office can be accomplished by using an ethylene oxide sterilization unit (Figure 11-15). There are two different types: the heated unit, which is fairly expensive, and a unit that can be used at room temperature. Both units are reliable for sterilization, but with all equipment, always follow the manufacturer's directions for use. Most heated units sterilize at 120°F (49°C) for two to three hours. Plastics and other instruments can be sterilized in this low-temperature unit. The room-temperature unit takes twelve hours to complete sterilization. It is less expensive but not as efficient as the heated unit. One disadvantage, besides the long processing time, is the toxicity of the ethylene oxide gas. Adequate ventilation is required, and any porous materials require an additional twenty-four hours for the gas to dissipate from it prior to use.

Hot (Glass) Bead or Salt Sterilization

A small sterilizer positioned at the dental unit is the hot (glass) bead or salt sterilizer (Figure 11-16). This unit operates at temperatures of approximately 450°F

TABLE 11-3   Sterilization Methods

Sterilization	Temperature/Time	Ability to Monitor	Special Considerations
Liquid chemical sterilization	Room temperature/6–10 hours	Difficult	Proper ventilation required Does not remain sterile after process
Ethylene oxide sterilization	Heated unit 120°F/2–3 hours Room temperature/12 hours	Difficult	Proper ventilation Additional twenty-four hours to dissipate gas after sterilization
Glass bead sterilizer	450°F/20–30 seconds	Not available	Limited size and use Special beads or salt required
Dry heat sterilization	340°F/1 hour	Easily monitored	Limited rust or corrosion of equipment Not for use with plastics/paper
Chemical vapor sterilization	270°F/20 minutes	Easily monitored	Proper ventilation Special solution required
Steam under pressure sterilization	250°F/30 minutes wrapped	Easily monitored	Requires distilled water May corrode instruments Not for use with many plastics
Steam (flash) autoclave sterilization	270°F/3 minutes unwrapped	Easily monitored	Requires distilled water May corrode instruments Not for use with many plastics

FIGURE 11-15 Ethylene oxide sterilizer. *(Courtesy of 3M Health Care, St. Paul, MN)*

FIGURE 11-16 Glass bead sterilizer.

(234°C) and sterilizes burs and endodontic instruments immersed in the glass beads or salt for twenty seconds and larger instrument tips for thirty seconds. The electrically heated cup that contains numerous 2-mm glass beads or salt conducts the high heat temperature. The

disadvantage of this sterilizer is its size and limited use. The advantage is that contaminated root-canal instruments and burs can be quickly sterilized. Monitors for effectiveness are not yet available (see "Biological Monitors" section in this chapter).

Dry Heat Sterilization

A sterilization unit that requires little maintenance and is easy to use is the dry heat sterilization unit (Figure 11-17). Other advantages are that dry instruments placed in the unit do not experience corrosion or rust. Instruments that are very delicate or have movable joints will not become rusty and lose their cutting edges as rapidly. After an initial pre-heat time of twenty minutes, this unit uses heat at 340°F (171°C) for one hour to sterilize. Several units are on the market, some using the long electromagnetic waves of radiation, the heated moving air/convection, or conduction (direct contact with the source of heat). Be sure to follow the manufacturer's directions to ensure proper sterilization. This unit can be monitored for effectiveness and is very reliable.

The high heat of the dry heat sterilizer can be a disadvantage, because plastic items and some solder joints melt and fabric chars. Instruments can be placed in this unit loose or wrapped. It requires that loads be carefully organized in the unit to allow circulation of the air and complete sterilization.

Chemical Vapor Sterilization

The chemical vapor sterilizer uses gaseous vapor of formaldehyde and alcohol under pressure to sterilize (Figure 11-18). The unit must be at 270°F (132°C) for twenty minutes to sterilize either loose or wrapped instruments. It is very reliable, and the effectiveness of the unit can be monitored. It is used frequently in the dental office due to the efficient sterilization time and because it causes very little rust and corrosion on metals. A special solution must be purchased for use in the unit, and it requires good ventilation. The high temperature does cause plastic and some other materials to be destroyed during the sterilization process. Like all ster-

ilizers, the manufacturer's directions must be followed to ensure proper technique in the sterilization process.

Steam Under Pressure Sterilization

The steam under pressure sterilization unit (Figure 11-19) is easy to use and easy to monitor. It uses distilled water and in many of the units the reservoir fill port and drain tube are in the front of the sterilization unit for easy usage. The fill port notates the level of the fluid and if the fluid is low the LCD display will indicate it needs to be filled and it will not begin until the fluid is filled. The display at the top front of the unit prompts the user in selecting the proper sterilization process. It can be used with wrapped or unwrapped packs or handpieces. It has four pre-selected cycles that can be used. Unwrapped instruments can be sterilized at 270°F three minutes, pouched instruments at 270°F for 5 minutes, and packs for 250°F for 30 minutes and handpieces at 270°F for 6

FIGURE 11-18 Chemical vapor sterilizer. *(Courtesy of Barnstead/Thermolyne Harvey Chemiclave)*

FIGURE 11-17 Dry heat sterilizer.

FIGURE 11-19 Steam sterilizer.

minutes. The cycle choices are on the top/front of the unit. The LCD display will indicate the mode selected, where the unit is in the process, the remaining time, temperature and pressure of the unit, and the time for the drying cycle. When the cycle is completed the door automatically opens and the steam begins to escape and the drying cycle that goes for 60 minutes begins. If the door is not closed properly the unit will indicate the problem and will not start until the problem is corrected. Due to the steam, instruments may corrode if drying is not completed. It is not for use with many of the plastics; always check the manufacturer's directions.

Steam Autoclave (Flash) Sterilization

Most dental offices have a steam autoclave sterilizer (Figure 11-20). These units use steam under pressure to quickly sterilize items. The effectiveness of this unit can be monitored, and it is very reliable. Items can be loose or wrapped during the process. Items must be wrapped, bagged, or placed in pouches and sealed to remain sterile after removing them from the sterilizer. The unit takes fifteen minutes at 250°F (121°C) at fifteen pounds of steam pressure at sea level. Careful packing of the unit so that the steam can penetrate all areas is essential. The steam pressure, along with the temperature, allows for much more rapid sterilization to occur. When unwrapped at 270°F (132°C) at fifteen pounds of steam pressure, sterilization for immediate use can be accomplished in three minutes.

After repeated use, the high temperature, along with the steam, results in melted plastics, corrosion and rust, and dull instruments. Most dental offices sterilize only dental handpieces in the steam sterilizer. The handpieces should be properly lubricated

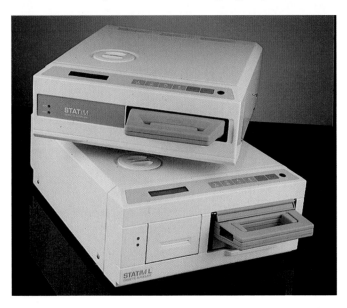

FIGURE 11-20 Steam (flash) sterilizer by Statium.
(Courtesy of Sci-Can)

and wrapped prior to sterilization if they are going to be stored. Improper care of the dental handpiece diminishes its useful life. Because dental equipment is relatively expensive, a rapid sterilization turnaround time is beneficial so that multiple handpieces do not need to be purchased. Many of the steam sterilization units require distilled water to be used in the machine. Always read the manufacturer's directions when using any sterilization equipment.

Equipment Maintenance

Sterilization equipment, like all equipment, must be maintained to function properly. The chambers should be cleaned out monthly, if not more frequently. Some sterilizers have special cleaners that must be used for this process. Other sterilizers require that the used solution be drained at the end of each day. A removable tray or drainage hose facilitates this process. Some sterilizers indicate when solutions are low; others must be checked frequently to ensure that they are full. *Making sure that the right solution is used in the appropriate machine is essential.* Using the wrong solution may cause the machine to break down, resulting in costly repair charges.

Many of the machines have gaskets around the door to seal the chamber during the sterilization process. If the machine is losing pressure and/or making a hissing sound, the dental assistant should check the gasket. This is an inexpensive item, and it can be replaced quite easily.

Continued maintenance allows equipment to work at capacity longer. The dental assistant can set up a maintenance program so that each item is routinely checked.

Handpiece Sterilization

Dental handpieces are very expensive, and it is important that they are sterilized properly and that the sterilization procedure does not extensively shorten the life of the handpieces. Always read the manufacturer's directions for sterilizing handpieces, and then form a protocol for sterilizing handpieces after each patient. After a patient has been dismissed, attach the handpiece to the unit with the bur in place, wipe all visible debris from the handpiece, and run it for twenty to thirty seconds to flush any debris, water, and air from the inside lines. Remove the bur from the handpiece, remove the handpiece from the unit, and take it to the sterilization area. The handpiece should be scrubbed with water, manufacturer-recommended soap, and a brush. For some handpieces, manufacturers recommend that parts or entire handpieces are cleaned in an ultrasonic unit. If the manufacturer notes that the ultrasonic should be used, do so, but do so only when recommended by the manufacturer.

The next step is lubricating the handpiece. Not all manufacturers recommend this step. It is critical that the manufacturer's recommendations be followed or the warranty may be invalid. If lubrication is recommended, use the proper lubricant for the handpiece. Never use the lubricant from another handpiece.

After lubricating, place the handpiece back on the unit with a blank bur in the chuck and run the handpiece to remove any excess lubrication from the handpiece.

Dental Fiber Optics. Clean the dental fiber optics of the handpiece with a swab moistened with isopropyl alcohol. This removes any film or debris from the optic surfaces and helps keep the fiber optic bundle bright and clear. To complete sterilization of the handpiece, dry the handpiece if moist, place it in a sterilization pouch, and sterilize it according to the manufacturer's directions.

Packaging and Loading Sterilizers

Most of the sterilizers can be loaded with loose instruments and obtain effective sterilization. Problems occur after the instruments come out of the sterilizer and are stored. There they may become contaminated. If they are sterilized in a labeled bag, then after the steriliza-

tion cycle is completed the instruments can stay in the labeled and sealed bag until used, therefore maintaining the sterile condition. Labeling of the bag is normally done in pencil so that when moisture occurs (in the steam and chemical sterilizers), the information remains readable. Special preprinted indicator tape is designed for identification of instrument setups in the sterilizing bag. Tape with such preprinted labels as exam, amalgam, and prophy could be used (Figure 11-21).

Many dental offices use the cassette instrument sterilizing system. The instruments from a procedure are kept in a cassette during the ultrasonic cleaning, rinsing, and drying and then the cassette is wrapped in penetrable paper or biofilm/paper pouches, sealed, and sterilized. The bags are heat sealed or taped because staples or pins make holes, thereby allowing microorganisms to enter. This cassette, often labeled or color coded for the procedure, is removed after the sterilization cycle and is ready to be placed on a treatment tray to be opened at the chairside for use on the next dental procedure. This keeps the instruments in a sterile state, ready for immediate use at the dental chair.

The dental assistant must ensure that the sterilization bags are not overfilled, hampering proper steril-

FIGURE 11-21 Cassette instrument sterilizing system. (A) Cassettes wrapped for sterilization. (B) Autoclave monitor tape. (C) Instrument Management System tape. *(Courtesy of Hu-Friedy Mfg. Co., Inc.)*

ization to be accomplished throughout. It is important also that the sterilizing units are not overpacked for the cycle. Use **sterilization indicators** routinely to ensure that errors in this area are not happening.

Instrument Storage

The best way to store instruments is in the packages in which they were sterilized. Limit the amount of package handling after sterilization. If packages become torn, wet, or contaminated in any manner, they need to be reprocessed. It is also important that "clean" and "dirty" areas in the sterilization room be identified. To avoid contamination, nothing from the dirty side should be placed on the clean side. This helps maintain sterilization integrity.

Sterile packs should be stored in a dry, cool (up to room temperature) area that has protection from recontamination. Normally, instruments used in dentistry have a quick turnaround time due to high cost and limited quantities. The shelf life of packages is indefinite as long as the packaging material remains intact and uncontaminated.

Sterilization Monitoring

Heat sterilizers are normally very reliable. It is important, however, that the sterilization process be monitored continually due to many factors that can diminish effectiveness. For example, the dental assistant could wrap instruments improperly, overload the unit, improperly set the time and temperature, or the sterilizer could malfunction.

Ongoing monitoring of the sterilization process is important to ensure proper technique and operation. The date that monitoring was concluded and the outcome must be documented. Records for each sterilizer should be maintained. Several types of monitors are available: biological monitors, process indicators, and dosage indicators.

Biological Monitors

Commercially prepared biological monitors offer the most accurate way to assess whether sterilization has occurred (Figure 11-22A). In the form of paper strips or sealed glass ampules of bacterial endospores, biological monitors are placed in the sterilizer along with the instrument load being sterilized. After completion of the cycle, the spores are cultured to determine if any has survived. Many dental offices have incubators for culturing. If one is not available, the processed monitors can be sent to a laboratory for culturing and results data. Both incubation processes will take several days to obtain results, so this must be an ongoing procedure, normally done weekly.

Process Indicators

Process indicators are normally heat-sensitive tapes or inks printed on packaging materials for sterilization or on the sterilization tape that can be placed on any packaging (Figure 11-22B). They contain dyes that change color upon quick exposure to sterilizing cycles. They indicate whether the packages have been exposed to heat but not whether sterilization has taken place. Process indicators should be used with biological monitoring to ensure effectiveness of the sterilization process.

Dosage Indicators

Dosage indicators work in much the same manner as process indicators. Dyes are placed in the sterilization packing, and they change color when exposed to dry heat, chemical vapor, or steam for a specific amount of time. They indicate whether correct conditions were present for sterilization to take place. Dosage indicators also must be used with biological monitoring.

FIGURE 11-22 (A) Biological monitors. (B) Process indicators used for dental sterilizers.

Techniques and Aids for Infection Control

Several techniques and aids are effective in infection control if practiced routinely. The dental office can continue to seek means to help reduce the exposure to microorganisms during invasive procedures. Staff training is essential to ensure that all procedure guidelines are followed.

Preprocedure Antiseptic Mouth Rinses

Using a preprocedure antiseptic mouth rinse is not a regulation but a recommendation. A patient who rinses before treatment reduces the total number of microorganisms in the oral cavity. Reducing the microorganisms in the mouth leads to fewer microorganisms coming from the mouth during indirect contact through splatter and aerosols. Patient mouth rinse helps prevent diseases from passing from the patient to dental team members.

The antimicrobial rinse often used is 0.12 percent chlorhexidine gluconate, which is effective up to five hours. Some procedures benefit from the rinse more than others. For instance, prophylaxis cleaning and ultrasonic scaling allow microorganisms to splatter mist in the air, unlike restorative procedures in which a dental dam (which is a barrier) can be used.

High-Volume Evacuation

The high volume evacuator (HVE) is an extremely effective way to minimize the spray coming from the high-speed rotary handpiece and the air-water syringe. (See Chapter 17, Introduction to the Dental Office and Basic Chairside Assisting, for correct placement of the HVE for maximum efficiency.) Evacuation systems use tips that are sterilizable or disposable. Most evacuation units have disposable traps that need to be cleaned routinely. Dental assistants must wear PPE while performing the cleaning procedure. Running water and specialized detergent deodorizers through the HVE at the end of each day helps reduce microorganisms in hoses and the trap.

Dental Dam Usage

The dental dam is used routinely as a barrier to the fluids and microorganisms in the oral cavity. If placed correctly, contact with saliva and oral debris is greatly reduced. However, the dental dam does not act as a perfect seal; thus, the use of gloves, glasses, and mask is required. Using the dental dam with the HVE significantly minimizes dental splatter and aerosols during dental procedures.

Disposable Items

Many disposable or single-dose use items are available for the dental office. These items are manufactured for a single use. They are disposed of after one use to prevent microorganism transfer from one patient to another. These disposable items should not be reused under any circumstances. They are not designed to be sterilized and often do not tolerate heat or chemicals. Disposable items are usually made from plastic, paper, or low-grade metals. From the infection-control standpoint, they are the most effective way to eliminate cross-contamination; however, functionally they may not be as efficient as reusable items, and they are more expensive overall.

Clinical Asepsis Protocol

Routine steps should be followed in all treatment areas to maintain clinical asepsis. Shortcuts should never be an option for asepsis in dentistry. The dental assistant must ensure that infectious diseases are not spread from patient to patient, health care worker to patient, patient to health care worker, or health care worker to family members.

Treatment Area Protocol for Disinfecting and Cleaning

As stated earlier, surfaces in the treatment area can be protected with barriers, disinfected, or both. When a barrier is dislodged or torn, microorganisms are allowed to pass through to the surface beneath the barrier. This surface must then be disinfected. Procedures 11-2 through 11-5 highlight the steps involved in preparing the treatment room, as well as disinfection and sterilization procedures to follow after treatment.

Dental Unit Waterlines

Dental unit waterlines are the small tubes that connect the water supply to the air-water syringe, high-speed dental handpieces, and ultrasonic cleaners. Water normally contains bacteria and fungi. Over time they form thin layers on practically any surface. For instance, they can be found in showerheads, fountains, and sink faucets, as well as in dental unit waterlines. Microbes attach themselves to the sides of the tubes and grow. A buildup of these slime layers of microbe becomes an ideal environment for the growth of **biofilms**, microscopic communities that allow bacteria, fungi, and viruses to multiply. When biofilms are passed to the patient, they increase disease susceptibility.

In the United States, water quality is measured by the number of coliform bacteria. The ADA set a goal in 1995 that all dental offices by 2000 would provide no more than 200 CFU/ml (colony-forming units per milliliter) in unfiltered water. Quality can be monitored using a water quality indicator (WQI). The ADA recommends that dental offices follow CDC, OSHA, and ADA guidelines for infection control for dental waterlines. These guidelines include flushing waterlines at the start of each day and between patients and recommend installing and maintaining antiretraction devices.

Preventing cross-contamination or potential aspiration of oral fluids through the high-speed handpiece or the air-water syringe (backflow) is another concern. The risk of backflow contamination is extremely low, but the ADA agrees that backflow prevention devices should be considered in the dental office.

Each handpiece should be flushed with air-water for twenty seconds between patients to help reduce patient-borne microbes that may have been sucked back into the handpiece during use in the oral cavity. Also, waterlines should be disinfected weekly to remove biofilms. Disinfection can be done using one part household bleach to nine parts water. After the lines are purged with air and the handpieces removed, the lines can be

PROCEDURE 11-2

Preparing the Dental Treatment Room

The procedure is performed by the dental assistant prior to seating the dental patient in the treatment room. By following a routine procedure that meets regulations and protocols set forth by the dentist and regulatory agencies discussed earlier in the chapter, the dental assistant prepares the operatory and equipment.

EQUIPMENT AND SUPPLIES

- Patient's medical and dental history (including dental radiographs)
- Barriers for dental chair, hoses, counter, light switches, and controls
- PPE for dental assistant (protective eyewear, mask, gloves, and overgloves)
- Patient napkin, napkin chain, and protective eyewear
- Sterile procedure tray

PROCEDURE STEPS (Follow aseptic procedures)

1. Wash hands.

2. Review the patient's medical and dental history, place the radiographs on the viewbox, and identify the procedure to be completed at this visit. Patient's medical and dental history can be placed in a plastic envelope barrier or under a surface barrier.

3. Place new barriers on all surfaces that can be contaminated (e.g., dental chair, hoses, counter, light switches, and controls) (Figure 11-23).

4. Bring the instrument tray with packaged sterile instruments into the operatory with patient's napkin and protective eyewear.

5. Place PPE (protective eyewear, mask, gloves, and overgloves).

6. Ensure that handpieces and three-way syringe are working properly.

FIGURE 11-23 Dental assistant placing barriers.

PROCEDURE 11-3

Completion of Dental Treatment

The procedure is performed by the dental assistant at the completion of dental treatment. By following a routine procedure that meets the regulations and protocols set forth by the dentist and regulatory agencies discussed earlier in the chapter, the dental assistant completes the procedure and dismisses the patient.

EQUIPMENT AND SUPPLIES

- Patient's medical and dental history (including dental radiographs)

- Barriers for dental chair, hoses, counter, light switches, and controls

- Dental handpiece

- Air-water syringe tip (disposable)

- Patient napkin

- Contaminated instruments on tray, including HVE tip

PROCEDURE STEPS *(Follow aseptic procedures)*

1. Remove handpieces, HVE tip, and air-water syringe tip and place on treatment tray.

2. Put on overgloves to document information on the chart or via computer and assemble radiographs and chart, preventing cross-contamination (Figure 11-24).

3. Remove patient napkin and place over the treatment tray prior to dismissing patient (see Chapter 17).

4. With glove in place, complete Steps 5 through 11.

5. Place the handpiece, HVE, and air-water syringe back on the unit and run for twenty to thirty seconds to clean the lines or flush the system. Remove handpiece and air-water syringe and return to treatment tray.

6. Place sharps in puncture-resistant sharps disposal container if disposal containers are kept in the dental treatment room (waist level). Sharps should be discarded in the treatment room or sterilization area.

7. Remove the chair cover from the patient dental chair, inverting it so that any splatter or debris remains on the inside of the bag.

8. Remove all barriers and place them in the inverted bag. All disposables can be placed in the bag as well (Figure 11-25).

9. Carry treatment tray with all items from treatment area to sterilizing area. All items to be sterilized are removed from the operatory at this time.

10. Remove treatment gloves and place them in the inverted bag. Dispose of the bag.

11. Wash hands.

FIGURE 11-24 Dental assistant wearing overgloves while writing on a patient's chart.

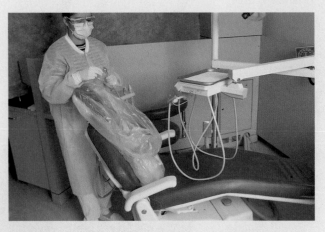

FIGURE 11-25 Postdental treatment, barriers being removed and placed in an inverted bag for disposal.

PROCEDURE 11-4

Final Treatment Room Disinfecting and Cleaning

The procedure is performed by the dental assistant after the treatment has been completed and the patient has been dismissed. This routine procedure meets the regulations and protocols set forth by the dentist and regulatory agencies discussed earlier in the chapter.

EQUIPMENT AND SUPPLIES

- Utility gloves
- Necessary disinfecting solutions (intermediate level)
- Wiping cloths
- 4 × 4 gauze

PROCEDURE STEPS *(Follow aseptic procedures)*

1. Wash hands, pull on utility gloves.

2. Bring the necessary solutions and wiping cloths, including 4 × 4 gauze, to the operatory.

> Use a small utility carry tote to hold and transport items such as disinfecting solutions, HVE solution, 4 × 4 gauze, towels, and chair disinfectant.

3. Have a routine procedure established for disinfection to ensure that nothing is missed. All surfaces need to be sprayed and cleaned first, then wiped to remove debris (Figures 11-26A and B). The surfaces are then sprayed a second time and the solution is left on surfaces for a designated time according to the manufacturer's directions (normally about ten minutes). After ten minutes, wipe the surfaces again.

4. Another method to accomplish the initial spray wipe is to use saturated "wiping devices." Lay out several pieces of 4 × 4 gauze on the counter, spray them with disinfectant, and wipe each surface carefully.

5. Spray on the disinfectant and leave it for the correct time to accomplish disinfection (normally ten minutes).

6. Rewipe all surfaces.

7. It is critical that all surfaces that could have been contaminated are disinfected. Areas that are sometimes missed include the amalgam cradle (holding device for amalgam capsule in the triturator), chair adjustments, curing light, and radiographic viewbox switch. (Take care when spraying disinfectants near switches.)

Disinfecting Procedure

- Spray.
- Wipe. (The "spray and wipe" technique also can be accomplished by wiping with a disinfectant-saturated "wiping device.")
- Spray and leave (normally ten minutes).
- Rewipe.

FIGURE 11-26 (A) Spraying the area. (B) Wiping and spraying the area with disinfectant again.

PROCEDURE 11-5

Treatment of Contaminated Tray in Sterilization Center

The procedure is performed by the dental assistant in the sterilization center. By following a routine procedure that meets the regulations and protocols set forth by the dentist and OSHA regulatory agencies discussed earlier in the chapter, the dental assistant completes the procedure.

EQUIPMENT AND SUPPLIES

- Utility gloves
- Necessary disinfecting solutions
- Wiping cloths
- 4 × 4 gauze
- Contaminated procedure tray

PROCEDURE STEPS *(Follow aseptic procedures)*

1. Place the treatment tray in the contaminated area of the sterilization center immediately following dental treatment. Sterilization can be taken care of immediately or after the operatory is disinfected and prepared for another patient.

2. If a long time will elapse before the tray is decontaminated, immerse the instruments in a disinfecting holding solution. This prevents debris from drying, begins the process of killing the microorganisms, and prevents airborne microorganisms from being transmitted.

3. Wear utility gloves during the entire procedure.

4. Sharps are disposed of in a sharps container if not already done while in the dental operatory (Figure 11-27).

5. All disposable items are discarded. If they are biohazard waste, they must be placed in an appropriately labeled waste container. (See Chapter 12 for further information.)

6. Place instruments in the ultrasonic cleaner using either open method or in a cassette. A small strainer is used for items that may become lost. Normally, burs, dental dam clamps, and other such items are

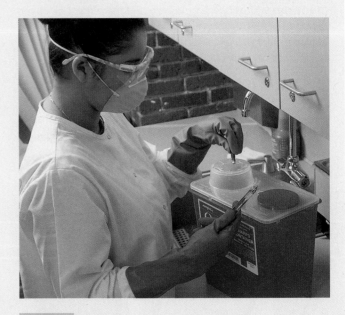

FIGURE 11-27 Dental assistant placing sharps in a sharps container.

placed in this small container. After the timed cleaning is accomplished in the ultrasonic unit (three to ten minutes), rinse the items thoroughly.

7. After instruments are rinsed, towel dry, bag, and place in the appropriate sterilizer (Figures 11-28A and B). Remember that if they are in a cassette, they can be dipped in an alcohol bath and left to air dry before being placed in a sealed bag and in the sterilizer.

8. Rinse off or wipe off the dental high-speed handpiece with isopropyl alcohol. Then it must be lubricated, bagged in an instrument pouch with indicator tape, and placed in the sterilizer (follow manufacturer's directions). The steam under pressure sterilizer is normally used due to the quick turnaround time.

9. The tray and other items on the tray need to be spray wiped, sprayed again, left for ten minutes or a time designated by the manufacturer of the disinfectant,

(continues)

PROCEDURE 11-5 *(CONTINUED)*

and wiped again before assembling them for another tray setup.

10. Clean up the area, wash and dry the utility gloves, remove them, and wash and dry hands.

11. After the sterilizer indicates that the time has lapsed and that the instruments are sterile, they can be removed from the sterilizer with forceps.

PPE for a Contaminated Tray

- Utility gloves are required when handling contaminated trays.

- Protective eyewear is required when handling contaminated trays.

- Masks are only required if cleaning will cause splash, aerosols, and/or splatter.

(A)

(B)

FIGURE 11-28 (A) Dental assistant placing bagged instruments in a sterilizer. (B) Sliding tray with bagged instruments into the sterilizer.

filled with disinfectant. Allow the bleach to remain in the lines for at least ten minutes but never more than thirty minutes. When using other disinfectants, follow manufacturer's directions. For instance, there is a pink solution that is run through the system until the pink solution appears at the end of the air-water syringe and handpiece lines. This solution can remain in the lines overnight. Early the next day, the solution can be discarded and flushed with hot water until the pink color is gone. If using the bleach solution, after ten to thirty minutes, purge the unit with air. If not using the unit, leave after purging; if ready to use the unit, install on the unit a disinfected bottle filled with treatment water. Run the unit for twenty or thirty seconds with a steady stream of treatment water that comes from the handpiece and syringe. After running the unit, it will be ready for use.

Dental Radiography Room and Equipment

So much attention is paid to treatment rooms that often separate radiography rooms and radiography darkrooms, among other rooms, are missed during infection control. When dental assistants expose and process radiographs, infection control practices must be followed. The room first must be prepared, much like a treatment room with appropriate barriers. Upon completion of the procedure, the radiography room must be disinfected in the same manner, disinfecting all surfaces that were contaminated. (See Chapter 21, Introduction to Dental Radiology and Equipment, for further information.) The radiographs that were placed in the mouth must be cared for properly and all the equipment must be disinfected. Procedure 11-6 outlines infection control procedures for the radiography room.

Dental Laboratory

The dental laboratory should be disinfected in the same manner as other rooms. Use the spray-wipe-spray-wipe technique on all surfaces. If the dental assistant is polishing with pumice on the rag wheel, PPE should be worn. Extra care is necessary when wearing gloves while using the rotary equipment for polishing, because gloves can easily become caught in the wheels or motors.

PROCEDURE 11-6

Dental Radiology Infection Control Protocol

The procedure is performed by the dental assistant in the dental radiography room if it is a separate area or at the dental unit if radiographs are taken in the same location as dental treatment. By following a routine procedure that meets the regulations and protocols set forth by the dentist and the regulatory agencies discussed earlier in the chapter, the dental assistant completes the procedure.

EQUIPMENT AND SUPPLIES

- Utility gloves
- Barriers
- Necessary disinfecting solutions
- Wiping cloths
- 4 × 4 gauze

PROCEDURE STEPS *(Follow aseptic procedures)*

1. Wash hands and place the barriers. The x-ray head fits into one of the dental chair bags. Using this type of barrier is much easier than trying to get into all areas to disinfect. It will also not be as hard on the equipment (spraying the disinfecting solution can destroy electrical equipment over time).

2. The x-ray room must have a lead-lined door and walls. Both sides of the door handle need barriers. Sandwich bags work well for this type of barrier. If the switches for use of the dental radiography machine are located in another area, place a barrier over them. The chair can be covered, although no splatter or spray is anticipated (unless the patient vomits).

3. Dental x-rays can be placed in barriers at this time. (See Chapter 21, Introduction to Dental Radiology and Equipment, for more information about dental x-ray barriers.)

4. Put on PPE as the patient is seated. Place the lead apron on the patient.

5. After each of the x-rays is taken, place it in a disposable cup outside the x-ray room.

6. After the procedure is completed and the patient is dismissed, remove the barriers and dispose of them, along with treatment gloves. If the x-rays have been in a barrier, remove the barrier carefully while allowing the untouched x-rays to fall into a clean disposable cup. Then, remove the treatment gloves.

7. Disinfect any areas not covered by barriers.

   NOTE: The lead apron is often missed during disinfection.

8. X-rays are then processed. If barriers on the dental x-ray packets have not been used, special attention should be taken not to cross-contaminate. Either new gloves must be donned as the x-rays are removed from the infected packets or a two-cup method must be used. Careful attention to aseptic techniques will ensure that x-rays are not recontaminated prior to putting them through the processor.

9. One frequently contaminated area are the sleeves of the daylight processor. Place two cups inside the processor (one with contaminated x-rays in it and one with nothing in it). Don new gloves prior to placing hands through the sleeves of the processor. Open the contaminated x-rays and place them in the clean cup. Remove the gloves and place them in the contaminated cup before using clean hands to place the uncontaminated dental film through the processor. Take clean hands out of the sleeves of the daylight processor and lift the lid. Remove the two cups from the daylight loader, touching only the outside of each cup. There are a number of other ways to accomplish this task without cross-contaminating, such as using overgloves and packet barriers.

After polishing, discard the pumice and disinfect the pan. (Some dental offices mix the pumice with disinfectant.) Rinse off the rag wheel and cycle it through the autoclave. Many disposable buffing wheels are now available, and can be discarded after use.

Thoroughly disinfect any contaminated dental laboratory cases before being handled in the office or sent to an outside laboratory. One effective way to achieve this is to place all acrylic appliances in a diluted sodium hypochlorite disinfection solution. Cases with any metal parts need to be placed in another solution, such as glutaraldehyde. Check the manufacturer's directions to identify solutions that will meet the criteria for this process.

Dental impressions also must be disinfected prior to sending them out. Check the manufacturer's directions regarding the correct procedure to accomplish this task. Alginate impressions cannot be immersed in any solution, because this can cause distortion. Alginate impressions must be sprayed and then placed in a sealed bag.

Final impression materials such as polysulfide and silicone can be immersed in most disinfecting solutions according to manufacturer's directions without distortion. Procedures for disinfecting polyether and polysiloxane impression materials vary. Some of the polyether impressions cannot go through the disinfecting procedure until a final set time of thirty minutes has elapsed. If the impression has not been disinfected prior to sending it to the dental laboratory, place it in a leak-proof bag with a biohazard label for transport and to indicate that it has not been disinfected.

CHAPTER SUMMARY

Staff must be trained for a safe workplace. Compliance with all regulations must be accomplished to ensure that the process of infection control will be adequate. Training will occur at initial employment, when job tasks change, and annually thereafter.

Case Study

Lisa Scott, a dental assistant, received a personal telephone call during patient dental care. She left the dental treatment room, removed her latex gloves, and answered the telephone in the sterilization area. While in the area, she looked up another telephone number in the phone book, put instruments from the ultrasonic unit in water to rinse and then into the sterilizer, and then returned to the treatment room. Knowing that leaving the treatment area during patient care is not advocated and focusing on asepsis, answer the following questions.

Case Study Review

1. What (if any) areas were contaminated?

2. What procedures should have been followed to prevent cross-contamination?

3. Identify the glove(s) that should have been used during each procedure.

REVIEW QUESTIONS

Multiple Choice

1. Ultimately, the responsibility for infection control lies with the
   a. patient.
   b. dentist.
   c. dental hygienist.
   d. dental assistant.

2. A regulating body that enforces that employers protect their employees from exposure to blood and OPIM is the
   a. Centers for Disease Control.
   b. Environmental Protection Agency.
   c. Food and Drug Administration.
   d. Occupational Safety and Health Administration.

3. Dental assistants fall into which category of job classification for exposure determination?
   a. 1
   b. 2
   c. 3
   d. 4

4. Personal protective equipment includes all the following except
   a. face masks.
   b. eyewear.
   c. ear plugs.
   d. uniforms.

5. The gloves most frequently used during dental patient care are
   a. latex.
   b. overgloves.
   c. utility.
   d. rubber.

6. The term that refers to all patients being treated as if they are infectious is:
   a. asepsis
   b. aseptic technique
   c. standard precautions
   d. universal precautions

7. The federal regulatory agency involved in the safety and effectiveness of disinfecting and sterilizing solutions is the:
   a. Food and Drug Administration.
   b. Environmental Protection Agency.
   c. Organization for Safety and Asepsis Procedures.
   d. Occupational Safety and Health Administration.

8. The antimicrobial handwashing agents that are the most beneficial include:
   a. chlorhexidine digluconate.
   b. triclosan.
   c. para-chlorometaxylenol.
   d. all of the above.

9. The symptoms of redness, initial itching, and vesicles that appear in areas of contact to latex within twenty-four to forty-eight hours, followed by dry skin with fissures and sores, are related to a condition known as:
   a. irritant contact dermatitis.
   b. Type IV hypersensitivity (delayed hypersensitivity).
   c. immediate-type hypersensitivity.
   d. Type I hypersensitivity.

10. The type of gloves that are used during disinfection and clean up procedures are called:
   a. overgloves.
   b. latex gloves.
   c. vinyl gloves.
   d. utility gloves.

Critical Thinking

1. If a small dental office with only four employees routinely follows infection control guidelines, would a surprise OSHA inspection be anticipated?

2. If a problem develops after a dental assistant misuses a dental solution, with whom does the liability lie?

3. During use of the high-speed handpiece, the dental assistant should be concerned with what primary route of microbial transmission?

Web Activities

1. Go to www.epa.gov and find the listing of registered tuberculocide or antimicrobial products. For three of them, write down product name, EPA registration number, manufacturer name, approval date, and active ingredients.

2. Go to www.osha.gov and identify the bloodborne pathogen standards. Read the section that addresses PPE and be prepared to discuss in class.

3. Go to www.ada.org and read the article under oral health topics about dental waterlines and biofilms and be prepared to discuss in class.

MANAGEMENT OF HAZARDOUS MATERIALS

SPECIFIC INSTRUCTIONAL OBJECTIVES

The student should strive to meet the following objectives and demonstrate an understanding of the facts and principles presented in this chapter:

1. Identify the scope of the OSHA Bloodborne/Hazardous Materials Standard.

2. Identify physical equipment and mechanical devices provided to safeguard employees.

3. Demonstrate safe disposal of sharps.

4. Describe MSDS manuals.

5. Demonstrate the use of the colors and numbers in hazardous chemical identification.

6. Describe employee training required to meet the OSHA standard for hazardous chemicals.

KEY TERMS

National Fire Protection Association's color and number method *(245)*

Needlestick Safety and Prevention Act *(234)*

parenteral *(239)*

INTRODUCTION

Infection control and the standards that relate to it are discussed in Chapter 11, Infection Control. This chapter discusses the requirements of the Occupational Safety and Health Administration (OSHA) Bloodborne/Hazardous Materials Standard, such as engineering controls, labeling, material safety data sheets (MSDSs), housekeeping, laundry, and the disposal of hazardous materials. Dental assistants must understand the entire standard and how compliance is accomplished (Figure 12-1). Dental assisting students do not fall under OSHA guidelines because they are not employees; however, following the same safety standards that are practiced in the workplace is preparation for employment. The scope of the standard covers:

- Employee training, safety, and documentation requirements
- Exposure determination

- Infection control, universal precautions, and standard measures used to control possible exposures
- Postexposure follow-up
- Labeling/MSDSs
- Housekeeping/laundry
- Disposal of biohazardous waste

OSHA's Bloodborne Pathogen Standard Revision

In 1991, OSHA published the Occupational Exposure to Bloodborne Pathogens Standard. At present, needle sticks and other sharps injuries still occur frequently and continue to initiate serious health effects. In 2001, according to OSHA, the CDC estimated that health care workers sustain nearly 600,000 percutaneous injuries annually involving contaminating sharps. Due to this information, the U.S. Congress passed the **Needlestick**

Scope and Application

- The Standard applies to all occupational exposure to blood and other potentially infectious materials (OPIMs) and includes part-time employees, designated first aiders, and mental health workers, as well as exposed medical personnel.
- OPIMs include saliva in dental procedures, cerebrospinal fluid, unfixed tissue, semen, vaginal secretions, and body fluids visibly contaminated with blood.

Methods of Compliance

- General—Standard precautions.
- Engineering and work practice controls.
- Personal protective equipment.
- Housekeeping.

Standard Precautions

- *All* human blood and OPIMs are considered infectious.
- The *same* precautions must be taken with all blood and OPIMs.

Engineering Controls

- Whenever feasible, engineering controls must be the primary method for controlling exposure.
- Examples include needleless IVs, self-sheathing needles, sharps disposal containers, covered centrifuge buckets, aerosol-free tubes, and leak-proof containers.
- Engineering controls must be evaluated and documented regularly.

Sharps Containers

- Readily accessible and as close as practical to work area.
- Puncture resistant.
- Labeled or color coded.
- Leak proof.
- Closeable.
- *Routinely replaced* so there is no overflow.

FIGURE 12-1 Understanding OSHA's Bloodborne/Hazardous Materials Standard.

(continues)

(continued)

Work Practice Controls

- Handwashing following glove removal.
- No recapping, breaking, or bending of needles.
- No eating, drinking, smoking, and so on in work area.
- No storage of food or drink where blood or OPIMs are stored.
- Minimize splashing, splattering of blood, and splashing of OPIMs.
- No mouth pipetting.
- Specimens must be transported in leak-proof, labeled containers. They must be placed in a secondary container if outside contamination of primary container occurs.
- Equipment must be decontaminated before servicing or shipping. Areas that cannot be decontaminated must be labeled.

Personal Protective Equipment

- Includes eye protection, gloves, protective clothing, and resuscitation equipment.
- Must be readily accessible and employers must require their use.
- Must be stored at work site.

Eye Protection

- Is required whenever there is potential for splashing, spraying, or splattering to the eyes or mucous membranes.
- If necessary, use eye protection with a mask, or use a chin-length face shield.
- Prescription glasses may be fitted with solid side shields.
- Decontamination procedures must be developed.

Gloves

- Must be worn whenever hand contact with blood, OPIMs, mucous membranes, non-intact skin, or contaminated surfaces/items or when performing vascular access procedures (phlebotomy).
- Type required:
    —Vinyl or latex for general use.
    —Alternatives must be available if employee has allergic reactions (e.g., powderless).
    —Utility gloves for surface disinfection.
    —Puncture resistant when handling sharps (e.g., Central Supply).

Protective Clothing

- Must be worn whenever splashing or splattering to skin or clothing may occur.
- Type required depends on exposure. Prevention of skin and clothes contamination is the key.
- Examples:
    —Low-level-exposure lab coats.
    —Moderate-level-exposure, fluid-resistant gown.
    —High-level-exposure, fluid-proof apron, head and foot covering.
- *Note:* If personal protective equipment (PPE) is considered protective clothing, then the *employer must launder it.*

Housekeeping

- There must be a written schedule for cleaning and disinfection.
- Contaminated equipment and surfaces must be cleaned as soon as feasible for obvious contamination or at end of work shift if no contamination has occurred.
- Protective coverings may be used over equipment.

Regulated Waste Containers (Non-Sharp)

- Closeable.
- Leak proof.
- Labeled or color coded.
- Placed in secondary container if outside of container is contaminated.

FIGURE 12-1 Understanding OSHA's Bloodborne/Hazardous Materials Standard. *(continues)*

(continued)

Laundry

- Handled as little as possible.
- Bagged at location of use.
- Labeled or color coded.
- Transported in bags that prevent soak-through or leakage.

Laundry Facility

- Two options:
  1. Standard precautions for all laundry (alternative color coding allowed if recognized).
  2. Precautions only for contaminated laundry (must be red bagged or biohazard labeled).
- Laundry personnel must use PPE and have a sharps container accessible.

Hepatitis B Vaccination

- Made available within ten days to all employees with occupational exposure.
- Free to employees.
- May be required for student to be admitted to a college health program, as well as to an externship.
- Given according to U.S. Public Health Service guidelines.
- Employee must first be evaluated by a health care professional.
- Health care professional gives a written opinion.
- If the vaccine is refused, the employee signs a declination form.
- Vaccine must be available later if initially refused.

Postexposure Follow-up

- Wash thoroughly with antimicrobial soap.
- Have a blood draw as soon as possible or within two hours.
- Document exposure incident.
- Identify source individual (if possible).
- Attempt to test source if consent is obtained.
- Provide results to the exposed employee.

Labels

- Biohazard symbol and word *Biohazard* must be visible.
- Fluorescent orange/orange-red with contrasting letters may also be used.
- Red bags/containers may be substituted for labels.
- Labels are required on:
  —Regulated waste.
  —Refrigerators/freezers with blood of OPIMs.
  —Transport/storage containers.
  —Contaminated equipment.

Information and Training

- Required for all employees with occupational exposure.
- Training required initially, annually, and if there are new procedures.
- Training material must be appropriate for the employees' literacy and education levels.
- Training must be interactive and allow for questions and answers.

Training Components

- Modes of HIV/HBV transmission.
- Explanation of exposure control plan.
- Explanation of engineering, work practice controls.

FIGURE 12-1 Understanding OSHA's Bloodborne/Hazardous Materials Standard. *(continues)*

(continued)

Training Components *(continued)*

- Explanation of bloodborne standard.
- Epidemiology and symptoms of bloodborne disease.
- How to select the proper PPE.
- How to decontaminate equipment, surfaces, and so on.
- Information about hepatitis B vaccine.
- Postexposure follow-up procedures.
- Label/color code system.

Medical Records

Records must be kept for each employee with occupational exposure and include:
- A copy of employee's vaccination status and date.
- A copy of postexposure follow-up evaluation procedures.
- Health care professional's written opinions.
- Confidentiality must be maintained.
- Records must be maintained for thirty years, plus the duration of employment.

Training Records

Records are kept for three years from date of training and include:
- Date of training.
- Summary of contents of training program.
- Name and qualifications of trainer.
- Names and job titles of all persons attending.

Exposure Control Plan Components

- A written plan for each workplace with occupational exposure.
- Written policies/procedures for complying with the standard.
- A cohesive document or a guiding document referencing existing policies/procedures.

Exposure Control Plan

- A list of job classifications where occupational exposure control occurs (e.g., medical assistant, clinical laboratory scientist, dental hygienist).
- A list of tasks where exposure occurs (e.g., medical assistant who performs venipuncture).
- Methods/policies/procedures for compliance.
- Procedures for sharps disposal.
- Disinfection policies/procedures.
- Procedures for selection of PPE.
- Regulated waste disposal procedures.
- Laundry procedures.
- Hepatitis B vaccination procedures.
- Postexposure follow-up procedures.
- Training procedures.
- Plan must be accessible to employees and be updated annually.

Employee Responsibilities

- Go through training and cooperate.
- Obey policies.
- Use universal precaution techniques.
- Use PPE.
- Use safe work practices.
- Use engineering controls.

FIGURE 12-1 Understanding OSHA's Bloodborne/Hazardous Materials Standard.

(continues)

(continued)

Employee Responsibilities

• Report unsafe work conditions to employer.
• Maintain clean work areas.

Cooperation between employer and employees regarding the Standard will facilitate understanding of the law, thereby benefiting all persons who are exposed to HIV, HBV, and OPIMs by minimizing the risk of exposure to pathogens.

Meeting the OSHA standard is not optional, and failure to comply can result in a fine that may total $10,000 for each employee.

FIGURE 12-1 Understanding OSHA's Bloodborne/Hazardous Materials Standard.

Safety and Prevention Act that directs OSHA to revise the bloodborne pathogens standard. The standard was revised and became effective in April 2001.

Exposure Control Plan Additions

Two new requirements were added to the standard. First, the employer must solicit input from employees involved in direct patient care. These employees should be nonmanagerial, and the selection should be from a wide range of direct patient care interaction. Annually, the representative number of employees will give input after requested from the employer.

The employer must document this input in the exposure control plan and who and how they solicited said input. The dentist can show they are meeting the standard by (according to the *Revision to OSHA's Bloodborne Pathogens Standard, Technical Background and Summary*):

■ Listing the employees involved and describing the process by which input was requested; or

■ Presenting other documentation, including references to the minutes of meetings, copies of documents used to request employee participation, or records of responses received from employees.

The employer must also:

■ Consider innovations in medical procedure and technological developments that reduce the risk of exposure; and

■ Document consideration and use of appropriate, commercially available, and effective safer devices used to evaluate those devices.

The employer must select devices that, based on reasonable judgment:

■ Will not jeopardize patient or employee safety or be medically inadvisable; and

■ Will make an exposure incident involving a contaminated sharp less likely to occur.

Another addition to the Standard is that, in addition to maintaining a log of occupational injuries and illnesses, the employer under the new revision must maintain a sharps injury log. This log must be kept as all other employee records, in protection of the employee's privacy. The sharps injury log must contain the type and brand of the device involved in the incident, the location of the incident, and the description of the incident. The format of the log is set by the employer and may contain additional comments as long as the privacy of the employee is maintained.

Under engineering controls in the OSHA standard, the revision now specifies that "safer medical devices, such as sharps with engineered sharps injury protections and needle-less systems" constitute an effective engineering control and must be used where feasible.

"Sharps with engineered sharps injury protections" is a new term that includes non-needle sharps or needle devices containing built-in safety features that are used for collecting fluids or administering medications or other fluids or other procedures involving the risk of sharps injury. This covers such devices as syringes with a sliding sheath that shields the attached needle after use and needles that retract into the syringe after use.

"Needleless systems" is a new term for devices that provide an alternative to needles for various procedures. This term is currently used more in medicine than dentistry. It refers to devices like a jet injection system or an IV medication system in which a port is used instead of a needle.

OSHA Compliance Directive

OSHA will continue to revise and create compliance directives to further protect employees and clarify new standards for employers. These directives are a way to clarify the intent of the standard and the enforcement procedures for compliance. Employers and employees should continue to stay abreast of standards and requirements. The OSHA (www.OSHA.org) and ADA (www.ADA.org) Web sites are good sources of information pertinent to dentistry.

Engineering/Work Practice Controls

The physical equipment and mechanical devices that employers provide to safeguard and protect employees at work are known as engineering and work practice controls. Examples of these would be splash guards on model trimmers, puncture-resistant sharps containers, and ventilation hoods for hazardous fumes. The employer must provide this equipment to meet OSHA standards and to provide a safe environment for employees. The employer must ensure that employees wash their hands immediately after gloves are removed and flush their eyes with water at an eye-wash station if contact with microorganisms or hazardous materials is suspected (Figure 12-2). The employer must ensure that employees flush any mucous membranes immediately if there has been possible contact with blood or other potentially infectious materials (OPIMs) in the office.

The employer sets up work practice controls to diminish harmful occupational exposure. OSHA defines occupational exposure as reasonably anticipated eye, skin, mucous membrane, or parenteral contact with blood or other OPIM that may result from the performance of an employee's duties. It further defines **parenteral** as a means of piercing mucous membranes or the skin barrier through such events as needlesticks, cuts, and abrasions.

Sharps

The dentist may purchase needle guards for dental needles to protect employees from unnecessary sticks. Several types are available. Needles should never be recapped using the two-hand technique, because it is easy to stick the opposing hand or the other person's hand. Instead, a scoop method using one hand must be followed during the recapping procedure (see Chapter 20, Anesthetic & Sedation).

Upon completing a procedure, contaminated sharps and needles must be placed immediately in a labeled, leak-proof, puncture-resistant container (Figure 12-3). Other sharps that are placed routinely in the sharps disposal container are blades from knives used in surgery, broken glass, anesthetic capsules, and orthodontic wires. When the sharps disposal containers are full, they are sealed, sterilized using an autoclave if possible, and sent to an outside biohazard agency for safe disposal.

Occupational Exposure to Bloodborne Pathogens

Any employee who has an occupational exposure incident must report it immediately (Figure 12-4). The employer must make available immediately to the exposed employee a confidential medical evaluation and follow-up. The medical evaluation and follow-up are made available to the employee at no cost. The dentist refers the exposed

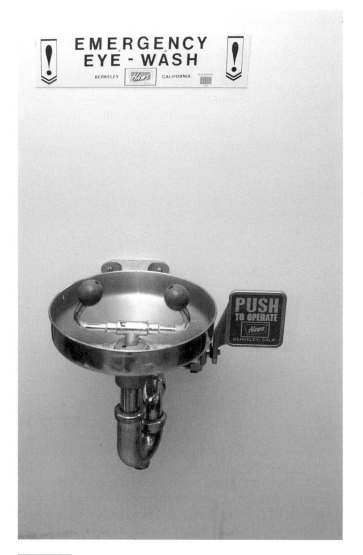

FIGURE 12-2 Flushing eyes at an eye-wash station.

FIGURE 12-3 Puncture-resistant sharps containers.

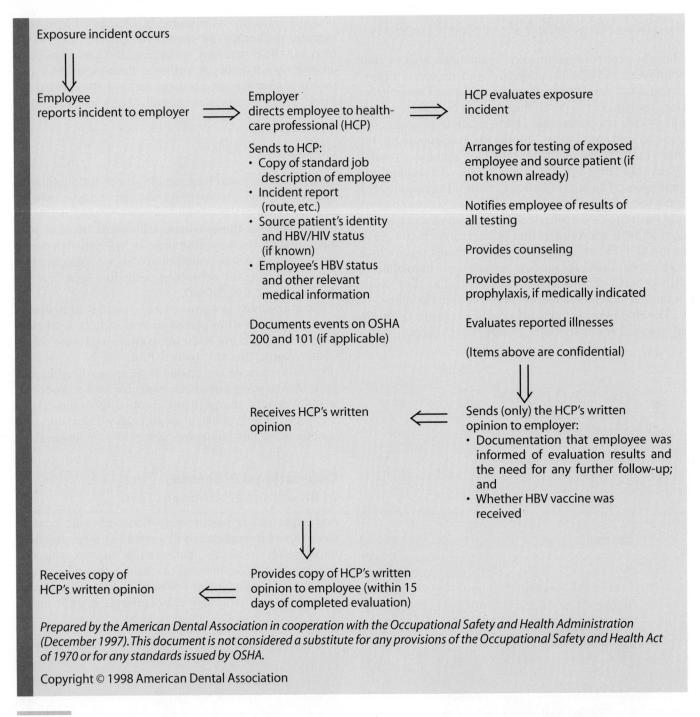

Exposure incident occurs

Employee reports incident to employer → Employer directs employee to health-care professional (HCP) → HCP evaluates exposure incident

Sends to HCP:
- Copy of standard job description of employee
- Incident report (route, etc.)
- Source patient's identity and HBV/HIV status (if known)
- Employee's HBV status and other relevant medical information

Documents events on OSHA 200 and 101 (if applicable)

Arranges for testing of exposed employee and source patient (if not known already)

Notifies employee of results of all testing

Provides counseling

Provides postexposure prophylaxis, if medically indicated

Evaluates reported illnesses

(Items above are confidential)

Receives HCP's written opinion ← Sends (only) the HCP's written opinion to employer:
- Documentation that employee was informed of evaluation results and the need for any further follow-up; and
- Whether HBV vaccine was received

Receives copy of HCP's written opinion ← Provides copy of HCP's written opinion to employee (within 15 days of completed evaluation)

Prepared by the American Dental Association in cooperation with the Occupational Safety and Health Administration (December 1997). This document is not considered a substitute for any provisions of the Occupational Safety and Health Act of 1970 or for any standards issued by OSHA.

Copyright © 1998 American Dental Association

FIGURE 12-4 Flowchart for occupational exposure to bloodborne pathogens. *(Courtesy of the American Dental Association)*

employee to a licensed health care professional to have the most current medical evaluation and procedures performed that are in accordance with the U.S. Public Health Service. OSHA standards do not dictate the procedures to be performed but allow for the most current recommendations to be applied. Reporting the incident immediately allows the dentist to carefully evaluate the circumstances surrounding the incident and to find ways to prevent the situation and exposure incident from happening again.

Documentation of Exposure Incident. The dentist documents the information of the exposure incident on a report. This report includes the route(s) of exposure, the circumstances that surrounded the exposure incident, and (if known) the identity of the source patient. The exposure incident report is placed in the employee's confidential medical record and a copy of this report is provided to the health care professional who is providing the evaluation.

The employer is required to provide the licensed health care professional with a description of the employee's job duties and their relation to the incident; information about the route of the exposure; the circumstances surrounding the incident; relevant employee medical records, including vaccination status; a copy of the bloodborne pathogen standard; and the results of the source patient's blood testing (if available).

If the employer has eleven or more employees, the employer may be required to complete the OSHA forms 200 (Log and Summary of Occupational Injuries and Illnesses) and 101 (Supplemental Record of Occupational Injuries and Illnesses) to meet the "recordable occupation injury" requirement.

In a bloodborne pathogen exposure, the dentist must identify and document in writing the source patient, if known. Further, the dentist must contact the source patient and request his or her consent to be tested for HBV and HIV and then further to disclose the results of these tests to the exposed employee. If the source patient does not give consent for the testing, the dentist must document this on the report of the exposure incident. If the source patient agrees to be tested, the tests should be completed as soon as feasible. When the results are disclosed to the exposed employee, information regarding the source patient's rights to disclosure must be discussed.

Exposed Employee Blood (Collection and Testing). The employee has the right to decline testing after an exposure incident or to delay the testing for up to ninety days. The employee may consent to have a baseline blood test that will determine the HBV and HIV serological status. The employee may choose to be tested only for HBV and not give consent for HIV testing at that time. The employee's blood sample must be saved for ninety days in case the employee elects to consent to the HIV testing. All tests must be performed by an accredited laboratory at no cost to the employee. The health care professional will notify the employee directly of all test results.

Postexposure Follow-up Procedures. The employer must provide to the exposed employee counseling, prophylaxis to prevent sexual transmission of any possible infection, and evaluation of reported illnesses. The counseling provided will aid the employee in interpretation of all tests and discussions about the potential risk of infection and the need for further postexposure prophylaxis. The employee should also be counseled on the necessary use of protection during sexual contact.

Postexposure prophylaxis is provided according to current recommendations of the U.S. Public Health Service. OSHA did not define this procedure in the bloodborne standard due to ongoing changes that have developed in this area.

Treatment may include, but is not limited to, HBV vaccine if the employee has not had it or chemoprophylaxis for high-risk cases of HIV transmission.

The health care professional also evaluates any reported illnesses that the exposed employee develops. The health care professional can evaluate the symptoms in relation to the HBV and HIV infection. This allows the exposed employee to have immediate medical evaluation and referral for medical treatment to take place so that the treatment can be started as soon as possible. This does not mean that the employer is responsible for any costs associated with the treatment of the disease.

The health care professional sends the dental employer a written opinion about the evaluation and notification that the employee was informed of the test results of the evaluation and of the further follow-up. The dentist provides the employee with a copy of this written opinion and evaluation of the exposed employee within fifteen days of the completion of the evaluation. The original document is placed in the employee's confidential record. The employer must maintain employee records in a confidential manner for the duration of employment plus thirty years in accordance with OSHA's standard on Access to Employee Exposure and Medical Records, 29 CFR 1910.20.

Employee Work Site

The employer must provide a work site that is clean and sanitary. Each office must have a written schedule for infection control and decontaminating procedures for each area. Wastepaper baskets, floors, and all other surfaces that may have been contaminated with blood or OPIM must be included. The assistant must wear utility gloves while cleaning contaminated surfaces. All disposable items that are contaminated, including gloves, must be discarded in a biohazard container.

Broken Glass. Broken glass must be cleaned up with a broom (or brush) and dust pan (or cardboard). Dental assistants must never touch broken glass with hands or gloved hands, therefore risking a puncture. Broken glass must be placed in a leak-proof sharps container, labeled biohazard.

Laundry. Contaminated laundry must be handled as little as possible. Gloves must be used when placing it in a biohazard container or a red bag that is labeled with a biohazard symbol (Figure 12-5). If the laundry is damp or wet, it must first be placed in a plastic bag to prevent blood or OPIM from seeping through it.

Laundry that is sent off-site for cleaning is placed in a red biohazard bag for transportation. Dental assistants should take special care when removing the protective clothing, especially items that are taken over the head. The chance for contamination of the face can take place if the outside surface of the clothing makes contact with it.

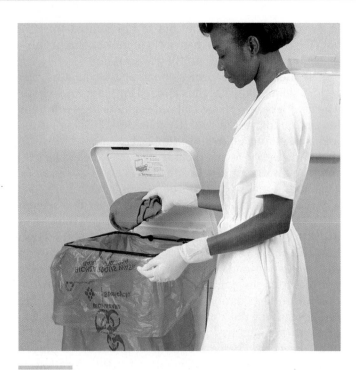

FIGURE 12-5 Proper disposal of contaminated laundry.

SAFETY TRAINING FORM

All employees receive safety training before those employees assume responsibilities that involve exposure to body fluids or chemicals or within thirty days of employment.
Items that must be covered in the training session are:
- Overall explanation of OSHA laws
- Explanation of the epidemiology and symptoms of HBV and HIV/AIDS
- Discussion about who is at risk in the dental office
- Transmission modes of microorganisms
- Methods of infection control in the workplace
- Universal/Standard Precautions
- Personal protective equipment
- Handwashing
- How spills are to be cleaned
- Postexposure incident procedure
- Coverage of the Hazardous Communication Standard
- Chemical labels and how to read them
- How to read MSDSs, how to get MSDSs, where MSDSs are kept in the office, and interpretation of warning signs on MSDSs
- How chemicals are to be stored and inventoried
- Hazardous waste laws and how to comply
- How to use sharps containers
- How and who keeps records
- Medical consent forms
- HBV forms
- Engineering control records
- Safety training certification and when training is to take place

FIGURE 12-6 Safety training form.

Hazardous Chemicals

The OSHA hazard communication standard is set up so that employees receive training about the risks of using hazardous chemicals and the safety precautions required when handling them. Employees must be trained in identification of hazardous chemicals and personal protective equipment to be utilized for each chemical. This training must occur within thirty days of employment or prior to the employee using any chemicals, and annually thereafter (Figure 12-6).

Employees must have a certificate available or in their personnel files that shows they have had the proper training. The certificate must identify that the employer has trained the employee in the proper handling of hazardous substances in the dental office (Figure 12-7).

As with the Bloodborne Pathogen Standard, a written plan identifying employee training and detailing specific control measures used in the workplace must be compiled for hazardous chemicals. If the office is not in compliance, penalties may be imposed on the employer.

All hazardous chemicals must be identified on a written form, such as a chemical inventory form (Figure 12-8). Other information required about the chemicals includes the quantity stored (each month or year), the physical state of the substance (liquid, solid, or gas), the hazardous class (health problem, fire hazard, reactive), what PPE is required, and the manufacturer's name, address, and phone number.

SAMPLE

OSHA HAZARD COMMUNICATION AND BLOODBORNE PATHOGEN STANDARD TRAINING CERTIFICATE

This certificate indicates your successful completion of the OSHA Hazard Communication and Bloodborne Pathogen Standard Training in the office of _____. The program instructed you of your rights as a worker, the responsibilities of your employer, and the proper knowledge and handling of hazardous substances and bloodborne pathogens in this dental office.

Date of employment _____

Date of training _____

Instructor's signature _____

Employee's signature _____

Employer's signature _____

FIGURE 12-7 Sample training form.

SAMPLE

CHEMICAL INVENTORY FORM

Date updated _____

Dental office _____

Chemical Name	Hazard Class				Physical State	Manufacturer	Comments
	(H)	(F)	(R)	(P)			

(H) Health
0—Minimal
1—Slightly
2—Moderate
3—Serious
4—Extreme

(F) Fire Hazard
0—Will not burn
1—Slight
2—Moderate
3—Serious
4—Extreme

(R) Reactivity
0—Stable
1—Slight
2—Moderate
3—Serious
4—Extreme

(P) Protection
A—Goggles
B—Goggles/gloves
C—Goggles/gloves/clothing
D—Goggles/gloves/clothing/mask
E—Goggles/gloves/mask
F—Gloves
G—Face shield/gloves

FIGURE 12-8 Sample chemical inventory form.

Material Safety Data Sheets

Every office must have a material safety data manual that is alphabetized, indexed, and available to all employees. These manuals can be in hard copy or on a computer. The manual contains the MSDSs (Figure 12-9). These sheets come from the manufacturer. If MSDSs are unavailable, the employer or a designated employee (the safety assistant) must request it from the manufacturer.

Material Safety Data Sheet

I—Product Identification

Company Name: We Wash Inc.

Address: 5035 Manchester Avenue
Freedom, TX 79430

Product Name: Spotfree
Synonyms: Warewashing Detergent

Tel. No.: (314) 621-1818
Nights: (314) 621-1399
CHEMTREC: (800) 424-9343

Product No.: 2190

II—Hazardous Ingredients of Mixtures

Material:	(CAS#)	% by Wt.	TLV	PEL
According to the OSHA Hazard Communication Standard, 29 CFR 1910.1200, this product contains no hazardous ingredients.		N/A	N/A	N/A

FIGURE 12-9 Sample MSDS. *(Courtesy of POL Consultants)*

(continues)

(continued)

III—Physical Data

Vapor pressure, mm Hg: N/A
Evaporation rate (ether=1): N/A
Solubility in H_2O: Complete
Freezing point F: N/A
Boiling point F: N/A
Specific gravity H_2O=1 @25C: N/A   Odor: Mild chemical odor

Vapor density (air=1) 60–90F: N/A
% Volatile by wt.: N/A
pH @ 1%   Solution 9.3–9.8
pH as distributed: N/A
Appearance: Off-white granular powder

IV—Fire and Explosion

Flash point F: N/AV   Flammable limits: N/A

Extinguishing media: The product is not flammable or combustible. Use media appropriate for the primary source of fire.

Special firefighting procedures: Use caution when fighting any fire involving chemicals. A self-contained breathing apparatus is essential.
Unusual fire and explosion hazards: None known.

V—Reactivity Data

Stability: Conditions to avoid: None known.

Incompatibility: Contact of carbonates or bicarbonates with acids can release large quantities of carbon dioxide and heat.

Hazardous decomposition products: In fire situations, heat decomposition may result in the release of sulfur oxides.
Conditions contributing to hazardous polymerization: N/A

Spotfree
VI—Health Hazard Data

Effects of overexposure (medical conditions aggravated/target organ effects)
A. Acute (primary route of exposure)   Eyes: Product granules may cause mechanical irritation to eyes.
     Skin (primary route of exposure): Prolonged, repeated contact with skin may result in drying of skin.
     Ingestion: Not expected to be toxic if swallowed; however, gastrointestinal discomfort may occur.
B. Subchronic, chronic, other: None known.

VII—Emergency and First Aid Procedures

Eyes: In case of contact, flush thoroughly with water for fifteen minutes. Get medical attention if irritation persists.
Skin: Flush and dry Spotfree from skin with flowing water. Always wash hands after use.
Ingestion: If swallowed, drink large quantities of water and call a physician.

VIII—Spill or Leak Procedures

Spill management: Sweep up material and repackage, if possible.
Spill residue may be flushed to the sewer with water.
Waste disposal methods: Dispose of in accordance with federal, state, and local regulations.

IX—Protection Information/Control Measures

Respiratory: None needed.   Eye: Safety glasses.   Glove: Not required.

Other clothing and equipment: None required.

Ventilation: Normal.

FIGURE 12-9 Sample MSDS. *(Courtesy of POL Consultants)*

(continues)

(continued)

X—Special Precautions

Precautions to be taken in handling and storing: Avoid contact with eyes. Avoid prolonged or repeated contact with skin. Wash thoroughly after handling. Keep container closed when not in use.
Additional information: Store away from acids.

Prepared by: D. Martinez   Revision date: 04/11/__

Seller makes no warranty, expressed or implied, concerning the use of this product other than indicated on the label. Buyer assumes all risk of use and/or handling of this material when such use and/or handling is contrary to label instructions.

While Seller believes that the information contained herein is accurate, such information is offered solely for its customers' consideration and verification under their specific use conditions. This information is not to be deemed a warranty or representation of any kind for which Seller assumes legal responsibility.

FIGURE 12-9 Sample MSDS. *(Courtesy of POL Consultants)*

The **National Fire Protection Association's color and number method** is used to easily identify information about various hazardous ingredients on the MSDS and product labels.

Chemical Warning Label Determination. The National Fire Protection Association's color and number method is used to signify a warning to employees using the chemicals (Figure 12-10). Four colors are used:

1. Blue identifies the health hazard.

2. Red identifies the fire hazard.

3. Yellow identifies the reactivity or stability of a chemical.

4. White indicates the PPE needed when using this chemical.

RED: FIRE HAZARD

4 = Danger: Flammable gas or extremely flammable liquid

3 = Warning: Flammable liquid

2 = Caution: Combustible liquid

1 = Caution: Combustible if heated

0 = Noncombustible

YELLOW: REACTIVITY

4 = Danger: Explosive at room temperature

3 = Danger: May be explosive if spark occurs or if heated under confinement

2 = Warning: Unstable or may react if mixed with water

1 = Caution: May react if heated or mixed with water

0 = Stable: Nonreactive when mixed with water

BLUE: HEALTH HAZARD

4 = Danger: May be fatal

3 = Warning: Corrosive or toxic

2 = Warning: Harmful if inhaled

1 = Caution: May cause irritation

0 = No unusual hazard

WHITE: PPE

A   Goggles

B   Goggles, gloves

C   Goggles, gloves, apron

D   Face shields, gloves, apron

E   Goggles, gloves, mask

F   Goggles, gloves, apron, mask

X   Gloves

FIGURE 12-10 The National Fire Protection Association's color and number method. *(Courtesy of POL Consultants)*

The level of risk for each category is indicated by the use of numbers 0–4. The higher the number, the greater the danger. Letters are used to identify the PPE needed.

A chemical warning label, a diamond-shaped symbol, displays the four colors with a place for the numbers to be written on each (Figure 12-11). The employee quickly can identify the hazard category, the risk for each, and the PPE equipment required. All hazardous chemicals must be labeled unless they are poured into separate containers for immediate use (Figure 12-12).

Chemical Warning Label Determination

The Hazard Communication Act contains specific labeling requirements. Labels must be on all hazardous chemicals that are shipped to and used in the workplace. Labels must not be removed. Material safety data sheets for all chemicals will be available to employees.

Manufacturer Requirements: Chemical manufacturers are required to evaluate chemicals, determine status as hazards, provide material safety data sheets (MSDSs), and label all shipped chemicals properly. Manufacturer labels must never be removed. The best way to determine the hazards of the chemical is to read the MSDS, obtain an OSHA designated list or State Hazardous Substance list. For most mixed chemicals, it is necessary to contact the manufacturer for MSDS.

Office Chemicals: Search through your office and write down all chemicals you have in the office. Most pharmaceuticals and common household products do not come under this standard. Ingredients can then be compared to a list of regulated substances or MSDSs will provide necessary information.

Employer's Responsibility: Any hazardous chemical used in the workplace that is not in its original container **must** be labeled with the identity of the chemical and hazards. "Target Organ" chemical labels may be used. The label must include the chemical and common name, warnings about physical and health hazards, and the name and address of the manufacturer. The employer is to compile a chemical inventory list that is to be updated as needed. MSDS information should be located in a place where it is accessible to all employees. Label and MSDS information should be provided during the safety training program.

Identity: The term *identity* can refer to any chemical or common name designation for the individual chemical or mixture, as long as the term used is also used on the list of hazardous chemicals and the MSDS.

Note: If a chemical is poured into another container for immediate use, it does not need to be labeled.

_____
Chemical name

_____
Common name

_____
Manufacturer

FIGURE 12-11 A chemical warning label. *(Courtesy of POL Consultants)*

FIGURE 12-12 Containers with chemical warning labels. *(Courtesy of POL Consultants)*

CHAPTER SUMMARY

OSHA regulations, including the hazard communication standard, are intended to require the employer to provide a safe work environment for all employees. The dental assistant must understand the complete standard and how compliance is accomplished. Staff must be trained for a safe workplace. Compliance with all standards must be accomplished to ensure a safe workplace.

Case Study

Rebecca Thomas, a twenty-five-year-old, is a newly hired employee in the office of Dr. Charles. She is working as a chairside dental assistant. She will be completing her first month of employment. A fellow employee is discussing a case with Rebecca and accidentally knocks over a glass container. It breaks into several pieces.

Case Study Review

1. What training should Rebecca have completed?

2. What records of the incident must be kept by Rebecca's employer? For how long must they be kept?

3. What must be used to clean up the broken glass?

4. Where should the pieces of broken glass be disposed of?

REVIEW QUESTIONS

Multiple Choice

1. The Bloodborne/Hazardous Materials Standard covers all the following *except*
   a. housekeeping.
   b. laundry.
   c. hours of employment.
   d. material safety data sheets.

2. An example(s) of engineering/work practice controls is (are)
   a. personal protective equipment.
   b. splash guards on model trimmers.
   c. gloves, masks, glasses.
   d. dental uniform.

3. After an exposure incident, the employer provides a copy of the health care professional written opinion within ____ days of a completed evaluation.
   a. 5
   b. 10
   c. 15
   d. 30

4. The color and number method often used to label various chemicals was developed by the
   a. Occupational Safety and Health Administration.
   b. American Dental Association.
   c. Environmental Protection Agency.
   d. National Fire Protection Association.

5. The color blue on the chemical warning label indicates
   a. health hazard.
   b. fire hazard.
   c. reactivity or stability of chemical.
   d. PPE needed.

6. Broken glass must be cleaned up and placed in ___.
   a. plastic bag
   b. leak-proof sharps container
   c. cardboard container
   d. garbage container

7. Yellow on the chemical warning label determination identifies the:
   a. fire hazard
   b. health hazard
   c. PPE needed
   d. reactivity or stability of a chemical

8. The OSHA hazard communication standard is set up so that ____ receive training about the risks of using hazardous chemicals and the safety precautions.
   a. employee
   b. employer
   c. patient
   d. both a. and b.

9. The following are accepted work practice controls *except:*
   a. no recapping
   b. no bending of needles
   c. mouth pipetting
   d. handwashing, following glove removal

10. The housekeeping area of the OSHA Bloodborne/Hazardous Materials Standard shows that all of the following must be done *except:*
    a. written schedule for cleaning and disinfection
    b. protective covering may be used over equipment
    c. carpets in all operatories
    d. If no contamination has occurred, the equipment and surfaces must be cleaned at the end of the work shift.

Critical Thinking

1. Would the scope of the OSHA Bloodborne/Hazardous Materials Standard cover the employee while traveling to the place of employment?

2. Employees have a lunch room that becomes untidy and disorderly. The dentist never uses the lunch room. If one of the employees has an accident in the room, who is responsible?

3. Standard precautions are issued by whom? To protect whom?

Web Activities

1. Go to www.osha.gov and find information on MSDSs and print the two pages of requirements for the OSHA 174 document.

2. Go to www.osha.gov and find information about biohazardous waste. Have there been any changes in this area since the publication of this textbook? If so, note these changes and bring information to class for discussion.

3. Go to the Web and identify a source with a list of MSDSs. Find two chemicals that are used in the school clinic. Were they on the list you found? What information did you find on the MSDSs for the two identified chemicals?

CHAPTER 13

PREPARATION FOR PATIENT CARE CDA

SPECIFIC INSTRUCTIONAL OBJECTIVES

The student should strive to meet the following objectives and demonstrate an understanding of the facts and principles presented in this chapter:

1. Help the patient complete the patient history.

2. Review the medical and dental history. Alert the dentist to any areas of concern.

3. Perform or assist the dentist in an oral evaluation including lips, tongue, glands, and oral cavity.

4. Perform vital signs on the patient, including temperature, pulse, respiration, and blood pressure.

5. Read the vital signs. Alert the dentist if the signs are abnormal.

KEY TERMS

antecubital space *(257)*

antipyretic *(254)*

asymmetric *(251)*

baseline vital signs *(253)*

brachial artery *(256)*

bradycardia *(255)*

bradypnea *(256)*

Celsius *(254)*

commissures *(251)*

diastolic blood pressure *(258)*

exhalation *(256)*

Fahrenheit *(254)*

fever *(254)*

hypertension *(258)*

hypotension *(258)*

hypothermic *(254)*

inhalation *(256)*

palpate *(251)*

smile line *(251)*

sphygmomanometer *(256)*

stethoscope *(257)*

symmetric *(251)*

systolic blood pressure *(258)*

tachycardia *(255)*

tachypnea *(256)*

vermilion border *(251)*

vital signs *(253)*

INTRODUCTION

Preparing for patient care is an important part of providing quality dental service to each patient. The dental assistant can begin the process of patient preparation by obtaining personal, medical, and dental history from each patient. After history forms are completed, the dental assistant reviews the information and alerts the dentist to any areas of concern.

Once the patient is in the treatment room, the dental assistant performs or assists the dentist in an evaluation of the patient. This clinical evaluation includes obtaining vital signs and performing both an internal and an external evaluation.

Patient History

Dental team members must thoroughly review a patient's medical history in order to treat the patient effectively. The information must be reviewed and updated at each visit. Most dental offices have a questionnaire for patients to complete. The information is confidential and should be as thorough as possible so that the best possible care is rendered. Sensitive topics may be discussed, such as medications being taken, medical treatment, and other factors contributing to the patient's health. Certain patients may be identified for "premedication" status before dental treatment.

Personal Information

One of the first steps in caring for patients is to have them complete a patient history. The patient is requested to fill out a personal history that includes the following: full name, address, phone number, Social Security number, insurance, emergency contacts, and physician's name and his or her phone number (Figure 13-1). (See Chapter 3, Ethics, Jurisprudence and Health Information Portability and Accountability Act (HIPAA).

Medical Information

The patient is also requested to fill out a medical history. The medical history contains questions about past surgeries, systemic diseases, injuries, and/or allergies. It is critical for the dental team to know about any allergies that may affect treatment. Normally, the allergies of concern are related to anesthetics, latex, and/or antibiotics. The patient also should disclose any medical concerns such as epilepsy, diabetes, or a heart condition. Allergies and medical alerts are to be noted on the chart and highlighted to bring them to the attention of dental team members. Any drugs the patient has taken recently or is currently taking should be recorded on the medical history. Often, a variety of questions are asked to gain the information needed. The assistant should tactfully

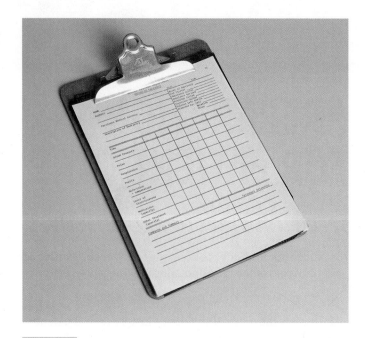

FIGURE 13-1 Health and medical history.

question any abnormalities. Usually, any "yes" answers on a questionnaire require further inquiry. Computerized software programs automatically print copies of the medical alert when the daily schedule prints. This provides added notification of patients who may require special accommodations.

Dental Information

Questions regarding the patient's dental history are included in the patient's history. This information alerts the dental assistant to any concerns the patient has regarding his or her current dental health. It also gives insight into any concerns the patient may have had regarding previous dental care. The last dental examination is noted, as well as the patient's last dental appointment and how often the patient seeks dental treatment. Some questions are asked regarding the patient's attitude toward dentistry and how he or she maintains his or her own personal oral health care.

Upon completion of the patient history, the patient signs and dates the form. This record provides the dentist and staff with useful information so that they may provide better care for the patient. The dentist and/or dental assistant will review the answers prior to initiation of treatment. The personal and medical history should be reviewed prior to each treatment series. It is the dentist's ethical and legal responsibility to gain information about the patient's medical history prior to dental treatment. The highest degree of confidentiality must be maintained by the dental team regarding the patient's history.

After thoroughly reviewing the patient's personal and medical/dental history and collecting the appropriate data, the patient is seated.

Clinical Observation

The dental assistant observes patients as they are escorted into the treatment room. If the patient displays any deviation from normal, such as walking with an abnormal gait, further probing into the health history may be required. The assistant may notice speech or behavior problems that should be brought to the dentist's attention. Looking at the patient's face for symmetry is the first step in the oral inspection. Although most individuals do not have faces that are totally **symmetric** (meaning that if the face was divided in half, the other half would be a mirror image), each side of the face should look fairly similar. If one eyelid droops, for example, or if the face is **asymmetric**, this should be noted on the patient's chart. The dental assistant also evaluates the patient's eyes and facial skin for any scars or abnormalities in color or texture.

Clinical Evaluation

Examine the lips for cracking and dryness. The dental assistant also observes the **smile line** (where the lips are when the patient smiles), the **vermilion border** (the line around the lip), and the **commissures** (the corners of the lips) (Figure 13-2). Any deviations from normal are noted on the patient's chart.

The assistant may place a lip lubricant (petroleum jelly) on the patient's lips prior to the examination to ensure the patient's comfort.

The next area to be examined is the external floor of the mouth and the cervical lymph nodes. The floor of the mouth is examined with the patient's mouth closed. The dental assistant palpates the soft tissues in the area with the fingers, checking for any abnormalities (Figure 13-3).

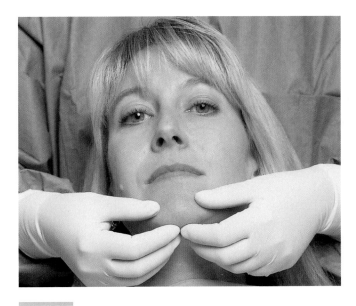

FIGURE 13-3 Examining the external tissues of the mandible and the floor of the mouth.

The cervical lymph nodes are examined by having the patient turn his or her head to the side. The dental assistant gently feels the chain of lymph nodes from the ear to the collar bone. This is done on the opposite side of the neck as well (Figure 13-4).

The last external area to be examined is the temporomandibular joint (TMJ). The dental assistant sits behind the patient's head to **palpate** the joint as the patient opens and closes his or her mouth. Also, the dental assistant places a finger from each hand just anterior to the tragus of each ear and has the patient open and close his or her mouth (Figure 13-5). The operator listens for any noise in the TMJ, such as clicking, and feels for any catching as the patient's mouth

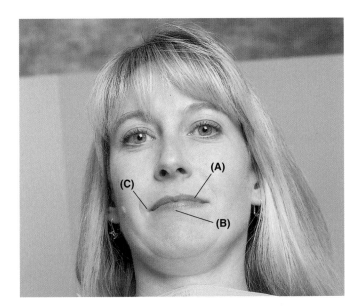

FIGURE 13-2 Visually examining (A) the smile line, (B) the vermilion border, and (C) the commissures of the lip.

FIGURE 13-4 Examining the cervical lymph nodes.

FIGURE 13-5 Examining the temporal mandibular joint as the patient opens and closes her mouth.

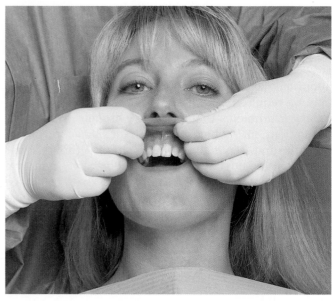

FIGURE 13-7 Examining the oral mucosa and the frenum.

opens. Any symptoms, pains, or tenderness is noted on the patient's chart.

At the beginning of the internal oral examination, the operator first does a quick visual assessment, looking for any obvious problems. Problems could include lesions in the mouth, abscessed teeth, or color changes in the oral mucosa. The operator examines the tissues of the floor of the mouth. This is accomplished by supporting the mandible with one hand while gently palpating with the fingers of the other hand on the ventral sides of the tongue and the floor of the mouth (Figure 13-6). The mucosa and the frena of the upper and lower lips are examined by gently

pulling the lips out and inspecting the area (Figure 13-7). The mouth mirror is used in the maxillary and mandibular buccal area. Using the mirror, the palate and the posterior of the tongue are examined visually (Figure 13-8).

The last area in the oral cavity to be examined is the tongue. A gauze sponge is needed to grasp the tongue. Placing the gauze around the tip of the tongue, the operator pulls to the side to visually inspect the posterior area on each side and then lifts to examine the underportion of the tongue (Figure 13-9). During this time, the patient is asked to say "ah-ah," therefore allowing the operator to examine the uvula and the tissues of the oropharynx.

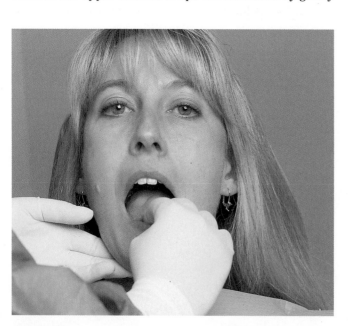

FIGURE 13-6 Operator (dentist or dental assistant) performing an intraoral examination of the floor of the mouth.

FIGURE 13-8 Examining the palate and the posterior of the tongue using a mouth mirror.

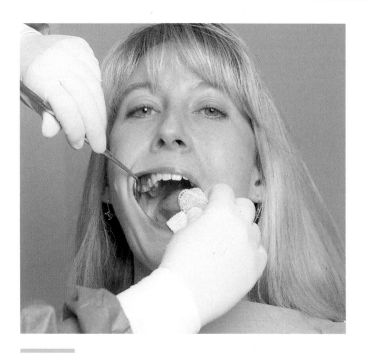

FIGURE 13-9 Examining the tongue using a gauze sponge on the tip of the tongue.

Vital Signs

The measuring and recording of vital signs is an important part of the health evaluation, and should be done with every patient before starting any dental treat-ment. After the patient's history is completed and the patient is seated, the dental assistant can obtain vital signs. Vital signs give the dental operator specific infor-mation about the physical and emotional condition of the patient. They may point out previously undetected abnormalities. Vital signs aid in planning the patient's dental treatment and are essential during emergency treatment.

Vital signs are the basic signs of life. They include body temperature, pulse, blood pressure, and respira-tion rate. Baseline vital signs are the initial measure-ments of vital signs. Baseline vital signs help the dentist compare subsequent measurements with the initial measurements.

Body Temperature

Measurement of body temperature is an essential component of every patient's health evaluation (Fig-ure 13-10). Body temperature is compared to the nor-mal body temperature range and, if higher or lower, it should be further investigated. A range is used when identifying the normal body temperature, because tem-perature varies from person to person and throughout the day. It is well known that after exercise, emotional excitement, and even eating, temperature rises. A person's face may turn red and blush due to excite-ment, increasing body temperature. Temperature in young children and young infants will vary more than in adults.

FIGURE 13-10 Fahrenheit and Celsius thermometers with the normal range indicated.

Normal Temperature Ranges

- Normal range in Fahrenheit 99.5°

    98.6° (average)

    96.0°

- Normal range in Celsius 37.5°

    37.0° (average)

    35.5°

On the Fahrenheit scale, the freezing point of water is 32°F and the boiling point of water is 212°F. On the Celsius scale, the freezing point of water is 0°C and the boiling point of water is 100°C.

The patient has a fever if he or she is above the normal range. An antipyretic, often used to reduce fever, could include cold packs, alcohol rubs, or an aspirin. A patient is said to be hypothermic if the body temperature is below normal. Hypothermia could be caused from prolonged exposure to cold and/or an overdose of antipyretic drugs, such as aspirin.

 There are a number of new digital thermometers on the market for measuring temperature in an expedient manner. Procedure 13-1 presents an overview of how to measure temperature using a digital thermometer. If the manual thermometer is used, place it under the tongue to remain in place with the lips closed for five minutes. The manual thermometer is mercury filled, which is a hazardous chemical, and if breakage occurs, it must be disposed of properly. If a digital thermometer is used to obtain temperature, dispose of the probe cover in a biohazard waste container.

Pulse

The pulse is the intermittent beating sensation felt when the fingers are pressed against an artery. A pulse rate is determined by palpation (feeling with the fingers or

PROCEDURE 13-1

Taking an Oral Temperature Using a Digital Thermometer

This procedure is performed by the dental assistant in order to obtain the patient's body temperature.

EQUIPMENT AND SUPPLIES

- Digital thermometer
- Probe covers
- Biohazard waste container

PROCEDURE STEPS *(Follow standard precautions)*

1. Wash hands.

2. Assemble the thermometer and probe cover.

3. Seat patient in the dental treatment room and position him or her comfortably in an upright position.

4. Verify that the patient has not had a hot or cold drink or smoked within the last half hour. (This may give a false temperature reading.)

5. Explain the procedure to the patient.

6. Position the new probe cover on the digital thermometer (Figure 13-11).

7. Insert the probe under the tongue to either side of the patient's mouth.

8. Instruct the patient to carefully close his or her lips around the probe without biting down on it (Figure 13-12).

9. Leave the probe in position until the digital thermometer beeps.

10. Remove the probe from the patient's mouth.

11. Read the results from the digital thermometer display window.

12. Dispose of the probe cover in a hazardous waste container.

13. Wash hands.

14. Document the procedure and record the results on the patient's chart.

(continues)

PROCEDURE 13-1 *(CONTINUED)*

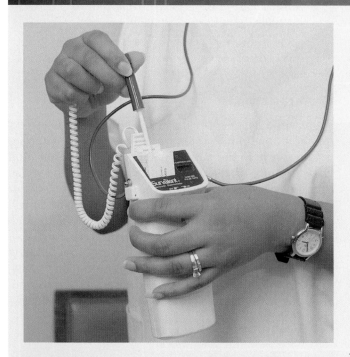

FIGURE 13-11 Slide the probe into the disposable cover, adjusting if necessary.

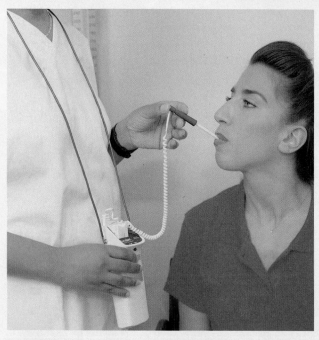

FIGURE 13-12 Insert the thermometer under the tongue to enter the mouth.

hand). Do not use the thumb to palpate, because it has a pulse of its own and could throw off the readings. Pulse may be palpated on one of several arteries: radial, carotid, or temporal. The dental assistant most commonly uses the radial artery.

Radial Pulse Site. The radial pulse site is located on the radial artery, on the thumb side of the wrist (Figure 13-13). It can be found approximately one inch above the base of the thumb. This is the most common site used for obtaining pulses in the dental office.

Carotid Pulse Site. The carotid pulse site is located on the carotid artery in the neck just below the angle of the mandible (Figure 13-14). It is normally large and therefore easy to locate.

Temporal Pulse Site. The temporal pulse site is over the smaller temporal artery located in the temporal fossa, which is a slight depression about the level of the eyebrow just in front of the ear (Figure 13-15). The temporal pulse is more difficult to locate than the radial or carotid.

After locating the pulse site, the dental assistant determines the number of beats per minute. This varies depending on the patient's age, sex, and physical and mental conditions. It is expressed in a range without an absolute number. Tachycardia is an abnormally rapid resting pulse rate, and bradycardia is an abnormally slow resting heart rate.

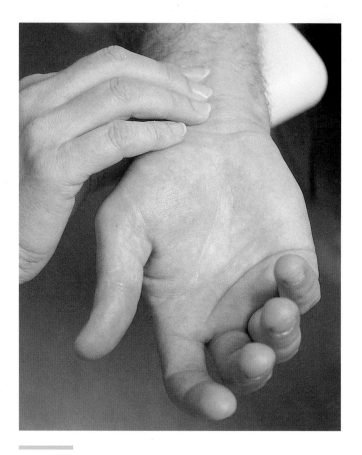

FIGURE 13-13 Radial pulse site.

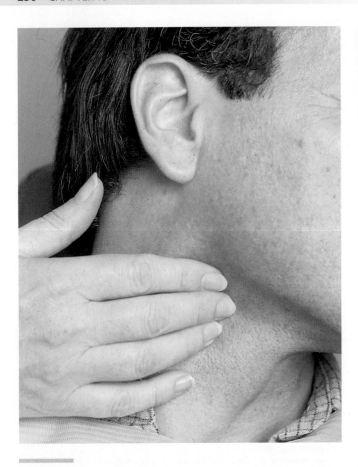

FIGURE 13-14 Carotid pulse site.

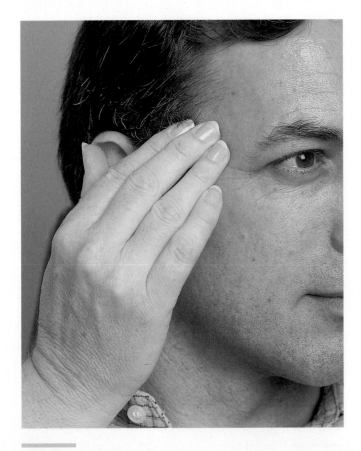

FIGURE 13-15 Temporal pulse site.

Normal Pulse Rates	
▪ Normal pulse rate for adults	Sixty to ninety beats per minute
▪ Normal pulse rate for children	Ninety to one hundred twenty beats per minute

Respiration

Respiration is one breath taken in (**inhalation**) and one breath let out (**exhalation**). To ensure an accurate reading—where the patient is unaware that respiration is being measured—take it after obtaining the pulse rate. Leave the fingers over the pulse site and count the breaths in and out for one minute. The patient will assume that the pulse is still being taken. **Tachypnea** is an abnormally rapid resting respiratory rate and, **bradypnea** is an abnormally slow resting respiratory rate. There are similarities in respiration and pulse rates. Children have a more rapid respiration rate; generally, as with the pulse rate, the younger the child, the faster the rate.

Normal Respiration Rates	
▪ Normal respiration rate in adults	Twelve to eighteen respirations per minute
▪ Normal respiration rate in children	Twenty to forty respirations per minute

Procedure 13-2 overviews the steps used in obtaining a pulse and a respiration rate.

Blood Pressure

Blood pressure is an important indicator of the health of a patient's cardiovascular system. A patient may have heart disease and still feel good and look outwardly healthy. However, the fear of dental treatment may be stressful enough to induce a heart attack. Therefore, taking and recording a patient's blood pressure are very important. It is not done in all offices today, because often the dental assistants have not been trained to perform this skill. Take time to learn this skill!

Some dental offices have purchased automatic blood pressure machines that record blood pressure digitally. A number of models on the market today require very little training. One that works well is placed on the wrist and inflates and records readings readily.

Blood pressure is measured by placing a **sphygmomanometer**, a "blood pressure apparatus," around the **brachial artery** (Figure 13-16). This apparatus is a cloth-covered inflatable rubber bladder used to control the flow of blood in the artery. There is a rubber hand bulb and pressure control valve attached to one tube and a pressure gauge attached to the other tube. The brachial artery is palpated. It is located at the inside of the elbow

FIGURE 13-16 Aneroid sphygmomanometer.

in the **antecubital space**, the indented area, as the arm is stretched straight.

Position the arm at the patient's heart height. After the brachial artery is located, the cuff of the sphygmomanometer can be placed one inch above the bend in the elbow and secured. The dental assistant then uses the **stethoscope**, an instrument used to hear and amplify the sounds produced by the heart (Figure 13-18). The stethoscope has two earpieces that must be placed in the ears in a forward position. At the end piece of the stethoscope is a diaphragm, which does the amplification and sends the sounds up the tubing to the ears. The dental assistant pumps up the cuff and closes off the blood in the artery and then slowly lets the air escape.

Before taking the patient's blood pressure, the assistant should estimate the systolic pressure using the "palpate, inflate, obliterate, deflate" method. While listening with the stethoscope, the assistant places the cuff on the patient's arm above the antecubital space

PROCEDURE 13-2

Taking a Radial Pulse and Measuring the Respiration Rate

This procedure is performed by the dental assistant in order to obtain the patient's pulse and respiration rate.

EQUIPMENT AND SUPPLIES

- Watch with a second hand

PROCEDURE STEPS *(Follow standard precautions)*

1. Wash hands.

2. Position the patient in a comfortable position, upright in the dental chair (same position used for taking the temperature).

3. Explain the procedure.

4. Have the patient position the wrist resting on the arm of the dental chair or counter.

5. Locate the radial pulse by placing the pads of the first three fingers over the patient's wrist.

6. Gently compress the radial artery so that the pulse can be felt.

7. Using the watch with the second hand, count the number of pulsations for one full minute (Figure 13-17).

8. Record the number of pulsations.

FIGURE 13-17 Taking patient's radial pulse and respiration.

(continues)

PROCEDURE 13-2 *(CONTINUED)*

9. Note any irregular rhythm patterns.

10. While still keeping the finger pads placed on the radial pulse, count the rise and fall of the chest wall for one minute. This allows the patient to breathe normally due to the fact that he or she believes the pulse is still being recorded.

11. Record the number of respirations. Note any irregularities in the breathing.

12. Wash hands.

13. Document the procedure and the pulse and respiration rates on the patient's chart.

FIGURE 13-18 A single-head stethoscope, which is used with a sphygmomanometer to measure blood pressure.

and palpates the radial pulse. Then the assistant slowly inflates the cuff just until the pulse is obliterated, memorizes the number (mm Hg), and releases the pressure in the bulb. Next the assistant adds 30 mm Hg to the number representing the pulse obliteration point. This number is an estimate of the systolic pressure and gives a point to inflate the cuff. It is best not to over-inflate the cuff and cause any additional discomfort to the patient's arm. The dental assistant should then wait one minute before reinflating. (For example, if the pulse obliterates at 120 mm, add 30 for estimated inflation of 150. This technique is accurate about 95 percent of the time.)

The dental assistant is now ready to begin taking the blood pressure and inflates the cuff to the estimated pressure. While listening carefully to the sounds, the assistant slowly deflates the cuff.

The assistant listens to the first pulsation sound and notes where the needle is indicating on the pressure gauge. This first sound indicates **systolic blood pressure**, which is created when the heart contracts and

forces blood through the arteries. Listening carefully, the dental assistant then watches the pressure gauge until the pulsation sound disappears. This reading is noted on the gauge as the **diastolic blood pressure**. The diastolic blood pressure is created as the arteries return to their original state when the heart relaxes between contractions. Two measurements are always recorded when taking blood pressure. They are recorded as a fraction—the systolic pressure is the upper figure and the diastolic pressure is the lower figure. They are always recorded in even numbers (the gauge has indications for even numbers only). There is no absolute number for normal blood pressure; it is recorded in ranges, much like other vital signs. Children normally have lower pressure and, as adults age, the blood pressure goes up. Some, however, use 120 over 80 as an average for an adult. This means 120 systolic over 80 diastolic pressure, recorded as 120/80. Normal blood pressure range is as follows:

Normal systolic pressure	100 to 140 mm Hg
Normal diastolic pressure	60 to 90 mm Hg

A higher-than-normal blood pressure is called **hypertension**, and lower-than-normal blood pressure is **hypotension**. An increase in the diastolic pressure is more significant than an increase in the systolic pressure, because it indicates that the heart is working harder. Procedure 13-3 presents the steps involved in measuring a blood pressure.

Normal Blood Pressure Readings	
Child 10 years of age	100/66
Adolescent 16 years of age	118/76
Adult	Systolic below 140
	Diastolic below 90

PROCEDURE 13-3

Measuring Blood Pressure

This procedure is performed by the dental assistant in order to obtain the patient's blood pressure.

EQUIPMENT AND SUPPLIES

- Stethoscope
- Sphygmomanometer
- Disinfectant and gauze

PROCEDURE STEPS *(Follow standard precautions)*

1. Wash hands.

2. Assemble the stethoscope and sphygmomanometer and disinfect the earpieces of the stethoscope.

3. Position the patient in a comfortable position, upright in the dental chair (same position used for taking the temperature).

4. Explain the procedure.

5. Have the patient position the arm resting at heart level on the counter or the arm of the dental chair.

6. Have the patient remove any outer clothing that is restrictive to the upper arm. Bare the upper arm and palpate the brachial artery (Figure 13-19).

7. Center the bladder of the cuff securely, about one inch above the bend of the elbow. Inflate the cuff slowly and palpate the radial pulse until the pulse is obliterated. Release the pressure. Add 30 mm Hg to the number representing the pulse obliteration point. Wait one minute before reinflating the cuff.

8. Position the earpieces of the stethoscope in a forward manner into the ears.

9. Place the diaphragm of the stethoscope over the brachial artery and hold it in place with a thumb. Place other fingers under the elbow to hyperextend the artery. (By extending the elbow, the artery can be accessed more easily and enable better reading of the blood pressure.)

10. Inflate the cuff using the bulb and the control valve on the sphygmomanometer. If the cuff is not inflat-

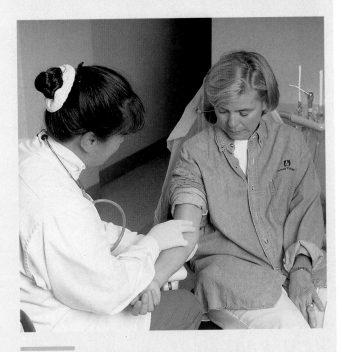

FIGURE 13-19 Palpating patient's brachial artery.

ing, recheck the control valve on the sphygmomanometer to ensure that it is closed. Air should not be escaping. The inflation should be to a level identified in Step 7 during the palpate, inflate, obliterate, and deflate technique.

11. Deflate the cuff at a rate of two to four millimeters of mercury per second by rotating the control valve just slightly (Figure 13-20).

12. Listen for the first sound and note its measurement on the scale.

13. Continue to deflate the cuff and listen to the pulsing sounds. Note when all sounds disappear. Continue deflating for another ten millimeters to ensure that the last sound has been heard.

(continues)

PROCEDURE 1 3 - 3 (CONTINUED)

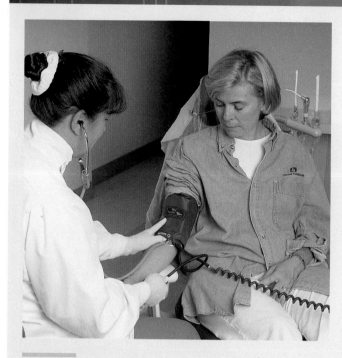

14. The cuff can then be deflated rapidly and removed from the patient's arm.

15. Disinfect the earpieces of the stethoscope.

16. Wash hands and record the procedure and the measurement on the patient's chart. (Remember that blood pressure is recorded in even numbers in a fraction format with the systolic measurement on top.)

FIGURE 13-20 Taking a patient's blood pressure.

CHAPTER SUMMARY

The health condition of a dental patient must be private, confidential, and updated at each visit. To treat a patient effectively, the patient's chart should include personal history, medical information, dental history, clinical observation, clinical evaluation, and vital signs.

Case Study

Dwayne Allen, a fifty-year-old male, was in the dental office for a dental examination. Upon taking his blood pressure, the dental assistant documented that Dwayne had a systolic pressure of 150 and a diastolic pressure of 90.

Case Study Review

1. Is Dwayne's blood pressure within the normal range?

2. Should the blood pressure be retaken to ensure that it was completed accurately?

3. Should this reading be brought to the attention of the dentist?

REVIEW QUESTIONS

Multiple Choice

1. The line around the lip is called the
   a. commissure.
   b. smile line.
   c. vermilion border.
   d. frenum.

2. The corners of the lips are called the
   a. commissures.
   b. smile lines.
   c. vermilion borders.
   d. frena.

3. The initial measurements of vital signs are the
   a. pulse.
   b. respiration.
   c. fever.
   d. baseline.

4. The normal range in body temperature, in Fahrenheit, is
   a. 95–100°.
   b. 96–99.5°.
   c. 97–99°.
   d. 96.5–98.5°.

5. An average range for a child's pulse rate is
   a. 60 to 90 beats per minute.
   b. 70 to 100 beats per minute.
   c. 80 to 110 beats per minute.
   d. 90 to 120 beats per minute.

6. An antipyretic is used to:
   a. evaluate pulse rate
   b. evaluate blood pressure
   c. locate the temporal pulse site
   d. reduce fever.

7. If a patient is said to be hypothermic the body temperature is:
   a. above normal
   b. below normal
   c. not affected
   d. none of the above

8. Bradypnea is abnormally:
   a. rapid resting respiratory rate.
   b. slow resting respiratory rate.
   c. higher than normal blood pressure
   d. lower than normal blood pressure

9. The normal range for systolic blood pressure is:
   a. 100 to 140 mm Hg
   b. 100 to 120 mm Hg
   c. 60 to 90 mm Hg
   d. 80 to 100 mm Hg

10. The normal range for diastolic blood pressure is:
    a. 120 to 140 mm Hg
    b. 100 to 120 mm Hg
    c. 60 to 90 mm Hg
    d. 80 to 100 mm Hg

Critical Thinking

1. What temperature would constitute a fever for a child? What effects on dental treatment would a fever pose?

2. A patient has had a negative experience with his or her teeth in the past. What impact could this have on the current treatment? What role can the dental assistant play in making this a positive experience for the patient?

3. If a dental assistant observes a patient walking with an unsteady gait to the dental treatment room but finds no indication of this symptom in the patient's medical and dental history, what should the assistant do?

Web Activities

1. Go to http://www.ada.org, click on A-Z Public Topics, and locate common mouth sores. Be prepared to come to class and discuss the differences of the canker sores and the cold sores.

2. Go to the Web and complete a search for medical thermometers. Identify several new models on the market and bring this information back to class for a discussion on what one would be best utilized in the dental office.

3. Go to http://www.ada.org, click on A-Z Public Topics, and locate the topic of Temporal Mandibular Joint (TMJ) and identify what percent of American adults suffer from chronic facial pain.

DENTAL CHARTING

SPECIFIC INSTRUCTIONAL OBJECTIVES

The student should strive to meet the following objectives and demonstrate an understanding of the facts and principles presented in this chapter:

1. Explain why charting is used in most dental practices.

2. Identify charts that use symbols to represent conditions in the oral cavity.

3. List and explain the systems used for charting the permanent and deciduous dentitions.

4. Define G. V. Black's six classifications of cavity preparations.

5. List common abbreviations used to identify simple, compound, and complex cavities.

6. Describe basic dental charting terminology.

7. Explain color indicators and identify charting symbols.

KEY TERMS

abscess *(269)*

abutment *(269)*

bridge *(269)*

cantilever bridge *(269)*

caries *(267)*

crown *(269)*

denture *(269)*

diastema *(269)*

drifting *(269)*

Fédération Dentaire
Internationale
(FDI) system for
numbering *(264)*

gold foil *(269)*

incipient *(269)*

Maryland bridge *(269)*

mobility *(269)*

overhang *(269)*

Palmer System for
numbering *(264)*

partial dentures *(269)*

periodontal
pocket *(270)*

pontic *(269)*

restoration *(270)*

root canal *(270)*

sealant *(270)*

Universal/National
System for
numbering *(263)*

INTRODUCTION

CDA Recording the conditions in the patient's oral cavity on a dental chart using symbols, numbers, and colors is a shorthand technique called charting. Charting is used in most dental offices. Numerous symbols and various charts are used, and the dental assistant must identify the doctor's preferred system to ensure accurate charting. Charting is part of the patient's legal record maintained in the office. As with all legal and medical records, each patient's chart should be complete and correct. The initial charting is normally accomplished during the patient's first examination. Dentists dictate their findings to dental assistants, who chart them on a tooth diagram or by computerized charting. The doctor indicates existing conditions, dental services that have been completed, and dental services that have not been completed. The patient's dental record (chart) is used for billing purposes, diagnosis, and consultation. Forensic dentistry also uses the patient's dental record to provide information and to identify individuals involved in homicides, abuse, or other tragedies.

Dental Charts

There are several types of dental charts. Each chart has an area designed for dental charting and an area in which to record treatment. The most commonly used chart is one with diagrams of the teeth that may show an anatomic or a geometric representation of the teeth. Most charts show both the permanent and the primary dentition. The anatomical charts show the crown of the tooth, the crown and a small portion of the root, or the crown and the complete root. The geometric charts show the teeth as circles. Each circle represents one tooth and is sectioned into five areas indicating the corresponding surfaces of the tooth. Each dental office chooses the chart deemed best for current needs.

Numbering Systems

Dental offices have several numbering systems available for their use, and dentists indicate the preferred systems to be used in their offices. All patient records in a given office are documented according to a single numbering system to prevent confusion.

Universal/National System for Numbering

In 1968, the American Dental Association (ADA) adopted the Universal/National System for numbering. This numbering system is currently the most commonly used in the United States (Figure 14-1). Each permanent tooth has its own number, starting from the maxillary right third molar as #1 and moving clockwise

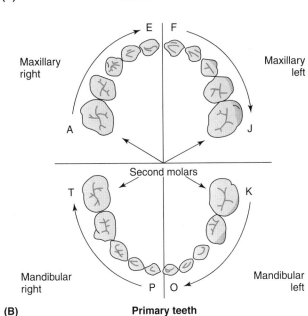

FIGURE 14-1 (A) Permanent and (B) primary dentition showing the Universal/National numbering and lettering system.

to the maxillary left third molar as #16. The mandibular left third molar is #17, and the mandibular right third molar is #32. Therefore, #1 and #32 occlude together and #16 and #17 occlude together. Always remember that it is the patient's right side where tooth #1 and

#32 are located, so that they are not reversed during charting. The primary teeth are each given a letter or a "d" with a number. The maxillary right deciduous second molar is lettered "A" or "d-1," and this continues across the maxillary arch, with the maxillary left second deciduous molar as "J" or "d-10." The mandibular left second deciduous molar is "K" or "d-11," and this continues across the mandibular arch, with the mandibular right second deciduous molar lettered as "T" or "d-20." Most standardized charts in the United States come with diagrams of the primary and permanent teeth using the Universal System for numbering (Figure 14-2).

Fédération Dentaire Internationale (FDI) System for Numbering

The International Standards Organization (ISO) TC 106 designated a system for teeth and areas of the oral cavity. It is widely used in Canada and European countries. This system is designed to provide an international system for coding teeth and the oral cavity. In 1996, the ADA adopted this system and the Universal System for tooth numbering. The **Fédération Dentaire Internationale (FDI) system for numbering** can be adapted easily to the computer and is widely used in most other countries (Figure 14-3). With this system, each quadrant is assigned a number. The oral cavity is given two digits. If two 00s are noted, the whole oral cavity is designated. If 01 is used, it designates the entire maxillary arch; 02 designates the entire mandibular arch. For example, a full denture on the upper (maxillary) arch is noted as denture 01.

The permanent dentition is identified by a 1 for the upper right quadrant, 2 for the upper left quadrant, 3 for the lower left quadrant, and 4 for the lower right quadrant. The deciduous dentition is assigned 5 through 8 for the corresponding quadrants. Each quadrant is numbered from 1 to 8, starting with the centrals and ending with the molars. The primary teeth are numbered from 1 to 5 in the same manner (Figure 14-4). When the FDI system is used, the quadrant number is recorded first. For example, the maxillary right lateral incisor is numbered 12 in the permanent dentition, and the maxillary right lateral incisor in the deciduous dentition is 52.

Palmer System for Numbering

The **Palmer System for numbering** and lettering the teeth is used in some dental offices (Figure 14-5). With this system, the permanent teeth are numbered 1 through 8 in each quadrant: The centrals are 1 and the third molars are 8. With each number, a quadrant bracket is used to denote which quadrant it is referring to. For example, the maxillary right first bicuspid is charted as 4⌋. The deciduous teeth are identified in a similar manner except that the teeth are lettered "A" through "E" for each quadrant. "A" represents the central incisors and "E" represents the primary second molars. Again, the quadrant bracket is used to denote which quadrant it is referring to (Figure 14-6). For example, the deciduous mandibular right central incisor is charted as $\overline{A|}$.

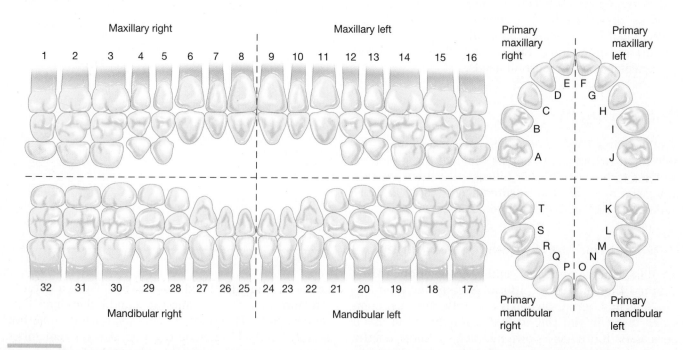

FIGURE 14-2 Universal numbering system for both permanent and deciduous teeth with identifying numbers and letters.

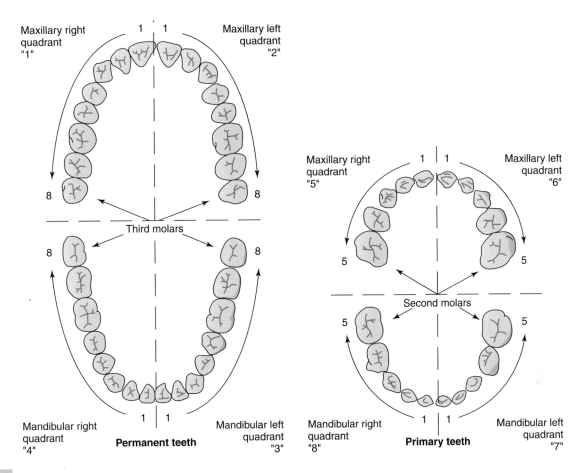

FIGURE 14-3 Permanent and primary dentition showing the International Standards Organization (ISO) TC 106 Designation System/ Fédération Dentaire Internationale system.

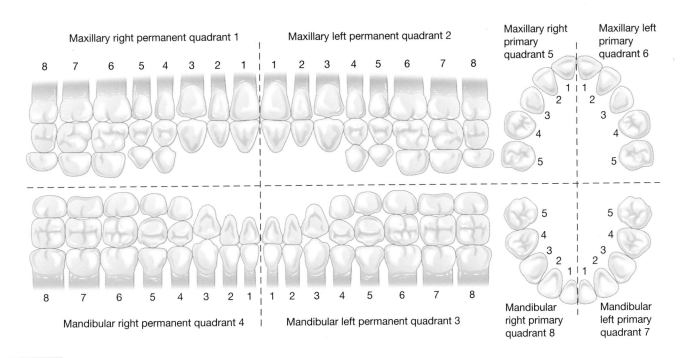

FIGURE 14-4 International Standards Organization (ISO) TC 106 Designation System/Fédération Dentaire Internationale numbering system for both permanent and deciduous teeth with identifying numbers.

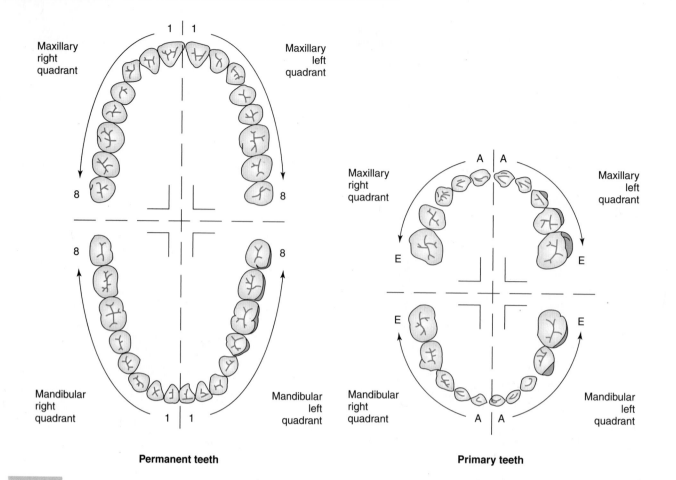

Permanent teeth

Primary teeth

FIGURE 14-5 Permanent and primary dentition with the Palmer numbering and lettering system.

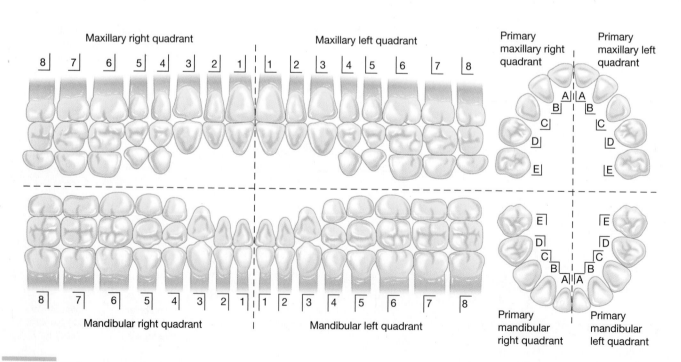

FIGURE 14-6 Palmer numbering system for both permanent and deciduous teeth with identifying numbers and letters and brackets shown.

Cavity Classifications

Five standard cavity classifications were developed by G. V. Black (the "grand old man of dentistry"), and a sixth class was added later. These classifications aid in recording the type of dental **caries** (cavities) on a patient's chart.

Class I

Class I caries include the following three types of developmental cavities in the pit and fissures of teeth (Figure 14-7).

- Occlusal surfaces of the posterior teeth (premolars and molars)
- Buccal or lingual pits on the molars
- Lingual pit near the cingulum of the maxillary incisors

Class II

Class II caries are on the proximal (mesial or distal) surfaces on the posterior teeth (premolars and molars) (Figure 14-8).

Class III

Class III caries are on the interproximal surface (mesial or distal) of anterior teeth (canines, lateral incisors, and central incisors) (Figure 14-9).

Class IV

Class IV caries are on the interproximal surface (mesial or distal) of anterior teeth and include the incisal edge (Figure 14-10).

MO restoration   MOD restoration

FIGURE 14-8 (A) Class II caries on the proximal surface of a premolar and a molar and (B) restorations on the MO surface of a premolar and the MOD surfaces of a molar.

(A)

(B)

(C)

FIGURE 14-7 Class I caries on the (A) occlusal surfaces of the premolars and molars, (B) buccal surface on the molar, and (C) lingual surface on the maxillary incisors.

FIGURE 14-9 Class III caries on the proximal surfaces of an incisor and a cuspid.

FIGURE 14-10 Class IV (A) fractured area on the proximal incisal surface of the incisor and (B) a completed restoration on the central incisor.

Class V

Class V caries occur on the cervical third of the facial or lingual surface of the tooth (Figure 14-11). Often, Class V caries occur because the patient regularly sucks on sweets. Additionally, the dental assistant may see several Class V caries in one quadrant because the patient takes medications, chews gum, or drinks sodas over long periods of time.

Class VI

Class VI caries were not part of the original standard classification of cavities developed by G. V. Black (Figure 14-12). They were later identified to more clearly label cavities that involve the incisal or occlusal surface that has been worn away due to abrasion.

FIGURE 14-12 Class VI caries on the occlusal surface of a mandibular incisor due to abrasion.

Abbreviations of Tooth Surfaces

Terms like simple, compound, and complex are used in cavity classification. A simple cavity involves only one tooth surface, a compound cavity involves two surfaces, and a complex cavity involves more than two surfaces (Table 14-1).

When documenting the chart to record the surfaces of the teeth that need to be restored or that have been restored, the dental assistant abbreviates the notations. Each surface is abbreviated using the first letter of the surface, capitalized. For instance, an abbreviated form of a mesial restoration on tooth #8 is #8 M. If two or more surfaces are restored, then a combined word is used. The "al" is normally dropped and "o" is substituted on the first word. For example, to identify the restoration on the distal and occlusal surfaces, the term is disto-occlusal restoration or DO restoration. If three surfaces are combined, the same principle is applied to the second word as well. If the tooth has a mesial-occlusal-distal restoration, the correct term is mesio-occluso-distal or MOD restoration. If a mesial surface of the tooth is restored with another surface, it is always used first. Occlusal and lingual normally fall in the last position.

FIGURE 14-11 Class V caries on the gingival buccal areas of the teeth.

TABLE 14-1 Abbreviations for Cavity Restorations

Abbreviations for Single-Surface Restorations (Simple Cavity Restorations)	
I	Incisal
M	Mesial
D	Distal
B	Buccal
O	Occlusal
F	Facial
Abbreviations for Two-Surface Restorations (Compound Cavity Restorations)	
OB	Occlusobuccal
MO	Mesio-occlusal
DO	Disto-occlusal
DI	Disto-incisal
DL	Disto-lingual
MI	Mesio-incisal
LI	Linguo-incisal
Abbreviations for Three or More Surface Restorations (Complex Cavity Restorations)	
MOD	Mesio-occluso-distal
MODBL	Mesio-occluso-disto-bucco-lingual

Basic Charting Terms

- **Abscess**—Localized area of infection.

- **Bridge**—Prosthetic device placed in the mouth where a tooth is missing, normally attached on each side and covering the space created by the missing tooth. The attaching sides are called **abutments** and the middle area is called the **pontic**. A **cantilever bridge** is attached on only one side. This kind is useful in an area that has little stress, such as a missing lateral. The abutment side could then be on the canine, which is a strong support. The **Maryland bridge** has wings on the pontic, and they are attached to the lingual sides of the adjacent (abutment) teeth.

- **Crown**—Often called a cap by the patient but not usually by dental professionals. Some crowns are cast in a laboratory and made to fit the patient's tooth exactly. They are made of several types or combinations of materials, such as gold, porcelain and gold, or porcelain. Crowns can be permanent or temporary or made for the anterior or posterior. Preformed (temporary) crowns are manufactured in quantities. The dentist sizes and forms the crown to fit the tooth. These crowns are usually made from stainless steel or plastic. All crowns are "fixed" or cemented into place in the patient's mouth and are not removable like partial and full dentures. Crowns cover the complete tooth, as in a full crown, or three-quarters of the tooth, as in a three-fourths crown.

- **Denture** (complete and partial)—A full denture replaces the complete arch of a patient's dentition. Patients sometimes refer to full dentures as their upper or lower plates. If all the natural teeth in one arch are missing, a full denture is needed. If some of the natural teeth are missing, a partial denture (artificial teeth mounted on a metal framework) can be used.

- **Diastema** (di-a-**STE**-ma)—The space between the maxillary central incisors in humans. The word *diastema* could also be used to denote a space between two adjacent teeth in the same dental arch.

- **Drifting**—All teeth are supported by each other in the dentition. If a maxillary tooth is removed, then the opposing mandibular tooth may drift, or overerupt, into the space. Also, the teeth adjacent to the space created by the removed tooth can drift into the space.

- **Gold foil**—A restoration created when several layers of pure gold are placed in the preparation. This restoration is not commonly used today.

- **Incipient**—Beginning decay that has not broken through the enamel. Incipient appears as a chalky area on the tooth. It is not yet decay, but the surface has begun to decalcify. Some doctors note this on the chart by placing the word "watch" on that area. Other doctors use a series of red dots, a symbol that represents an incipient area.

- **Mobility**—When the tooth moves in the socket, normally due to periodontal disease or trauma. A numbering system is used to indicate how many millimeters the tooth moves and is recorded in Roman numerals, or 0 to 4.

- **Overhang**—Excessive restorative material normally found interproximally near the gingiva.

- **Partial dentures**—Prosthetic devices that replace missing teeth. They have a metal framework and artificial teeth.

■ **Periodontal pocket**—The space in the gingival sulcus created by periodontal disease. It is measured by a periodontal probe in millimeters. A healthy sulcus depth is 1–3 millimeters; beyond this depth it is a periodontal pocket. See Chapter 29, Periodontics.

■ **Restoration**—An agent that is effective in replacing missing tooth structure. Patients may refer to these as fillings. A number of different materials are used in dental restorations, including gold, amalgam, and composite.

■ **Root canal**—When the pulp is removed and replaced with a filling material.

■ **Sealant**—An enamel sealant is a resin material used to seal pits and fissures to prevent decay.

Charting Color Indications and Symbols

Colors and symbols are used in charting to indicate the condition of the patient's teeth and surrounding tissues and the restorative services required (Table 14-2 and Figure 14-13). Some symbols allow for common references when interaction takes place between dental professionals.

Red represents the dentistry that needs to be done, and blue indicates the work that has been completed. Some symbols can be charted in either color. For instance, if a tooth is fractured but causing no discomfort to the patient or not affecting the patient's appearance, the dentist may decide not to restore it. A notation is made on the chart that nothing is to be done at this time and it is charted in either color.

Many offices are now using computerized or automated dental charting instead of, or in addition to, manual charting. Computerized dental charting increases efficiency and fosters standardization. Some offices will use voice-activated systems with their software. These systems are designed to recognize a voice and record the information. Often, voice systems confirm findings before charting them. This helps prevent mistakes. When not using a voice-activated system, the dental assistant can enter the information into the computer by keyboard or light pen. When keyboarding, the keyboard must be covered so that cross-contamination does not occur. The light pen can also be covered with a barrier for use. The light pen looks like a writing pen and is sometimes attached by a cord to the monitor. It is touched to the screen to activate a command. If, for example, the dental assistant wanted to note a composite restoration that was placed in the mouth, the assistant would touch the light pen to the screen over the tooth, highlighting the tooth. After highlighting the tooth, the assistant would move the light pen to the side of the screen and select composite restoration and the surfaces to be included. Finally, the dental assistant would touch the light pen to "existing" or "needs to be completed." The computer program would then put the color coding and/or symbol on the dental chart on the correct tooth and make a

TABLE 14-2   Color Indications and Charting Symbols of Completed Work

• Amalgam restoration (outlined and filled solid blue when complete or red when to be done)	▰
• Composite restoration (outlined in red when to be done or blue when complete)	▭
• Gold restoration (area outlined with diagonal lines, red when to be done or blue when complete)	⧄
• Porcelain restoration (outlined with red when to be done or blue when complete and/or *P* inside the outline)	P
• Sealant (*S* on occlusal surface, red when to be done or blue when complete)	S
• Stainless steel (outlined with swervy lines through it or two *S*s inside it, red when to be done or blue when complete).	〰

Missing teeth (removed or never erupted)		Teeth that are drifting / overerupted	
Multiple missing teeth		Teeth that are drifting / mesial inclination	
Teeth to be extracted		Teeth that are drifting / distal inclination	
All teeth missing		Teeth that need root-canal therapy	
Tooth with root canal treatment, apicoectomy, and silver amalgam retrofilling		Tooth with an abcess	
Teeth impacted or unerupted		Tooth with a completed root canal	

FIGURE 14-13 Charting symbols.

(continues)

(continued)

Tooth with full gold crown	Fixed bridge (abutment 3/4 gold crown-pontic-full gold-abutment full gold)
Tooth with a 3/4 gold crown	Fixed bridge (porcelain fused to metal abutment-pontic-porcelain fused to metal-abutment full gold crown)
Tooth with an MOD onlay crown	Maryland bridge
Tooth with a DO inlay crown	Supernumerary tooth
Tooth with a porcelain crown	Tooth with a temporary restoration
Tooth with a porcelain fused to metal crown	Periodontal pocket

FIGURE 14-13 Charting symbols.

(continues)

(continued)

Overhang on a restoration	Occlusal caries
Food impaction	Occlusal amalgam restoration
Open contacts	Occlusal composite restoration
Decalcification	Enamel sealant
Heavy calculus	Disto-occlusal (DO) caries
Mesio-occluso-distal (MOD) amalgam restoration with recurrent decay	Class IV MI composite restoration

FIGURE 14-13 Charting symbols.

(continues)

(continued)

Class V facial caries

Class I lingual amalgam restoration

Class III M composite restoration

Gingival recession / furcation involvement

Mobility

Partial denture

Full denture

Rotated tooth

Diastema

FIGURE 14-13 Charting symbols.

(continues)

(continued)

Fractured tooth or fractured root	Porcelain veneer
Stainless-steel crown	Dental implant

FIGURE 14-13 Charting symbols.

notation on the patient's chart under findings or treatment plan (Figure 14-14).

Dental software programs work differently but are learned easily. Offices evaluate which systems meet their needs before purchase. Many offices have computers or computer monitors in each operatory for the auxiliary to chart findings and complete the notations and services rendered. (For more information about computer use in the dental office, see Chapter 36, Dental Office Management.)

Dental assistants can become very proficient at computer charting. The software programs for computer charting can record perio charting (see Chapter 29, Periodontics, for periodontal charting), conditions of the dentition, tissue, occlusion or any notations the dentist or auxiliary would like.

CHAPTER SUMMARY

Dental charting provides legal documentation of the patient's oral cavity. The correct numbering system and charting symbols ensure proper documentation. Therefore, accuracy in charting is critical.

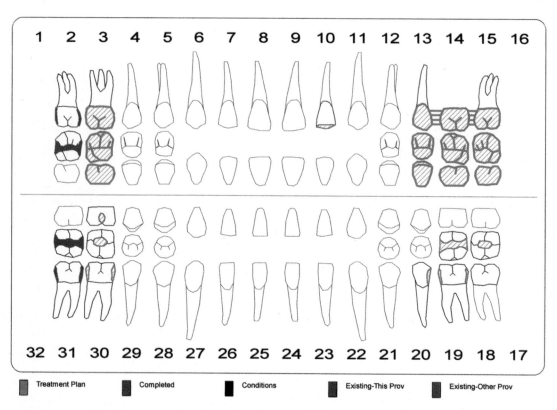

Chart

Patient: Patricia Abbott

Birthdate: 09/30/1963

Provider: Dennis D. Smith D.D.S.

Phone: (801)763-9300

Office: 732 E. Utah Valley Drive # 500
American Fork, UT 84003

Chart #: ABB102

Date: 01/22/2003

SS#:

Treatment Plan Completed Conditions Existing-This Prov Existing-Other Prov

Treatment Plan Estimate

Tooth	Description	Amount	Pat.	Dental Ins.
3	Crown-porc fuse high noble mtl	613.00	306.50	306.50
3	Crown buildup, includ any pins	149.00	29.80	119.20
3	Permanent Insert	0.00	0.00	0.00
10	Resin-one surface, anterior	71.00	14.20	56.80
13	Retainer crn-porc fused-hi nob	613.00	306.50	306.50
14	Pontic-porcelain fused to hnob	613.00	306.50	306.50
15	Retainer crn-porc fused-hi nob	613.00	306.50	306.50
18	Resin-1 surface, post-permanent	80.00	16.00	64.00
19	Resin-3 surface +, post-perm	146.00	29.20	116.80
20	Resin-1 surface, post-permanent	80.00	16.00	64.00
30	Resin-3 surface +, post-perm	146.00	29.20	116.80
	Treatment Plan Totals	3124.00	1360.40	1763.60

* Treatment Plans Are Estimates Only

FIGURE 14-14 Sample computer chart. *(Courtesy of Dentrix)*

Case Study 1   Charting Using the Anatomical Representation of the Teeth and the Universal System for Numbering (Figure 14-15)

Tooth	#1	Impacted
	#2	Class II DO amalgam restoration present
	#4	Class II MOD amalgam restoration present
	#6	Class III M composite restoration present
	#8	Class IV MI composite restoration present
	#8 #9	Diastema present
	#9	Class III M decay
	#13	Class II MOD amalgam restoration with recurrent decay
	#14	Class II MO amalgam restoration present; food impaction between 13 and 14
	#16	Has been removed
	#17	Partially impacted and must be removed
	#19	Bridge present, abutment full gold crown
	#20	Bridge present, pontic porcelain with gold
	#21	Bridge present, abutment porcelain with gold
	#24	Mobility of III , periodontal pocket on M and D of 4 mm each, heavy calculus from mandibular left cuspid to mandibular right cuspid
	#25	Periodontal pocket on M and D of 3 mm each
	#28	Needs a full gold crown with a porcelain facing
	#28	Has a completed root canal
	#30	Class I O decay
	#31	Class II MO amalgam restoration present
	#32	Has been removed

Case Study Review

1. Which tooth has a class III M caries?

2. How many teeth are restored?

3. Which tooth is a pontic?

(continues)

Case Study 1 *(continued)*

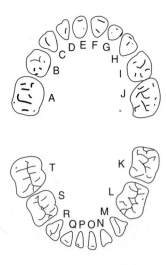

FIGURE 14-15 Charting using the anatomical teeth and the Universal/National System for numbering.

Case Study 2 — Charting Using the Geometric Representation of the Teeth and the ISO System for Tooth Identification (Figure 14-16)

Tooth	#18	Impacted
	#16	Full porcelain with gold crown present
	#15	Class II MO amalgam restoration present
	#14	Class I O sealant present
	#12	Class III M composite present with recurrent decay
	#11	Class I L composite present
	#24	Bridge present, abutment full porcelain with gold
	#25	Bridge present, pontic full porcelain with gold
	#26	Bridge present, abutment full porcelain with gold
	#28	Has been removed
	#38	Has been removed
	#36	Has a full gold crown
	#34	Has an abscess and needs a root canal
	#33	Is missing and the deciduous tooth is retained
	#31	Class IV MI composite restoration present
	#42	Has a fracture on the MI edge
	#45	Class II DO amalgam restoration with an overhang
	#47	Has been removed
	#48	Mesial inclination

Case Study Review

1. Which tooth has an enamel sealant?

2. Which primary tooth is in the patient's mouth?

3. Which tooth needs endodontic therapy?

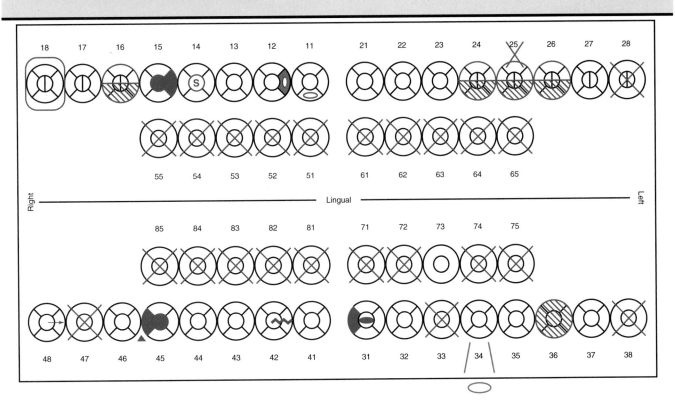

FIGURE 14-16 Charting using the geometric representation of the teeth and the ISO TC 106 designation system for the teeth.

REVIEW QUESTIONS

Multiple Choice

1. Which of the following charting systems uses brackets?
   a. Universal System for numbering
   b. Nationale System for numbering
   c. International Fédération Dentaire
   d. Palmer System for numbering

2. Cavities on the interproximal surface of the anterior teeth that do not include the incisal edge are
   a. Class I.
   b. Class II.
   c. Class III.
   d. Class IV.

3. Excess restorative material found near the gingival tissue is
   a. sealant.
   b. overhang.
   c. drifting.
   d. gold foil.

4. Restorations that need to be completed are charted in which color?
   a. Yellow
   b. Black
   c. Red
   d. Blue

5. Gold crowns are charted with which symbol?
   a. Diagonal lines
   b. Crosshatch lines
   c. Multiple dots
   d. Swervy lines

6. The charting system that uses only numbers is the _____
   a. Universal System for numbering.
   b. Nationale system for numbering.
   c. International Fédération Dentaire.
   d. Palmer System for numbering.

7. A ____ bridge is only attached to one side.
   a. Maryland
   b. pontic
   c. abutment
   d. cantilever

8. The space between the maxillary central incisors in humans is the _____.
   a. sealant
   b. diastema
   c. bridge
   d. overhang

9. Teeth that are impacted or unerupted have the symbol of ____
   a. circle around the tooth.
   b. "X" over the tooth.
   c. arrow pointing in the apical direction.
   d. with a small circle at the apex of the tooth.

10. The dental implant is noted on charting by ____.
    a. swervey lines on the crown of the tooth
    b. root area completely filled in
    c. parallel lines across the crown of the tooth
    d. parallel lines across the root of the tooth

Critical Thinking

1. The five surfaces on a posterior tooth are mesial, distal, occlusal, lingual, and buccal. What are the five surfaces on an anterior tooth? Which of these surfaces is the same for both anterior and posterior?

2. A young adult broke his upper teeth at a drinking fountain, from the middle of the biting edge to the middle of each front tooth in an upside-down V pattern. Which surfaces, classifications, and teeth numbers would be involved if using the Universal System for numbering? The ISO or FDI system? The Palmer System?

3. If an anterior tooth is fractured and does not need to be restored, which color would it be charted in and why?

Web Activities

1. Go to www.softdent.com and look at the new features in dental charting available on the Softdent computer software for dentistry.

2. Go to www.delmarhealthcare.com and find out what books are available on dental charting. Evaluate how the textbooks would help you as a dental assistant.

3. Go to www.ezdent.com and look at the charting examples. Contrast these with the information on the www.softdent.com site. Which software program provides the most complete information on dental office charting? What are the positive features of each program?

CHAPTER 15

PRACTICE

PHARMACOLOGY

SPECIFIC INSTRUCTIONAL OBJECTIVES

The student should strive to meet the following objectives and demonstrate an understanding of the facts and principles presented in this chapter:

1. Identify terms related to drugs, pharmacology, and medicines.

2. Identify the difference between drug brand names and generic names.

3. Identify the parts of a written prescription.

4. Identify the texts pertinent to pharmacology.

5. Give the English meanings of the Latin abbreviations used for prescriptions.

6. Specify the drug laws and who enforces them.

7. Identify the schedules for the Comprehensive Drug Abuse Prevention and Control Act of 1970.

8. Identify the routes through which drugs can be administered.

9. Summarize the uses and effects of tobacco, caffeine, alcohol, marijuana, and cocaine.

10. Summarize information about heroin, morphine, and codeine.

11. Supply information about amphetamines.

12. Demonstrate an understanding of hallucinogenic drugs such as LSD, PCP, and mescaline.

13. Demonstrate an understanding of barbiturates.

14. Demonstrate an understanding of the drugs used in dentistry and the ways in which they are used.

OUTLINE

KEY TERMS

addiction *(282)*

analgesic *(291)*

anesthesia *(295)*

brand names *(282)*

broad spectrum *(292)*

cirrhosis *(290)*

closing *(284)*

Comprehensive Drug Abuse Prevention and Control Act of 1970 *(285)*

Controlled Substances Act *(285)*

Council on Dental Therapeutics *(283)*

depressant *(290)*

drug *(282)*

drug abuse *(288)*

Drug Enforcement Agency (DEA) number *(283)*

drug interaction *(282)*

enteric-coated *(283)*

Food and Drug Administration (FDA) *(285)*

generic names *(282)*

habit forming *(282)*

(continues)

KEY TERMS (continued)

hallucinate (291)

heading (284)

inhalation (287)

inscription (282)

intradermal (288)

intramuscular (287)

intravenous (287)

medicine (282)

oral (287)

over-the-counter (OTC) drugs (282)

pharmacology (282)

Physician's Desk Reference (PDR) (283)

prescription (282)

psychologically dependent (282)

The Pure Food and Drug Act (285)

The Pure Food, Drug, and Cosmetic Act (285)

rectal (287)

scored (283)

side effect (282)

stimulant (289)

subcutaneous (288)

sublingual (287)

subscription (284)

substance abuse (288)

superscription (284)

tolerance (291)

topical (287)

transdermal (288)

ulcer (289)

withdrawal (282)

INTRODUCTION

The terms *pharmacology* and *drugs* are normally associated with treating a disease, but in reality they cover a much broader aspect of chemically induced changes in the body. **Pharmacology** is the study of all drugs, their properties, how they react with each other, and the actions of the drugs within the body. Pharmacology is constantly changing due to the constant information and knowledge gained about drugs, new drugs being created, and drugs being altered. A **drug** is a substance that can change life processes within the body. **Medicines** are drugs that are used to treat diseases.

Drugs have never been as widely used/misused as they are today. The dental assistant needs to pay attention to patients' medical and dental histories and carefully document the drugs used by each patient. The dental assistant must have knowledge about pharmacology, the side effects of drugs, and the interactions that take place when more than one drug is used. When a drug causes an unintended result, this result is called a **side effect**. For example, if a patient is taking antihistamines and decongestants to clear up the symptoms of a cold and the patient becomes tired, fatigue is a side effect.

At times, it is necessary to take more than one drug at a time. This can be dangerous and should be avoided if the patient taking the drugs is not knowledgeable about the interaction. **Drug interaction** occurs when one drug changes the effect of another drug by increasing or decreasing the intended result. The risk of combining the drugs (synergistic effect) is much greater to the person than the risk of taking either one of the drugs alone.

Some drugs are addictive. When a person has an **addiction**, he or she is physically dependent on a drug. Being physically dependent means that the addict must continue to take the drug in order to avoid withdrawal symptoms. The symptoms that occur when the person addicted to the drug stops taking it are called **withdrawal**. Nervousness, stomach cramps, diarrhea, shaking, and depression are symptoms of withdrawal.

Some people become **psychologically dependent** on a drug. This means that the person taking the drug has developed a strong emotional need to take that drug. It is similar to a craving. This person may not have any physical need for the drug but becomes psychologically dependent on it. The drugs that cause psychological dependence are referred to as **habit forming**.

Legal drugs are classified according to their availability to the public and their potential for abuse. Drugs with the **inscription** "Federal law prohibits dispensing without prescription" must be prescribed by a licensed medical professional and dispensed by a pharmacist. Drugs without the inscription are referred to as **over-the-counter (OTC) drugs**.

Drug Names

When filling a **prescription** for a dentist, the pharmacy identifies whether the drug is to be filled with a drug brand or with a generic substance. The generic substance has a similar composition to the drug brand and often does not affect the outcome for the patient.

Brand Names

Brand names of drugs are assigned to the drug by the manufacturer. These brand names, often referred to as trade names, are always capitalized and have registered trademarks. These names are controlled by the manufacturer. For example, Bayer™ is a brand name for aspirin.

Generic Names

Generic names of drugs are not capitalized and are not patent protected. They refer to the chemical composition of the drug, and are less expensive than brand-name drugs. For example, acetylsalicylic acid (aspirin) is a generic name.

Prescriptions

Only physicians, dentists, and physician assistants are legally allowed to write prescriptions. This limits the dispensing of controlled substances to those trained and licensed to provide patients with drugs. The drugs are dispensed only when a customer gives the pharmacist a correctly written prescription signed by a doctor with his or her **Drug Enforcement Agency (DEA) number** on it. In the past, a prescription had a form of recipe for the drug needed on it. Today's medicines are packaged in correct dosage amounts preformulated for dispensing. Oral drugs come in numerous forms. They can be scored or unscored, **enteric-coated** (coating that resists breaking down by the gastric juices and dissolves in the intestines) or not, gelatin or in timed-released capsules (Figure 15-1). When a capsule is **scored** (cut superficially to allow it to separate or break apart more easily) the patient can divide the dosage if directed to do that by the provider. Therefore, the doctor can simplify the prescription, asking for the number of tablets, pills, capsules, or liquid amount and not indicating dosage amounts. This ensures that the patient receives the proper dosage each time the drug is taken, and the correct packaging saves time for the doctor and the patient.

All dentists have the legal obligation to use "due care" while treating their patients. They must have a complete health history on the patient and must be knowledgeable about the drug they prescribe to the patient. The American Dental Association **Council on Dental Therapeutics** gathers information about the drugs used in dentistry, and this information is given to the dentist to assist him or her in gaining necessary information about the use of new therapeutic agents. A recent publication of accepted dental therapeutics can be obtained from the ADA. The dentists can call the ADA with questions concerning accepted dental therapeutics or if questions arise regarding any drug or chemical used in the office. Dentists can also obtain information about drugs from several texts. The most commonly used in the dental office is the *Physician's Desk Reference (PDR)*. The *PDR* is printed annually and has the drugs listed by trade or product name, generic and chemical names, and by category. The *PDR* is available both in book form and as a CD-ROM. Information about the drug includes the chemical description, indications and use of the drug, contraindications of using the drug, warnings and precautions related to the use of the drug, and adverse drug reactions. Information about the recommended drug dosages and how the drug is supplied is also listed in the *PDR* (Figure 15-2). Many of the drugs are packaged with inserts that list the same information

FIGURE 15-1 Tablets and capsules come in different colors, sizes, shapes, and forms. (A) Scored and un-scored tablets; (B) enteric-coated tablets; (C) gelatin capsules; and (D) time-release capsules.

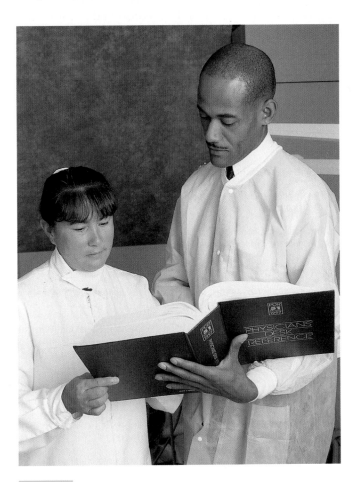

FIGURE 15-2 Dentist and dental assistant using the *Physician's Desk Reference* (PDR) to obtain information about a medication.

contained in the *PDR* about the drug. These inserts usually are not given to the patient but are retained by the pharmacist. Many drugs now have inserts that give clear instructions to the patient as well as warnings. These are given to the patient with the prescription unless the doctor specifies on the written prescription not to do so. Pharmacists use two main references that have detailed information about each drug. These are the *United States Pharmacopoeia (USP)* and the *National Formulary (NF)*.

Parts of a Prescription

A prescription is written in several parts (Figure 15-3). All information must be completed to ensure that the correct drug is being dispensed in the correct manner according to the directions of the dentist. Being thorough and writing clearly will assist in accuracy and quality control. It is recommended that a copy of the prescription be placed in the patient's chart for future reference.

Heading. The **heading** includes the doctor's name and degrees, office address, and phone number. The dentist's DEA number must be printed in this area or near the signature. This number was assigned to the doctor and must be used every time a controlled substance is prescribed.

Superscription. The **superscription** is directly below the heading. This area has blank lines where the dentist can fill in the name and address of the patient. Included in this area is a space for the date that the prescription was written. Other information, such as the patient's

phone number, age, and gender, is also helpful to the pharmacist. Patients do not always fill the prescriptions immediately and may in fact not need them at a later date. Having the date filled in aids the pharmacist in obtaining pertinent information about the need for the drug. The age and gender give further information as to the dosage amount needed by the patient. The pharmacist has extensive training about each drug and is a helpful member of the health care team. The pharmacist may call the dentist and consult about a prescription or about a patient obtaining prescriptions from numerous offices. Health care providers must work together in discouraging drug abuse.

Body of the Prescription. The body of the prescription is labeled with the Rx symbol and has both the **inscription** area and the **subscription** area. In this area, the doctor inscribes or writes the name and strength of the drug being prescribed, the dose, and in what form the drug is to be dispensed. He or she subscribes or specifies the number of doses and directions on how the drug should be taken. Special directions to the pharmacist are written in this area as well. The writing of the body of the prescription is often done in abbreviated format. Many Latin abbreviations are used for this. For example, the prescription might read as follows: Sig: 1 tab qid for 2 wks. This means take one tablet four times a day for two weeks. When the prescription is dispensed by the pharmacist, it is a law that the name of the drug and directions be put on the label of the drug container.

Closing of the Prescription. The **closing** of the prescription is where the dentist signs his or her name, authorizes whether the prescription can be refilled and how

Parts of a Prescription

1. The heading includes the dentist's name, address, telephone number, and registration number.

2. The superscription includes the patient's name, address, and the date on which the prescription is written.

3. The *subscription* that includes the symbol Rx ("take thou").

4. The *inscription* that states the names and quantities of ingredients to be included in the medication.

5. The *subscription* that gives directions to the pharmacist for filling the prescription.

6. The *signature* (Sig) that gives the directions for the patient.

7. The dentist's signature blanks. Where signed, indicates if a generic substitute is allowed or if the medication is to be dispensed as written.

8. REPETATUR 0 1 2 3 p.r.n. This is where the dentist indicates whether or not the prescription can be refilled.

9. ☐ LABEL Direction to the pharmacist to label the medication appropriately.

[1]

LEWIS & KING, DDS
2501 CENTER STREET
NORTHBOROUGH, OH 12345

[2] Name___Juanita Hansen_____

Address ___143 Gregory Lane, Apt. 43___ Date _4/7/--_

[3] Rx

[4] Amoxicillin   500 mg

[5] Disp. #40

[6] Sig   1 cap quid x 10 days

[7] Generic Substitution Allowed ___Susan Lewis___
                                                    D.D.S.

Dispense As Written_____
[8] REPETATUR 0 1 2 3 p.r.n.   D.D.S.

[9] ☐ LABEL

FIGURE 15-3 Prescription with parts identified.

many times, and checks whether a generic brand of this medication can be dispensed in place of the one written.

Latin Abbreviations and English Meanings of Prescriptions	
Latin Abbreviation	**English Meaning of Latin Abbreviation**
a.a.	Of each
a.c.	Before meals
b.i.d.	Twice a day
t.i.d.	Three times a day
q.i.d.	Four times a day
q.h.	Every hour
q.4.h.	Every four hours
q.8.h.	Every eight hours
Sig	Take
p.c.	After meals
p.r.n	When necessary or as needed

Many offices have prescription pads that are numbered sequentially and the information regarding the office and doctor's name and address is preprinted on them. They may have them printed in triplicate so that a copy of each written prescription can be kept in the corresponding patient's chart or on the pad according to the number. Either way, a notation should be written on the patient's chart about the prescription and instructions given. The prescription pads must be kept in a secure place to prevent theft.

Drug Laws

In 1906, the U.S. government passed the **Pure Food and Drug Act**. This law was enacted to control and regulate the composition, sale, and distribution of drugs. Prior to 1906, drugs were not regulated and drugs of varying compositions and purity were sold. Many of these drugs were harmful for human consumption.

Other laws were passed to control the sale of narcotic drugs in the early twentieth century. The **Pure Food, Drug, and Cosmetic Act** was passed in 1938. This allowed only the United States **Food and Drug Administration (FDA)** to have control of all food, cosmetics, and drugs sold. The drugs and cosmetics must pass standards set by the FDA and obtain approval prior to sale. The FDA also controls the advertising for all food, drugs, and cosmetics. This act was amended in 1951 and 1965 to establish additional regulations to prevent tampering with foods, drugs, and cosmetics. It also required that warning labels are present on certain preparations such as: "This product may cause drowsiness," or "do not drive while taking this product." This act also covered a clause that any nonprescription or prescription drugs must be shown to be effective as well as safe. Products may note, on their packaging, that they have met the rigid standards set by the FDA.

The **Comprehensive Drug Abuse Prevention and Control Act of 1970** was established to identify drugs according to five schedules of abuse potential. Title II of this act deals with the control and enforcement of drugs. The **Controlled Substances Act** gives the power of enforcement of this act to the DEA, which is part of the U.S. Department of Justice. Individuals who dispense drugs must have DEA-issued numbers to prescribe drugs. Dentists who dispense controlled substances improperly can have their offices closed and their licenses revoked. The dental assistants and the dentist must carefully check the patient's medical and dental histories prior to writing the prescription.

Drug Schedule for the Comprehensive Abuse Prevention and Control Act of 1970

Schedule number "I" has a higher abuse potential and is more dangerous than schedule number "V." Drugs are added and subtracted to this schedule (Table 15-1) as well as moved from one schedule number to another. This is dependent upon incidences of overdose or if a drug becomes more of a societal problem. The schedule numbers are referenced with the Roman numerals and often these Roman numerals are inside the capital C. These schedule numbers appear on drug packages and drug inserts as well as other drug information resources (Figure 15-4).

■ Schedule I drugs have a high potential for abuse and no accepted medical use. Drugs in this schedule include mescaline, heroin, and hallucinogens, such as LSD.

■ Schedule II drugs have a high potential for abuse but also have accepted medical uses. These drugs lead to physical and psychological dependence. Drugs in this schedule include narcotics such as morphine, codeine, barbiturates such as tranquilizers, and amphetamines. Prescriptions in this schedule cannot be refilled.

■ Schedule III drugs have a lower potential for abuse than those in Schedule II and have accepted medical uses. Compounds from this category are used in several of drugs routinely prescribed in the dental office. The drugs in this category may lead to chemical dependence and include barbiturates, stimulants, and depressants not in Schedule II and a number of compounds such as Tylenol III.

■ Schedule IV drugs have less potential for abuse than those in Schedule III and also have acceptable medical uses. Schedule IV drugs have limited dependence risk. Drugs in this schedule include antidepressants, anti-anxiety drugs, and sedative drugs not included in the first three schedules.

TABLE 15-1 Five Schedules of Controlled Substances

Schedule Number	Abuse Potential and Legal Limitations	Examples of Substances
1. Ⅰ	High abuse potential Not approved for medical use in the United States	heroin, LSD, mescaline
2. Ⅱ	High abuse potential May lead to severe dependence Written prescription only No phoning in of prescription by office health care worker No refills May be faxed, but original prescription must be turned in to pick up prescription In emergency, physician may phone in, but handwritten prescription must go to pharmacy within 72 hours	morphine, codeine, methadone, Percocet, Tylox, Dilaudid, Ritalin, cocaine, Oxycontin, meperidine (Demerol)
3. Ⅲ	May lead to limited dependence Written, faxed, or verbal (phoned in) prescription, by physician only May be refilled up to five times in 6 months	Marinol, Tussionex, Tylenol with codeine
4. Ⅳ	Lower abuse potential than above schedules Prescription may be written out by health care worker, but must be signed by the physician Prescription may be phoned in by health care worker or faxed May be refilled up to five times in 6 months	Valium, Ativan, Xanax, phenobarbital, Librium, Darvocet, Restoril, Ambien
5. Ⅴ	Low abuse potential compared to above schedules Consists primarily of preparations for cough suppressants containing codeine and preparations for diarrhea (e.g., paregoric and opium tincture)	Phenergan with codeine, Robitussin-A-C, Tussi-Organidin, N.R., Donnagel-PG, Lomotil

Note: Some states may have stricter schedules than the federal regulations. You must be aware of the regulations in your state.

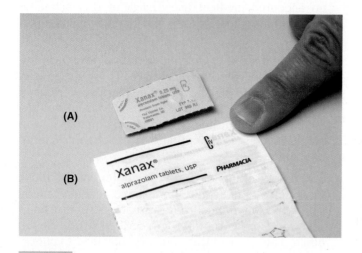

FIGURE 15-4 (A) Drug packages and (B) drug inserts showing the controlled substance schedule numbers. They are also found in numerous drug reference books.

■ Schedule V drugs have the least potential for abuse and may consist of a compound from other schedules in small amounts. The drugs in this schedule may be anti-diarrhea medicines or cough medicines. The drugs in this group are also called OTC drugs.

Dental Assistants and the Law

It is often the responsibility of the dental assistant to keep accurate records of the drugs dispensed and the information that was given to the patient should be recorded as well. Dental assistants will be involved in phoning or emailing in prescriptions when applicable. They may write many of the prescriptions manually or on the computer that the doctor reviews and signs, obtaining the forms that the prescriptions are written on and insuring that the prescription pads are not left out in the open. They may also be involved in placing controlled substances in locked cupboards and insuring that some medications are kept on stock. Dental assistants play a large role in making sure that drug samples are left in a designated area when the pharmaceutical representatives leave these for the dentist to try. It may also be the dental assistant who is the professional representative of the office whom the pharmacist gets to know the best. This relationship can be valuable in insuring that abuse does not occur and as a resource to the dentist in prescribing the most current and relevant drug for patient use. It is important that the following guidelines are followed in the dental office.

1. Controlled substances, if used in the office, must be locked and kept secure at all times. Records

of these substances must be maintained. These records should show what was received by the office and when this occurred and what and to whom this substance was dispensed. There must be notation of any substance that was destroyed by the office. These records, and the records of the past two years, have to be available to the DEA at any time when requested.

2. A current drug reference should be available at all times. There are a number of books available that pertain primarily to dentistry as well as a DVD and online service that is updated regularly.

3. Update knowledge on any changes in the scheduled drugs. Check with the DEA, FDA, and the ADA for updates in drug usage and routes of administration.

4. Get to know the pharmacist who is recommended by the office and other pharmacists in the area. Establish a working rapport with them and utilize their knowledge to aid the dentist in dispensing prescriptions. The pharmaceutical sales representative is also a tremendous resource on information about drugs and their usage in patient care.

5. Place prescription pads, computer-generated prescription applications, and the dentist's DEA registration number out of the public areas. Keep this information concealed and safe to ensure that fraud and drug tampering do not occur.

6. Keep accurate records! In most cases it is advisable to make a copy of the prescription for the patient's records. It must also be noted along with the date after the treatment that the patient received. Many of the computer software programs allow for this information to be attached to the patient's computer record.

FIGURE 15-5 Devices used to deliver medication via inhalation. (A) Small volume aerosol nebulizer. (B) Metered dose inhaler.

Drug Administration Routes

Drugs can be administered in a number of ways. The dentist will evaluate and decide the most beneficial route for the patient to take the drug.

■ **Oral** administration is the most common method of taking medications. Tablets, capsules, pills, and liquids are taken in this manner. The patient swallows the dispensed amount of the drug with a glass of water.

■ The ointment, lotion, gel, or cream is applied **topically** to the skin surface or mucosa. Dentistry uses a topical drug to prepare for local anesthesia. It is applied on the oral mucous membrane to numb the area prior to injection.

■ **Inhalation** means to breathe in the gas or aerosol (Figure 15-5A and B). This allows the drug to be taken quickly into the lungs. One of the drugs used in dentistry by inhalation is nitrous oxide.

■ **Sublingual** administration involves placing the medication under the tongue until it dissolves. For example, if a patient is experiencing angina pectoris, a nitroglycerin pill or spray is administered sublingually. Drugs are seldom administered by this route in the dental office.

■ **Rectal** route of administration for drugs used in the dental office is nonexistent. Patients can administer enemas or suppositories in this manner to obtain the effects of drugs in this class. This route is used when an oral route is not recommended.

■ **Intravenous** route of administration means to inject the substance directly into the vein. This route is used for immediate drug response (Figure 15-6).

■ **Intramuscular** route of administration means to inject the substance into the muscle tissue (Figure 15-7). This route gives a slower response than intravenous administration but has a longer-lasting effect.

FIGURE 15-6 Administering a drug through the intravenous route.

(A)

(B)

Epidermis
Dermis
Subcutaneous
Muscle

FIGURE 15-9 (A) The needle is held almost flat against the skin with the bevel up during the intradermal injection. (B) The injection must be done slowly so that the skin does not bubble up. It is under the epidermis of the skin just slightly.

Epidermis
Dermis
Subcutaneous
Muscle

FIGURE 15-7 Administering an intramuscular injection.

- **Subcutaneous** route of administration means to inject the substance just under the skin, above the muscle (Figure 15-8).
- **Intradermal** route of administration means to inject the substance under the epidermis (top layer of skin) (Figure 15-9A and B).
- **Transdermal** route of administration means to deliver medications from a drug reservoir in a patch applied to the skin in a consistent, controlled manner (Figure 15-10A, B, and C).

Drugs

The following section covers both illegal and prescription drugs. Dental assistants are concerned with prescribed drugs but must have knowledge about illegal drugs that patients may be using and must understand what can happen if the drugs interact. There is an increased rise in **substance abuse/drug abuse** (using drugs for other than medicinal purposes) in today's society. More and more individuals are seeking drugs for thrills or for coping with daily life. It is important that the caregiver pay special attention to the patient and listen to the information that the patient provides. It is also important

Epidermis
Dermis
Subcutaneous
Muscle

FIGURE 15-8 Administering a subcutaneous injection.

FIGURE 15-10 Transdermal administration of nitroglycerin ointment. (A) Ointment is applied on an application ruler on the paper. (B) The application paper is then inverted and the ointment contacts the skin and it is attached with paper tape. (C) Nitro-Dur® is a transdermal system of delivering medication (nitroglycerin) to manage angina pectoris. It is also available in pre-dispensed sealed application.

to know the signs and symptoms that individuals may experience if under the influence of drugs. Having background knowledge about drugs and their effects helps the dental assistant provide better patient care.

Tobacco

People often do not associate tobacco with drugs, but tobacco contain nicotine. Nicotine is a **stimulant**; it speeds up metabolic activities. The drug nicotine is not used for any purpose to treat disease and therefore is not a medicine. It has been shown that tobacco is harmful to the health of smokers as well as to others who may breathe in the secondary smoke. Cancer, lung, and heart disease are much more prevalent in smokers than nonsmokers. A smoker has ten times the risk of developing lung cancer than nonsmokers. Tobacco smoke contains carbon monoxide (the same gas found in car exhaust). This gas does not allow the blood to obtain the correct amount of oxygen in the cells and therefore the heart and circulatory system have to work harder. This leads to heart disease, the number one cause of death in the United States today. Federal law requires that every package of cigarettes carry a warning indicating the health hazards of smoking.

Smokeless tobacco (chewing tobacco) causes some of the same problems that smoking does. Chewing tobacco adds a high risk factor for oral cancer. Both smoking and chewing tobacco are causative factors in tooth staining, periodontal disease, and halitosis.

Many dental offices are reluctant to hire a dental assistant who smokes. The dental office is a health facility where the promotion of good health habits is essential. Dental assistants should seriously consider smoking cessation. A number of measures are currently available to aid in smoking cessation.

Caffeine

Caffeine is a habit-forming stimulant. It can be found in a number of sources, including coffee, espresso, tea, soft drinks, chocolate, and cocoa. This habit-forming drug also has side effects that may be harmful. Because it is a stimulant, caffeine causes the heart to work harder and may affect the nervous system. It may cause or irritate open sores (**ulcers**) in the wall of the stomach. Teeth are often stained by caffeine use. Too much caffeine can be toxic. If an individual were to drink thirty double "shots" of espresso or seventy to 100 cups of coffee, the result could be fatal. However, under normal use, coffee and espresso are safe to drink.

Caffeine Count	
Source	**Mg of Caffeine**
Cocoa (1 cup)	13
Tea (1 cup)	30–45
Coffee (1 cup)	40–150
Espresso (1 shot)	60–175
Carbonated diet soft drink (1 8-oz glass)	30–50
Carbonated regular soft drink (1 8-oz glass)	35–65

Alcohol

One of the oldest known drugs is ethyl alcohol, which is found in alcoholic beverages such as wine, beer, and whiskey. Alcohol is a **depressant**, a drug that slows down body processes. This habit-forming drug has the opposite effect of stimulants. It affects the body functions rapidly because it is absorbed directly into the blood and then carried throughout the body. A 0.08 to 0.10 percent alcohol level is considered legal intoxication in most states. At 0.05 percent, an individual experiences loss in judgment and coordination and exhibits slowed reactions and slurred speech. More than 20,000 people are killed each year by drunken drivers unable to respond to situations while behind the wheel of a car. This statistic represents about half of automobile accidents.

A person can become both physically and psychologically dependent on alcohol. Some people cannot stop at one drink and become alcoholics, unable to control their drinking. Some people are more likely to experience this disorder than others. Genetics and body weight play a role in the likelihood of alcoholism. One side effect of this drug is liver deterioration, called **cirrhosis**. The liver eventually stops working and death results. A pregnant woman who drinks large amounts of alcohol may cause birth defects in the fetus. Patients may take alcohol to overcome the fear of dentistry. Dental assistants must be alert to this because of possible harmful interaction between alcohol and other drugs used in dentistry. Alcoholics feel full and satisfied and do not seek a well-balanced diet, often resulting in malnutrition.

Marijuana

Assistants should watch for signs of drug abuse, and must have a basic knowledge of drugs and how they affect body functions in order to help if an emergency should arise. One illegal drug that acts as both a stimulant and a depressant is marijuana. Marijuana contains a number of drugs, one of the most active being tetrahydrocannabinol (THC). Some side effects of marijuana use include increased heart rate (as much as 50 percent), lung tissue damage due to the smoking, and reproductive system disorders (abnormal hormonal levels, abnormal sperm production, and, in some cases, defects in the developing fetus).

The nervous system of regular marijuana users is affected. They are not able to speak and think as clearly, coordination is deteriorated, and they seem to lose the motivation to be productive without marijuana use. Individuals who use the drug daily have 10 percent more THC in their body tissues than monthly users. A person is unlikely to become physically dependent on marijuana but often becomes psychologically dependent.

A marijuana derivative is used as a medicine to treat patients taking other drugs in cancer therapy. It seems to decrease nausea and regurgitation. Another application is medicine used to treat eye conditions such as glaucoma.

Cocaine

Cocaine, a very habit-forming drug, makes the user feel in control, as if he or she has tremendous power. This drug is often referred to as the "rich man's drug" because a day's "dosage" can cost hundreds or thousands of dollars. Side effects of this stimulant are heart problems, mental disorders, violent behavior, and death. Long-term users suffer from great anxiety and are restless and irritable.

Cocaine is often mixed with other drugs to boost the high. Sometimes, a mixture of heroin and cocaine (called a speedball) is injected intravenously. The result can be fatal. Purified cocaine that resembles a crystalline rock is called crack. This substance is smoked in a pipe or sprinkled on tobacco and smoked. The powder form of cocaine is inhaled into the nose or rubbed into the mucosa. Intraorally, this may appear much like toothbrush abrasion but over a wider area, because the substance is abrasive and wears on the tooth structure as it is rubbed back and forth into the tissue. If the person inhales cocaine, permanent damage occurs to the nasal mucosa over time.

Due to abuse of this drug, its use as medical treatment has been reduced. Cocaine causes both a physical and a psychological dependency. Physical dependency may occur after only one or a few uses. This dependency varies with each individual according to the quantity used, frequency, and sensitivity of the person to the drug. If the person tries to stop usage, withdrawal symptoms such as craving the drug, intense anxiety, and mental illness such as depression are common.

Narcotics

Narcotics are addictive depressants used to relieve pain. They have been in use for about 7,000 years. For centuries, they were the most useful painkillers available to physicians. Morphine and codeine are made from the opium poppy plant. Heroin is made from morphine. All drugs in this classification cause strong psychological and physical dependency and have been replaced for medical use by drugs less addictive.

Heroin. An individual who uses heroin regularly and tries to stop will become sick within twelve hours. Symptoms include hot and cold flashes with goose bumps, stomach cramps, vomiting, diarrhea, nervousness, shaking, muscle and bone pain, and an intense craving for the drug. The intensity of the withdrawal is dependent on how much the individual has been using. It does not take long for a person who uses heroin to develop a **tolerance** to the drug. This tolerance causes the person to need larger amounts of the drug in order to produce the same effect. The desired effect is loss of pain, highness, or a feeling of euphoria and drowsiness.

Side effects include addiction, loss of appetite, constipation, and decreased respiratory and heart rates. The drug can be taken intravenously, injected subcutaneously, or inhaled. Drug users who share needles run the risk of contacting contagious diseases such as hepatitis B and HIV (human immunodeficiency virus).

Heroin is the most addictive of the narcotic drugs. A person may become addicted the first time he or she uses the drug. Overdoses cause the user to vomit and experience diarrhea and decreased respiratory and heart rates, followed by symptoms of shock and possible coma. The patient should be taken immediately to a hospital for treatment. If heroin overdose is diagnosed, the narcotic antagonist will be given to reverse the effects of the heroin. An untreated overdose can be fatal. Newborns of addicted mothers show symptoms of addiction and will die if not treated properly.

Morphine. Morphine is one of the best-known narcotic **analgesic** (pain killer) drugs. Medically, it is given intravenously to relieve severe pain caused by myocardial infarction (heart attack). It is administered intramuscularly to control postoperative pain. It also can be given orally to patients who are terminally ill. Possible side effects include constipation, nausea, vomiting, and confusion. Long-term use leads to addiction and an increased level of tolerance. Due to physical dependence, if the drug is stopped suddenly, the person experiences symptoms of withdrawal, such as sweating, stomach and body cramping, and flu-like manifestations.

Codeine. Used since the early 1900s, codeine is an effective analgesic drug (painkiller). Dentistry uses it in combination with other drugs to relieve mild to moderate pain. Other medical uses for codeine are as a cough suppressant (because it suppresses the part of the brain that triggers coughing) and as an antidiarrheal drug (one that acts in the intestinal wall to slow down muscle contractions).

Codeine induces drowsiness, especially if taken with alcohol. Other side effects are constipation if taken over a long period of time and physical and psychological dependence.

Amphetamines

Amphetamines are stimulants that increase the heart and respiratory rates and blood pressure. They were used in the past to treat obesity because they cause a loss of appetite along with side effects of nervousness and restlessness. The street name for these drugs is "uppers." Taking amphetamines leads to violent behavior and poor judgment. Prolonged use causes physical dependence and tolerance to the drug.

Medically, amphetamines are used to treat narcolepsy (abnormal daytime sleeping) and children with attention deficit hyperactivity disorder (ADHD). Amphetamines have an opposite effect on hyperactive children. Rather than causing restlessness, the drug has a calming effect. There are few other medical uses for amphetamines.

Hallucinogens

Hallucinogens are drugs that cause people to see and hear images and sounds (**hallucinate**) that do not exist. An individual using a hallucinogen may experience a mild effect where colors change or more severe ones causing emotional extremes such as terror. Sometimes, a person under the influence of a hallucinogen becomes so frightened that he or she reacts in an extreme manner—doing anything to "escape" the hallucination. This loss of control over emotions or actions is due to a change in brain activity. Hallucination is a major symptom of schizophrenia. The symptom may also be caused by bipolar affective disorder.

Hallucinogenic "recreational" drugs, also called psychedelic drugs, include LSD, PCP, mescaline, and psilocybin. Marijuana and alcohol taken in large amounts have also been reported to cause hallucinogenic symptoms.

Lysergic Acid Diethylamide. LSD is a synthetic drug made from ergot, a fungus that grows on rye and wheat. LSD has a high potential for abuse and no medical uses. Minute amounts of LSD can produce a "bad trip," where the user has a serious personality breakdown (including violence), which may last up to twelve hours. Flashbacks from these bad trips may occur up to several years after the user has taken LSD. There is no scientific evidence proving that LSD causes mental illness, but it is thought that it may induce psychosis, and thus predispose the user to mental illness. A habitual user may become both physically and psychologically addicted to the drug. Psilocybin is a hallucinogenic drug similar to LSD that originates from mushrooms.

Phencyclidine. One of the most dangerous hallucinogenic drugs is phencyclidine, called PCP. This drug is often given the name of "angel dust" because users often think they can fly when under its influence. It is ingested by eating, smoking, or sniffing, and is either a stimulant or a depressant. As it scrambles the brain's messages, it causes the user to become violent. Adverse side effects include violent behavior, respiratory depression, agitation, nausea, vomiting, and convulsions. Memory loss that can last for weeks often results from PCP drug use.

Mescaline. The hallucinogenic drug mescaline is obtained from the peyote cactus. It produces psychosis and effects similar to LSD that last for four to eight hours. The likelihood of "bad trips" is not as prevalent with mescaline. However, this addictive drug may leave the user with permanent psychosis and a constant craving for the drug.

Barbiturates

Barbiturates are sedative drugs that depress brain activity. If used over a long period of time, physiological and physical dependency develops, along with tolerance for the drug. If withdrawal occurs after four weeks of use, the user experiences stomach cramps, nausea, vomiting, twitching, convulsions, weakness, and insomnia. An overdose of the drug can result in delirium and a comatose state; it can also be fatal. If barbiturates are used with alcohol, the outcome is particularly harsh.

Barbiturates such as amobarbital, pentobarbital, and secobarbital are used today to treat sleeplessness and anxiety. Phenobarbital sometimes is given to dental patients who exhibit severe anxiety to dental treatment. This is especially true in treating children. It is dispensed in a liquid and taken orally. Pentobarbital also is used in the treatment of epilepsy because it reduces the sensitivity of the brain to abnormal electrical activity that brings on seizures.

Prescribed Drugs

Dentists take great care in administering drugs. After discussing the condition with the patient, the dentist may prescribe or administer certain medications to alleviate treatment anxiety and discomfort. The patient's dental record must show all prescriptions given to the patient, the route administered, and the information the doctor and assistant gave orally to the patient at the time of dispensing. A copy of the prescription should be placed in the patient's record indicating the dosage amount. Any OTC drugs the dentist recommended to the patient should be noted on the patient's record as well. The dentist must understand all of the drugs, their classifications, the uses of the drug, and the side effects of each. Table 15-2 has some drugs, uses, and some possible side effects noted.

Analgesics. Analgesic drugs (anesthesia) cause loss of pain but not a loss of all sensation. Drugs that relieve pain can be non-narcotic, such as aspirin, ibuprofen, and acetaminophen, or narcotic, such as codeine and morphine. The non-narcotic analgesics are useful in the treatment of mild or moderate pain. If severe pain persists, a stronger narcotic analgesic is prescribed. Aspirin normally is not prescribed after a dental extraction because of its ability to thin blood and inhibit clotting. This effect is contraindicated for healing the socket area following an extraction. Other side effects of aspirin are stomach irritation and nausea. Patients must be instructed to take aspirin with a large glass of water to ensure that the pill dissolves and does not irritate the stomach lining in a concentrated form.

Side effects of narcotic analgesics, such as nausea, vomiting, constipation, and breathing difficulties, are minimal but may still occur.

Tranquilizers. Drugs that provide a sedative effect are called tranquilizers. Tranquilizers relieve anxiety and allow the patient to undergo the procedure with reduced tension. Valium (diazepam) is often given orally a half-hour before the procedure to calm and relax the patient.

Antibiotics. Antibiotics—aminoglycosides, cephalosporins, penicillins, tetracyclines, and others—are given to patients to treat infection. These drugs are derived from fungi and molds or are manufactured synthetically. Some of the antibiotics are broad spectrum, meaning they are effective against a wide range of bacteria, while some treat only one type of bacteria. More than one type of antibiotic may be prescribed to increase the probability of success in disease treatment. A culture can be taken to further identify the specific type of bacteria to be treated. Antibiotics are ineffective against viruses.

Normally, antibiotics are taken to treat infections, but they are often prescribed as a prophylactic measure to prevent infection. Any patient who has had rheumatic fever, joint replacement, heart valve replacement, or a heart murmur should take a dose of antibiotics prior to dental treatment to reduce the risk of endocarditis (inflammation of the lining of the heart).

Resistance to antibiotics can develop. This often occurs when the user fails to take the antibiotic drug as directed. The patient begins to feel better and stops taking the antibiotic before all the disease-causing bacteria have been killed. The bacteria then return stronger and more resistant to the antibiotic.

Adverse side effects of antibiotics include nausea, diarrhea, and an allergic rash. They can also kill normal body flora, causing oral, intestinal, or vaginal candidiasis (thrush). Some people also have severe allergic reactions with a rash, itching, swelling, and difficulty in breathing. If this happens, an antihistamine is used to counteract the reaction of the allergen.

- **Penicillin** was the first group of antibiotic drugs to be discovered. It is still used in the treatment of many diseases, including tonsillitis, bronchitis, and pneumonia. Side effects of the drugs in this category are allergic reactions. If an individual becomes allergic

TABLE 15-2 Drug Classifications

Drug Type	Examples	Some uses of the Drug	Action of Drug	Some Possible Side Effects
analgesic	Acetaminophen, aspirin, Dilaudid, Percodan, Tylenol, Bufferin, Panadol	Control pain	Pain therapy	GI distress, bleeding and bruising
antibody	Keflex, amoxicillin, tetracycline, penicillin G	Treatment of infection	Treat streptococcal, some staphylococcal and meningococcal infections	Electrolyte imbalance, hypersensitivity reaction
Anti-cholinergics	Atropine Propantheline bromide	Treatment to reduce secretions	Treat bradycardia, dilate the pupil for ophthalmic examination, inhibit the flow of saliva	Mouth dryness, Blurred vision
Anti-coagulant	Coumadin Aspirin Heparin	Prevent formation of blood clots	Embolism control	Hemorrhage Blood in urine Minor bleeding
Anti-convulsant	Zarontin, Klonopin, Depakene, Dilantin	Reduce the number and severity of seizures	Epileptic seizure control	Irritability, GI distress, sedation
Anti-diabetic	Glucophage Avandamet Dymelor Glucotrol	Regulation of blood sugar	Diabetes control	GI distress Dermatological effects
Anti-depressant	Prozac, Tofranil Elavil	Treat depression, stabilize moods	Elevates mood	Mouth dryness Increased appetite Drowsiness Constipation Confusion
antifungal	Mycostatin Mycostain nystatin	Used as a fungicide	Treat candidiasis, Thrush	Rare, nausea
antihistamine	Benadryl, Tavist Allergy, Phenergan	Provide relief of allergic symptoms caused by histamine release	Treat allergies, conjunctivitis and rash	Drying of secretions, Sedation
Anti-hypertensive	Tenormin Methyldopa Hydralazine	Slows heart rate Inhibits arteries from closing	Treat hypertension and elevated blood pressure	Hypotension GI symptoms
anti-inflammatory	Motrin, Advil, prednisone, cortisone	Inflammation	Reduce inflammation process	GI ulceration or bleeding, heartburn, headache,
Anti-lipemic	Lipitor, Zocor, Advicor, Niaspan	Transport cholesterol and other fats through the bloodstream	Treatment of high cholesterol levels	Muscle weakness, Mild GI distress, headache, elevated liver enzymes
Anti-thyroid	Synthroid, Levoxyl, Levothroid	Used to relieve symptoms of hyperthyroidism	Treat symptoms of hyperthyroidism	Rare: Rash, fever

(continues)

TABLE 15-2 Drug Classifications *(continued)*

Drug Type	Examples	Some uses of the Drug	Action of Drug	Some Possible Side Effects
bronchodilator	Abuterol sulfate Primatene Volmax	Relax the smooth muscles of the bronchial tree	Relieve bronchospasm treat asthma	Hypoventilation GI distress Hypertension
contraceptive	Provera Ovrette Progestin	Prevent ovulation	Birth control	Fluid retention Weight gain or loss, migraine headaches
decongestant	Afrin, Allerest, Sudafed	constrict blood vessels in respiratory tract	Treat congestion Open airways	Anxiety, Hypertension
diuretic	Lasix, Aldactone Dyrenium	Increase excretion of water, sodium, chloride and potassium	Treat edema, Electrolyte imbalance	Fluid and electrolyte imbalance, dehydration, Hypotension
hemostatic	Gel Foam	Induce clotting	Used for dry socket	Rare
Hormone replacement	Estrogen Estratest Humulin	Hormone regulator	Maintain hormone level treats menopause symptoms	Hypertension GI effects Skin disorders
MAOIs	Marplan, Nardil, Parnate	Anticonvulsants and Antiparkinsonian drugs	Control convulsing behavior	Interact with many foods and other drugs Nervousness, headache, hypertension tachycardia
Nitrates	Nitrostat, Nitroglycerin, Nitrolingual spray	Used to dilate blood vessels	Treat angina pectoris and chest pain	Headache, hypotension, dry mouth
Tranquilizer/ anti-anxiety	Xanax, Librium, Valium (diazepam) Serax	Promote relaxation	Calming effect, minor tranquilizer	Drowsiness Dizziness

to one type of penicillin, others in this group or any derivatives must be administered with great caution.

- **Penicillin V** or phenoxymethyl-penicillin is limited to gram-positive bacteria, such as ulcerative gingivostomatitis and streptococcal infections.
- **Penicillin G benzathine** is often the drug chosen for a variety of infections, including pneumococci, gonorrhea, syphilis, streptococci, and meningococcal meningitis.
- **Amoxicillin** is another broad-spectrum antibiotic. Like most antibiotics, it is important to take the entire prescription to avoid antibiotic resistance. Watch for any allergic reaction as with penicillin.
- **Ampicillin**, also a broad-spectrum antibiotic, is often used for dental patients at risk for bacterial endocarditis, and is given prior, during, and after an invasive dental procedure.

- **Cloxacillin**, **nafcillin**, and **oxacillin** are primarily used to treat *Staphylococcus aureus* infections.
- **Erythromycin** is an antibiotic much like penicillin that can be used by individuals who are allergic to penicillin and by children as a substitute for tetracycline. It is a coated tablet so that it is not destroyed by the acid in the stomach when taken orally. It can be given in capsule or liquid form, injected, and by ointment. Side effects include stomach pain, nausea, vomiting, and diarrhea. It can produce a rash if the individual becomes hypersensitive to the substance.
- **Tetracycline** is a broad-spectrum drug, killing a wide range of bacterial microorganisms. It must be taken with care, taking one tablet one hour before meals or two hours after a meal. The drugs become useless if taken with some foods or dairy products. Tetracycline must not be given to children under twelve or

to pregnant women because it discolors developing teeth. People with poor kidney function should not take tetracycline antibiotics, because they may cause kidney failure.

Side effects of tetracycline are much like those of other antibiotics: nausea, vomiting, diarrhea, and possible rash, if allergic.

Antifungal Agents. Drugs prescribed to treat infections caused by fungi are antifungal agents. They are available in a number of forms, such as tablets, suspensions, creams, injections, and vaginal suppositories. Preparations applied to the skin may show adverse reactions by increasing the irritation. Preparations taken orally may, in rare cases, show serious side effects of liver or kidney damage.

- *Nystatin* is an antifungal drug used in dentistry to treat candidiasis (oral thrush). The suspension administered orally is held in the mouth prior to swallowing. It is safely taken during pregnancy. Patients should continue to take it forty-eight hours after the last sign of infection is apparent. Extremely high doses taken orally may cause nausea, vomiting, and diarrhea. Nystatin ointment can be used for Angular cheilitis (see Chapter 26, Oral Pathology). The ointment is applied to the lesion four times a day until healed.

- **Other Pathologic Conditions.** Flucinonide gel is applied by a cotton swab to affected areas twice daily to treat mild to moderate lichen planus, a condition in the oral cavity that often presents as a lacy network of white spots covering the lining of the cheeks (see Chapter 26, Oral Pathology). Mild allergic reactions may be treated with diphenhydramine HCl, 50 mg, which is dispensed every four hours as needed. Herpetic infections are often treated with a drug called penciclovir 1-percent cream, which is applied to affected areas every two hours while awake.

Anticholinergics. Anticholinergic drugs are used as premedications before general anesthesia to reduce secretion from the lungs and as emergency drugs to treat people with abnormally slow heart rates (bradycardia). They are also used to dilate the eyes during an ophthalmology examination.

- *Atropine sulfate* and propantheline bromide are anticholinergic drugs used in dentistry to inhibit the flow of saliva. A patient who produces excessive saliva may make it difficult for the dental team to obtain a good impression for crown or bridge treatment. If atropine is taken a couple of hours prior to treatment, the patient will have a dry mouth, which allows for a clearly defined impression to be obtained. This effect will disappear in four to six hours after the drug is administered.

Herbal and Other Alternative Medications

Dental assistants may be asked about herbal or other alternative medications. If this occurs it is advisable to consult the dentist and it may be prudent to refer the patient to some reliable sources for further information. There are herbal and alternative medications that can be helpful for patient care but much of the information is not based on facts. Patients should be cautioned in taking medications that are not approved by the FDA and the ADA. The FDA has published a report entitled *An FDA Guide to Dietary Supplements.*

This guide helps answer many of the questions that the patients may have. The dietary supplements such as herbal and other alternative medications do not have to follow the same regulations as other medications and so the labeling may lead the individual astray. For instance, if a label says natural it does not guarantee that this product is safe. Consumers have to seek out factual information and then evaluate if it meets their needs. There are several online sources that provide scientific data for consumers to review. The FDA Consumer (1998) is available at: http://www.cfsan.fda.gov. A free online database of herbs providing scientific data behind the use of herbs for health from HerbMed (2001) is available at www.herbmed.org. Patients can be given these sites for their review and evaluation.

CHAPTER SUMMARY

At no other time have drugs been so widely used/misused as they are today. The dental assistant will need to pay attention to the patient's medical and dental history and carefully document the drugs used by the patient. The dental assistant will have to become knowledgeable about pharmacology, the side effects of drugs, and drug interactions. Dental assistants are concerned with prescribed drugs, but they must also have knowledge about illegal drugs that patients may be using and what will happen if the two types of drugs interact. It is also important to know the signs and symptoms that individuals may experience if under the influence of drugs. Background knowledge about drugs and their effects aids the dental assistant in providing better patient care.

Case Study

Jordan Taylor, a twenty-year-old male, comes in because an upper anterior tooth is abscessed. He is a smoker and has just had four shots of espresso (coffee) in a drink. He seems nervous about the upcoming treatment. Further information obtained from Jordan is that he also had two regular soft drinks and a candy bar in the past two hours.

Case Study Review

1. What reaction should the dental team expect from Jordan due to the drugs he has ingested recently?

2. Are these drugs stimulants or depressants?

3. Would giving other drugs to Jordan be a problem?

REVIEW QUESTIONS

Multiple Choice

1. The most commonly used resource to obtain information about drugs in the dental office is [the]
   a. *United States Pharmacopoeia.*
   b. *National Formulary.*
   c. *Dental Therapeutics.*
   d. *Physician's Desk Reference.*

2. Dental ointment that is placed on the mucosal surface is administered by which route?
   a. Sublingual
   b. Oral
   c. Topical
   d. Intravenous

3. A form of addictive depressants used to relieve pain are
   a. narcotics.
   b. amphetamines.
   c. hallucinogens.
   d. barbiturates.

4. The legislation that was established to identify drugs according to five schedules of abuse potential is the
   a. Pure Food, Drug, and Cosmetic Act.
   b. Comprehensive Drug Abuse Prevention and Control Act of 1970.
   c. Occupational Safety and Health Act.
   d. Controlled Substances Act.

5. If an antibiotic is said to be broad spectrum, it means that
   a. a culture can be taken to identify the type of microorganism.
   b. many microorganisms resist it.
   c. it causes side effects, such as nausea or an allergic rash.
   d. it is effective against a wide range of bacteria.

6. The drug schedule number that has the higher abuse postential and is more dangerous is
   a. Schedule I.
   b. Schedule II.
   c. Schedule III.
   d. Schedule IV.

7. The route of administration of a drug that is delivered right under the skin level is
   a. intravenous.
   b intramuscular.
   c. subcutaneous.
   d. intradermal.

8. Tylenol with codeine is under which schedule numbers of controlled substances:
   a. Schedule I
   b. Schedule II
   c. Schedule III
   d. Schedule IV

9. Percodan is an _____ drug type.
   a. antibody
   b. analgesic
   c. anti-cholinergic
   d. anti-coagulant

10. A drug used to treat thrush or candidiasis could be _____.
   a. Prozac
   b. Benadryl
   c. glucophage
   d. nystatin

Critical Thinking

1. How does knowledge of illegal drugs help the dental assistant's career?

2. What are some of the side effects of tetracycline and when is it contraindicated?

3. If a patient has a heavy flow of saliva, what drug classification and which specific drug may be used during the impression phase of a crown preparation procedure?

Web Activities

1. Go to www.ada.org, and then find "Dental Therapeutics." Read the prescription tips and be prepared to discuss them in class.

2. Go to www.rxlist.com and look up tetracycline. Write down the drug's indications, dosage, side effects, drug interactions, warnings, and precautions.

3. Go to www.fda.gov and read the "Hot Topics." Report on one hot topic of interest to you.

PRACTICE

EMERGENCY MANAGEMENT CDA

SPECIFIC INSTRUCTIONAL OBJECTIVES

The student should strive to meet the following objectives and demonstrate an understanding of the facts and principles presented in this chapter:

1. Describe several emergency situations that may take place in the dental office. Explain how dental assistants can be prepared for these possibilities.

2. Describe the ABCs of CPR and demonstrate the associated skills.

3. Define the terms and anatomy used in CPR delivery. Determine if the patient is unconscious and demonstrate knowledge of opening the airway and when and how to deliver chest compressions.

4. Identify several causes of airway obstructions in the dental office. Demonstrate the ability to open the airway and to perform the Heimlich maneuver, manual and chest thrusts, and the finger sweep.

5. Identify the causes, signs, and treatments for syncope, asthma, allergic reactions, anaphylactic reaction, hyperventilation, epilepsy, diabetes mellitus, hypoglycemia, angina pectoris, myocardial infarction, congestive heart failure, and stroke/cerebrovascular accident.

6. Identify several dental emergencies that a patient may have, such as abscessed tooth, alveolitis, avulsed tooth, broken prosthesis, soft tissue injury, broken tooth, and loose crown

KEY TERMS

abscessed tooth *(316)*

alkalosis *(312)*

allergens *(311)*

allergic reactions *(312)*

allergy *(311)*

alveolitis *(316)*

anaphylactic shock *(312)*

angina pectoris *(314)*

angioedema *(312)*

antibodies *(311)*

antigens *(311)*

antihistamines *(311)*

arteriosclerosis *(314)*

avulsed tooth *(316)*

bronchioles *(311)*

cardiopulmonary resuscitation (CPR) *(301)*

cerebral embolism *(315)*

cerebral hemorrhage *(315)*

cerebral infarction *(315)*

congestive heart failure *(315)*

convulsion *(313)*

diabetes mellitus *(313)*

diabetic acidosis *(314)*

edema *(312)*

epilepsy *(312)*

erythema *(312)*

fistula *(316)*

foreign body airway obstruction (FBAO) *(305)*

gingival hyperplasia *(313)*

grand mal seizure *(313)*

Heimlich maneuver *(305)*

hemiplegia *(316)*

hyperglycemia *(314)*

hypersensitive *(311)*

hyperventilation *(312)*

(continues)

KEY TERMS *(continued)*

INTRODUCTION

Emergencies can happen at any place and any time. Even though members of the dental profession try to make dentistry as comfortable as possible, patients feel stress about dental care, and this can increase the possibility of an emergency occurring in the dental office. Other factors that did not exist in the past to the same degree that may increase the incidence of an emergency are advancements in medical care, increase in drug therapy, increase in street drugs, elderly patients seeking dental treatment, and longer dental appointments.

Advances in medical care have allowed treatments that were not available in the past. A patient seeking dental treatment may have a heart or liver transplant or pacemaker or be taking any number of drug therapies. Many patients, especially older patients, take more than one drug. Other patients take one or more street drugs prior to dental treatment. Any drugs given in the dental office for treatment may interact with the drug therapy or street drugs taken by the patient, therefore causing an emergency situation. Another contributing factor to the increased likelihood of emergencies is the length of appointments. Most patients would rather sit for longer appointments and have more complex dentistry completed at one time to accommodate their busy schedules. The dental offices are also more productive when longer appointments are scheduled, because less time is wasted removing barriers and practicing aseptic techniques before and after several shorter appointments. These lengthy appointments may overtax the patient's ability to remain comfortable, therefore causing more anxiety and stress, leading to an emergency situation.

Even though the number of emergencies is not high in a dental office, the dental assistant must always be observant of the patient and be prepared to deal with emergencies. Additionally, emergencies may happen to the dentist and to other dental assistants and staff.

Routine Preparedness for Dental Team Members

When an emergency arises, the dental team must react with an automatic response. Any hesitation at such a time could cost a life. A routine response should be established. Details such as who should call for emergency help and written directions on how to locate the office should be predetermined and posted close to the phone. Providing medical response teams with specific directions regarding the office location, including which door to enter, will save valuable time during the emergency response.

The Dental Assistant's Role in Emergency Care

The dental assistant has a vital role in prevention of emergencies and emergency care. First, the assistant closely observes the patient while escorting him or her from the waiting room to the dental treatment room. Does the patient have difficulty moving? Do the patient's eyes respond to light? Is the patient's speech slurred? Does the patient indicate anxiety about the dental treatment? Look for signs of concern the patient has or seems to have. Many of these signs will be covered up after the patient is seated, the anesthetic is given, and the dental dam is placed. Any areas of concern should be reported to the dentist prior to starting dental care. The patient's medical history should be reviewed as a matter of routine procedure. It is crucial that the dental team have knowledge of any changes in the patient's health. The dental assistant must be alert to any area of concern, because he or she will more than likely be the first one to suspect a possible emergency.

Another role of the dental assistant is to stay well trained for an emergency. Ideally, the dentist and dental assistants will establish a definitive plan to render treatment in an emergency situation. Often, this training takes place in a staff meeting or at a seminar. All members of the dental team should have current cardiopulmonary resuscitation (CPR) cards and have continuing training and updated knowledge of emergency situations. The dental assistant should know the answers to the following questions in order to ensure competency in dealing with emergencies:

- Where is the emergency kit and who will retrieve it?
- Who will take and monitor vital signs?
- Who will retrieve and administer oxygen?
- When will the call for help be placed and by whom?
- Who will perform basic life support, if needed?
- Who will review the medical history of the individual?

If any of these questions cannot be answered quickly by the dental team, training is needed. Once the emergency takes place, attention to the patient's condition will take precedence. All personnel must perform their tasks in a timely manner to ensure that the best treatment is administered.

Dental Office Emergency Kit

Every dental office should have an up-to-date emergency kit (Figure 16-1). A dentist may choose to design his or her own. This kit must be arranged for the specific needs of the practice. Other kits are manufactured for use in dental offices and can be obtained from a dental supply company. These are normally color coded for easy equipment and drug access. All dental emergency kits should include:

- Sterile syringes, tourniquets, tracheotomy needle, barrier devices for delivery of CPR, and several oral airway devices

- Oxygen inhalation equipment, if office does not have nitrous/oxygen equipment in each treatment room (Figure 16-2)

- Stimulants (ammonia inhalants, thin glass vials of ammonia covered with a strong gauze fabric that can be broken easily)

- Vasodilators that will increase oxygenated blood supply to heart (such as nitroglycerin, translingual nitroglycerin, or amyl-nitrite inhalants)

- Antihistamine drugs (such as adrenaline-epinephrine, Benadryl-antihistamine, solu-corticosteroid, or aminophyline-bronchodilator). An epi-pen (a two-dose syringe of epinephrine) is recommended for quick and easy delivery

- Vasopressor to increase blood pressure (such as Wyamine™)

- Analgesics for pain (such as Talwin™)

- Depressants for convulsions (such as diazepam)

- Vagal blockers to increase pulse rate (such as atropine)

This kit should be labeled and located in an easily accessible place so that it can be quickly obtained. A crash cart with oxygen and emergency equipment can be utilized for quick access. If the emergency kit contains controlled substances, it must be kept locked up and have a log that indicates when substances were delivered and used. This log should also note if any substances were lost or stolen. Time is an extremely

FIGURE 16-1 Sample dental office emergency kit.

FIGURE 16-2 Oxygen inhalation equipment for use in dental emergencies. *(Courtesy of Mada Medical Products, Inc.)*

PROCEDURE 16-1

Administration of Oxygen

Many dental assistants may routinely administer oxygen in conjunction with the nitrous oxide gas under the supervision of the dentist. This system is most often brought into the dental treatment room through a wall-piped system. In some instances, the tanks may be on a mobile unit that is brought into the treatment area. The dental assistant should know where the system is located and how to administer oxygen during an emergency.

EQUIPMENT AND SUPPLIES

- Oxygen tank with gauge at top or gauge in the dental treatment area

- Oxygen mask and tubing

PROCEDURE STEPS *(Follow aseptic procedures)*

1. Position the patient comfortably in a supine or **Trendelenburg position**.

NOTE: The Trendelenburg position is a supine position with the feet elevated above chest level.

2. Explain the procedure to the patient and reassure the patient that everything is being taken care of (if an emergency should occur).

3. Place the oxygen mask over the patient's nose and drape the tubing on either side of the face. The mask may need to be adjusted so that it is secure over the nose.

4. Start the flow of oxygen immediately. It should flow at two to four liters per minute.

5. Instruct the patient to breath through his or her nose and have the mouth remain closed.

6. Continue to calm the patient by talking softly in reassuring tones.

important factor in treating emergencies. The kit should be well organized so that the assistant or dentist can find the necessary items at a glance. All items should be labeled with information pertinent to their uses and dosages. A periodic inspection of the emergency items is essential. Many of the drugs have limited shelf lives and need to be replaced annually. A sphygmomanometer and stethoscope are essential parts of the emergency kit to monitor vital signs.

Oxygen inhalation equipment must be readily available as well. The oxygen tanks are green and must be stored upright and secure. Administration of oxygen may be the most important factor in caring for the patient until medical help arrives. The steps for administering oxygen are presented in Procedure 16-1. Even though the dental team is well trained to act in emergencies, a medical response team should be contacted immediately if the patient becomes unconscious.

Cardiopulmonary Resuscitation

If the patient has a sudden cardiac arrest or progresses to this condition, **cardiopulmonary resuscitation (CPR)** is necessary to help the person survive. If the patient becomes unconscious, the first step is to immediately call for emergency medical care. *Phone first and phone fast!* After calling for help, start CPR. The technique of CPR is easy to remember if you follow the ABCs.

Note: Dental assistants must take a formal CPR training program every two years from the American Red Cross or the American Heart Association (AHA) at the health care provider level to be proficient in emergency management.

The ABCs of CPR

"A" stands for **airway**. After determining that the patient is unconscious and calling for help, the airway must be opened. In 2005, the Basic Life Support for Health Care Providers guidelines recommended several changes that were designed to simplify CPR. It recommended that lone health care providers should tailor their sequence of actions for the most likely cause of arrest in victims of all ages. The provider should "Phone first" and get the Automated External Defibrillation unit for any individual presenting with a sudden collapse. The provider may need to try several times to reopen the airway and deliver effective breaths (ones that visibly raise the chest). The provider wants to make sure not to give too large breaths or too many breaths per minute because this may be harmful. If the patient is in a supine position on a firm surface, CPR can be administered more effectively. If the patient is in the dental chair, adjust the chair so that the operator has the access needed (clear pathway and correct height). Tilt the head backward and lift the chin. This process lifts the tongue and epiglottis from the back of the throat and opens the airway.

The rescuer places his or her ear and face close to the adult patient's mouth while looking for the patient's chest to rise and fall. The rescuer *looks* for the chest to rise and fall, *listens* for air exchange, and *feels* for any breath. **"B"** stands for **breathing**. The patient may begin breathing, but, if not, the rescuer administers two slow breaths (two seconds per breath for an adult and one to one-and-one-half seconds per breath for a child). The rescuer watches for the chest to rise and waits for the exhalation between breaths. The proper steps for administering rescue breaths are outlined in Procedure 16-2.

PROCEDURE 16-2

Rescue Breathing for Adults

If an emergency occurs, the dental assistant must be prepared to respond to a patient who ceases breathing and/or to assist the dentist in rescue breathing for a patient.

EQUIPMENT AND SUPPLIES

- Resuscitation mouthpiece
- Gloves (latex or vinyl—optional)

PROCEDURE STEPS *(Follow aseptic procedures)*

1. Determine if the patient is responding. Ask, "Are you okay?"

2. If the patient gives no response, have someone call emergency services. (If alone, call quickly and return to the patient.)

3. Don gloves (if possible). Look, listen, and feel for breathing.

4. If the patient is not breathing, tilt back the head, lift the chin, position the resuscitation mouthpiece, and close the nose by pinching it together (Figure 16-3).

5. Give two slow breaths. Watch the chest gently rise while the breaths are being given. Turn your face to the side and listen and watch for air to return.

6. Check the pulse on the carotid artery, the side closest to you. Use the forefinger and the middle finger to palpate the pulse.

7. If a pulse is present but the patient is not breathing, give one slow breath every five seconds. Continue to do this for one minute (twelve times).

8. Recheck the pulse and breathing after each twelve breaths or each minute.

9. Continue rescue breathing for as long as the pulse remains. If the pulse ceases, begin CPR. If the pulse remains, continue rescue breathing until breathing is restored or until someone else arrives and takes over.

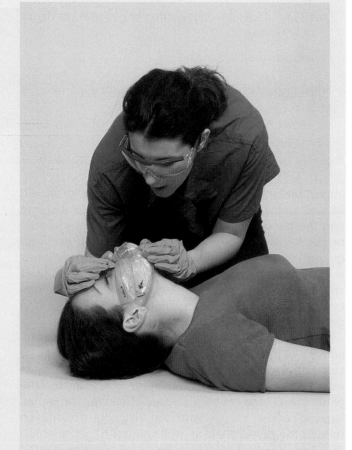

FIGURE 16-3 Tilt the patient's head back, lift the chin, and pinch the nose closed. Use the forefinger and middle finger to check the patient's pulse at the carotid artery.

10. Dispose of the resuscitation mouthpiece in a biohazard container. Remove gloves and wash hands.

11. Document what was done on the patient's chart.

"C" is for **circulation**, which is the next step in CPR. The rescuer checks the carotid pulse. If the patient has a pulse, the rescuer continues breathing at a rate of one breath every five seconds or about twelve breaths per minute (one breath every three seconds or about twenty per minute for a child one to eight years of age). If the patient does not have a pulse, a cycle of thirty chest compressions are given at a rate of 100 per minute. According to the new guidelines for Basic Life Support, health care providers should use a 30:2 compression-to-ventilation ratio for a one-rescuer CPR for victims of all ages and for two-rescuer CPR for adults. Health care providers should use a 15:2 compression-to-ventilation ratio for two-rescuer CPR for infants and children. For unresponsive infants and children, the health care provider should provide CPR first. This means that the providers should give 5 cycles or 2 minutes of CPR before activating the emergency response number. The likelihood of children and infants responding in the first 2 minutes is greater than with adults. The lower third of the sternum (breastbone) is located, the heels of the rescuer's hands (one on top of the other with the fingers interlocked) are placed on the lower third of the sternum and compressions begin. The breastbone must be compressed downward about 1.5 to two inches (one-third to one-half depth of the chest for a child aged one to eight). Counting one and, two and, three and, and so on helps establish a rhythm and a total count. After every thirty compressions, deliver two more slow breaths. Repeat this cycle four times and then check the pulse. If no pulse is found, continue another four cycles of thirty compressions and two breaths and then recheck the pulse. This process continues until medical help arrives. Procedure 16-3 presents an overview of the proper method to deliver CPR to an adult patient by one health care provider.

With recent advances in technology, a "D" is being added to the ABCs of CPR. **"D"** stands for **defibrillation** and requires additional equipment (Figure 16-5). If the site has an automated defibrillator, it increases the chances of survival for patients who have cardiac arrest. AED's are available in many sites. Airlines, shopping centers, schools, and other sites have AED's available. It is advisable to check the sources close to the dental office or purchase one to have it available when needed. It has been found to be extremely helpful in successful basic life support. The equipment guides the user. The equipment's voice system indicates when and where the electrodes are to be placed. The electrodes are placed only if the patient is unconscious, not breathing, and has no pulse. The steps required for AED use are outlined in Procedure 16-4.

PROCEDURE 16-3

CPR for an Adult, One Rescuer

If an emergency occurs, the dental assistant must be prepared to respond to breathing and/or cardiac arrest and perform CPR or to assist the dentist in performing CPR.

EQUIPMENT AND SUPPLIES

- Resuscitation mouthpiece
- Gloves (latex or vinyl)

PROCEDURE STEPS *(Follow aseptic procedures)*

1. Assess the patient's condition. Ask the patient, "Are you okay?"

2. If he or she gives no response, have someone call emergency services. (If no one is available, call for emergency services immediately and return to the patient.)

3. Wash hands (if possible). Put on gloves (if possible).

4. Look, listen, and feel for breathing. If the patient is not breathing, continue to Step 5.

5. Tilt the head back and lift the chin. Insert the mouthpiece and pinch the nose closed (Figure 16-3).

6. Give two breaths and watch the chest rise.

7. Check the pulse (for ten to fifteen seconds) at the carotid artery.

8. If the patient does not have a pulse, start chest compressions.

9. Position hands on top of each other and position your shoulders over your hands. Compress the chest thirty times at a rate of eighty to 100 per minute (Figure 16-4).

10. Follow with two breaths.

(continues)

PROCEDURE 16-3 *(CONTINUED)*

11. Continue for four cycles of breaths and compressions.

12. Check the pulse at the carotid artery. If no pulse is apparent, continue for four cycles and then repeat.

13. Continue until the patient is revived or another person takes over.

14. Dispose of the resuscitation mouthpiece in a biohazard container.

15. Document the emergency information and procedure on the patient's chart.

FIGURE 16-4 Position the hands on top of each other, and position your shoulders over your hands. Compress the chest fifteen times. Follow with two slow breaths.

FIGURE 16-5 An automated defibrillator increases the chances of survival for patients who experience cardiac arrest. (A) Transportable defibrillator. (B) Machine with electrodes ready for placement. *(Courtesy of Medtronic Physio-Control.)*

PROCEDURE 1 6 - 4

Operating an Automated External Defibrillation (AED) Unit

Health professionals may have a defibrillator available within the facility for emergencies.

EQUIPMENT AND SUPPLIES

- Gloves (latex or vinyl—optional)
- Automated external defibrillation (AED) unit (Figure 16-5)

PROCEDURE STEPS *(Follow aseptic procedures)*

- If there is no pulse, follow the ABCs of CPR.
- Perform CPR until the defibrillator is attached.

1. Press "analyze" on the defibrillation unit.

2. Follow each step as the unit instructs.

3. Attach the AED to the patient as indicated by instructions on the lid of the unit.

4. State loudly, "Everybody clear of the patient!" Verify that everyone is clear of the patient and press the analysis control switch on the AED. The assessment takes ten to twenty seconds depending on the brand of AED. Everyone should remain clear during this time.

5. If the device indicates that a shock is not advised, resume CPR.

6. Once the unit begins charging, a synthesized voice message or light indicator indicates that it is charging. Assume that ventricular fibrillation (VF/VT) is present and that the AED will indicate the need to deliver a shock.

7. Verify that everyone is clear of the unit. The AED delivers shocks without additional actions from the operator. It may indicate "shock now."

8. Give three consecutive shocks.

9. Check the pulse.

10. If a pulse is present, assess the vital signs, support airway, and breathing.

11. If no pulse is present, give CPR for one minute.

12. Check the pulse. If it is not present, press "analyze" on the AED.

13. Defibrillate up to three times.

14. If VF persists after nine shocks, repeat sets of three stacked shocks with one minute of CPR between each set until the "no shock indicated" message is received on the AED or until the patient is revived.

Foreign Body Airway Obstruction

The body depends on oxygen availability to function. Oxygen is an odorless, tasteless, and colorless gas that is essential for life. In the dental office, incidents of airway obstruction are more likely than other possible emergencies. The patient is lying in a supine position, therefore allowing objects to be propelled naturally down the throat. The moisture from saliva and blood makes objects more slippery and harder to hold. Also, the use of a number of items and materials in the mouth allows for a greater possibility of **foreign body airway obstruction (FBAO)**. A patient may take a breath at a time when a tooth is being removed, thereby dislodging it from the forceps and allowing it to fall directly into the airway. Other items causing FBAO are crowns, amalgam, composite, cotton rolls, gauze, endodontic instru-ments, and impression material. The person may begin choking and clutch the throat with the hands, which is the **universal distress signal** (Figure 16-7). Ask, "Are you choking?" The first action is to stop treatment, sit the patient upright, and encourage him or her to cough. If the patient cannot expel the foreign body, the rescuer goes behind the patient and wraps his or her arms around the patient's waist. Tightly wrap one hand over the other fisted hand and, with a quick movement, give upward thrusts into the patient's abdomen. This procedure is referred to as the **Heimlich maneuver** (subdiaphragmatic thrusts); the proper steps for performing this maneuver are outlined in Procedure 16-5. If the patient is in the final stages of pregnancy or obese, the rescuer stands behind, wraps his or her arms under the patient's armpits, and gives quick, inward chest thrusts. If the rescuer is unable to do this technique and the patient is

PROCEDURE 16-5

Heimlich Maneuver (Subdiaphragmatic Thrusts) for a Conscious Adult

If an adult is conscious and has a blocked airway, the rescuer can talk to him or her and perform the Heimlich maneuver to open up the blocked airway.

EQUIPMENT AND SUPPLIES

■ No equipment required

PROCEDURE STEPS *(Follow aseptic procedures)*

1. Verify that the patient is choking. Ask, "Are you choking?"

2. If the patient is standing, tell him or her what the procedure is going to be, position yourself behind the patient, and proceed to wrap arms around the patient's abdomen.

3. Place the thumb side of a fisted hand against the middle of the abdomen, just above the umbilicus.

4. Grasp hands together, keeping one hand fisted and the other wrapped on top of it.

5. Give quick, upward thrusts with hands against the abdomen (Figure 16-6).

FIGURE 16-6 Place the thumb side of your fist against the middle of the person's abdomen, just above the umbilicus. Give quick, upward thrusts against the person's abdomen.

6. Repeat the procedure until the patient expels the object or until the patient becomes unconscious.

7. Wash hands.

8. Document the procedure.

FIGURE 16-7 Holding hands to the throat is the universal distress signal for choking.

still unconscious, have the patient lie over a chair back to force air from the abdomen and help him or her expel the foreign body.

If the patient becomes unconscious, lay the patient on the floor and immediately activate emergency medical services (EMS). Look into the oral cavity of the patient and, with a hooked finger, sweep deeply from one side to the other in order to remove the foreign body. Attempt to give the patient two slow breaths. If unable to do this, reposition the head and chin to see if rescue breathing can be accomplished. If the airway remains obstructed, perform the chest thrust maneuver on the patient by straddling the patient's thighs and pressing into the abdomen with quick, upward thrusts. Place hands below the tip of the xiphoid notch (lowest portion of the sternum) and above the patient's navel. Place the heel of one hand on the victim's abdomen and the second hand on top of the first to deliver the thrusts. If this is not successful after three to five thrusts, repeat the sequence. The steps for performing abdominal thrusts on an unconscious adult are presented in Procedure 16-6.

PROCEDURE 1 6 - 6

Abdominal Thrusts for an Unconscious Adult with Airway Obstruction

If an adult is unconscious and has a blocked airway, the rescuer performs abdominal thrusts to open up the blocked airway.

EQUIPMENT AND SUPPLIES

- Gloves
- Resuscitation device

PROCEDURE STEPS *(Follow aseptic procedures)*

1. If the patient is unconscious, activate EMS immediately.

2. Lay the person on his or her back.

3. Perform the tongue-jaw lift followed by a finger sweep to remove the object (Figure 16-8A).

4. Open the airway, place the resuscitation device, and try to ventilate (Figures 16-8B and C). If the airway is still obstructed, reposition the patient's head and try to ventilate again.

(B)

(C)

(A)

FIGURE 16-8 (A) Perform the tongue-jaw lift, followed by a finger sweep to remove the object. (B) Open the airway. (C) Attempt to ventilate.

(continues)

PROCEDURE 16-6 *(CONTINUED)*

5. Place the heel of hand against the person's abdomen just above the navel and well below the breastbone (Figure 16-8D).

6. Kneel astride the patient's thighs. Give up to five abdominal thrusts in a motion toward the diaphragm (Figure 16-8E).

7. Repeat Steps 3 through 6 until effective or help arrives.

(D)

(E)

FIGURE 16-8 (D) Place the heel of your hand against the person's abdomen. (E) Apply five abdominal thrusts.

Causes, Signs, and Treatment of Emergencies

If an anxious or a fearful patient has heart problems, his or her heart may be beating rapidly and working harder, precipitating a heart attack. Patients may become light-headed as they see instruments in the dental treatment room and anticipate the procedures. These patients may react by **syncope** (fainting) (see Table 16-1).

Dental assistants may use preventive measures to render patients less likely to exhibit syncope. It is important that assistants are aware of anxiety-provoking events and ensure that patients do not encounter them. Talk to patients, and assure them that everything is all right. Help them overcome the apprehension and fear of treatment. In addition, keep instruments, needles, and blood out of the patient's sight. If patients are undergoing long treatments, make sure they have eaten and allow them to get up occasionally. Patients may complain of feeling flushed, having upset stomachs, and racing heart rates, and appear to have pale skin. Blood pressure may also decrease. Be aware of the signs and symptoms and try to prevent a syncope through close observation of the patient and preventive techniques.

Syncope

The most common and least life-threatening emergency that may occur in the dental office is the vasodepressor syncope, commonly known as fainting. This loss of consciousness is caused by a decrease in blood flow to the brain. Syncope is normally caused by some form of stress, emotional, physical, or both. When a patient experiences stress, the body reacts by pumping large amounts of blood to the arms and legs. This response (often referred to as the "fight or flight syndrome") occurs so that the patients can quickly respond by moving their bodies. Dental patients often remain motionless, so their blood pools in the arms and legs and the cerebral blood flow is diminished. As a result, the brain is deprived of oxygenated blood and the patient becomes unconscious (unable to respond to any sensory stimulation).

TABLE 16-1 Emergency Conditions, Symptoms, and Treatments

Condition	Symptom(s)	Treatment
Syncope	Loss of consciousness	Lower the head to increase blood flow to the brain
Asthma	Breathlessness	Administer patient's bronchodilator (inhaler)
Allergic reaction	Edema, erythema, urticaria	Remove irritant, administer an antihistamine if needed
Anaphylactic reaction	Blood pressure drops, airways constricted	Injection of epinephrine
Hyperventilation	Quick breathing, nervousness, faintness	Calm patient, have patient breathe in paper bag or cupped hands
Epilepsy Grand mal	Seizure lasting two to five minutes, body jerking, twitching	Remove items that harm patient, make patient comfortable after seizure
Status epilepticus	Continuous seizures	Summon emergency services
Petit mal seizure	Blank stare	No treatment necessary
Partial seizures	Simple/patient conscious, complex/patient unconscious, involuntary twitching	No treatment necessary
Type I diabetes mellitus	Thirst, frequent urination, disorientation, nausea/vomiting, abdominal pain	Administer patient's insulin
Type II diabetes mellitus	Same symptoms as Type I but not as severe	Normally controlled by diet, may need to administer oral hypoglycemics
Hypoglycemia	Nervousness, trembling, weakness, cold sweats	Administer orange juice or other source of sugar, such as cake icing gel, in buccal mucosa or administer injection of glucagon
Angina pectoris	Pain in chest/base of neck	Administer nitroglycerin pills or spray
Myocardial infarction	Possible pain in chest, ashen color, diaphoresis (sweating profusely)	Position patient with head slightly elevated, administer oxygen and nitroglycerin pills, summon medical services
Congestive heart failure	Difficulty breathing, swollen ankles and legs	Elevate the head and heart, allow frequent restroom breaks
Stroke	Loss of speech, dizziness, weakness on one side of body	Administer oxygen, take vital signs, summon medical services
Orthostatic hypotension	Loss of consciousness when standing upright, light-headed	In the dental office, have the patient sit upright initially before standing*

*If it is a fall in blood pressure from other underlying issues, the patient needs to consult a physician.

The patient may feel dizzy, nauseated, or extremely weak prior to syncope. The patient appears pale and clammy and breathes in shallow gasps. If the patient indicates that he or she is feeling faint, remain calm, quickly sit the patient down, and lean his or her head forward and place it between the knees. If a fainting person is **unconscious** and breathing normally, lay him or her down in the Trendelenburg position (Figure 16-9). This position allows the blood to flow back to the head. If the patient is not breathing normally, establish an airway by tipping the head back and performing a chin lift. At this time, any tight, constricting clothing or jewelry can be loosened or removed around the neck area.

FIGURE 16-9 The Trendelenburg position (supine position with the feet elevated slightly).

Administer oxygen and monitor vital signs. The patient will normally resume breathing in less than ten seconds. If the patient becomes unconscious, break a vial of spirits of ammonia and pass it under the patient's nose. The strong odor of the ammonia causes the patient to quickly inhale, which stimulates breathing. This gauze-covered ammonia vial is very strong, so only pass it under the patient's nostrils a couple of times and *do not* leave it in a place where it can cause irritation to the nasal passage membranes. The patient normally will revive totally within a couple of minutes but may remain weak. It is best to reschedule dental treatment and contact someone to drive the patient home. If the patient does not revive from the unconscious state, call for emergency help, closely monitor breathing, and begin CPR, if necessary, until help arrives. Procedure 16-7 presents the steps to follow in the event that a patient has a syncopal event in the dental office.

PROCEDURE 16-7

Treatment of a Patient with Syncope

Dental assistants must be prepared to treat syncope in the dental office. Often, patients will have syncope in the treatment room while in the dental chair, but it may happen anywhere in the office. The dental assistant should keep the patient in the Trendelenburg position.

EQUIPMENT AND SUPPLIES

- Oxygen tank with gauge at top or gauge in the dental treatment area
- Oxygen mask and tubing
- Spirits of ammonia

PROCEDURE STEPS *(Follow aseptic procedures)*

1. Position the patient in a supine or Trendelenburg position (supine with feet elevated to increase blood flow to the brain). If the patient is wearing a dress or other garments that are misplaced during the syncope, attend to modesty issues as soon as possible.

2. Establish that the airway is open. If it is not, perform the head-tilt, chin-lift to open the airway.

3. Breathing normally begins spontaneously within the first ten to fifteen seconds.

4. Administer oxygen as a precautionary treatment only.

5. If the patient has not revived within the first fifteen seconds, remove the oxygen mask (if one has been placed) and pass a broken ammonia gauze sponge under the patient's nose for one or two seconds only. (Holding the ammonia for a long period of time under the patient's nose may cause undue irritation.)

6. The patient will normally respond rapidly to the pungent odor of the ammonia and take in a breath of air, therefore receiving oxygen.

7. Full revival of the patient should occur within a minute or two.

8. If revival of the patient does not occur, follow the guidelines of CPR.

9. Postpone dental treatment and call for patient transportation.

Orthostatic Hypotension

Orthostatic hypotension is when an individual loses consciousness or a level of consciousness when he or she sits in an upright position rapidly. This condition is also known as postural hypotension. It happens often in the dental office if the patient has been lying in a prone position for a long period of time during dental treatment and then tries to sit up rapidly or rises to the feet immediately. It occurs from a lack of blood flow to the brain. Patients may say that they feel "light-headed." This feeling lasts only a few seconds and the patient is feeling better.

It is advisable to have the patients rise up with the chair and sit in that position for a few minutes before standing. Often the dental assistant can write on the chart and then dismiss the patient and during this time the patient's blood flow to the brain will return to normal. Patients who are given nitrous oxide or oxygen, have been in the dental chair for long periods in a prone position, pregnant women, and patients who have had intravenous sedation are more prone to having orthostatic hypotension.

Asthma

Recurrent attacks of breathlessness accompanied by wheezing while breathing out and often a dry cough are symptoms of asthma. The wheezing and breathlessness are due to the narrowing of small airways in the lungs (**bronchioles**). When a patient with asthma exhales, the lungs collapse to expel the air, causing the bronchioles to further narrow and making it more difficult to breathe. If the lining of the bronchioles is inflamed, sputum (phlegm) is produced, making the bronchioles further obstructed, increasing difficulty breathing.

Asthma is becoming more prevalent. Normally, the disease occurs during childhood, but the symptoms improve in adulthood. Approximately one in ten children in the United States has asthma. Heredity is a major factor in development of the disease. Asthma may be caused by an allergy to a substance. An **allergy** is an exaggerated reaction of the immune system to an offending agent. Upon the first contact with the agent, the body becomes sensitized to it and develops **antibodies** (also called immunoglobulins) to fight these **antigens** (foreign bodies). The second or subsequent time that the body has contact with these offending agents, it overreacts in a **hypersensitive** manner. The most common **allergens** (the antigens that trigger the allergic reaction) responsible for asthma are animal fur, house dust, pollens, tobacco smoke, feathers, food, and drugs.

Asthma attacks are more frequent in the morning and vary from slight breathlessness to respiratory failure. There is no cure for asthma, but tests are available to identify what causes the most severe reactions in an individual so the individual can avoid it. **Immunotherapy** (injection of the allergen) can be a treatment choice, and corticosteroid drugs also provide successful therapy.

Antihistamines are often used to treat the physical symptoms produced by the antigen. These drugs counteract the body's production of histamine. They are administered with an **inhaler**, a pressurized canister with a mouthpiece (Figures 16-10A and B). The patient carries an inhaler and, when an asthma attack is anticipated, the drug can be dispensed. The patient should bring an inhaler to any dental treatment appointment. If the patient has an attack and an inhaler is unavailable, the dentist may use the bronchodilator from the emergency kit. The drug of choice in this bronchodilator (inhaler) is albuterol, because it widens the bronchioles and improves air flow but does not stimulate the cardiovascular system like the drug epinephrine would. To use the bronchodilator, the patient exhales first, then takes a slow, deep breath while releasing the drug as the canister is depressed. After two dispensed amounts are taken, breathing should improve within fifteen minutes. If the patient does not improve, the inhaler is used again. If this does not alleviate the condition, emergency services should be deployed to take the patient to the hospital. While waiting for the emergency services, the dental office team should administer oxygen and reassure and calm the patient. The patient should also be instructed to see his or her general physician.

FIGURE 16-10 (A) Inhalers or nebulizers. (B) Inhalation of bronchodilator drug from inhaler.

Allergic Reactions

A number of other **allergic reactions** may take place in the dental office. The body may react to drugs, toothpaste, latex protein, or a number of the dental materials. Keep in mind that these exaggerated reactions of the immune system occur only subsequent to exposures to the offending antigen. The hypersensitive reaction may vary in symptoms and severity. It may be localized or cover the entire body. It could occur immediately or several hours after exposure to the antigen. Dermatitis, or skin reaction, may occur. If a skin reaction is apparent, dental treatment ceases until the irritant is removed.

Examples of skin reactions include:

- **Edema** (eh-**DEE**-mah), or swelling
- **Erythema** (er-ih-**THEE**-mah), or redness
- Vesicle formation
- **Urticaria** (ur-tih-**KAY**-ree-ah), or hives
- Giant urticaria, or **angioedema** (an-jee-oh-eh-**DEE**-muh), poorly defined, single swollen areas

Treatment for both urticaria and angioedema is to remove the irritant. In some cases, the dentist will administer an antihistamine to reduce the edema.

Anaphylactic Reaction

Anaphylactic shock is a severe allergic reaction that is life threatening. It occurs in people who are extremely sensitive to a particular allergen. This may happen to a patient who has been administered local anesthetic or has taken penicillin. Once the allergen is in the bloodstream, the body produces large amounts of histamine and other chemicals. The blood pressure drops, bronchospasm (constriction of the airways in the lungs) occurs, the tongue and throat swell, and the person experiences stomach pain. All of these symptoms come on rapidly and an injection of epinephrine must be administered immediately to save the patient's life. Patients who know they are extremely sensitive to some allergens (bee sting venom, for example) may carry antihistamine drugs and take immunotherapy treatment to desensitize for the allergen.

Hyperventilation

Dealing with the patient's anxiety prior to treatment alleviates fear and distress and, hopefully, reduces the chance of **hyperventilation**. Children normally do not experience hyperventilation because they can more readily express their concerns about dentistry. However, because adult patients may try to hide their fears, their anxiety can result in hyperventilation. They start to breathe deeply and rapidly, not realizing that they are breathing differently. When they continue in this manner, they experience a numbness in the extremities, faintness, and a sense of inability to take a full breath.

A loss of carbon dioxide from the blood occurs, causing **alkalosis** (increase in blood alkalinity). The patient panics and breathing speeds up. This is hyperventilation.

To treat the patient, first stop all dental treatment. Sit the patient upright to allow easier breathing and then calm him or her. Tell the patient what is happening and encourage him or her to breathe in and hold it several seconds before exhaling. This process allows more carbon dioxide to enter the bloodstream. If the patient is too agitated to follow instructions, instruct the patient to breathe into cupped hands or a paper sack (Figure 16-11). This allows the levels of carbon dioxide and oxygen to return to normal.

Epilepsy/Seizure Disorder

Human emotions and thoughts normally occur in an organized, methodical, electrical excitation of nerve cells in the brain. With **epilepsy**, an unorganized and chaotic electrical discharge occurs. Seizures may appear spontaneously or as a result of a stimulus, such as a flashing light. Symptoms of the seizures may range from insignificant to severe. It is estimated that one person in every 200 suffers from epilepsy. Many wear bracelets or carry identification cards. Epileptics should advise colleagues about what to do in the case of a seizure.

The dentist will utilize fixed appliances, if feasible, when treating patients who experience seizures due to epilepsy. During an epileptic seizure, the muscles tighten and the person has no control over movements.

FIGURE 16-11 Patient breathing in a paper bag to increase carbon dioxide in the body.

A loose dental appliance may become dislodged or broken, obstructing the airway during a seizure.

Some identified causes of epilepsy are head injury, infections, fever, brain tumor, strokes, metabolic imbalance, and drug and alcohol withdrawal states. However, the causes of the majority of cases are unknown. Heredity is known to play a role. Types of seizures are classified in three general categories: grand mal, petit mal, and partial seizures.

Grand Mal Seizure. The grand mal seizure (tonic clonic seizure) is the most common. During this seizure or convulsion, which lasts two to five minutes, the person becomes unconscious and the body jerks, twitches, and stiffens. Breathing is often irregular. Once the seizure subsides, bladder and bowel control may be lost as the muscles relax. The person may be disoriented and exhausted, normally with no memory of the seizure. He or she may want to sleep. After the seizure, reassure the patient. If the patient experiences one seizure after another, called status epilepticus (continuous seizures), emergency services should be summoned.

> *Note:* About 10 percent of patients experiencing status epilepticus will die due to the body's inability to deal with this overexertion.

Petit Mal Seizure. The petit mal seizure (absence seizure) is where a person experiences a momentary loss of consciousness. The patient may exhibit a blank stare or blinking of the eyes that lasts five to ten seconds. Others around the person may not be aware of the seizure because of the lack of abnormal movements. The person may appear inattentive or seem to be daydreaming. Absence seizures occur in children and normally decrease in frequency with age. The absence seizure may occur several times a day and with other forms of seizures. Often, before a grand mal seizure, a petit mal seizure may be experienced first, as a warning. A person then can alert someone prior to the loss of consciousness.

Partial Seizure. Partial seizures can be classified into two categories: simple (person remains conscious) and complex (person becomes unconscious). The simple partial seizure is referred to as Jacksonian epilepsy. As a twitching occurs and spreads slowly from one part of the body to another on one side, the person remains conscious and is able to recall details of the event. During the complex seizure, a person remembers very little and exhibits involuntary actions, such as lip smacking, as the twitching spreads from one part of the body to another on one side. If the seizure develops into total body, it is then referred to as a grand mal seizure.

To prevent seizures, a person should try to eliminate extreme stress and fatigue. Anticonvulsant drugs are the first line of treatment for epilepsy and may minimize seizures. Side effects of the drugs are fatigue and loss of concentration. Some of the drugs (such as dilantin) cause gingival hyperplasia, or overgrowth of gingival tissue. This thick, granular tissue may cover the teeth and have to be surgically removed.

Treatment for Patients Who Experience Seizures. When patients experience seizures, stop dental treatment and remove everything from the oral cavity. Also, remove items from the area that could harm the person. Normally, no further action is necessary. The seizure runs its course. Do not restrain the person or place anything in the patient's mouth. Once the seizures have ceased, place the patient in the recovery position (on the right side with the airway open). Always be cognizant of the person's dignity and treat him or her in a considerate manner. The patient may feel embarrassed and reassurance is important. If the seizures continue for more than five minutes or continue one after another, summon emergency help and reassure the patient.

Diabetes Mellitus

The cause of diabetes mellitus was discovered in the 1920s: the pancreas produces an insufficient amount of or no insulin (the hormone responsible for absorbing glucose into the cells for energy and into the liver and fat cells for storage). Therefore, the level of glucose in the blood becomes too high, which causes thirst and excessive urination. In addition, the body cannot store glucose for the vast number of cells in the body that need glucose to survive. The body normally experiences weight loss and fatigue. Diabetes mellitus is classified in two categories: Type I and Type II.

Type I Diabetes Mellitus. Type I diabetes mellitus, the more severe, normally occurs in people between the ages of ten and sixteen. Type I is often termed juvenile diabetes due to the age at which it commonly affects people. However, the condition also can occur in older people. It is known that heredity is a factor in the disease; diabetes can pass from one generation to another or miss a generation. There is a theory that the mumps virus may damage the cells of the pancreas, thereby bringing on diabetes. Insulin-dependent diabetes mellitus (Type I) develops rapidly when the insulin-secreting cells in the pancreas become ineffective. If the person does not have regular injections of insulin, he or she could lapse into a coma. Individuals with Type I diabetes mellitus (about 10 percent of diabetes cases) experience the most medical complications because they have the disease for long time periods. Thus, the disease has to be monitored very carefully.

Type II Diabetes Mellitus. Type II diabetes mellitus was called adult-onset diabetes until it also was identified in the younger population. Type II, making up 90 percent of diabetes mellitus cases, normally is diagnosed in obese, middle-aged people. It can be controlled with diet and oral hypoglycemics (medications that lower blood sugar levels) and does not require insulin injections.

Disturbances in the balance of glucose intake and insulin can result in hyperglycemia (too much glucose in the blood). The onset is slow and the person experiences early symptoms days prior to the onset, such as increased thirst, increased urination, nausea/vomiting with abdominal pains, loss of appetite, fatigue, and pain. If these patients (possibly undiagnosed diabetics) are having dental treatment, they could go into diabetic comas. If a patient reacts in this manner, stop dental treatment; if the patient is conscious, have him or her administer an insulin shot. If the patient becomes unconscious, call for emergency help and transfer him or her to a medical facility as soon as possible. One of the most serious consequences of hyperglycemia, a condition in which the patient goes into a coma and dies if not treated, is diabetic acidosis. This condition occurs when the patient has too much sugar (glucose) and not enough insulin. The body in this condition produces acids, and the body's pH is lowered. The body's pH range is 7.35 to 7.45. If the body's pH drops below 7.0, diabetic acidosis may occur.

Today, more is known about diabetes, and patients are diagnosed more readily and therefore deal with the symptoms before the diabetes gets to the later stage, such as diabetic coma. Some patients have insulin pens or portable pumps that inject insulin if needed (Figure 16-12). Individuals can test their urine and blood for glucose levels.

Hypoglycemia

Too little glucose or sugar causes a person to experience hypoglycemia. This condition comes on rapidly and the patient becomes nervous, shows signs of trembling and weakness, and has cold sweats. The patient becomes hungry and shows signs of a personality change. If the person remains conscious, stop dental treatment and give him or her a sugar source, such as orange juice.

If the person becomes unconscious, terminate dental treatment, summon medical assistance, perform basic life support, and if necessary, give him or her an injection of glucagon or a sugar source such as cake icing gel placed in the buccal mucosa. If this condition happens frequently, the individual's physician may prescribe antidiabetic drugs to stimulate the pancreas to produce more insulin. Normally, however, the condition arises only when the person misses a meal, is overexerted, or is in a situation that causes emotional stress. Due to the stress patients experience regarding dentistry and long appointment times, most dental offices have orange juice or other sources of sugar available for patients feeling changes in their blood sugar levels. Severe hypoglycemia causes insulin shock, manifested by tremors, sweating, and nervousness, and is soon followed by delirium, seizure-like jerkings, and collapse. Treatment requires administration of glucose intravenously.

Cardiovascular Emergencies

An emergency involving the heart may occur in the dental office, so it is important to understand the anatomy of the heart. (Refer to Chapter 6.) The heart can be required to work harder due to physical and emotional stress. If the heart is healthy, the vessels dilate and pump more oxygen-rich blood into it. If the heart is diseased and unhealthy, this process cannot take place. Arteriosclerosis (commonly referred to as hardening of the arteries) is one condition that will not allow the heart to get more oxygenated blood. This condition evolves over a number of years. The arteries build up plaque deposits on the inside of the artery wall (Figure 16-13). This narrows the diameter of the artery, therefore restricting blood flow. In the later stages, a patient may experience angina pectoris and, if the vessel is totally occluded, the patient may experience a myocardial infarction.

Angina Pectoris

A Latin phrase meaning "strangling the chest," angina pectoris causes pain in the chest area. Pain may radiate into the jaw area from the base of the neck; this continuous jaw pain may be the first indication of heart disease. The chest pain normally lasts for five minutes. During that time, the person wants to remain motionless and stop all activity. The person may experience an increase in blood pressure and pulse rate, have a feeling of impending doom, and become pale and clammy. If this is not the first indication of the disease, the patient may be under the care of a physician. If the patient is under the care of a physician, he or she has nitroglycerin pills or spray. The small nitroglycerin pills are placed sublingually (under the tongue) to allow them to dissolve and be absorbed rapidly. Nitroglycerin spray (sprayed translingually into the oral cavity) also can be used. Nitroglycerin helps dilate the coronary

(A)

Insulin pen

Refill cartridge

Spare needles

Portable pump

Cannula

Pump

(B)

FIGURE 16-12 (A) Insulin pen. (B) Portable insulin pump.

arteries, allowing the heart to receive more oxygenated blood. This rapid-action drug is the accepted remedy for angina pectoris. Each patient is given a very specific dosage, because some individuals are more susceptible to the drug. If the condition arises in a dental office, all dental treatment stops. The dental team remains calm and reassures the patient. Any items that may increase stress for the patient are removed from sight. Oxygen can be administered while the patient takes the first dosage of nitroglycerin. A second dose can be administered within three to five minutes if the patient is feeling no relief while at rest. A final, third dose can be administered three to five minutes following the second dose. If the pain is not alleviated, the dental team can assume that the patient is experiencing myocardial infarction and emergency help should be summoned to transport the patient to a medical facility.

Myocardial Infarction

A condition known as **myocardial infarction**, commonly known as a heart attack, occurs when the coronary arteries are blocked or severely narrowed (Figure 16-13). It causes sudden death of part of the heart tissue and may be precipitated by angina pectoris or may occur in a person who never had any prior symptoms. In about one-third of the cases, the person will die from myocardial infarction. The signs of a heart attack are similar to those of angina pectoris, but the pain may be increased and is not alleviated by nitroglycerin pills. A number of risk factors for the disease can be identified:

- Males are more likely to exhibit heart attacks than females.
- Smokers have a higher incidence of heart attacks than nonsmokers.
- Increased age, specific diseases such as diabetes mellitus, and heredity are uncontrollable factors.
- Diet, stress level, high blood pressure, and exercise levels are controllable factors.

The dental team should remain calm, stop all dental treatment, reassure and reposition the patient in a comfortable position (normally the head is elevated slightly), and remove any items that may increase stress. Administer oxygen and nitroglycerin pills or spray and summon medical emergency help immediately.

Congestive Heart Failure

As the heart weakens, the person may experience **congestive heart failure.** The weakened heart is not able to pump the fluids around the body as it should. When the person stands or sits for long periods, this fluid collects around the ankles and legs. The person may appear with swollen ankles and legs and report indigestion and difficulty breathing. Many older patients show signs of the heart getting weaker. When they lie in bed, these patients report difficulty breathing and need to have large pillows to keep the head and heart elevated. This occurs because the fluids from the feet, legs, and other parts of the body gravitate toward the heart and lungs. The medical treatment for this patient is diuretic drugs to rid the body of excess fluid by increasing the output of urine. In some cases, these patients take other drugs to strengthen the contractions of the heart. In the dental office, be sure that these patients are seated with their heads elevated to eliminate discomfort, and reduce undue stress. Allow them to visit the restroom as needed.

Stroke/Cerebrovascular Accident

Stroke is a leading cause of disability and death for Americans. This condition has a sudden onset and is caused by a **cerebral infarction**, or the blood supply to the brain being interrupted by a blockage such as a **cerebral embolism** (blood clot), or a **cerebral hemorrhage** (rupture of a blood vessel). Strokes happen to people of all ages but occur primarily in older people. The person may have an intense headache,

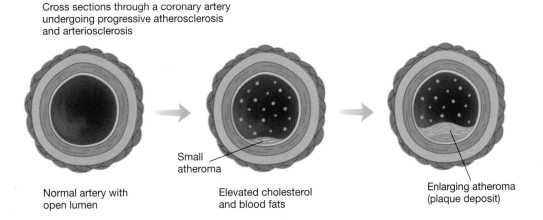

Cross sections through a coronary artery undergoing progressive atherosclerosis and arteriosclerosis

Normal artery with open lumen

Elevated cholesterol and blood fats

Small atheroma

Enlarging atheroma (plaque deposit)

FIGURE 16-13 The progression of coronary heart disease.

loss of speech, unexplained dizziness, hemiplegia (weakness, numbness, or paralysis on one side of the body), and loss of consciousness. An average of 200 people per 100,000 suffer strokes annually in the United States and Canada, according to the Centers for Disease Control (CDC). This figure rises with age; men have more strokes than women, and African Americans suffer more strokes than Caucasian Americans. If the person has diabetes mellitus or if the person has had a prior stroke, the risk is greater. Heredity is also a risk factor. Controllable risk factors are cigarette smoking, high blood pressure, heart disease, and a high red blood cell count. Some people experience transient ischemic attacks (stroke-like symptoms that disappear within twenty-four hours). They should seek medical attention, because these are strong predictors of an impending stroke. A person may be given blood thinner to prevent blood clots from forming and thus the onset of a stroke.

Damage to an area of the brain may impair body sensation, function, or movement. The cerebral hemisphere in the brain on the left side controls the functions on the body's right side and vice versa. This one-sided weakness or paralysis is known as hemiplegia and it is one of the most common effects of a stroke. If a patient has had a stroke the dental assistant may observe the patient walking with an abnormal gait or a way of walking that doesn't seem to be normal. If the patient has not indicated anything on the medical history about this, the dental assistant can request information from the patient. The patient may not think that it is important to the dental treatment and feel that he or she is making a strong recovery and it is insignificant to the dental medical history. It is important that the dental assistant obtain the information from the patient but also that the dental assistant is observant when seating the patient. The doctor does not have this opportunity to view the patient as he or she is coming in for treatment.

If a patient has a stroke in the dental office, stop all dental treatment and remove any items from the patient's mouth. Position the patient so that his or her head is slightly elevated. Administer oxygen and monitor vital signs while emergency medical help is summoned. Calm the patient and provide CPR as needed.

Dental Emergencies

Patients may call the office about any number of dental emergencies. Most offices will reserve time in the schedule for emergencies. Some emergencies require rescheduling other patients and giving specific instructions for the patient seeking dental treatment. Several possible patient emergency situations are mentioned here. After the dentist sees each patient, a diagnosis is made and treatment rendered.

Abscessed Tooth

One of the most common emergencies for which patients seek dental care is an abscessed tooth. The patient's symptoms include pain from pressure, swelling, and severe responses to heat. The tooth has become infected, and as the abscess grows, it places a great deal of pressure in the area because fluid has no place to escape in the bone. If the abscessed tooth goes untreated long enough in this painful state, the infection process may create a fistula in the bone and through the oral mucosa near the root end of the tooth. This fistula, an abnormal, tube-like passage at the end of the tooth to the outside surface in the oral cavity, allows the fluid to be discharged and the pressure to be released slightly. The fistula normally closes after the tooth is treated and the infection is reduced/eliminated.

Alveolitis

Alveolitis (al-vee-o-**LIGH**-tis; alveolar osteitis), a condition commonly known as a dry socket, happens after a tooth has been removed. This condition occurs when a blood clot does not form or is washed out of the socket, allowing the nerve endings over the bone to become exposed. This condition increases the chance of infection in the area. Alveolitis causes great discomfort. It is treated by gently rinsing the socket with saline solution to remove any debris and packing a medicated iodoform gauze strip that is cut in a sufficient length into the socket. The medicated iodoform gauze treatment, which is only palliative, may have to be repeated every day or two until the pain diminishes. The patient may be given analgesics to relieve additional discomfort.

Avulsed Tooth

A patient may call the dental office and report that one tooth has been forcibly misplaced (avulsed). This avulsed tooth (also spelled evulsed) can be replanted into the socket and have a fairly high success rate if handled quickly. The patient should immediately wrap the tooth in clean, wet gauze, place it in the mucosa between the teeth and the lip, or place it in milk while transporting it to the office. The area where the tooth came out can be packed with gauze and pressure applied to control the bleeding. The outcome correlates greatly with the time that has elapsed. Getting the patient to the office and under the dentist's care quickly is essential. The dentist replants the tooth in the socket and secures it to the adjacent teeth. The dentist may perform immediate root canal therapy on the avulsed tooth prior to replanting it in the socket or complete the endodontic treatment six to eight weeks after reimplantation. Follow-up care is necessary until the tooth is reattached. There are individual emergency tooth avulsion kits available through dental suppliers and pharmacies.

Broken Prosthesis

A patient may call with a broken prosthesis. Normally, the patient is not in any physical pain but needs help due to appearance concerns and loss of function. The broken prosthesis can be repaired in the office by the dentist or sent to the dental laboratory. Additional treatment is scheduled at a convenient time for the patient and dental office. The length of time for prosthesis repair varies. It may be necessary to perform temporary repairs in the interim, until the permanent treatment can be completed.

Soft Tissue Injury

Patients experience a number of soft tissue injuries. Running with sharp or blunt objects or falling down with something in their mouth may cause a number of oralfacial injuries. Electrical burns in the oral cavity can result from an individual biting into an electrical cord. Children can also fall and push newly erupted teeth back down/up into the sockets, called **traumatic intrusion**. Sports injuries result in soft tissue damage. The dental office should be contacted when such soft tissue injuries occur.

Soft tissue injury can occur in the dental office during any intraoral dental procedure. The oral cavity is moist and slippery, the patient may move suddenly, and dental instruments and equipment can easily become displaced, causing injury.

Broken Tooth

A patient may call with a broken tooth. Anterior teeth are commonly fractured at drinking faucets, on steering wheels, or on diving boards. The dental receptionist discerns whether the patient needs to be scheduled immediately by gaining information from the patient as to the level of discomfort, whether there are sharp edges, and how extensive the broken area is. In most offices, the patient is seen for an initial appointment on an emergency basis to determine the treatment needed.

Loose Permanent or Temporary Crown

A patient's crown may become loose or come off, requiring recementation. The patient may be in discomfort if the pulp is exposed or if the restoration has sharp edges. If the patient is out of town and unable to get dental care, petroleum jelly or orthodontic wax can be used to temporarily keep the crown in place. The patient will have to exercise extreme care while eating. If the patient can get to the dental office, treatment consists of recementing the crown with temporary or permanent cement, as indicated.

CHAPTER SUMMARY

Even though the number of emergencies is not high in a dental office, the dental assistant must always observe the patient and be prepared to deal with emergencies. Emergencies may also happen to the dentist and to other dental auxiliaries.

When an emergency arises, the dental team must react automatically. Any hesitation at such a time may cost a life. It is best if a routine is established so that everyone can ensure that everything is addressed. The assistant has a vital role in the prevention of emergencies and in emergency care. Patient observation at all times assists in the prevention evaluation.

Case Study

Thelma Lynd, a forty-six-year-old woman, is seated in the dental treatment room. She indicates that recently she has not been feeling well. As she continues to talk, she experiences loss of speech, dizziness, and weakness on one side of her body. Her vital signs are elevated and she cannot respond.

Case Study Review

1. What probable condition is Thelma experiencing? *Stroke*

2. What should the dental assistant do in this situation? *Stop all treatment, remove items from mouth, head sl. elevated, get med. help, oxygen, vital signs, CPR if needed*

3. Is reassurance for the patient important in this case? Why?

REVIEW QUESTIONS

Multiple Choice

1. An exaggerated reaction by the immune system is called an
   a. allergy.
   b. antibody.
   c. antigen.
   d. allergen.

2. Asthma attacks are more frequent in the
   a. late evening.
   b. afternoon.
   c. morning.
   d. nighttime hours.

3. A medical term for giant hives is
   a. edema.
   b. erythema.
   c. urticaria.
   d. angioedema.

4. A seizure in which a person experiences a momentary loss of consciousness is called a
   a. grand mal seizure.
   b. petit mal seizure.
   c. partial seizure.
   d. status epilepticus.

5. Type _____ of diabetes mellitus is more severe.
   a. I
   b. II
   c. III
   d. IV

6. Traumatic intrusion is the term for a newly erupted tooth being _____.
   a. removed
   b. pushed back into the socket
   c. decayed
   d. knocked out

7. Angina pectoris causes pain in the ____.
   a. legs
   b. left arm
   c. stomach
   d. chest

8. An average of ____ people per 100,000 suffer strokes annually in the United States and Canada.
   a. 100
   b. 200
   c. 300
   d. 400

9. A continuous seizure is called _____.
   a. grand mal seizure
   b. status epilepticus
   c. petit mal seizure
   d. partial seizure

10. A condition commonly known as a dry socket is called _____.
    a. alveolitis
    b. avulsed
    c. angina pectoris
    d. abcessed

Critical Thinking

1. A patient is having extensive dental work completed. The patient's health history includes epilepsy. The patient becomes nervous and then unconscious as the body begins to jerk, twitch, and stiffen. How should the dental team respond?

2. The disease in which an individual has too little glucose or sugar is called hypoglycemia. What are the steps for treating a patient experiencing hypoglycemic symptoms? *Give sugar*

3. A patient has heart disease that continues to progress over the years. He has a condition that will not allow the heart to receive the oxygenated blood that it needs. What is the condition and what is it commonly called? *Arterial sclerosis*

Web Activities

1. Look up the chain of survival at http://www.americanheart.org. List the four steps in the chain of survival.

2. Go to http://www.redcross.org and find the address and phone number of the Red Cross closest to you.

3. Go to http://www.americanheart.org and look up recent discoveries supported by the AHA. Complete a one-page report on one recent discovery.

SECTION

V

CLINICAL DENTAL PROCEDURES

INTRODUCTION TO THE DENTAL OFFICE AND BASIC CHAIRSIDE ASSISTING CDA

SPECIFIC INSTRUCTIONAL OBJECTIVES

The student should strive to meet the following objectives and demonstrate an understanding of the facts and principles presented in this chapter:

1. Describe the design of a dental office, explaining the purpose of each area.
2. Describe the equipment and function of the equipment in each area.
3. Explain basic concepts of chairside assisting.
4. Describe the necessary steps to prepare a patient for treatment.
5. Describe the daily routine to open and close the dental office.
6. Identify the activity zones and classifications of motion.
7. Explain the necessary steps to seat the patient for treatment.
8. Describe the ergonomics of the operator and the assistant at chairside.
9. Describe the necessary steps to dismiss the patient after treatment is concluded.
10. Identify the special needs of certain patients.

KEY TERMS

(continues)

INTRODUCTION

Dental offices have numerous designs, including a single building, a medical/dental complex of individual units, a remodeled home, a suite in an office building, or space in a mall. Dental professionals go to great lengths to ensure that their offices are clean and convenient and offer pleasant settings for patients. The dentist's vision and expectations are reflected in the office design, which should always consider the patients the dentist serves. The practice may serve families, primarily children, or primarily adults and may be in a rural or an urban setting. The most successful practices encompass all facets into a welcoming atmosphere where dental treatment can be provided.

The appearance of the dental office makes a statement about the dentist, the dental staff, and the quality of the dental care. The following information describes the rooms in the dental office, the specific equipment used by dental professionals, and the concept of chairside assisting.

The Dental Office Design

The dental office has several basic components designed to meet the dentist's individual preferences and needs. The office may be small with two or three treatment rooms or it may have a clinic setting with any number of treatment rooms (Figure 17-1). Most offices are designed with a reception area, a business area, treatment rooms, a sterilizing area, a laboratory, an x-ray processing room, a restroom, and the dentist's office. The sizes and numbers of these rooms vary (Figure 17-2). Dental offices may also include the following: consultation rooms/areas, staff lounge, prevention and/or patient education area, storage area, office for the office manager, space for panoramic radiograph machine, shower/change room, and laundry room. OSHA requirements have changed the office by

FIGURE 17-1 Small dental office blueprint. *(Courtesy of Burkhart Dental Supply).*

FIGURE 17-2 Large office blueprint. *(Courtesy of Burkhart Dental Supply.)*

requiring a room for staff to change and store uniforms. Some offices have added laundry facilities. In addition, dental offices are requiring more space in the business office to accommodate high-technology equipment and to facilitate increased dental insurance processing.

Innovations in dental offices include more open designs with partial walls and greater access to the treatment rooms, sterilizing area, and so on. Higher ceilings, open doorways, and more windows also create the feeling of openness for the patient and the dental team. The office should have a climate-control system that remains at a comfortable temperature throughout the year, regardless of the weather conditions. Architects and decorators often work with dental professionals to achieve the look the dentist desires.

The Reception Room

The **reception room** is the area the patient initially enters and therefore gives the first impression of the office. It is important that this room be pleasing and comfortable as well as neat and clean (Figure 17-3). The dental staff should tidy this room regularly. Magazines should be current and appropriate for the dentist's clientele. Often, there is an area designed specifically for children with a table, chairs, and activities to keep them occupied while they wait.

The reception room is an excellent place to provide patient education materials for all age groups. The decor of this room should be changed as often as needed to keep the atmosphere friendly and positive for the patients as they enter the dental office.

The Reception Desk and Business Office

The reception desk and business office is often part of or adjacent to the reception room, so patients can be greeted as they enter the office. This area is where appointments are made, telephone calls are received, and patient records are updated and stored (Figure 17-4). This area includes counter space, desk space, adequate lighting, accessible filing system, access to computer terminals, and telecommunication systems. The counter space allows some privacy for the business office staff and provides a space for patients to pay bills and schedule appointments. Often there is a conference

FIGURE 17-3 Reception areas can be designed to appeal to the client population the dentist serves. *(Courtesy of Dr. Charles Regalado and Dr. Jay Enzler.)*

FIGURE 17-4 Business area. *(Courtesy of Dr. Charles Regalado and Dr. Jay Enzler.)*

room or an area somewhere close to the business office for private conversations with patients. Because this area is where the staff makes the first and last contacts with the patient, it should reflect a positive image of the qualities of the dental practice.

Sterilizing Area

The **sterilizing area** should be near the **treatment rooms** and should be neat and clean at all times (Figure 17-5). The sterilizing room should have good air circulation to protect everyone from the chemical fumes and exhaust from the sterilizers. In this area is a sink, counter space for the ultrasonic equipment, and sterilizing units. Infection control protocol is accomplished in the sterilizing area for the patient treatment tray and equipment. Upon completion of sterilization, trays are set up and sometimes stored in this area. Infection control, procedure supplies, and hazardous waste supplies are stored in the sterilization area. (The sterilizing equipment is discussed in Chapter 11, Infection Control.)

Dental Office Laboratory

The dental office **laboratory** is a separate area that is also well vented (Figure 17-6). The amount of lab work done in the office depends on the dentist's preference. If the dentist's practice includes a number of patients needing prosthodontic treatment, a lab technician and a lab is set up in the office. In other offices, the dental lab may be used for finishing or adjusting crowns, bridges, partials, or dentures and for pouring impressions, trimming models, polishing removable appliances, and making custom trays.

The dental laboratory may contain a vibrator, a model trimmer, a laboratory handpiece, a vacuum former, a sink, an exhaust fan, plaster and stone storage bins, a heat source, and a dental lathe. Cupboards provide stor-

FIGURE 17-6 Laboratory area. *(Courtesy of Drs. Rodney Braun and Chris Chaffin.)*

age for instruments such as lab knives, spatulas, and rubber bowls. All aseptic precautions must be followed when working in this setting, because often the materials have been in the patient's mouth before coming to the lab. The staff should wear protective glasses and masks to prevent dust and debris from causing injuries when working with the equipment.

X-Ray Processing Room

The x-ray processing room or **darkroom** is a small room near the treatment rooms (Figure 17-7). This room contains a sink, a manual processing tank, drying racks, space for storage, safelights, and counter space for processing and mounting radiographs. With the use of automatic processors with daylight loading, the need for this space has changed. The automatic processor may be in the processing room or in treatment rooms, the steril-

FIGURE 17-5 Sterilizing area with sink, counter space, storage, ultrasonic unit, and sterilizing unit. *(Courtesy of Dr. Jay Enzler.)*

FIGURE 17-7 X-ray processing area with sink, counter space, storage, and automatic processing unit with daylight loader.

izing area, or an open area in a hall space. (This room and the equipment are described in detail in Chapter 21, Introduction to Dental Radiology and Equipment.)

Radiography Room

In most dental offices, radiograph machines are in each treatment room for intraoral x-rays. The extraoral radiographic equipment is in a radiography room. This room must provide occupational safety from ionizing radiation and be large enough to house this equipment. Guidelines come from the state health department, and periodic inspections may be required by state agencies (Figure 17-8).

Optional Rooms in the Dental Office

Optional rooms in the dental office are dictated by the dentist's preference, patient usage, amount of space available, and practice budget. Any or all of the following rooms may be included in the dental office design. Often the office is built with additional rooms available for later growth in the practice.

Dentist's Private Office. The dentist's private office is designed according to the individual taste of the doctor. The dentist's private office is where the dentist conducts personal and professional business. This office may be used to consult with patients privately or for staff meetings.

Staff Lounge. A staff lounge is a place for staff to have lunch, meet, and relax. In the staff lounge are a sink, refrigerator, microwave, coffee machine, table and chairs, storage cupboards, and countertop space. A washer and dryer may also be in this area.

Patient Education Area. A patient education area is a very functional and diverse area in the dental office. With each type of practice, its use may vary; for example, in

the orthodontic office, the space may be furnished with mirrors and sinks where patients can practice home-care techniques. The patient education area may be an information center containing a variety of information on dental care and treatments available to patients, such as bleaching treatments or dental implants.

Often this room has a sink, a counter or table with chairs, and multimedia equipment including a television and DVD equipment. This area is also used for consultations with the patient or for the patient to wait, if necessary.

The Treatment Rooms and Dental Equipment

Dental treatment rooms are also called **operatories** (Figures 17-9 and 17-10). Each dentist usually has a minimum of three treatment rooms. The type and size of practice

FIGURE 17-9 Dental treatment area: counter space and storage, patient chair, operator and assistant chairs, dental light, dental unit with handpieces, air-water syringe, HVE, and rheostat.

FIGURE 17-8 Panoramic machine area.

FIGURE 17-10 Two treatment rooms with the open concept. *(Courtesy of A-dec, Inc., Newberg, Oregon, USA.)*

dictate the number of operatories. The treatment rooms in a general practice are usually designated for operative dentistry or hygiene and are equipped accordingly. They can be individual rooms or open spaces divided by walls and/or equipment. The rooms need to be large enough to contain the necessary equipment while still allowing for easy access to it. The treatment rooms should be designed for maximum efficiency.

A dental treatment room contains a dental chair, dental unit, operating stools, cabinets, sinks, x-ray machine, x-ray viewbox, and mobile carts. There are many manufacturers and designs of equipment to choose from to meet office requirements. Dental equipment is expensive and, with careful maintenance, is meant to last for years. Someone in the office often is assigned to perform the routine maintenance of the equipment. A dental equipment technician is called when more substantial problems occur.

The Dental Chair

The dental chair is the center of all clinical activity (Figures 17-11 and 17-12). The chair is designed for the operator and the assistant to provide patient treatment comfortably and efficiently. The dental chair supports the patient's entire body, in an upright, **supine position** (reclined position with the nose and knees on the same plane) or a **subsupine position** (reclined position with the head lower than the feet) (See Figure 17-31).

The dental chair is designed to accommodate children and adults. The head rest is narrow to allow the dentist and the assistant to be close to the patient's head and is adjustable to provide support. The dental chair has arm rests that are designed to lift or move out of the way when the patient is being seated or dismissed. It also has controls to move the chair up and down, recline the back rest, and raise the seat and a combination button that automatically reclines or raises the patient. The controls are on the sides of the chair back or on the floor (the floor controls are becoming more popular because they eliminate the need for infection control barriers). The chair also has a control on the floor that allows it to be rotated left and right. To prevent cross-contamination, the head rest and controls on the chair are covered with barriers.

The dental chair is upholstered in a material that is comfortable, easy to clean, and coordinates with the office color theme. The base of the chair is sometimes secured to the floor. The chair base should be cleaned and disinfected routinely.

FIGURE 17-11 Digital controls for adjusting the dental chair position.

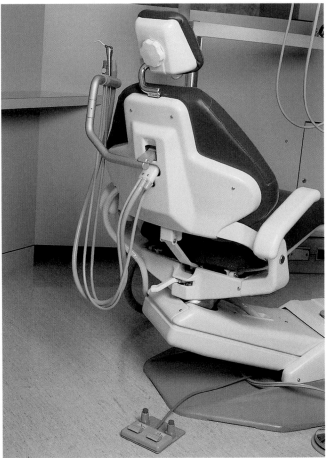

FIGURE 17-12 Dental chair with foot controls for adjusting the chair.

The Dental Unit

The **dental unit** consists of handpieces, an air-water syringe, a saliva ejector, an oral evacuator (HVE), an ultrasonic scaling unit, and numerous other options. The dental unit may be fixed to the wall, the cabinets, or on mobile carts. The unit is positioned according to the preference of the dentists, whether the dentists are left- or right-handed, if they routinely work with assistants, and according to the design of the treatment room. The dental unit is available in three basic modes of delivery:

1. The **rear delivery system** is designed with the equipment behind the patient's head (Figure 17-13).

2. The **side delivery system** is designed with the equipment on the dentist's side. The unit is mounted to a moveable arm or mobile cart (Figure 17-14).

FIGURE 17-13 Rear delivery system. *(Courtesy of A-dec, Inc., Newberg, Oregon, USA.)*

FIGURE 17-14 Side delivery system. *(Courtesy of A-dec, Inc., Newberg, Oregon, USA.)*

3. The **front delivery system** is designed so that it can be pulled over the patient's chest and is between the dentist and the assistant (Figure 17-15).

Mobile Carts. Sometimes, **mobile carts** are used to hold delivery systems, including the air-water syringe, oral

FIGURE 17-15 Front delivery system. *(Courtesy of A-dec, Inc., Newberg, Oregon, USA.)*

evacuator, handpieces, and saliva ejector (Figure 17-16). One cart may be used by both the operator and the dental assistant with the instrumentation on the appropriate side. Two carts, one on each side of the dental chair, may be equipped and used. The **operator's cart** is usually set up for two or three dental handpieces plus an air-water syringe (Figure 17-16A). The **assistant's cart** is usually set up with the air-water syringe, saliva ejector, and HVE (Figure 17-16B). Carts are designed to be

FIGURE 17-16 (A) Operator's cart with dental handpieces and air-water syringe. (B) Assistant's cart with saliva ejector, HVE, and air-water syringe. *(Courtesy of A-dec, Inc., Newberg, Oregon, USA.)*

FIGURE 17-17 Air-water syringe. (A) Handle. (B) Air-water controls. (C) Removable and disposable tips.

FIGURE 17-18 Dental unit. (A) Dental handpieces. (B) Air/water syringe, saliva ejector, high volume evacuation (HVE).

moved easily, provide a work space and some storage, and hold basic instruments.

Air-Water Syringe. The **air-water syringe** provides air, water, or a combination spray of air and water (Figure 17-17). The tip of the syringe is removable and made of disposable plastic or autoclavable metal. New barriers are placed on the syringe handle and the tubing for each patient. The controls for the syringe are on the handle and should be easy to operate with the thumb of one hand. Air, water, and the combination spray help keep the oral cavity clean and dry and protect the tooth from the heat produced by the handpieces. For easier use, the syringe tips come in several lengths and are slightly angled. To reduce the risk of retaining oral fluids, flush the air-water syringe with water between patients and at the beginning and end of the day.

Dental Handpieces. There are usually two dental **handpieces**: low and high speed (Figure 17-18A). The handpieces are attached to hoses that are part of the dental unit. It is important that these hoses are not bent or tangled. Each handpiece has two controls. First, the hose attachment has an on/off switch to prevent more than one handpiece from running at once. Second, the speed of the handpiece is controlled by a foot pedal called a **rheostat** (REE-oh-stat). The rheostat is the round disk as seen on the floor in Figures 17-15 and 17-16A. The dental handpieces are removed after each patient's treatment and are sterilized. (Before removal from the unit, like the air-water syringe, caution should be taken to flush oral fluids from the handpieces.) There are ways to test handpieces to see whether they retract fluids when they stop running and manufacturers are designing means to prevent this from occurring. At the beginning and end of the day, the handpiece should be flushed for several minutes. Between patients, run the handpieces for at least one minute to flush the system. Some dental manufacturers provide a self-contained water system. Each unit has a water reservoir that supplies water for the dental handpieces and the air-water syringes. The **water reservoir** is maintained daily. Distilled water is often used to prevent tap-water deposits from building up in the water lines. (Water line maintenance is discussed in Chapter 11, Infection Control.)

Ultrasonic Scaler. The **ultrasonic scaler** is attached to the dental unit. The scaler is used during prophylaxis and periodontal procedures. Small tips attach to the ultrasonic scaler. The scaler has a vibrating action that removes hard deposits, such as calculus, and other debris from the teeth. (The ultrasonic scaler is also discussed in Chapter 29, Periodontics.)

Saliva Ejector. The **saliva ejector** is used to remove saliva and fluids from the patient's mouth slowly. It has a low volume suction that is used during certain pro-

FIGURE 17-19 Saliva ejector.

FIGURE 17-20 High volume evacuation disposable trap.

cedures, such as fluoride treatments and under rubber dams. The saliva ejector tip is a thin, flexible, plastic tube that is disposed of after each patient's treatment (Figure 17-19). This plastic tip slides into the opening of the saliva ejector hose that is part of the dental unit. There is a small trap in the saliva ejector that must be cleaned routinely.

High Volume Evacuation (HVE). The **high volume evacuation (HVE)** is also called the oral evacuator. It is used by the assistant to remove fluids from the patient's mouth. Evacuation tips are wider tubes that are often beveled at both ends. Some of the tips are metal and can be sterilized, but most offices use plastic tips that can be sterilized or disposed of. The evacuation tips fit into the handle of the hose, which is covered with a protective barrier during procedures. The on/off control for the HVE is on the handle. Each unit has a trap that collects debris from the evacuator (Figure 17-20). This trap must be changed or cleaned weekly or as needed. The HVE is flushed after each patient and there are cleaning systems available to flush and to do a thorough cleaning of the HVE at the end of the day and week.

Dental Stools

Dental stools are required by the operator and the assistant during most procedures. Ergonomic studies have resulted in the improved design of dental stools to provide comfort and prevent fatigue during dental procedures. When selecting stools, the dentist and staff should try a variety of stools to find the one that meets their requirements, provides good support, and is comfortable. There is more information on ergonomics and the dental team later in this chapter. The operator's and assistant's stools have some similarities but also have several differences (Figures 17-21 and 17-22).

Operator's Stool. The operator's stool has the following ergonomic characteristics:

- **Adjustable height**—The stool should have adjustment for height so that the operator's feet can be flat on the floor and the thighs can be parallel to the floor when seated.

- **Adjustable back rest**—The stool should have a back rest that is adjustable, both vertically and horizontally, to provide support and comfort. The back rest should support the **lumbar** region (lower region of the back) of the operator's back.

- **Comfortable seat**—The stool seat should be broad with firm padding and have no seams or edges to restrict circulation in the legs and feet. The seat also should be covered with a material that is easy to clean.

- **Mobility**—The stool should move easily on four to five casters and freely, even on floors with carpet.

- **Broad base**—The stool should have a broad, heavy base to prevent tipping, especially during movement. The base stabilizes the stool for the operator.

Dental Assistant's Stool. The dental assistant's stool has the following ergonomic characteristics:

- **Adjustable height**—The stool should adjust to a variety of different levels to accommodate the height of the assistant. The assistant is positioned four to eight inches higher than the operator, with feet resting on the foot ring and thighs parallel to the floor.

- **Adjustable back rest/Extended arm**—The stool back rest should provide support for the lumbar region and be easily adjustable. Some stools have an extended arm for support of the abdomen or side areas. The arm moves easily into place and locks to stabilize the assistant when leaning or reaching.

FIGURE 17-21 Operator's stool with back support, broad base, comfortable seat, and casters. *(Courtesy of KaVo Dental Corporation.)*

FIGURE 17-22 Assistant's stool with front arm support, comfortable seat, broad base, foot rest, and casters. *(Courtesy of KaVo Dental Corporation.)*

- **Comfortable seat**—The seat of the stool has the same criteria as the operator's stool: a broad, flat surface with no seams or hard edges.

- **Mobility**—The assistant's chair should be designed to move freely. Usually, five casters are recommended to provide stability.

- **Broad base**—The base of the stool should be broad and well balanced. It should be heavy and stable to prevent tipping.

- **Foot rest**—The assistant is usually positioned higher than the operator, so it is difficult to sit correctly on the stool and rest feet flat on the floor. The foot rest gives the assistant support so that good circulation is maintained.

- **Easy to adjust**—All parts of the assistant's stool should be easy to adjust. Adjustments should be made quickly between patients.

Operating Light

The **operating light** is attached to the dental chair or mounted to the ceiling (see Figures 17-13, and 17-14). Both the operator and the assistant should be able to adjust the position of the light. Operating lights have improved in many ways—they are easier to move, more flexible, and direct less heat onto the patient. The light has a control switch for high and low intensities, an on/off switch, and handles on both sides. The light is attached to extension arms for positioning over the patient's face to view the maxillary or mandibular arch.

The handles and on/off switch are covered with barriers during procedures. The barriers are changed between each patient. Maintenance includes changing the lightbulb occasionally and keeping the heat shield clean. It is important to follow the manufacturer's instructions for both of these procedures.

Cabinetry

Most treatment rooms have some type of cabinetry for storage of supplies and materials used during treatment. Some dental units are designed in fixed cabinets that surround the patient, operator, and assistant. These units include cupboards that open from the front and the back for treatment trays, drawers for materials frequently used, and sinks for the operator and the assistant (see Figures 17-13 and 17-14). The amount of cabinetry depends on the size of the room and the dentist's preference.

Mobile cabinets are also used in the treatment room. These cabinets come in a variety of designs and are used for storage and as work spaces. The mobile cabinet is stored against the wall and then pulled into position after the patient is seated.

Sink

The treatment room should be designed with sinks in convenient locations for the dentist and the assistants. Some treatment rooms have two sinks, one on each side of the dental chair. Other treatment rooms have one sink that is located centrally behind the dental unit for both the dentist and assistant to use.

The water controls on the sink should be operated by wrist, foot, or knee controls (this prevents the hands from becoming contaminated after handwashing by turning off the water controls). There are light and motion sensor devices that turn the water on and off automatically when standing in front of the sink.

The sinks should be easy to clean and have an area nearby for soap and towel dispensers.

Dental X-Ray Unit

A dental x-ray unit used to expose intraoral radiographs is part of most treatment rooms. Sometimes the x-ray tubehead is housed between two rooms with doors on both sides for the x-ray tubehead to slide out into either room. The controls are found outside the room so that the dental assistant is not exposed to radiation. (Further information about the x-ray unit can be found in Chapter 21, Introduction to Dental Radiography and Equipment.) The panoramic machine for exposing extraoral radiographs is usually in a separate area outside the treatment room.

Small Equipment Found in the Treatment Room

There may be a variety of small equipment in the treatment room depending on the primary use of the room. Most rooms have an x-ray viewbox, a curing light, an amalgamator, a communication system, a computerized intraoral dental camera, and (typically) a computer linked to the office local area network.

X-Ray Viewbox. The x-ray viewbox is used to read radiographs (Figure 17-23). The viewbox may be placed on a counter or in a wall or cabinet. It consists of a bright light source covered with a frosted surface. X-rays are placed on the frosted surface for clear viewing.

Dental Curing Light. A dental **curing light** is used to "cure" or "set" light-cured materials (Figure 17-24A). Many dental products are now light cured. There are various types of curing lights dentists may choose from depending on the types of materials they use and their preferences. Dentists evaluate the characteristics of curing lights needed according to the intensity and spectrum of the light, the speed of the cure, the heat that is generated, and whether they are lightweight and ergonomic in design, quiet, portable, durable, and reliable. Most curing lights have small motors or sometimes fans, wands, or tips; some have filters, protective shields, handles, and triggers to activate the light. Some have digital display countdown timers and preset curing times. In some offices, curing lights are mounted on the sides of counters or integrated into dental units to conserve counter space.

Light curing units have advanced a great deal over the years and continue to do so as the technology for the curing lights and materials evolve. Curing light technologies include the **tungsten halogen**, **argon laser**, **plasma arc (PAC)**, and **light emitting diode (LED)**.

The traditional curing light uses a tungsten halogen bulb. This curing light has been around for a while and is durable, less expensive, cures relatively quickly, and is fairly effective. It does give off some heat, uses a filter to remove useless energy emitted by the halogen bulb, and the unit is not portable.

FIGURE 17-23 X-ray viewbox.

(A)

(B)

FIGURE 17-24 (A) Dental curing light. (B) LED curing light.

The halogen curing lights do have a fan to cool the unit; thus it is important to remember not to turn off the unit until the fan has stopped. Light intensities can vary and change with use. To determine if the light is working at full capacity, the curing light should be tested monthly.

Curing Light Radiometer. Curing lights should be tested periodically with a **radiometer (light meter)** because the light bulbs will deteriorate over time and not produce an adequate cure. Small hand-held meters are available to test the halogen curing lights. The light guide is positioned over a small area on the meter and then turned on. A reading is given to determine the intensity of the light and the need to replace the bulb. Some curing light units now have light meters built in, so the light can be tested more conveniently (Figure 17-25).

The argon laser (light amplification by stimulated emission of radiation) technology produces a relatively high-intensity light that does not generate noticeable heat. The speed of curing ranges from moderate to fast.

The argon laser lights are not compatible with some dental materials. The laser light will not cure some materials due to the type of photoinitiator used in the materials. The argon laser curing lights are much more expensive than other types of curing lights. (*Note:* The photo-initiator is the substance added to a dental material that reacts to light and acts as a catalyst to initiate the setting [polymerization] process.)

The PAC curing lights, ultrafast and powerful, are more expensive. Some are large units that are not portable. Because these lights produce significant amounts of light that are not useful in the curing process, many of the PAC lights offer multiple setting tips that are filtered. The light tips filter the light to match that of the photo-initiator in the dental material. The PAC units produce a high level of heat that is a concern in some cases.

The LED curing lights are lightweight; some are ergonomically designed and have cordless portability. Some curing lights are mounted on the sides of counters or integrated into the dental unit to conserve counter space. These units are durable, produce minimal heat, have no bulbs, and are quiet because there is no need for a fan. This technology is rapidly changing to improve light performance (Figure 17-24B).

It is not as important to check the corded LED light units with a radiometer as it is with the halogen lights. But the cordless LEDs that are battery powered need to be checked according to the manufacturer's recommendations. The batteries wear down and the light output decreases.

The LED lights are still changing and improving. These lights are so convenient that more and more dental offices are purchasing them. As with all the curing lights there are pros and cons so before an office purchases a new light they should check the manufacturer for procedures the lights are most effective with.

FIGURE 17-25 Curing light being tested for accuracy with a radiometer.

Curing light technology is rapidly changing to improve curing intensities and speed. Materials manufacturers are evaluating their photo-initiator systems. One initiator for photo-curable dental materials being reevaluated is Camphorquinone (CPQ). This photo-initiator system works with a variety of curing lights.

If light guides come in contact with any materials during the curing process immediately wipe them off or the dental assistant can place a sleeve cover over the light guide to protect it or use some acetone to remove any residue that may have formed on the end of the guide.

Amalgamator. The amalgamator is a small machine that mixes (triturates) dental amalgam and some dental cements. It is placed near the assistant, either on the counter or in a drawer (Figure 17-26). (The amalgamator is discussed further in Chapter 34, Restorative Materials Dental Dam, Matrix and Wedge.)

Communication System. The communication system is a color-coded light system or intercom system the office uses as a method for the staff and the dentist to communicate with each other. Usually, the system is found on the walls in the treatment rooms, sterilization area, laboratory, and staff lounge. It is made of a series of colored buttons that light up when pushed or an intercom/phone system. (Refer to Figure 17-2, the layout of the dental treatment room.) The system can designate a specific message or call a member of the dental team. For example, the hygienist lets the dentist know the patient is ready for examination or the receptionist tells everyone that the next patient has arrived. These systems can be customized for the individual needs of an office.

Computerized Equipment. Computerized equipment includes an intraoral camera and a computer terminal. The intraoral wand contains a small camera that transmits to the computer monitor (Figure 17-27). The wand is placed in the patient's mouth, and the image is displayed on the monitor. The computer freezes a picture on the screen or prints it out. The intraoral camera allows the patient to see areas and conditions in their mouth while the dentist is discussing them.

Many offices are computerized with terminals in the treatment rooms as well as the business office. Computer systems allow the office to be "paperless" and to be more efficient at completing specific tasks, such as billing. Some systems allow the dentist and staff to enter treatment plans, chart the condition of the patient's mouth, make the patient's next appointment, bill the insurance

(A)

(B)

FIGURE 17-27 (A) Intraoral camera. (B) Pictures inside the oral cavity using the intraoral camera. *(Courtesy of Gendex Dentsply International.)*

FIGURE 17-26 Dental amalgamator.

company, and give information and instructions. The number of computers and the programs/systems used in the office are determined by the dentist. To use the computers efficiently and effectively, additional training and cooperation of all staff members are required.

Digital radiography equipment is also part of the technology found in the dental office. (Digital radiography equipment is discussed in Chapter 22, Extra Oral and Digital Radiography.)

Dental Air Compressor and Central Vacuum System

The **air compressor** provides compressed air for the handpieces and air for the air-water syringes. The size of the air compressor depends on the number of dental units used by the office. Usually, the compressor is stored away from the main office because of its size and noise level.

The **central vacuum system** provides suction for saliva ejectors and oral evacuators at each dental unit. The filters or traps must be cleaned regularly to keep this system working to capacity. This system is also stored away from the main office.

Dental office staff and dental service companies must follow manufacturer instructions for maintenance and repairs on the air compressor and the vacuum system. Both units may be set up on time clocks to run only when the office is open and operating.

Routine Office Care

With the amount of equipment being operated in the dental office, a routine schedule needs to be in place to ensure proper maintenance control. Often this responsibility is given to the dental assistants. Usually, the office is cleaned professionally, but the assistant should periodically check the overall appearance of the office.

Daily, weekly, or monthly maintenance tasks might include changing x-ray processing solutions, cleaning the inside of the sterilizers, changing ultrasonic solutions, performing monitoring activities to check the effectiveness of the sterilizers, and making miscellaneous repairs. It is necessary to keep replacement parts on hand for equipment that needs routine care (e.g., the O-rings in the air-water syringe, which must be changed when air or water leaks).

Opening and Closing the Dental Office

The daily routine of opening and closing the dental office usually falls to the dental assistants. These tasks are sometimes divided with one assistant opening the office and the other closing the office. If there are numerous staff members often these responsibilities are divided by the week or month.

Whoever is responsible to open the office in the morning usually arrives a half hour to forty-five minutes early and completes the routine (Procedure 17-1) before the other staff members arrive.

To close the office the responsible person stays after the last patient and makes sure everything is turned off and the office is ready for patients the next day (Procedure 17-2).

Concepts of Dental Assisting

Originally, the dentist and the dental assistant worked standing on either side of the dental chair. Although some dentists still may stand occasionally, both the dentist and assistant now sit during procedures most of the time. Many studies and research in ergonomics found that sit-down dentistry was the best for both the dentist and the assistant, creating less strain and increasing efficiency. When the dentist and assistant are working at the dental chair together, it is called **four-handed dentistry**. The assistant assists the dentist throughout the entire procedure, passing instruments, mixing materials, and watching the patient. Sometimes, an additional assistant is needed to bring items to the treatment room, assist the assistant in mixing materials, or help with a patient. This is called **six-handed dentistry**. Four- and six-handed dentistry have proven to be efficient and effective in providing patients with quality care.

Activity Zones

When the dentist and the assistant are positioning themselves around the patient, the following are vital:

- Good visibility of the patient's mouth
- Easy access to all areas of the patient's mouth
- Easy access to dental equipment, instruments, and materials
- Safety and comfort for the patient, the operator, and the assistant

The area around the patient's mouth is divided into four **activity zones**: **operating zone**, **assisting zone**, **static zone**, and **transfer zone**. These activity zones are determined by visualizing the patient's head as the center of a clock (Figure 17-28 and 17-29).

The operating zone is the area where the operator is positioned to access the oral cavity and have the best visibility. For right-handed operators, this area extends from the 7 to 12 o'clock position. For left-handed operators, this area extends from the 12 to 5 o'clock position. The operator moves within the zone depending on which arch, quadrant, or surface of the patient's teeth the operator is working on.

The assisting zone is the area in which the assistant is positioned to easily assist the dentist and access instruments, evacuator, and dental unit or cart without interference. The assistant's zone for a right-handed

PROCEDURE 17-1

Daily Routine to Open the Office

These tasks are done by the assistant each morning. The assistant arrives at the office early to open the office and prepare for the day's schedule.

PROCEDURE STEPS

1. Turn on master switches to lights, each dental unit, the vacuum system, and the air compressor.

2. Check the reception room, turn on lights, straighten the magazines and the children's area, and unlock the patients' door to the office.

3. Turn on the communication system, check the answering machine or the answering system, start the computers, unlock the files, and organize the business area.

4. Post copies of patient schedules in designated areas throughout the office.

5. Turn on all equipment in the x-ray processing area. Change the water in the processing tanks and replenish solutions, if necessary.

6. Change into appropriate clinical clothing, following OSHA guidelines.

7. Review the daily patient schedule.

8. Prepare treatment rooms for the first patients. Check supplies, place barriers, fill water reservoirs, and review patient records. Then, prepare the appropriate trays and lab work for the first patients.

9. Turn on any sterilizing equipment and check solutions levels. Prepare new ultrasonic and disinfection solutions. Complete overnight sterilization procedures.

10. Replenish supplies needed for the day.

PROCEDURE 17-2

Daily Routine to Close the Office

These tasks are done by the assistant at the end of the day. The office evening routine includes closing the office for the evening and preparing for the next day. As with the opening routine, the assistants usually share the responsibility of closing the office. Each office has specific details, but the following are general tasks.

PROCEDURE STEPS

1. Clean the treatment rooms. This may include an in-depth cleaning of the dental chair and dental unit. Flush the handpieces and air-water syringes, run solutions through the evacuation hoses, clean traps/filters, and maintain water reservoirs.

2. Position the dental chair for evening housekeeping.

3. Turn off all master switches.

4. Process, mount, and file x-rays. Follow manufacturer instructions to shut down automatic processors. Turn off water supply to manual processing tanks.

5. Wipe counters and turn off the safe light.

6. Sterilize all instruments and set up trays for the next day. Empty ultrasonic solutions and turn off all equipment. Restock supplies.

7. Make sure all laboratory cases have been sent to the lab and early-morning cases have been received from the lab.

8. Confirm and complete appointment schedule for the next day, insurance forms, and daily bookkeeping responsibilities. Pull charts for the next day.

9. Turn off business office equipment and turn on the answering machine or service. Lock patient and business office files.

10. Straighten the reception room. For the security of the office, all doors and windows should be locked.

11. Change from uniform to street clothes, following OSHA guidelines.

12. Turn off machines in the staff lounge and clean tables and counters.

FIGURE 17-28 Activity zones for a right-handed operator, with the assistant on the left.

FIGURE 17-29 Activity zones for a left-handed operator, with the assistant on the right.

operator is 2 to 4 o'clock and for a left-handed operator 8 to 10 o'clock.

The static zone extends from 12 to 2 o'clock for a right-handed operator and from 10 to 12 o'clock for a left-handed operator. Rear delivery systems are found in the static zone, along with dental instruments and equipment used at the chair.

The transfer zone is the area below the patient's nose where instruments and materials are passed and received. Usually, the operator and the assistant transfer instruments between the area that is below the patient's nose and above the upper chest. To follow the clock concept, this would be between 4 and 7 o'clock for a right-handed operator and 5 and 8 o'clock for a left-handed operator.

Classifications of Motion

There are five **classifications of motion** to describe the dental team's range of motion:

1. **Class I motion** involves only finger movement.

2. **Class II motion** involves movement of the fingers and wrist.

3. **Class III motion** involves finger, wrist, and elbow movement.

4. **Class IV motion** involves movement of the entire arm and shoulder.

5. **Class V motion** involves movement of the arm and twisting of the body.

Ideally, for proper ergonomics the operator and the assistant should be positioned to stay in class I, II, and III motion ranges. The dental unit, counter space, instruments, and equipment should all be close enough to avoid classes IV and V.

Preparing the Treatment Room

The dental assistant prepares the treatment room for each patient. The room is cleaned and disinfected after each patient, and new barriers are placed on the dental unit, dental chair, counters, and dental light switches (see Chapter 11, Infection Control). After all the barriers are placed, the room is tidied so that no obstacles are in the patient's path upon entering the treatment room. The rheostat is placed behind the dental chair, and the operator and dental assistant's chairs are moved out of the way. Mobile carts are pulled out of the patient's path, and the dental light is raised out of the patient's way as he or she sits in the chair. The arm of the dental chair is raised or turned for easy access for the patient. The dental chair is positioned about 15 to 18 inches from the floor, and the chair is tilted back slightly.

Patient records are reviewed to double-check the procedures to be done, and the medical/dental history for each patient is examined for any previous problems or alerts. The x-rays are placed on the viewbox, and the charts/records are located away from the treatment area or covered with a barrier. Any model or lab work is brought into the treatment room. The tray is set up, and accessory items for specific procedures are prepared.

Seating the Dental Patient

One of the roles the dental assistant plays is to put the patient at ease and to begin to establish a rapport with the patient. This begins when the dental assistant seats the patient in preparation for treatment.

Greet and Escort the Patient

Greet the patient by stepping into the reception area and identifying him or her by name. Then, tell the patient that you are ready for him or her now. If you have not met the patient before, introduce yourself, and, before leaving the reception area, ask the patient if he or she wants to hang up his or her coat. Then, ask the patient to follow you into the treatment room.

When escorting the patient back to the treatment room, it is a good idea to identify the room by number, color, or location. Make sure that all obstacles are out of the way, and offer assistance if the patient appears to need it. For example, patients who have trouble getting up out of chairs or patients who walk with canes or walkers may need assistance.

Once in the treatment room, as a courtesy to the patient and for infection control, ask the patient if he or she would like to rinse his or her mouth with mouthwash before he or she sits down. Then, offer to store any personal items, such as a purse or briefcase, on a counter or shelf. These items should be placed where they are in the patient's view but not interfering with the treatment.

It is important to establish rapport with the patients and make them feel welcome and at ease. Remember to talk to the patients and show an interest in what they have to say. Ask them about subjects they are involved with and are comfortable discussing. People like to talk about themselves, their families, work, vacations, and hobbies. Note points of interest on the treatment chart so continued reference can be made. Often, patients will ask questions about dental concerns. General information can be given by the dental assistant. The dentist can answer specifically when he or she comes into the treatment room. Communication with patients begins when they walk into the office and should continue until they leave.

Seat and Prepare the Patient

Ask the patient to be seated in the dental chair. The patient's back should be against the back rest and his or her legs completely supported. Once the patient is in the chair, lower the arm of the chair and offer a drink of water, tissue to remove lipstick, and lip lubricant. Place the napkin or bib on the patient and secure it with the napkin chain (bib clips). Make sure more of the napkin/bib is on the operator's side of the patient. Give the patient safety glasses for protection during the procedure.

Before reclining the patient, review the medical history and ask if the patient has any questions. Then, inform the patient that you are going to recline the chair. Recline the patient to the supine position, with the patient's nose and knees at about the same level (Figure 17-31A). After the dentist has been seated sometimes he or she will lower the patient's head beyond the supine position, this is called the subsupine position (Figure 17-31B). In this position the patient's head is back further and slightly tilted up toward the dentist, making it easier for the dentist to see. Sometimes the chair height will need to be adjusted so the patient is at the height of the operator's elbow; this is about eight inches above the seat of the operator's chair. Adjust the head rest and ask the patient if he or she is comfortable (Figure 17-32).

Position the dental light for maximum illumination of the area where the dental procedure is being performed. This is accomplished by bringing the light about three to five feet from the patient's mouth and tilting the light downward toward the patient napkin. Then, turn the light on (this is to avoid shining the light in the patient's eyes). After the light is on, slowly raise it to the arch being treated.

- For the mandibular teeth, the light is raised and the beam is directed downward (Figure 17-33).
- For the maxillary teeth, the light is lowered and the beam is directed upward (Figure 17-34).

After the light is adjusted, the assistant turns the light off until the operator is seated. During the procedure, the light may need to be adjusted periodically. The assistant must be observant to keep the field of operation well lit.

Ergonomics for the Operator and the Assistant

As individuals stay in the profession of dentistry for many number of years and seek to improve the working environment and reduce stress, dental ergonomics has become an important issue. Ergonomics is the study and analysis of human work, including the anatomic and psychological aspects of people and their work environments. Ergonomics must be learned and then applied to benefit individuals. All members of the dental team should be involved in applying ergonomic concepts in the dental office.

PROCEDURE 17-3

Seating the Dental Patient

This procedure is performed by the dental assistant to prepare the patient for the dental treatment. The dental assistant has reviewed the patient's medical and dental records, cleaned and prepared the treatment room with appropriate barriers, readied the tray setup, and removed any possible obstacles from the patient's pathway. After being greeted by name in the reception area, the patient is escorted to the treatment room by the dental assistant.

EQUIPMENT AND SUPPLIES

- Patient's medical and dental records (updated)
- Basic setup: mouth mirror, explorer, and cotton pliers
- Saliva ejector, evacuator (HVE), and air-water syringe tip
- Cotton rolls, cotton-tip applicator, and gauze sponges
- Lip lubricant
- Patient napkin and napkin clip
- Tissue
- Safety glasses

PROCEDURE STEPS *(Follow aseptic procedures)*

1. Greet and escort the patient to the treatment room. Show the patient where to place personal items, such as a purse, backpack, or coat. Some offices offer mouthwash to the patient at this time.

2. Seat the patient in the dental chair. Have the patient sit all the way back in the chair. (At this time, the dental assistant may offer the patient a tissue to remove lipstick and ask if he or she would like lubricant for his or her lips.)

3. Place the napkin on the patient, and give the patient safety glasses to wear during the procedure (Figure 17-30).

4. Review the patient's medical history for any changes since his or her last visit. Ask the patient if he or she has any questions, and give a brief explanation or confirmation of the dental treatment to be completed at this appointment. Place x-rays on the viewbox.

5. Position the patient for treatment, adjust the head rest until the patient's head is well supported and the patient is comfortable, and adjust the dental light for the appropriate arch.

6. Position the operator's stool and the rheostat.

7. Position the assistant's stool. Put on mask and protective eyewear, and then wash hands and place on gloves before being seated at chairside.

8. Position the tray setup. Prepare the saliva ejector, evacuator tip, air-water (three-way) syringe tip, and dental handpieces.

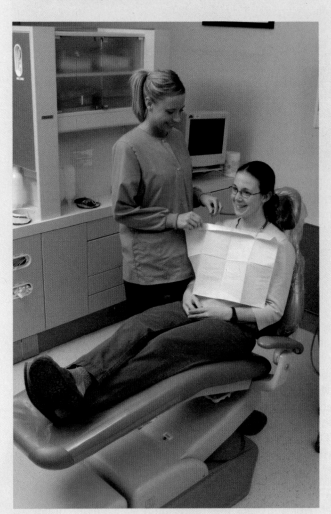

FIGURE 17-30 Dental assistant placing napkin and eyewear on the patient once he or she is seated in the dental chair.

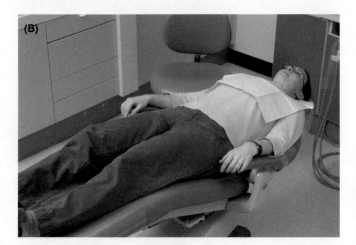

FIGURE 17-31 (A) Patient in the supine position with nose to knees level. (B) Patient in the sub-supine position with the head below the plane of the nose to knees.

FIGURE 17-32 Patient prepared for treatment with protective glasses and napkin in place.

FIGURE 17-33 Patient seated and light adjusted for mandibular arch.

Correct ergonomic practices for the operator and the assistant can save time and prevent muscle strain and fatigue. In four-handed, sit-down dentistry, it is ideal when the equipment and materials are as close as possible to the operator and the assistant. This allows the dental team to function as a coordinated and organized unit. Both the operator and the assistant are seated according to the operating zones previously discussed. (For additional information see Chapter 36, Dental Office Management.)

To prevent back strain and fatigue evaluate the comfort and function of the operator's and dental assistant's stool. The stools should be well padded and easy to adjust to different positions. The material should be easy to clean and maintain.

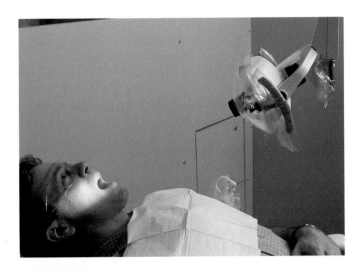

FIGURE 17-34 Patient seated and light adjusted for the maxillary arch.

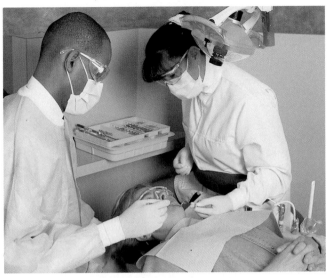

FIGURE 17-35 Operator and assistant positioned for proper ergonomics with patient reclined and ready for treatment.

Ergonomics for the Operator

The operator's position is key to the arrangement of the patient, assistant, and equipment. The operator must be seated in a comfortable position to perform the dental procedure efficiently, with easy access to the oral cavity and clear vision of the operating field. The following are characteristics for proper positioning for the operator:

- The operator is positioned squarely on the seat of the operator's stool, with his or her weight evenly distributed.

- The operator's thighs are parallel to the floor and the feet are flat on the floor. The stool should be adjustable to accommodate varying heights.

- The operator's back is supported in the lumbar region. The back and neck are in an upright position with the top of the shoulders parallel to the floor.

- The operator's elbows are close to the body.

- The patient's chair is lowered over the operator's thighs, to about the same level as the operator's elbow.

- The distance between the operator's face and the patient's oral cavity is approximately fourteen to eighteen inches.

- The operator moves freely in the operator's zone (Figure 17-35).

Ergonomics for the Assistant

The assistant is positioned across from the operator on the opposite side of the patient. The assistant must also have good visibility and easy access to the oral cavity. The tray setup and other necessary instruments should

be close at hand. The following are characteristics of proper positioning for the dental assistant:

- The assistant's stool is positioned 4 to 6 inches above the operator's for good visibility (Figure 17-36).

- The assistant is positioned on the stool so that his or her weight is distributed evenly over the seat.

- The front edge of the assistant's stool is even with the patient's mouth.

- The assistant's feet are resting on a flat ring or tabular bar around the base of the stool just above the casters (wheels), and his or her thighs are parallel to the floor.

- The assistant is positioned as close as possible to the side of the patient.

- The assistant's back is straight, with support in the lumbar region; on some assistant's chairs there is a side support that extends around in front of the assistant. This extension supports the assistant when he or she leans forward slightly or when reaching. The side support is adjusted to fit the assistant at the level of the abdomen.

- After the assistant is correctly positioned on the chair, the cabinet top or mobile cart is placed over the thighs as close as possible for convenience and efficiency.

Dismissing the Patient

After the treatment is completed, the light is turned off and moved out of the way. The dentist leaves and the assistant begins the process of dismissing the patient. The assistant raises the dental chair to an upright posi-

FIGURE 17-36 Dental assistant properly positioned on a stool with feet resting on foot rest, thighs parallel to the floor and back upright.

tion. The patient is asked to remain seated for a minute, in case he or she is a little light-headed from being in the supine or subsupine position during treatment.

The HVE tip, saliva ejector, and syringe tip are removed and placed on the tray. During this time, the assistant wipes any debris from the patient's face and removes the napkin. The tray can be covered with the patient's napkin.

The dental assistant should put on overgloves or remove treatment gloves and wash hands before documenting the procedure and escorting the patient to the reception area.

The rheostat and the operator's chair should be moved out of the patient's way. The right arm of the chair is raised so the patient can stand easily. Ask the patient if he or she has any questions, and give postoperative instructions at the dentist's directions. Return any personal items to the patient, and escort him or her to the reception area.

The dental assistant gathers the patient's records, including the x-rays, to give to the receptionist. The receptionist can make future appointments and complete financial arrangements (Figure 17-38).

Patients with Special Needs

Although most patients can be seated in a routine manner, some patients need special considerations. With most of these patients, planning and preparing before their appointments eliminate problems.

Child Patients

Many of the skills in seating a child patient are the same as when seating an adult. However, some changes are needed to adapt to the child's size, maturity, and age.

PROCEDURE 17-4

Dismissing the Dental Patient

This procedure is performed by the dental assistant after the dental procedure has been completed.

EQUIPMENT AND SUPPLIES

The following items were set up for the procedure and now must be handled as the assistant dismisses the patient.

- Patient's medical and dental records

- Basic setup: mouth mirror, explorer, and cotton pliers

- Saliva ejector, evacuator (HVE), and air-water syringe tip

- Cotton rolls, cotton-tip applicator, and gauze sponges

- Lip lubricant

- Patient napkin and napkin clip

(continues)

PROCEDURE 17-4 *(CONTINUED)*

- Tissue
- Safety glasses

PROCEDURE STEPS *(Follow aseptic procedures)*

1. When the operator is finished with the procedure, rinse and evacuate the patient's mouth thoroughly. The dental light is positioned out of the patient's way.

2. The patient is positioned in an upright position and asked to remain seated. Remove any debris from the patient's face. (The patient can double-check in a mirror before leaving the office.)

3. The napkin is removed from the patient and is placed over the tray setup. The patient's safety glasses are removed (Figure 17-37).

4. The evacuator (HVE) tip, saliva ejector, and air-water syringe tip are removed and placed on the tray.

5. The operator's stool and the rheostat are moved out of the patient's way.

6. After removing treatment gloves and washing hands or donning overgloves, the procedure is documented on the patient's chart or in the computer terminal. The patient's chart and x-rays are gathered.

7. Postoperative instructions are given to the patient.

8. The patient's personal items are returned and the patient is escorted to the reception area.

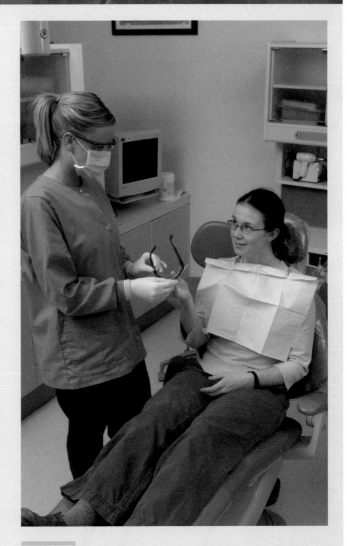

FIGURE 17-37 Dismissing the dental patient after treatment.

Preparing the patient's records is the same, except the child's parent or guardian should be consulted when reviewing the medical history. The dental chair is lowered to accommodate the child. A booster chair, pillow, or cushion may be used to elevate the child in the chair. If the child is too small to reach the head rest, some operators just remove or reposition it so that it does not interfere with treatment or the patient's comfort. To prevent the child from sliding down in the dental chair, have him or her sit with legs crossed (Figure 17-39).

When the dental assistant steps into the reception room, it is important to greet both the parent and the child, but the focus should be on the child. Kneel down to the same level as the child and greet him or her. Escort the child to the treatment room, and assist him or her into the dental chair, if necessary. Answer questions the child has, using language appropriate to his or

FIGURE 17-38 Patient making final arrangements at reception desk before leaving the office.

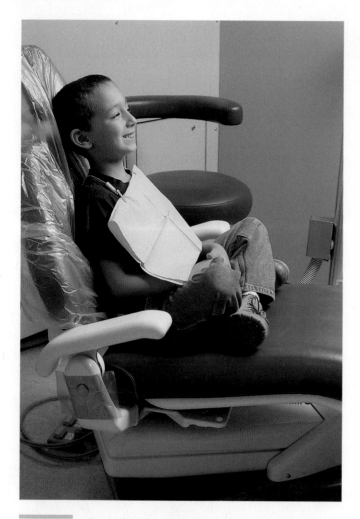

FIGURE 17-39 Child patient seated with legs crossed to prevent sliding down in the chair.

her level of understanding. More information on dealing with the child patient appears in Chapter 28, Pediatric Dentistry.

Once the procedure is completed and the child is dismissed, escort him or her to the reception area and inform the parent/guardian about the treatment performed. Postoperative instructions for the child should be repeated to the parent/guardian.

Senior Patients

With senior patients, assistance may be needed. The dental assistant should be careful not to offend these patients by challenging their ability to take care of themselves. Usually, the older patient will ask for help if it is needed. Review the medical history for any changes in health and medication. Treatment can be broken into shorter segments to accommodate restroom and stretching breaks. The senior patient may not be comfortable in the reclined position for long periods, so

the dental assistant should position the patient upright whenever possible.

Pregnant Patients

When a pregnant woman is sitting in a reclined position, it may be difficult for her to breathe. The dental assistant can allow her to sit upright until the dentist is ready to begin the procedure. During the first trimester of pregnancy, women may find dental treatment uncomfortable because of nausea. The safest and most comfortable time to schedule dental appointments is during the second trimester of pregnancy. Restroom breaks may become more necessary for women in the third trimester of pregnancy.

Hearing-Impaired or Blind Patients

When a patient has hearing difficulties, the dental assistant must be in a position where the patient can observe lip movement and facial expression. Remove the mask and speak normally but slowly; make eye contact and ask questions to be sure the patient understands. To make the patient feel comfortable and show that the assistant really cares about him or her, the assistant may consider learning a few words in sign language.

The patient who is blind may be escorted by someone, but he or she is often very independent. Good communication requires information about his or her abilities and concerns. Talk to the blind patient throughout the procedure, explaining what is happening or what is about to be done.

Patients with Wheelchairs or Walkers

If a patient comes into the office in a wheelchair or using a walker, he or she may need some assistance getting into the dental chair. The pathway to the treatment room should be cleared as much as possible. If the patient is using a walker, give assistance when needed. Usually, the patient has a routine and will tell you if help is needed. The wheelchair patient often needs someone to lift or move him or her from the wheelchair to the dental chair (Figure 17-40).

Patients with special needs know their abilities. Communicate with them to understand their needs and treat them the same as all other patients.

Patients Who Speak No English

Some dental practices have patients who neither understand the procedures nor do they speak English. The dental staff needs to assist these patients in any way they can. Sometimes an interpreter, a relative, a friend, or someone from a church or social agency comes with the patient. This is very helpful, especially during the first several visits. The staff may try to learn key words in the patient's language to assist in communication as well as show that the office cares and is making an effort to understand the patient. The dental staff may research and find information about the patient's country or culture to identify something in common with the patient. Pictures help when trying to make the patient understand what is involved in a procedure and what to expect.

Finding means of communicating with patients from other cultures who speak languages other than English is important. Placing yourself in that situation should help you imagine how you would feel if you have a dental problem when traveling or living abroad. Think of ways to work with these patients.

CHAPTER SUMMARY

Dental health professionals go to great lengths to ensure patient and employee safety and an ergonomic work environment. It is therefore extremely important to understand the dental setting according to facility design, employee role responsibility, and job description by procedure.

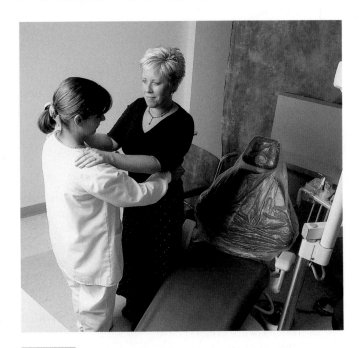

FIGURE 17-40 Patient being transferred from wheelchair to the dental chair.

Case Study

Mrs. Maxine Rose, age 77, had several restorations completed during her hour-long appointment. She is in good health but was in the supine position for most of her appointment.

Case Study Review

1. What can the dental assistant expect will happen once the procedure is complete and the patient is again seated upright?

2. How can the assistant aid Maxine before escorting her to the reception area?

3. Is there anything the dental assistant can do to prevent patients from experiencing discomfort resulting from positioning during treatment?

REVIEW QUESTIONS

Multiple Choice

1. In which of the following areas would a dental unit be located?
   a. Reception area
   b. Dental treatment room
   c. Sterilizing area
   d. Processing room

2. When seating a dental patient, where does the dental assistant place the patient's personal items?
   a. In the reception area
   b. In the treatment room where the patient can see them
   c. In the lounge
   d. In the dentist's office

3. The ultrasonic equipment would be located in which of the following areas?
   a. Treatment room
   b. Sterilizing area
   c. Laboratory area
   d. X-ray processing area

4. The patient is in the supine position when:
   a. The patient is sitting upright
   b. The patient is reclined so the head is lower than the rest of the body
   c. The patient's nose and knees are on the same plane
   d. The patient's nose is a foot above the feet

5. The front delivery systems are:
   a. Pulled over the patient's chest and between the dentist and the assistant
   b. Located behind the patient's head
   c. Located on the dentist's side of the dental unit
   d. Located on the assistant's side of the dental unit

6. The function of the rheostat is to:
   a. Control the air-water syringe
   b. Regulate the water reservoir
   c. Control the speed of the dental handpieces
   d. Control the overhead light

7. The saliva ejector is used:
   a. During fluoride treatments
   b. Under rubber dams
   c. For low volume suction
   d. All of the answers are correct

8. All of the following are true statements about the assistant's stool EXCEPT:
   a. The height is adjustable
   b. There is an extended arm for support
   c. There is a foot rest for the dental assistant to rest his or her feet
   d. There are two arm rests one on each side of the chair

9. Tungsten halogen, argon laser, plasma arc, and light emitting diode are:
   a. Dental amalgamators
   b. Dental curing lights
   c. Computer communication systems
   d. Intraoral cameras

10. The light is raised and the beam is directed downward when working on the _____.
    a. Maxillary teeth
    b. Mandibular teeth

Critical Thinking

1. List ways a dental assistant can create an atmosphere that would put patients at ease and give them the impression that this office is competent and provides quality dentistry.

2. Explain what is necessary when the dentist and the assistant are positioned around the patient to be effective and efficient.

3. Identify methods to ensure comfort for a patient having dental treatment while in the third trimester of pregnancy.

Web Activities

1. Go to http://www.ada.org and search for the ADA's stand on OSHA's ergonomics regulations.

2. Go to http//www.Adec.com and view a line of dental chairs, units, and accessories.

3. Visit www.hspinc.com, and click on the link for the four-handed dentistry training manual. Review the benefits and concepts behind the technique.

CHAPTER 18

INSTRUMENT TRANSFER AND MAINTAINING THE OPERATING FIELD

SPECIFIC INSTRUCTIONAL OBJECTIVES

The student should strive to meet the following objectives and demonstrate an understanding of the facts and principles presented in this chapter:

1. Describe the transfer zone.

2. Define a fulcrum and tactile sensation.

3. Describe the grasps, positions, and transfer of instruments for a procedure.

4. List the eight rules for instrument transfer.

5. Understand instrument transfer modification.

6. Describe and demonstrate how to maintain the oral cavity.

7. Explain the equipment used in the treatment of the oral cavity.

8. Describe techniques for moisture control and isolation.

KEY TERMS

air-water syringe *(360)*

dry angles *(362)*

high-volume evacuation (HVE) *(356)*

fulcrum *(348)*

modified pen grasp *(348)*

mouth props *(361)*

palm grasp *(349)*

palm-thumb grasp *(349)*

pen grasp *(348)*

reverse palm-thumb grasp *(349)*

saliva ejector *(360)*

tactile *(348)*

thumb-to-nose grasp *(349)*

transfer zone *(348)*

INTRODUCTION

In this chapter the dental assisting student will learn the "bread and butter" skills needed when assisting the dentist. Maintaining the operating field and transfer of instruments are very important aspects to four-handed, sit-down dentistry. It is the responsibility of the assistant to think ahead and have everything ready for the dentist as the procedure progresses.

The dental assistant will learn how to grasp the different instruments and then how to transfer the instruments to the dentist. Instruments can be transferred with one or two hands. Both of these methods are discussed as well as modifications when passing two instruments at a time, hinged instruments, dental handpieces, and the air-water syringe.

To maintain the operating field the assistant must adjust the dental light, evacuate the area with the HVE and the saliva ejector, use mouth props, retract the cheeks, lips, tongue, and tissue and know when and where to place cotton rolls and dry angles.

These skills take practice and knowledge of how the dentist wants things. Once the assistant has mastered the basic skills, he or she can adapt to different dentists and/or hygienists fairly easily. By being organized and comfortable with maintaining the operating field and transferring instruments the assistant can make the procedure go smoother and faster.

Instrument Transfer

Instrument transfer or exchange is one of the basic functions in four-handed, sit-down dentistry. The assistant must learn to pass and receive instruments to the operator with confidence and skill. Efficient instrument transfer allows the operator to keep his or her eyes focused on the oral cavity and requires little movement of the operator's hand. A smooth transfer of instruments and materials occurs when the assistant is able to anticipate the operator's needs. This takes practice and cooperation between the operator and the assistant. Once the transfer skills are accomplished, the operator and assistant work as one. The following occurs when proper instrument transfer is accomplished:

- The operator's view remains on the oral cavity.
- Stress and fatigue for the operator and the assistant are reduced.
- Safety and comfort are maintained for the patient.
- Production is increased in less time and with less motion.

The transfer of instruments between operator and assistant takes place in the **transfer zone**, the area just below the patient's nose, near the chin. The assistant brings the instrument to the operator so that the operator will not have to move his or her hand from the established **fulcrum** to exchange the instrument. The **tactile** sensation allows the operator to know that the exchange has taken place without his or her eyes moving from the area. The assistant should pass the instrument with pressure firm enough for the operator to feel the instrument in his or her hand.

Fulcrum

A fulcrum is a point of rest on which the fingers are stabilized and can pivot from. For example, when working on the mandibular first molar, the fingers rest on the occlusal surface of the mandibular bicuspids, providing the fulcrum.

Tactile Sensation

Tactile sensation is the feeling sensed by touch. For example, the pressure of the instrument exchanged during an instrument transfer is tactile sensation.

Transfer Hand

To aid the assistant in the delivery of instruments, the fingers and thumb of the hand are identified as follows: the thumb, the index finger or the first finger, the middle finger or the second finger, the ring finger or the third finger, and the little finger or the fourth finger (Figure 18-1).

The assistant passes and receives instruments with the left hand when working with a right-handed dentist and with the right hand when assisting a left-handed operator. Using one hand for instrument transfer frees the other hand for evacuation and retraction.

Instrument Grasps

The way an instrument is held influences how efficiently the instrument can be used. Selecting the correct grasp allows the operator control of the instrument and greater tactile sensitivity, and reduces fatigue to the operator's fingers and hand. The way an instrument is grasped also dictates how it is exchanged. Several different instrument grasps are commonly used in operative dentistry: pen, modified pen, palm, palm-thumb, and reverse palm-thumb.

Pen Grasp. The **pen grasp**, as the name indicates, is when an instrument is grasped in the same manner as a pen or pencil (Figure 18-2). The instrument is held between the pad of the thumb and the pad of the index finger, with the side of the middle finger on the opposite side of the thumb. With the pen grasp, the instrument is held at the junction of the shank and handle of the instrument (see Chapter 19, Basic Chairside Instruments and Tray Systems). The pen grasp is used to hold instruments that have angled shanks.

Modified Pen Grasp. The **modified pen grasp** is similar to the pen grasp. The instrument is held with the same

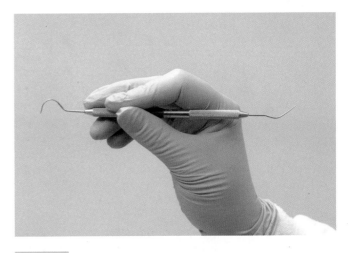

FIGURE 18-3 Modified pen grasp.

T	Thumb	3	Ring finger
1	Index finger	4	Little finger
2	Middle finger		

FIGURE 18-1 Fingers of the hand labeled for instrument transfer reference.

FIGURE 18-2 Pen grasp.

fingers as the pen grasp, except that the pad of the middle finger is placed on the top of the instrument with the index finger (Figure 18-3). The modified pen grasp is preferred by some operators and provides more control and strength in some procedures. This grasp also lessens operator fatigue. The modified pen grasp is used with the same instruments as the pen grasp—those with angled shanks.

Palm Grasp. With the palm grasp, the operator holds the instrument in the palm of the hand and fingers grasp the handle of the instrument (Figure 18-4). The palm grasp is used with surgical pliers, rubber dam forceps, and other forceps. In some procedures, the palm is up when the operator is working on the maxillary teeth and the working end of the instrument is pointed upward. The palm is down when working on the lower teeth and the working end of the instrument is pointed downward.

Palm-Thumb Grasp. For the palm-thumb grasp, the operator grasps the handle of the instrument in the palm of the hand with the four fingers wrapped around the handle while the thumb is extended upward from the palm (Figure 18-5). The palm-thumb grasp is used with instruments having straight shanks and blades, such as the straight chisel or the Wedelstaedt chisel.

Reverse Palm-Thumb Grasp. The reverse palm-thumb grasp is a variation of the palm-thumb grasp that is frequently used to hold the evacuator tip in the patient's mouth. The reverse palm-thumb grasp is sometimes called the thumb-to-nose grasp. With this grasp, the evacuator tip is held in the palm of the hand with the thumb directed toward the assistant instead of toward the patient, as with the palm-thumb grasp (Figure 18-6).

Instrument Transfer Methods

The assistant selects the next instrument and holds it ready for transfer until the operator signals for the

FIGURE 18-4 Palm grasp.

FIGURE 18-5 Palm-thumb grasp.

FIGURE 18-6 Reverse palm-thumb grasp.

exchange. Usually, this signal occurs when the operator tilts the instrument back away from the patient while still maintaining the fulcrum. The assistant removes the used instrument from the operator's hand and places the new instrument in it.

Eight Basic Rules for Instrument Transfer

1. With angled-shank instruments, the primary working end should be placed away from the assistant on the tray.

2. With straight-shank instruments, the primary working end should be placed toward the assistant on the tray.

3. With hinged instruments, the beaks are placed toward the assistant. Once the instrument is picked up, it is rotated so the beaks are up for the maxillary arch and down for the mandibular arch.

4. Hold the instrument between the thumb and the index finger and the middle finger (Figure 18-7).

5. With pen grasp instruments, pick up the instrument from the tray near the end closest to the assistant. This is the end opposite from the one that the operator uses.

6. The assistant's hand is placed on the instrument opposite from the end the operator uses to allow the operator to receive the instrument (Figure 18-8).

7. Rotate the working end of the instrument until it is directed toward the dental arch being treated, positioned upward for maxillary and downward for mandibular.

8. Hold the instrument to be passed parallel to the instrument held by the operator. Instruments are held as close to one another as possible, without becoming tangled during the transfer.

One-Handed Transfer. The one-handed transfer is the most common transfer. It saves time and allows the

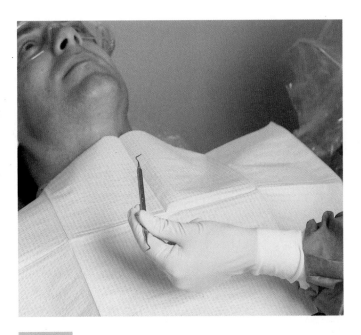

FIGURE 18-7 Instrument correctly held for transfer.

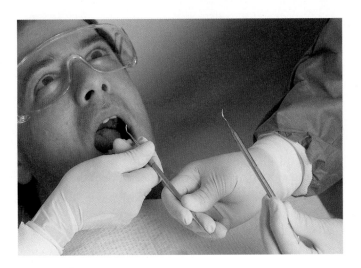

FIGURE 18-8 Two-handed transfer. Assistant uses one hand to receive instrument from the operator and the other hand to pass a new instrument.

assistant to use the evacuator or the air-water syringe at the same time. With the one-handed transfer, the assistant picks up the next instrument to be transferred with one hand and with the same hand receives the instrument the operator is finished using. Immediately after receiving the used instrument, the dental assistant rotates the new instrument into the operator's hand.

With the one-handed transfer, the assistant can also receive an instrument from the operator and then rotate the instrument for use with the opposite working end. A sequence for instrument transfer includes the following movements: the approach, the retrieval, and the delivery (Procedure 18-1).

Two-Handed Transfer. With the two-handed transfer, the assistant uses both hands for the transfer. One hand receives the instrument from the operator and the other passes the next instrument. This transfer is used most commonly for surgical forceps or when both hands are free. For the two-handed pass, the assistant picks up the instrument from the tray and positions it for delivery with one hand. When the operator signals for an exchange, the assistant retrieves the instrument from the operator with one hand and delivers the new instrument with the other hand. This transfer is also used for dental handpieces and the air-water syringe.

The two-handed exchange follows the same steps as the one-handed exchange: the approach, followed by the retrieval, and then the delivery (Figure 18-8). The two-handed transfer requires the assistant to use both hands for the exchange—one to receive the used instrument and one to pass the new instrument to the operator.

Instrument Transfer Modifications

There are times when the transfer must be modified. The operator may have to move away from the mouth to receive some instruments, or the size or weight of some instruments may require the transfer to be modified.

The Mirror and Explorer Transfer. At the beginning of the procedure, the operator needs the mirror and the explorer to examine the area to be treated. The assistant picks up the mirror in the right hand and the explorer in the left hand to transfer to a right-handed operator. The operator signals readiness by putting his or her hands in position. The assistant then simultaneously places both instruments in the operator's hands (Figure 18-9).

The Cotton Pliers Transfer. When nonlocking cotton pliers are used to transfer small items, a one-handed

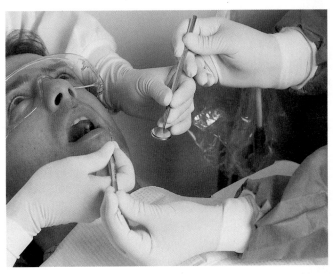

FIGURE 18-9 Mirror and explorer being transferred to the operator at the same time.

One-Handed Instrument Transfer

This procedure is performed at the dental unit by the dental assistant and the operator. In this procedure, the dental assistant uses his or her left hand to transfer instruments for a right-handed dentist. This is reversed for a left-handed operator. The dental assistant's free hand may hold the evacuator or retract oral tissues.

EQUIPMENT AND SUPPLIES

- Basic setup: mouth mirror, explorer, and cotton pliers

- Spoon excavator (for pen or modified pen grasp)*

- Straight chisel, forceps, or elevators (for palm grasp)*

*Any instrument combination can be used to provide a variety of instrument grasps and transfers.

PROCEDURE STEPS *(Follow aseptic procedures)*

Approach

1. Lift the instrument from the tray using the thumb, index finger, and second finger, holding it near the nonworking end (Figure 18-10).

2. Turn the palm upward into passing position, rotating the nib toward the correct arch (Figure 18-11).

3. Move toward the operator's hand.

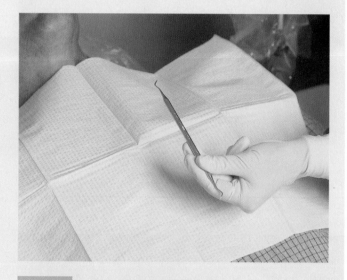

FIGURE 18-11 The assistant carries the instrument and approaches the operator for the exchange.

Retrieval

4. Extend the little finger and/or the ring finger and close around the handle of the instrument the operator is holding (Figure 18-12).

FIGURE 18-10 Instruments on tray in order of the procedure sequence. The assistant picks up the instrument at the end closest to the edge of the tray.

FIGURE 18-12 The operator signals when ready for an exchange. The assistant retrieves the instrument.

(continues)

5. Lift the instrument out of the operator's hand and pull this instrument toward the assistant's palm and wrist.

Delivery

6. Rotate the hand toward the operator and place the instrument in the operator's fingers (Figure 18-13).

7. Once the operator has the new instrument, rotate it to the delivery position for use again or return it to the tray.

FIGURE 18-13 The assistant places the new instrument in the operator's hand.

---

transfer can be accomplished with slight modifications. The assistant must hold the pliers closer to the working end; this way, the item remains secure in the pliers during the transfer. When the pliers are returned to the assistant, he or she receives them at the working end to avoid dropping any materials (Figure 18-14).

Scissors Transfer. Modifications are required of both the assistant and the operator when transferring scissors. The assistant picks up the scissors, slightly open, at the hinge near the working end. The operator's hand is moved away from the oral cavity and positioned with thumb and fingers apart to receive the scissors. The operator's hand comes away from the oral cavity. When finished with the scissors, the assistant receives the scissors near the hinge and the working area (Figure 18-15).

Dental Handpieces. Dental handpieces are bulky, but they can be transferred with the one-handed transfer. The assistant picks up the handpiece near the hose attachment, away from the working end. Handpieces are heavier and, with the hose attachment, are difficult to transfer, but with time and practice the transfer will be smooth and

FIGURE 18-14 Cotton plier transfer. (A) Cotton roll in non-locking cotton pliers ready for transfer. (B) Operator receiving cotton pliers. (C) Operator returning cotton pliers to the assistant.

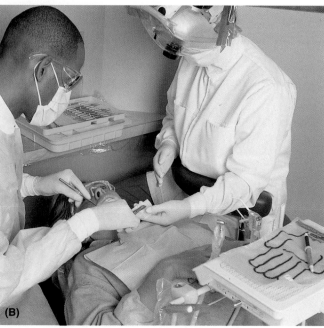

FIGURE 18-15 Scissors transfer. (A) The operator receives the scissors. (B) The operator comes away from the oral cavity to return the scissors to the assistant.

manageable. If both hands are free, use the two-handed pass to transfer the handpieces (Figure 18-16).

Air-Water Syringe Transfer. To pass the air-water syringe, the assistant holds the end of the syringe covering the nozzle and tip with the palm of the hand. The handle of the syringe is projected toward the operator for easier grasping. The operator receives the syringe at the handle. For the return transfer, the assistant receives the syringe in the same manner it was passed, by covering the nozzle and tip with the palm of the hand. This process can be accomplished with both the one- and two-handed exchanges (Figure 18-17).

Miscellaneous Items. The dental assistant transfers dental materials close to the operator's reach, usually near the patient's chin. If the material is on a paper pad, the assistant holds the pad near the patient's chin and holds a gauze for the removal of any excess material (Figure 18-18).

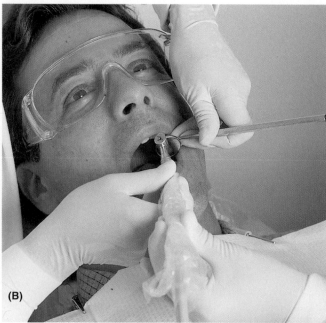

FIGURE 18-16 Dental handpiece transfer. (A) The dental handpiece is prepared for transfer. (B) The operator receives the handpiece.

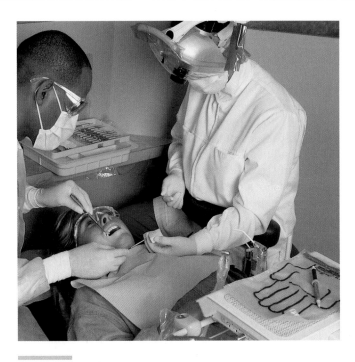

FIGURE 18-18 The dental assistant holds a paper pad with mixed cement close to the patient's chin, ready for the operator's use.

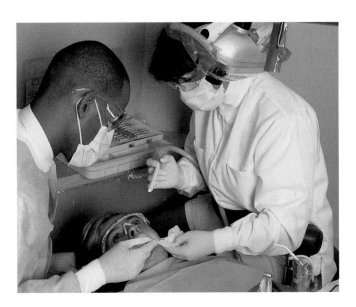

FIGURE 18-19 The assistant holds 2 × 2 gauze open to receive the instrument with debris on the working ends.

Materials that come in a syringe are passed like scissors, with the assistant holding the syringe near the working end. The operator grasps the handle to complete the transfer.

Any time the operator passes an instrument or material back to the assistant with blood and debris on the working end, the assistant should have a gauze ready to place over the working end as the instrument is received (Figure 18-19). This prevents the patient from viewing the blood and debris and contains them.

FIGURE 18-17 Air-water syringe transfer. (A) The assistant holds the air-water syringe near the handle in transfer position. (B) The operator receives the syringe handle with the tip in position for use.

Maintaining the Operating Field

Maintaining the operating field is the process of keeping the area directly involved in the treatment clean, visible, as accessible as possible, and comfortable for the patient. A well-maintained field is essential for the procedure to be performed safely.

The requirements of maintaining the operating field are determined by the type of procedure, the tooth or teeth being treated, the oral anatomy of the patient, and the preferences of the operator. The dental assistant is primarily responsible for ensuring that:

- The operator's vision and access are not obscured by oral tissues, moisture, or debris
- Fluids do not interfere with the application of dental materials
- There are no fluids or materials for the patient to swallow or aspirate
- There is no interference with the manipulation of the handpiece and the instruments being used by the operator

Maintaining the operating field is accomplished by a combination of the following techniques:

- Use of the dental dam or cotton rolls to isolate the field
- Use of high-volume evacuation and the air-water syringe to rinse and clean the oral cavity
- Retraction of oral tissues for clear vision

The following items are used by the dental team for maintaining the operating field:

- Dental lighting
- High-volume evacuator
- Low-volume saliva ejector
- Air-water syringe
- Retractors and mouth props

Lighting

The operator must be able to see the area of the oral cavity that is receiving treatment. Part of the dental assistant's responsibility is maintaining the operating field by positioning the dental light throughout the procedure. The dental light, the illuminated dental mouth mirror, and the fiber optics on the dental handpiece provide the lighting needed to illuminate the oral cavity. (For more information, refer to the section on the dental lighting in this chapter and the fiber optic handpiece discussed in Chapter 19, Basic Chairside Instruments and Tray Systems.)

The Evacuation System

The evacuation system is designed to remove fluids and debris from the oral cavity. Dental handpieces require the use of a water coolant to reduce the frictional heat that is produced while cutting tooth structure. Because there is a considerable amount of water released from the handpiece during this phase of the procedure, a **high-volume evacuator (HVE)** is used to remove the water, saliva, blood, and debris. This system eliminates the need for the patient to sit up and empty his or her mouth.

Parts of High-Volume Evacuation System

- **Hose**—The hose is flexible tubing that connects to the unit at one end and to the handle at the other end. The hose must be long enough for the assistant to reach the patient's oral cavity without restrictions.

- **Evacuation tip**—The evacuation tip is a plastic or metal tip that fits into the handle/hose of the evacuation system. These tips come in a variety of lengths and shapes and can have beveled ends. They may be straight or slightly bent, and they are either disposable or can be sterilized (Figure 18-20A). Some procedures require a tip that is very narrow on one end. These are used during surgical procedures to allow evacuation in a restricted area.

- **Handle**—The handle is where the evacuation tip is inserted and the on/off controls are located. The control switch may be a dial, switch, or button—there are many variations. The assistant should be able to operate the control switch with the hand that holds the evacuator (Figure 18-20B).

(A)

The evacuator tip is placed on this end

(B) This end connects to the evacuation hose on the dental unit

FIGURE 18-20 (A) Several types of evacuator tips (curved metal tip and variety of plastic tips). (B) Evacuator (HVE) handle. *(Courtesy of A-dec, Inc., Newberg, Oregon, USA.)*

PROCEDURE 18-2

Specific Tip Placements for Evacuation of the Oral Cavity

This procedure is performed by the dental assistant during dental treatment. The oral cavity is maintained to keep the area clear and clean for the operator and for the comfort of the patient. Each area of the mouth requires different evacuator tip positioning. The following illustrates how to position the tip for each quadrant when assisting a right-handed operator.

EQUIPMENT AND SUPPLIES

- Basic setup: mouth mirror, cotton pliers, and explorer
- HVE tip and air-water syringe tip
- Cotton rolls
- Dental handpiece

PROCEDURE STEPS *(Follow aseptic procedures)*

1. Maxillary right posterior tip placement (Figure 18-21).

FIGURE 18-22 Evacuator tip in position with cotton rolls. Also, the handpiece and mouth mirror are in position with the air-water syringe tip. The evacuator tip is positioned parallel to the buccal surface of the teeth and is resting on a cotton roll.

FIGURE 18-21 The tip is placed near the lingual surface, just distal to the tooth being worked on. The bevel of the tip is parallel to the lingual surface of the teeth. Notice that the tip is resting on the teeth in the maxillary left quadrant.

2. Maxillary left posterior tip placement (Figure 18-22).

3. Mandibular right posterior tip placement (Figure 18-23).

FIGURE 18-23 Evacuator tip in position with handpiece and mouth mirror. The tip comes across the mandibular left teeth and is positioned between the lingual surface of the teeth and the tongue. The tip is parallel to the lingual surface of the teeth. A cotton roll is used to retract the tongue.

(continues)

PROCEDURE 18-2 (CONTINUED)

4. Mandibular left posterior tip placement (Figure 18-24).

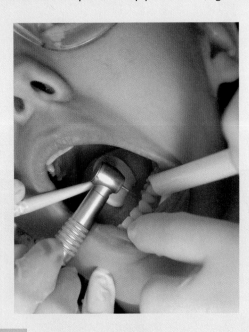

FIGURE 18-24 The evacuator tip is placed and the handpiece is positioned. The tip of the bevel of the evacuator tip is positioned parallel to the buccal surface of the teeth.

5. Maxillary anterior facial tip placement (Figure 18-25).

FIGURE 18-25 The evacuator tip is placed with the handpiece positioned. For the anterior facial tip placement, the operator is positioned on the facial. The evacuator tip is placed near the lingual surface of the maxillary anterior teeth with the beveled tip rotated to catch the water near the facial surface with the bevel of the tip rotated toward the incisal edge of the maxillary teeth.

6. Maxillary anterior lingual tip placement (Figure 18-26).

FIGURE 18-26 The evacuator tip is placed with the handpiece, mouth mirror, and air-water syringe tip. The tip is placed on the lingual, out of the operator's way. Optional tip placement would be from the facial surface.

(continues)

PROCEDURE 18-2 *(CONTINUED)*

7. Mandibular anterior facial tip placement (Figure 18-27).

FIGURE 18-27 The tip is placed and the handpiece is in position. The evacuator tip is positioned on a cotton roll near the facial surface of the teeth. The lip is retracted and the bevel is parallel to the facial surface.

8. Mandibular anterior lingual tip placement (Figure 18-28).

FIGURE 18-28 The tip is placed and the handpiece and the mouth mirror are positioned. The evacuator tip is positioned with the bevel parallel to the lingual surface of the teeth.

In Which Hand Is the Evacuator Positioned?

The evacuator is held in the assistant's right hand when assisting a right-handed operator and in the left hand when assisting a left-handed operator.

Grasps for Oral Evacuation. There are several ways to grasp an evacuator tip. Which grasp to use is determined by where the tip is placed, whether it is used to evacuate fluids or retract tissue or both, and how comfortable the assistant feels with the grasp. The grasps most commonly used are the pen, modified pen grasp, thumb-to-nose, and the reverse palm-thumb. The pen grasp or the modified pen grasp are used when working on the anterior maxillary and mandibular teeth or when using the narrow surgical tip. The thumb-to-nose grasp is used for maxillary and mandibular posterior teeth. When using the thumb-to-nose grasp, the assistant has greater control and better retraction of the cheeks and tongue, and causes less strain on the assistant's hand.

General Guidelines for Oral Evacuation Tip Placement

- Carefully place the evacuator tip in the patient's mouth. Avoid bumping the teeth, lips, or gingiva.

- Place the evacuator tip in the mouth, and position it before the operator positions the handpiece or an instrument.

- Place the evacuator tip approximately one tooth distal to the tooth being worked on.

- Hold the bevel of the evacuator tip parallel to the buccal or lingual surface of the teeth.

- The middle of the evacuator tip opening should be even with the occlusal surface. Position the tip far enough away from the handpiece so that it does not draw the water coolant away from the bur.

- Hold the evacuator tip still while the handpiece or instrument is being used. Any movement may startle the operator or the patient and may cause the handpiece or instrument to be bumped.

- Rest the tip on cotton rolls, not the gingival tissue. Cotton rolls are placed in the vestibular area near the tooth being worked on before the evacuator tip is placed.

- Avoid placing the evacuator tip on the soft palate, the back of the tongue, or the anterior pillar/tonsilar area. Allowing the tip to contact any of these areas could cause the patient to gag.

- Keep the evacuator tip far enough away from the mucosal tissue to prevent it from being sucked into the tip and making a noise. If this does occur, either turn it off or rotate the tip to break the seal, and avoid saying "Oops" or "I'm sorry." Just go on with the procedure.

Refer to Chapter 11, Infection Control, for a review on how to maintain the HVE and saliva ejector. It is important for the dental assistant to establish a routine for maintaining these systems

Saliva Ejector

The **saliva ejector** is the low-volume evacuation system. It is a flexible, plastic tube about one-third the size of the high-volume evacuation tube. The saliva ejector is bent and then positioned between the tongue and the mandibular teeth or between the cheek and the mandibular teeth.

Parts of the Saliva Ejector

- **Plastic tube** or a metal "shepherd's hook" tube—The plastic tube is the most common, although stainless-steel tubes are available. The plastic saliva ejectors are less expensive and are disposable. The end placed in the patient's mouth has a guard cover to prevent large particles of debris from becoming lodged in the tube.

- **Handle**—The plastic tube is inserted in the handle, which is connected to the hose. The handle has an on/off control and also a small screen that acts as a filter, located near the tube end of the handle.

- **Hose**—The hose end attaches to a low-volume vacuum source in the unit.

The saliva ejector is used during procedures that do not require removal of large amounts of fluids, such as during fluoride treatments, under the rubber dam, or during a coronal polish (Figure 18-29).

The Air-Water Syringe

The **air-water syringe**, also referred to as the three-way syringe, emits water, air, or a combination of both in a spray. The patient's mouth is rinsed with the air-water syringe and simultaneously evacuated. The assistant can dry an area or keep the mirror clean with air for the operator to have clear vision. The air-water syringe is held in the assistant's left hand for a right-handed operator and in the right hand for a left-handed operator.

Parts of the Air-Water Syringe

- **Handle**—The handle is connected to a hose which in turn is connected to the unit. The top of the handle is called the nozzle area and has buttons for the water and the air. If the buttons are pressed simultaneously, a spray of water and air is released (Figure 18-30A). In the handle, there are O-rings that may have to be changed if the syringe begins to leak.

- **Syringe tip**—The syringe tip directs the air, water, or spray. The tips are either metal and can be removed and sterilized or plastic and disposable. The tips can be rotated for positioning toward the maxillary or mandibular teeth (Figure 18-30B).

FIGURE 18-29 (A) Saliva ejector hose, control, and several different types of saliva ejectors. (B) Saliva ejector in the patient's mouth. Notice the handle control on the hose and the flexibility of the saliva ejector, bent to stay in the patient's mouth.

FIGURE 18-30 Parts of the air-water syringe: (A) handle, (B) syringe tip, (C) air control, (D) water control. Both controls are pressed simultaneously for air-water spray. *(Courtesy of A-dec, Inc., Newberg, Oregon, USA.)*

Guidelines for Use of the Air-Water Syringe

1. The most effective way to use the air-water syringe is with the air-water spray. A spray is effective and easier to control (Figure 18-31A). However, the spray creates aerosal and so some dentists prefer water followed by air.

FIGURE 18-31 (A) Assistant using the air-water syringe. (B) Assistant using the HVE and the air-water syringe.

2. When rinsing a patient's mouth, use the evacuator tip to follow the spray. The patient's mouth is rinsed in quadrants, and the evacuator tip and the air-water syringe tip are rotated for correct placement (Figure 18-31B). Rinsing and evacuating the patient's mouth requires practice to achieve efficiency and control.

3. When the operator is using the handpiece and a mirror for indirect vision, water from the handpiece falls onto the mirror and distorts the operator's view. The assistant will be expected to keep the mirror surface dry and free from debris. To accomplish this, the assistant places the tip of the air-water syringe close to the edge of the mouth mirror and directs air across the surface of the mirror without interfering with the operator's view.

4. When the operator stops the handpiece, the assistant completes a quick "rinse and dry" to give the operator a clean, dry mirror for good vision. This is accomplished by using the spray, followed by air.

Retraction of Tissues

Retraction of the tongue, cheeks, lips, and tissue is used to increase the field of vision in the oral cavity. There are several types of retractors used, including the mouth mirror, the rubber dam, the evacuator tip, cotton rolls, cotton gauze, and specially designed tissue retractors. Retractors are used during any procedure to allow for better access and lighting and to prevent injury to the tissues (Figures 18-32A and B).

Mouth Props. Mouth props are used to assist the patient in keeping his or her mouth open during treatment (Figure 18-33A). Mouth props are available in several different wedge-shaped designs and materials such as rubber, plastic, and styrofoam. Another distinctive type

FIGURE 18-32 (A) Retraction using a mouth mirror. (B) Retraction using cotton gauze.

FIGURE 18-33 (A) Examples of mouth props. (B) Mouth prop in a patient's mouth.

of mouth prop is a metal adjustable prop, with rubber tubing over the area where the teeth rest and a handle to adjust the opening. To place the prop between the maxillary and mandibular teeth, ask the patient to open wide, insert the prop, and instruct the patient to close on the prop. After placing the prop, ask if the patient is comfortable and adjust the prop, if necessary (Figure 18-33B).

Techniques for Moisture Control and Isolation

We have discussed the use of the saliva ejector and the HVE to control the moisture in the oral cavity and the importance of removing fluids and keeping the area dry and free of debris. Several other techniques can assist in keeping the field dry during a procedure. These techniques include the use of cotton rolls, dry angles (absorbent wafers), and the placement of the dental dam. (Dental dam techniques are described in Chapter 34, Restorative Materials, Dental Dam, Matrix, and Wedge.)

Cotton Rolls

Cotton rolls come in a variety of sizes and designs. They are used to isolate an area, rest the evacuator (HVE) on, place materials with, or serve as something for the patient to bite on. Cotton rolls are flexible for easy placement. They can be placed using cotton pliers or directly placed in the mouth by the dentist or the dental assistant. To place the cotton rolls on the buccal side (cheek side) of the teeth (for both the

maxillary and mandibular arches), the cheek is gently pulled away from the teeth. The cotton roll is then placed in the vestibule area (the pocket formed by the soft tissues of the cheeks and the gingiva, sometimes referred to as the mucobuccal fold). To place cotton rolls on the lingual side of the mandible, the tongue is gently retracted and then the cotton roll is placed between the lingual surfaces of the teeth and the base of the tongue.

To remove the cotton rolls from the mouth, again either use cotton pliers or directly remove from the mouth. When cotton rolls are moist, they remove easily. When they are dry, they should be *moistened with water* from the air-water syringe before removal. When cotton rolls are dry, they stick to the mucosal tissues and need to be moistened to prevent tissue irritation.

Dry Angles

Saliva from the parotid gland enters the mouth through the Stenson's duct. As discussed in Chapter 7, Head and Neck Anatomy, the Stenson's duct is on the buccal mucosa around the maxillary second bicuspid area. To help control the moisture from this area, **dry angles** are used. Dry angles are triangular, absorbent pads that absorb the flow of saliva and protect the cheek (Figure 18-34A). Dry angles are placed directly on the buccal mucosa and absorb moisture as well as provide a surface for cheek retraction (Figure 18-34B). Like cotton rolls, they need to be moist before removal. Use the air-water syringe to wet the dry angle, then remove with cotton pliers. Dry angles may need to be changed during the procedure if they become too saturated with moisture.

FIGURE 18-34 (A) Dry angles. (B) Dry angles placed in a patient's mouth against the cheek.

CHAPTER SUMMARY

Four handed, sit-down dentistry has changed the role of the dental assistant. Working right at the chair with the dentist or dental hygienist the assistant has become an important aspect of performing dental procedures on patients. Transferring instruments and evacuation are skills the dental assistant will use every day with every patient. Learning how to correctly perform these tasks and understanding what needs to be done during a procedure will enable the dental assistant to be a great asset to the operator and a comfort to the patient.

Case Study

Dr. Danton and his assistant, Kaitlin, are placing a composite filling on Chance Garrett. Kaitlin wants to prove her skills and efficiency during the procedure by having instruments ready and keeping the operating field clean and dry.

Case Study Review

1. What can Kaitlin do to prepare for the procedure that will keep everything moving smoothly during the procedure?

2. Describe how Kaitlin should transfer instruments.

3. What is involved in maintaining the operating field?

REVIEW QUESTIONS

Multiple Choice

1. There are four activity zones. Which zone extends from 12 to 2 o'clock for a right-handed operator?
   a. Operating zone
   b. Assisting zone
   c. Static zone
   d. Transfer zone

2. All of the following are instrument grasps except the
   a. pen grasp.
   b. modified pen grasp.
   c. palm grasp.
   d. palm-index finger grasp.

3. Which of the following is used to remove small amounts of fluid and debris from the oral cavity?
   a. The saliva ejector
   b. The oral evacuator
   c. The HVE
   d. The air-water syringe

4. Which grasp is generally used with instruments that have plier-like (hinged) handles?
   a. Pen grasp
   b. Modified pen grasp
   c. Palm-thumb grasp
   d. Palm grasp

5. The three procedure steps in instrument transfer are:
   a. Approach, delivery, and return
   b. Pick-up, retrieval, and return
   c. Approach, pick-up, and retrieval
   d. Approach, retrieval, and delivery

6. When a pen grasp instrument is received by the dentist, the dentist grasps it:
   a. In the middle of the handle
   b. Near the working end
   c. Near the non-working end
   d. None of the above

7. Which of the following is used to assist the patient to hold his/her mouth open during treatment?
   a. The evacuator tip -HIV
   b. A bite block
   c. A saliva ejector
   d. An air-water syringe

8. The evacuator tip (HVE) is usually positioned:
   a. One tooth posterior to the tooth being treated
   b. One tooth anterior to the tooth being treated
   c. On the opposite side of the mouth from the area being treated
   d. Always near the most posterior tooth in the arch

9. To work on tooth #29 for an MO, the evacuator tip (HVE) placement on the mandibular right quadrant is:
   a. The bevel on the lingual surface of tooth #30
   b. The bevel on the buccal surface of tooth #31
   c. The bevel on the lingual surface of tooth #19
   d. The bevel on the buccal surface of tooth #18

10. Water and debris that is suctioned from the mouth through the evacuator tip (HVE) goes into:
    a. The cuspidor
    b. The filter
    c. The sink
    d. A recycling center

Critical Thinking

1. How can contamination buildup in the evacuator and air-water syringe be prevented?

2. Identify ways to control moisture and isolation methods in the oral cavity. List the location of the salivary glands and ducts to locate areas that need moisture control.

3. How does the dentist steady his or her hand when working with a dental instrument to ensure control?

Web Activities

1. Go to http://osap.org. Find the dental waterline fact sheet. Look under "How" for what you can do to prevent contamination of dental unit waterlines.

CHAPTER 19

BASIC CHAIRSIDE INSTRUMENTS AND TRAY SYSTEMS

SPECIFIC INSTRUCTIONAL OBJECTIVES

The student should strive to meet the following objectives and demonstrate an understanding of the facts and principles presented in this chapter:

1. Identify the parts of an instrument.
2. Describe how instruments are identified.
3. Identify the categories and functions of dental burs.
4. Describe the types and functions of abrasives.
5. Explain the various handpieces and attachments.
6. Describe the types of tray systems and color-coding systems.

KEY TERMS

abrasives *(382)*

acrylic bur *(381)*

air abrasion *(386)*

amalgam carrier *(374)*

amalgam condenser *(374)*

amalgam gun *(374)*

angle former *(371)*

bevel *(366)*

bi-beveled *(366)*

binangle *(367)*

Black's formula *(368)*

blade *(366)*

bur block *(383)*

burnisher *(375)*

burs *(378)*

carborundum disc *(382)*

carver *(374)*

cement spatula *(376)*

chisel *(369)*

chuck *(384)*

composite instrument *(373)*

contra-angle *(384)*

cotton plier *(373)*

crown and collar (bridge) scissors *(376)*

cutting edge *(366)*

electric handpiece *(385)*

excavator *(371)*

explorer *(372)*

fiberoptic light source *(384)*

file *(375)*

finishing knife *(375)*

frictional heat *(383)*

friction-grip shank *(379)*

gingival margin trimmer (GMT) *(370)*

hatchet *(370)*

high-speed handpiece *(384)*

hoe *(370)*

Jo-dandy disc *(382)*

laboratory spatula *(376)*

latch-type shank *(379)*

low-speed handpiece *(384)*

mandrel *(382)*

manufacturer's number *(368)*

microetcher *(386)*

monangle *(367)*

mouth mirror *(372)*

periodontal probe *(373)*

plastic filling instrument *(373)*

plastic spatula *(376)*

(continues)

KEY TERMS *(continued)*

preset tray system *(387)*

revolutions per minute (rpm) *(384)*

rheostat *(384)*

rotary instrument *(378)*

separating disc *(382)*

shaft *(367)*

shank *(367)*

straight shank *(379)*

vulcanite bur *(381)*

working end *(366)*

INTRODUCTION

Dental instruments are continually developing as technology changes and dental materials require instruments of specific designs or materials. Most instruments are made of stainless steel, and a few consist of a high-tech plastic/resin or anodized aluminum. Manufacturers of dental instruments provide many designs and sizes and make improvements as new materials become available. Dentists select the instruments that they feel the most confident and comfortable using. Each procedure requires special instruments to accomplish the task. For example, when examining the pits and grooves of the teeth, the dentist uses an explorer. The ends of all explorers are pointed and sharp but designed with different angles to reach all surfaces of the tooth.

The dental assistant is responsible for keeping the instruments sterilized and in working condition. The dental assistant orders new instruments as needed and keeps the instruments in sequence while assisting during the procedure.

Instruments are generally categorized into hand instruments and rotary instruments. Hand instruments are manually operated and are categorized by procedure. In this chapter, the basic instruments used in general dental procedures are discussed, including common cutting and noncutting instruments.

Instruments for Basic Chairside Procedures

Learning the parts of dental instruments will aid in the understanding of how and where the instrument is used. Dental instruments are also classified in several different ways including number of working ends, their function, manufacturer's number, and Black's formula. The classifications make it easier to remember each instrument's name and function.

Instruments for basic chairside procedures include the basic setup found on all trays. This basic setup includes the mouth mirror, explorer, and cotton pliers. Sometimes a periodontal probe is included in this setup. Instruments that are found on restorative tray setups such as composite and amalgam procedures will also be discussed in this section. Instruments used for

specialty procedures will be found in the specific specialty chapters, such as the root canal instruments will be found in the Endodontic chapter.

Basic Structural Parts of Dental Hand Instruments

The dental instrument is generally six inches long and is single- or double-ended. The parts of the dental hand instrument include the working end, shank, and handle (Figure 19-1).

The Working End of an Instrument. The working end performs the specific function of the instrument. The working end may be a point, blade, or nib. A point is sharp and is used to explore, detect, and reflect materials. The blade may be flat or curved and have a rounded or cutting edge. The cutting edge is formed by a bevel (slanted edge or side) on the working end of the instrument. The blade may also be bi-beveled (beveled on both sides of the blade). A nib is a blunt end that is serrated or smooth (Figure 19-2).

The working ends of instruments may also be beaks or rounded ends. The beaks may be smooth, serrated, or grooved, depending on their functions. The rounded

FIGURE 19-1 Parts of the single-ended dental instrument. *(Courtesy of Miltex Instrument Co., Inc., Lake Success, NY.)*

FIGURE 19-2 Various working ends. (A) Point. (B) Blade. (C) Nib. *(Courtesy of Miltex Instrument Co., Inc., Lake Success, NY.)*

FIGURE 19-3 (A-E) Various instrument handle styles. (F-I) Ergonomically designed handles.

ends come in different sizes and shapes and are used to smooth surfaces.

The Handle (Shaft). The handle, or shaft, of an instrument is where the instrument is held by the operator. The handle may be serrated or smooth. It is usually hexagonal (six sided), which provides for a better grip. Some handles are ergonomically designed, which means they are made larger and designed with finger rests and grooves. Other handles are covered with a soft, rubber-like material that makes the instruments easier to hold and grip. These instruments are sterilizable and durable. A few instruments are designed with cone socket handles, which allow the working ends to be replaced (Figure 19-3).

The Shank. The shank connects the handle to the working end. It narrows or tapers from the handle to the working end. The shank may be angled to reach particular areas of the mouth. Usually, instruments that are used in the posterior areas of the oral cavity have more angles, while instruments with fewer angles are used in anterior areas. Shanks of dental instruments are formed in the following ways: straight (no angles), curved (slightly bent), monangle (one angle), binangle (two angles), or triple angle (three angles) (Figure 19-4).

FIGURE 19-4 Instrument shanks. (A) Straight. (B) Curved. (C) Monangle. (D) Binangle. (E) Triple angle.

Basic Classification of Dental Instruments

Dental instruments are classified in many ways, including by number of working ends, function, manufacturer's name and number, and Black's number formula.

Number of Working Ends. The number of working ends on an instrument falls into two categories: single-ended and double-ended instruments (Figure 19-5). Single-ended instruments have only one working end and long handles. Double-ended instruments have two working ends in the following combinations:

- The two ends have similar functions, but one end is larger than the other (for example, an amalgam condenser).

- The two ends are paired right and left for preparing the right or the left side of a cavity preparation (for example, a gingival margin trimmer).

- The two ends have a combined function in which the ends are used for the same procedure but each end has a different use (for example, a plastic filling instrument).

Instruments Classified by Function. Instruments are classified by function. Operative hand instruments are categorized as **cutting** and **noncutting**. Other instruments are classified according to a specialty, use with a specific material, or a procedure.

Cutting and Noncutting Instruments

Cutting Instruments
- Angle formers
- Chisels
- Excavators
- Gingival margin trimmers
- Hatchets
- Hoes

Noncutting Instruments
- Basic instruments (mouth mirror, explorer, and cotton pliers)
- Burnishers
- Carriers
- Carvers
- Composite instruments
- Condensers
- Files
- Finishing knives
- Plastic filling instruments

Manufacturer's Number. The manufacturer's number is found on the handle of the instrument. This number, used when ordering the instrument, indicates the instrument's placement in a set of instruments. Some instruments are named or classified by the name of the individual who designed the instrument.

Black's Formula. Black's formula was developed by G.V. Black to standardize the exact size and angulation of an instrument. This formula minimizes discrepancies in the production of instruments from one manufacturer to another and simplifies ordering instruments. Black's formula for hand cutting instruments includes the size of the blade and the angle at which it is positioned to the handle. Some instruments, such as chisels, hatchets, and hoes, have series of three numbers and some, such as angle formers and gingival margin trimmers, have four numbers.

FIGURE 19-5 Working ends of (A) cotton pliers for transporting materials and (B) burnishers for smoothing materials. *(Courtesy of Miltex Instrument Co., Inc., Lake Success, NY.)*

Black's Three Number Formula
1. The first number (Figure 19-6) is the width of the blade in tenths of a millimeter. In the formula 20 9 14, the first number (20) indicates that the blade is 2.0 mm wide.
2. The second number is the length of the blade in millimeters. In the formula 20 9 14, the second number (9) indicates that the blade is 9 mm long.
3. The third number gives the angle of the blade to the long axis of the handle, in degrees centigrade. In the formula 20 9 14, the third number (14) indicates that the instrument has a blade at an angle of 14/100 of a circle.

FIGURE 19-6 Instrument with Black's three-number formula.

FIGURE 19-7 Instrument with Black's four-number formula.

Black's Four-Number Formula

1. The first number (Figure 19-7) is the same as that in the three-number formula, representing the width of the blade in tenths of a millimeter. In the formula 15 85 8 12, the first number (15) indicates that the blade is 1.5 mm long.

2. The second number differs from that in the three-number formula, representing the degree of the angle of the cutting edge of the blade to the handle of the instrument. In the formula 15 85 8 12, the second number (85) indicates that the cutting edge forms an 85-degree C angle with the handle.

3. The third number is the same as the second number in the three-number formula. Using the formula 15 85 8 12, the third number (8) indicates that the blade is 8 mm long.

4. The fourth number is the same as the third number in the three-number formula. Using the formula 15 85 8 12, the fourth number (12) indicates that the blade forms a 12-degree C angle with the handle of the instrument.

Cutting Instruments

Hand cutting instruments are used to assist in the design of the cavity preparation. They refine and define the cavity walls and margins. There are six hand cutting instruments: chisels, hatchets, hoes, gingival margin trimmers, angle formers, and excavators.

Chisels. Chisels are used to shape and plane enamel and dentin walls of the cavity preparation. The blade of the chisel is straight and has a cutting edge with a one-sided bevel. The chisel is usually a double-ended instrument—one end with a standard bevel on the blade and one end with a reversed bevel on the end of the blade (Figure 19-8). Chisels have several different shanks, which is where they get their names.

FIGURE 19-8 (A) Chisel with standard and reverse bevel. (B) Close-up view of the working end of the chisel. *(Courtesy of Hu-Friedy Mfg. Co., Inc.)*

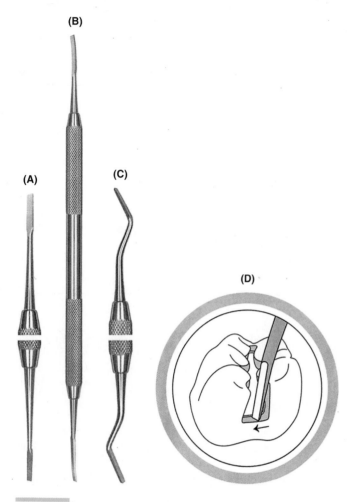

FIGURE 19-9 Chisels. (A) Straight. (B) Wedelstaedt. (C) Binangle. (D) Chisel being used to prepare cavity. *(Courtesy of Hu-Friedy Mfg. Co., Inc.)*

- *Straight chisels* have no angle in the shanks and are used on maxillary and mandibular teeth in class III or IV cavity preparations (Figure 19-9A). Straight chisels are used with a mallet to remove fixed prosthetics.
- *Wedelstaedt chisels* have slightly curved shanks and are used for class III and IV cavity preparations (Figure 19-9B and D).

- *Binangle chisels* have two angles in the shanks of the instruments and are used in Class II cavity preparations (Figure 19-9C).

Hatchets. **Hatchets,** sometimes called enamel hatchets, are similar to hatchets used to cut wood. There is an angle in the shank of a hatchet and the blade is flat. Hatchets are paired left and right, with a bevel on one side of the blade on one end of the instrument and on the reverse side of the blade on the other end. The hatchet is used in a downward motion to refine the cavity walls and to obtain retention in the cavity preparation (Figure 19-10). Sometimes, hatchets are marked with rings on the handles to indicate left and right ends.

Hoes. A **hoe** is an instrument that is used in a pulling motion to smooth and shape the floor of the cavity preparation. A hoe is shaped like a garden hoe, with straight and angled shanks. All hoes have blades that form cutting edges (Figure 19-11A and B).

Gingival Margin Trimmers. The **gingival margin trimmer (GMT)** is similar to the hatchet regarding the position of the blade to the handle, but there are two distinct differences. First, the blade on the GMT is curved, not flat like the hatchet. Second, the cutting edge is at an angle, not straight across like the hatchet. The GMT is a double-ended and paired instrument. With the double ends of the instrument, one end curves toward the left and the other end curves toward the right. A pair of GMTs is used during the cavity preparation, because one instrument is for the distal surfaces and another is for the mesial surface (Figures 19-12A and B). The GMTs are used to bevel the gingival margin wall of the cavity preparation.

Gingival Margin Trimmer Identification

To distinguish between the mesial and the distal GMT, consider the following:
1. *The number on the handle.* This is a Black's four-numbered instrument, so the second number in the series on the handle indicates the angle of the blade. If this number is 90 or above, it is used on the distal surface of the cavity preparation; if it is 85 or below, it is used on the mesial surface.

FIGURE 19-10 (A) Hatchet. (B) Close-up view of working end of the hatchet. *(Courtesy of Hu-Friedy Mfg. Co., Inc.)*

FIGURE 19-11 (A) Hoe. (B) Fracturing away the undermined enamel with a hoe. (C) Close-up view of working end of the hoe. *(Courtesy of Hu-Friedy Mfg. Co., Inc.)*

FIGURE 19-12 Gingival margin trimmers. (A) Distal GMT and (B) close-up view of working end of the Distal GMT. (C) Mesial GMT and (D) close-up view of working end of the Mesial GMT.

> 2. *Hold the instrument upright.* If the cutting edge forms a line that is parallel to the handle, it is used on the distal (down for distal). If the cutting edge does not form this line, it is used on the mesial.

Angle Formers. The angle former is used in a downward pushing motion to form and define point angles and to sharpen line angles. The angle former is similar to the hoe, except the cutting edge is angled like the gingival margin trimmer. Therefore, this also is a four-numbered instrument. This instrument is double-ended, so it can be used on either the left or right surfaces of a cavity preparation (Figure 19-13).

Excavators. Excavators, also known as "spoon excavators," are used to remove carious material and debris from the teeth. This instrument is also used for numerous other tasks, including removing excess dental cement, tucking rubber dam material, and packing gingival retraction cord. The excavator is similar to the GMT with the curved blade, but the difference is that the cutting edge of the excavator is rounded all the way around the periphery of the blade (Figure 19-14).

Noncutting Instruments

Noncutting instruments include basic examination instruments and instruments used to insert and finish amalgam and composite restorative materials. Examples of noncutting instruments include basic examination setup, plastic instruments, amalgam carriers, condensers, carvers, burnishers, files, and finishing knives.

FIGURE 19-13 Angle former. *(Courtesy of Hu-Friedy Mfg. Co., Inc.)*

FIGURE 19-14 Excavators. (A) Blade. (B) Close-up view of working end of Blade Excavator. (C) Spoon. (D) Close-up view of working end of Spoon Excavator. *(Courtesy of Miltex Instrument Co., Inc., Lake Success, NY.)*

Basic Examination Instruments. The basic examination setup instruments are used for examining the teeth but are also common to all tray setups. All procedures begin with the operator examining the teeth, so the mouth mirror, explorer, and cotton pliers are the first three instruments on a procedure tray setup. The periodontal probe is an optional instrument in the basic examination setup.

Mouth Mirrors. The **mouth mirror** is a single-ended instrument made of metal or plastic. It may have a handle with a "cone socket" for easy replacement of the mirror head or come in one piece. Mirrors are available in various sizes and types. The mirror sizes are identified by number; the most commonly used are numbers 4 and 5. The mouth mirror may be sterilized (by autoclaving, dry heat, or cold chemical sterilizing) or may be disposable. The types of mirrors are the plane surface, front surface, and concave surface.

- *Plane or regular surface mirrors* have reflective surfaces (silver coatings) on the backs of the glass (Figure 19-15A). This gives the image a "ghost image" as the light reflects from the glass and the silver layer.

- *Front surface mirrors* have reflective coatings (rhodium) on top of the glass. This coating eliminates the "ghost image"; it reflects only once to give a clear view free of distortion (Figure 19-15B).

- *Concave surface mirrors* magnify the image.

Uses of Mouth Mirror

- *Indirect vision*—When the operator uses a mirror to view areas of the oral cavity not seen with direct vision

- *Reflection of light*—Illumination of an area being examined or treated

- *Retraction*—When the cheeks or tongue is retracted for better visibility and for protection of the tissues

- *Transillumination*—Reflection of light through the tooth surface to detect fractures

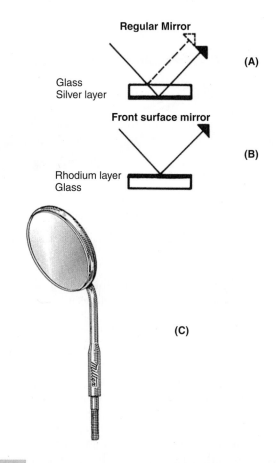

FIGURE 19-15 (A) Plane (regular) surface mirror. (B) Front surface mirror. (C) Cone socket mirror. *(Courtesy of Miltex Instrument Co., Inc., Lake Success, NY.)*

Explorers. **Explorers** are single- or double-ended instruments. The working end is a thin, sharp point of flexible steel. This allows the operator to examine surfaces of the teeth to detect any irregularity. There are a variety of angles of explorers, and often the ends are different so that the operator can access various areas of the mouth. Several common shapes include the pig tail, shepherd's hook, right angle, and #17 (Figure 19-16).

FIGURE 19-16 Types of explorers. (A) Pigtail. (B) Shepherd's hook and #17. *(Courtesy of Miltex Instrument Co., Inc., Lake Success, NY.)*

Uses of Explorers

- *Examination of the tooth structure* for defects or areas of decay

- *Examination of restorations* to check for faulty margins or fractures

- *Removal of excess materials* from around the margins of restorations or from bases and liners in the cavity preparation

Cotton Pliers. **Cotton pliers** are shaped like large tweezers with smooth surfaces or serrations on the ends of the beaks. They are available with locking or nonlocking handles, and the tips may be straight or angled. They are made of stainless steel and can be sterilized. The pliers are used frequently during a procedure by the operator and the dental assistant to transport and manipulate various materials (Figure 19-17).

Uses of Cotton Pliers

- *To place* and remove items from the oral cavity, such as cotton rolls, cotton pellets, wedges, and large pieces of debris

- *To grasp* and transfer materials to and from the oral cavity

- *To retrieve* materials from drawers, cupboards, and so on to avoid contamination

Periodontal Probes. **Periodontal probes** are used to measure the depth of the gingival sulcus. They may be single- or double-ended instruments. The working end of the probe is a blade that is rounded or blunted and is marked in millimeters (mm). There are variations in the indication of calibrations, including color coding (Figure 19-18A). A combination instrument that has an explorer tip on one end and a periodontal probe on the other end is known as an expro. It is very functional and reduces the number of instruments on the tray (Figure 19-18B) (also see Chapter 29, Periodontics).

(A)

(B)

FIGURE 19-17 (A) Cotton pliers. (B) Locking cotton pliers.

Plastic Filling Instruments. **Plastic filling instruments** are used to place and condense pliable restorative materials and to place cement bases in the cavity preparation. These instruments are made of plastic or metal and are usually double-ended. One of the most common plastic instruments has a paddle on one end and a small condenser on the other end (Figure 19-19A).

Composite Instruments. **Composite instruments** are very similar to plastic filling instruments in use and shape. They are also double-ended. The main difference

FIGURE 19-18 (A) Periodontal probe. (B) Expro with explorer (1) and periodontal probe (2). (B. *Courtesy of Miltex Instrument Co., Inc., Lake Success, NY.*)

FIGURE 19-19 (A) Plastic filling instrument. (B) Woodson instrument. (C) Composite instrument.

is that the composite instruments are made of a high-grade thermoplastic material or anodized aluminum to prevent discoloration of the composite or glass ionomer restoration materials (Figure 19-19C).

Amalgam Carriers. Amalgam carriers are designed to carry and dispense amalgam or composite into the cavity preparation. The carriers may be single- or double-ended with small and large ends. Most carriers are made of stainless steel, and some have Teflon or coated barrels to prevent clogging. The dental assistant loads both ends of the carrier with the restorative material and either passes it to the operator or places the amalgam in the cavity preparation and then refills the carrier as needed (Figure 19-20A).

A spring-action amalgam gun is used to carry and place composites, glass ionomers, and amalgam alloys. It is single-ended and made of high-grade plastic (Figure 19-20B).

Amalgam Condensers (Pluggers). Amalgam condensers, or pluggers, are used to pack amalgam into the cavity preparation. There are hand condensers and mechanical condensers. The hand condensers are usually double-ended and are available in a wide variety of working ends. The locations and designs of cavity preparations have required condensers to be diverse in design. The working ends may be plain (smooth) or serrated. They may be round, ovoid, rectangular, diamond, or cone shaped (Figure 19-21). The shanks of condensers may be monangled, binangled, or triple angled.

Mechanical condensers, sometimes called amalgam packers or vibrators, are used to pack and condense amalgam through vibrations into the cavity preparation. These condensers are attached to the dental unit and operated with compressed air. Packing points come in a variety of shapes and sizes. The action of the condenser is like a woodpecker, with short, quick movements.

Carvers. Carvers are used to remove excess restorative material and to carve tooth anatomy in the res-

FIGURE 19-20   (A) Double-ended amalgam carrier. (B) Amalgam gun. *(Courtesy of Miltex Instrument Co., Inc., Lake Success, NY.)*

FIGURE 19-21   Various shapes of condensers. *(Courtesy of Hu-Friedy Mfg. Co., Inc.)*

toration before the material hardens. Carvers are also used to carve wax inlays, onlays, and crowns. There are a wide variety of working ends on carvers, including long-bladed pointed ends and rounded and oval shapes. Usually, carvers are double-ended, with some ends having sharp edges and others rounded blades similar to excavators. The operator usually has several favorite carvers, which often include the Hollenback and the cleoid-discoid. The Hollenback is a long-bladed carver used to shape the restoration, and the cleoid-discoid carver is used to shape amalgam restorations. The cleoid end looks like a claw, and the discoid end is shaped like a round disc (Figures 19-22A through D).

Burnishers. Burnishers are used to smooth rough margins of the restoration and to shape metal matrix bands. Burnishers are blunt, rounded instruments that come in a variety of shapes, including ball shaped, T-ball, and the acorn. The acorn burnishers are very popular to smooth composite and amalgam restorations. Burnishers may be single- or double-ended instruments (Figure 19-23).

Files. Files are used to trim excess filling material and to smooth the restoration, especially the margins. They come in a variety of shapes, with a serrated surface on one side of the blade. The working end is often thin and small enough to reach interproximal spaces. Files are available as single- or double-ended instruments (Figure 19-24).

Finishing Knives. Finishing knives are used to trim excess filling material. The working ends of the finishing knives have sharp, knife-like blades. Finishing knives

FIGURE 19-22 Carvers. (A) Hollenback. (B) 1. Cleoid. 2. Discoid. (C) Ward's. (D) Frahm. *(Courtesy of Hu-Friedy Mfg. Co., Inc.)*

come in a variety of shapes and angles to access restoration margins (Figure 19-25).

Miscellaneous Instruments

Additional instruments found on restorative trays include spatulas, articulating forceps, and scissors.

Spatulas. During restorative procedures, **cement spatulas** may be used. These spatulas are single-ended and made of stainless steel. They come in a variety of sizes and strengths. Spatulas are used to mix cements, bases, and liners (Figure 19-26). **Plastic spatulas** are used to mix composite resin materials. These spatulas are usually double-ended and may be disposable. **Laboratory spatulas** are used to mix impression materials and plaster. These spatulas are larger and have longer, wider blades. Laboratory spatulas are made entirely of plastic or with metal blades and wooden handles.

Articulating Forceps. Articulating forceps are used to hold articulation paper, a colored paper used to check the patient's occlusion after the filling material has been placed. The forceps are made of stainless steel or disposable plastic and are opened and closed by placing pressure on the handle (Figure 19-27). Sometimes, cotton pliers, especially locking cotton pliers, are used in place of articulating forceps.

Scissors. The scissors used most commonly with restorative procedures are **crown and collar (bridge) scissors.** These scissors have short blades that may be straight or curved. Crown and collar scissors are used to trim matrix bands, to cut retraction cord, and in a variety of other ways (Figure 19-28).

Instrument Care, Maintenance, and Sterilization

All dental instruments must be properly cared for, maintained, and sterilized to ensure that the instruments will last a long time, function as designed, and be used safely. Instruments should be cleaned as soon as possible after use. When this cannot be done, the instruments should be placed in a presoak solution to prevent blood and debris from drying on the instruments.

To properly clean the instruments, place them in an ultrasonic bath or another instrument washer for a designated amount of time. The instruments should be covered with the ultrasonic solution and spread out as much as possible. Instrument cassettes enhance handling of the instrument by reducing the possibility of damage to the instrument and providing more organization and efficiency. The cassettes also reduce the risk of injury to the dental assistant during the cleaning and sterilization of the instruments.

Hinged instruments should always be cleaned and sterilized in the open position, because doing so prevents debris from gathering in the hinges and keeps the instruments functioning smoothly. Following manufacturer's directions when lubricating hinged instruments after cleaning but before sterilizing will increase the longevity of the instruments.

When instruments are removed from the ultrasonic bath, they should be rinsed thoroughly under running water and then dried before being prepared for sterilization. After sterilization, instruments should be dried completely before being stored. When instruments are not dried before being stored, corrosion and staining could occur. When the sterilization bags in which the

FIGURE 19-23 (A) Burnisher. (B) Ball burnisher. (C) Football burnisher. (D) Beaver tail burnisher. (E) T-Ball burnisher. (F) Acorn burnisher. *(A. and F. Courtesy of Miltex Instrument Co., Inc., Lake Success, NY.)*

FIGURE 19-24 File. *(Courtesy of Hu-Friedy Mfg. Co., Inc.)*

FIGURE 19-25 Finishing knife. *(Courtesy of Hu-Friedy Mfg. Co., Inc.)*

FIGURE 19-27 (A) Articulating forceps. (B) Disposable articulating forceps. *(A. Courtesy of Miltex Instrument Co., Inc., Lake Success, NY.)*

FIGURE 19-28 Straight crown and collar (bridge) scissors. *(Courtesy of Miltex Instrument Co., Inc., Lake Success, NY.)*

FIGURE 19-26 Cement spatulas. *(Courtesy of Miltex Instrument Co., Inc., Lake Success, NY.)*

instruments are processed are not completely dry, they become a source of bacterial contamination and they also tear more easily. In some cases, this would mean that the instruments should be resterilized.

The dental assistant should examine all instruments carefully. Check for corrosion, stains, broken tips, and sharpness. See if hinged instruments open and close smoothly and have no excess lubricant near the hinges. This evaluation step allows time for manufacturer's maintenance and/or replacement instruments to be ordered.

Dental Rotary Instruments

Dental **burs** are part of a group of instruments referred to as **rotary instruments**. Rotary instruments include discs and stones and are designed to be used with dental handpieces. They are used in handpieces that operate at various speeds, both at chairside and in the dental laboratory. Burs are used for cavity preparations, finishing and polishing restorations, surgical procedures, and dental appliance adjustments.

Burs are made of steel or tungsten carbide materials. The steel burs are not used as often as the carbide burs because they become dull very fast. Bur groups include cutting, diamond, surgical, laboratory, and finishing.

Parts of the Bur

All burs have three basic parts: shank, neck, and head (Figure 19-29A).

FIGURE 19-29 (A) Parts of a bur. (B) Different shanks: straight, latch type, and friction grip.

Shank. The shank of the bur is inserted into the handpiece. To accommodate various dental handpieces, there are three styles of bur shanks (Figure 19-29B). The **straight shank** (designated HP when ordering), or long shank, functions with the straight, low-speed handpiece. The **latch-type shank** (designated RA) is shorter than the straight-shanked burs. On the latch-type shank is a notch that fits into the contra-angle/right-angle handpiece and latches securely in place. The **friction-grip shank** (designated FG) is short, small, and smooth. These burs are used in friction-grip, high-speed handpieces.

Neck. The neck of the bur is the tapered connection of the shank to the head.

Head. The head is the working end of the bur. There are many shapes and sizes of heads on dental burs. A variety of burs are needed to perform the multiple tasks in restoring teeth and specialty procedures.

Cutting Burs

There are nine basic cutting bur shapes, including round, inverted cone, plain fissure straight, plain fissure cross-cut, tapered fissure straight, tapered fissure cross-cut, end cutting, wheel, and pear. These burs are identified by number ranges. The bur numbers describe the shape, size, and variation of the bur. It is important to know the number ranges, because dentists often will ask for a bur by its number. Cutting burs have six to eight cutting blades or surfaces (Table 19-1 and Figure 19-30).

Burs also vary in both head and shank design. An example of a change in the head (working end) of the bur is on the fissure burs. Normally, the fissure burs are flat on the end, but some fissure burs have rounded or dome-shaped working ends. The number range for these burs differs from that for the regular fissure burs.

The lengths of the three bur shanks vary and are designated by an *L* for longer length, an *S* for short shanks, or *P* for pedodontic shanks. The letter designation follows the number of the bur.

Diamond Burs

Diamond rotary instruments are categorized as diamond burs or stones. They are used for rapid reduction of tooth structure during cavity preparation, polishing and finishing composite restorations, and occlusal adjustment. Diamond burs are also used for bone and gingival contouring during surgical procedures.

Diamond burs come in a wide variety of shapes, sizes, and grits. Diamond particles are embedded in the bur head through an electroplating or a bonding process. The burs are either color coded for easy grit identification or have letters following the bur numbers to indicate the grit (Figures 19-31A and B). These burs may be specifically designed for a certain procedure, such as finishing, trimming, and composite restorations.

TABLE 19-1 Burs and Their Functions and Number Ranges

Name	Function
Round bur	Used first to open the cavity and remove carious tooth structure.
Inverted cone bur	Removes caries and makes undercuts in the preparation.
Plain fissure straight bur and Plain fissure cross-cut bur	Forms the cavity walls of the preparation.
Tapered fissure straight bur and Tapered fissure cross-cut bur	Forms divergent walls of the cavity preparation.
End cutting bur	Forms the shoulder for crown preparations.
Wheel bur	Forms retention in preparations.
Pear bur	Opens and extends the cavity preparation.

FIGURE 19-30 Bur shapes and number ranges. *(Courtesy of Miltex Instrument Co., Inc., Lake Success, NY.)*

Finishing Burs

Finishing burs smooth, trim, and finish metal restorations and natural-tooth-colored materials. Finishing burs can have up to thirty blades for ultra-fine finishing. These burs come in a variety of shapes and sizes, similar to the cutting burs. They are identified by the manufacturer's number. Some are color coded for easy identification. A red band indicates 8 and 12 blades on the finishing bur. A yellow band indicates 16 and 20 blades, and a white band indicates a 30-blade finishing bur (Figure 19-32).

Surgical Burs

Surgical burs are used in a low-speed handpiece to reduce and contour the alveolar bone and tooth structure. The heads of surgical burs come in various sizes and shapes and have long shanks (Figure 19-33).

Laboratory Burs

Laboratory burs are used to adjust acrylic materials, such as partials, dentures, and custom trays. They are also used on plaster, stone, and metal materials. Labo-

FIGURE 19-32 Finishing burs in various shapes.

FIGURE 19-31 (A) Diamond bur with color coding for size of grit. (B) Various shaped diamond burs in: coarse, fine, and extra fine. (C) Variety of diamond burs. (B. *Courtesy of Miltex Instrument Co., Inc., Lake Success, NY.*)

FIGURE 19-33 Surgical burs.

ratory burs have long shanks and large working ends. These burs come in a variety of sizes and shapes. Sometimes they are referred to as **vulcanite** or **acrylic burs** (Figure 19-34).

Fissurotomy Burs

Fissurotomy burs are extremely small (0.33 mm). Made of carbide, they are used to explore the occlusal surface and to allow for effective diagnoses and treatment while preserving healthy tooth structure. These burs cut quickly, leaving a smooth, minimally invasive groove in suspicious pits and fissures. Fissurotomy burs are designed as depth gauges, allowing the burs minimal access to the fissures that permit virtually pain-free fissure cavity preparation.

FIGURE 19-34 Laboratory burs. (*Courtesy of Miltex Instrument Co., Inc., Lake Success, NY.*)

Abrasives

Abrasives are nonbladed instruments used to finish and polish restorations and appliances. Some abrasives also are used for cutting. Abrasives come in a wide variety and are categorized by their shapes, such as discs, points, and wheels. Abrasives also are categorized by the materials they are made of, such as rubber, stone, and sandpaper. Some restorative materials come with select abrasives that are designed to give the restoration a premium finish.

Mandrels

Mandrels are rods of various lengths that are used in low-speed handpieces with various abrasives. The abrasives are either permanently attached (mounted) to a mandrel or separate and placed on a mandrel (unmounted). Mandrels are available in three shanks: latch, friction grip, or straight. The head of the mandrel, where the abrasives attach, is available in snap on, screw on, or pin (Figure 19-35).

Discs

Discs are used to polish, smooth, and adjust restorative materials and dental appliances. Discs are circular, abrasive instruments that are usually designed to be mounted to mandrels. The abrasive agents are bonded on one or both sides of paper, metal, or plastic. The discs may be rigid or flexible, and are available in a variety of sizes and grits. The abrasive material may be made of several different materials, such as garnet, diamond, quartz, sand, and carborundum. When ordering abrasives, size, grit, abrasiveness, and mandrel type must be specified.

Sandpaper Discs. Sandpaper discs are used to finish and polish all types of restorations and appliances. They are available in a wide variety of sizes, grits, and abrasive materials, including garnet, sand, emery, and cuttlefish. These materials are mounted on one side of the paper disc. Sandpaper discs are flexible and are applied to surfaces on one side only. They come with metal or pinhole centers (Figure 19-36).

Diamond Discs. Diamond discs have diamond particles or chips bonded to both sides of steel discs. They are used for rapid cutting.

Carborundum Discs. **Carborundum discs**, also known as **Jo-dandy discs** and **separating discs**, are thin, brittle discs that break easily. They are double-sided and are used primarily in the dental laboratory to cut and finish gold restorations, but they can be used intraorally as well (Figure 19-37A).

Stones

Stones are available in many sizes, shapes, and grits, similar to discs. They are used for cutting, polishing, and finishing amalgam, gold, composite, and porcelain restorations. Stones are used in the laboratory to adjust and polish appliances and custom trays. The type of abrasive material and the grit control the cutting or polishing action of the stone. The abrasive materials

FIGURE 19-36 Sandpaper discs in various sizes, types, and grits. *(Courtesy of 3M ESPE Dental.)*

FIGURE 19-35 Mandrels with different heads and shanks. (A) Screw-type mandrels. (B) Snap-on mandrels. *(Courtesy of Miltex Instrument Co., Inc., Lake Success, NY.)*

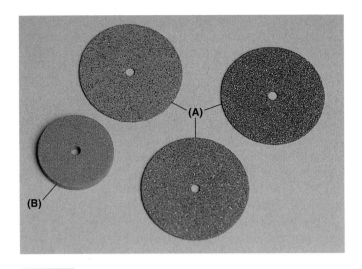

FIGURE 19-37 (A) Carborundum discs. (B) Rubber wheel.

FIGURE 19-38 (A) Various types and grits of stones, wheels, and points. (B) Various points, cups, and wheels to define, polish, and finish composite restorations.

include silicon carbide, garnet, and aluminum oxide. Stones may be mounted or unmounted. Some stones are considered heatless, thereby allowing the operator to polish a restoration without creating frictional heat (Figure 19-38).

Rubber Wheels

Wheels are made of rubber material impregnated with an abrasive agent (Figures 19-38 and 19-39). They come mounted and unmounted and are available in various grits. They are used for finishing and polishing.

Rubber Points

Rubber points come in a variety of sizes and grits. They are made of rubber material impregnated with abrasive agents. Points are used to polish and are especially adaptable when defining anatomy in the restoration (Figures 19-38 and 19-39).

FIGURE 19-39 Wheel and points.

Sterilization, Maintenance, and Storage

Rotary instruments are sterilized or disposed of after each use in the oral cavity. Burs that are sterilized are first scrubbed or placed in an ultrasonic unit to remove debris from the blades; when debris remains between the blades, a wire brush is used to remove embedded materials. The burs are then rinsed and sterilized according to the manufacturer's instructions.

Bur Blocks. Rotary instruments are stored in a bur block. There are many variations and designs, such as round or rectangular shapes. Bur blocks come with covers and may be magnetic. Both friction-grip and latch-type burs can be stored in bur blocks. They are made of metal or plastic (Figure 19-40).

FIGURE 19-40 Bur block with covers, magnetized and made of metal. *(Courtesy of Hu-Friedy Mfg. Co., Inc.)*

Some bur blocks can be sterilized with the burs they hold. If the bur blocks cannot be sterilized, the burs are placed in a mesh holder that looks like a tea strainer. The burs are placed in this holder and run through the ultrasonic cleaner, and then placed in the sterilizer.

Dental Handpieces

A wide variety of dental handpieces are available to meet the needs of dental procedures, both in the oral cavity and in the laboratory. Handpieces are used to remove dental decay and to prepare the tooth for a restoration; to polish the teeth; to polish and finish dental restorations; and to cut, finish, and polish dental appliances, models, and trays.

The Parts of the Dental Handpiece

All dental handpieces have the following basic parts (Figures 19-41A and B):

- *Working end (head)*—Where burs, discs, stones, and other rotary instruments and attachments are held and the cutting and polishing are accomplished.
- *Shank*—The handle portion of the handpiece.
- *Connection end*—Where the handpiece attaches to the power source. The forward and reverse controls may be located here.

Dental handpieces are often divided into two categories: **high-speed handpieces** and **low-speed handpieces**. The high-speed handpieces operate at 400,000 revolutions per minute (rpm) and higher (Figure 19-41A). The low-speed handpieces operate under 30,000 rpm (Figure 19-41B).

High-Speed Handpiece

The high-speed handpiece is used to rapidly cut tooth structure and finish restorations. Because of the high speed of this handpiece, frictional heat is produced. Frictional heat can cause pulpal damage to the tooth, so to reduce the frictional heat of the handpiece, a coolant such as air, water, or an air-water spray is used.

The high-speed handpiece design is a smooth, one-piece design, usually a **contra-angle**, with the head slightly angled to the shank of the handpiece (Figure 19-42A). The high-speed handpiece does not hold any attachments but does hold burs and other rotary instruments. To hold these rotary instruments, the head of the handpiece has a small, metal cylinder called a **chuck**. The chuck holds the shank portion of the bur in place. To tighten or loosen the chuck, either a bur tool/wrench or a button/release lever on the back of the head of the handpiece is used. The manufacturer provides the specific bur tool with the handpiece (Figure 19-42C). The head of the handpiece comes in standard and pediatric sizes. The pediatric handpiece is used for easier access with children and adults with small mouths.

The power source for the dental handpiece comes from the unit. The compressed air drives the turbines in the handpiece. To activate and control the speed of the handpiece, a **rheostat** (foot control) is operated, much like the accelerator on a car.

High-speed handpieces are available with **fiberoptic light sources**. Fiberoptic systems greatly improve visibility of the treatment area for the operator. The fiberoptic light is carried along optical bundles in the tubing of the handpiece. The light source is either a separate control box or a bulb behind the handpiece in the dental unit.

Low-Speed Handpiece

The low-speed handpiece is often referred to as the straight handpiece because the shank and head are in a straight line. These handpieces are used in both the dental operatory and the laboratory. At the dental unit, the low-speed handpiece is used to polish teeth and restorations, remove soft carious material, and define cavity margins and walls.

In the dental laboratory, this handpiece is used to adjust, finish, and polish appliances. Usually, the low-speed handpiece does not have or need a water supply, but in some procedures the dental assistant periodically applies air or water to the tooth or restoration to prevent any heating of the tooth.

The low-speed handpiece is a little bulkier than the high-speed handpiece. The straight handpiece is used with long-shank rotary instruments, such as burs, discs

(A)

(B) Slow-speed with prophyangle

Straight slow-speed nose cone

Slow-speed motor

FIGURE 19-41 (A) High-speed handpiece. (B) Low-speed handpieces. *(Courtesy of A-Dec, Inc., Newberg, OR.)*

(A)

(B)

(C)

FIGURE 19-42 (A) High-speed handpieces with fiberoptics. (B) High-speed handpieces with pushbutton back to place and remove burs. (C) Handpiece with a bur tool to place and remove the bur. (A. *Courtesy of Midwest Dental Products Corporation, a division of DENTSPLY International.*)

and stones, and attachment heads such as the contra-angle and the right-angle (Figure 19-43).

- The contra-angles are usually latch type, but they also come in friction grip. The contra-angles hold burs, discs, stones, rubber cups, and brushes for intraoral and extraoral procedures.

FIGURE 19-43 (A) Low-speed handpiece with nose cone and attachments for the low-speed handpiece: (B) Contra-angle with and without a disc. (C) Right-angle or prophy angle, with rubber cup. (D) Round bur with long shank to be place in nose cone of the straight low-speed handpiece.

- The right angles or prophy angles are used to polish the teeth with rubber cups or brushes.

On the shank of the low-speed handpiece is a mechanism to lock the rotary instrument or the attachment onto the handpiece. This may be a tightening knob or a snap-on apparatus. Also on the shank near the connecting end there may be a reverse and forward control. The power source for controlling the speed of the low-speed handpiece is the rheostat.

Electric Handpiece

Electric handpieces are an alternative to the air-driven handpieces mainly used by dentists today. The electric handpieces have greatly improved and are becoming more popular in the dental office. The units can be calibrated to be used with existing air pressure and rheostats. They can be used for all high- and low-speed needs operating at a speed range of 27-200,000 rpm with various attachments. Procedures they are used for include cavity preparation, endodontic procedures, contouring and trimming provisional crowns and bridges, adjusting crowns, bridges, permanent restorations, prophylaxis, and composite polishing. There is also an interproximal head for interproximal polishing, cleaning, and preparation. The electric handpieces are quiet, vibration free, efficient and sterilizible.

FIGURE 19-44 Electric handpiece. *(Courtesy of KaVo.)*

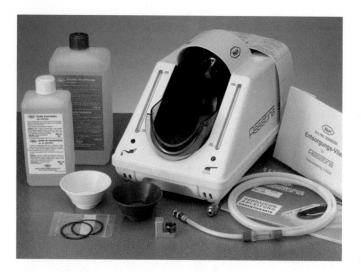

FIGURE 19-45 Handpiece cleaner and lubricant maintenance unit. *(Courtesy of A-dec, Inc., Newberg, Oregon.)*

The high-speed electric handpiece has a pushbutton auto chuck that firmly grips the bur, cellular optic rod delivers illumination that reduces eye fatigue and is light weight. The low-speed electric handpiece has several attachments and is available in the contra-angle or straight handpiece style (Figure 19-44).

Maintenance and Sterilization of Dental Handpieces

The manufacturer's directions for maintaining and sterilizing the handpiece should be followed carefully. Handpieces that are used for patient treatment must be sterilizible; disinfecting handpieces is not acceptable. General guidelines include:

- While the handpiece is attached to the tubing and a bur is still in the handpiece, flush the handpiece by running it for twenty to thirty seconds. Follow the manufacturer's instructions for specific flushing and for the use and maintenance of waterlines and check valves.

- Scrub the handpiece to remove debris. Rinse and dry it if manufacturer instructions include this step.

- Lubricate the handpiece if it is not lube free. Use only the manufacturer's suggested lubricants. This must be done before the handpiece is sterilized.

- Sterilize the handpiece as directed.

- Lubricate if instructed to do so.

Some units clean and lubricate handpieces. The maintenance units (Figure 19-45) are located in the sterilizing area and require electrical and air pressure connections and water. Some of the units also sterilize the handpiece.

Air Abrasion Unit

Air abrasion technology is becoming increasingly popular. Air abrasion reduces or eliminates the use of anesthetics and drilling with dental handpieces. This shortens and/or reduces the number of patient appointments. The technology allows various types of cavities to be prepared for restoration, special repairs in restorations to be accomplished, and the insides of restorations to be roughened before bonding.

Air abrasion base units (Figure 19-46) come in movable floor models or small countertop units. They consist of the base unit, control panel, foot switch, air pressure gradient (varies the pressure in small increments), handpiece and handpiece nozzler, abrasive flow control, and external suction device. Each unit requires an air pressure source (most can use air lines to the dental unit) and the abrasive. The abrasive is aluminum oxide. The particle size varies, with 27 or 50 microns most commonly used, but more variations are being developed for specific tasks.

During use, the dental team and the patient should wear protective eyewear. The dental assistant uses the HVE in addition to external suction to remove debris.

Routine maintenance is important and the manufacturer's directions should be followed.

Microetcher

The **microetcher** is a smaller version of the air abrasion units. They are used for intraoral sandblasting and dentin bonding. Microetchers are used for many procedures including:

- Removal of occlusal stains from deep occlusal grooves

- Pit and fissure sealant preparation

- Denture repairs

FIGURE 19-46 Air abrasion unit. *(Courtesy of Midwest Dental Products Corporation, a division of DENTSPLY International.)*

FIGURE 19-47 Microetcher with hose, abrasive reservoir.

- Etching of existing amalgam, composites, and porcelain restorations
- Roughening the surface for bonding of orthodontic bands and brackets
- Roughening the surface of crowns, bridges, and posts for maximum bonding

The microetcher looks like and is about the size of a pen and it has an abrasive reservoir with an interchangeable jar. The reservoir is attached to the microetcher and holds the abrasive. The microetcher comes with several different tips called nozzles (Figure 19-47). It can be hooked up in an operatory or a lab where there is an air line for compressed air of 40 to 100 psi.

Microetcher Abrasives

The abrasives used with the microetcher should be dry and clean. Since abrasives are hygroscopic (water loving) they should be kept in a tightly sealed container to keep them dry and clean. Some of the abrasives used include:

- Aluminum oxide, 90 micron, tan for rapid removal of cements and etching of metals to prepare for bonding
- Aluminum oxide, 50 micron, white for preparation of amalgam, composite, and porcelain bonding

- Microprophy B, white for stain removal
- SA-85 to remove resin
- Glass beads, 90 micron, white to clean dentures

The jar on the microetcher should be filled about three-quarters to allow the abrasive to move easily in the jar.

Operation, Safety, and Sterilization. When using the microetcher the dentist and assistant should wear protective eyewear and a mask. The patient should have protective eyewear on and a rubber dam should be placed on the patient.

The microetcher can be sterilized if used intraorally. A plastic barrier can be placed over the microetcher with only the tip exposed to avoid contamination by the patient. To prepare for sterilization remove the abrasive jar and then allow the compressed air to flow through the unit. Remove any debris from the microetcher and the nozzle and then sterilize.

Tray Systems

A **preset tray system** is most commonly used in dental offices. It provides an efficient means of transporting instruments to the treatment room, which saves time for the dental assistant. With this system, instruments and auxiliary items are placed on a tray in the order of their use during the procedure. Then the tray is covered and carried to the treatment room when the patient is seated. There are many varieties of systems to choose from, including plastic or metal trays, tubs, or the cassette system. Trays, tubs, and accessories can be color coded for efficient handling and storage. Plastic or paper barriers are used before placing instruments on the tray, especially for ribbed trays. These barriers help with tray disinfection.

Positioning on Trays

Every operator has preferences on the instrumentation for a procedure. However, there are some basic considerations:

- Tray barriers may be placed.
- Instruments are placed in order of use, beginning on the left and moving to the right.
- The basic tray setup (mouth mirror, explorer, cotton pliers) is placed first on the left side.
- Instruments should be grouped according to functions; for example, all the carvers are placed together.
- Cotton supplies are usually arranged across the top of the tray.
- Scissors, hemostats, or other hinged instruments are placed on the far right of the tray for easy access.
- Return instruments to their original positions after receiving them from the operator. This ensures that an instrument can be found easily if the operator needs to use it again.
- Keep instruments clean and free of debris before returning them to the tray. Gauze sponges on the tray aid with the immediate removal of cement, blood, or debris, which will harden on the instrument after use.

Cassette System for Instruments

Cassette systems are designed to carry instruments for use in treatment rooms, through the cleaning and sterilizing processes, and then into storage (Figure 19-48). Instruments for a certain procedure are color coded and then placed in a cassette. The cassette provides an efficient and safe means for handling instruments. Also, when the cassette is open, it provides its own tray. After being used for a procedure, the cassette is carried to the sterilization area. Here the instruments are reorganized and placed in the cassette. When the cassette is closed, the instruments remain securely in place. The cassette is then placed in the ultrasonic or instrument washer. When this process is complete, the cassette is rinsed thoroughly, and then wrapped or packaged and labeled, sterilized, and stored until needed. In the treatment room, the cassette is unwrapped on the counter top or cart, ready for use. The wrap acts as a barrier between the tray and the counter (Figure 19-48).

The cassette system efficiently keeps instruments together at all times. It increases safety by reducing the possibility of puncture injuries during cleaning and sterilizing. The cassettes come in different sizes and can be stored vertically or horizontally because the instruments are held into position. The wrapped cassettes are labeled with tape that is premarked for all procedures performed in the office. This makes it easy to identify the tray set that is needed in the treatment rooms. For more information, refer to Chapter 11, Infection Control.

Color-Coding Systems

Color coding is a method for easily identifying instruments and trays (Figure 19-49). The color coding may be set up to indicate the following:

- Procedures, such as amalgam or composite.
- Treatment rooms, where the instruments are stored or used.

FIGURE 19-48 Cassette system. Cassettes are wrapped in paper and taped with label tape and then placed in sterilizer. *(Courtesy of Hu-Friedy Mfg. Co., Inc.)*

FIGURE 19-49 Tub, tray, and instruments, all color coded.

(A)

(B)

(C)

FIGURE 19-50 Color-coding materials. (A) Plastic rings. (B) Tape. (C) Tray, instrument mat, mouth mirror, bur block, and colored rings all coordinated.

- Additional sets of instruments (there may be four composite setups, each marked for the procedure and then a second color for the set).

- Individual operators. The dentist may have two tray setups for prophylaxis and the hygienist may have four additional prophylaxis tray setups. Color coding keeps the dentist and the hygienist tray setups separate.

- Sequence. Instruments can be color coded diagonally to indicate the sequence of use.

- Any combination of these.

Types of Color Coding Materials

There are several different types of materials used to color code dental instruments, including plastic rings and colored coding tape. Color coding tape may also be used to color code tubs and trays, bur blocks, and tray mats. Also available are color-coded systems where the tubs, trays, tray mats, bur blocks, and mouth mirrors are all one color. Color-coding materials must be autoclavable and durable (Figure 19-50).

CHAPTER SUMMARY

The basic instruments used in general dental procedures include common cutting and noncutting instruments. Instruments are generally categorized as hand instruments and rotary instruments. Each procedure requires special instruments to accomplish specific tasks. The assistant is responsible for keeping the instruments sterilized, organized, and in working condition.

Case Study

Dr. Charles Thomas has been practicing dentistry for five years, and his practice has grown to the point where his tray setup system must be changed. Dr. Thomas has three treatment rooms and one hygiene room. He is willing to finance the necessary updating and would like to color code his instruments, trays, and so on.

Case Study Review

1. Before deciding on a system, what factors must be considered?

2. Suggest some color-code combinations.

3. What are the benefits of an office in which a color-coding system is effectively used?

REVIEW QUESTIONS

Multiple Choice

1. The part of the dental instrument that is straight, curved, monangle, binangle, or triple angle is called the
   a. handle.
   b. shank.
   c. working end.
   d. shaft.

2. Which of the following instruments has a four-number formula?
   a. Chisel
   b. Angle former
   c. Spoon excavator
   d. Hoe

3. Mouth mirror uses include all of the following except
   a. indirect vision.
   b. light reflection.
   c. retraction.
   d. direct vision.

4. The instrument used to carve an amalgam restoration before it hardens is the
   a. Hollenback.
   b. gingival margin trimmer.
   c. Wedelstaedt chisel.
   d. T-ball burnisher.

5. The rotary instrument also known as a "Jo-dandy" is the
   a. diamond bur.
   b. sandpaper disc.
   c. carborundum disc.
   d. rubber wheel.

6. Which of the following handpiece types would accept a notched bur?
   a. Friction-grip
   b. Screw-on right angle
   c. Snap-on right angle
   d. Latch contra-angle

7. The end of the handpiece where cutting or polishing instruments are attached is called the:
   a. Working end of the handpiece
   b. Shank of the handpiece
   c. Connecting end of the handpiece
   d. Plunger

8. The shank of a chisel may be:
   a. Straight only
   b. Straight or curved only
   c. Straight, curved, or binangle
   d. Binangle

9. The manufacturer's number on an instrument may indicate:
   a. The section the instrument is found in the catalog
   b. The instrument's placement in a set of instruments
   c. The length of the cutting edge in millimeters
   d. The date of the manufacture of the instrument

10. Egg shaped, t-ball, football, acorn, and beavertail are all shapes of _____.
    a. Finishing knives
    b. Burnishers
    c. Plastic filling instrument
    d. Gingival margin trimmers

Critical Thinking

1. What information does a bur number provide about the bur?

2. Which handpiece would the dental assistant select if the procedure included polishing the patient's teeth? Would an attachment be required?

3. List the basic hand instruments that would be necessary for an amalgam restoration procedure.

Web Activities

1. Go to http://www.agd.org and find out if air abrasion is suitable for everyone.

2. Dental rotary instruments can be ordered from numerous sources. Visit http://www.dental-burs.net and look up the price of diamond burs and carbide burs.

3. Go to http://www.thedentalnet.com and find out how to care for dental handpieces between patients and weekly or as needed.

ANESTHESIA AND SEDATION

SPECIFIC INSTRUCTIONAL OBJECTIVES

The student should strive to meet the following objectives and demonstrate an understanding of the facts and principles presented in this chapter:

1. Describe the methods used to manage the pain and anxiety associated with dental procedures.

2. Explain various topical anesthetics and their placements.

3. Describe types of local anesthetics.

4. List the steps for preparing for the administration of local anesthetic.

5. Identify the injection sites for the maxillary and mandibular arches.

6. Describe the equipment and materials needed to administer local anesthetic.

7. Identify supplemental techniques to administer anesthetics.

8. Discuss the role of nitrous oxide in the care of the dental patient.

9. Demonstrate the ability to assist in the administration of nitrous oxide.

KEY TERMS

aspirating syringe *(397)*
carpules *(395)*
cartridges *(395)*
computer-controlled local anesthesia *(408)*
conscious sedation *(393)*
electronic dental anesthesia *(408)*
epinephrine *(396)*
field block anesthesia *(396)*
general anesthesia *(394)*

infiltration anesthesia *(396)*
inhalation sedation *(393)*
intramuscular sedation *(393)*
intraosseous anesthesia *(404)*
intrapulpal injection *(408)*
intravenous conscious sedation (IV) *(393)*
local anesthesia *(394)*
lumen *(400)*

National Institute of Occupational Safety and Health (NIOSH) *(409)*
nerve block anesthesia *(396)*
nitrous oxide *(409)*
oral sedation *(393)*
paresthesia *(396)*
periodontal ligament injection *(407)*
topical anesthetic *(394)*
toxic reaction *(395)*
vasoconstrictors *(396)*
Wells, Horace *(409)*

INTRODUCTION

One of the biggest fears for patients visiting the dentist is the injection. People have shared their "experiences with the needle" for generations. Over the years, though, many advances have been made to control patients' pain and anxiety. Improved administration techniques and equipment for managing patients' pain and anxiety continue to be focuses of research.

Because most procedures require some form of anesthesia, the dentist may select one or a combination of methods to control pain, depending on the patient and the procedure to be completed.

Anesthetics and Sedation

Depending on the formal education a dentist has received determines the type of anesthesia and sedation he or she can administer. Guidelines are set by the American Dental Association for various levels of training and clinical experience required. Some specialties include the necessary training to administer conscious sedation, deep sedation, and general anesthesia (e.g., oral and maxillofacial surgery and periodontics). If a general dentist wishes to use conscious sedation, deep sedation, or general anesthesia, he or she must complete specific courses and programs to achieve this credential. Some dentists hire a nurse anesthetist or anesthesiologist to administer general anesthetic to their patients.

Sedation and anesthesia in dentistry include the following: conscious sedation, IV sedation, oral sedation, inhalation anesthesia, intramuscular sedation, general anesthesia, topical anesthesia, local anesthesia, and nitrous oxide.

Conscious Sedation

With **conscious sedation** the patient is placed in an altered state of consciousness. Pain relievers and sedatives are used to lower pain and discomfort for the patient. Trained professionals administer and closely control the patient who is under conscious sedation. The patient can communicate any discomfort and respond to questions or comments. The patient may experience a headache, nausea, and brief periods of amnesia after conscious sedation. But this is a very safe means for patients to be free of any pain and discomfort during dental procedures.

Intravenous Conscious Sedation (IV Sedation)

Intravenous conscious sedation is when sedative drugs are administered directly into the patient's blood system. An IV is set up in the vein and remains throughout the procedure. A specially trained person monitors the patient's pulse and oxygen levels. IV sedation allows the patient to be conscious but in a deep relaxed state. Often the patient does not remember what took place from the time the IV drug was started until the drug starts to wear off.

This is a very common means to keep patients relaxed, comfortable, and pain free during dental procedures. More about IV sedation will be discussed in Chapter 25, Oral and Maxillofacial Surgery.

Oral Sedation

Oral sedation is taken before the dental appointment to relieve anxiety about the dental procedure the patient is going to have done. The dentist prescribes the oral sedation drug to be taken the night before the appointment. This relieves stress for the patient and helps the patient get a good night's rest.

Benzodiazepine is a commonly prescribed drug that can be used in a couple of ways: one is as a sedative hypnotic and the other is as an anti-anxiety drug. If benzodiazepine is used as a sedative hypnotic the patient is calm and drowsy. If benzodiazepine is used as an anti-anxiety drug the patient will be very calm and relaxed.

Inhalation Sedation

The dentist may use **inhalation sedation** when IV sedation is difficult to administer. These potent inhalation agents are odorless and colorless gases that provide general anesthesia.

Inhalation sedation is easy to administer through a facemask, a laryngeal mask airway, or an endotracheal tube. Inhalation anesthetics relieve pain and cause sleepiness and the patient doesn't remember much of the procedure. Patients are closely monitored, and because the agent is not long-lasting, a local anesthetic may also be administered to relieve pain after the general anesthetic wears off.

Intramuscular Sedation

With **intramuscular sedation** a needle is used to inject the sedative drug into the muscle of the upper arm or thigh. This is not a very common form of sedation, but may be used in the pediatric dental office with children more than the general dental practice that treats mainly adults. The effect of intramuscular sedation is to ease a fearful or anxious patient's concerns or apprehension when visiting the dentist. The patient will be totally relaxed and will remember little of the appointment. They lapse into a dreamy state and have an attitude of indifference toward their dental treatment. The injection is given at the office into either the muscle of the upper arm or thigh.

Intramuscular drugs take longer to take effect, usually about 20 to 30 minutes before the procedure can begin.

General Anesthesia

When **general anesthesia** is administered, the patient goes into an unconscious state which is carefully controlled by an anesthetist. The anesthetic temporarily alters the central nervous system so that sensation or feeling is lost. General anesthetic is ideal for some patients for various dental surgeries and treatments.

General anesthesia is accomplished with a mixture of very potent drugs to ensure major surgeries are accomplished without pain to the patient. With general anesthesia the patient's vital signs and fluids are closely monitored and a ventilator breathes for the patient while the patient is unconscious. The ventilator remains on until after the surgery and the patient recovers enough to breathe on his or her own.

Usually general anesthesia is given in a hospital setting but some oral and maxillofacial surgeons have "mini" operating rooms that are fully equipped to administer general anesthesia. Some dentists have received the necessary training to administer general anesthesia but often an anesthesiologist or nurse anesthetist performs this task so the dentist can concentrate on the surgery.

The dental assistant is not involved with the administration of the general anesthetic but does assist during the surgery and is responsible for dismissing and monitoring the patient during recovery. Refer to Chapter 25, Oral and Maxillofacial Surgery, for more information.

Definitions

Analgesia is defined as the absence of pain.

Analgesic is a drug that relieves pain.

Anesthesia is defined as partial or complete loss of sensation with or without the loss of consciousness caused by disease, injury, or injection or inhalation of an anesthetic agent.

Sedation is defined as a state of calmness or process of reducing nervous excitement.

Topical Anesthesia

Before the local anesthesia is injected, the area is numbed with **topical anesthetic**. This material desensitizes the oral mucosa for a brief period so that the patient will not feel the pinch of the needle. Topical anesthetics affect the small nerve endings in the surface of the skin and mucosa. Dental assistants must be aware of the various topical anesthetic solutions and possible patient reactions. They must know application sites and how to apply the anesthetic. In some states, the dental assistant can apply the topical anesthetic for the dentist before an injection.

Local Anesthesia

Local anesthesia produces a deadened or pain-free area while the dentist performs a procedure that may cause the patient uncomfortable sensations if no anesthetic were used. Sensory impulses, such as pain, touch, and thermal change, are temporarily blocked. Local anesthesia only works when it contacts the nerve fibers carrying impulses to the brain or the small nerve endings picking up sensations in the tissue.

The dental assistant must be aware of the various anesthetic solutions and techniques used when administering local anesthetic. The dental assistant is responsible for preparing, safely transferring, and caring for the anesthetic syringe and accessories.

Topical Anesthetics

Topical anesthetics are placed on the surface of the oral mucosa to eliminate sensation, but they have several other uses in dental procedures, such as decreasing pain sensation for subgingival scaling, root planing, seating crowns, placing matrix bands, and performing periodontal probing. Sometimes topical anesthetic is used to depress the gag reflex that occurs when taking intraoral x-rays or impressions.

Topical anesthetics are available in gels, ointments, liquids, or metered sprays (Figure 20-1). The gels, ointments, and liquids are applied in small amounts to specific areas. The sprays are metered to control the amount of solution sprayed and to confine it to the desired area. Topical anesthetic gels are also available in single dose packaging, where there is a swab and topical gel in a single package. There is also a gel patch for specific placement. The patch can be trimmed and shaped.

FIGURE 20-1 Examples of topical anesthetic, metered spray, gel, gel patch, and single dose.

The composition of topical anesthetics is classified as the ester or amide local anesthetics. Benzocaine is an example of an ester, and lidocaine is an example of an amide topical anesthetic. These classifications are according to chemical linkages, which define several properties of the anesthetics, including how the materials are absorbed into the system. The concentration of solution for topical anesthetics is greater than the concentration of solution used for local anesthetics. For example, lidocaine topical anesthetic is a 5- or 10 percent concentration, while the lidocaine used as a local anesthetic is a 2 percent concentration. Due to the higher concentrations of the topical anesthetics, there is a greater risk for allergic and/or toxic reactions to occur than there is with local or general anesthetics.

An allergic reaction is a hypersensitive reaction to the anesthetic solution. The reaction can range from mild to severe and can occur up to twenty-four hours or more after the application. Clinical manifestations include swelling, redness, ulcerations, and difficulty swallowing and breathing. Topical anesthetics may also contain flavorings that patients may be allergic to, such as banana flavor, mint, or cherry.

Toxic reactions are symptoms that appear to result from overdose or excessive administration of the anesthetic solution. The first symptom is the stimulation of the central nervous system (CNS). The patient becomes more talkative, apprehensive, and excited, with an increased pulse rate and blood pressure. This is followed by depression of the central nervous system (CNS) as the drug dissipates.

To avoid either of these reactions, review and revise the patient's medical history at each visit, taking special care to note any allergies or allergic reactions.

The ADA recommends that topical anesthetics be left on the mucosa for one minute for the solution to be most effective. The dentist considers the type, concentration of the anesthetic solution, treatment location, and manufacturer's directions when applying topical anesthetic. The procedure for typical placement is described later in this chapter.

Local Anesthetics

Local anesthetics are used to manage pain for most dental procedures. The solution is injected into the soft tissues. To be effective, it must contact the sensory nerve fibers. Once the anesthetic solution anesthetizes the nerve, sensations cannot pass through to register the feeling of pain in the brain. The tissues and teeth in the affected area can be operated on without the patient experiencing pain.

The local anesthetics used for injection are available in liquid form and supplied in premeasured carpules or cartridges (Figure 20-2). They come in cans or blister packs.

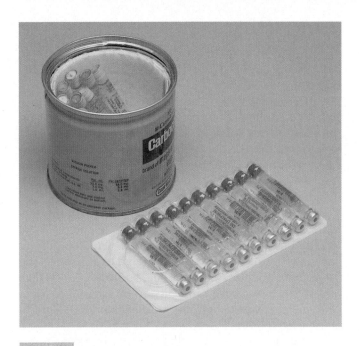

FIGURE 20-2 Various anesthetic cartridges (they come in a can or sealed package).

Local Anesthetic Agents

There are two local anesthetic solutions used for injections in dental procedures. They are amide or ester chemical compounds. Some of the available agents are:

- *Amides:* lidocaine, mepivacaine, prilocaine, articaine, bupivacaine, and etidocaine
- *Esters:* propoxycaine and procaine

Patients may react to one type of local anesthetic but not to another. Specific notations should be made on the patient's chart regarding the type of anesthetic, type of injection, percent of solution, number of cartridges administered, and any reaction the patient experienced.

Duration. Most patients want as much dental treatment completed at one time as possible. This requires an anesthetic that lasts for a long period of time. The duration of the local anesthetics, which can be divided into the three following sections, depends on the presence or absence of a vasoconstrictor.

1. *Short-duration* solutions last about thirty minutes and contain no vasoconstrictor.
2. *Intermediate-duration* solutions last about sixty minutes and usually contain a vasoconstrictor. Most anesthetics fall into this category.
3. *Long-duration* solutions last longer than ninety minutes and contain a vasoconstrictor.

Vasoconstrictors

Vasoconstrictors are drugs that are added to anesthetic solutions to constrict the blood vessels around the injection site and reduce blood flow in this area. Vasoconstrictors slow the absorption of the anesthetic into the bloodstream, thereby affecting the intensity and duration of the solution in the area. Adding vasoconstrictors to the anesthetic lowers the level of local anesthetic solutions in the bloodstream, which decreases the risk of a toxic reaction. Vasoconstrictors also decrease bleeding at the operating site.

The most common vasoconstrictor used in dentistry is epinephrine. Epinephrine is added to local anesthetics in very small amounts. The dilution of vasoconstrictors is commonly referred to as a ratio. The most common ratios are 1 : 20,000, 1 : 50,000, 1 : 100,000, and 1 : 200,000. These ratios, listed on cartridges, indicate one part vasoconstrictor to 20,000 or 100,000 parts anesthetic solution.

Sometimes, other drugs that patients are taking interact with the vasoconstrictor and cause reactions. Again, this information should be highlighted on the patient's medical/dental history.

Possible Complications of Local Anesthetics

A toxic reaction is a complication that also occurs with local anesthetics. Anesthetics used for dental procedures are very safe, but the possibility exists for a toxic reaction. Reactions to the anesthetic depend on the following:

- Type of anesthetic solution
- Amount of anesthetic injected
- Rate at which the solution was injected and absorbed
- Patient's characteristics

Another complication of local anesthetic is paresthesia, the sensation of feeling numb. Paresthesia can last for hours or days beyond the temporary numbness experienced after an injection. Most patients who experience paresthesia regain sensation within eight weeks without treatment. Paresthesia may be caused by:

- Trauma to the nerve sheath (covering) during the injection
- Hemorrhage into or around the nerve sheath, causing pressure on the nerve
- Injection of local anesthetic contaminated by alcohol or disinfecting solution near a nerve

Paresthesia can be permanent if the damage to the nerve is severe enough, but this rarely occurs. If the patient calls the office following a dental procedure and complains of extended numbness, the patient should speak to the dentist and be scheduled for an examination as soon as possible. In most cases, paresthesia is limited. The major concern of short-term numbness is that patients may injure themselves by biting the tongue, cheeks, or lips.

Types of Injections

Three types of injections are given for dental procedures: (1) local infiltration, (2) field block, and (3) nerve block. The type of injection is determined by the injection site and the innervation of the area or specific tooth.

Local Infiltration. Local infiltration anesthesia is an injection method that places anesthetic solution into the tissues near the small terminal nerve branches for absorption (Figure 20-3). The local infiltration injections are used for various dental treatments, including root planing, soft tissue incision for a biopsy, gingivectomy, or frenectomy.

Field Block Anesthesia. Field block anesthesia is commonly referred to as local infiltration anesthesia but with the field block anesthesia, the anesthetic is deposited near larger terminal nerve branches (Figure 20-4). This prevents impulses from passing from the tooth to the CNS. This anesthesia is used most often for dental procedures involving the teeth or bone on the maxillary and mandibular anterior regions. Field block anesthetic injections are given near the apex of the tooth and involve one or two teeth. Usually, the patient feels numb within two to three minutes.

Nerve Block Anesthesia. Nerve block anesthesia is injected near a main nerve trunk (Figure 20-5). The anesthetic prevents any pain sensation from passing from the site to the brain, including any branches of the nerve trunk. These injections eliminate sensations over a larger area than infiltration or field block anesthesia. Some nerve block injections numb from the posterior region

FIGURE 20-3 Local infiltration. Anesthetic is placed in area of treatment. *(Courtesy of Dr. Gary Shellerud.)*

FIGURE 20-4 Field block anesthesia. Anesthetic is injected near the larger terminal nerve ending at the apex. *(Courtesy of Dr. Gary Shellerud.)*

FIGURE 20-5 Nerve block anesthesia. Anesthetic is injected close to the main nerve trunk. *(Courtesy of Dr. Gary Shellerud.)*

of a quadrant to the midline. The nerve block injection usually takes effect within four to five minutes.

Injection Sites

To assist effectively or place the topical anesthetic correctly, the dental assistant must know the injection sites. The sites are divided between the maxillary and mandibular arches (Figures 20-6 and 20-7 and Tables 20-1 and 20-2).

Anesthetics, Syringes, and Needles

The equipment needed to administer local anesthetic includes a syringe, a needle, and an anesthetic carpule.

The Syringe

Various types of syringes are used for dental procedures, but the most common is the **aspirating syringe**. The aspirating syringe, recommended by the ADA, is designed to allow the operator to check the position of the needle before depositing the anesthetic solution. The aspiratory syringe has a harpoon on the end of the piston. The harpoon penetrates the rubber end of the anesthetic cartridge. Once the needle is placed in the tissues, the operator retracts the thumb ring, creating negative pressure (Figure 20-8). If the needle has penetrated a blood vessel, a thin line of blood is drawn into the cartridge. The operator then repositions the needle to avoid injecting the anesthetic into the blood vessel and retests until there is evidence that the needle is not placed in a blood vessel. The aspirating syringe allows the operator to place the anesthetic for maximum benefit.

Syringes may be metal (stainless steel) or nonmetal (plastic). Metal syringes are autoclavable, while nonmetal syringes may be disposable or autoclavable.

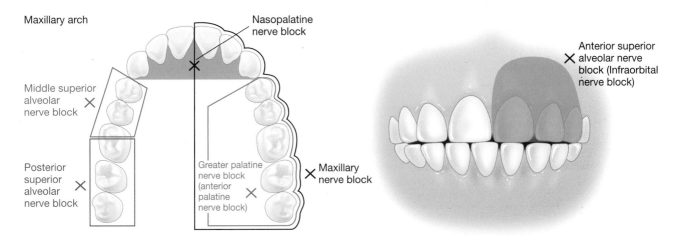

FIGURE 20-6 Maxillary arch injections and site locations.

FIGURE 20-7 Mandibular arch injections and site locations.

TABLE 20-1 Maxillary Local Anesthesia Injection Sites

Name of Injection	Affected Teeth/Tissues	Location of Injection
Infiltration (field block)	Individual teeth.	Near the apex of the tooth; most commonly used on the maxillary anteriors.
Anterior superior alveolar nerve block (also referred to as the infraorbital nerve block)	Maxillary central and lateral incisors and cuspid in a single quadrant.	Height of the mucobuccal fold at the maxillary first premolar.
Middle superior alveolar nerve block	Maxillary premolars in one quadrant and mesial of maxillary first molar.	Height of mucobuccal fold at the maxillary second premolar.
Posterior superior alveolar nerve block	The maxillary second and third molars, the distobuccal and palatal roots of the first molar. The buccal tissues adjacent to these teeth.	Apex of the second molar toward the distobuccal root.
Greater palatine nerve block	The hard palate and soft tissues covering the hard palate from the distal of the canine posteriorly.	Anterior to the greater palatine foramen, middle of the maxillary second molar on the palate.
Nasopalatine nerve block	The anterior one-third of the hard palate from canine to canine.	The lingual tissue adjacent to the incisive papilla.
Maxillary nerve block	The buccal, palatal, and pulpal tissues in one quadrant. Skin of the lower eyelid, side of nose, cheek, and upper lip.	Height of the mucobuccal fold above the distal of the maxillary second molar.

TABLE 20-2 Mandibular Local Anesthesia Injection Sites

Name of Injection	Affected Teeth/Tissues	Location of Injection
Infiltration (field block)	Individual teeth.	Near the apex of the individual tooth.
Inferior alveolar nerve block (commonly referred to as the mandibular block)	A mandibular quadrant including the teeth, mucous membrane, anterior two-thirds of the tongue and floor of the mouth, lingual soft tissues, and periosteum.	Inside of the mandibular ramus, posterior to the retromolar pad, below and anterior to the mandibular foramen.
Buccal nerve block	Buccal tissue adjacent to the mandibular molars only.	Mucous membrane to the distal and toward the buccal of the last mandibular molar tooth in the arch.
Lingual nerve block	The lingual tissues and side of the tongue. Mandibular teeth to the midline.	Lingual to mandibular ramus and adjacent to maxillary tuberosity.
Mental nerve block	The mandibular premolars, canines, and facial tissues adjacent to these teeth.	Anterior to the mental foramen, between the apices of the roots of the mandibular premolars.
Incisive nerve block	Premolars, canine, lateral, and central incisors. Buccal mucous membrane from the mandibular second premolar, the lips, and chin.	At the height of the mucobuccal fold in front of the mental foramen.

FIGURE 20-8 Aspirating syringe with parts labeled. (A) Needle adapter. (B) Piston with harpoon. (C) Finger grip. (D) Thumb ring. (E) Syringe barrel.

Parts of the Aspirating Syringe

- *Thumb ring*—Located at one end of the syringe. A ring for the operator's thumb allows the operator to aspirate and apply force during the injection. The thumb ring loosens and should be checked and tightened as needed before every use.

- *Finger grip/bar*—Supports the index and middle fingers of the operator as the anesthetic solution is administered into the oral tissues.

- *Syringe barrel*—Holds the cartridge. One side of the barrel is open so that the cartridge/carpule can be loaded, known as a breech-loading syringe. Opposite the open side is a "window" for the operator to view the solution left in the cartridge.

- *Plunger* or *piston rod*—Located inside the syringe barrel. It is a rod with the harpoon on the end. The rod is used to apply force to the rubber stopper in the anesthetic cartridge to expel the solution.

- *Harpoon*—A barbed tip at the end of the piston rod that engages the rubber end in the cartridge. The harpoon allows the operator to aspirate with the syringe. When the operator pulls the thumb ring back, the engaged harpoon pulls the rubber end of the cartridge.

- *Threaded end of the syringe*—Where the needle attaches to the syringe. This end must be checked to be sure it is secure on the syringe. Also, sometimes the needle attaches so tightly to the threaded end that this end loosens with the needle and can be discarded mistakenly.

Care and Handling of the Anesthetic Syringe. Follow manufacturers' recommendations for the care and handling of autoclavable syringes. After each use, the harpoon is cleaned with a brush and the syringe is prepared for sterilization like other autoclavable instruments. Some syringes need periodic lubrication in the threaded joints and where the thumb ring meets the finger bar. The harpoon may need to be replaced if it becomes bent or dull and does not remain embedded in the rubber stopper.

The Needle

The needle is used to penetrate the tissues and to direct the local anesthetic solution from the carpule into the surrounding tissues. Most needles are made of stainless steel and are disposable.

One factor to consider when selecting a needle for a dental procedure is needle length. Dental needles are available in two lengths: short (one inch) and long (one and five-eighths inch) (Figure 20-9). The selection usually depends on the operator's preference, the approximate depth of the soft tissues to be penetrated, and the aspiration potential. The short needle is used for injections that require little penetration of the soft tissues, such as infiltration and field block injections, and the following nerve block injections: posterior superior alveolar, incisive nerve block, and mental nerve block. Periodontal ligament injections are also often administered with a short needle.

The long needle is used for injections that require the penetration of several layers of soft tissue. The long needle is used for nerve block injections, such as the infraorbital, buccal, and maxillary and mandibular nerve blocks.

Another consideration when selecting a needle is the needle gauge or diameter. The needles used in dentistry are 25, 27, and 30 gauge. The smaller the gauge, the larger the diameter of the needle. Both long and short needles come in all sizes. The 25-gauge needle is used when there is a high risk of positive aspiration. The internal opening of the needle, where the anesthetic solution flows through, is called the **lumen**.

Parts of Needle

- *Bevel*—The slanted tip of the needle that penetrates the soft tissues.
- *Shank*—The length of the needle from the hub to the tip of the bevel. It is sometimes referred to as the shaft. Along the inside of the shank runs the lumen.
- *Hub*—The part of the needle that attaches to the threaded end of the syringe. The hub may be a plastic or metal piece. The hub is normally prethreaded.
- *Syringe end*—The end of the needle that punctures the diaphragm end of the anesthetic cartridge.

Care and Handling of Dental Needle. The needle is used on a patient and then disposed of in a sharps container. If the operator penetrates the tissue with the needle more than four times during a procedure, the needle should be changed, because disposable needles become dull. When opening the needle package, a seal must be broken; if the seal is already broken, do not use the needle and dispose of the needle as if it had been used. Always be aware of the location and position of the uncovered needle tip to minimize the risk of a needlestick. Keep protective covers on needles when they are not being used. Dispose of needles following OSHA guidelines with protective coverings and in a sharps container.

Needle Stick Protection. There are many types of guards to protect the operator and the assistant from a needle stick. Needle sticks can occur during the transferring of the syringe or during the recapping procedure. Most devices are easy to use with one hand and involve the needle cap being securely held in position for the needle to be placed back in the cap. The devices are plastic or metal and not large in size. They are located near the operator and assistant for easy placement.

A stick shield may also be used for protection against a needle stick. The shield is a rectangular piece of cardboard that slips onto the needle cap. With the shield in place the assistant is protected when handling the syringe with a contaminated needle (Figure 20-10). (In the case of a needle stick, begin treatment and report the incident immediately to the dentist. Follow guidelines discussed in Chapter 11, Infection Control.)

FIGURE 20-9 Needle parts labeled; short and long needles. (A) Syringe end. (B) Hub. (C) Shank. (D) Bevel.

Procedure if needlestick occurs

1. Immediately squeeze the area of the needlestick or puncture to make it bleed.
2. Go to a sink and wash the wound area with an antimicrobial soap.
3. Notify the dentist and find out which patient the instrument was used on.
4. Review the patient's chart and medical history.
5. Follow OSHA protocol for occupational exposure to bloodborne pathogens. (Refer to Chapter 12, Occupational Safety and Health Administration Standards (OSHA).

FIGURE 20-10 Needle stick protection.

The Anesthetic Cartridge

The anesthetic cartridge, also called the carpule, is a glass cylinder that contains the anesthetic solution (Figure 20-11).

Parts of Anesthetic Cartridge

■ *Glass cartridge*—Contains the anesthetic solution. A thin, plastic label covers all glass cartridges. This

FIGURE 20-11 (A) Anesthetic cartridge with parts labeled. (1) Rubber diaphragm. (2) Aluminum cap. (3) Neck. (4) Glass cylinder. (5) Rubber stopper. (B) Anesthetic cartridge and Mylar plastic label with information identified.

provides protection to the patient, the dentist, and the assistant should the glass break. In addition, manufacturers place pertinent information on the label. This information includes the following: volume of anesthetic, brand name, solution concentration, vasoconstrictor ratio (if the anesthetic has vasoconstrictor added), lot number, and expiration date. Each anesthetic cartridge contains 1.8 ml of solution. In a 2% solution the volume or amount of anesthetic is 36 mg and in a 3% solution the volume or amount of anesthetic is 54 mg.

■ *Rubber stopper* or *plunger*—Located in the harpoon end of the cartridge. Most stoppers are treated with silicone so that they can move along the inside of the glass more smoothly. The stopper should be slightly indented from the edge of the glass cartridge.

■ *Aluminum cap*—Located at the opposite end of the cartridge from the rubber plunger. It is a silver-colored aluminum cover that fits tightly around the neck of the glass cartridge. In the center of the end is a thin diaphragm.

■ *Diaphragm*—Where the syringe end of the needle penetrates the anesthetic solution. The diaphragm is made of a latex rubber.

Color Coding of Local Anesthetic Cartridges. Manufacturers of local anesthetics that want to carry the ADA seal of acceptance are adopting a uniform cartridge color-coding system for identifying local anesthetics and local anesthetic/vasoconstrictor combinations. This color-coding, which will standardize local anesthetics and local anesthetic/vasoconstrictor combinations from manufacturer to manufacturer, will include a band near the stopper end of the cartridge. The cap may match the ADA color-coding system or be silver. Stoppers will not be color coded and will not indicate the drug or the color code. The lettering on the cartridge is black and is durable print that is not removed with normal handling (Figure 20-12).

Care and Handling of the Anesthetic Cartridge. Carefully examine cartridges before using them. Things to look for include:

■ expired shelf-life dates,

■ large bubbles,

■ extruded plungers (caused by the solution being frozen),

■ corrosion (caused by immersion in disinfecting solutions),

■ cracks around the neck region and the rubber stopper,

■ rust on the aluminum caps (caused by a broken or leaking anesthetic cartridge).

If you find any of these conditions, the cartridges should be discarded.

Product	PMS Color Code		
Lidocaine 2% with epinephrine 1:100,000	Red: 185, 186, 199 or 200		Red 185
Lidocaine 2% with epinephrine 1:50,000	Green: 347, 348, 355, or 356		Green347
Lidocaine plain	Light Blue: 279		L. Blue 279
Mepivacaine 2% with levonordefrin 1:20,000	Brown: 471, 477, 478, 498, or 499		Brown 471
Mepivacaine 3%	Plain Tan: 466, 467, or 468		Tan 466
Prilocaine 4% with epinephrine 1:200,000	Yellow: 108, 109, 110, 115, or 116		Yellow 108
Prilocaine 4%	Plain black		Black
Bupivacaine 1.5% with epinephrine	Blue: 300 or 301		Blue 300
Articaine 4% with epinephrine 1:100,00	Gold: 871, 872, 873, 874, or 875		Gold 871

FIGURE 20-12 ADA color coding of local anesthetic cartridges. *(Copyright 2002 American Dental Association. All rights reserved.)*

The anesthetic cartridge is discarded after use on each patient. Be aware of the expiration date indicated by the manufacturer. The cartridges should be stored at room temperature and in a dark place. The cartridge need not be heated before use.

Anesthetic cartridges are stored in their original containers until they are used. The cartridges are sterilized and often come in sealed units called blister packs (refer back to Figure 20-2). Many dentists feel the need to wipe the diaphragm with a solution before use. A 2 × 2 gauze sponge moistened with 91% isopropyl alcohol or 70% ethyl alcohol is used. A single day's supply of cartridges can be stored in a dispenser with alcohol gauze sponges in a separate container.

Charting Anesthetic Administration. Like other aspects of dental treatment, anesthetic administration should be charted carefully and in detail. The charting may be completed by the dentist, or the hygienist or the dental assistant under the dentist's supervision. Most dentists will want a comprehensive description of the anesthetic given to the patient.

In the charting include the following:

- The type of injection given
- Type of topical and local anesthetic administered
- If the anesthetic contains vasoconstrictor
- Percentage of solution
- Number of carpules used
- Any reactions by the patient

Some dentists also want to record the needle(s) used and the volume (in milligrams) of the solutions used.

Example of a chart notation: *R-PSANB, 2% lidocaine with 1:150,000epi, 25-short, 1 carpule (36 mg). No complications*

Procedure 20-1 outlines the proper steps for preparation of an anesthic syringe. Procedure 20-2 provides the steps required for assisting with the administration of local or topical anesthesia.

PROCEDURE 20-1

Preparing the Anesthetic Syringe

The dental assistant prepares the syringe out of the patient's view. A topical anesthetic is applied by the dentist or the dental assistant. The equipment and materials are on the procedure tray or stored at the dental unit.

EQUIPMENT AND SUPPLIES (Figure 20-13)

- Sterile syringe
- Selected disposable needle
- Selected anesthetic cartridge
- Needlestick protector
- 2 × 2 gauze sponge moistened with 91% isopropyl alcohol or 70% ethyl alcohol

FIGURE 20-13 Equipment and supplies needed to prepare an anesthetic syringe.

PROCEDURE STEPS (Follow aseptic procedures)

NOTE: It is common in dentistry to first attach the needle to the syringe before placing the cartridge. Precautions should be followed with this technique, because pressure is required on the thumb ring to engage the harpoon into the rubber plunger, which can break the cartridge. Also, if the plunger is not retracted fully while placing the cartridge into the syringe, the needle can bend easily. If this happens, a new needle must be placed before the syringe can function.

This procedure is described for a right-handed person.

1. Following aseptic procedures, select the disposable needle and the anesthetic the dentist has specified for this procedure.

2. Remove the sterilized syringe from its autoclave bag or pouch. Inspect the syringe to be sure it is ready for use. Tighten the thumb bar or ring, as this sometimes is loose.

3. Hold the syringe in the left hand and use the thumb ring to fully retract the piston rod (Figure 20-14).

FIGURE 20-14 Left-hand retraction of the piston rod of an aspirating anesthetic syringe.

4. With the piston rod retracted, place the cartridge in the barrel of the syringe. The plunger end (rubber stopper end) goes in first (Figure 20-15). To prevent contamination, do not place a finger over the diaphragm while placing the cartridge in the syringe. Once the cartridge is in place, release the piston rod.

5. With moderate pressure, push the piston rod into the rubber stopper until it is engaged fully (Figure 20-16). Do not hit the piston rod to engage the harpoon, and do not hold your hand over the cartridge while engaging the harpoon.

(continues)

PROCEDURE 20-1 *(CONTINUED)*

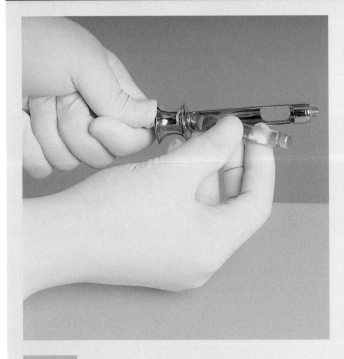

FIGURE 20-15 Technique for placing a cartridge in an aspirating syringe.

FIGURE 20-16 Engage the harpoon with pressure on the finger ring (bar).

6. Remove the protective plastic cap from the syringe end of the needle, and then screw or press the needle onto the syringe depending on the type of needle hub. Make sure that the needle is secure but not too tight (Figure 20-17). A disposable needle guard is often placed on the protective cap covering the needle.

7. Carefully remove the protective cover from the needle. Holding the syringe upright, expel a few drops to ensure that the syringe is working properly. Replace the cap and place on the tray, ready for use.

FIGURE 20-17 Open the cap on the needle.

Supplemental Anesthetic Techniques

Various techniques for administering anesthetics supplement the infiltration and block injection techniques or can be used as the only anesthetic injection technique.

Intraosseous Anesthesia

Intraosseous anesthesia places local anesthetic directly into the cancellous bone (spongy bone). This injection is used for anesthesia in a single tooth or multiple teeth in a quadrant. The bone, soft tissue, and root of a tooth/teeth are anesthetized by the intraosseous injection. This type of anesthetic injection is useful for patients

PROCEDURE 20-2

Assisting with the Administration of Topical and Local Anesthetics

The dental assistant checks with the dentist for instructions on the type of anesthetic and needle for the procedure. The equipment and materials are on the procedure tray or stored at the dental unit.

EQUIPMENT AND SUPPLIES *(Figure 20-18)*

- Patient's medical dental history and chart
- Basic setup: mouth mirror, explorer, and cotton pliers
- Air-water syringe tip and evacuator tip (HVE)
- Cotton rolls, cotton-tip applicator, and 2 × 2 gauze sponges
- Topical anesthetic
- Aspirating syringe
- Anesthetic cartridge
- Selection of needles

PROCEDURE STEPS *(Follow aseptic procedures)*

Placing Topical Anesthetic (by the dentist or the assistant)

1. After seating the patient, review and update the medical dental history.

2. Prepare the patient for the procedure and explain what you are doing and the tastes and sensations the patient may experience. (Explain briefly and avoid such words as "pain," "shot," and "injection.") Explain that the topical anesthetic is being applied to make the patient more comfortable during the procedure.

3. Place a small amount of topical anesthetic on a cotton-tip applicator.

4. Prepare the oral mucosa by drying with a sterile 2 × 2 gauze sponge. Keep the tissue retracted.

5. Place the topical anesthetic on the site of the injection and leave in place for one minute (Figure 20-19).

Administering the Local Anesthetic

6. While waiting for the topical anesthetic to take effect, prepare the syringe, if this has not been completed. Assemble the syringe, cartridge, and needle as described previously.

7. When the operator indicates, take the cotton-tip applicator and prepare to pass the syringe.

8. Check the needle bevel so that it is directed toward the alveolar bone, and then loosely replace the cap on the needle. The protective cap is placed on the hub of the needle so that it is secure but can be removed easily.

FIGURE 20-18 Equipment and supplies needed to place the topical anesthetic and pass the prepared syringe.

(continues)

PROCEDURE 20-2 (CONTINUED)

FIGURE 20-19 (A) Dry the tissue with a gauze. (B) Place the topical anesthetic on the maxillary injection site. (C) Place the topical anesthetic on the mandibular injection site.

9. Pass the syringe below the patient's chin (or behind the patient's head), placing the thumb ring over the dentist's thumb (the dentist grasps the syringe at the finger rest and takes the syringe) (Figure 20-20). As the dentist takes the syringe, remove the protective guard. During the injection, watch the patient for any adverse signs or reactions.

NOTE: There are different methods to safely remove the cap and complete the transfer. It is important for the dentist and the assistant to establish a routine. The assistant can hold the operator's hand until they have cleared the needle.

10. The operator recaps the syringe with one of two methods. The technique for recapping without a

recapping device is called a one-hand scoop technique. With this technique the operator slides the needle into the protective guard. The second technique uses a mechanical recapping device. If a second injection is given, remove the cartridge, insert a new cartridge, test the syringe by expelling a few drops, check the bevel, and position the needle for the dentist to retrieve.

NOTE: At this time, the syringe is contaminated. Most needlesticks occur during recapping. To prevent this from happening, the dentist should recap the needle and retrieve it after the assistant has replaced the cartridge and has repositioned the syringe on the tray or counter. A variety of needle holders are available. These devices hold the needle cap so that the needle can be recapped while protecting the hand.

(continues)

PROCEDURE 20-2 (CONTINUED)

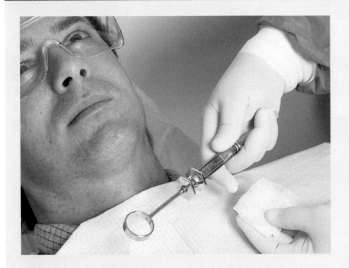

FIGURE 20-20 Pass the prepared anesthetic syringe.

11. The recapped syringe is placed on the tray, out of the way for the rest of the procedure but close in case more anesthetic is needed.

12. Rinse the patient's mouth with the air-water syringe and evacuate to remove the water, saliva, and taste of anesthetic solution.

Unloading the Anesthetic Syringe

1. After the procedure is completed and the patient is dismissed, don utility gloves, take the syringe apart, and prepare it for sterilization.

2. Retract the piston to release the harpoon from the cartridge (Figure 20-21A).

3. Remove the cartridge from the syringe by retracting the thumb ring enough to release the cartridge. Turn the syringe until the cartridge is free (Figure 20-21B).

4. Carefully remove the needle with the protective cap in place. Carefully unscrew the needle. A hemostat can be used to hold the needle while it is being

(A)

(B)

FIGURE 20-21 (A) Retract the piston to release the harpoon from the cartridge and (B) remove the cartridge from the syringe.

removed from the syringe. Also, there are mechanical devices that cut the needle from the hub; after being cut, the needle falls into a closed container. The needle is discarded in the sharps container.

NOTE: The needle can also be removed before the cartridge.

5. Prepare the syringe for sterilization.

---

who do not like the feeling of numb lip and tongue. It is immediate in action and is atraumatic for patients.

The intraosseous injection requires a special system for administration. This technology has been modified with two parts:

1. A perforator, which is a solid needle that attaches to a slow-speed handpiece. The needle perforates the cortical plate of bone.

2. An 8-mm, 27-gauge needle that is inserted into the predrilled hole for administration of the anesthetic (Figure 20-22).

To ensure that this is a "painless" injection, a topical anesthetic is first placed on the tissues. Once the perforator (solid needle) is injected into the tissues, a small amount of anesthetic is administered to numb the nerve endings in this area.

Periodontal Ligament Injection

The **periodontal ligament injection**, or intraligamentary injection, is used for pulpal anesthesia of one or two teeth in a quadrant and sometimes as an adjunct to another injection where the patient is only partially anesthetized.

FIGURE 20-22 Stabident system (Lasystem). *(Courtesy of Fairfax Dental Inc., 1-800-233-2305, e-mail: Fairfax@stabident.com.)*

FIGURE 20-23 Periodontal ligament injection syringe and selection of needles.

It also is used as an aid for diagnosing abscessed teeth and when a patient does not want the lip and tongue numb.

This technique involves inserting the needle into the gingival sulcus along the long axis of the tooth to be treated on the mesial or distal or the root. The original pressure syringe used for the periodontal ligament injection was developed in 1905. This technique has become popular again, mainly because manufacturers have designed pressure syringes for easier administration (Figure 20-23).

Intrapulpal Injection

The **intrapulpal injection** technique deposits the anesthetic directly into the pulp chamber or root canal of the involved tooth. This injection may be used when there is difficulty in securing pain control. A 25- or 27-gauge short or long needle is used; sometimes, the needle is bent to access the pulp canal.

Electronic Anesthesia

Electronic dental anesthesia has been used for a long time with low to moderate levels of success. When used with nitrous oxide inhalation sedation, the effectiveness is improved. It has been used in many dental procedures, such as placing restorations, muscle relaxation, and determining the patient's centric occlusion. Electronic dental anesthesia may be used when local anesthetics are contraindicated, such as with patients who are allergic to local anesthetics or are extremely fearful of the injection.

Computer-Controlled Local Anesthesia Delivery System

Computer-controlled local anesthesia delivery systems promise pain-free injections. These systems can be used to administer all traditional infiltration and block injections. The computer-controlled system is a microprocessor that delivers a controlled pressure and volume of anesthetic solution at a rate that is commonly below the pain threshold. The microprocessor adjusts the pressure for low-resistant tissues to high-resistant tissues and can be used for injections on the palate and periodontal ligament.

Standard anesthetic cartridges and any size or gauge Luer Lock needle can be used with the system. On the microprocessing unit, the cartridge is twisted into place with the diaphragm end of the cartridge down and the rubber plunger up; a plastic microtubing is linked from the plunger to the "handpiece," where the needle is attached. A foot control is used to activate the delivery of the anesthetic (Figure 20-24).

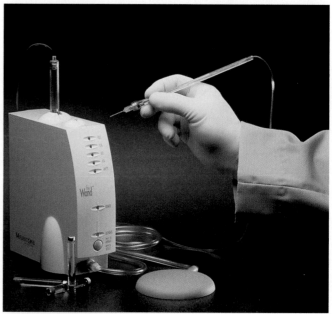

FIGURE 20-24 Computer-controlled local anesthetic delivery system (The Wand). *(Courtesy of Milestone Scientific.)*

Nitrous Oxide Sedation

Nitrous oxide and oxygen gases are combined to provide relaxation and to relieve apprehension for patients during dental treatment. These two gases used together allow a safe method of sedation for patients who experience great fear during dental care. This gas allows patients to maintain consciousness while taking the "edge" off the pain so that relaxation can occur. Patients report a floating sensation, tingling fingers, and the feeling that time is passing quickly. Used safely, nitrous oxide can be a wonderful aid to allow patients to be comfortable and relaxed while receiving dental treatment.

Nitrous oxide is a stable, nonflammable gas. When used with oxygen, nitrous oxide is one of the safest anesthetic agents available. It is administered through a small nosepiece to the patient and has very little offensive odor. As the patient breathes in the gas, it travels through the nasopharynx and oropharynx, then down the larynx to the trachea. From the trachea, it continues into the right and left bronchi. The gas then travels through the smaller tubes, called the bronchioles, to the alveolar sacs, which consist of alveoli (see Chapter 6, General Anatomy and Physiology). The gases are then transferred across the alveoli in the lungs and blood plasma and red cells of the circulatory system. The blood carries the gas in the blood plasma and red cells to the brain, where the nitrous oxide analgesic agent takes effect. This process is much the same as breathing atmospheric air in which the body takes oxygen through the lungs and into the blood, and the blood carries the oxygen to the brain and throughout the body. The pharmacologic actions of nitrous oxide and oxygen are mild and mainly affect the central nervous system. Nitrous oxide raises the pain threshold without the loss of consciousness so that the patient can talk and follow directions.

Nitrous oxide gas was first discovered by Joseph Priestly in the early 1770s. It was thought the gas would cure diseases. Horace Wells (1815–48) (Figure 20-25), a Connecticut dentist, was the first to use nitrous oxide as an anesthetic during dental surgery. He immediately recognized that it could be used to reduce pain during dental procedures.

FIGURE 20-25 Horace Wells (1815–48), artist unknown, c. 1838, oil. *(Courtesy of Menczer Museum of Medicine and Dentistry.)*

Safety and Precautions

The use of nitrous oxide needs to be monitored for both the safety of the dental health team and the patient. Excessive exposure to nitrous oxide or exposure for specific populations of patients may result in adverse health effects.

Dental Office Personnel Safety. The ADA has been monitoring and pursuing information about the safe use of nitrous oxide for many years. In addition, the **National Institute of Occupational Safety and Health (NIOSH)**, which has continued activities relating to safe nitrous oxide concentrations in the dental office, in 1994 reported that the recommended exposure limit of 25 ppm can be controlled with leak-free delivery units, better-fitting masks, proper exhaust rates, and additional exhaust ventilation. The ADA convened an expert panel and made a number of recommendations to ensure safe usage of nitrous oxide for dental personnel. They suggested that twice a year chairside personnel exposed to nitrous oxide be checked with diffusive samplers (dosimeters) or with infrared spectrophotometers, for example.

Patient Safety. Safety and precautions must be practiced with patients because of problems associated with nitrous oxide. Women in the first trimester of pregnancy, infertile people using in vitro fertilization procedures, immunocompromised people at risk of bone marrow suppression, and people with neurological complaints need special consideration. Nitrous oxide may cause fertility problems for those who work with and around nitrous oxide sedation long term.

Indications for Use of Nitrous Oxide Sedation

Patients who would benefit from nitrous oxide analgesia follow:

- Fear dental treatment
- Have a very sensitive gag reflex
- Can breathe through their nose

- Have a heart condition (they benefit because of oxygen and stress reduction)
- Have a long appointment

Contraindications for Use of Nitrous Oxide Sedation

- Patients unable to breathe through their nose
- Patients involved in drugs or psychiatric treatment
- Women in the first trimester of pregnancy
- Immunocompromised people at risk of bone marrow suppression
- Infertile people using in vitro fertilization procedures
- People with neurological complaints

Equipment

Nitrous oxide is delivered to the patient through tubing connected to a nosepiece and tanks of nitrous oxide and oxygen. The gases flow through a unit with a flow meter and adjustment. After the adjustments are made, the gas flows through the breathing tubes to the mask. The excess gas and air exhaled from the patient flows through the scavenging nasal hood, which is a mask inside another mask. Each mask has two tubes connected to it. The inside mask receives the nitrous oxide that flows directly to the patient and the outside mask. The outside mask is connected to the reservoir bag and the vacuum system, which carries away exhaled and additional gases from the treatment area, the patient, and dental team members.

Nitrous oxide units can be portable or wall mounted and distributed throughout the office (Figures 20-26 and 20-27). Cylinders of nitrous oxide gas are blue, those of oxygen are green. When a wall-mounted nitrous oxide unit is used, the gas is sent from the cylinders through pressure lines to outlets in the treatment rooms.

Procedure 20-3 outlines the steps for administration of nitrous oxide.

FIGURE 20-26 Portable nitrous oxide-oxygen unit.

FIGURE 20-27 Example of a wall-mounted nitrous oxide-oxygen unit with gas cylinders in remote storage area. *(Courtesy of Accutron, Inc., Phoenix, AZ.)*

PROCEDURE 20-3

Administration and Monitoring of Nitrous Oxide Sedation

Some states allow dental assistants to perform this task under the supervision of the dentist; in other states, assistants assist dentists in administering nitrous oxide and/or monitoring nitrous oxide.

EQUIPMENT AND SUPPLIES

- Nitrous oxide unit with controls and gauges
- Tanks of nitrous oxide and oxygen
- Patient nitrous nosepieces (sterile)

PROCEDURE STEPS *(Follow aseptic procedures)*

Preparation

1. Check all equipment to verify that it is working properly.

2. Check the levels of gases to determine that the tanks are full.

Administration

1. Seat the patient and place him or her in a supine position.

2. Explain the effects, sensation, and potential hazards of nitrous oxide to the patient.

3. Have the patient give informed consent, allowing administration to continue.

4. Attach a sterile nitrous scavenger mask to the tubing (Figure 20-28).

5. Place the nosepiece mask over the nose of the patient, ensuring a proper fit, with the tubing draped to each side.

6. Instruct the patient to breathe through the nose slowly.

7. Begin the flow of oxygen (five plus liters per minute) and nitrous oxide. (Many offices begin with the flow of oxygen for a minute before the nitrous oxide. This allows the patient to become accustomed to the mask and the situation before adding the effects of the nitrous oxide.)

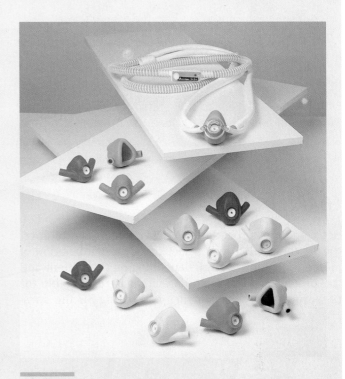

FIGURE 20-28 Nitrous oxide nasal hoods with scavenging circuit. *(Courtesy of Accutron, Inc., Phoenix, AZ.)*

8. Sit with the patient and monitor for any effects as the nitrous oxide is administered. Watch for Guedel's signs, stage I. Talk with the patient and ask how he or she is feeling. (This allows the baseline nitrous oxide to be identified for the patient. Adjustments are made until a comfortable level of sedation is achieved. The patient does not lose consciousness and dialogue is ongoing.)

9. Watch the patient's chest and the reservoir bag rise and fall during the breathing.

10. The local anesthetic solution is administered within a few minutes of nitrous oxide application. The patient is comfortable and the procedure can continue.

(continues)

PROCEDURE 20-3 *(CONTINUED)*

Recovery

1. When the dental procedure is nearing completion, turn off the nitrous oxide.

2. The patient will breathe oxygen for a minimum of five minutes or until all signs of the nitrous oxide sedation have disappeared.

3. Remove the nosepiece from the patient's nose.

4. Turn off the oxygen at the unit. The flow meters for the nitrous oxide and oxygen will be at zero.

5. Seat the patient upright and ask how he or she feels.

6. Ask the patient to stay seated for a minute or two until his or her head clears. (Even without nitrous oxide, rising from the supine position may make the patient feel lightheaded.)

7. Dismiss the patient when he or she feels normal.

8. Complete all documentation on the patient's chart, including notation about the administration of nitrous oxide.

9. The patient nosepiece is given to the patient for later use or disposed of. Some offices provide plastic bags for patients to save their nitrous oxide masks for repeated use to reduce disposables. Patients then bring their masks back for future appointments.

10. Disinfect the tubing.

CHAPTER SUMMARY

Because most procedures require some form of anesthesia, the dentist may select one or a combination of methods to control pain, depending on the patient and the procedure. The dental assistant is responsible for preparing, safely transferring, and caring for the anesthetic syringe and accessories. During this time, the assistant must be aware of the various topical solutions, the application sites, how to apply the topical anesthetic, and possible patient reactions. In addition, the assistant follows the dentist's directions for the administration of sedation and monitoring requirements.

Case Study

Chuck Thompson, forty-five years old, was scheduled for a crown preparation. Topical anesthetic was placed, and Chuck became very talkative and excited. His pulse rate increased.

Case Study Review

1. Which items in the patient's medical history could be related to or cause this reaction?

2. What kind of reaction is Chuck experiencing?

3. Are there any other symptoms to watch for?

REVIEW QUESTIONS

Multiple Choice

1. Anesthetic that produces a deadened or pain-free area is called _____ anesthetic.
   a. general
   b. local
   c. topical
   d. sedation

2. Topical anesthetics are available in all of the following forms except
   a. powders.
   b. gels.
   c. ointments.
   d. metered sprays.

3. An injection that deposits anesthetic near a large terminal nerve branch, and is mainly used for treatment on the maxillary or mandibular anterior regions is a(n) _____ injection.
   a. infiltration
   b. field block
   c. block
   d. periodontal ligament

4. All of the following are parts of the dental needle except the
   a. bevel.
   b. syringe end.
   c. plunger.
   d. hub.

5. A drug that is added to anesthetic solutions to reduce blood flow around the injection site is called
   a. paresthesia.
   b. vasoconstrictor.
   c. infiltration.
   d. nitrous oxide.

6. Which of the following best describes the injection site for the mental nerve block?
   a. the lingual tissue adjacent to the incisive papilla.
   b. halfway between the apices of the roots of the mandibular premolars.
   c. the mucofacial fold adjacent to the root apex of the maxillary premolars.
   d. distal to the maxillary second molar.

7. All of the following are *allergic reactions* a patient might experience *except*:
   a. swelling.
   b. difficulty breathing and/or swallowing.
   c. talkativeness.
   d. redness.

8. Before passing the anesthetic syringe the dental assistant adjusts the bevel of the needle:
   a. toward the alveolar bone.
   b. away from the alveolar bone
   c. either way—it really doesn't make a difference
   d. none of the above

9. Patients report a floating sensation, tingling fingers, and the feeling that time is passing quickly when _____ is administered to them before a dental procedure.
   a. topical anesthetic
   b. local anesthetic
   c. nitrous oxide sedation
   d. general anesthetic

10. The first dentist to use nitrous oxide as an anesthetic during dental surgery was
   a. Joseph Priestly.
   b. Pierre Fuchard.
   c. Wilhelm Roentgen.
   d. Horace Wells.

Critical Thinking

1. Which anesthetic solution would dentists select to administer to a patient if they wanted a stronger ratio of the vasoconstrictor?

2. What should be noted on the patient's chart regarding the local anesthetic?

3. Which types of patients benefit most from nitrous oxide analgesia?

Web Activities

1. Go to http://milesci.com and look up clinical studies on the benefits of computerized anesthetic.

2. Go to http://aamgpaloalto.com and research the role of an anesthesiologist in the dental office.

3. Go to http://www.library.uchc.edu and search for historical information about Horace Wells.

4. Go to http://www.resouree4dentistry.com and look up sedation dentistry.

SECTION VI

DENTAL RADIOGRAPHY

INTRODUCTION TO DENTAL RADIOGRAPHY AND EQUIPMENT CDA

SPECIFIC INSTRUCTIONAL OBJECTIVES

The student should strive to meet the following objectives and demonstrate an understanding of the facts and principles presented in this chapter:

1. Explain the history of radiation and the use of the Hittorf-Crookes and Coolidge tubes.

2. List the properties of radiation and explain the biological effects of radiation exposure.

3. Identify the components of a dental x-ray unit and explain the function of each component.

4. Describe safety precautions when using radiation.

5. Explain how an x-ray is produced.

6. Describe the composition, sizes, types, and storage of dental x-ray film.

KEY TERMS

as low as reasonably achievable (ALARA) *(422)*
anode *(417)*
basal cells *(421)*
cathode *(417)*
central beam *(424)*
collimator *(424)*
contrast *(423)*
control panel *(423)*
density *(423)*
electromagnetic energy *(418)*
focal spot *(424)*
focusing cup *(424)*
gray (GY) *(421)*
halide crystals *(427)*
hard radiation *(420)*

intraoral *(418)*
ionization *(419)*
kilovoltage (kV) *(423)*
latent period *(422)*
leakage radiation *(421)*
long wavelength *(420)*
maximum permissible dose (MPD) *(422)*
milliamperage (mA) *(423)*
milliamperage seconds (mAs) *(423)*
milliroentgen (mr) *(421)*
mitosis *(421)*
position indicator device (PID) *(418)*
primary radiation *(420)*
radiation absorbed dose (rad) *(421)*

radiolucent *(427)*
radiosensitive *(421)*
relative biological effectiveness (rbe) *(421)*
roentgen equivalent man (rem) *(421)*
roentgen *(421)*
scatter radiation *(421)*
secondary radiation *(421)*
short wavelength *(420)*
sievert (Sv) *(421)*
soft radiation *(420)*
thermionic emission *(427)*
tubehead *(423)*
x-ray *(417)*
x-ray tube *(424)*

INTRODUCTION

Wilhelm Conrad Roentgen (rent'-gun) discovered **x-rays** in 1895 (Figure 21-1). Roentgen was a professor of physics at the University of Wurzberg in Germany. At that time, he was performing experiments with a cathode ray tube called the Hittorf-Crookes tube. This glass vacuum tube had an electrical circuit connected to each end. Roentgen, as well as a number of other physicists at this time, was interested in the stream of bluish colored light that passed from one end of the tube to the other when the electrical circuit was connected. The colored light was later discovered to be a stream of electrons that traveled from the **cathode** end to the **anode** end of the tube.

Roentgen placed an aluminum sheet with a window opening on the side of the tube to study the properties of the cathode ray. The room was darkened and a number of fluorescent screens were placed around the laboratory. While conducting his experiments, Roentgen noticed that a fluorescent screen on the other side of the room was glowing. Because Roentgen knew that the cathode rays (negatively charged particles) could travel only a short distance outside the cathode tube in the air, he knew he was observing a new phenomenon, an unknown ray that he identified as an "x" ray, noting the unknown in mathematics.

Roentgen continued his experiments with the x-ray. He placed various objects in front of the beam and observed the images that were made on the fluorescent screen. For instance, when he placed metal in front of the beam, there was no visible image on the fluorescent screen. The metal blocked the beam. However, paper and wood allowed the x-ray to pass through, and the glow on the fluorescent screen changed according to the density of the object. It was while placing the objects in front of the screen that Roentgen noticed that he could see a shadow of the bones of his hand. The soft tissues of the hand allowed the x-rays to pass through, but the harder tissue of the bones stopped the x-rays.

Roentgen furthered his experiments with the x-ray and produced images on photographic plates. A couple of the first radiographs made were those of Roentgen's shotgun barrel and his wife Berta's hand (Figure 21-2).

FIGURE 21-1 Wilhelm Conrad Roentgen (1845–1923) discovered x-rays in 1895. *(Courtesy of the American College of Radiology, Reston, VA.)*

FIGURE 21-2 Early radiograph, thought to be Mrs. Bertha Roentgen's hand. *(Courtesy of the American College of Radiology, Reston, VA.)*

News of the discovery of the x-ray was soon heard around the world. Roentgen was awarded the first Nobel Prize in physics in 1901 for his work. Today, units of x-ray exposure are still expressed in roentgens in his honor.

In Germany in 1895, Dr. Otto Walkoff was the first to take a dental radiograph, just two weeks after the discovery of the x-ray. He used a small glass plate coated with photographic emulsion and an exposure time of about twenty-five minutes to obtain his desired result.

In 1896, Dr. C. Edmond Kells, a New Orleans dentist, took the first intraoral radiograph using his own equipment and techniques. Later he presented a clinical demonstration of dental x-rays at a dental association meeting in North Carolina. Dr. Kells used a method for adjusting the x-ray beam he called "setting the tube." In this technique, he placed his hand between the tube and the screen and adjusted the beam until he could see the bones of his hand clearly. He was unaware of the dangerous effects of radiation. Kells experienced pain and erythema (redness of the skin) on his hands from continued radiation exposure. Ongoing exposure resulted in the subsequent loss of three fingers, Kells's hand, his arm, and eventually his life, at age seventy-two.

The inventor of the first dental x-ray unit was Dr. William Rollins of Boston, Massachusetts, in 1896. He reported effects of radiation exposure, noting burning of the skin on his hands. He was an early advocate of cautious use of "x" radiation.

Dr. William D. Coolidge, a physicist, invented the hot cathode x-ray tube in 1913. This hot filament replaced the need for the residual gas of the older model and established a standard for producing x-rays that were more uniform and therefore more predictable. The first American-made x-ray machine was manufactured around this time as well.

In 1923, the Victor X-Ray Corporation, which later became known as the General Electric Corporation, developed a dental x-ray machine using the Coolidge tube in the machine head, which was cooled by oil immersion. Although the x-ray machine has been enhanced with numerous modifications to meet current application and safety requirements, this basic prototype is still used today.

Around 1905, Dr. Howard Rober and A. Cieszyski, an engineer, developed the bisecting technique. This technique applies a geometric principle. This principle is known as the rule of isometry (discussed later in this book).

In 1920, Frank McCormack developed an additional technique for exposing dental x-rays called the paralleling technique. This technique is often called the right-angle technique. To further improve the paralleling technique, Gordon M. Fitzgerald and William J. Updegrave developed the long cone technique and devices for positioning x-rays and refined information on how to expose the x-ray properly. Over the years, the long cone technique has become simpler due to the change in the shape of the cone. Open-ended cylinders or rectangular tubes have replaced the pointed cone, allowing the operator to direct the x-rays more accurately. The open-ended tube, called the position indicator device (PID), is still commonly called the cone.

Several doctors researched the concept of rotational panoramic machines. The desired outcome was an x-ray of the entire dental arch on one film. To accomplish this, some machines rotated the film, others rotated the patient, and some rotated the x-ray beam. In 1959, the panoramic technique was developed. Dr. Paatero was credited with developing the first orthopantomograph unit that would take acceptable panoramic radiographs. Over the next ten years, a number of advances were made, and in 1980 the Panorex II was developed by Dr. Charles Morris. This machine allowed the operator to make a split or continuous image of the oral cavity.

Current radiographic technology uses the principles of tomography, whereby mouth structures can be visualized in a chosen layer or plane while intentionally blurring structures in other planes. This technique is not routinely used in dental offices.

X-ray film also has changed throughout history. At first, glass photographic plates were used. Later, film was cut to size in the darkroom and wrapped in paper and a rubber coating; this process was very time consuming. In 1913, Kodak developed the first prewrapped film packets. Today's x-rays come in easy-to-use sizes and of a quality we have come to expect. They require minimal patient exposure to achieve results.

Digital imaging, introduced in dentistry in 1987, is currently used in many offices. Images are computer generated, and thus are not processed. The term "digital" comes from the use of "digits" (numbers) that are sent to the computer to produce an image. This technology permits numerous image adjustments without retaking and additional processing, as well as rapid transfer during consultations. Because the images are computerized, they may be integrated into "paperless charts," are easily stored, and require much less storage space. Digital imaging is also used at chairside to help patients understand diagnoses. (See Chapter 23, Extraoral and Digital Radiography, for additional information on digital imaging.)

Radiation Physics and Biology

Radiation is a type of electromagnetic energy. The most familiar forms of electromagnetic energy are radio and television waves and visible light. All electromagnetic energy has some similar properties. First, the energy travels in waves that move in straight lines at the speed of light (186,000 miles per second). Second, the waves consist of energy only. Therefore, energy can be sent through lines to a receiver, such as a television. No mass is involved, only energy. Third, electromagnetic energy travels through space in the form of transverse waves. The wavelength, the distance between the peaks of adjacent waves, is called a cycle (Figure 21-3).

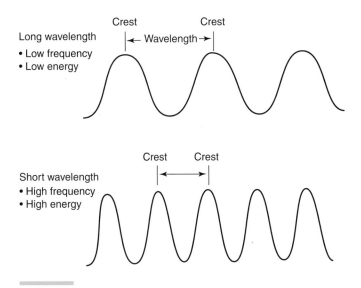

FIGURE 21-3 Wavelengths as they relate to energy, frequency, and x-rays. In dentistry, the shortest wavelength with high frequency and energy is used to expose dental film.

The length of the wavelength is the characteristic that categorizes electromagnetic energy. Examples of electromagnetic radiation with longer wavelengths are visible light, television, and radio waves. Forms of electromagnetic radiation with shorter wavelengths are x-rays and gamma rays. The electromagnetic scale identifies the relationship between type of energy and length of wave (Figure 21-4). The more cycles that pass a point in a given time, the higher the frequency. Therefore,

■ Short wavelength with high frequency = more energy

■ Long wavelength with low frequency = less energy

It is important that individuals working with radiation understand the behavior and nature of x-rays. Visible light is the only wavelength that is detectable with human senses. Invisible x-rays, used for diagnosis in dentistry, carry 10,000 times more energy than visible light. X-rays travel in a straight line and can be deflected off an object and scatter. They can penetrate matter, whereas visible light is absorbed or reflected.

The Structure of an Atom and Ionization

Understanding the composition of an atom helps the dental assistant understand the process of **ionization**, in which atoms change into negatively or positively charged ions during radiation. Atoms make up all matter. An atom is composed of a nucleus (the inner core that is positively charged) and electrons (negatively charged particles that orbit the nucleus). The nucleus is composed of protons (positively charged), neutrons (not charged), and subatomic particles that are divided into hadrons, leptons, and quarks.

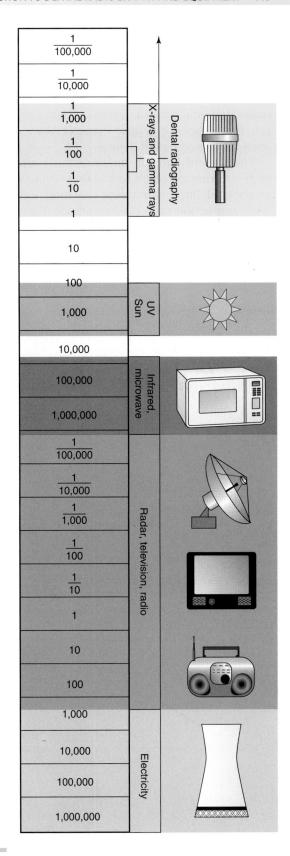

FIGURE 21-4 Electromagnetic energy spectrum and applications.

Unless disturbed, electrons remain stable as they orbit the nucleus. If they are disturbed, for example, when x-ray photons collide with the atoms, electrons are lost and the atoms that have lost electrons become positive ions (Figure 21-5). These positively charged ions can then react with atoms in tissues and other matter. This process can alter living cells and tissues and even cause permanent damage.

The patient and the operator must always be protected during exposure to ionizing radiation. Following safety guidelines, monitoring radiation, and using lead-lined protection protects individuals from the harmful effects of radiation.

Radiation Types

The wavelengths desired in dental radiographs are **short wavelengths**, or **hard radiation**. These have high frequency, high energy, and high penetrating power. **Soft radiation**, or **long wavelengths**, have low energy, low frequency, and low penetrating power. They are unsuitable for exposing dental radiographs. These soft radiation rays are often called Grenz rays.

The four types of radiation (Figure 21-6) follow:

1. **Primary radiation** is the central beam that comes from the x-ray tubehead. It consists of high energy, short wavelength x-rays traveling in a straight line.

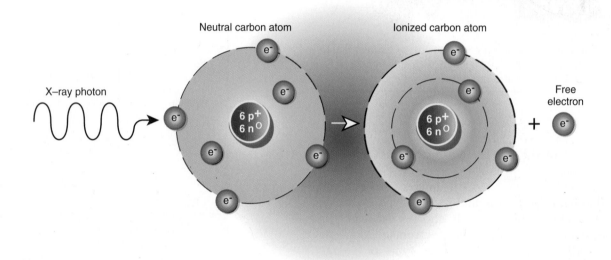

FIGURE 21-5 Protons (+ charge) and neutrons (no charge) comprise the nuclei of atoms. Virtual clouds of electrons (– charge) orbit nuclei at different energy levels (sometimes called "shells"). When an x-ray beam interacts with electron clouds, ionization of atoms occurs.

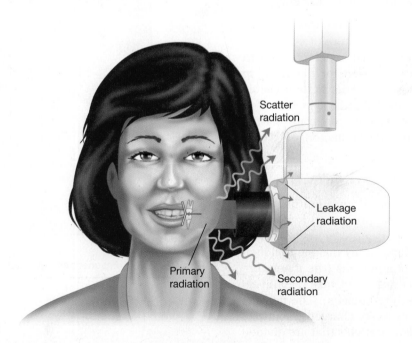

FIGURE 21-6 Primary, secondary, and leakage radiation identified on an x-ray tube and a patient's face.

Primary radiation, often called the primary beam, is the useful x-ray that produces the diagnostic image on the x-ray film.

2. **Secondary radiation** forms when primary x-rays strike the patient or contact matter (any substance). The waves are often transformed into longer wavelengths that lose their energy.

3. **Scatter radiation** is deflected from its path as it strikes matter. Often, secondary and scatter radiation are used interchangeably. This radiation scatters in all directions and therefore presents the most serious danger to the operator. Due to scatter radiation, the operator must stand at least six feet from the patient while exposing x-ray film or behind structural shielding and out of the path of the primary beam.

4. **Leakage radiation** escapes in all directions from the tube or tubehead. The x-ray machine must be checked for leakage and should not be used until the problem is addressed. Leakage radiation is not useful to the diagnostic process; the long wavelengths only cause harm.

Radiation Units of Measurement

The terminology for measurement of radiation has changed. Several new terms are replacing older, more familiar ones (Table 21-1).

In 1937, the International Committee for Radiological Units established the official definition of radiation quantity. A **roentgen (R)** equals the amount of radiation that ionizes one cubic centimeter of air. A **radiation absorbed dose (rad)** or **gray (GY)** is the amount of ionizing radiation absorbed in a substance. A **roentgen equivalent man (rem)** or **sievert (Sv)** is the dose at which body tissues are exposed, measured in terms of estimated biological effects in relation to an exposure dose of one R of x or gamma radiation. A **milliroentgen (mr)** is one one-thousandth (1/1,000) of an R.

Relative biological effectiveness (rbe) is the measurement unit used to compare the biological effects of various tissues irradiated by different forms of energy.

Dental x-rays have arbitrarily been assigned an rbe unit of one.

Determine the rem by multiplying the rad by the rbe. Therefore, 100 rads times one equals 100 rems. The rad and the rem are considered equal for dental x-rays; a rad is an absorbed dose, not the amount coming from the machine.

Biological Effects of Radiation

X-rays can damage body tissues. Some of these injuries heal, but some do not. If the cell is affected by direct radiation, the cell may die immediately, change immediately, change at **mitosis** (cell division in the sex cells in which the number of chromosomes in each is reduced to one-half), or remain unaffected.

Somatic and Genetic Effects of Radiation

The cells in the body are divided into two groups: somatic and genetic. The somatic group includes all cells except the reproductive cells. The genetic group includes all the reproductive cells, such as the ova and the sperm. The biological effects of radiation are classified according to the type of cell affected by the radiation, that is, somatic or genetic.

The somatic effects of radiation leave the individual in poor health, with cataracts, cancer, or leukemia. The effects are not passed to the next generation; the consequence of the radiation exposure remains with the primary individual. Genetic effects, in contrast, may not involve the primary individual exposed to the radiation. Genetic effects cannot be repaired and are passed to future generations.

Radiosensitive Cells

Some cells are more **radiosensitive** than others. The more sensitive cells are immature cells, rapidly dividing cells, and cells that do not perform specialized functions. Examples of rapidly dividing cells are the **basal cells** of the skin. They are sloughed off and continuously

TABLE 21-1 Radiation Measurement Terms

	Standard System (Traditional)	Metric Equivalent or Système Internationale (SI)
Exposure (C/kg)	Roentgen (R) 3.88 × 10 R =	Couloumb per kilogram 1 c/kg
Dose	Radiation absorbed dose (RAD) 100 rads =	Gray (GY) 1 Gy
Dose equivalent	Radiation equivalent man (REM) 100 rems =	Sievert (Sv) 1 Sv

replaced. Therefore, a person may develop skin cancer due to prolonged exposure to sunlight, a high dosage of radiation, and/or frequent radiation exposure.

Today, people are more informed about the effects of radiation. Most patients request protection from radiation during pregnancy, because individuals understand that the embryo is very sensitive to it. Radiation of an embryo may cause death, congenital malformations, or growth retardation. The effects of radiation depend on the stage of the developing embryo and radiation dosage. Therefore, when pregnancy is suspected, as with every patient receiving x-rays, every precaution is taken. All patients should receive protection with lead aprons with thyroid collars during radiation exposure.

Mature cells that rarely undergo cell divisions are radioresistant or less sensitive to radiation. Examples of radioresistant cells are nerve and muscle cells. Table 21-2 shows the levels of sensitivity of different cells.

Low-level radiation normally does not cause damage that cannot be repaired within cells. Tissues that are radiosensitive in the dental region are the lens of the eye and the thyroid gland. Because of their location near the oral cavity, the tissues may be exposed to the primary beam (central beam) of the x-ray. Very high radiation dosages (not used in dentistry) have been known to cause cataracts in the eye and thyroid carcinoma. It is unlikely that dental x-rays cause one of these serious effects, but it is always necessary to use the least amount of radiation possible. All dental personnel use the **as low as reasonably achievable (ALARA)** concept for radiation protection. Dental offices use a thyroid shield extension on the lead apron to further protect patients.

TABLE 21-2 Tissue and Organ Radiation Sensitivity

Most sensitive	Lymphoid Reproductive cells Bone marrow Intestinal epithelium Thyroid
Moderately sensitive	Skin Intestinal tract Oral mucosa
Sensitive	Connective tissue Growing bone
Less sensitive	Mature bone Salivary glands Liver
Least sensitive	Kidney Muscle Nerves

Occupational Exposure

Individuals who routinely use ionizing radiation in their occupations are regulated by the dose limitations defined by the National Council on Radiation Protection and Measurements. The **maximum permissible dose (MPD)** is the maximum dose of radiation that, in light of present knowledge, would not be expected to produce any significant radiation effects in a lifetime. The MPD calls for the dose limit of occupational exposure to be at 0.05 Sv (5.0 rems) per year or 100 mrem per week for radiation workers; nonoccupational and pregnant workers are regulated at one-tenth that limit. Most resources recognize the 0.05 Sv per year maximum; however, recommendations by the International Commission on Radiological Protection call for the occupational exposure dose limits to be 20 mSv (2 rems).

Daily Radiation Exposure

The general population is exposed to two major categories of radiation daily: natural and artificial. Annually, a person encounters an average 3.6 mSv (360 mrem) of radiation from all sources. Natural sources make up about 55 percent of radiation exposure. It comes from the earth (radon, for instance), the sun, and the atmosphere.

About 41 percent of radiation exposure comes from artificial radiation, such as x-rays used for diagnosis, as well as from consumer products, such as television, airline travel, tobacco, and smoke alarms.

Accumulation of Radiation

The effects of radiation are cumulative, meaning that the effects of exposure increase every time the individual is exposed to radiation. This is often called the "long-term effect."

The normal aging process tends to accelerate due to radiation accumulation. Most adults know that the skin of individuals who have (or had) high exposure to the sun ages at an increased rate. The higher the doses, the more rapid the effects. This period between direct exposure and the development of biological effects (or symptoms) is called the **latent period**.

Components of the Dental X-Ray Unit

The dental assistant should know and understand the components in a dental x-ray unit. The assistant may be responsible for obtaining x-rays, as well as for the care and maintenance of equipment used to obtain patient x-rays.

Control Panel

The **control panel** is where the circuit boards and controls that allow the operator to adjust the correct setting for each patient are located (Figure 21-7). It is where the on/off switch is located, along with the selection for the milliamperage (mA) and kilovoltage (kV) and the electronic timer.

The operator chooses settings according to the individual (for example, children need less radiation), the area of the oral cavity needing diagnostic x-rays, exposure technique, and film speed.

Milliamperage. Milliamperage (mA) determines the amount or quantity of electrons. Milli (1/1,000) amperage is a measurement unit for electrical current. The higher the mA, the greater the amount of radiation.

Some dental x-ray machines use 10 or 15 mA. Many machines are set up with selectors for 10 or 15 mA on the control panel. This milliamperage selector also acts as the on/off switch for the machine. Often, 10 mA is used with this type of dental x-ray machine. Radiation is not produced until the electronic timer is pushed. Some newer units are preset at 7 mA for all x-rays; they have separate on/off switches.

Kilovoltage. Kilovoltage (kV) determines the quality or penetrating power of the central beam. The higher the kV, the greater the penetration power of the x-rays and the less exposure time required. Therefore, there is less patient radiation. The speed that radiation goes through the tissues, the higher the quality of the radiograph (showing a longer range of the Gray scale). A longer range of the Gray scale would show varying tissue density and provide greater diagnostic quality.

The kilovoltage meter is on the control panel. The operator adjusts the kilovoltage selector to the desired setting. The most common settings for kilovoltage are

FIGURE 21-7 Control panel.

from 70 to 90 kV. On many of the digital machines, the kilovoltage is set automatically according to the area to be x-rayed.

Electronic Timer. The electronic timer controls the total time that rays flow from the x-ray tube. It is a rotating dial with which the dental assistant selects how many fractions of a second or impulses are needed to produce the x-ray. Thirty impulses equal one-half a second. The operator determines the number of impulses or exposure time after evaluating the technique to be used, the type of x-ray film, the target film distance, and which tissues are going to be radiographed. Again, this may be preset on the digital machines. The digital machines have touch pads and/or switches with simple drawings of adults or children on which to select patient size. By indicating patient size, the amount of kV, and the area to be radiographed, the machine sets the timer automatically.

The switch to the timer is outside the room or behind a lead barrier. The operator pushes the switch, and the timer allows the electrons to flow from the x-ray tube for the indicated time. Then it resets. The milliamperage, kilovoltage, and electronic timer components control the image quality factors of mAs, contrast, and density.

Milliamperage Seconds. Milliamperage seconds (mAs) determine the amount of radiation exposure the patient receives. To determine mAs, the dental assistant calculates the milliamperage times the exposure time. Once set, most offices do not change the kVp and mAs, except for child and adult variations.

Contrast. An x-ray is a black-and-white picture that also shows shades of gray. Contrast is the difference between shades of gray. The black, white, and shades of gray on an x-ray reflect the densities of the subject and the film. The kV, the developing process (if the developing solution is old or exhausted), film fog (possibly caused by a light leak in the darkroom), and distortion (patient or cone moving) control contrast.

Density. Density is the degree of darkness on an x-ray. Contrast is basically the difference between the densities of adjacent areas on a film. Several factors affect the density of a film, including distance from the x-ray tube to the patient, patient tissue thickness, and amount of radiation reaching the film. Density is controlled by mAs, developing techniques, kV, and film fog.

Arm Assembly and Tubehead

The arm assembly is attached firmly to the wall in the x-ray room (Figure 21-8). The flexible extension of the arm allows the operator to freely position the tube head for the various positions required for dental radiography exposures.

The **tubehead** is where the x-ray vacuum tube and step-up and step-down transformers are located (Figure 21-8). The high voltage (step-up transformer) provides

(A)

(B)

FIGURE 21-8 Parts of dental arm assembly. (A) 1. Control panel. 2. Extension arm. 3. Tubehead. 4. Position indicator device (PID). (B) 1. Tubehead. 2. PID. 3. Vertical indicator scale.

FIGURE 21-9 X-ray tube. *(Courtesy of Dunlee, Division of Philips Medical Systems.)*

the kV needed to propel the electrons, and the low voltage (step-down transformer) adjusts the voltage down to the amount of power needed to heat the filament of the cathode and produce the milliamperage. It is where x-rays are generated. The tubehead is made of a metal casing that is lead lined or made of lead to limit the amount of radiation leakage. An oil bath surrounds the components in the tubehead to provide cooling as heat is given off. The heat is derived from production of the cloud of electrons and then manufacturing of the x-rays.

The **x-ray tube**, approximately six inches long and one-half inch in diameter, is often called a Coolidge tube (Figure 21-9). The tube is made from leaded glass and has a window (aperture window) of unleaded glass in the side where the x-rays exit. The tube is a vacuum tube (all air has been removed from the tube), so the electrons are free to travel at the speed of light and not collide with air or gas molecules. On the cathode (–) side of the tube, a **focusing cup** made of molybdenum with a filament of tungsten is positioned. This is where the electrons originate. Tungsten is used because it has a high melting point, high ductility so it can be made into a fine wire, and a high atomic number so that a large number of electrons are ejected when it is heated. The focusing cup is designed to direct the stream of electrons to the anode. The anode (+), which is opposite the cathode, is made of a tungsten target set at an angle to direct the flow of x-rays. The small spot on the tungsten target where the electrons hit is called the **focal spot**. After the electrons hit, a great deal of heat is generated. The anode tungsten target is attached to a copper stem and then to a heat radiator to conduct the heat away from the focal spot. The heat dissipates through the copper stem and then is cooled by the heat radiator and the surrounding oil bath.

After leaving the anode, the x-rays go through the aperture or non-leaded window and encounter a solid metal filter, usually made of aluminum. The aluminum filter, known as the inherent filter, is placed in the path of the x-rays to eliminate the soft x-rays (those with low penetrating power). The hard x-rays with short wavelengths, called the **central beam**, continue through the filter to the **collimator** (lead diaphragm). This collimator is a lead disc with an opening in the middle that restructures the beam and filters out additional weak rays. The opening limits the size of the x-ray beam that is allowed to pass through the open cone and out the PID. The x-ray beam cannot exceed 2.75 inches in diameter. Approximately 1 percent of the kinetic energy (energy of motion) created during the x-ray process is converted to useful x-rays. The remaining 99 percent is dissipated as heat.

Bremsstrahlung radiation is the primary type of radiation in the x-ray beam going from the tubehead. Bremsstrahlung originates from a German word meaning "braking." This braking action takes place when the electrons strike the anode target. Bremsstrahlung also refers to the specific characteristics of the beam.

Safety and Precautions

 It is the responsibility of manufacturers, dental team members, and patients to follow safety and precaution measures when using radiography equipment. Steps must be taken to minimize risk to the patient and all dental personnel.

Manufacturer's Responsibilities

The federal government has set up safety specifications that all manufacturers of dental x-ray units must meet.

- The machine must have a separate control switch to cut off electricity to the machine. The exposure switch must have an electronic timer to stop the electricity automatically when the control switch is released. This "deadman" switch ensures that the exposure ends when the preset time has passed and not when the button is released.

- The PID must be lead lined, and the x-ray tube must be sealed in an oil-immersed casing.

- The control panel must have indicators that display mA, kV, and impulses per exposure time. Some models display the preset number for mA and only two choices for kV. On a digital control panel, the timer is preset, and changes on the digital panel display according to the chosen exposure area.

- The collimator, fitted directly over the opening where the x-ray beam exits the tubehead, is made of a lead plate. The opening or a hole in the middle of the lead plate of the collimator is regulated to ensure that the useful beam does not exceed 2.75 inches in diameter.

- Filtration of 2.5 mm of aluminum is required and built into the head of all x-ray machines operating at a kV higher than 70. Total filtration of 1.5 mm is required for x-ray units operating at or below 70 kVp (peak kilovolts).

Dentist's Responsibilities

- The dentist is responsible for having all x-ray equipment installed safely and to maintain it properly. The office design must provide occupants with lead filtration protection from radiation. The location of the x-ray room and the protective lead barriers must meet specific requirements for safety that allow at least six feet in the opposite direction of the primary ray. X-ray machines must be inspected regularly, usually once a year, by the state regulatory agency, x-ray control section, to ensure proper functioning.

- The dentist must prescribe x-rays for patients responsibly, remembering that only x-rays for a proper diagnosis are necessary. The dentist is responsible for adhering to the "Guidelines for Prescribing Radiographs" (see ADA Web site www.ada.org to download chart or purchase hard copy). These guidelines indicate that the dentist is responsible for ensuring treatment of each patient for her or his individual radiographic needs and thus avoiding prescription of routine x-rays for every patient.

- It is the dentist's responsibility to repair x-ray equipment when necessary and to stop usage immediately when a problem is apparent.

- The dentist is responsible for having dental assistants properly credentialed and trained to expose and process radiographs. The dentist is also responsible for supervising dental assistants in these tasks.

In 1981, the Consumer Patient Radiation Health and Safety Act was enacted. This federal law requires each state to inform the Secretary of Health and Human Services how compliance with the act is accomplished.

Dental Assistant's Responsibilities

- The dental assistant must be trained in aseptic techniques, radiation hygiene, and maintenance of quality assurance and safety.

- Dental assistants must obtain proper education in exposure and processing techniques. They must understand the physics and biological effects of ionizing radiation and use their understanding during every radiographic exposure.

- The dental assistant must understand the ALARA principle and use a lead apron with thyroid cervical collar for the patient's safety every time an x-ray is taken.

- Dental assistants must label and store patient x-rays properly to prevent loss.

Patient's Responsibilities

The patient is responsible for notifying the office of any changes in health (pregnancy, for instance). Patients are also responsible for presenting, to the best of their abilities, radiation histories as part of their dental records.

Additional Notes on Reducing Radiation Exposure

- Using E-type film instead of D-type film reduces the time of radiation exposure to the patient by up to 50 percent. There has been some resistance to changing from the standard D film because of quality control, but recent studies have demonstrated that E film is of comparable quality.

- Kodak InSight dental film is an F-speed film that reduces radiation exposure up to 20 percent compared to Kodak Ektaspeed plus intraoral dental film, and up to 60 percent compared to D-speed films.

- A patient having an eighteen-film series (full mouth) using a long, round PID without a lead apron results in a genetic exposure of 0.5 mrad; with a lead apron, the genetic exposure is approximately 0.01 mrad. If a thyroid collar is used, a 50 percent reduction is noted in the thyroid area.

- A patient having an eighteen-film series using a rectangular PID instead of a round PID reduces the radiation exposure to the patient by approximately 60 percent (Figure 21-10).

- The National Council on Radiation Protection and Measurements (NCRP) makes recommendations on radiation protection and measurements and disseminates information and guidance. In a recent report titled, "Radiation Protection in Dentistry" (report 145), the Council stated that a lead apron is not necessary if a dental office is using F-speed film and rectangular collimation. Staying current on changes and recommendations via the ADA and NCRP is critical for a dental team using ionizing radiation. The NCRP works with the Centers for Disease Control and Prevention. To contact the NCRP, access NCRPpubs@NCRPonline.org or phone 1-800-229-2652, ext. 25.

- The *best* way to reduce a patient's radiation exposure is to use "faster" film and "rectangular" collimation. "F"-speed film is currently the fastest, and many manufacturers offer cone attachments available for the dental position indicator device (PID).

- Proper filtration can reduce somatic (all tissues) exposure by 50 percent. A number of rare earth filters are being used to further reduce radiation exposure in extraoral radiography. Contact the Radiation Health and Safety Board or the Kodak Company for updated information on approved filters.

A dosimeter badge should be worn at all times at the heart level, on outside clothing in the dental office by any dental assistant producing radiographs (Figure 21-11). This badge monitors an individual's radiation exposure in the office. It is important that the badge not be worn outside the office, because it will produce an inaccurate reading. The badges are normally read monthly, and each

FIGURE 21-11 Operator wears a film badge to detect radiation exposure.

employee should be apprised of the outcome immediately and corrective measures taken.

A quality assurance (QA) program should be developed for the production and processing of radiographs in the dental office.

Radiation Production

X-rays are produced when the operator depresses the exposure switch and starts generating electricity (Figure 21-12). The electricity passes to the control panel by way of the step-down and step-up transformers, where specified instructions on the quantity and the quality of x-rays have been selected. From the setting of the mA, time, and kV circuits, the electricity travels to the cathode filament. This current passes through

FIGURE 21-10 Compared to the rectangular collimator, the round collimator exposes the patient to greater excess radiation.

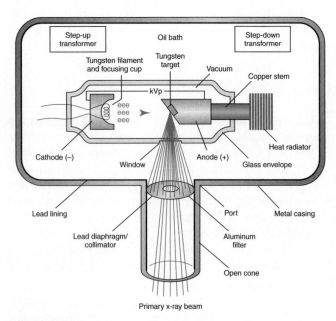

FIGURE 21-12 X-ray production in the tubehead.

the filament and heats it to an extremely high temperature. This process is called **thermionic emission**. When the filament reaches a certain temperature, electrons are ejected. Electrons are negatively charged, and therefore are attracted to the positively charged anode side of the tube. The electrons rapidly travel toward the anode. The focusing cup on the cathode directs the electrons to a small area (about 1 mm^2 in size), called the focal spot, on the anode tungsten target. The precise moment of contact occurs when the x-rays are produced due to forceful collision of the electrons. At the time of collision, the x-rays "bounce" off the tungsten target and weaker rays go in all directions. The useful x-rays travel through the filters and collimator and out the PID opening.

The excess heat generated by the collision is dissipated by a heavy copper stem that takes the heat from the tungsten target and cools it in oil in the tubehead. In addition to the copper stem cooling, a bulb also takes heat into the oil bath chamber of the tubehead to increase cooling.

Dental X-ray Film

Proper care and handling of the dental x-ray film is critical to the quality of the x-rays produced. It is important to understand the qualities of the film. A sound understanding of the quality and characteristics of the film will allow the dental assistant to maintain high quality radiographs.

Composition of Dental X-ray Film

The film used in dental radiography is composed of a flexible, thin, polyester plastic base (about 0.2 mm thick). This semi-clear base (cellulose acetate) has a slightly bluish tint to enhance the quality of the image. The primary function of the base is to support the emulsion. It permits easy handling during the processing and makes viewing

FIGURE 21-13 Composition of dental x-ray film.

the image less difficult. The base is coated on each side by the emulsion and is attached firmly by an adhesive (Figure 21-13). The adhesive ensures that the emulsion is distributed uniformly over the base. The emulsion is made of a homogeneous mixture of silver **halide crystals** suspended in a gelatin. Halides are halogen compounds, such as chlorine, bromine, and iodine, that combine with another element, such as silver. In dental films, silver is combined most frequently with bromine. During radiation exposure, the silver halide crystals store the energy to which they have been exposed and react with the chemicals in the processing tank to form a black (**radiolucent**) region on the film. The silver halide crystals that have not been struck by the radiation are not energized and wash off the film when it processes.

This energy or latent image does not become visible until the film has been exposed to chemicals for a given time at a given temperature. If a film has been totally exposed to visible light, it appears black after the processing. If the film was not exposed to light or radiation, the film appears clear after processing. The emulsion washes off and appears as a semi-clear blue base. The emulsion is placed on both sides of the base to reduce the amount of radiation needed, and it means that the x-ray can be read from either side. On top of the emulsion is a protective coating that is used to protect the emulsion, especially from the rollers in an automatic processor.

Film Speed

Crystal size in the emulsion regulates the speed of the film. The larger the crystals, normally the faster the film. Dentists typically use one of three dental x-ray films: D-speed film, called Ultraspeed, E-speed film, called Ektaspeed, or F-speed film, called InSight. Ektaspeed film requires approximately 40% less exposure time than Ultraspeed, and InSight requires 60% less exposure time than D-speed and 20% less exposure time than E-speed. InSight film is the highest-speed dental film for the greatest reduction in radiation exposure for the patient.

Film Sizes

Dental intraoral film packets come in five basic sizes (Figure 21-14). Each size is used for a specific radiographic exposure, depending on the size of the patient's oral cavity and the area to be radiographed (Table 21-3). The film that produces the best radiographic results with the least radiation exposure for the patient is selected.

Dental Film Packet

The intraoral film packet has a sealed outer plastic wrap (Figure 21-15). Inside the wrapper, black paper is folded around the film and a lead foil backing is placed away from the x-ray tube. The lead foil absorbs any unused

FIGURE 21-14 Sample dental x-ray films showing sizes and numbers. (Size no. 1, narrow anterior film size, and Size no. 3, long bite-wing film size, are not shown.)

FIGURE 21-15 Film packet.

TABLE 21-3 Intraoral Film Sizes and Uses

Film Size	Description/Use
No. 0	Child size
No. 1	Narrow anterior film size
No. 2	Adult size
No. 3	Long bite-wing film size
No. 4	Occlusal film size

radiation and the scattering of secondary radiation and helps prevent film fogging. The outer plastic or paper wrap is completely sealed to prevent moisture from getting to the film.

The film packets also come in double packets. These film packets contain two films per packet. They take slightly more radiation for exposure but allow both the doctor and the specialist to have an original film. Package color and numbering may differ from one manufacturer to another. Kodak numbers on the film and packet denote film speed, size, and single- or double-packet film. An example is Kodak EP-22, which indicates that the film speed is EP (E-Speed or Ektaspeed Plus), #2 size film, and two packets or double-packet film. Single-packet film of the same size and speed would be labeled EP-2.

Dental Film Storage

Before use, dental x-ray film should be stored carefully. It is sensitive to stray radiation, high temperatures, and chemicals. Ideally, unexposed film should be stored at 50 to 70°F (10 to 20°C). Many dental offices store the film in the refrigerator. Dental assistants take only the needed films to the area and use disposable cups to collect and transfer exposed radiographs.

The dental assistant should pay careful attention to the expiration date on the boxes of film. Placing the boxes of film in the storage area so that the oldest film is used first will prevent any film from expiring. Using expired film for a patient's radiographs may inhibit diagnostic quality.

After the film has been exposed and processed, it should be mounted and placed in a protective envelope. All x-rays should be handled with care so that they are not scratched and the integrity of the radiograph is not compromised. Radiographs are records of the patient's conditions at that time and may be used as legal documents.

CHAPTER SUMMARY

Dental assistants must understand the physics and biological effects of ionization radiation, use their understanding during every radiographic exposure, understand the ALARA principle, and use the lead apron with cervical collar for the patient's safety every time an x-ray is taken. The assistant must label and store patient x-rays properly to prevent loss and thereby avoid the need for x-rays being retaken.

Case Study

In 1910, dentist Deziree Scott was very interested in radiography and had obtained a unit for her office. Every time she used it, she would test the machine by focusing it on her hand to ensure that bones could be viewed and to focus the x-ray tube. Her hand started turning red after a few weeks of using it this way.

Case Study Review

1. What is the damage to Dr. Scott's hand called?

2. Should Dr. Scott continue with this procedure?

3. What will occur if Dr. Scott continues to adjust the x-ray tube in this manner?

4. Would it be possible to lose her hand due to this procedure?

5. Would it be possible to lose her life from this procedure?

REVIEW QUESTIONS

Multiple Choice

1. Physics professor _____ discovered x-rays in 1895.
   a. Dr. C. Edmond Kells
   b. Dr. Otto Walkoff
   c. Dr. William Rollins
   d. Wilhelm Conrad Roentgen

2. _____ film requires less exposure time.
   a. D-speed
   b. E-speed
   c. F-speed
   d. Ultraspeed

3. The polyester plastic base of dental x-ray film has a slightly _____ tint.
   a. green
   b. blue
   c. red
   d. orange

4. _____ invented the hot cathode x-ray tube.
   a. William Rollins
   b. Dr. Howard Rober
   c. Frank McCormack
   d. Dr. William Coolidge

5. The hot cathode x-ray tube was developed in
   a. 1895.
   b. 1896.
   c. 1913.
   d. 1920.

6. All of the following are examples of electromagnetic radiation with longer wavelengths *except*
   a. visible light.
   b. radio waves.
   c. television.
   d. x-rays.

7. _____ radiation escapes in all directions from the tube or the tube head.
   a. Primary
   b. Secondary
   c. Scatter
   d. Leakage

8. Identify the most sensitive tissue or organ to radiation.
   a. Reproductive cells
   b. Muscle
   c. Nerves
   d. Mature bone

9. The amount of ionizing radiation absorbed by a substance is called a
   a. rem.
   b. sievert.
   c. milliroentgen.
   d. gray.

10. The quality or penetrating power of the central beam is determined by
    a. Milliamperage
    b. Kilovoltage
    c. The electronic timer
    d. The collimator

Critical Thinking

1. A patient has been exposed to a large number of radiographs due to other health issues. The dental assistant is going to take a necessary radiograph as requested by the dentist. In order to minimize radiation exposure, the dental assistant decides to reduce the kilovoltage. Is this sound thinking? Name some practices that would reduce the patient's exposure.

2. If the film badge that the dental assistant wears during radiograph exposures comes back registers a high exposure reading, what should be done initially? What questions should be directed to the dental assistant? Besides a defective x-ray machine, what could have caused the high readings?

3. A dental assistant's friend is outdoors sunbathing. After she went indoors, the sun worshipper tells the assistant that she had been in the sun for several hours and tanned very little. A few hours later the friend is in a great deal of pain and her "sun lines" are extremely red. How would you explain minimal change in her skin tone earlier in the day and her subsequent discomfort? Does ongoing exposure to the sun cause aging?

Web Activities

1. To find questions that patients frequently ask about dental x-rays, go to http://www.ada.org and search under x-rays.

2. Go to http://www.nrc.gov, locate the radiation protection topic, and find sources of radiation. Be prepared to share five sources of radiation with the class and instructor.

3. At the site http://www.osha.gov, click on Safety and Health Topics, and then in the topics index, choose Radiation. Find the scale that shows both nonionizing radiation and ionizing radiation. Be prepared to discuss in class.

PRODUCTION AND EVALUATION OF DENTAL RADIOGRAPHS

SPECIFIC INSTRUCTIONAL OBJECTIVES

The student should strive to meet the following objectives and demonstrate an understanding of the facts and principles presented in this chapter:

1. Explain intraoral and extraoral x-ray production.

2. Describe a diagnostic quality x-ray.

3. Identify the means of producing quality radiographs on various patients.

4. Explain the bisecting principle and technique.

5. Explain the paralleling principle and technique.

6. Describe manual film processing equipment and technique.

7. List and explain the composition of processing solutions.

8. Describe automatic processing equipment and explain the technique.

9. Explain and demonstrate how to mount dental x-rays.

10. List common radiographic errors that occur during exposure and processing of x-ray films.

11. Explain how to duplicate dental radiographs.

12. Describe the storage of final radiographs and legal implications concerning dental radiographs.

13. List standardized procedures and state policies that dental offices follow to ensure quality radiographs.

KEY TERMS

acetic acid (462)

automatic processing (462)

bisecting technique (435)

bite-wing radiograph (435)

blurred image (468)

clear film (468)

cone cutting (467)

cross-section technique (448)

developer solution (460)

double exposure (468)

duplication technique (471)

elon (462)

elongation (467)

fixer solution (462)

fogged film (470)

foreshortening (467)

herringbone pattern (469)

horizontal angulation (436)

hydroquinone (462)

(continues)

KEY TERMS *(continued)*

interproximal *(440)*

manual processing *(458)*

occlusal radiograph *(435)*

overlapping *(467)*

paralleling technique *(435)*

partial image *(470)*

periapical radiograph *(435)*

potassium alum *(462)*

potassium bromide *(462)*

quality radiograph *(432)*

radiopaque *(469)*

reticulation *(471)*

sodium carbonate *(462)*

sodium sulfite *(462)*

sodium thiosulfate *(462)*

topographic technique *(448)*

underexposed *(469)*

vertical angulation *(435)*

Producing Quality Radiographs

Producing a **quality radiograph** involves many steps, which are grounded in the dental assistant's skills in exposing the radiograph, and knowledge of what the dentist needs to read the x-rays and make a diagnosis. Careful attention must be focused on preparation of the x-ray room and setting up the x-rays, film holders, and barriers for each patient. The patient is prepared in the chair and the protective apron is placed. Films are positioned for correct exposure.

What Is a Quality X-ray?

- Desired teeth and surrounding area are on the film.
- Images are dimensionally accurate.
- The contacts between the teeth are open.
- The teeth are not elongated or foreshortened.
- The entire length of the tooth is visible, including 1 to 2 mm beyond the cusps and 4 to 6 mm beyond the apex.
- The film has enough contrast and density to show good detail of all anatomy.
- The radiograph is free of spots, stains, handling marks, and other artifacts (black lines).

Preparing for X-ray Exposure

The dental chair should be covered with a plastic bag or at least have a barrier on the head rest and chair controls. The x-ray units should have barriers covering the dials, the exposure buttons, the cone, the tubehead, areas of the extension arm that would be touched, and any other areas that may be contaminated (Figure 22-1A and B). If there is a door the dental assistant needs to open and close, a barrier should be placed on the door knob (plastic sandwich bags work well to barrier this area). An area for clean and contaminated films should be prepared. The procedure for infection control is outlined in Procedure 22-1.

(A)

(B)

FIGURE 22-1 (A) Control panel. (B) Tubehead with barriers.

Set up the materials needed. For example, assemble the parts of the sterile Rinn XCP instruments and select the appropriate x-ray films. Also, have a tissue available for the patient and gauze and cotton rolls for x-ray film positioning. X-ray film that is going to be used should be prepared, and kept close to the room where the x-rays will be taken, but not in the same room.

During Film Exposure

During film exposure, the dental assistant should wear gloves, protective eyewear, and masks. After removing the exposed film from the patient's mouth, wipe the saliva from the film and place it in a paper cup or on a covered surface. Film can be purchased with a plastic barrier or separate plastic barriers can be purchased to place on the individual film packets before exposure.

PROCEDURE 22-1

Radiography Infection Control

This procedure is performed by the dental assistant. The dentist designates which radiographs are needed for diagnosis. The dental assistant prepares the patient and area, takes the radiographs, and processes and mounts the films for viewing according to infection control protocol.

EQUIPMENT AND SUPPLIES

- Barriers for the x-ray room
- X-ray film (size selected accordingly)
- Rinn XCP materials (assembled for use) or other paralleling technique aids
- Film barriers (optional)
- Lead apron with thyroid collar
- Container for exposed film

PROCEDURE STEPS *(Follow aseptic procedures)*

1. Wash and dry hands.
2. Place appropriate barriers on the dental chair, film, and x-ray equipment (Figure 22-9).

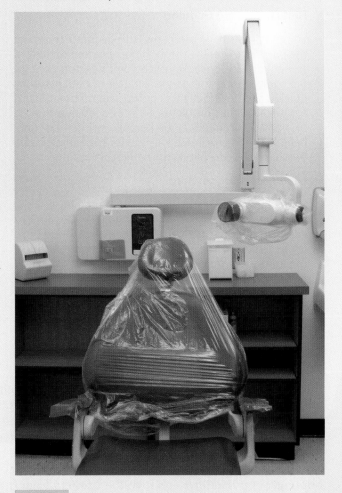

FIGURE 22-9 Room prepared with barriers: on the chair, film, tubehead, and switches.

(continues)

PROCEDURE 22-1 (CONTINUED)

3. Prepare equipment and supplies needed for the procedure, including sterile Rinn XCP instruments, tissue or paper towel, and a cup or container with the patient's name on it.

4. After the patient is seated and positioned, wash and dry hands. Don treatment gloves. (Glasses and mask may also be worn.)

5. After the x-rays are exposed and removed from the patient's mouth, wipe off the x-rays and place them in a cup/container or on a covered surface.

6. When all x-ray exposures are complete, remove the lead apron from the patient. There are sev-

eral ways this is done to follow aseptic protocol. The lead apron can be removed once the contaminated gloves are removed or overgloves can be placed over the treatment gloves and the lead apron removed. If the lead apron is removed with contaminated gloves, it must be disinfected following the procedure.

7. After the patient is dismissed, remove and dispose of all barriers.

8. Any areas that were not covered with a barrier must be disinfected, including the x-ray film.

Patient Exposure

Before the patient is seated, prepare the room following aseptic techniques. Review the patient's medical history and check the dental chart to confirm the number and types of x-rays the dentist has requested for diagnosis.

Establish a routine to check the x-ray machine. Check the settings for the kV, mA, and exposure time. (Note that some x-ray machines are pre-set and require no changes.) Select the x-ray unit if the control panel operates more than one tubehead.

Escort the patient into the room, seat the patient in an upright position, and position the head rest to secure the head. Ask the patient to remove eyeglasses, partials, or any metal objects that will interfere with the x-rays (Figure 22-2). Place a lead apron with a thyroid collar on the patient, making sure that it is secured and covers the patient. Explain the procedure to the patient and indicate how the patient can assist during the exposure

FIGURE 22-2 Barriers on a dental x-ray unit, and a lead apron with a thyroid collar on a patient.

of the x-rays. Bring the tubehead close to the working area and proceed.

Hints to Prevent Gagging

Some patients have problems with gagging. Try to get the patient to breathe through the nose and to think of something else, because psychological factors contribute to triggering the gag reflex. Talk to patients, work quickly, and have patients concentrate on breathing. If a patient still has problems, an anesthetic mouth rinse or a throat lozenge may be helpful. Position the tubehead in the approximate location for the film exposure before placing the film in the patient's mouth.

Lead Apron Suggestions

After exposing the x-ray film, remove the film, pull the x-ray tubehead out of the way, and place the film in a cup/container or on a barrier. After all films have been taken, remove the lead apron from the patient, disinfect the apron, and then place the lead apron over a bar or hang it on a hook to prevent creases or folds. If the lead apron is creased routinely, the lead may be damaged and protection from x-ray exposure would be incomplete in these areas.

After Films Are Exposed

After films are exposed, dental assistants remove their gloves or place overgloves on, remove the lead apron from the patient, and make chart notations. Films are then taken to the processing area for processing. After films are processed, they are reviewed by the dentist. The patient is dismissed. Following appropriate infection control procedures, remove the barriers from the dental chair, x-ray unit, and control buttons. Dispose of barriers after each patient and disinfect the area. When handling contaminated films without barriers, wipe or spray them with a disinfectant, and leave for ten minutes. If film barriers are used, remove them, along with other contaminated barriers.

Types of Film Exposures

Three types of film exposures/radiographs are used most commonly in the dental office: the periapical, bitewing, and occlusal. The type of film used and the number of x-rays taken are determined by the dentist.

Periapical Radiographs. The **periapical radiograph** pictures the entire tooth and surrounding area (Figure 22-3A). The periapical radiographs are used to assess the health of the teeth, bone, and surrounding tissues. Tooth development and eruption stages also are seen on periapical radiographs. Abnormalities and pathological conditions are diagnosed by the dentist using these radiographs. The size of the patient's mouth usually determines the size of the x-ray film and the number of exposures.

Bite-Wing Radiographs. The **bite-wing radiograph** pictures the crowns, the interproximal spaces, and the crest area of the alveolar bone of both the maxillary and the mandibular teeth (Figure 22-3B). Bite-wing radiographs, usually taken only on the posterior teeth, are used to detect caries, faulty restorations, and calculus, and to examine the crestal area of the alveolar bone. The size of the patient's mouth determines the size of the film used for the bite-wing x-ray.

Occlusal Radiograph. The **occlusal radiograph** pictures large areas of the mandible or maxilla (Figure 22-3C).

These radiographs can be used alone or to supplement periapical or bite-wing films. For adults, a No. 4 film is used; for children, a No. 2 film may be used.

Intraoral Techniques for Film Exposures

There are two basic techniques used for film exposures in dentistry: the **bisecting technique** and **paralleling technique**. The bisecting technique, which is used for more specific or unique radiographs rather than the routine, is the oldest technique. The paralleling technique is widely accepted because the detail of the image is more accurate. The American Association of Dental Schools and the American Academy of Oral and Maxillofacial Radiology recommend the paralleling technique.

Bisecting Technique

The bisecting technique is used to expose periapical, bite-wing, and occlusal radiographs (Figure 22-3A through C). In the bisecting technique, a film holder is used to secure the film close to the tissue/tooth without bending the film. In this technique, the central ray is directed at an imaginary line that bisects the angle created by the length (long axis) of the tooth and the film packet. The central ray must be perpendicular to this bisecting line (the rule of isometry). The direction of the central ray creates **vertical angulation**. An average for the vertical angulation has been predetermined for this technique. The angulation works with most patients, but operators should determine the appropriate angle after the patient has been positioned and the film is in place (Figure 22-4) (Table 22-1).

FIGURE 22-3 (A) Periapical radiograph showing crowns, roots, and supporting bone. (B) Bite-wing radiograph showing crowns of teeth on both arches. (C) Occlusal radiograph showing entire dental arch.

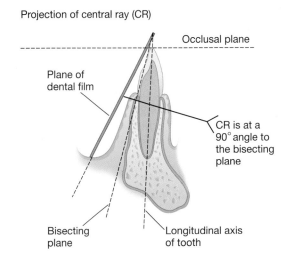

Projection of central ray (CR)

Occlusal plane

Plane of dental film

CR is at a 90° angle to the bisecting plane

Bisecting plane

Longitudinal axis of tooth

FIGURE 22-4 Principle of the bisecting technique. The central ray is directed at a right angle to the bisecting plane (imaginary bisector). The image on the film will be equal to the length of the tooth when the central ray is directed at a 90° angle to the bisecting plane.

TABLE 22-1 Vertical Angulation Table

Area	Maxillary	Mandibular
Incisor/lateral	+40°	−15°
Cuspids	+45°	−20°
Bicuspids (premolars)	+30°	−10°
Molars	+20°	−5°

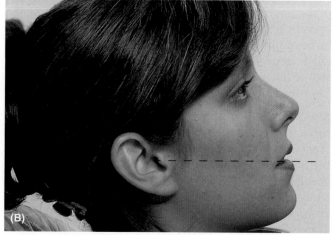

FIGURE 22-5 When exposing radiographs using the bisecting technique, the patient's head is positioned as shown for (A) the maxillary regions (tragus of the ear to the alla of the nose) and (B) the mandibular regions (tragus of the ear to corner of the mouth).

Principles of Bisecting Technique. The principles of the bisecting technique include the following:

- The patient's head must be in the correct position for each arch. For the maxillary arch, seat the patient in an upright position and support the head so the occlusal surfaces of the maxillary teeth are parallel to the floor and the patient's nose is positioned slightly downward (Figure 22-5A). For the mandibular arch, seat the patient in an upright position and support the head slightly tilted back so the occlusal surfaces of the mandibular teeth are parallel to the floor and the patient's nose is positioned slightly upward (Figure 22-5B).

- The film is placed in the patient's mouth as close to the lingual surface of the tooth as possible without bending the film.

- Various kinds of film holders can be used to hold the film. Examples include the Stabe, Snap-a-Ray, Rinn XCP, Precision, and bite-blocks. As a last resort, the patient's finger can be used to hold the film in position. Be sure that the patient's finger pressure is adequate to prevent film movement during exposure, but not so firm as to cause the film to bend.

- Set the appropriate vertical angulation using the vertical angulation degree guide on the x-ray tubehead (Figure 22-6). **Horizontal angulation** is determined by directing the central ray at the teeth to be exposed, aiming the beam directly through the interproximal spaces (Figure 22-7).

- The film is placed in the patient's mouth so that only an edge of the film, one-eighth of an inch, can be seen beyond the occlusal surface or the incisal edge. The cone must cover the x-ray film completely. As with other techniques, the patient and the tubehead should be still during exposure.

- Exposure time, mA, and kVp selections are determined according to the type of film, area of exposure, and dental x-ray machine being used.

Disadvantages of Bisecting Technique. Disadvantages include image distortion, guesswork with the technique, patient positioning, and increased exposure to the patient's finger and hand.

The technique is still used, however, on small children, adults with small or tender mouths, for selected endodontic exposures, and on patients who have conditions or oral anatomies that make it difficult to use the parallel positioning instruments.

Paralleling Technique

The paralleling technique is the technique most commonly used in exposing periapical and bite-wing radiographs and is highly recommended by the American Dental Association. It is accurate and produces excellent diagnostic-quality radiographs. There is less exposure to the patient's head and neck, and the technique is easier and requires less guesswork. However, the paralleling technique can be uncomfortable for small children, adults with small or sensitive mouths, or for patients with low palatal vaults. Practice helps the operator gain the skills and confidence needed to use the paralleling technique with all patients.

The paralleling technique requires the film packet and the long axis of the teeth to be parallel. The x-ray beam is directed perpendicular to this parallel line formed by the teeth and the film packet (Figure 22-8). The anatomy

FIGURE 22-6 Example of cone positioning for vertical angulation (up and down rotation). Numerical degree guide on the side of the tubehead is also shown.

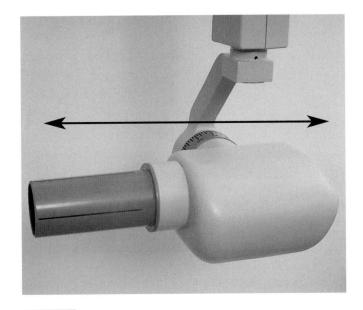

FIGURE 22-7 Example of cone positioning for horizontal angulation (left and right rotation).

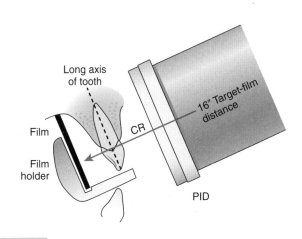

FIGURE 22-8 Position of film for paralleling technique.

FIGURE 22-10 Film-holding devices for the paralleling technique.

of the oral cavity requires the film to be placed toward the center of the mouth, with the exception of the mandibular molars, to keep the film packet flat and have the film parallel to the long axis of the teeth. A film holder is used for ease of technique and correct alignment.

Holders for Paralleling Technique. Various film holders are available for use with the paralleling technique. The function of the holder is to secure the film away from the lingual surfaces of the teeth and parallel with the long axis of the teeth. Some holders have supports to prevent the film from bending. One example is the Rinn XCP. Also, several holders have positioning rings that assist the operator in correct cone placement and allow the patient to be in varied positions for x-ray exposure. The film holders (Figure 22-10) may be simple one-piece bite-blocks (snap-a-rays), hemostats with rubber bite-blocks, or they may come with several pieces, such as the Rinn XCP kit or the Precision paralleling device (Figure 22-11). It is important to be familiar with these to allow for quick and accurate assembly.

Film Positioning. When using the paralleling technique, the film should be placed in the patient's mouth with care to keep the patient relaxed and cooperative for the film and holder placement. Place the film in the film

FIGURE 22-11 Rinn XCP components assembled correctly for (A) anterior exposures, (B) bite-wing exposures, and (C) posterior exposures.

holder evenly and allow no more than one-eighth inch to extend beyond the edge of the occlusal plane once the film/film holder is placed in the patient's mouth. The dot on the x-ray film should be toward the occlusal/incisal surface. The film packet/film holder should be parallel to the long axis of the teeth, covering all teeth to be exposed. Keep the film packet flat and away from the lingual surface of the teeth. Vertical and horizontal angulation is obtained by keeping the cone end even with the positioning ring or following the guide of the handle with the other film holders (Figure 22-12). The positioning ring guides the cone for correct placement to ensure that the film is covered. Without the ring to act as a guide, the operator needs to visually check the film placement and direct the cone to cover the entire film.

Full-Mouth Radiographic Survey

A full-mouth radiographic survey (FMX) is composed of periapical and bite-wing radiographs (Procedure 22-2). This survey includes a number of radiographs that collectively display all the teeth and surrounding structures and areas. The dentist determines what is needed for diagnosis and for the patient's records.

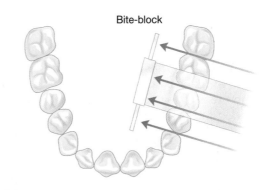

Bite-block

FIGURE 22-12 Correct placement of premolar bite-wing film using a film-holding device. The film is positioned such that the x-rays pass directly through the interproximal spaces to prevent overlapping of the teeth. The curve of the patient's arch is evaluated when placing the dental film.

PROCEDURE 22-2

Full-Mouth X-ray Exposure with Paralleling Technique

This procedure is performed by the dental assistant. The dentist requests a full-mouth set of radiographs. The dental assistant prepares the equipment (Rinn XCP instruments), the area, and the patient; takes the radiographs; and processes and mounts the films for viewing according to infection control protocol.

This procedure explains film placement and exposure for the central incisors in each arch and one-half of the maxillary arch and one-half of the mandibular arch. The same technique would be used to expose the opposite arches.

EQUIPMENT AND SUPPLIES

- Barriers for the x-ray room and equipment
- X-ray film (appropriate size and number of films)
- X-ray film barriers (optional)
- Cotton rolls (optional)
- Rinn XCP materials (assembled for use) or other paralleling technique aids
- Lead apron with thyroid collar
- Container for exposed film
- Paper towel or tissue

PROCEDURE STEPS *(Follow aseptic procedures)*

1. Review the patient's chart.

2. Wash and dry hands.

3. Place appropriate barriers on dental chair, film, and x-ray equipment.

4. Prepare equipment and supplies needed for the procedure, including sterile Rinn XCP instruments, tissue or paper towel, and cup or container with patient's name on it.

5. Turn the x-ray machine on and check the mA, kV, and exposure time.

6. Seat and position the patient in an upright position.

7. Have the patient remove all removable appliances, earrings, facial jewelry, or eyeglasses that may interfere with the exposing process.

8. Place the lead apron with the thyroid collar on the patient.

9. After the patient is prepared, wash and dry hands and don latex treatment gloves.

The number and the size of radiographs taken depend on several factors, including what the dentist needs to view on the radiograph, the size of the patient's mouth, the number of teeth in the oral cavity, conditions that may interfere with film placement, and the patient's ability to cooperate. A full-mouth survey for an adult routinely includes fourteen periapical and four bite-wing films. This number may vary depending on the factors listed and the dentist's directions.

When exposing any radiographs, an order should be followed to prevent double-exposing the patient. There is no recommended sequence, so dental assistants should decide what order they are comfortable with and can follow routinely. Once films are exposed, they should be placed in a cup or on a barrier away from the unexposed film.

Bite-Wing Series

Bite-wing radiographs are a routine part of the dental exam. They are taken as part of the full-mouth series and also at six- to twelve-month intervals. These radiographs are used specifically for caries detection but also assist in the evaluation of restorations, calculus detection, assessment of the alveolar crestal bone, tooth eruption, occlusal relationships, and some pulpal pathology. Bite-wing radiographs, also known as **interproximal** radiographs, are taken of the premolar area and the molar area. The film is placed most often in a horizontal position, but when the dentist wants to see more of the tooth root and alveolar bone, the film is placed vertically.

- **Horizontal Positioning**
  With adults, four No. 2 size films are taken (one premolar and one molar on each side). Some dentists choose to use the longer No. 3 size film and take one on each side, but care must be used when selecting this film size because different horizontal angulations are needed on the premolars and molars to open the contacts. With children, the size of the child's mouth determines the number and size of films. Older children may need only one No. 2 size film on each side of the mouth, while younger children or children with small mouths may need two No. 0 or No. 1 size film on each side of the mouth.

- **Vertical Positioning**
  Vertical bite-wing radiographs are requested by the periodontist as well as the general dentist. With the increase in periodontal disease, dentists are requiring bite-wing radiographs that show more of the root area. Root caries, advanced periodontal pockets, and bone loss can be seen to a greater extent on bite-wing radiographs if the film is placed vertically instead of horizontally. The vertical bite-wing can be used in both the posterior and anterior areas. An adhesive tab or film-holding device is used to hold the film in the correct position. The film placement and vertical and horizontal angulation remain the same as with the horizontal bite-wing radiograph (Figure 22-13).

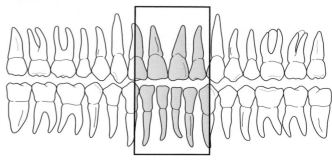

FIGURE 22-13 Anterior vertical bite-wing.

Positioning for Maxillary Arch

- **Maxillary Incisors** (Figure 22-14)

  1. To prepare the maxillary incisors for exposure, tilt the back of the film holder slightly and insert the film vertically into the slot on the bite-block. Adjust the ring on the metal rod to cover the film. Pull the positioning ring backward on the metal rod, away from the bite-block.

  2. Bring the tubehead near the area of exposure.

  3. Tilt the film/film holder downward to place in the patient's mouth. Position in the mouth away from the lingual surfaces and centered behind the incisors. Have the patient close slowly and evenly on the bite-block.

  4. Holding on to the metal rod, slide the positioning ring close to the patient's face. Position the cone parallel to the metal indicating rod and place to within one-half inch of the positioning ring. The cone end should be at an equal distance from the positioning ring. This directs the central ray

FIGURE 22-14 Maxillary incisors.

perpendicular to the film. The patient may help hold the metal rod to secure the film holder in position.

5. The incisal edges rest on the flat portion of the bite-block.

6. The diagram shows the film, tooth, positioning ring, and open end of the cone parallel to each other. The central ray will be perpendicular to the film. (No. 2 size film will show all four incisors. Teeth are centered on the radiograph, showing the apices, roots, and crowns. The bite-block may be seen as a radiopaque area near the incisal edge of the film.)

■ **Maxillary Cuspids** (Figure 22-15)

1. For the maxillary cuspids, tilt the film/film holder, place it in the patient's mouth, and position it away from the lingual surfaces. The film is placed in the mouth, directly behind the center of the cuspid and toward the midline.

2. Have the patient close slowly and center the cuspid on the bite-block. Holding the metal rod, slide the positioning ring toward the patient's face.

3. Bring the tubehead toward the ring, placing the cone end evenly around the positioning ring.

4. All planes are parallel so that the central ray will be directed perpendicular to the film plane. Because of the curvature of the maxillary arch, the distal of the cuspid is overlapping the first bicuspid on many cuspid radiographs. Note that the central ray is directed at the center of the cuspid.

■ **Maxillary Premolars** (Figure 22-16)

1. For the maxillary premolars, tilt the film/film holder, place it in the patient's mouth, and position it away from the lingual surfaces, toward the middle of the palate.

2. Place the anterior edge of the film behind the middle of the cuspid to ensure that the film will cover the area of the two premolars.

3. While holding the film in place, have the patient close slowly on the bite-block. Hold the metal rod and slide the positioning ring toward the patient's face.

4. Bring the tubehead toward the ring, placing the open cone evenly around the ring. Note the angle of the film and the film holder, positioned so that the central ray will pass through the contact point of the first and second premolars.

5. The bite-block is centered on the premolars. On this radiograph, the distal of the cuspid is visible and the first and second bicuspids show that the contact between them is open.

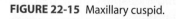

FIGURE 22-15 Maxillary cuspid.

FIGURE 22-16 Maxillary bicuspids (premolars).

■ **Maxillary Molars** (Figure 22-17)

1. For the maxillary molars, tilt the film/film holder so that it is less vertical when entering the patient's mouth. Place the film in the patient's mouth and position it away from the lingual surfaces of the molars.

2. Center the bite-block on the second molar. Have the patient close slowly on the bite-block.

3. Bring the tubehead toward the ring, placing the open end of the cone evenly around the positioning ring.

4. The diagram shows the film, tooth, and cone lined up for correct direction of the central ray. This radiograph shows the open contact between the first and second molars. The distal of the second premolar is seen. Note that the film angles are parallel to the lingual surface of the molars and placed near the middle of the palate.

Use of Cotton Rolls during X-ray Exposure

Cotton rolls are often placed between the teeth and the bite-block of the arch that is not being exposed. This technique makes it easier for the patient to close on the bite-block and stabilize it to prevent movement. The cotton roll is placed over the teeth in the arch that is not going to be exposed and then the bite-block is placed on top of it. The patient is asked to close and secure the Rinn in place. This is an optional technique, and may be used for all exposures or only those in areas where the patient is having difficulty closing.

Positioning for Mandibular Arch

■ **Mandibular Incisors** (Figure 22-18)

1. The film holder is assembled in the same way for mandibular and maxillary positions. For the mandibular incisors, tilt the film/film holder and place it in the patient's mouth, gently pressing the film on the floor of the mouth behind the incisors and away from the lingual surface.

2. Have the patient close slowly on the bite-block. Holding the metal rod, slide the positioning ring close to the patient's face.

3. Bring the tubehead close and place the cone parallel to the metal rod. The open end of the cone should be even with the ring.

4. The diagram in Figure 22-18 shows how far the film needs to be placed in the mouth to see the entire length of the tooth. Sometimes the tongue is moved when the film is being placed. Being gentle with the placement will encourage patient cooperation.

FIGURE 22-17 Maxillary molars.

FIGURE 22-18 Mandibular incisors.

5. The mandibular incisors are centered on the bite-block. The incisal edges of the teeth are one-eighth inch from the top of the film.

6. The central ray is directed between the two central incisors to open contact areas. The curve of the arch will cause some overlapping on the distal of the lateral incisors.

7. The drawing illustrates the film placed directly behind the incisors and as far into the mouth as the tongue attachment allows.

■ **Mandibular Cuspids** (Figure 22-19)

1. For the mandibular cuspids, tilt the film/film holder, place it in the patient's mouth, and position it away from the lingual surface.

2. Center the bite-block on the cuspid and have the patient slowly close. Move the positioning ring close to the patient's face, bring the cone parallel to the metal rod, and position the open end of the cone flat with the ring.

3. Insert the film toward the floor of the mouth enough to ensure that the film covers the entire length of the cuspid.

4. The film, tooth, and the plane of the open end of the cone are all parallel. The central ray will be directed perpendicular to the film plane.

5. In the diagram, the film is angled on the center of the cuspid. As with the incisors, place it toward the base of the tongue, away from the alveolar bone.

■ **Mandibular Premolars** (Figure 22-20)

1. For the mandibular premolars, tilt the film/film holder and place the film in the patient's mouth, gently positioning it between the lingual surface of the teeth and the tongue.

2. Place the anterior edge of the film at the middle of the cuspid to ensure that the film covers the area of the two premolars.

3. Have the patient close on the bite-block.

4. Note the position of the film as it is placed in the space between the tongue and the mandibular arch.

5. The film, teeth, and plane of the open end of the cone are all parallel. The first and second premolars are seen on this film with the contact points open.

■ **Mandibular Molars** (Figure 22-21)

1. For the mandibular molars, tilt the film/film holder and place the film holder with the film in the patient's mouth, positioning it between the tongue and the lingual surfaces of the teeth.

FIGURE 22-19 Mandibular cuspid.

FIGURE 22-20 Mandibular bicuspids (premolars).

FIGURE 22-21 Mandibular molars.

2. Center the bite-block over the second molar. Hold it in the desired position, and have the patient close to secure it in place.

3. Gently place the patient's cheek over the bite-block, if this is more comfortable for the patient.

4. Align the positioning ring and cone.

5. Note how close the film is to the lingual surface. Move the tongue toward the center of the mouth to make this placement more comfortable for the patient.

6. The edge of the film is positioned only one-eighth inch above the occlusal edge.

7. The first, second, and third molars are seen on this film with the contacts open. The third molar may not be erupted into the oral cavity, but it will be seen on the film.

8. During placement, to prevent the film and film holder from moving forward, hold the bite-block in position until the patient closes firmly on it.

■ **Premolar Bite-Wing** (Figure 22-22)

1. To position bite-wing radiographs, a tab or positioning instrument is used. Tabs come with adhesive backs or with loops to surround the film. The positioning instrument comes with a bite-wing holder, an indicator rod, and a positioning ring.

2. Holding the film horizontally, place the tab in the center of the film or, if using a positioning instrument, make sure the film is centered on the bite-wing holder with the smooth side of the film directed toward the positioning ring.

3. The drawing/radiograph illustrates the position of the film covering the premolars with the front edge of the film to the middle of the cuspid while the back edge of the film may be to the mesial of the second molar.

4. Hold the tab and place the film near the lingual surface of the teeth in the patient's mouth, positioning the film to cover the mandibular premolars.

5. While holding the tab in place, have the patient close and slowly rotate fingers out of the way.

6. When using a positioning instrument, place the bite-wing holder in the patient's mouth, away from the lingual surface of the teeth. Position the film to cover the premolars and to be parallel to them. Have the patient close slowly on the bite-wing holder to secure it in place.

7. The cone positioning for the premolar bite-wing begins with the vertical angulation set between +5° to +10°, depending on the slant of the film as it is positioned in the patient's mouth.

FIGURE 22-22 Premolar bite-wing using bite-wing tab.

8. The horizontal angulation is positioned so that the beam is aimed directly between the contacts of the premolars and the cone is perpendicular to the film. This film placement is sometimes uncomfortable for the patient because of the alveolar ridge curvature near the cuspid. Gentleness when positioning this exposure will be rewarded with patient cooperation. When using the positioning instrument, first hold the indicator rod, and then bring the positioning ring close to the patient's face.

■ **Molar Bite-Wing** (Figure 22-23)

1. Position the film to cover the molars and the distal half of the second premolar. Place the front edge of the film at the distal of the second molar.

2. Holding the tab, place the film in the patient's mouth, away from the lingual surfaces, gently moving the tongue toward the middle of the mouth.

3. When using the positioning instrument, place it in the patient's mouth, pushing the tongue away from the lingual surfaces.

FIGURE 22-23 Molar bite-wing using Rinn XCP.

4. The vertical angulation for the molar bite-wing is set at 0° so the cone is perpendicular to the film. The horizontal angulation is directed so that the beam is between the contacts of the first and second molars. Place the cone near the patient's face, covering the film and perpendicular to the film. Look at the curve of the patient's arch rather than the patient's face to position the cone.

Producing Special Radiographs

Special radiographs include a type of radiograph, the occlusal radiograph; radiographs on children and edentulous patients; endodontic radiographs; and radiographs on special needs patients or compromised patients. Each situation requires additional skills in working with the patient, and knowing how to correctly position the radiograph to achieve the desired results.

Occlusal Radiographs

Occlusal radiographs show a large area of the dental arch. They are used with children when periapicals are difficult to expose and with patients who have difficulty opening the mouth or controlling muscular movement. The films are placed on the occlusal surface and then the patient closes gently on the film to hold it in place. Occlusal radiographs are used to locate or define the following: fractures, impacted teeth, foreign bodies in the bone or floor of the mouth and to identify the location of other artifacts, changes in the size and shape of the arches, supernumerary teeth, cleft palate, root fragments, cysts, malignancies, tumors (odontomas), osteomyelitis, stones in the ducts of the salivary glands, unerupted teeth, and malpositioned teeth.

Two techniques are used to expose occlusal radiographs: the **topographic technique** and the **cross-section technique** (Procedure 22-3). Technique selection is determined by the view the dentist needs for diagnosis. With

---

PROCEDURE 22-3

Exposing Occlusal Radiographs

This procedure is performed by the dental assistant at the direction of the dentist. The dental assistant prepares the equipment and supplies, the area, and the patient. The occlusal films are exposed using the topographic or cross-sectional technique.

EQUIPMENT AND SUPPLIES

- Barriers for the x-ray room
- Occlusal film (No. 2 for children and No. 4 for adults)
- Lead apron with thyroid collar
- Container or barrier for exposed film

PROCEDURE STEPS *(Follow aseptic procedures)*

1. Wash and dry hands.
2. Place appropriate barriers.
3. Prepare film, tissue or paper towel, and cup or container with patient's identification on it.
4. Seat the patient in an upright position and place the lead apron on the patient.
5. Wash and dry hands and don treatment gloves.

Topographic Technique

6. For the *maxillary view,* positioning is similar to that used for the bisecting technique. The patient is positioned so that the maxillary arch is parallel to the floor.
7. The film is placed in the mouth with the smooth/plain side toward the cone.
8. Have the patient close on the film, leaving about 2 mm of an edge beyond the incisors.
9. Move the cone to a vertical angulation of +65° to +75°.
10. Direct the cone over the bridge of the nose, with the lower edge of the cone covering the incisors (Figure 22-24).
11. For the *mandibular view* using the topographic technique, the patient's head is tilted back.
12. Place the smooth side of the film on the occlusal surfaces of the teeth with the central incisors at the front edge of the film.
13. Have the patient close gently on the film.
14. The vertical angulation will vary with each patient between −40° and −55°.

(continues)

PROCEDURE 22-3 *(CONTINUED)*

FIGURE 22-24 Topographic occlusal radiograph of the maxillary arch. (A) Vertical film placement. (B) Horizontal film placement.

15. Center the cone over the film, directing the central ray at the middle and tip of the chin (Figure 22-25).

Cross-Section Technique

1. For the *maxillary view* using the cross-section technique, the patient should be in an upright position with the head tilted backward slightly.

2. The film placement is the same as with the topographic technique. The cone is positioned over the top of the patient's head with the central ray directed perpendicular to the film.

3. Be sure the cone covers the maxillary area to be exposed (Figure 22-26).

4. For the mandibular view, the patient's head should be tilted backward.

5. The film placement is the same as with the topographic technique.

6. The cone is positioned under the patient's chin with the central ray directed perpendicular to the film. The patient may have to lift the chin up in order to position the cone (Figure 22-27).

(continues)

PROCEDURE 22-3 (CONTINUED)

FIGURE 22-25 Topographic occlusal radiograph of the mandibular arch.

FIGURE 22-26 Cross-sectional occlusal radiograph of the maxillary arch.

(continues)

P R O C E D U R E   2 2 - 3   *(C O N T I N U E D)*

(A)

(B)

FIGURE 22-27 Cross-sectional occlusal radiograph of the mandibular arch. (A) Horizontal film placement. (B) Vertical film placement.

the topographic technique, the rules of bisecting are followed. The central ray is directed perpendicular to the bisecting plane. With the cross-section technique, the central ray is perpendicular to the film.

Pediatric Radiographs

Radiographs play an important role in the dental health of children. They are used to detect caries, abscesses, cysts, anodontia, and fractures, and to evaluate eruption stages and growth patterns. Technique suggestions associated with pediatric radiographs follow:

1. Because developing tissues are sensitive to radiation, the exposure time should be reduced and the number of radiographs should be kept to a minimum.

2. The oral mucosa of young children in eruption stages is sensitive to the slightest pressure, so carefully examine the mouth for loose or erupting teeth, any parulis, pulp polyps, cold sores (herpes simplex), canker sores (aphthous ulcers), or any deviation from the normal.

3. Talk to the child and demonstrate what is going to happen.

4. Evaluate the child's behavior and cooperation. Having the child help often reduces apprehension.

5. Work quickly and confidently, because children move constantly and become bored easily.

6. Evaluate the child's mouth to determine the number and size of x-ray film to be used. Select the smallest film you can to minimize discomfort and

still obtain the view needed. For preschool children, No. 0 film is most often used. Older children will vary from a No. 0 film to Nos. 1 and 2, depending on the size of the mouth, the tenderness of the tissues, and the depth of the palate and the floor of the mouth. For occlusal views, No. 2 film is used. The number of films and the size of the film used can be tailored to the child and the dentist's needs (Figure 22-28).

7. Take anterior films first to encourage the child's cooperation.

8. The paralleling technique is most frequently used; all guidelines are the same as for adults. Procedure 22-4 outlines the steps involved in taking a pediatric full mouth exposure.

Edentulous Radiographic Survey

A series of radiographs on the edentulous (ee-**DENT**-you-lous), or toothless, or partially edentulous patient may be indicated to show cysts, impacted teeth, retained root tips or bone fragments, other pathological conditions, and normal landmarks, such as the mental foramen, mandibular canal, maxillary sinuses, and alveolar bone. As part of the routine examination, radiographs are taken before dentures

and partials are made; if abnormal pathology or sensitivity is found, the patient can receive treatment before the removable prosthesis is made. Technique suggestions associated with treatment for the edentulous patient follow:

1. A routine full-mouth survey consists of six anterior and eight posterior films, but these numbers can be reduced by taking fewer anterior films in smaller arches, thus eliminating bite-wing radiographs.

2. Either the paralleling or the bisecting technique can be used, but both will need to be modified. In the paralleling technique, cotton rolls are used with the film holder to position the film parallel to the alveolar ridge. If the patient has dentures or partials, leave the appliance in the opposing arch for better support. In the bisecting technique, the film will be almost flat. Just extend the edge of the film one-quarter inch beyond the crest of the alveolar ridge.

3. The vertical angulation will be increased. Reduce exposure time by one-quarter of the normal time to prevent overexposure of an area where teeth are missing and the bone is thinner.

4. Try using occlusal film and exposing individual quadrants and/or arches, take a panoramic film

FIGURE 22-28 Pedodontic full-mouth surveys of a child three to five years. (A) Includes two bite-wings and two occlusals. *(continues)*

FIGURE 22-28 *(continued)* (B) Includes two bite-wings, two occlusals, and four periapicals. This is a pedodontic full mouth-mouth survey of a child three to five years old. (C) Includes two bite-wings, six anterior incisors, and four posterior periapicals. This is a pedodontic full mouth-mouth survey of a child six to twelve years old.

PROCEDURE 22-4

Full-Mouth Pediatric X-ray Exposure

This procedure is performed by the dental assistant. The dentist requires that a pediatric full-mouth set of radiographs be taken and identifies the eight films. The dental assistant prepares the equipment (Rinn XCP instruments), the area, and the patient; takes the radiographs; processes the films; and mounts the films for viewing according to infection control protocol.

This procedure explains film placement and exposure for the two occlusal films (maxillary and mandibular), two bitewing x-rays, and four periapical x-rays.

EQUIPMENT AND SUPPLIES

- Barriers for the x-ray room and equipment
- X-ray film, six No. 0 films and two No. 2 size films
- X-ray film barriers (optional)
- Cotton rolls (optional)
- Rinn XCP materials (assembled for use) or other paralleling technique aids
- Lead apron with thyroid collar
- Container for exposed film
- Paper towel or tissue

PROCEDURE STEPS *(Follow aseptic procedures)*

1. Review the patient's chart.
2. Wash and dry hands.
3. Place appropriate barriers on the dental chair, film, and x-ray equipment.
4. Prepare film No. 2 for children.
5. Assemble sterile Rinn XCP instruments and prepare tissue or paper towel and cup or container with patient's name on it.
6. Turn on the x-ray machine and check the mA, kV, and exposure time.
7. Seat the patient in an upright position.
8. Place the lead apron with the thyroid collar on the patient.
9. After the patient is prepared, wash and dry hands and don latex treatment gloves.
10. Explain the procedure to the patient.

Maxillary Occlusal Film/Topographic Technique

1. For the maxillary view, positioning is similar to that used for the bisecting technique. The patient is positioned so that the maxillary arch is parallel to the floor.
2. Place the film in the mouth with the smooth/plain side toward the cone.
3. Have the patient close on the film, leaving about 2 mm of an edge beyond the incisors.
4. Move the cone to a vertical angulation of +65° to +75°.
5. Direct the cone over the bridge of the nose with the lower edge of the cone covering the incisors.

Mandibular Occlusal X-ray/Topographic Technique

For the mandibular view using the topographic technique, the patient's head is tilted backward to allow for correct placement for the bisecting technique until the mandibular arch is parallel to the floor.

1. Place the smooth side of the film on the occlusal surfaces of the teeth with the central incisors at the front edge of the film.
2. Have the patient close gently on the film.
3. The vertical angulation will vary with each patient between −40° and −55°. Center the cone over the film, directing the central ray at the middle and tip of the chin.

Deciduous Bite-Wings

1. To position bite-wing radiographs, a tab or positioning instrument is used. Tabs come with adhesive backs or with loops to surround the film. The positioning instrument comes with a bite-wing holder, an indicator rod, and a positioning ring.

(continues)

2. While holding the film horizontally, place the tab in the center of the film or, if using a positioning instrument, make sure the film is centered on the bite-wing holder with the smooth side of the film directed toward the positioning ring.

3. Position the film covering the deciduous first and second molars with the front edge of the film to the middle of the cuspid.

4. Hold the tab and place the film near the lingual surface of the teeth in the patient's mouth, positioning the film to cover the mandibular deciduous molars.

5. While holding the tab in place, have the patient close and slowly rotate the fingers out of the way.

6. When using a positioning instrument, place the bite-wing holder in the patient's mouth, away from the lingual surface of the teeth. Position the film to cover the deciduous molars and be parallel to them. Have the patient close slowly on the bite-wing holder and hold it in place.

■ The cone positioning for the premolar bite-wing begins with the vertical angulation set at 0°.

Positioning for Maxillary Deciduous Molars

1. For the maxillary deciduous molars, tilt the film/film holder, place it in the patient's mouth, and position it away from the lingual surfaces, toward the middle of the palate.

2. Place the anterior edge of the film behind the middle of the cuspid to ensure that the film will cover the area of the two molars.

3. While holding the film in place, have the patient close slowly on the bite-block. Hold the metal rod and slide the positioning ring toward the patient's face.

4. Bring the tubehead toward the ring, placing the open cone evenly around the ring. Note the angle of the film and the film holder, positioned so that the central ray passes through the contact point of the first and second deciduous molars.

5. Center the bite-block on the deciduous molars. On this radiograph, the distal of the cuspid is seen and the first and second deciduous molars have the contact between them open.

Positioning for Mandibular Deciduous Molars

1. For the mandibular deciduous molars, tilt the film/film holder, place the film in the patient's mouth, and gently position it between the lingual surface of the teeth and the tongue.

2. Place the anterior edge of the film at the middle of the cuspid to ensure that the film covers the area of the two deciduous molars.

3. Have the patient close on the bite-block.

4. Note the position of the film as it is placed in the space between the tongue and the mandibular arch. The film, teeth, and plane of the open end of the cone are all parallel. The first and second deciduous molars are seen on this film with the contact points open.

that includes both arches and surrounding area on one film, or use periapical films if areas are of a suspicious condition (Figure 22-29).

Endodontic Radiographic Technique

Radiographs are taken periodically during the endodontic procedure. The radiographs allow the dentist to check the progress of the procedure and take the necessary measurements. Technique suggestions associated with endodontic procedures are:

1. Use the paralleling technique to reduce distortion whenever possible.

2. Place film in a hemostat, snap-a-ray, or special endodontic positioning device. The endodontic film-holding device is made of plastic and aids in positioning the film while keeping the patient's mouth open. The patient needs to hold the mouth open during this time, because there is a reamer in the root canal that extends beyond the tooth. The endodontic film holder is like the Rinn film holder in that there is also a ring to line up the cone.

3. Loosen the dental dam from the frame on one side and position the film on the lingual, parallel to the tooth. If a plastic frame is not used, the metal frame may have to be removed to prevent the frame from being exposed on the radiograph and possibly distorting the image.

4. The film should cover the entire length of the tooth and the surrounding area at the apex of the root.

Maxillary anterior region

Maxillary posterior region

Mandibular anterior region

Mandibular posterior region

FIGURE 22-29 Radiographs of a full-mouth series of an edentulous patient. Cone and film-holding device positioned in four areas. (Note: An additional bite-block is secured to the Rinn bite-block to provide the height that the teeth would normally provide. A cotton roll is placed on the opposite side to assist the patient in holding the bite-block securely.)

5. Center the tooth on the film and direct the central ray perpendicular to the tooth. The patient must keep the mouth open because of protruding endodontic instruments and materials, so work quickly (Figure 22-30).

Special Needs Patients/ Compromised Patients

Patients come to the office with a wide variety of special needs. Consideration and creativity often are required to obtain desired radiographs. The wheelchair patient is one example where advance preparation is needed to have the treatment room ready (Figure 22-31). When there is a plan in place to expose the x-ray, the procedure is much easier for everyone involved. With other special needs patients, a parent or guardian may be asked to assist in holding the patient or the x-ray steady; however, every

attempt should be made to expose the x-ray by another means. Work as quickly as possible. If it is impossible to expose a periapical film, an occlusal or a panoramic film may be substituted. Technique suggestions associated with treatment for special needs patients follow:

1. Before treating special needs patients, discuss how to best handle the patients with the entire office. A good time to do this is office meetings. The entire staff needs to work together to make these patients' visits as simple and comprehensive as possible.

2. Prepare all areas in the office that the patient will be in before the appointment, including the reception and treatment rooms. For example, have extra radiation protection in the treatment room for the parent or guardian in case he or she has to hold the film in the patient's mouth.

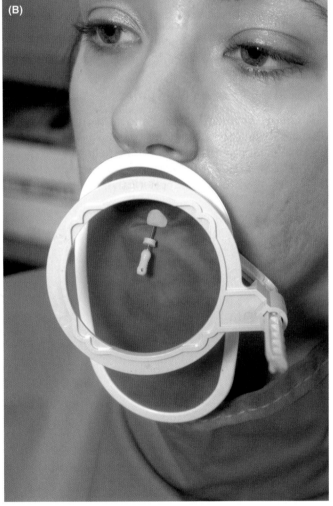

FIGURE 22-30 (A) When an x-ray is positioned for an endodontic radiograph, the patient does not close on the film holder because of the reamer in the root canal. Radiograph shows the reamer. (B) Patient with tray positioned for endodontic exposure.

3. Call the patient, caregiver, or guardian in advance and ask for suggestions on how to best accommodate the patient's needs.

4. Read about patients' conditions to better understand and communicate with them. For example,

FIGURE 22-31 Wheelchair patient having intraoral radiographs taken.

when working with a deaf patient, learn a few words in sign language.

Processing Quality Radiographs

CDA Normally, the darkroom is in the center area of the dental office or near the x-ray units for easy accessibility by dental assistants. It is a small room where x-ray processing (develop, fix, and wash) can be accomplished. This room needs to be well ventilated and of an adequate size.

One of the main concerns of the darkroom is that it exclude all white light. It is important that there are no light leaks from around doors, fans, and vents, because light harms the sensitive film emulsion during processing. Safelights must be used when the film packets are opened, when attaching the film to the racks, and during processing procedures. A safelight will not affect the film emulsion because it is in the red-orange spectrum. The film is much more sensitive to the blue-green spectrum (wavelengths are shorter). Safelight filters must be free of scratches and fit precisely. The safety lights should be mounted at least four feet from the counter surface where the films are unwrapped. A 15-watt incandescent bulb should be used. If the safelight must be mounted closer to the counter, a lower-watt bulb, such as 7.5 watts, needs to be used. When using indirect lighting (facing the light toward the ceiling), a 25-watt bulb may be used with the proper filters. It was once thought that the walls of the room should be painted black, but it is currently recommended that they be a light color to reflect the safe light. It is more important that the walls be washable because of the spills and splashes that take place during processing.

When processing films where an intensifying screen has been used, a filter that eliminates more light must be used (a red filter should be used in place of the orange). Films that have been exposed with intensifying screens are more sensitive to light. Therefore, orange filters for the safelight should never be used for extraoral films. A good safelight filter to use with both intraoral films and extraoral screen films is the GBX-2 safelight filter manufactured by Kodak.

There are no recommendations for the overhead white light. It is, however, important that it provide proper illumination for the whole room, and that the switch not be placed where it could be turned on accidentally.

Many offices have view boxes in their darkrooms so x-rays can be read while still wet. This box also should be in an area where the switch cannot be turned on accidentally.

There may be a warning light outside the darkroom that indicates when x-ray processing is taking place. Also, it is advisable to have a lock on the door to prevent light exposure if the door is opened accidentally. A rotational darkroom door that allows access for individuals while maintaining darkness in the room can be used.

The darkroom must have a hot and cold water source, along with a drainage line. Thermostatic water controls are also necessary to control the intake waterline and to enable adjustment of the water to maintain constant temperatures in the processing solutions. A large sink with a gooseneck faucet is recommended for use in replenishing and changing the processing solutions (Figure 22-32).

Manual Processing Equipment

The **manual processing** tanks should be made of stainless steel. The processing tank contains a large tank for the water bath and two one- or two-gallon insert tanks (Figure 22-33). The water bath has an inlet valve where the water flows in and an outlet valve or overflow pipe

FIGURE 22-32 Manual processing room with equipment. (A) Thermostatic water gauge. (B) Thermostatic water control. (C) Disinfectant solution. (D) Timer. (E) Silver recovery unit. (F) Manual tank. (G) Floating thermometer. (H) X-rays on rack. (I) Dryer. (J) Storage for stirring rod, solutions view box, and cleaning supplies. (K) Safelight is above manual tanks.

FIGURE 22-33 (A) Typical manual processing tank showing developer and fixer insert tanks in the water bath. (B) Line drawing of manual processing tank.

Other items needed in the darkroom are a thermometer, a timer, processing racks, stirring rods, a dryer, and brushes or sponges with long handles (Figure 22-32). The thermometer is designed so that it can be suspended in the developing solution. It is critical that the solution is checked before developing a set of x-rays. The dental assistant must know the precise temperature of the developer rather than of the water surrounding the tanks or the incoming water. Because it takes time for the developer and the surrounding water temperature to equalize, it is important to check the developer solution each time.

No darkroom is complete without a timer. The correct monitoring of processing time is critical in producing quality x-rays. An accurate timer that can be set easily and has a loud alarm must be used.

Processing racks, sometimes called intraoral film hangers, come in a number of sizes, ranging from one to twenty clips. They are made of stainless steel and, except for the single film hanger, have equal numbers of clips on each side. If the film hanger has defective clips, it should be discarded. It causes films to be lost or it may scratch films on other racks.

Stirring rods or paddles are used first thing in the morning and first thing in the afternoon to stir the developer and fixer solution. They should be marked according to solution and not used interchangeably.

Dental x-ray dryers are used after the processing is complete. The x-rays are left on the racks and placed in the dryer, suspended from a rod over a fan and heat element to dry. This process takes between fifteen and twenty minutes. An alternative to this procedure is to hang the x-rays from a towel rack or rod and to let them air dry. It is important that the x-rays not touch and that the drying is out of the way in a clean area to prevent dust and other debris from collecting on the x-ray.

Long-handle brushes or sponges are used to clean the inside of the processing tanks. There should be one brush for the developing tank and one for the fixing tank. These brushes should be marked and never be interchanged. After use, they should be rinsed and stored separately.

Processing Preparation

The developing and fixing solutions are normally prepared from liquid concentrates, following the manufacturer's instructions. They come in two-packs with color-coded lids and labels. Verify that the correct solution is placed in the proper tank to prevent chemical cross-contamination. After checking the date on the solution, carefully open the top and pour the developer into the developing tank. Add water, about 68° or slightly cool to the touch, to the indicator line at the top of the tank. The fixer is prepared the same way. After the insert tanks are in the processing tank, start the water coming through the inlet valve. The water can run in fairly quickly during this time. When it is up to the point where it is flowing out the outlet or overflow

where the water escapes the tank. The tank comes with a tank cover that must be kept on at all times, except when placing or removing films, to prevent the solution from oxidizing or evaporating. Many newer insert tanks come with film retrievers that slide into the insert tanks and have bars across their tops for use in placement and removal. The film retriever is used to bring the x-ray from the bottom of the tank upward so that it can be retrieved if it has mistakenly loosened from the x-ray rack. Normally, when facing the processing tank, the developer is on the left side of the processing tank and the fixer is on the right side. The insert tanks should never be interchanged due to the sensitivity of the processing solutions.

pipe, adjust the water to a slow, steady flow. Then stir each insert tank with the appropriate stirring paddle to mix the chemicals completely. Check the temperature of the developing solution; if it is around 68°, it is ready to process x-rays. A time/temperature chart appears on every developer/fixer solution package. Have the chart available in the darkroom for review. Charts may vary slightly from manufacturer to manufacturer.

Temperature (°F)	Time in Developer (minutes)
80	2½
75	3
70	4
68	4½
60	6

The optimal temperature is from 68° to 70°. If the temperature goes 20° up or down from the optimum, the chemicals in the solutions may be destroyed and will have to be discarded. It is necessary to change the solutions every three to four weeks to maintain optimal processing, under normal use. With heavy use, change solutions more often.

Each day, a test film should be processed to compare to the film that was processed the first day the solutions were changed. If a change is seen in the processed films, then the solutions may not be effective. It is important to keep a log of the date that you last changed the solution. Also, check the solution visually to ensure that it is not cloudy or dark. This also may indicate that the solution must be changed.

Replenishing Processing Solutions. Processing solutions may need to be replenished periodically. The solutions may be low before the time of changing the solutions. If this happens, open a pack of the concentrated developer solution and add a fifty/fifty consistency of developer and water. In other words, add the same amount of developer as water to the developer insert tank. The fixer is different because water comes from the water bath of the processing tank on the x-rays into the fixer during each processing sequence. Therefore, add straight fixer to the fixer insert tank to replenish it.

Manual Film Processing Technique

After the solutions are stirred with the appropriate stirrers and the temperature in the developer is checked, it is ready to process x-rays (Procedure 22-5). The work area must be clean and dry. Obtain the correct processing rack and write the patient's name, date, and number of x-rays on the identification tab at the top with a pencil. The x-rays themselves may be in a cup. If they have come directly from the patient's mouth, wear gloves while the x-rays are carefully unwrapped and placed on the racks. Do not touch any portion of the film directly. Other ways to handle the aseptic technique are to dis-

infect the x-rays before bringing them into the darkroom or use preplaced protective coverings on the films themselves, which are removed, and place the uncontaminated films in a cup ready for processing. It is not important which technique is used, but a standard policy must be followed so that cross-contamination does not take place.

The overhead light is turned off and the safety light is turned on. The door is locked, when possible. When the eyes are accustomed to the safety light, unwrap the film; pull back the plastic coating, the black paper, and the lead foil; and attach the film to the hanger. Hold the film by the edges to confirm that it is securely on the hanger. Place each film on the x-ray rack in the same manner. When this process is completed, lift the lid off the processor, and place the rack in the developer solution. Be sure to agitate the films in the solution by quickly raising and lowering the films several times into the solution before attaching the rack to the side of the tank. This ensures that the films are bathed totally in the solution and that no bubbles are on the surface of the film. Place the lid on the processing tank and wait four minutes if the temperature is at 70°. The timer should be set immediately after the lid is on. When the time is up, open the lid cover (safety lights only) and lift the rack from the developer. Carefully shake off excess solution and then place the rack in the water bath solution. The x-ray films must be rinsed for at least thirty seconds in the running water (middle portion of the tank). The rinsing stops the process of the developing solution. After thirty seconds, raise the rack and let the excess water drain off. Place the film in the fixer insert tank. The tank cover is then replaced over the tank and the timer is set again. The time for processing in the fixer is twice that of the developer; therefore, process for eight minutes at 70°. After the fixing time is complete, the films are removed from the fixer solution and placed in the wash bath in the center of the tank for the final rinse. The films are rinsed by clear running water for about twenty minutes. When this is complete, the films are removed and hung from a towel rack or placed in an electric dryer for fifteen to twenty minutes. The films are then ready for mounting.

Composition of Processing Solutions

Film processing involves a series of steps that convert an invisible latent image on the dental x-ray film to a visible permanent image on the dental radiograph. The diagnostic quality of the radiograph image depends on following the detailed steps involved in processing these films. In this section, the role of film processing solutions will be discussed, and manual and automatic processing equipment and techniques identified.

The Developer. The **developer solution** has a pH above 7 and chemically reduces the exposed area of the emulsion, making it visible to the naked eye. The pH scale

PROCEDURE 22-5

Processing Radiographs Using a Manual Tank

This procedure is performed by the dental assistant. The assistant prepares the equipment, supplies, and area. The exposed radiographs are taken to the darkroom by the dental assistant to process.

EQUIPMENT AND SUPPLIES

- Barriers for the darkroom counter
- Exposed radiographs
- X-ray rack
- Processing tank
- Safelight(s)
- Timer
- Thermometer
- Pencil
- Electric film dryer

PROCEDURE STEPS *(Follow aseptic procedures)*

1. Wash and dry hands (gloves must be worn if the x-rays are contaminated).

2. Make sure the area is clean and free of splashes. Place barriers on the counter in the darkroom.

3. Check the temperature of the developer with the thermometer. Also, check the processing chart for the corresponding temperature and time information.

4. Check the volumes of the processing solutions to ensure that they do not need replenishing. Replenish if necessary.

5. Stir the developer and fixer when the first processing is being completed that morning or afternoon. Stir the solutions with the corresponding stirring rods. Do not interchange.

6. Check the x-ray rack to ensure that the clips are in working order.

7. Label the x-ray rack in pencil with the patient's name, date of exposure, and the number of x-rays taken.

8. Turn on the safelights and turn off the white lights.

9. Remove the films from their wrappers and place on the x-ray racks. Use gloves if the x-rays are contaminated.

10. Check each film to make sure it is attached securely and placed in a parallel manner so that it is not touching the adjacent film.

11. Place in the developer tank and agitate the rack slightly in the developing solution to eliminate bubbles on the surface of the emulsion.

12. Place the tank cover on the processing tank. Set the timer for four minutes if the temperature of the developer is at 70°. The area can be cleaned up and the barrier and x-ray wrappers are disposed of.

13. When the timer goes off, remove the x-ray rack from the developer, letting the excess solution drip into the developer prior to placing the rack in the running water (the middle area in the processing tank). Let it rinse for thirty seconds.

14. Remove the x-ray rack from the rinsing, let the excess water drip off, and then immerse the rack in the fixing solution for eight minutes. If the dentist must view the patient's x-rays, they can be removed after three minutes, then returned to the fixer for the remaining time.

15. Replace the processing lid and set the timer for ten minutes.

16. After the eight minutes, remove the x-ray rack from the fixer and place it in the running water at the center of the processing tank. The final wash takes twenty minutes to complete.

17. The rack of x-rays can be removed from the water after twenty minutes and placed in an x-ray dryer for an additional fifteen to twenty minutes or until drying is complete.

18. When the x-rays are dry, remove them from the rack and place them in a labeled x-ray mount.

is from 0 to 14, with 7 as neutral. Anything below 7 is considered acidic and anything above 7 is considered alkaline.

The following components make up the developing solution: hydroquinone, elon, sodium carbonate, sodium sulfite, potassium bromide, and water. **Hydroquinone** is extremely sensitive to changes in temperature, and is inactive when the temperature is below 60°. Hydroquinone is a reducing agent, or a chemical that blackens exposed silver halide crystals. Even though this chemical acts slowly, the image gains density steadily during the developing process. Hydroquinone is responsible primarily for the film contrast. **Elon** is a reducer that also blackens the exposed silver halide crystals. Elon is not affected greatly by temperature changes. It acts quickly, and is responsible for giving detail to the film. Reducers develop only in an alkaline medium. **Sodium carbonate** is often used as the alkaline medium in the developer. It softens and swells the emulsion so that the reducers can reach the silver crystals. If the solution has too much alkaline medium, overswelling of the emulsion takes place, causing blisters on the film.

The reducer and alkaline medium are affected by oxygen. The oxygen in the air and solution can spoil the developer. Therefore, a preservative is used to slow this process. **Sodium sulfite** prevents oxidation and increases the life span of the developing solution by two to four weeks.

If the chemicals work too fast, a film fog appears and the x-rays are unclear. A restrainer such as **potassium bromide** is used to slow the developing process to a practical speed and prevent film fog.

The last ingredient used to mix all these chemicals is water. Distilled water is recommended so that no additional chemicals are brought into the developing solution.

Fixer Solution. The **fixer solution** removes the unexposed and undeveloped crystals from the film emulsion as well as stops the developing process. The following components make up the fixer solution: sodium thiosulfate, acetic acid, potassium alum, and water. **Sodium thiosulfate**, or hyposulfite, is known as the "hyp" agent. It is responsible for removing the unexposed and undeveloped crystals from the film. The chemical that stops the developing action and provides the required acidity for sodium thiosulfate to work is **acetic acid**. The third chemical in the fixer is sodium sulfite, and it works much as it does in the developer, by preserving the solution and preventing oxidation. **Potassium alum** is the chemical that shrinks and hardens the emulsion gelatin. This hardening process protects the film from abrasion and helps the films dry more quickly. The final ingredient is water. It is used as a medium to incorporate the chemicals. It is not as critical to have distilled water in the fixer as it is in the developer.

Used fixer solution stains clothing; the silver salts accumulate in it and form spots that may not show up until after the garment is laundered. If the fixer solution has spotted the clothing before being washed, rinse it first in unused fixer solution and then thoroughly with water before laundering. There are several products on the market for treating stains on dental uniforms.

Disposing of the Fixer and Developer (OSHA Guidelines). Disposal of the fixer and developer solution must follow OSHA hazardous waste guidelines. Silver is in the fixer solution and must be disposed of properly. It cannot be washed down the sink. Both the used developer and fixer solution should be put in a leak-proof container and disposed of by a company specializing in biohazard waste. The solutions also can be treated in dental offices that have silver recovery units, which take the silver from the solutions. The treated solutions can then be disposed of properly.

The lead in the film packet is also a hazardous material. The lead can be saved in a container and sold along with the recovered silver to a metal recycling company.

The dental office should retain receipts of developer and fixer solution disposal to prove proper disposal of hazardous wastes.

Automatic Processing

Automatic processors are used in most dental offices (Figure 22-34). Automatic processors are easy to use and reduce processing time. The x-rays are consistently of a good quality. Most processors are compact and require minimal darkroom space. If space in the darkroom is a problem, some processors have daylight loading units that can be added (Figure 22-34A). With the daylight loading units, the processors can be placed wherever they are convenient to use. One important factor to consider when using automatic processors is that maintenance of the units and daily chemical control is essential.

Although **automatic processing** follows the same basic sequence as manual processing, the order in which the film is placed in solutions differs (Procedure 22-6). With automatic processors, a series of rollers or guides move the x-ray film through the developing compartment, the fixing compartment, the water compartment, and, last, the drying compartment before depositing it onto a tray (Figure 22-35).

The rollers/guides are moved by gears, belts, or chains that must be lubricated and maintained according to the manufacturer's instructions. The x-ray film is processed in four to seven minutes depending on the temperature of the developing solution. The temperature also determines the speed at which the rollers/guides are set. Automatic processing is done between 82°F and 95°F. This increase in temperature greatly reduces total processing time. The rollers/guides move the film through each compartment and also "squeeze" off the excess solution between compartments. This prevents processing chemicals from being carried into the next stage of processing.

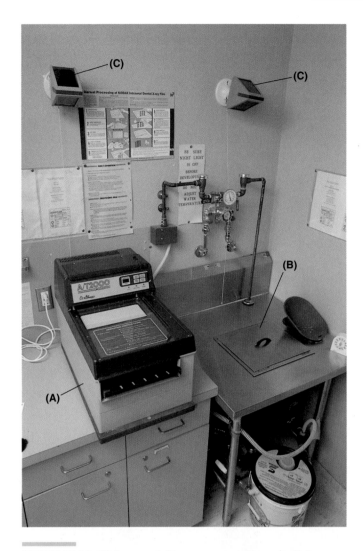

FIGURE 22-34 (A) Automatic film processor without daylight loader. (B) Manual processing tank in darkroom. (C) Safelights.

Automatic Processing Solutions. Automatic processing solutions are designed specifically for automatic processors and are not interchangeable with solutions used for manual processing. In automatic processing solutions, the developer has chemicals added to prevent the emulsion from becoming soft and sticking to the rollers. The solution also has an agent that reduces the swelling of the emulsion so that the films will not absorb too much developing solution. Automatic processing solutions are used to replenish solutions daily. Some machines have the ability to replenish the solutions automatically each time a film is fed into the unit.

Care of Automatic Processor. Proper care of automatic processors is critical. To ensure quality x-ray film processing, daily and weekly maintenance must be followed. Read the manufacturer's instructions and set a schedule for maintenance. Designate a staff member to be the "quality assurance controller" for x-ray processing. A few general guidelines follow:

- Every morning, check the solution levels and add solutions where needed. Turn the water on so that fresh water is running continuously, or place fresh water in the units without a water hookup. Place on the lid securely and run a film through the processor to remove any debris.

- Turn off the water every night. Lift off the lid and place it slightly ajar to prevent fumes from accumulating and condensing (which can cause films to fog), and processor motor problems.

- Weekly, rinse the rollers with warm water, and then soak them as recommended by the manufacturer.

- Solutions should be changed between two and six weeks depending on use and how often the solutions were replenished. Cleaning solutions rec-

---

PROCEDURE 22-6

Processing Radiographs Using an Automatic Processor

This procedure is performed by the dental assistant. The dental assistant prepares the equipment, supplies, and work area. The exposed radiographs are taken to the automatic processor by the dental assistant to process.

EQUIPMENT AND SUPPLIES

- Exposed radiographs

- Automatic x-ray processor with daylight loader

PROCEDURE STEPS *(Follow aseptic procedures)*

1. Turn on the automatic x-ray processor at the beginning of each day. This ensures that it is warmed up and ready to process after the x-rays are exposed. (The chemicals must be heated to the correct temperatures or the x-rays will appear light and the diagnostic quality will be diminished.)

(continues)

PROCEDURE 22-6 (CONTINUED)

2. Wash and dry hands.

3. Place exposed radiographs in the daylight loader with two additional containers/cups.

4. Don gloves, and position gloved hands through the sleeves of the daylight loader.

5. Remove each radiograph from its packet, and place the film in one uncontaminated container. Be careful not to touch and contaminate the film as the packet is removed.

6. Place the empty packets in the other container/cup.

7. After all x-rays are unwrapped, remove the gloves and place them in a contaminated container with the empty packets.

8. With clean hands, feed the unwrapped films into the machine *slowly*. Start on one side of the processor and rotate to the other side. Repeat. If using a film holder, place all films in the holder and release for processing. Continue until all films are placed in the processor.

9. Remove processed films from the outlet area and place in a labeled x-ray mount.

FIGURE 22-35 (A) Automatic film processor. (B) Drawing of the inside of a typical automatic film processor. *(Courtesy of Air Techniques, Inc.)*

ommended by the manufacturer should be used routinely.

■ Rinse the rollers completely before replacing them in the compartments. Each compartment has a plug that needs to be secure before the tanks are filled.

Mounting Radiographs

Each radiograph has a raised dot to facilitate the mounting process. The film pack is placed in the patient's mouth so that the raised dot, or convex side, is toward the x-ray cone. Mounting the radiographs so that the dot is toward the operator means that the operator is looking at the film as if the operator were facing the patient. The patient's left side would be on the operator's right side facing the film mount. This type of mounting is called labial mounting (Pro-

cedure 22-7). The ADA recommends that dental offices use labial mounting. An x-ray viewbox may be used to mount dental radiographs. A viewbox is a lighted box that has a white, frosted surface so that x-rays can be viewed easily for diagnostic purposes.

In the other type of mounting, called lingual mounting, the depressed dot (concave side) is toward the operator, and therefore the operator views the films from the inside out, or from a position inside the oral cavity looking outward. This type of mounting has the patient's left side on the operator's left side. Both systems of mounting are used in the dental offices today; however, the labial system is more common.

A number of different mounts are available (Figure 22-36). The size range follows: 1, 2, 4, 7, 14, 16, 18, 20, and 28 windows. Bite-wing x-ray mounts normally come in 2 or 4 windows. The 14- or 16-window mounts are used most commonly for periapical mounts. The 18- or

PROCEDURE 22-7

Mounting Radiographs

This procedure is performed by the dental assistant. A viewbox may be utilized when mounting the radiographs.

EQUIPMENT AND SUPPLIES

- Radiographs
- Lighted viewbox
- X-ray mount (using full-mouth, 18 x-ray mount)
- Clean, dry surface

PROCEDURE STEPS *(Follow aseptic procedures)*

1. Wash and dry hands.

2. Label the x-ray mount with the patient's name and the date of the exposure (in pencil).

3. Turn on the viewbox (optional).

4. Place the radiographs on a clean surface so that all dots are convex or outward to viewing.

5. Categorize all x-rays into three groups: bite-wings (four in number), anterior (six in number), and posterior (eight in number).

6. Place the bite-wing x-rays in the mount, making sure the dots remain convex, the molars are toward the outside, and the bicuspids (premolars) are toward the inside. Make sure that the x-rays are mounted according to the curve of the spee.

7. Put the anterior x-rays in place, with the maxillary on the upper and the mandibular on the lower. The incisal edges should be closest to each other in the mount and the roots positioned as they grow. The centrals are placed in the middle with the cuspids on the outer sides. (The maxillary centrals are much larger than the mandibular centrals.)

8. Place the remaining posterior x-rays. The molars should be placed toward the outside and the bicuspids (premolars) toward the inside. The maxillary molars have three roots and the mandibular molars have two roots. Both should be placed according to their position in the mouth, with the roots opposite each other and the biting surfaces more closely positioned.

9. Review the mounted x-rays to verify that they have been placed properly.

FIGURE 22-36 Various full-mouth, bite-wing, and single-film mounts.

20-windows are used most often for full-mouth (both periapical and bite-wing) mounting.

Mounts can be purchased in a number of different materials. They should be stiff enough to keep the films rigid and hold them securely in place. The most commonly used mounts are made from plastic or cardboard. The plastic mounts come in clear, frosted, or dark colors. The advantage of plastic mounts is that they are water repellant and can be reused. Disadvantages are that the plastic mounts can crack or split and, if the operator uses the clear mounts, they can give off a glare around the films and inhibit diagnosis (the frosted and dark mounts cut glare).

The cardboard mount is normally less expensive than the plastic mounts and blocks out any glare around the film. It can be reused if a pencil is used to write in the patient's name. The cardboard mounts have an area for each film to slide into place. Some operators prefer one type of mount over another. The disadvantages of a cardboard mount are that it is not water resistant and it bends and breaks easily. The operator can determine which mount to use.

After selecting the correct mount, place the x-rays on a clean counter in front of a viewbox. If mounting a full-mouth set of x-rays, divide the x-rays into three groups: bite-wings, anterior periapicals, and posterior periapicals. It is easy to identify the bite-wing x-rays because they have both the crowns of the mandibular and the maxillary teeth on them. Individuals may find it easier to mount the bite-wing x-rays first to reference them for the placement of the periapicals. However, there is no set pattern for which x-rays should be mounted.

The four bite-wing x-rays are mounted so that the molar x-rays are on the outside and the corresponding bicuspid x-rays are on the inside, just as if looking directly at the patient (Figure 22-37). Note the curve of Spee (or formation of a smile pattern), which comes from the curvature of the mandible on correctly mounted x-rays. Check carefully that the dots are convex, the molars are on the outside, the bicuspids are on the inside, and the occlusal plane is curved in a smile pattern.

Now mount the anterior periapical x-rays. The maxillary anterior teeth are always larger and wider than the mandibular anterior teeth. The maxillary central teeth are normally the easiest to identify. Locate them and place them in the full-mouth mount in the center upper portion. They should be placed as they are positioned in the mouth, with the incisal edge in the middle of the mount and the roots toward the outside of the mount. Find the mandibular central x-rays (they will appear to have the smallest teeth on them). Place them directly below the maxillary teeth with the incisal edges toward each other. There are four cuspid x-rays (two maxillary and two mandibular) left to mount. Look for the maxillary cuspids first. They will appear larger and may show the maxillary sinuses near the distal side of the apex of the roots. Remember that the roots always tend to curve distally. Mount both the maxillary and the mandibular cuspid x-rays in the correct position with the lateral sides toward the centrals and the bicuspid sides outward. Make sure that all the incisal edges come together in the middle, just like the mouth does.

The mandibular and maxillary posterior films are differentiated from each other on the basis of root and crown shape, along with anatomic landmarks. The maxillary posterior x-rays may show the nasal cav-

FIGURE 22-38 Full-mouth x-rays mounted with correct placement references.

ity or sinuses. The maxillary premolars usually have two roots and the molars have three roots. The roots of the maxillary molars may look unclear because of the lingual root showing through the mesial and distal roots. Mount the maxillary molars on the upper part of the mount toward the outside. The bicuspids will be placed between the molars and the anterior cuspids. The bicuspid and molar x-rays that have been placed in the mount must match each other as well as the corresponding crowns of the bite-wing x-rays. Identify the same restoration in several x-rays (it may be from different angles but still should appear similar). The mandibular periapical x-rays should be mounted in much the same manner as the maxillary. The molars will have two roots that are more clearly defined than the maxillary; the bicuspids will have one root. After all the x-rays are in the mount, do a quick check to see whether all the x-rays are mounted similar to the position of the teeth in the mouth (Figure 22-38). Several practices may be necessary to be able to quickly identify any incorrectly mounted x-rays and to replace them correctly.

Common Radiographic Errors

Errors during exposure and processing of radiographs are inevitable, especially when learning. Understanding basic principles and practices helps to produce quality diagnostic x-rays. Practice on manikins to gain experience and prevent errors. Perfect x-ray technique skills to reduce the number of unnecessary retakes, which expose the patient to more radiation and require more time for everyone. To avoid common radiographic errors, it is necessary to understand what constitutes a quality x-ray.

Correct assembly of the film-holding device eliminates many errors. Be sure the bite-block is in the correct position for the corresponding arch. Also, be sure that the film is centered in the indicating ring. Select the correct size film to cover the area to be exposed. If the film is too small, the apex may be cut off. If the film is too large, it may be difficult for the patient to hold and the x-ray may be distorted. When the film is placed properly in the mouth, a 1- to 3-mm edge of the film should show beyond

FIGURE 22-37 Full-mouth mount with bite-wing x-rays in place.

the occlusal/incisal surface of the tooth. If a hemostat or snap-a-ray film holder is used, be sure to hold the film at the edge, touching it just enough to hold the film secure.

Common Exposure Errors

Common exposure errors involve positioning of the film in the patient's mouth or the position of the cone in relationship to the teeth and the film. Other errors are nonexposure of the film or double-exposing the film. The patient needs to remain immobile during exposure to prevent a blurred image, and the x-ray machine must be set correctly to match the type of film being exposed.

Distortion. Sometimes the film will bend or curve on the palate and in the cuspid area on the mandible; when the film bends, the image distorts. During film placement, the film may crease. These crease marks show on the processed film as black lines (artifacts). Adjust the film position farther into the mouth, toward the midline of the palate of the maxillary, and push the tongue gently so that the film is between the tongue and the mandible (Figures 22-39 and 22-40).

Elongation. Elongation, a vertical angulation error, is caused by too little angulation, meaning that there is too little positive angulation on the maxillary or negative angulation on the mandibular. This error occurs more often when using the bisecting technique. In the paral-

leling technique, elongation is minimized if the cone end is positioned evenly against the indicating ring and the film is placed correctly.

> Paralleling instruments are aids, but evaluate each cone placement. Sometimes the angulation may need to be slightly increased or decreased from the guides (Figure 22-41).

Foreshortening. Foreshortening is also a vertical angulation error. Foreshortening is the opposite of elongation and is caused by too much angulation. This error also occurs more often with the bisecting technique and can be corrected by decreasing the vertical angulation. If the paralleling technique is used, align the cone with the film holder (Figure 22-42).

Overlapping. Overlapping is caused by incorrect horizontal angulation. When the cone is angled toward the mesial or the distal surfaces of the teeth instead of the interproximal areas, overlapping occurs. The cone/central ray should be directed straight at the teeth and at a 90° angle to the film in order to keep the contacts open. Remember to evaluate the film placement in regard to the curve of the arch, not the contour of the patient's face (cheeks) (Figure 22-43).

Cone Cutting. Cone cutting means that the x-ray beam missed part of the film, causing the film to be only partially exposed. Because the cone is lead-lined, the shape of the cone cut on the film will match the shape of the

FIGURE 22-39 A curved film distorts radiograph images.

FIGURE 22-40 A bent film appears as a black crease or thin, dark, radiolucent line.

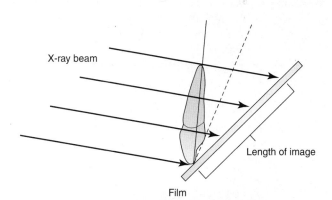

X-ray beam

Length of image

Film

FIGURE 22-41 Elongation on a radiograph. Diagram shows how a film is elongated.

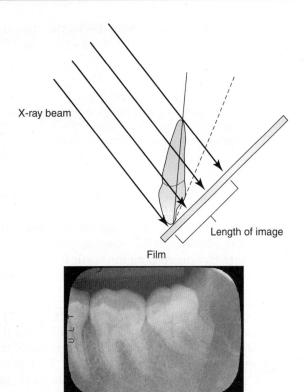

FIGURE 22-42 Foreshortening on a radiograph. Diagram shows how a film is foreshortened.

FIGURE 22-43 Overlapping. Diagram shows the position of an x-ray beam to prevent overlapping.

cone (either round or rectangular). Be sure that the x-ray film is placed in the center of the cone (Figure 22-44).

Clear Film. A **clear film** indicates that the film was exposed to no radiation. Check your machine to verify that it was turned on. If it was, then it is malfunctioning. If the exposure routine was interrupted, an unexposed film may have been placed in the cup with exposed films (Figure 22-45).

Double Exposure. Sometimes, inadvertently, film is exposed twice. This can be avoided by keeping exposed film separate from unexposed film. A **double exposure** results in indistinct images or dark x-rays. Examine the film closely and two images can be seen. Establishing a routine can help avoid double-exposed films (Figure 22-46).

Blurred Image. **Blurred images** result from movement of the patient's head or tubehead or from the x-ray film moving in the patient's mouth. The images are undefined and unclear. Be sure the patient can hold the film

FIGURE 22-44 Cone cut. Diagram shows correct and incorrect positions of a cone to prevent cone cutting.

FIGURE 22-45 Clear film. This film has not been exposed to x-rays.

FIGURE 22-46 Double exposure. Film was exposed twice with each exposure shown on the x-ray film.

FIGURE 22-49 Sample radiopaque image on an x-ray. Full-gold crown on lower first molar.

in place and hold still for the exposure. Also, make sure the tubehead is still before leaving the room.

Underexposed Film. When the film appears light and has a thin image, it may be **underexposed**. Check the mAs, kVs, and exposure times for the type of film being used, the size of the patient, and the x-ray machine. Another reason for this outcome is that the cone may not have been positioned close enough to the patient's face (Figure 22-47).

Overexposed Film. When the film has a dark image, it is overexposed and too dark (dense) to see any structures clearly and accurately for a diagnosis. Use the same checks used for the light film image (Figure 22-48).

FIGURE 22-50 Film was placed in the patient's mouth backward. Note the herringbone pattern on the molars.

Radiopaque Film Images. Often, such metal objects as eyeglasses, earrings, and partial appliances show as **radiopaque** (not transmitting light) objects on the processed x-ray (Figure 22-49). Check for and remove objects before exposing the film.

Backward Film. Placing the film in the mouth backward or reversed causes the images on the film to be light and a **herringbone pattern** (tire track) appears. The white, plain side of the film is always placed facing the tubehead. If the film is reversed, the amount of x-rays that reach the film are reduced by the lead foil. The herringbone or tire track pattern on the foil is seen on the sides of the processed x-ray (Figure 22-50).

Common Film Processing Errors

Common film processing errors involve how the film is handled during the processing stage and the maintenance and setting of film processing equipment. Dental x-ray film is sensitive to temperature of the processing solutions, and films must be handled carefully when they are being unwrapped and placed in the processing machine. Maintenance of the processing machine is necessary to ensure clean films without streaks or stains.

Light Film Image. Light and dark film images can occur while exposing the film and during processing. A light film is said to be underprocessed. If the film is underprocessed, the developing time was too short, the developer temperature was lower than recommended,

FIGURE 22-47 On underexposed film, the image appears light.

FIGURE 22-48 On overexposed film, the image appears dark.

or the developing solution was "exhausted" (too weak from overuse and needs to be changed).

Another cause is the fixing process. If the film is not fixed completely, the emulsion will not be sufficiently hardened and will wash off in the water. With overfixation, the film is left too long in the fixer and the image bleaches out. Also, if the film was placed in the mouth backward, the result is a lighter film (Figure 22-51).

Dark Film Image. The dark film images can be caused by overdeveloping, the developing solution temperature being too high, the developing solution being too strong, or the film being left in the developer too long. Routinely check solutions and adjust processing times accordingly (Figure 22-52). Refer to x-ray film processing section discussed later in this chapter for more detail on how to check the temperature of processing solutions. Several methods of monitoring film quality are discussed later in this chapter.

Fogged Film. Fogged films have a gray appearance, image detail is lost, and contrast is lessened. It is like viewing a film image through a dense fog. Fog on films can be caused by improper storage conditions, outdated films, light leaks in the processing room, or light leaks from loose fittings on automatic processors and daylight loaders. Also, safelights (lights with filters under which the film can be manipulated without exposing it) may need to be adjusted or changed; for example, they may be too close to the processing area, too bright, or faulty (Figure 22-53).

Partial Image. A partial image on the film is the result of film placement in the processing tanks when the solution levels are low. The film is not completely immersed and a partial image results. Always check the levels of the processing solutions. Daily, some evaporation takes place and the films absorb some developer, so replenish the developer regularly (Figure 22-54). To avoid the chance of a partial image, do not use the top clips on the x-ray racks.

Film Artifacts. Film artifacts result from not handling the films carefully or not keeping the area around the processing tanks clean. Examples of artifacts include water spots on unprocessed film, which leave clear areas on the film, fixer on unprocessed film, which leaves a white area on the film, and developer, which leaves black spots. If the film is not washed/rinsed properly, a yellowish brown stain is left on the film. Black film artifacts can occur from a small charge of electricity, such as a lightning streak, when you pull the x-ray film from the packet in a dry climate. Fluoride ions on gloves that are transferred to the film during handling leave dark fingerprint smudge marks (Figure 22-55). X-rays that overlap (touch) during processing leave an artifact on the films (the artifact is in the shape of the edge or corner of the film).

FIGURE 22-51 Light image due to film processing error.

FIGURE 22-53 Fogged film.

FIGURE 22-52 Dark image due to film processing error.

FIGURE 22-54 Partial image due to low levels of processing solution.

FIGURE 22-55 Sample fingerprint from processing solutions on an x-ray.

FIGURE 22-57 Films that are agitated poorly when placed in processing solutions leave air-bubble artifacts on the processed film.

Torn or Scratched Film. Rough handling of the film can lead to the emulsion on the film being torn or scratched, which leaves a white area or mark on the processed film. Films can be scratched and torn if they are not handled carefully in overcrowded tanks or during retrieval if lost off the film racks (Figure 22-56).

Air Bubbles on Film. Air bubbles are trapped on the film if it is not agitated when placed in the processing solutions. The air bubbles leave round, white spots where they were attached to the film (Figure 22-57).

Reticulation. Reticulation occurs when a film has been exposed to a high temperature followed by a low temperature. The film emulsion swells and then shrinks. The film looks like it is dried and has tiny cracks. The temperature of the solutions and the water should be monitored to ensure that they are within the recommended temperature ranges.

Streaks. Streaks on films may result from unclean rollers when using automatic processors or from unclean x-ray racks. Debris is picked up as the films pass through the rollers, leaving a streaked appearance on the film. Streaks from unclean x-ray racks occur during the processing procedure; debris, including processing solutions, runs from the racks onto the film.

Duplicating Radiographs

Dental x-rays can be duplicated so that the originals never have to leave the office. The need for duplication is increasing, because more patients have dental insurance, patients request that x-rays be sent to specialists, and requests are made to forward x-rays when patients change residence. Also, malpractice suits have increased, which require radiographs for defense support. Copies of x-rays can be made by a duplication process in the darkroom. These copies offer protection for the dentist as well as reference sources for the patient.

The duplication technique requires the purchase of duplicating film and a duplication machine. The film comes in a variety of sizes and can be processed manually or with an automatic processor (Procedure 22-8). Duplicating film has emulsion on one side only and is coded with a notch in the upper right corner, when the emulsion side is facing you. Duplicating film is a direct positive film; thus, if an increase in film darkness (density) is desired, exposure time is reduced.

Duplicating machines have light sources with glass over them. The lid closes with a latch to prevent light leaks. There is a setting for viewing the x-rays and a timing selector. These machines are not large and fit conveniently on a counter top.

Storage of Patient Radiographs

Patients' radiographs are stored in the treatment record. If they are removed from the mount, they are placed in a small envelope with the patient's name, date, and number of x-rays enclosed labeled on the outside. Each state has regulations on the length of time radiographs must be saved (because they are considered legal records). Dental assistants should inquire about the pertinent statutes of limitation in their states.

FIGURE 22-56 Radiograph with torn or scratched emulsion.

PROCEDURE 22-8

Processing Duplicating Technique

This procedure is performed by the dental assistant. The dental assistant prepares the equipment, supplies, and work area. The radiographs to be duplicated are taken to the darkroom by the dental assistant to duplicate.

EQUIPMENT AND SUPPLIES

- Duplicating film and radiographs to be duplicated
- X-ray duplicating machine
- Automatic x-ray processor with daylight loader

PROCEDURE STEPS *(Follow aseptic procedures)*

1. Place the x-rays in the desired position on the duplicator (Figure 22-58). Make sure the dot on the film is upward (convex).

2. If the machine has a viewing light, turn it on to assist during placement of the x-rays.

3. Turn off the viewing light, and, under safelight conditions, place the duplicating film over the x-rays with the emulsion side facing downward so it contacts the x-rays (the notch will be in the upper left corner).

4. Cover with the lid and latch tightly. Set the timer to four to five seconds (this may vary with machines).

FIGURE 22-58 Duplicating machine and duplicating film used to duplicate full-mouth series and panoramic exposures.

5. Activate the machine to expose the film.

6. When completed, remove the duplicating film under safelight conditions and process the film.

Legal Implications of Radiographs

 As stated above, x-rays are legal records and should not be destroyed. They belong to the dentist and should not be given to the patients. If a patient switches to another dentist, send a duplicate of the x-rays to the new dentist; keep the original for the office files.

Quality Assurance

A quality assurance (QA) program refers to routine procedures that have been developed to ensure the highest quality and minimal risk to the patients in radiation exposure. Under this program, equipment, solutions, and procedures are tested to ensure that consistent high quality is maintained.

Several aspects of the equipment should be checked each year by state regulatory agencies:

- kV output
- mA output
- Exposure timer working properly
- Half value layer (HVL)
- Focal spot size
- Beam alignment and beam size
- X-ray output and reproducibility of exposure
- Stability of tubehead

These recommendations were published in the *Recommendations for Quality Assurance in Dental Radiography* by the American Academy of Dental Radiology. It is important that the date of the test, the type of the test performed, the name of the person performing the test, and the results be kept in a service log. Include documents of any service work in the log. Radiographic units are like any equipment and must be calibrated occasionally to work optimally.

Implementation of a QA program and assessment of the variables that affect x-ray quality greatly benefit patients and operators. The tests used for routine assessment give the accuracy needed to provide good diagnostic x-rays.

- One of the most important aspects of a QA program is monitoring film processing. Make sure your lighting conditions in the darkroom are safe. Use the proper filters for the films currently in use. If the faster films are used, then the red filter is correct. If in question, check with a state regulatory representative.

- Another area of concern are the white light leaks in the darkroom. A simple way to evaluate the darkroom for possible light leaks is to do a "coin test." On the counter in the immediate processing area, place a coin on an unwrapped, unexposed x-ray film under the safelight for two to three minutes. Then, process the film using standard procedures. If the outline of the coin is evident on the film after processing, then the safelight illumination is inadequate or a white light leak is possible (Figure 22-59). Document the results in a log and date it. Correct any problems and do the test again. This test should be performed monthly.

A technique for monitoring the quality of the processing solutions is to use a step wedge. Use a commercial step wedge or make a step wedge by placing several lead foil pieces, from x-ray film packets, together in a stair-step manner and soldering them (Figure 22-60). Expose twenty x-rays the first day the processing solution is changed. Make sure it is stirred, and check the temperature. Then, process one of the x-rays. This pro-

FIGURE 22-60 (A) Manufactured step wedge. (B) Step wedge made from lead foil from x-ray film packets.

cessed film will become a standard for evaluating other films. Choose a density in the middle of the film to be used for comparison. Store the other nineteen exposed x-rays in a cool, dry place. Every day or two process another of the x-rays and compare it to the first one. The same middle density on these later films should be comparable to the first one. If the later film differs from the standard by two or more steps, check the processing solution.

Other areas to be checked include the last time the solution was changed or replenished, water temperature, processing time, and whether the solutions have been contaminated. After checking all possibilities and correcting the problem, process an additional test x-ray to compare to the standard film.

- Monthly, the x-ray machine can be checked by using several additional equipment items. To test the timer, a spin top is needed (Figure 22-61A). Place the film (normally size No. 4) on the sitting area of the x-ray chair. Select the mA and kVp values and the number of impulses to be tested. Place the spin top on the film, place the PID over the top and film, set it to spin, make the exposure, and process the film. Count the number of dots visible on the film to interpret the results (Figure 22-61B). The number should correspond to the number of impulses selected on the machine.

- To evaluate the effectiveness of the milliamperage, use the step wedge and place it on a size No. 2 film,

FIGURE 22-59 Unexposed film with a coin on it for the safelight test.

FIGURE 22-61 (A) Spin top used in checking time accuracy and exposed x-ray showing results of the spin top test. (B) Impulses indicated by markings on the x-ray.

and position the PID so that it covers the film. Then expose the film. Do this each month; if the appearance of the corresponding shade varies more than two steps, the mA should be checked and adjusted by a qualified service person (Figure 22-62).

■ To measure the kVp, a dosimeter and charger are needed (Figure 22-63). Make sure the dosimeter is

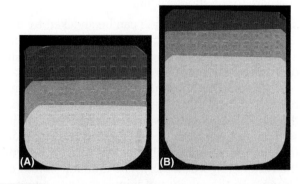

FIGURE 22-62 Comparison of two x-rays exposed using the step wedge. (A) Standard processed when the solution was first prepared. (B) Standard processed after solution replenishment.

FIGURE 22-63 A dosimeter used to evaluate kilovoltage. (A) Dosimeter charger. (B) Dosimeter.

charged and at the 0 reading. Place the dosimeter on a surface, place the PID over it, and expose the dosimeter. It should show a reading of the appropriate kVp. If it does not, have it checked by a qualified service person.

If a problem is apparent, it is important that no radiographs be taken until the problem is fixed. Quality control cannot be overlooked. Each step of the procedure must be followed carefully, including storage of unexposed films, use of a lead apron with a thyroid collar, proper placement of the film and cone to reduce retakes, and correct, final labeling of the film mount from which the diagnosis is to be made. All the steps in between are important to minimize radiation to the patient. It is important that each dental assistant has proper training to take x-rays. Every patient deserves competent, quality service.

1. Set high standards for quality assurance.
2. Follow a consistent procedure to maintain control.
3. Check equipment, solutions, and procedures often.
4. Keep a log of daily, monthly, and yearly procedures used to maintain quality radiographs.

CHAPTER SUMMARY

The dentist uses both intraoral films placed in the patient's mouth for exposure, and extraoral films placed outside the patient's mouth to produce quality radiographs used in diagnosing dental conditions. Simply, a quality radiograph facilitates accurate diagnosis.

The two techniques used to expose radiographs are bisecting and paralleling. Both techniques are described in this chapter, but the paralleling technique and equipment required for this technique are demonstrated in each area of the mouth for adults and children.

Once the radiographs have been exposed, they must be processed. Manual and automatic processing equipment and techniques are described and compared. Chemical components of the developing and fixing solutions are listed, and the role they play in converting the latent image into a visible permanent radiograph is discussed.

Radiographs are then mounted for viewing. There are various types of dental x-ray mounts to choose from, and helpful hints to determine the order the x-rays are mounted, especially when learning, are addressed.

Common radiographic errors during processing and exposing x-rays are listed and examples provided. Care-

ful attention to positioning during x-ray exposure and detailed step-by-step procedures for processing can assist in the elimination of errors.

Patient radiographs are needed for many reasons. For instance, insurance companies require copies of the patient's x-rays to determine insurance coverage, and other dental offices require a copy of the patient's x-rays for their own diagnoses. Radiographs can be duplicated so that the original radiographs never have to leave the office. The special film and equipment needed for this process are discussed. Dental offices are required to properly store final radiographs to prevent losses, and thereby avoid the need for x-rays to be retaken.

Case Study

Dr. David Candell has requested that Coral Nicolus have a full-mouth series of x-rays. Coral is a new patient and has had no x-rays taken for over five years. Dr. Candell wants radiographs to view the condition of the teeth and supporting bone. Coral is in good health except for having difficulty opening her mouth very wide. It would be uncomfortable for a periapical size No. 2 film to be placed in her mouth for exposure.

Case Study Review

1. What alternatives to periapical exposures does the dental assistant have?

2. Would the information the dentist requested be visible on the panoramic exposure?

3. Does the patient have any limitations that would alter this procedure?

4. Must the dentist be informed of changes before the radiographs are exposed?

REVIEW QUESTIONS

Multiple Choice

1. Which error results in interproximal spaces overlapping on a radiograph?
   a. Vertical angulation
   b. Horizontal angulation
   c. Improper film placement
   d. Improper film processing

2. When processing film in an automatic processor, what is the sequence of the solutions?
   a. Developer, fixer, water
   b. Developer, water, fixer
   c. Water, developer, fixer
   d. Fixer, developer, water

3. What is the optimal temperature for processing x-rays in the automatic processor?
   a. 85° to 95°F
   b. 70°F
   c. 100°C
   d. 75°F

4. When viewing properly mounted x-rays, where or how is the dot on the film mounted?
   a. So that it is raised or convex
   b. So that it is depressed or concave
   c. In the middle of the film
   d. In any position

5. The entire tooth and surrounding area are seen on the
   a. periapical x-ray.
   b. bite-wing x-ray.
   c. occlusal x-ray.
   d. None of the above.

6. Which one of the two exposure techniques listed below uses a vertical angulation table for proper positioning of the cone?
   a. Paralleling technique
   b. Bisecting technique

7. Occlusal radiographs are used to locate or define all of the following *except*
   a. fractures.
   b. impacted teeth.
   c. changes in size and shape of arches.
   d. a facial view of entire mandibular arch.

8. A full-mouth survey of a child aged three to five years includes
   a. two bite-wings, six anterior incisors, and four posterior periapicals.
   b. four bite-wings, six anterior incisors, and two posterior periapicals.
   c. two bite-wings, two anterior incisors, and four posterior periapicals.
   d. four bite-wings, six anterior incisors, and eight posterior periapicals.

9. All of the following are exposure errors *except*
   a. distortion.
   b. elongation.
   c. torn or scratched film.
   d. overlapping.

10. Duplicating film is the same film used to expose x-rays of the teeth.
    a. True
    b. False

Critical Thinking

1. If the radiographs were dark after processing, what areas would the dental assistant want to check to correct the problem?

2. List three primary errors that may be apparent on routine bite-wing x-rays, and explain how they can be corrected.

3. Discuss how taking radiographs on children is different from exposing radiographs on adults.

Web Activities

1. To find questions that patients frequently ask about dental x-rays, go to http://www.ada.org and look under x-rays.

2. Check http://www.Kodak.com under dental products, learning center for tutorials on dental radiology subjects.

3. To identify three different duplicating machines, go to http://www.Rinncorp.com.

CHAPTER 23

EXTRAORAL AND DIGITAL RADIOGRAPHY

SPECIFIC INSTRUCTIONAL OBJECTIVES

The student should strive to meet the following objectives and demonstrate an understanding of the facts and principles presented in this chapter:

1. Identify extraoral films and describe exposing techniques.

2. Identify normal and abnormal radiographic landmarks.

3. Identify imaging systems used for dental purposes.

4. Describe digital radiography.

5. Identify the components of digital radiography.

6. Explain the procedure for using digital radiography.

KEY TERMS

analog image *(494)*

axial plane *(494)*

cassette *(478)*

cephalometric
    radiograph *(488)*

charge-coupled device
    (CCD) *(497)*

computed tomography
    (CT scanning) *(493)*

digital image *(494)*

digital imaging
    technology *(493)*

digital radiology *(494)*

direct digital
    imaging *(496)*

extraoral film *(480)*

focal trough *(479)*

Frankfort plane *(483)*

ghost image *(481)*

gray scale *(495)*

indirect digital
    imaging *(496)*

intensifying
    screens *(480)*

lateral jaw
    radiograph *(488)*

lead apron
    artifact *(484)*

magnetic resonance
    imaging (MRI) *(493)*

midsagittal plane *(483)*

panoramic
    radiography *(478)*

pixels *(494)*

radiolucency *(495)*

radiopacity *(495)*

"rare earth"
    phosphors *(480)*

rotational center *(479)*

storage phosphor
    imaging *(496)*

tomography *(479)*

tragus of the ear *(488)*

transcranial
    temporomandibular
    joint
    radiograph *(488)*

trismus *(478)*

INTRODUCTION

Extraoral radiography is standard practice in the dental office; both panoramic and cephalometric radiographs are taken routinely as part of patient records. Panoramic radiographs are used in general and specialty dental offices, while the cephalometric radiographs are mainly taken by orthodontists. The lateral jaw radiograph and the transcranial temporomandibular joint radiograph are the other extraoral radiographs discussed in this chapter.

The dental assistant should become familiar with radiograph interpretation, because it will help them take quality radiographs, and to be more prepared for selected treatment. Interpretation involves learning the terminology, and then identifying the landmark on a radiograph.

Digital radiography is becoming standard in many dental offices, and it is likely that all dental offices in the future will take and store digital radiographs. Digital equipment and techniques and their advantages and disadvantages will be discussed. Digital radiography equipment is changing and improving, while the technique is made easier for the dentist and dental staff to learn and incorporate into their office routine.

Extraoral Radiographs

Extraoral radiographs are used by the dentist to identify large areas of the skull on one radiograph. These radiographs give the dentist an overall view and are used most often in conjunction with periapical, bite-wing, and occlusal radiographs. Orthodontists and oral maxillofacial surgeons routinely use extraoral radiographs, especially panoramic and cephalometric exposures.

Panoramic Radiography

Many dental offices have **panoramic radiography** machines (Figure 23-1). Panoramic machines take a radiograph that shows the entire maxilla and mandible on one film (Figure 23-2). Panoramic radiography is commonly known and named after the brand name of the panoramic x-ray machine. There are many types of panoramic machines, but most use the same techniques. The film holder (**cassette**) and the x-ray head rotate opposite each other around the patient's head. Because they are connected by bars extending from the top of the machines, they rotate at the same speed. The result is an x-ray that extends from the condyle on one side of the patient's head to the condyle on the other side. There is some overlapping and loss of detail, but panoramic radiographs are valuable when an overall assessment of the patient is needed. Panoramic x-rays can be taken on adults, children, edentulous patients, patients who have **trismus** (lack the ability to open the mouth very wide), and patients in wheelchairs.

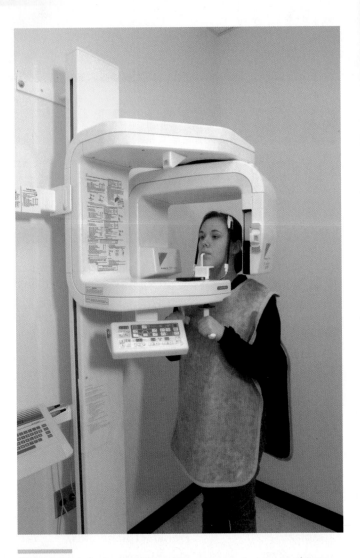

FIGURE 23-1 Patient positioned in a panoramic x-ray machine.

FIGURE 23-2 A panoramic radiograph.

Panoramic x-rays give the dentist a general view of the following:

- The entire dentition
- Nasal and orbital areas
- Alveolar bone

- Carious lesions
- Fractures, cysts, tumors
- Malocclusion
- Maxilla and mandible
- Sinuses
- Unerupted teeth
- Dental appliances and restorations
- Periodontal disease
- Temporomandibular joint

Fundamentals of Panoramic Radiography

As mentioned previously, the x-ray tubehead and film move around the patient in panoramic radiography. Panoramic radiography is based on the principle of tomography (*tomo* means section). Tomography shows the imaging of one layer or section of the body while blurring images from other areas. In panoramic radiography, the image conforms to the curve of the dental arches. The patient is positioned, and when the panoramic exposure button is pushed, the tubehead rotates in one direction around the patient while the cassette that holds the x-ray rotates in the opposite direction. The patient may stand or sit in a stationary position during the exposure. The rotation is synchronized from rotational centers. Rotational centers vary in number and location, depending on the manufacturer of the panoramic machine. They also influence the shape and size of the focal trough. The focal trough (Figure 23-3) (also known as the image layer or sharpness) is a three-dimensional curved zone in which the dental arches are positioned to achieve the sharpest image. The panoramic machine will expose this selected plane of tissue, while the areas outside the selected plane will be blurred. The size and shape of the focal trough varies from one panoramic machine to another, but each machine is designed to accommodate the average person. The quality of the panoramic radiograph depends on precise positioning of the patient's teeth within the focal trough, and if the patient resembles the average person design of that specific machine. The manufacturer provides specific instructions for positioning the patient, and how to work with "non-average" patients.

Panoramic Unit

Panoramic units are constantly being updated and improved (Figure 23-4). They differ by size and shape of the focal trough, number and location of rotational centers, and type of cassette (holder) for the x-ray film. All units, however, include the following basic components:

- Exposure controls
- Head positioner

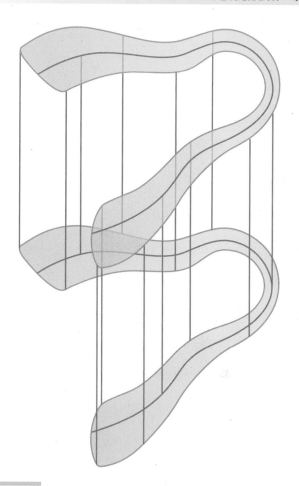

FIGURE 23-3 Focal trough or image layer.

- X-ray tubehead
- Cassette holder

Exposure Controls. The exposure controls are usually located outside the x-ray room; in cases where the controls are part of the unit, but the exposure control button is located outside the room. The manufacturer determines many exposure factors, such as exposure time, but kilovoltage and milliamperage can be adjusted. The instruction manual provides information on variations for different exposures.

Head Positioner. The head positioner consists of lateral head supports or guides, chin rest, notched bite-block, and forehead rest. There are also handles for the patient to hold onto for support located near this area. Each panoramic machine is slightly different, and the operator must follow the manufacturer's instructions on how to correctly position the patient.

X-ray Tubehead. The x-ray tubehead is similar to an intraoral x-ray tubehead in producing x-rays; however, the collimator shape is different. The collimator used in panoramic machines has a narrow vertical slit, in contrast to the small round or rectangular shape of intraoral machines. The x-ray beam is emitted from the panoramic tubehead through the narrow slit that forms

FIGURE 23-4 Panoramic unit.

FIGURE 23-5 (A) 1. Hard cassette for a panoramic x-ray. 2. Intensifying screens on the inside of a cephalometric cassette. (B) Soft cassette.

a vertical band of x-rays which pass through the patient and exposes the panoramic film through a vertical slit in the cassette holder. The patient receives minimal radiation exposure due to the collimator shape and the amount of x-rays emitted from the x-ray tubehead.

Cassette Film Holders. Cassettes are used to hold the film during exposure. They are flat, hard containers that open on the back or flexible, thin sleeves that open on one end (Figure 23-5). Both prevent light from coming through but allow x-rays to pass through. The cassettes must be marked to distinguish left or right because there is no raised dot on the film. With some panoramic machines, the films are labeled with the patient's name, dentist's name, date, and so on. The assistant enters the information digitally before exposure. After exposure under safelight conditions, the film is run through a marking device. The film is then processed, and the information appears on the film.

In addition, care must be taken to avoid scratching the screens, and to keep them free of stains and debris. Cassettes usually are lined with **intensify-**

ing screens. The action of the x-rays on the film is increased or "intensified"; therefore, the exposure to the patient is decreased. A substance called phosphor is used on the screens. The phosphor emits light when struck by x-rays. Some phosphors emit blue light and others emit green light. It is important to use film that is sensitive to the kind of light the phosphor emits. The green-light phosphors are known as **"rare earth" phosphors** and are faster; thus, the patient receives fewer x-rays during exposure. Calcium tungstate phosphors emit blue light. These screens are not as fast and require more x-rays to make a radiograph than the rare earth screens.

Extraoral Film. The **extraoral film** comes in a variety of large sizes, ranging from 5×12 for the panoramic to 8×10 for the cephalometric exposure. The film is not wrapped individually; it comes in a box of fifty or more (Figure 23-6). Therefore, the film must be loaded into the cassettes in the darkroom under safelight conditions. The box must be closed carefully to prevent light exposure to the remaining film in the box.

Extraoral film is screen film, requiring the use of screens for exposure. The film is placed between two intensifying screens in the cassette holder. Screen film is sensitive to the light emitted from the intensifying screens rather than to radiation. The film must be sensitive to the type of light emitted by the screen particles. It

FIGURE 23-6 Extraoral film. (A) Panoramic film. (B) Cephalometric film.

is important to have extraoral film that is designed specifically for the type of intensifying screens being used.

Film-Holding Devices. Panoramic machines have cassette holders attached to them. With other extraoral exposures, the cassette holder may be attached to a wall or the patient may hold the cassette. For some extraoral exposures, the cassette is placed on a flat surface and the patient rests her or his face on it.

Panoramic Exposure Technique Suggestions

There are many types of panoramic machines, and each machine has specific instructions provided by the manufacturer for successful exposures on a variety of patients. Be sure to read and follow these instructions. A few guidelines for all panoramic exposures follow:

- The patient always should wear a lead apron *without* a thyroid collar. The collar interferes with the image and, because the x-ray beam is directed upward, the x-ray exposure to the thyroid gland is minimal.

- The patient needs to be still during the entire exposure. Every machine is equipped with some type of chin rest, bite-block, and head positioner to prevent movement.

- Explain the procedure to the patient, including rotation of the machine and what to do during the exposure. Remove bulky sweaters, coats, hair clips, or anything that may interfere with the rotation of the x-ray tubehead. Remove earrings, necklaces, and dental appliances as well.

- Place the cassette in the machine, prepare your patient, carefully take the readings, set the machine, and take the exposure. Release the patient and remove the cassette for processing and reloading (Procedure 23-1).

Common Panoramic Radiography Errors

Errors in preparation and positioning of the patient are discussed in this section.

Preparation Errors. When preparing the patient, make sure that the patient has removed all metal objects that might cast a **ghost image** on the film. A ghost image is a radiopaque artifact seen on the panoramic film that is caused by double-exposure of a dense object by the x-ray beam. A ghost image is similar to the real image but is cast on the opposite side of the x-ray, and is larger, higher, and blurred. A common ghost image is produced by an earring left in one ear. All metal objects (e.g., earrings, eyeglasses, hairpins, necklaces, facial piercing,

PROCEDURE 23-1

Exposing Panoramic Radiographs

This procedure is performed by the dental assistant at the direction of the dentist. The assistant prepares the cassette, panoramic machine, and patient for exposure.

EQUIPMENT AND SUPPLIES

- Mouth mirror
- Panoramic film
- Cassette
- Bite-block
- Barrier for the bite-block
- Lead apron without thyroid collar
- Panoramic machine

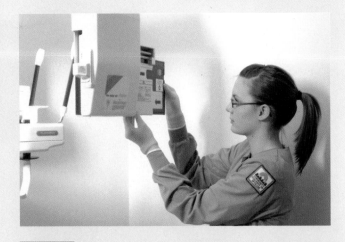

FIGURE 23-7 Placing a cassette into the panoramic machine.

PREPARATION FOR PANORAMIC RADIOGRAPHIC EXPOSURE

1. Under safelight conditions, load the cassette in the darkroom. The cassettes are lined with two intensifying screens, and the panoramic film is placed between them. The cassette must be securely closed to prevent light leaks. With some cassettes, information can be added such as left and right, and the patient's name, date, and dentist's name.

2. Place the cassette into the cassette holder of the panoramic machine (Figure 23-7).

3. Prepare the bite-block. A protective barrier can be placed on the bite-block (such as plastic wrap). The bite-blocks should be sterilized between patients.

4. Adjust the machine to the patient's approximate height, and set the kilovoltage and milliamperage according to the manufacturer's guidelines.

PREPARE PATIENT FOR PANORAMIC EXPOSURE

1. Explain the procedure to the patient, and answer any questions.

2. Ask the patient to remove eyeglasses, earrings, tongue bars, facial piercing, hairpins and clips, necklaces, hearing aids, partial and full dentures, and any-

thing else that may interfere with the film exposure or cast a shadow on the film.

3. Place and secure the lead apron on the patient. The lead apron used for the panoramic exposures is double-sided and *without* a thyroid collar (Figure 23-8). This apron is placed with one side on the front of the patient and one side on the back to protect the patient as the machine rotates around during the exposure. The thyroid collar is not recommended for panoramic exposures because it may interfere with the exposure and block part of the x-ray beam.

4. Guide the patient into position, whether sitting or standing. Ask the patient to stand/sit up as straight as possible so that the spine is perfectly straight. If the spinal column is not straight, it will cast a white shadow in the middle of the radiograph.

5. Raise the machine to the appropriate level so that the patient can easily bite on the bite-block. Have the patient move forward until the upper and lower teeth are secured in the groove on the bite-block. The groove aligns the teeth in the focal trough. If the patient is edentulous, the alveolar ridges should be positioned over the grooves of the bite-block.

(continues)

FIGURE 23-8 Patient with lead apron on ready to be positioned in the panoramic machine.

FIGURE 23-9 Patient biting on bite block correctly positioned for panoramic exposure. Horizontal line highlighted on patient's face indicates the midsagittal plane and the vertical line shows the Frankfort plane.

7. The **midsagittal plane** is the imaginary line that evenly divides the face into right and left halves. This midsagittal plane must be perpendicular to the floor, so that the head is not tilted; otherwise, the image will be distorted (Figure 23-10A).

8. The **Frankfort plane** is the imaginary line drawn from the middle of the ear to just below the eye socket across the bridge of the nose. This line must be parallel with the floor, which will place the occlusal plane at the correct angle (Figure 23-10B).

9. Before taking the exposure, have the patient swallow, place the tongue at the roof of the mouth, and close the lips around the bite-block. Reassure the patient and instruct him or her to remain still during the exposure.

10. After the exposure is complete, guide the patient away from the panoramic machine and remove the lead apron.

11. Remove the cassette and proceed with film processing as described in Chapter 22, Production and Evaluation of Dental Radiographs.

Cotton rolls can also be used to assist in positioning (Figure 23-9).

6. Some panoramic machines have lights to assist in positioning of the midsagittal plane and the Frankfort plane. At this point, turn the light on and adjust the patient accordingly.

(continues)

PROCEDURE 23-1 (CONTINUED)

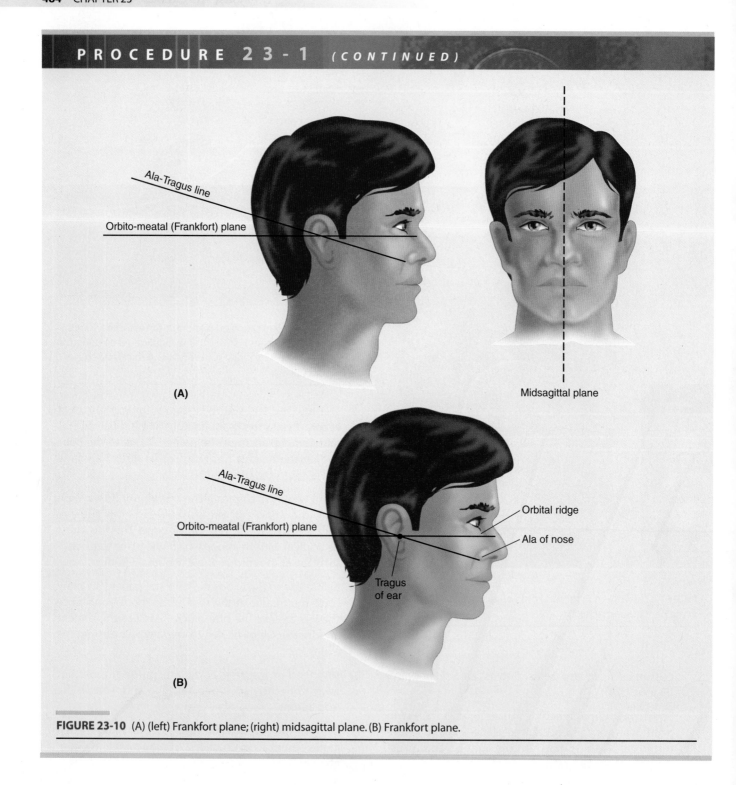

FIGURE 23-10 (A) (left) Frankfort plane; (right) midsagittal plane. (B) Frankfort plane.

partial or removable dentures, hearing aids, orthodontic retainers) must be removed before exposure to ensure that the radiograph is of adequate quality for diagnosis.

Adjust the lead apron correctly so that it lies flat around the patient and below the cassette and x-ray tubehead as they rotate around the patient. A **lead apron artifact** will also occur if a lead apron with a thyroid collar is used. The collar on most people is large and closes around the chin.

Positioning Errors. The patient must be positioned correctly to expose the clearest and most accurate image possible. Panoramic radiographs show the dentist the entire dentition and related structures, from one condyle to the other condyle. The dental assistant must pay attention to every detail of positioning the patient. See Table 23-1 for common errors in positioning the patient.

TABLE 23-1 Patient Positioning Errors

Problem	Correction
Patient positioned too far forward on the bite-block. The anterior teeth are not in the grooves on the bite-block, but are biting forward of the grooves. The anterior teeth will be out of the focal trough, so they will be blurred. The spine is superimposed on the ramus areas of the mandible; the bicuspids appear overlapped (Figure 23-11).	Have the patient bite in the grooves of the bite-block and hold in this position. The head supports might need to be adjusted to prevent the head from moving forward.
Patient is positioned too far back. The anterior teeth are not in the grooves on the bite-block but are biting too far back of the grooves. The anterior teeth will be out of the focal trough, and thus will be blurred and appear wide. Ghost images of the mandible and spine will also appear (Figure 23-12).	Have the patient bite in the grooves of the bite-block and hold in this position. The head supports might need to be adjusted to prevent the head from moving backward.
Frankfort plane/patient's head is tilted downward. Apices of the lower incisors are blurred, mandibular condyles may not be seen, a shadow of the hyoid bone is superimposed over the center of the mandible, and the curve of the arch is exaggerated in an upward direction (Figure 23-13).	Carefully position the patient with the Frankfort plane parallel to the floor.
Frankfort plane/patient's head is tilted upward. Maxillary incisors are blurred, hard palate and floor of the nasal cavity appear superimposed over the apices of the maxillary teeth, and the curve of the arch is exaggerated in a downward direction (Figure 23-14).	Carefully position the patient with the Frankfort plane parallel to the floor.
Patient's tongue was not resting on the roof of the mouth during exposure. This will cause a dark radiolucent area above the apices of the maxillary teeth (Figure 23-15).	Instruct and watch the patient as she or he swallows, and raises the tongue to of the roof the mouth and holds it there during the exposure.
Patient was not standing or sitting up straight, resulting in a ghost image of the spine superimposed in the center of the x-ray (Figure 23-16).	Position the patient so that the midsagittal plane is perpendicular to the floor and the midline is centered on the bite-block.

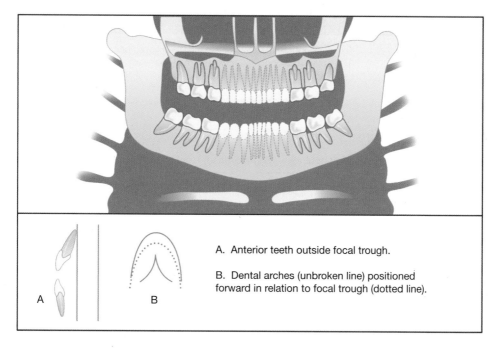

A. Anterior teeth outside focal trough.

B. Dental arches (unbroken line) positioned forward in relation to focal trough (dotted line).

FIGURE 23-11 Panoramic film of patient positioned too far forward.

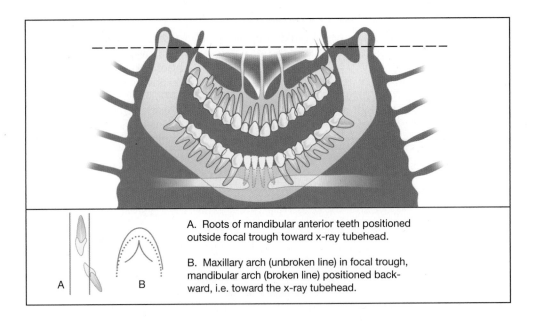

A. Anterior teeth outside focal trough.

B. Dental arches (unbroken line) positioned backward in relation to focal trough (dotted line).

FIGURE 23-12 Panoramic film of patient positioned too far back.

A. Roots of mandibular anterior teeth positioned outside focal trough toward x-ray tubehead.

B. Maxillary arch (unbroken line) in focal trough, mandibular arch (broken line) positioned backward, i.e. toward the x-ray tubehead.

FIGURE 23-13 Panoramic film of patient's head tilted downward. Frankfort plane adjustment needed.

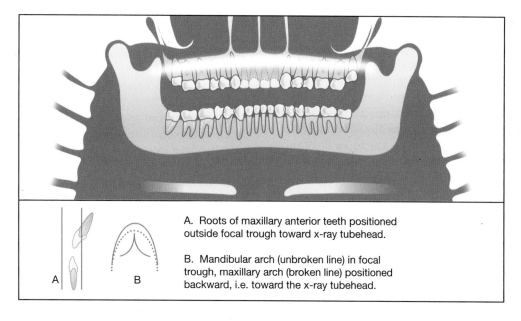

A. Roots of maxillary anterior teeth positioned outside focal trough toward x-ray tubehead.

B. Mandibular arch (unbroken line) in focal trough, maxillary arch (broken line) positioned backward, i.e. toward the x-ray tubehead.

FIGURE 23-14 Panoramic film of patient's head tilted upward. Frankfort plane adjustment needed.

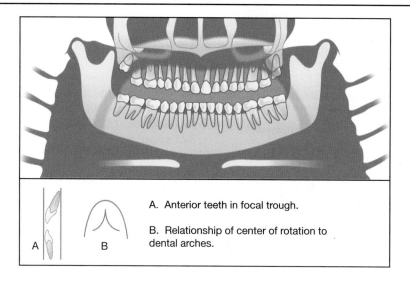

A. Anterior teeth in focal trough.

B. Relationship of center of rotation to dental arches.

FIGURE 23-15 Panoramic film of patient's tongue not against the roof of the mouth.

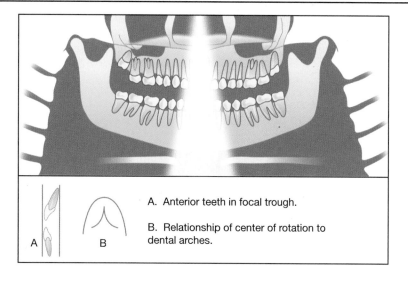

A. Anterior teeth in focal trough.

B. Relationship of center of rotation to dental arches.

FIGURE 23-16 Panoramic film of patient not standing up straight. Midsagittal plane error.

Cephalometric Radiographs

Cephalometric radiographs (*cephalo* means head and *metric* means measurement) are used to assess the patient's skeletal structure and profile (Figures 23-17 and 23-18). The cephalometric radiographs are used mainly by orthodontists in treatment planning for their patients, but some oral maxillofacial surgeons and general practitioners include these radiographs for patient assessment. The patient's bony structure as well as soft tissues are recorded on the cephalo-metric radiograph. Lateral (side) or posterior anterior (back to front) views are used for orthodontic measurements, examination of the sinuses, implant evaluation, and TMJ assessment. A cephalometric unit is a way to ensure that the patient is accurately positioned in a manner that can be duplicated as the patient grows and as repeated radiographs are needed for comparison. The unit consists of a cephalostat, or head-holding device; a cassette holder for an 8 × 10-inch cassette; and an x-ray tubehead.

For lateral views, position the patient by placing the left side of his or her head against the cassette, positioned so the midsagittal plane is parallel to the cassette. The Frankfort plane, or line from the **tragus of the ear** to the floor of the orbit, of the patient is parallel to the floor. The x-ray beam is directed perpendicular to the cassette.

For posterior anterior radiograph views, the patient faces the cassette with the Frankfort plane parallel to the floor and the x-ray beam directed at the occipital bone and perpendicular to the cassette (Figure 23-19A and B).

Lateral Jaw Radiograph. The **lateral jaw radiograph** can be used if the dental office does not have a panoramic x-ray machine. Large areas of the jaw can be radiographed by using a 5 × 7- or an 8 × 10-inch film cassette and having the seated patient hold the cassette next to his or her face and resting on his or her shoulder. The x-ray tubehead is positioned on the opposite side and directed so that the central ray is perpendicular to the patient's head and the cassette. The x-ray exposure time is increased because of the layers of tissue and bone. The patient's head is positioned differently depending on the area the dentist needs to view.

Transcranial Temporomandibular Joint Radiograph. The **transcranial temporomandibular joint radiograph** is taken with the patient holding a cassette against the side of the head and the cone/central x-ray positioned on the opposite side of the patient's head, slightly above and behind the external auditory meatus. Positioning devices assist in correctly aligning the head for the x-ray (Figures 23-20 and 23-21). The radiograph can be taken with the patient's mouth open or closed.

Radiographic Interpretation

Being familiar with the terminology used in radiographic interpretation will make the dental assistant better prepared to perform radiograph procedures (Table 23-2).

Learning landmarks makes radiographic interpretation much easier and more meaningful. The following structures are defined and identified on radiographs and/or in diagrams, showing both normal and abnormal landmarks. The dental assistant interprets radiographs to prepare for the dentist and the procedure.

FIGURE 23-17 Patient positioned for a lateral cephalometric radiograph.

FIGURE 23-18 A lateral cephalometric radiograph.

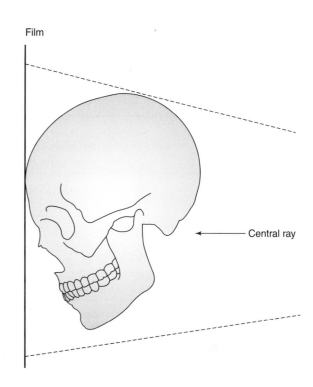

FIGURE 23-19 (A) Posterior anterior radiograph. (B) Line drawing of a posterior anterior radiograph, labeled.

FIGURE 23-20 Patient positioned for a transcranial lateral position TMJ radiograph with the mouth closed.

The terms begin with the tooth and the surrounding tissues, and then cover the maxilla and the mandible. Periapical, occlusal, and panoramic radiographs are used to show each term, but the landmark may be seen on more than one type of radiograph.

Tooth and Surrounding Tissues

Enamel: Radiopaque area on the crown of the teeth.

Dentin: Area just inferior to the enamel; it is less radiopaque than enamel.

FIGURE 23-21 Transcranial TMJ radiograph with the mouth closed, showing the relationship of the condyle to the glenoid fossa.

Cementum: Radiopaque like dentin; look for the thin covering on the root(s).

Pulp chamber: Radiolucent area surrounded by dentin. The pulp horns can be seen; these projections usually

TABLE 23-2   Terminology Used in Radiographic Interpretation

Terminology	Explanation
Anatomical landmarks	Anatomical areas that assist in identification for mounting x-rays and communicating with the dentist and the patient. (The dental assistant does not diagnose x-rays, but can interpret x-ray images and recognize what is normal and what is abnormal.)
Radiopaque	Structures that are dense and do not allow rays to pass through them. The x-rays are blocked or absorbed to varying degrees depending on the density of the structure. The structures show up in light gray to white shades on the x-ray, depending on the density.
Radiolucent	Show up on x-rays in shades of dark gray to black. The structure is not dense; x-rays penetrate in varying degrees.
Diagnosis	To know; the art or act of identifying disease.
Interpretation	To explain the meaning of something.
Superimposition	One structure lying over another.

Note: Radiopaque and radiolucent are comparative terms. They are used to compare one structure or substance to another.

correspond with the cusps of the tooth, as seen on the x-ray.

Pulp canals or root canals: Radiolucent areas in the root, which extend from the pulp chamber to the apex of the tooth.

Periodontal ligament/space: Radiolucent area that surrounds the root(s) of the tooth.

Lamina dura: Radiopaque line of cortical bone that surrounds the root(s) of the tooth and the periodontal ligament.

Cortical plate: Dense compact bone that forms the tooth socket.

Interradicular bone: Alveolar bone found between the roots of a tooth; it shows radiopaque on the x-ray.

Interdental bone: Alveolar bone found between two teeth; it shows radiopaque (Figure 23-22).

Mandibular Landmarks (Figure 23-23)

Mental foramen: A radiolucent area between the roots of the premolar.

Mandibular canal: Canal is radiolucent, but outlined by radiopaque lines that extend from the mandibular foramen to the mental foramen.

External oblique ridge: Ridge on the external surface of the mandible extending from the middle of the rami to beyond the molar area. This ridge runs in an oblique line but curves more to the middle third of the molars than the internal oblique ridge.

Trabecular patterns: Spongy/cancellous bone that surrounds the teeth and forms the mandible. The spongy bone pattern is shown as radiopaque with radiolucent spaces.

FIGURE 23-22 X-rays identifying the parts of a tooth and surrounding structures; (d) Dentin. (c) Cementum. (e) Enamel. (p) Pulp canal. (pch) Pulp chamber. (DEJ) Dentinoenamel junction. (pl) Periodontal ligament (black line). (ld) Lamina dura (white area of cortical bone). (irb) Interradicular bone. (idb) Interdental bone.

Alveolar crest: Compact edge of the cortical bone that shows as radiopaque between the teeth.

Mandibular retromolar area: Area behind the last mandibular molar; it shows varying tissues in this triangular space.

Lingual foramen: Radiolucent area on the lingual surface of the mandible at the midline/symphysis.

Genial tubercle: Raised areas of bone that surround the lingual foramen.

Internal oblique ridge: Ridge of bone on the mylohyoid ridge internal surface of the mandible that runs from the middle of the rami to the third molar region. Sometimes

FIGURE 23-23 (A) Panoramic radiograph identifying mandibular landmarks. (mf) Mental foramen. (mc) Mandibular canal. (eor) External oblique ridge. (ac) Alveolar crest. (c) Condyle. (cor) Coronoid. (bom) Border of mandible. (s) Symphysis. (mrp) mandibular retromandibular pad. (msn) medial sigmoid notch. (B) X-ray showing lingual landmarks of the mandible. (lf) Lingual foramen. (gt) Genial tubercles. *(Courtesy of Dr. Rodney Braun and Dr. Chris Chaffin.)*

it continues past the molars up to the cuspid area; this extension is known as the mylohyoid ridge and shows superimposed over the root area.

Mandibular foramen: Radiolucent area in the middle of the ramus of the mandible on the interior surface.

Condyle: Back projection on the top of the ramus; it shows radiopaque and is articulated in the glenoid fossa.

Coronoid process: Front projection of the tip of the ramus; it shows radiopaque.

Medial sigmoid notch: Indented area between the condyle and coronoid processes on the ramus; also known as the coronoid notch or the mandibular notch.

Ramus: Section of each side of the mandible that runs vertically.

Body of mandible: Section of the mandible that runs horizontally.

Border of the mandible: Lower edge of the body of the mandible that is made of compact bone.

Symphysis: "Chin" area, or anterior portion of the mandible.

Hyoid bone: "U"-shaped bone suspended by ligaments below the mandible but anterior to the larynx; it is occasionally seen on dental x-rays.

Nutrient canals: The radiolucent paths that extend toward the alveolar crest.

Maxillary Landmarks (Figure 23-24)

Hard palate: Radiopaque structure that forms the roof of the mouth.

Incisive foramen: Radiolucent area at the midline of the palate behind the central incisors.

Maxillary suture: Also known as median palatine suture, a radiolucent line that joins the right and left halves of the maxillary bone and palatine bones.

Zygomatic process: Process on the external surface, which begins around the first molar region.

Malar: Part of the zygomatic bone that forms the cheek.

Nasal septum: Radiopaque line that divides the nasal fossae.

Nasal cavities: Two side-by-side openings of the nose.

Nasal conchae: Bony, scroll-shaped plates in the lateral walls of the nasal cavity.

Maxillary sinuses: Left and right cavities above apices of the teeth, which can extend from the canines to the molar area.

Infraorbital foramen: Radiolucent area below the inferior border of the orbit (eye socket).

Orbit: Bone that circles the eyeball.

FIGURE 23-24 Panoramic and periapical radiograph identifying the maxillary landmarks. (EAM) external auditory meatus. (gf) Glenoid fossa. (HP) Hard Palate. (I.F) Incisive foramen. (M) mastoid process. (MS) Maxillary Sinus. (MT) Maxillary tuberosity. (NC) Nasal Conchae. (nf) nasal fossa. (NS) Nasal Septum. (O) Orbit. (zp) zygomatic process. (*Courtesy of Dr. Rodney Braun and Dr. Chris Chaffin.*)

Maxillary tuberosity: Radiopaque area behind the most posterior molar on the maxilla.

Glenoid fossa: Depression on the lower border of the temporal bone where the condyloid process of the mandible articulates as the temporomandibular joint.

Mastoid process: Process of the temporal bone that lies in the lower anterior section just behind the ear (auditory canal).

External auditory meatus: Radiolucent area in the temporal bone for the auditory canal.

Hamular process: Slender projection of bone that lies behind/posterior and medial to the maxillary tuberosity.

Styloid process: Projection of bone, larger than the hamular process, which comes from the temporal bone and lies behind the glenoid fossa.

Conditions or Artifacts on X-rays. Conditions or artifacts that may appear on x-rays (Figure 23-25):

- Dental caries
- Implants
- Impacted tooth
- Recently extracted tooth
- Root canal with reamer
- Periodontal pocket
- Fracture
- Mixed dentition
- Abrasion
- Drifting
- Supernumerary tooth
- Horizontal bone loss
- Orthodontic bands
- Overhang
- Calculus
- Attrition
- Abscesses
- Cysts
- Vertical bone loss
- Eyeglasses
- Amalgam shavings
- Vertebra
- Metallic restoration
- Bridge
- Earrings
- Edentulous patient
- Cement base/lining
- Root canal restoration
- Pins/posts
- Cervical burnout
- BB's or shrapnel
- Framework from reconstructive jaw surgery

Imaging Systems/ Digital Imaging Systems

Imaging systems are used frequently by dental professionals. The systems most commonly used are **computed tomography (CT scanning)** and **magnetic resonance imaging (MRI)**. These imaging systems are found in hospitals or specialized clinics.

Advances also are being made in **digital imaging technology**. These computerized systems are the future in dental radiology and will be in every dental office. Dental assistants continually need to be up-to-date concerning these systems as they are integrated into the dental office.

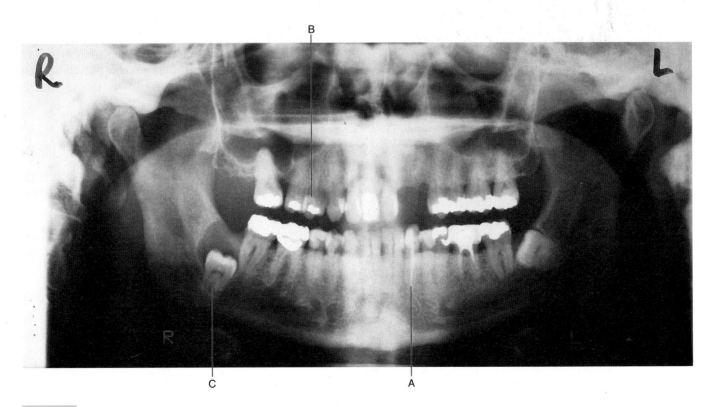

FIGURE 23-25 Panoramic radiograph showing artifacts that may appear, such as (A) root canal, (B) caries, and (C) impacted tooth. (*Courtesy of Dr. Rodney Braun and Dr. Chris Chaffin.*)

Computed Tomography (CT Scanning)

CT scanning is used to plan implant surgery and to locate and define lesions associated with the oral cavity. Computed tomography has eliminated the use of x-ray film but still uses ionizing radiation as the source of energy. Patients are placed in a CT unit, where the radiation and image detector rotate around them. The information is transmitted to a computer, which calculates an image and displays it on a monitor. The image can be transferred to a film for later study. The computer is able to produce images in all dimensions or planes, although the original image is taken in one plane, the axial plane. This is where the original CAT scan (computed axial tomography) came from. CT scanning is the accepted term for computed tomography (Figure 23-26).

Magnetic Resonance Imaging

MRI techniques are used mainly in diagnoses of temporomandibular joint (TMJ) disease. They enable the dentist and radiologist to view the soft tissues of the TMJ with very little risk to the patient. These techniques use low-energy electromagnetic radiation instead of ionizing radiation. The patient is placed in a unit that contains powerful primary and secondary coils. The primary coils produce the magnetic field, while the secondary coils maintain the magnetic field and alter the primary magnetic field to receive information from different planes of the body. The secondary coils also transmit and receive radio frequency pulses or magnetic signals.

Digital Radiography in the Dental Office

Digital intraoral imaging is one of many recent changes in dentistry. Digital radiography is expected to eventually replace all conventional film exposure. Digital radiology is a computerized system that allows the dentist to take an intraoral or extraoral radiograph, and then display the image on a computer screen without exposing and processing dental film (Figure 23-27). Table 23-3 provides definitions of terminology related to digital radiography.

Fundamental Concepts of Digital Radiography

Digital radiography breaks the radiographic image into electronic pieces and then displays them on the computer. The image can be digitized, enhanced, printed, stored, or sent to another office by fax or modem. In digital radiography systems, the term *image* is used to describe the picture produced instead of "radiograph" or "x-ray" film. Digital radiography is not limited to intraoral images; extraoral images such as panoramic and cephalometric images can be taken with some digital imaging systems.

In the traditional system, when the x-rays strike the film the information is recorded on the film. This is known as an analog image. Analog images depict a continuous spectrum of gray shades between black and white. The analog image is a smooth transition from one color/shade to another. In digital imaging, the sensor receives the analog information and converts it to a digital image in the computer. The digital image is like a mosaic, comprised of many small pieces known as pixels. Pixel is short for "picture elements"; each pixel is a small dot in a digital image. The more pixels,

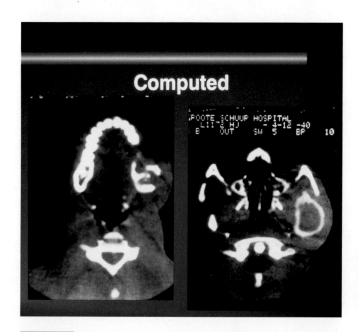

FIGURE 23-26 CT scan of the skull in the coronal plane. *(Courtesy of Dr. Kenji Higuchi.)*

FIGURE 23-27 Intraoral digitizing unit. *(Courtesy of Gendex Dentsply International.)*

TABLE 23-3 Digital Radiology Terminology

Term	Definition
Analog image	An image produced by traditional film, in which there is a continuous spectrum of gray shades between black and white.
Charge-coupled device (CCD)	Solid-state detector used in many common electronic devices such as video cameras, fax machines, and surgical microscopes. In digital radiography, the CCD is the image receptor in the intraoral sensor. This receptor converts x-rays into electrical charges, the intensity of which is related to a color (gray scale).
Digital radiography	Filmless imaging system that uses a sensor and computer to capture an image and convert it into pixels (electronic data). This image is enhanced, presented, and then stored as part of the patient's record.
Digital subtraction	This feature allows images taken at different times to be compared. The images are electronically merged with images that did not change, thereby canceling each other out. The images that did change will stand out. Another feature of digital subtraction is the ability to reverse the gray scale of the image; the *radiolucent* images (normally black) now are white and the *radiopaque* images (normally white) are now black.
Digitize	Conversion of an x-ray film image into a digital image that can be processed by the computer.
Direct digital imaging	A technique of exposing an intraoral sensor to radiation to obtain a digital radiographic image that can be viewed on a computer. This method uses an intraoral sensor, x-ray machine, computer monitor, and computer software program.
Gray scale	Shades of gray visible in an image.
Indirect digital imaging	Technique of exposing an intraoral sensor to radiation, scanning the x-ray image on the sensor, and converting the image to a digital format (i.e., electronic file). This method uses an intraoral sensor, x-ray machine, scanner, computer monitor, and computer software program.
Pixel	Derived from the plural of *picture* (pix) and the word *element* (el). Discrete units of information that comprise an image.
Sensor	Small electronic or specially coated plate that is sensitive to x-rays. When placed intraorally and exposed to radiation, the sensor captures the radiographic image.
Storage phosphor imaging	Indirect digital imaging method of obtaining a digital image. The image is recorded on a special phosphor-coated plate, and then placed in an electron scanner. A laser scans the plate and produces an image on the computer monitor.

the higher the resolution and the sharper the image. Each pixel has a distinct shade of gray, black, or white. The **gray scale** of the image is important for diagnosing the condition of the teeth, tissues, and surrounding bone. The dentist relies on the contrast—**radiolucency** and **radiopacity**—to determine the presence of disease. The computer monitor can display over two hundred shades of gray, but the human eye can only detect around 32 shades of gray. However, computer software is used to enhance gray shades to improve detailing and comparison.

A sensor or image detector takes the place of traditional x-ray film (Figure 23-28). This sensor is an electronic or specially coated plate that is positioned in the mouth and then exposed to x-rays. When the x-ray beam contacts the sensor, an electronic charge is produced on the surface of the sensor. This electronic form/signal is digitized, or converted into data that can be read and stored by the computer. Depending on the type of imaging system, the sensor may connect directly to the computer through a fiber optic cable or the sensor may be wireless.

Types of Digital Imaging

Currently there are direct and indirect methods of obtaining a digital image.

FIGURE 23-28 Top Left: Barrier. Bottom Left: Imaging plate. Right: Direct digital radiography sensor.

Direct Digital Imaging. Direct digital imaging systems include the following components: x-ray machine, sensor, and computer monitor and computer software (Figure 23-29). The sensor is placed in the patient's mouth and exposed to x-rays. The image is produced on the surface of the sensor, digitized, and then transmitted to the computer. Almost immediately, the image appears on the monitor. Software is then used to enhance the image and store the image as part of the patient's records.

Indirect Digital Imaging. Indirect digital imaging systems convert traditional film x-rays to digital images, which are then viewed and stored in the computer. The following components are necessary for indirect digital imaging: a scanner/CCD (charge-coupled device) camera and a computer and computer software. With this technique, an existing x-ray film can be digitized using the scanner. The scanner digitizes the image and then displays it on the computer monitor (Figure 23-30). Indirect digital imaging is not used as much in dentistry because the quality of the image is inferior to a direct digital image. However, this technique does offer a means to digitize existing x-rays.

Storage phosphor imaging, another type of indirect digital imaging, is a wireless system that uses specially coated plates instead of sensors to record the image. These plates are coated with phosphors and resemble an intensifying screen used to expose extraoral film in the way they convert x-rays into light, and must be cleared between uses by exposing them to viewbox light for several minutes. Once the image is erased, the plates are sterilized for use again.

The plates are covered with a barrier and then placed in the mouth. They are flexible and fit into the mouth much like intraoral film. Unlike the direct digital imaging sensors, there is no cable attached. Once the plate is exposed to x-rays, it is placed in a high-speed laser scanner to convert the information into electronic files. The scanner is an electronic processor, and produces

▌**Easy positioning and high definition imaging**

VisualiX eHD is a unique system developed to optimize positioning of the intraoral sensor in the oral cavity.

Due to its special drop-like shape, its smooth edges and round corners, the VisualiX eHD follows the anatomical shape of the oral cavity, simplifying sensor positioning and maximizing patient comfort.

VisualiX eHD also provides superior digital image quality due to the "High Definition" imaging technology developed by Gendex. The eHD technology optimizes the efficiency of the image capture process and provides excellent definition of the various anatomical details.

FIGURE 23-29 Direct digital imaging system *(Courtesy of Gendex Dentsply International)*.

an image that is transmitted to a computer monitor. Because of this extra step, which ranges from seconds to minutes, this type of digital radiography is more time consuming than direct digital imaging.

Digital Radiography Equipment

Equipment needed for digital imaging includes dental x-ray machine, sensor or image detector, and a computer and digital imaging software.

X-ray Machine. A conventional x-ray machine is used with digital radiography. The x-ray machine should be capable of producing 70 kV or less, and 5mA or less milliamperage. The timer must be adapted to allow exposure in a time frame of 1/100 of a second.

Sensor (Image Detector). As previously stated, the sensor is a small detector that takes the place of traditional x-ray film. It is placed in the patient's mouth and used to capture the image. Sensors are electronic or specially coated plates that are the same size as 0, 1, 2, and 4 x-ray film. Some of the sensors are thick, bulky, and rigid,

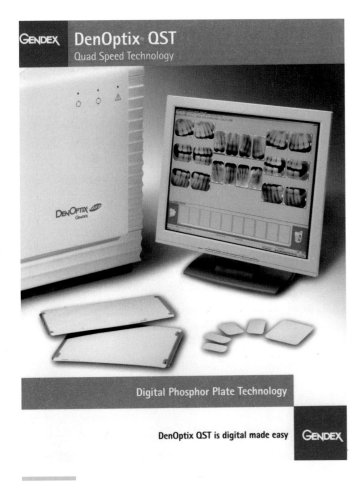

FIGURE 23-30 Indirect digital imaging sensors *(Courtesy of Gendex Dentsply International).*

while others are thin and flexible. The edges are sometimes too sharp to be very comfortable in the patient's mouth, but improvements are continually being made. The sensors are covered with barriers before being placed in a patient's mouth and some can withstand cold sterilization.

Intraoral sensors used in digital imaging may be *wired* or *wireless*. Wired sensors are attached to a fiber optic cable connected to a computer. The computer then records the signals sent as the sensor converts the x-rays into the electronic form. The cable varies in length from 8 to 35 ft (1.5 to 10.7 m); the shorter the cable the more limited the range of motion. Wireless sensors are not connected directly to the computer. They must be placed in a scanner after exposure for the information to be converted and then sent to the computer.

Charge-Coupled Device. The **charge-coupled device (CCD)** is one of the most common image receptors used in dental digital radiography. Developed in the 1960s, the CCD is used in many devices, such as fax machines, home video cameras, microscopes, and telescopes. The CCD is a solid-state detector comprised of a grid of small transistor elements that convert x-rays to electrons. The electrons produced by the x-ray are

deposited in a small box or "well" known as a pixel. A pixel is the digital equivalent of a silver halide crystal used in traditional radiology. The arrangement of the silver halide crystals is random unlike the pixels in digital radiography, which are structured in an ordered arrangement. The CCD is 640×480 individual pixels in size.

Once the elements are exposed to x-rays, they are read and the electron charges are converted to form the digital image.

Computer and Computer Software. The computer digitizes, processes, and stores information received from the sensor or scanner. Some requirements for this computer are adequate memory for rapid converting and storage of digital radiographs while simultaneously generating high-resolution images shown on a monitor. The computer must be conveniently located for easy viewing by the dentist and the patient, connected to a printer to generate hard copy as needed, and linked to the Internet for electronic transfer of patients' images to insurance companies, other dentists, or dental specialists.

Software is provided by manufacturers of digital imaging systems. They offer a variety of features to enhance the images for better detection and for improved patient understanding.

Advantages and Disadvantages of Digital Radiography

Although digital radiography is continually advancing, there are advantages and disadvantages to this technology.

Advantages

- Less exposure to radiation for the patient. Sensors are more sensitive and require less radiation, falling to 50% when using F-speed films.

- Results appear on the computer monitor almost immediately after exposure to x-rays. The dentist then can enhance, contrast, zoom, take exact measurements, make notes about the image, and alter color and brightness/contrast of the image right at chairside to better evaluate the patient's condition.

- Patients can view images when the dentist is discussing areas of concern.

- Because digital images are stored on computer media, much less space is required for storage.

- The darkroom, processing equipment, and solutions are eliminated, thereby eliminating maintenance of that equipment and the need to deal with storage of used chemicals.

- Digital images are quickly and easily sent via email attachment to other dental offices, insurance companies, patients, and so on. Thus, processing of insurance claims (for example) is faster.

PROCEDURE 23-2

Digital Radiology Techniques

This procedure serves as general guidelines when using digital radiology. Manufacturers of digital radiography systems provide detailed instructions on preparation of the equipment and the patient, taking the exposure, and using the software.

PREPARATION OF EQUIPMENT

1. Turn on the computer and load software to select the type of radiography to be exposed.

2. Enter the patient's identification information and the date.

3. Select a sensor that has been disinfected/sterilized, and then prepare by placing an approved barrier over the sensor (Figure 23-31).

4. Place the sensor in an appropriate x-ray film holder (Figure 23-32).

5. Prepare the x-ray machine and adjust settings. For most digital systems, the exposure settings are half those used for F-speed x-ray film exposures. (For suggestions on exposure settings, always follow the manufacturer's instructions.)

PREPARATION OF PATIENT

Patient preparation is virtually the same as for traditional radiograph exposure.

1. Seat the patient and have him or her sit so that the midsagittal plane is perpendicular to the floor.

2. Adjust the chair to a comfortable level.

3. Adjust the headrest to position the patient's head so that the occlusal plane is parallel to the floor.

FIGURE 23-32 Sensor being placed in the Rinn x-ray film holder.

FIGURE 23-31 Sensor that has been prepared with a barrier prior to placement in the patient's mouth.

(continues)

PROCEDURE 23-2 *(CONTINUED)*

4. Place the lead apron with thyroid collar on the patient.

5. Request that the patient remove eyeglasses and all objects from the mouth that might interfere with the procedure.

6. Quickly inspect the oral cavity for anything that may require alteration of sensor placement, such as tori or a shallow palate.

TAKING THE EXPOSURE

1. Place the sensor in the patient's mouth (Figure 23-33), and carefully move into position for exposure.

2. Align the x-ray cone and PID to direct the central rays, using the same technique for x-ray film exposure.

3. Using the keyboard or mouse, activate the sensor to exposure.

4. Press the exposure button to expose the sensor.

DIRECT DIGITAL IMAGING SYSTEM

1. Wait until the image appears on the monitor and evaluate it. If the image is what the dentist needs for a quality diagnosis, continue on with the next image to be exposed. If a positioning error has occurred, do not remove the sensor from the patient's mouth; determine what caused the error and correct the sensor position or realign the PID. (Note: Even though the amount of radiation that the patient is exposed to is reduced, retakes should be limited just as they are when taking traditional radiographs.)

2. When the image is satisfactory, remove the sensor or reposition it for additional exposures. Repeat until all exposures are acquired.

INDIRECT DIGITAL IMAGING SYSTEM

1. Remove the imaging plate from the patient's mouth.

2. Remove the imaging plate from the film holder and remove the plastic barrier.

3. Place the imaging plate in a dark container until all exposures have been taken.

4. After all exposures are complete, in a semi-dark room place the imaging plates on the scanner and activate.

FIGURE 23-33 Sensor being placed in the patient's mouth for correct alignment.

5. The images will begin to appear on the monitor. Evaluate the images according to requirements for quality diagnostic images. Retake any images that do not meet the dentist's needs by using the same technique listed above, but also including erasing the image from the plates and disinfecting them according to the manufacturer's instructions. Then replace the barrier and retake the exposure (Figure 23-34).

AFTER EXPOSURE

1. Save the patient's images and back up the file on the computer or a supplemental storage system.

(continues)

PROCEDURE 23-2 *(CONTINUED)*

The DenOptix Imaging Cycle

2. Load intraoral, panoramic or cephalometric imaging plates

1. Erase imaging plates for reuse

3. Take x-ray – intraoral, panoramic or ceph

5. Place in scanner and scan images

4. Mount intraoral, pan or ceph imaging plates in carousel

01:26

FIGURE 23-34 Indirect digital imaging cycle. *(Courtesy of Gendex Dentsply International.)*

Disadvantages

- The main disadvantage of digital imaging is the initial expense of the equipment and software. Prices vary according to manufacturer and system quality.

- Extra time is required to become proficient in using the digital imaging hardware and software. Correctly positioning the sensor/imaging plate is still a prerequisite for a detailed, quality radiograph. Positioning technique errors are similar to traditional x-ray exposures.

- There is a learning curve for dentists in reading and diagnosing from digital radiography, as the approach is different from that used in traditional radiography.

- Sensors are usually thicker than x-ray film packets. Placement is often uncomfortable for the patient, and sometimes causes the patient to gag. However, sensor design is improving, and these problems will sooner or later be eliminated.

- There are concerns about rapid and costly updating, computer viruses, and system failures.

- Infection control is a concern with digital radiography. The sensors are covered with barriers that can tear and are not always totally aseptic. The keyboard and mouse must also be covered and the covers changed with each patient. Some manufacturers suggest an intermediate-level disinfectant applied with gauze pads for cleaning and disinfecting the sensor, keyboard, and mouse as needed.

CHAPTER SUMMARY

Manufacturers, dental team members, and patients are responsible for following safety precaution measures when using radiography equipment. Steps must be used to minimize risk to the patient and all dental personnel.

The dentist is responsible for having dental assistants properly credentialed and trained to expose and process radiographs. The dentist is also responsible for supervising dental assistants in these tasks. In 1981, the Consumer Patient Radiation Health and Safety Act was enacted. This federal law requires each state to inform the Secretary of Health and Human Services how compliance with the act is accomplished.

Dental assistants must be trained in aseptic techniques, radiation hygiene, and maintenance of quality assurance and safety, and must obtain proper education in exposure and processing techniques. They must understand the physics and biological effects of ionizing radiation, utilize their understanding during every radiographic exposure, understand the ALARA principle, and use the lead apron with cervical collar for the patient's safety every time an x-ray is taken. The assistant must label and store patient x-rays properly to prevent loss and thereby avoid the need for x-rays being retaken.

Case Study

Dr. Danton is considering changing the way his office takes radiographs. His patients have been asking about reducing radiation exposure during x-rays. Dr. Danton has been practicing for about ten years and is comfortable with traditional x-ray film exposures for both intraoral and extraoral radiographs, but he also wants to keep up with technology and current trends in dentistry.

Case Study Review

1. Describe alternatives to traditional x-ray film exposures that Dr. Danton can explore.

2. Enumerate advantages and disadvantages of digital technology.

3. What factors must be considered by the dental team that decides to use a digital radiography system?

REVIEW QUESTIONS

Multiple Choice

1. Which of the following is considered extraoral film?
   a. Panoramic radiograph
   b. Occlusal radiograph
   c. Cephalometric radiograph
   d. Both A and C

2. A cassette is used to
   a. hold the film for extraoral radiographic exposures.
   b. act as a lining.
   c. intensify the x-rays.
   d. hold films during processing.

3. The _____ is the type of extraoral film primarily used by orthodontists.
   a. panoramic radiograph
   b. occlusal radiograph
   c. cephalometric radiograph
   d. lateral jaw radiograph

4. All of the following are true statements about panoramic exposure techniques *except*:
   a. Remove bulky sweaters, coats, and hair clips that may interfere with the rotation of the x-ray tubehead.
   b. The patient should always wear a lead apron without a thyroid collar.
   c. The film is placed in the patient's mouth and the patient gently closes on the film.
   d. The patient is positioned in the chin rest, biting on a bite-block, with the head properly positioned for the film exposure.

5. Dental assistants are allowed to diagnose dental disease by interpreting x-rays.
   a. True
   b. False

6. Which of the following quality assurance tests evaluates the darkroom for possible light leaks?
   a. Manufactured step wedge
   b. Placing a coin on unexposed film
   c. Spin top
   d. Dosimeter

7. How often should the quality assurance test be run?
   a. Daily
   b. Weekly
   c. Monthly
   d. Yearly

8. Which of the following radiology techniques is used mainly for diagnosis of temporomandibular joint disease?
   a. Computer tomography
   b. Magnetic resonance imaging
   c. Digital imaging
   d. None of the above

9. _____ allows the dentist and/or dental staff to take x-rays and then display the image on a computer monitor.
   a. Computer tomography
   b. Magnetic resonance imaging
   c. Digital imaging
   d. CT scanning

10. Both intraoral and extraoral radiographs can be taken with digital imaging.
    a. True
    b. False

Critical Thinking

1. The patient appears to have a fractured mandible. The dentist requests an x-ray. What type of x-ray would be the most beneficial for diagnosing a fractured mandible? Would the dental assistant be able to obtain this x-ray clinically?

2. Name the types of radiographs in which all of the following can be seen: alveolar crest, coronoid process, maxillary retromolar pad, and the mental foramen.

3. List some conditions or artifacts that may be misinterpreted.

Web Activities

1. At http://www.gendexxray.com, identify measures of satisfaction when using digital radiography equipment. Go to DenOptix, and then customer profile/satisfaction.

2. To study questions that patients frequently ask about dental x-rays, go to http://www.ada.org, go to Oral Health Topics A-Z, look under "X" for X-rays and then go to Additional Resources information on Digital Radiology

3. Check http://www.Kodak.com under dental products and look up the different types of film available for the panoramic and cephlometric exposures.

SECTION VII

DENTAL SPECIALTIES

ENDODONTICS

SPECIFIC INSTRUCTIONAL OBJECTIVES

The student should strive to meet the following objectives and demonstrate an understanding of the facts and principles presented in this chapter:

1. Define endodontics and describe what an endodontist does.

2. Describe pulpal and periapical disease.

3. Identify diagnostic procedures.

4. Identify instruments used in endodontic procedures and describe their functions.

5. Identify materials used in endodontics and describe their functions.

6. Describe endodontic procedures and responsibilities of the dental assistant.

7. Describe endodontic retreatment.

8. Explain surgical endodontic procedures and the instruments used.

KEY TERMS

abscess *(506)*

apex finder *(515)*

apexification *(524)*

apexogenesis *(524)*

apical periodontitis *(505)*

apicoectomy *(521)*

barbed broaches *(510)*

cellulitis *(506)*

chelating *(515)*

electronic pulp tester *(508)*

endodontic handpiece *(515)*

endodontics *(505)*

extirpate *(510)*

exudate *(505)*

files *(510)*

fistula *(506)*

flex files *(510)*

Glick #1 *(513)*

gutta percha *(507)*

heating unit *(515)*

Hedström files *(510)*

hemisection *(524)*

intracanal instruments *(510)*

irreversible pulpitis *(505)*

K-type files *(510)*

master cone *(520)*

nonvital pulp *(505)*

obturating *(513)*

osteomyelitis *(506)*

percussion *(507)*

periapical abscess *(506)*

pluggers *(513)*

pulpal necrosis *(505)*

pulpectomy *(521)*

pulpotomy *(521)*

reamers *(510)*

retrograde filling *(523)*

reversible pulpitis *(505)*

root amputation *(524)*

root canal sealer *(512)*

rubber stops *(512)*

selective anesthesia *(508)*

sodium hypochlorite *(515)*

spreaders *(513)*

transillumination test *(508)*

ultrasonic unit *(516)*

vital pulp *(505)*

vitality scanner *(508)*

INTRODUCTION

Endodontics comprises diagnosis and treatment of diseases of the pulp and periapical tissues. Endodontic procedures include diagnosis, root canal treatment, and periapical surgery.

The endodontist has advanced education and training in the field of endodontics. General dentists, who can also treat the pulp and periapical tissues, render the same standard of care within their education and experience, but then refer the patient to an endodontist for cases requiring advanced knowledge and training.

The general dentist sends written instructions and radiographs to the endodontist to prevent miscommunication. The endodontist also often communicates with the referring dentist concerning the patient's treatment and prognosis. The patient may return to the general dentist for the final restoration after the endodontic treatment is completed by the endodontist.

Endodontic Team

The staff in the endodontist's office shares responsibilities similar to those of the general dental office staff, except there is an increase in communication with other dental offices because most of the patients are referrals.

The endodontist is assisted by dental assistants who perform traditional assisting responsibilities in addition to expanded duties specific to endodontics as allowed by state dental practice acts.

Progress of Pulpal and Periapical Diseases

The healthy pulp is said to be a vital pulp. When the pulp or periapical tissues are irritated or injured, the result is inflammation. Advanced dental decay is one of the main sources of irritation. Other irritations or injuries include heat, impact trauma, fractures, invasive restorative procedures, and adverse reactions to dental materials. The degree of pulpal inflammation depends on the severity and duration of the irritation or injury and the ability of the tissues to respond. The patient may or may not have symptoms that indicate the degree of the inflammation of the nonvital pulp.

Pulpal Diseases

Pulpal diseases include reversible pulpitis, irreversible pulpitis, and pulpal necrosis.

- **Reversible pulpitis**—The pulp is inflamed but able to heal when the irritant is removed. Causes include incipient caries, enamel fractures, and occlusal attrition. Symptoms include sensitivity to hot and cold. Treatment involves removing the irritant and placing sedative materials to soothe and heal the pulp.

- **Irreversible pulpitis**—The inflammation continues until the pulpal tissue cannot recover. Symptoms include pain to the patient that may be short and sharp or dull and continual. The treatment for irreversible pulpitis is root canal therapy or extraction.

- **Pulpal necrosis**—The death of the pulpal cells often results from irreversible pulpitis. Symptoms and treatment for pulpal necrosis are similar to those for irreversible pulpitis. As the pulp inflammation progresses, exudate (**ECKS**-you-dayt), or pus, and gas form in the pulp chamber. If the tooth is sealed and the exudate cannot escape, pulpal necrosis is rapid. If the exudate drains through caries or exposure to the oral cavity, the process is slowed. A fistula is a tubelike passage that sometimes forms to drain an abscess from the apex of a tooth to the oral cavity. The exudate in the fistula may move from an area of high concentration to an area of low concentration, forming a "gumball" on the tissue.

Periapical Diseases

When the infection in the pulp reaches the apex of the tooth, it continues into the periapical area. The intensities of the inflammation and the host response determine the extent of the infection. Periapical disease includes apical periodontitis and periapical abscess.

- **Apical periodontitis**—Pulpal inflammation extends into the periapical tissues. This acute condition subsides if the irritation is removed. If the process continues and the irritant is not removed, the apical periodontitis becomes a chronic inflammation. A radiograph of the area shows an interruption of the lamina dura and destruction of the periapical tissues (Figure 24-1). The immediate area of chronic apical periodontitis is usually classified as a granuloma or a cyst. A granuloma consists of numerous cells of the inflammatory process. If a granuloma is left untreated and the irritation continues, a cyst forms. A cyst is filled with liquid and semisolid materials and is

FIGURE 24-1 Radiograph of tooth with apical abscess (dark shadow at the apex). *(Courtesy of Clifton O. Caldwell, Jr., DDS, FICD, FACD.)*

FIGURE 24-2 Patient with gingival abscess (red area above tooth #8 near frenum). *(Courtesy of Dr. Gary Shellerud.)*

partially lined with stratified squamous epithelium (**SKWAY**-mus ep-ih-**THEE**-lee-um) and surrounded by connective tissue.

■ **Periapical abscess**—A localized destruction of tissue and accumulation of exudate in the periapical region. The patient's reaction can range from moderate to severe discomfort and/or swelling. The treatment includes releasing the pressure by creating an opening into the pulp chamber, removing the necrotic pulp, and root canal therapy.

Related Terms

■ **Fistula** (**FIS**-tyou-lah)—A path to the external surface, created by the body to drain the **abscess** (Figure 24-2)

■ **Cellulitis** (sell-you-**LYE**-tis)—When the abscess spreads into the facial tissues, causing swelling and discomfort

■ **Osteomyelitis** (oss-tee-oh-my-eh-**LYE**-tis)—An advanced stage of periapical infection that spreads into and through the bone

Endodontic Diagnosis

Endodontic diagnosis includes patient medical and dental history; clinical examination, including pulp testing; and review of communication from the referring dentist about the case. Each office has a routine procedure that is followed carefully to ensure that all pertinent information is gathered.

Medical History

The first step is for the patient to fill out a medical history. Once completed, the history is reviewed and clarified to ensure that accurate and complete information is gathered. The medical history may reveal information that relates to previous treatment of the tooth pulp to be used in diagnosis.

Dental History

The dental history provides the endodontist dental experiences and the signs and symptoms of the current concern. The dental history opens the way for subjective examination (the problem explained in the patient's words). The patient should be allowed to describe the type of pain, sensitivity to heat and cold, duration of the condition, and any other symptoms.

Clinical Examination and Pulp Testing

The clinical examination, or the objective examination, includes evaluation of the extraoral tissues, such as facial asymmetry, swelling, redness, and external fistulas.

During the intraoral examination, the soft tissues are thoroughly evaluated and palpated, while searching for any abnormalities or signs of inflammation. Visual examination of the teeth may reveal caries, discoloration, or fractures, but clinical tests are usually performed to develop a complete diagnosis. Clinical tests are performed by the dentist to correctly diagnose the patient's situation. Selected testing procedures are described below.

Radiographs. Radiographs are often the most useful of the diagnostic tools. Radiographs are taken and processed immediately so that the dentist can refer to them. If the inflammation has extended beyond the apex of the tooth and has bone involvement, a radiolucent area will be apparent. Detailed periapical x-rays with accurate positioning and good contrasting qualities are necessary to view the area around the end of the tooth root.

Palpation. Palpation of the soft tissues is performed by the endodontist. Pressure is applied to the mucosal tissue near the apex of the root of the suspicious tooth. Normally, one or more additional teeth are palpated for comparison. Around the indicated tooth, the area may be soft and raised (pus filled).

Percussion. Percussion is performed by tapping on the occlusal or incisal surface of the tooth. The handle of a mouth mirror is often used (Figure 24-3). The tapping is first done on a control tooth and then on the symptomatic tooth. The control tooth should be the same tooth in the opposite arch. The patient may experience mild to moderate pain if there is periodontal inflammation, sharp pain if there is periapical inflammation.

Mobility. Mobility is evaluated to determine the condition and involvement of the supporting structures of the tooth. Teeth that move two to three millimeters should not have root canal therapy because they lack sufficient support. Mobility is tested by placing the handle of an instrument or a finger on the lingual surface and the handle of another instrument on the facial surface of the tooth and applying pressure (Figure 24-4).

Cold Test. Cold testing is accomplished using dry ice, ethyl chloride (Figure 24-5A), or a piece of ice (ice is the most common and easiest to use). The tooth is isolated and dried, and then the ice (usually the water that is frozen is a sterilized, anesthetic carpule) is applied to the facial surface of the tooth (Figure 24-5B). The ice test is more effective on the anterior teeth than the more insulated posterior teeth. A normal tooth will respond within a few seconds. If the response to the cold is intense and long lasting, irreversible pulpitis is indicated. Teeth with necrotic pulps will not respond to the cold test.

Heat Test. Heat testing uses several heat sources. Examples include a small ball of gutta percha heated by a flame, the heated end of a ball burnisher, or frictional

FIGURE 24-3 Percussion test with instrument handle.

FIGURE 24-4 Mobility test using the ends of two instruments.

(A)

(B)

FIGURE 24-5 (A) Endo Ice used to test the vitality of a tooth. *(Courtesy of Coltene/Whaledent Inc.)* (B) Cold test on patient's tooth with an ice stick.

heat from running a rubber cup on the tooth surface. Heat is applied to the tooth and, if the pain increases and lasts, there is a distinct chance of irreversible pulpitis (Figure 24-6).

> Gutta percha is a thermoplastic material used to fill the canal.

Electric Pulp Testing/Vitality Scanner. Electric pulp testing does not measure the degree of tooth vitality but indicates whether the tooth is vital or nonvital. Like

FIGURE 24-6 Heat test on patient with gutta percha ball.

other pulp tests, the **electronic pulp tester** can produce a false reading (Figure 24-7A). Therefore, other tests should be completed for comparison and thus determination of pulp vitality. Electronic pulp-testing units are usually battery operated and deliver high-frequency currents that can vary. The current creates an electrical stimulus to the tooth.

The **vitality scanner** allows the dentist to scan each tooth in minutes (Figure 24-7B). The scanner indicates endodontic problems in the early stages. The probe on the scanner records a reading and then automatically resets for the next tooth. Procedure 24-1 outlines the steps for electronic pulp testing.

Transillumination Test. The **transillumination test** involves the use of a strong fiberoptic light that transmits light through the crown of the tooth. The light produces shadows that may indicate vertical fractures.

Selective Anesthesia. Sometimes the patient cannot identify which tooth or which arch is causing the problem. In these cases, after talking with the patient and completing the clinical examination, **selective anesthesia** is used. One area of the patient's mouth is selected and an injection is given. If anesthetic in this area alleviates the discomfort, the problematic quadrant has been determined. Usually, selective anesthetic is used on the maxillary teeth beginning in the most suspicious anterior area, and then progressing to the posterior area.

Caries Removal. The removal of dental caries is necessary in some patients to evaluate the pulp condition. If the patient has no symptoms but the radiograph shows deep caries and the tooth responds positively to other tests, caries removal will further determine pulp status. The dentist uses the dental handpiece to remove the decay and to determine whether there is reversible or irreversible pulpitis. Depending on the prognosis for the tooth, the endodontist would place a temporary or permanent restoration.

FIGURE 24-7 (A) Electronic pulp tester. (B) Vitality scanner. *(Courtesy of Analytic Endodontics.)*

PROCEDURE 24-1

Electronic Pulp Testing

EQUIPMENT AND SUPPLIES

- Basic setup: mouth mirror, explorer, and cotton pliers
- Electronic pulp tester
- Conducting medium, such as toothpaste

PROCEDURE STEPS

Follow these steps to electronically test the pulp (test control tooth first):

1. Place a small amount of toothpaste on the tip of the electrode (the toothpaste acts as a conducting medium). Dry the tooth before using the electrode.

2. Ask the patient to signal when he or she notices a sensation, which is usually a tingling or hot feeling.

3. Place the tip on the facial surface of the tooth and gradually increase the power. **Caution:** Do not place the electrode on a metal restoration, a wet surface, gingiva, or artificial crowns.

4. If the patient feels any sensation, some degree of tooth vitality is indicated. If no sensation is felt, the pulp may be necrotic.

Treatment Plan

Once all the information has been gathered and the dentist has made a diagnosis for root canal therapy, the patient is informed of the necessary treatment. The patient must sign a consent form and make appointments and financial arrangements before treatment begins. To minimize anxiety and answer questions about the upcoming procedure, endodontic pamphlets or videos may be provided.

Endodontic Instruments

Procedures performed in endodontic treatments may require the use of specialized instruments. The dental assistant working in an endodontic office should be familiar with the various instruments used for endodontic treatment.

Characteristics of Intracanal Instruments

Endodontic **intracanal instruments** are made of stainless steel and nickel titanium alloy wire. They are flexible, fracture resistant, smooth, able to maintain sharp cutting edges, and corrosion resistant. The wire is twisted and tapered into instruments called files and reamers. To ensure consistency in the sizes and lengths of intracanal instruments, the ADA and manufacturers have standardized a number and color-code system (Figure 24-8). Intracanal instruments have precise diameters and lengths that are consistent from manufacturer to manufacturer. Intracanal instruments range in size from 08 to 140 and in length from 21 to 25 mm.

Barbed Broaches

Barbed broaches are made of fine metal wire with tiny, sharp projections or barbs along the instrument shaft. The barbs are angled to allow a smooth entry but to catch tissue when retracted. Broaches are used to remove soft tissue from the pulp canal (to **extirpate** the canal). The dentist selects a broach that is large enough to remove pulpal tissue but small enough so that it will not bind in the canal.

Barbed broaches are supplied in various diameters, ranging from xxx-fine to coarse. The handles are metal or plastic and are color coded (Figure 24-9).

(A)

(B)

FIGURE 24-9 (A) Barbed broach. *(Courtesy of Sybron Endo.)* (B) Close-up picture of a barbed broach.

Files

Endodontic **files** are used to enlarge and smooth the canal. They are long, tapered, twisted instruments that are moved up and down inside the canal, and are available in various diameters and types. The handles of the endodontic files are color coded according to standardized measurements. For example, a size-15 file is color coded white, and a 20 is yellow.

Standard files are known as **K-type files**. These tightly twisted files are used to scrape and widen the walls of the canal and to remove necrotic tissue. The K-type file is rotated in the canal and then removed from the canal (Figure 24-10A).

Hedström files are manufactured by a different process than the K-type files (Figure 24-10B). They are shaped like pine trees and resemble stacks of cones. The edges of Hedström files are very sharp and cut aggressively. These files are only used in a push-and-pull motion; they are not rotated like K-type files because they will bind in the canal due to their design.

Another group of files is available from many manufacturers: **flex files** (Figure 24-10C). Flex files are made of stainless steel or nickel-titanium and are crafted for an optimal balance of flexibility, strength, and sharpness. Used for curved and narrow canals that require flexibility to negotiate, flex files come in various sizes and in both the 21- and 25-mm lengths.

Reamers

Reamers are used with a "reaming" or twisting motion. They have long, twisted shanks like the files, but their

FIGURE 24-8 K-Flex files showing standardized numbers. *(Courtesy of Sybron Endo.)*

FIGURE 24-11 Close-up view of a reamer.

FIGURE 24-10 (A) K-type file. (B) Hedstrom file. (C) Flex files. *(Courtesy of Sybron Endo.)*

(B)

FIGURE 24-12 (A) Various intracanal instruments in an endodontic organizer for storage and sterilization, and a sponge holder/ring for use at the chair. (B) Another style of intracanal organizer. *(Courtesy of Hu-Friedy Mgf. Co., Inc.)*

blades are spaced much farther apart (Figure 24-11). The cutting action is completed as the reamer is revolved out of the canal. They are color coded and numbered according to size, similar to the files. Reamers are not used as frequently as files.

Rotary Intracanal Instruments. Broaches, files, and reamers are also available for use with an endodontic handpiece; they are called rotary or engine broaches, files, and reamers. These instruments have a notched end that attaches to a slow-speed handpiece that is specially designed for use in endodontic procedures. The rotary intracanal instruments are numbered and color-coded just like manual instruments.

Endodontic Organizers

Various methods are available to store and organize reamers and files. Some storage containers can be sterilized and are designed to hold a range of intracanal instruments. Large organizers often have built-in measuring gauges for setting stops. Finger rings are much smaller, holding only a few instruments at once (Figure 24-12). They come with disposable styrofoam pads.

Rubber Stops

Rubber stops (also called file stops, endo stops, or markers) are placed on reamers and files to mark the length of the root canal (Figure 24-13). These small, circular, silicone disks have prepunched holes in the center for easy application. The length is determined by holding a file with a rubber stop against a radiograph and adjusting the stop to match the incisal or cusp edge. The marked file is then measured on a small millimeter gauge. This number is recorded for reference and for marking other intracanal instruments.

Gates-Glidden Drills

Gates-Glidden drills are used with latch attachments on low-speed handpieces. These drills run in a clockwise direction and are long shanked and elliptically shaped

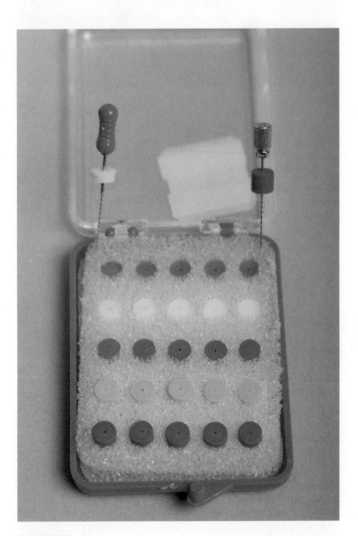

FIGURE 24-13 Examples of rubber stops and how they are positioned on files.

with blunt, football-shaped ends and they are supplied in six sizes, marked near the notch of the shank. For example, a #1 drill has one stripe and a #6 has six stripes. The #1 is equal to a size 50 K-type file, with each consecutive size increasing in diameter (Figure 24-14). Gates-Glidden drills are used in the upper portion of the canal to prepare access to the opening by removing obstructing dentin.

Peeso Reamers

Peeso reamers have parallel cutting sides rather than the elliptical shape of the Gates-Glidden drills (Figure 24-15). They are used with latch attachments on low-speed handpieces. Peeso reamers are supplied in various sizes, beginning at 0.70 mm for #1 and increasing 0.20 mm for every subsequent size, ending at #6. The handles are striped to indicate corresponding size. These instruments are supplied with or without safe tips. Peeso reamers are used to prepare the canal for a post and to reduce the curvature of the canal orifice for straight-line access.

Lentulo Spirals

The Lentulo spiral is a long, twisted, very flexible wire instrument used to spin root canal sealer, or cement, into the canal (Figure 24-16). The spirals are used with low-speed handpieces and latch attachments.

FIGURE 24-14 Gates-Glidden drills. The tip of the drill is elliptically shaped and has a noncutting end. *(Courtesy of Sybron Endo.)*

FIGURE 24-15 Peeso reamer. The blades are long and parallel with noncutting ends. *(Courtesy of Premier Dental Products Company.)*

FIGURE 24-16 Lentulo spiral used to place root canal sealer in the canal.

Endodontic Spoon Excavator

The spoon excavator has a very long shank that allows the instrument to reach into the coronal portion of the tooth. The spoon-ended excavator removes deep caries, pulp tissue, and temporary cement. The double-ended instrument has right and left ends (Figure 24-17A).

Endodontic Explorer

The endodontic explorer is designed to help locate canal orifices (openings). It is a double-ended instrument with long, tapered ends that have sharp points. This stiff-ended explorer is designed specifically for endodontic procedures (Figure 24-17B).

Endodontic Spreaders, Pluggers, and the Glick #1

Spreaders and pluggers (condensers) are instruments used to laterally condense materials when obturating (sealing/filling) the canal. Both these instruments have long, tapered working ends. The spreaders are pointed on the ends, while the pluggers are flat. Both these instruments have instrument metal handles or "finger-type" plastic handles (Figure 24-18). Spreaders are used to adapt the gutta percha into the canal (lateral condensation); pluggers are used to condense the filling material to provide space for additional gutta percha cones (Figure 24-18C).

The Glick #1 instrument is used to remove excess gutta percha from the coronal portion of the canal and to condense the remaining gutta percha in the canal opening (Figure 24-19).

(A)   **(B)**

FIGURE 24-17 (A) An endodontic spoon excavator. (B) An endodontic explorer. *(Courtesy of Hu-Friedy Mfg., Inc.)*

Endodontic Materials

Endodontic materials are substances used in endodontic procedures to dry, fill, or treat the root canal. The dental assistant should be aware of characteristics of the various types of materials used.

Absorbent Paper Points

Paper points are used to dry canals, place medications, and take cultures of the canal (Figure 24-20). Paper points are absorbent and are supplied in various sizes, from x-fine to coarse. Also available are color-coded paper points to match the color coding of reamers and files. The colors change when they absorb moisture. They come conveniently packaged and are supplied sterile or nonsterile. Locking cotton pliers are used to transport paper points to and from the tooth being treated endodontically.

FIGURE 24-18 Endodontic spreaders. (A) Finger spreader. (B) Handled spreader. (C) Endodontic pluggers. *(Courtesy of Sybron Endo.)*

FIGURE 24-19 Glick #1 endodontic instrument. *(Courtesy of Hu-Friedy Mfg. Co., Inc.)*

FIGURE 24-20 Examples of various sizes of paper points.

Gutta Percha

Gutta percha is used to obturate the canal. It is a thermoplastic material that is flexible at room temperature yet stiff enough to be placed in the root canal. Gutta percha cones are supplied in graduated sizes, from x-fine to large (Figure 24-21). Color-coded gutta percha is also available to match color-coded reamers and files.

Thermal gutta percha endodontic obturation systems (e.g., thermafil endodontic obturators) are also available. These systems include metal cores coated with gutta percha. The gutta percha and cores are heated with units specific to the system or with an open flame and then inserted by hand or with low-speed handpieces into the root canal (Figure 24-21).

Silver points are rarely used any more to obturate the canal. They are used much like the gutta percha but are not as flexible. However, the silver points may be removed and replaced with gutta percha.

Irrigation Solutions

During root canal treatment, the root canal is irrigated frequently to remove debris. Sterile water can be used for irrigating, but the most common biomechanical cleaner

FIGURE 24-21 Thermafil obturators and gutta percha points.

is **sodium hypochlorite**, which is household bleach. This solution is mixed with water (50/50) and loaded into a Luer-Lock syringe. The canal is irrigated with the sodium hypochlorite/water solution, which disinfects and dissolves necrotic tissue. The dental assistant places the evacuator close to the tooth to remove the debris and solution.

Besides sterile water and sodium hypochlorite, other solutions used to irrigate the root canal include hydrogen peroxide, saline solutions, alcohol, anesthetic solution, and chlorinated soda.

Root Canal Disinfecting, Cleaning, and Lubricating

Dentists may sometimes want to disinfect the root canal. A small amount of disinfectant is applied to the inside of the root canal walls with an applicator tip and left in between appointments.

Materials for cleaning the root canal come in paste or gel form. These specially formulated materials, a variety of which are available on the market, allow for a chemo-mechanical action that softens calcified deposits. Some materials also produce a bubbling action that flushes debris from the root canals.

A gel is sometimes used during the root canal treatment as a lubrication and **chelating** agent. Chelation is the process by which an agent encloses or grasps a toxic substance and makes it nontoxic. The lubricant acts as a conditioner to make the cleaning and shaping of the canals easier. Lubricating agents are typically available in a syringe and gel for easy application.

Root Canal Sealers/Cements

Root canal sealers used with obturating materials prevent microleakage in the canal. Various materials are used as sealers/cements, including zinc oxide-eugenol, calcium hydroxide, and glass ionomer. They are supplied in powder/liquid, paste, syringe, and capsule forms (Figure 24-22). Sealers are mixed to a thick consistency and then inserted into the canal using paper points, the Lentulo spiral, or files, or by placing the sealer directly on the gutta percha.

FIGURE 24-22 Root canal sealer. (A) Powder/liquid sealer. (B) Two paste system. (C) Capsules of powder and liquid sealer.

Equipment Used in Endodontic Procedures

 As technology advances, new equipment is being developed to assist in endodontic procedures.

■ The **apex finder** measures the distance to the apex of the tooth and displays the information on a digital readout (Figure 24-23A). Some apex finders/locators also display a graphic design of the endodontic file positioned in the root canal during treatment. The position of the file changes as the treatment progresses. As the file nears the apex, some units enlarge the image. The apex finders may have audio feedback—the unit produces a sound as it nears the apex of the root canal. The volume can be set and, on some units, the distance from the apex can be programmed.

■ The **heating unit** can be controlled or continuous. It has many applications, including heat for vitality testing, warming the gutta percha for obturation, and providing heat for bleaching procedures (Figure 24-23B).

■ The **endodontic handpiece** is an attachment to a low-speed handpiece. The handpiece supplies quarter-

(A)

(B)

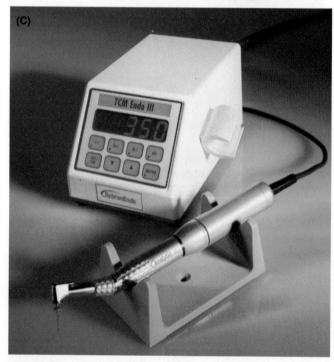

(C)

FIGURE 24-23 (A) Apex finder. (B) Touch'n Heat heating unit. (C) Endodontic handpiece. *(Courtesy of Sybron Endo.)*

turn motion consistently and evenly. It duplicates the manual motion needed during the cleaning and enlarging of the root canal. The endodontic handpiece can be used with all hand instruments (Figure 24-23C).

■ The **ultrasonic unit** is designed specifically for endodontic procedures. Microprocessors operate and control the unit to deliver the right amount of power and amplitude at the tip to complete a variety of endodontic procedures. Various tips are used to perform specific tasks. This unit is used for troughing (making a groove or channel) around a post and opening calcified canals, breaking away cement or calculus, and vibrating a post out of a canal or vibrating a crown or bridge off. Other uses include seating a crown, acting as a spreader in the root canal procedure, assisting in the retrieval of separated files that are lodged in the apical third of the canal, and preparation of root canals (Figure 24-24).

■ The endodontic bender is designed to carefully bend endodontic reamers, files, posts, pluggers, and spreaders to conform to the shape of the root canal. They are made of stainless steel, and are used instead of hemostats, cotton pliers, and fingers. The endodontic bender is autoclavable (Figure 24-25).

Sterilization Procedures

Endodontic instruments must be sterilized before they are used and during the cleaning and shaping of the canal. Sometimes instruments are sterilized at chairside, using a small glass bead or salt sterilizing unit (refer to Chapter 11, Infection Control). A flame may also be used at chairside to resterilize endodontic instruments and burs.

Reamers and files are fragile and should be examined closely before use. If there is any concern about the ability of the instrument to function properly, it should be discarded. Some manufacturers recommend one-procedure use for reamers and files.

Endodontic Procedures

Common endodontic procedures that the dental assistant should be familiar with are root canal treatment, endodontic retreatment, pulpectomy, and pulpotomy.

Root Canal Treatment

Root canal treatment is usually completed in two appointments, but this varies depending on the degree of infection and the dentist's judgment. The dentist may decide to postpone filling the canal to allow more time to treat the infection. When this occurs, the canal is irrigated, sometimes medicated, and a temporary filling is placed in the coronal portion of the tooth. The patient is rescheduled for a continuation of the procedure.

The procedure begins with the dentist opening the coronal portion of the tooth with a dental high-speed handpiece and burs. This is followed by cleaning and enlarging the canal. Restoration of the canal is also known as obturation. During this phase of treatment, the pulp canal is permanently filled and sealed. The steps involved in a root canal treatment are outlined in Procedure 24-2.

General Steps in Root Canal Therapy

The following general steps in root canal therapy can be divided into two or more appointments depending on dentist preference and the extent of the infection. Steps 1 through 8 would take place on the first appointment. Steps 6, 7, and 9 would be done at the second appointment. Once completed, the patient would follow Step 10.

1. Administer the anesthetic.
2. Isolate the area.
3. Gain access to the pulp.
4. Locate the canals.
5. Remove the pulpal tissues.
6. Enlarge and smooth the root canal.
7. Irrigate the root canal.
8. Place temporary filling.
9. Obturate (seal) the root canal.
10. Refer the patient to a general dentist for final restoration.

Endodontic Retreatment

In most cases, teeth that have been treated endodontically will last as long as natural teeth. However, patients continue to experience sensitivity to heat and pain in some teeth. This can happen immediately after treatment or years later. If the tooth fails to heal and the disease process continues or starts again, it can be retreated and have a second chance to heal.

Root canal treatment may fail for a variety of reasons:

- Abscess did not heal
- Narrow or curved canals were not treated during first treatment
- New decay along filling material
- Complicated canal anatomy, such as supplemental canals, went undetected
- Restoration was not placed soon enough after treatment
- Restoration became loose, cracked, or broken, and exposed the tooth to new infection

When the patient feels pain and discomfort with a tooth that has had root canal treatment, she or he should return to the endodontist and discuss treatment options. The endodontist will reopen the tooth to gain access to the root canal. This can be difficult to accomplish because

(A)

(B)

FIGURE 24-24 (A) Various tips to be used with the ultrasonic unit. (B) Ultrasonic unit. *(Courtesy of Sybron Endo.)*

FIGURE 24-25 Endodontic bender. *(Courtesy of Sybron Endo.)*

PROCEDURE 24-2

Root Canal Treatment

This procedure is performed by the dentist, who is assisted by the dental assistant. The following sequence will indicate steps involved in a root canal treatment that requires two appointments.

EQUIPMENT AND SUPPLIES *(Figure 24-26)*

- Basic setup: mouth mirror, explorer, and cotton pliers
- Endodontic explorer and spoon excavator
- Locking cotton pliers
- Saliva ejector, evacuator tip (HVE), air-water syringe tip
- Cotton rolls, cotton pellets, and gauze sponges
- Anesthetic setup
- Dental dam setup
- High-speed handpiece and assortment of burs
- Low-speed handpiece
- Irrigating syringe and solution (sodium hypochlorite or hydrogen peroxide)
- Barbed broach, assorted reamers and files, and rubber stops
- Paper points (assortment)
- Temporization materials
- Permanent obturating materials (gutta percha or silver points and root canal sealer)
- Heat source
- Endodontic spreaders, pluggers, and the Glick #1
- Articulating forceps and paper

PROCEDURE STEPS *(Follow aseptic procedures)*

Administer Anesthetic

1. Administer topical and local anesthetic for endodontic treatment in the same way as for restorative procedures in general dentistry.

2. Usually the dentist will anesthetize the patient at every appointment, but it is at the dentist's discretion. After the first appointment, when the pulp

FIGURE 24-26 Root canal treatment tray setup, opening appointment. (A) Mouth mirror. (B) Explorer. (C) Cotton pliers. (D) Endodontic explorer. (E) Endodontic spoon excavator. (F) Locking cotton pliers. (G) Cotton rolls. (H) Gauze sponges. (I) Anesthetic setup. (J) Dental dam setup. (K) High-speed handpiece. (L) Low-speed handpiece. (M) Millimeter ruler. (N) Irrigating syringe and solution. (O) Paper points. (P) Barbed broach, assorted reamers and files, with stops in endodontic organizer. (Q) Pesso reamers. (R) Gates-Glidden drills. (S) Glick endodontic instrument. (T) Temporary filling material.

chamber has been opened and the canals have been cleaned, the dentist may determine that anesthetic is unnecessary.

3. Prepare the syringe and assist during the administration of the anesthetic.

Isolate Area

1. Place the dental dam, isolating the tooth being endodontically treated. Besides isolating the tooth, the dam improves visibility and protects the tooth from saliva and solutions used in endodontic treatment. The dental dam also maintains an aseptic field and protects the patient's mouth and throat.

2. Once the dental dam is placed, wipe the area with a disinfectant to remove bacterial contaminants.

(continues)

P R O C E D U R E   2 4 - 2   *(C O N T I N U E D)*

Gain Access to Pulp

1. The dentist uses the high-speed handpiece and a round or fissure bur to access the pulp. The opening is made through the crown of the tooth and should be sufficient to expose the pulp chamber and permit access for intracanal instruments.

2. Evacuate and maintain good visibility for the dentist.

3. Once access to the pulp has been gained, the endodontic explorer is used to locate the main and accessory canals.

Remove Pulpal Tissues

1. The dentist inserts a barbed broach into the canal and withdraws the pulpal tissue to remove pulpal tissues.

2. Receive the barber broach in a gauze sponge.

Enlarge and Smooth the Root Canal

1. Using the periapical radiograph, the dentist estimates the length of the tooth root (Figure 24-27). The assistant should record the root length on the patient's chart for reference. An apex finder may also be used. Rubber stops are used to mark the tooth length on files and reamers. A series of small files are used to remove debris and enlarge the canals. Canals must be at least a #25 file before Gates-Glidden burs can be used. As the files enlarge, diameter of the canal, size of the files, and/or Gates-Glidden burs increase, respectively.

2. Prepare the stops on the files and reamers according to the dentist's instructions. This measurement must be precise for each hand instrument. (The duties of the assistant may vary greatly depending on the preferences of the dentist. For example, some dentists may want the assistant to sterilize the reamers and files at chairside, or they may want radiographs taken periodically.)

3. Keep the files and reamers in order and free of debris.

Irrigate Root Canal

1. Periodically, the canal is irrigated to remove debris (Figure 24-28). After the canal is flushed, it is dried with paper points.

2. Prepare the solution in the disposable syringe and transfer it to the operator. As the operator flushes the solution into the canal, evacuate the area. Then, transfer paper points in locking pliers to the operator and receive the used saturated points in a gauze sponge. To dry the canal, measure 1 mm short of the apex.

NOTE: At this time, the dentist may decide to place a temporary restoration and reappoint the patient in several days to two weeks.

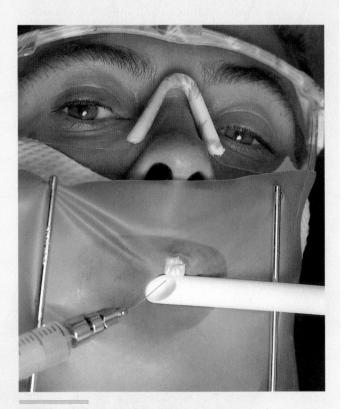

FIGURE 24-27 Measuring length of the root using a radiograph and reamer.

FIGURE 24-28 Irrigating the root canal.

(continues)

PROCEDURE 24-2 *(CONTINUED)*

3. Prepare the temporary restorative materials and place the temporary or assist the dentist in placement.

4. Remove the dental dam and dismiss the patient.

Obturate Root Canal *(Figure 24-29)*

1. Obturation of the root canal is routinely performed at the second appointment. After the patient is seated, the temporary is removed and the canal is flushed to remove debris.

2. Radiographs are taken periodically throughout the procedure for the dentist to evaluate the progress. Once the canal is adequately enlarged and free of disease, it is permanently filled to prevent debris, fluids, and bacteria from entering the canal. There are many materials and techniques available to fill the canal, but gutta percha materials are most common.

3. The dentist selects a gutta percha point as the **master cone**. The cone should be no more than 1 mm short of the prepared length. The dentist inserts the cone into the canal to check the fit. If the master cone is the correct length and fits snugly near the apex, the cone is removed and the root canal sealer is prepared.

4. The root canal sealer is mixed and then placed in the canal with a Lentulo spiral and/or a master cone dipped in the sealer and placed in the canal.

5. A spreader is used to create space for additional accessory gutta percha cones. Dip each accessory gutta percha cone into the root canal sealer and transfer it to the dentist for placement. Transfer the spreader to create space for the subsequent cones. Repeat this procedure until the canal is filled (Figure 24-30).

6. Once the canal is filled, the excess gutta percha in the crown of the tooth is removed with a hot Glick #1 or a heated plugger. The warm gutta percha is condensed vertically into the cervical portion.

7. Hold a 2 × 2 gauze to remove any excess gutta percha from the instruments.

8. A final radiograph is taken.

9. The coronal portion of the tooth is sealed with a permanent restoration or a temporary restoration if a fixed prosthesis is the treatment choice.

10. The dental dam is removed and the patient's mouth is rinsed.

11. The patient's occlusion is checked with articulating paper.

12. Give the patient postoperative instructions and dismiss him or her.

NOTE: The patient returns to the general dentist for the final restoration of the tooth. Follow-up radiographs may be taken at six-month and one-year intervals.

FIGURE 24-29 Root canal completion appointment tray setup. (A) Mouth mirror. (B) Endodontic explorer. (C) Locking cotton pliers. (D) Endodontic spoon excavator. (E) Irrigating syringe. (F) Burs. (G) High- and low-speed handpiece. (H) Spreaders. (I) Pluggers. (J) Spatula. (K) Glick instrument. (L) Gates-Glidden drills. (M) Absorbent sterile paper points. (N) Lentulo spiral. (O) Gutta percha. (P) Root canal sealer. (Q) Heat source.

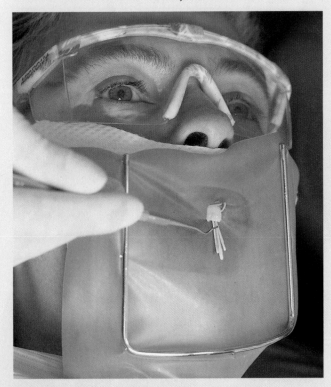

FIGURE 24-30 Root canal filled with gutta percha cones and sealer.

the tooth may have a crown, post, and core material, and all of these have to be removed to permit access.

After removing the restorative materials, the endodontist can clean the canal and carefully examine the inside of the canal. The problem could be supplemental canals and/or unusual anatomy. After cleaning, the canal will be filled and sealed, and a temporary filling will be placed. The patient will then return to her or his general dentist for the final restoration, which may include a new post, core build-up, and crown.

Sometimes the endodontist may believe that the problem is at the apex of the tooth, and will recommend an apicoectomy (discussed later in this chapter).

Pulpectomy

A **pulpectomy** is the removal of all pulpal tissues beginning in the coronal portion of the tooth and terminating 1 to 3 mm short of the apex in the root canal of a tooth. This procedure is used in the treatment of deep caries in permanent teeth. Pulpectomy is the first stage of root canal treatment; cleaning and enlarging the canal usually follow.

Pulpotomy

A **pulpotomy** involves removing the pulp in the coronal portion of the tooth, leaving the pulp in the root canal intact and vital.

A pulpotomy is indicated for the following:

- Primary teeth with pulp exposures
- Treatment in emergency situations where there is pulpal exposure
- Teeth with deep carious lesions
- Apexogenesis (ay-**PECKS**-oh-jen-ah-sis) (treatment of vital tooth where the root is incompletely developed)
- Fractured anterior teeth (Figure 24-31)

FIGURE 24-31 Fractured central incisor with pulp exposure indicates the need for a pulpotomy. *(Courtesy of George J. Velis, DDS.)*

Surgical Endodontics

Endodontic treatment has a high rate of success, but situations arise in which surgical endodontic treatment is necessary to prevent extraction of the involved tooth. Surgery is performed in the area surrounding the roots of the teeth. These surgeries involve a facial surface incision through the tissue to expose the underlying bone. An opening through the alveolar bone is made to expose the root area where surgical endodontic treatment is performed.

Surgical techniques include apicoectomy, root amputation, and hemisection.

Apicoectomy

One of the most common endodontic surgical procedures is an **apicoectomy** (a-pee-koh-**ECK**-toh-me) (see Procedure 24-3). In this procedure, the apex of the

---

PROCEDURE 24-3

Apicoectomy

This procedure is performed by the dentist, who is assisted by the dental assistant.

EQUIPMENT AND SUPPLIES *(Figure 24-32)*

- Basic setup: mouth mirror, explorer, and cotton pliers
- Endodontic explorer and spoon excavator
- Locking cotton pliers
- Saliva ejector, surgical evacuator tip, and air-water syringe tip
- Cotton rolls and gauze sponges
- Anesthetic setup

(continues)

PROCEDURE 24-3 *(CONTINUED)*

- Scalpel and blades

- Periosteal elevator and tissue retractors

- High-speed handpiece and assortment of burs (handpiece is specifically designed with a very small head)

- Surgical curettes

- Irrigating syringe and sterile saline solution

- Hemostat and surgical scissors

- Amalgam setup

- Suture setup

FIGURE 24-33 Apicoectomy procedure begins with a flap incision.

FIGURE 24-32 Apicoectomy tray setup.

FIGURE 24-34 Dental handpiece is used to remove the bone and expose the root tip.

PROCEDURE STEPS *(Follow aseptic procedures)*

1. Anesthetic is administered to the patient.

2. The dentist makes a flap incision with the scalpel and lifts the tissue away from the bone with a periosteal elevator (Figure 24-33). Retract the tissue for the dentist throughout the procedure.

3. Transfer instruments and keep the site clear and clean using the surgical evacuator and tissue retractors.

4. The high-speed handpiece is used by the dentist to gain access to the root apex through the bone (Figure 24-34).

5. The dentist removes debris and infection around the apex of the root with a surgical curette (apical curettage) (Figure 24-35).

6. Evacuate and remove debris from instruments with a gauze sponge.

7. Prepare handpiece and sterile saline irrigation syringe.

8. The high-speed handpiece and burs are used to remove a section of the exposed root tip (Figure 24-36). The root tip is beveled to enhance access. The

(continues)

PROCEDURE 24-3 *(CONTINUED)*

FIGURE 24-35 Apical curettage. Removing infection and debris with a surgical curette.

FIGURE 24-36 Opening the root apex in preparation for retrofill.

area is rinsed with the sterile saline to prepare the root to receive the **retrograde filling** material.

9. Retrograde filling material is placed in the prepared cavity (Figure 24-37). Amalgam is commonly used, but gutta percha, zinc oxide eugenol, and composites are also used.

10. Flap replacement and suturing are the final steps of this procedure. The flap is returned to position and held in place for a few minutes. The dentist then sutures the flap into place.

11. Prepare sutures and assist during placement. Once suturing is complete, give the patient postoperative instructions, a prescription for pain medication, and dismiss him or her.

Amalgam restoration

FIGURE 24-37 Retrofill being placed in the root canal at apex of the tooth.

root and infection surrounding the area are surgically removed. Indications for this treatment include the following:

- Extreme curvature of the root, preventing root canal instruments from reaching the apex
- Root canal is hypercalcified, obstructing root canal therapy
- Previous endodontic treatment did not adequately seal the canal due to additional canals, fractures, or other causes of endodontic failure
- Gaining access to the apex of the root canal for examination and treatment

Root Amputation

Root amputation is a surgical procedure to remove one or more roots of a multirooted tooth. The root is amputated where the root meets the crown. The most common indication for the root amputation procedure is extensive bone loss around the root or furcation of the tooth (Figure 24-38).

Hemisection

Hemisection is the surgical removal of one root and the overlying crown. The tooth is separated buccolingually through the bifurcation, and the affected or diseased portion of the tooth is removed. Surgical burs, chisels, elevators, and forceps are used in this procedure. Indications for a hemisection are the same as for root amputation (Figure 24-39).

Once the hemisection is complete, the remaining tooth and root are restored with a fixed prosthesis. The tooth may need a crown, or it may become part of a bridge.

FIGURE 24-38 Root amputation on a mandibular first molar. The crown is saved, but the diseased root is surgically removed. *(Courtesy of Dr. Gary Shellerud.)*

FIGURE 24-39 Hemisection on a mandibular first molar. One root and half the crown over the root are removed. *(Courtesy of Dr. Gary Shellerud.)*

Apexification

Apexification is treatment of the root canal apex in a tooth that is necrotic. Apexification creates a calcified barrier across the open apex of the tooth. The treatment involves cleaning and shaping the canal to remove debris and bacteria, which is followed by placing a material such as a drug or paste into the canal to the apex. Forms of zinc oxide, cresol, antibiotic paste, or calcium hydroxide have been used to temporarily obdurate the canal to stimulate apical calcification. Calcium hydroxide is commonly used because of its bactericidal properties and alkaline pH.

Apexogenesis

Treating the pulp of a young tooth with an open apex is called **apexogenesis**. The tooth is vital, but has a carious or traumatic exposure (reversible pulpitis) or irreversible pulpitis. It is treated with a pulp capping or pulpotomy to permit continued closure of the open apex and growth of the root. Calcium hydroxide preparation is again indicated in this treatment. In most patients, a calcified bridge will form across the exposure; the pulp will heal and stay vital and the apex will continue to develop and grow to maturity.

CHAPTER SUMMARY

Endodontics comprises the diagnosis and treatment of pulp and periapical tissue diseases. Procedures include diagnosis, root canal treatment, and periapical surgery.

The endodontist is assisted by dental assistants who perform traditional assisting responsibilities in addition to expanded duties specific to endodontics as allowed by state dental practice acts.

Endodontic diagnosis includes patient medical and dental history, clinical examination, including pulp testing, and review of communication if the patient is sent from a referring dentist.

Case Study

Gerold Frank, aged sixty-seven, had an appointment with Dr. Lamb for examination of his mandibular right side. He has been experiencing pain and inflammation in this area. Upon examination, Dr. Lamb suspects that the mandibular first molar is causing Mr. Frank's problem.

Case Study Review

1. What are the key indications for treatment?

2. What clinical tests should be prepared?

3. Identify a possible treatment.

4. What information should be given to Mr. Frank concerning his treatment?

REVIEW QUESTIONS

Multiple Choice

1. Which of the follow diseases is a localized destruction of tissue and accumulation of exudate in the periapical region?
   a. Periodontitis
   b. Apical periodontitis
   c. Osteomyelitis
   d. Periapical abscess

2. The clinical examination for endodontic diagnosis includes all of the following except
   a, radiographs.
   b. sweet test.
   c. mobility.
   d. cold test.

3. Which instrument is used to enlarge and smooth the root canals?
   a. Barbed broach
   b. Endodontic file
   c. Endodontic reamer
   d. Peeso reamer

4. Root canal treatment is most often completed in ___ appointments.
   a. two
   b. three
   c. four
   d. five

5. Which procedure is performed to gain access to the apex of the root canal?
   a. Pulpotomy
   b. Root canal treatment
   c. Apicoectomy
   d. Root amputation

6. Sodium hypochlorite is used to
   a. open the root canal at the beginning of the procedure.
   b. irrigate the canal to remove debris.
   c. fill the canal after it has been cleaned and enlarged.
   d. enlarge the canal.

7. All of the following are used in endodontic procedures, *except* the
   a. apex finder.
   b. vitality scanner.
   c. curing light.
   d. heating unit.

8. In which of the following procedures is one root and the overlying crown surgically removed?
   a. Hemisection
   b. Root amputation
   c. Pulpotomy
   d. Apicoectomy

9. Peeso reamers are used during the root canal procedure to
   a. prepare the opening access by removing the obstructing dentin in the upper portion of the canal.
   b. prepare the canal for a post and to reduce the curvature of the canal orifice for straight-line access.
   c. mark the reamers and files to the length of the root canal.
   d. spin root canal sealer or cement into the canal.

10. All of the following are true statements about absorbent paper points, *except* that they
    a. are used to dry the canals.
    b. come in various sizes.
    c. are used to place medication and take cultures.
    d. need to be heated and condensed into the root canal.

Critical Thinking

1. Differentiate among a pulpectomy, pulpotomy, and root canal treatment.

2. Is anesthetic always administered for root canal treatment? Explain.

3. What is the difference between K-type files and Hedström files?

Web Activities

1. To see more endodontic equipment and supplies, visit http://store.tulsadental.com.

2. For a Web site dedicated to patients with questions about endodontic treatment, go to http://www.aae.org, sponsored by the American Association of Endodontists.

3. To learn more about the newest endodontic instruments and apex finders, vitality testers, and endo handpieces, go to http://www.sybronendo.com.

CHAPTER 25

ORAL AND MAXILLOFACIAL SURGERY

SPECIFIC INSTRUCTIONAL OBJECTIVES

The student should strive to meet the following objectives and demonstrate an understanding of the facts and principles presented in this chapter:

1. Describe the scope of oral and maxillofacial surgery.

2. Identify the surgical instruments used in various types of surgery and describe their functions.

3. Explain the aseptic procedures followed in the oral surgeon's office.

4. Describe evaluation procedures for new patients.

5. Describe how to prepare the patient for surgical treatment.

6. Explain surgical procedures, including tray setups and assisting responsibilities.

7. List the postoperative instructions given to patients.

8. List and describe biopsy techniques.

9. Describe temporomandibular joint disease (TMJ).

10. List and describe the types of dental implants and explain the surgical procedures for placing the implants.

11. Explain the oral surgeon's relationship with the hospital.

ADVANCED CHAIRSIDE FUNCTIONS

12. Explain the function of sutures and when they are placed.

13. List the equipment and supplies needed for suture removal.

14. Determine and identify the location and number of sutures and how to evaluate the healing process.

15. Identify the following suture patterns: simple, continuous simple, sling, continuous sling, horizontal, and vertical mattress.

16. List the basic criteria for suture removal.

17. Explain the steps of removal for identified suture patterns.

18. Explain postoperative patient care.

KEY TERMS

apical elevators *(534)*   alveoplasty *(541)*   cheek retractors *(530)*

alveolitis *(553)*   biopsy *(542)*   *(continues)*

527

OUTLINE *(continued)*

KEY TERMS *(continued)*

INTRODUCTION

Oral and **maxillofacial** surgery is the branch of dentistry that focuses on the diagnosis and treatment of diseases, injuries, and malformations. It involves surgery for both functional and esthetic aspects of the face, jaws, mouth, neck, and head. This specialty is sometimes called oral surgery.

General dentists refer surgical cases that go beyond their scope of training to oral surgeons. Although the general dentist studies surgical procedures, the number of surgical procedures performed in the general dentist's office depends on preference and training. Upon graduating from dental school, a surgeon receives a minimum of four more years of advanced training in anatomy, anesthesia, pain control, and surgical procedures in and out of the hospital setting before receiving a degree in oral and maxillofacial surgery.

The Oral and Maxillofacial Surgeon's Office

There are various settings for oral surgeons' offices, just as there are for other dental offices. Some surgeons prefer to be close to a hospital if they routinely perform surgeries in a hospital. Oral surgeons have operating rooms in their offices for less complicated surgeries, which eliminates the need for the patient to go to the hospital. The oral surgeon brings to the office the staff needed to perform the surgery.

The oral surgeon's office includes areas similar to the general office, with the addition of a recovery area. Some offices have separate areas for patients recovering from general anesthesia. Often, there is a large reclining chair or bed in this area so that the patient can lie down. Postoperative instructions and prescriptions are given to the patient or the patient's support person in the recovery area.

The Oral and Maxillofacial Surgery Team

The oral surgery office team varies according to the surgeon's goals for the practice. In addition to the oral and maxillofacial surgeon, the team usually consists of the receptionist, the business office staff, the dental assistants, and, in some offices, a nurse anesthetist or an anesthesiologist.

Oral and Maxillofacial Surgeon

The oral and maxillofacial surgeon performs the following: patient examination; diagnosis; teeth extraction; cyst and tumor removal; temporomandibular joint treatment; biopsies; and emergency, reconstructive, and implant surgeries. The oral surgeon works mainly in the office setting but also goes into the hospital to perform complicated surgeries and to treat emergencies. Like all professionals, the oral surgeon continually attends seminars and courses to advance knowledge and skills.

Receptionist and Business Staff

The receptionist and the business staff perform many of the same duties in the oral surgery office as they would in the general dental office. Because most of the oral surgeon's patients are referred by other dental and medical offices, communication and recordkeeping responsibilities increase. The patient's x-rays and written information must be received in the surgeon's office before the patient's appointment. When patients first arrive at the office, they are given forms to fill out. Appointments for treatment are scheduled and insurance claims and financial arrangements are completed before the day of the surgery.

Surgical Dental Assistant

The surgical dental assistant's responsibilities often vary depending on the size of the practice. For example, a dental assistant may be responsible for sterilization and room preparation, the seating and dismissing of patients, pre- and postoperative care, and assisting the oral surgeon during all procedures.

Typical responsibilities of a surgical dental assistant follow:

- Perform traditional duties, such as instrument transfer and maintaining the operating field during the procedure
- Assist with the administration of intravenous sedation and analgesics
- Take and record vital signs
- Prepare the treatment rooms
- Sterilize instruments

- Ensure that all presurgery steps are completed and any materials or prosthetics required are ready
- Prepare the patient for treatment
- Maintain asepsis throughout the procedure
- Stabilize the patient's head and mandible during surgery, if necessary
- Provide postoperative care of the patient
- Clean the treatment room
- Remove sutures (if this is a legal expanded function)

During surgical procedures, six-handed dentistry is often practiced. The second assistant provides support in maintaining the patient's position and acts as a rover for off-tray items. The main assistant is then free to focus on assisting the dentist.

Nurse Anesthetist or Anesthesiologist

The oral surgeon makes the decision to have a nurse anesthetist or anesthesiologist as part of the surgical team. The nurse anesthetist may be a full- or part-time member of the surgical team, while an anesthesiologist is generally only part-time in the office and works with the oral surgeon with every patient in the hospital setting.

The responsibility of the nurse anesthetist varies but may include administering the anesthesia and maintaining the patient during the procedure; continuously monitoring the patient's vital signs; managing fluid therapy; providing or supervising postoperative recovery, postoperative follow-up, and patient evaluation and maintaining records.

The anesthesiologist is hired to perform preoperative evaluations and preparations, administer anesthetics, monitor patient reactions to the anesthetic and surgery, and advise the oral surgeon of adverse reactions. The oral surgeon communicates very closely with the anesthesiologist to ensure that both have all the information they need to ensure the safety of the patient and enable the oral surgeon to successfully accomplish the procedure. The anesthesiologist relieves the oral surgeon of anesthetizing the patient so that the surgeon can concentrate on the procedure to be performed.

Oral Surgery Instruments

 Surgical instruments are designed to apply adequate pressure in specific areas to remove bone tissue or teeth. Surgical instruments are made of stainless steel (so they can be sterilized after each use) or disposable plastics.

Scalpel

Surgical scalpels are surgical knives used to incise or excise soft tissue precisely with the least amount of trauma.

Scalpels are designed in two sections: the handle and the blade (Figure 25-1). The metal handle is slim and straight and is designed to accommodate detachable, disposable blades. A common handle is the Bard Parker style. This handle is flat and has a metric ruler. The blades are very sharp and are supplied in various lengths and designs. The blades are used once and then disposed of in the sharps container. Blades are made of surgical carbon steel and are numbered according to shape. Common blades are #15 for surgical procedures and #11 and #12 to incise and drain.

Disposable scalpels are also available. They have plastic handles with metal blades. Disposable scalpels are supplied in sterile packages and are disposed of after one use.

When removing or replacing blades on the scalpel handle, use cotton pliers, a hemostat, or a blade protector to avoid injury. Practice placing and removing the blades to familiarize yourself with the mechanics of this skill. Disposable surgical blade removers are available. The scalpel blade is placed in the plastic cap of the removers and removed from the handle. The blade is left in the cap and discarded.

Retractors

Retractors are used to deflect tissue from the surgical site so that the view is unobstructed. Careful handling of retractors is necessary to avoid traumatizing the tissue. There are several types of retractors: tissue retractors, cheek and lip retractors, and tongue retractors.

Tissue retractors are supplied in forceps (hinged) type (**tissue forceps**) or cotton-plier style. The working end of both types of retractors has small teeth to assist in grasping the tissue securely (Figure 25-2).

Cheek and **lip retractors** are used to hold the patient's cheeks away from the operating site. They increase visibility by retracting the cheeks and expanding the viewing area. Cheek retractors are made of metal or plastic (Figures 25-3 and 25-4).

Tongue retractors are placed between the border of the tongue and the lingual surfaces of the teeth. The dental assistant gently but firmly retracts the tongue from the operating site. Tongue retractors are spoon shaped or have long blades (Figures 25-3 and 25-4). Tongue retractors also are used to retract the cheeks. They are placed on the buccal mucosa and then the tissue is retracted for a clear view.

FIGURE 25-1 (A) Blade removal devices. (B) Metal scalpel handles. (C) Scalpel package and scalpel blade. (D) Scalpel blades #11, 12, and 15.

FIGURE 25-2 Tissue retractors. *(Courtesy of Miltex Instrument Co., Inc., Lake Success, NY.)*

FIGURE 25-3 (A) Tongue and cheek retractors. (B) Lip, tongue, and cheek retractors.

FIGURE 25-4 (A) Retracting the tongue with the University of Minnesota retractor. (B) Cheek retractor in patient's mouth.

Mouth Props

Mouth props are used to prevent the patient's mouth from closing during the procedure. Sometimes, appointment length, the type of anesthesia administered, or the physical condition of the patient requires the use of props. Mouth props are made of hard rubber, silicone, plastic, or stainless steel. They are supplied in child and adult sizes. The prop is inserted into the patient's mouth with the tapered end toward the posterior teeth. This allows the muscles to relax while keeping the mouth open.

Another type of mouth prop is the Molt mouth gag, which is hinged and has handles, a ratchet release, and beaks. Molt mouth gags are supplied in pediatric, child, and adult sizes. The beaks are closed when inserted into the patient's mouth, and the handle is gently squeezed, which opens the beaks and the patient's mouth. The forceps are locked in this position until the release is engaged (Figure 25-5).

Hemostats

Hemostats have multiple uses during surgical procedures. They are used to retract tissue, remove small root tips, clamp off blood vessels, and grasp loose objects. A hemostat is a forceps with working ends that are not

FIGURE 25-5 Molt mouth gags in patient's mouth.

sharp but long, serrated, or grooved beaks. They have locking handles that can be manipulated with one hand (Figure 25-6).

Hemostats are supplied in various sizes to accommodate the uses of the instrument. Tissue, bone, and tooth fragments are easily grasped and removed with the hemostat. There are various types, including the Kelly and the Halstead-Mosquito. Hemostats come with straight and curved beaks.

Needle Holders

Needle holders are similar to hemostats and function in much the same manner. They are forceps with straight beaks, but needle-holder beaks are shorter than hemostat beaks. The needle holder has fine serrations with a groove down the center of each beak to hold the suture needle. They are supplied in various sizes (Figure 25-6).

Surgical Scissors

Surgical scissors are used to cut sutures and to trim soft tissue. They are supplied in various sizes and shapes (Figure 25-7). They are made of stainless steel and should be used only for surgical procedures to maintain their sharp edges. The surgical scissors have pointed beaks with straight or angled blades.

Surgical Aspirating Tips

Surgical aspirating tips are made of metal or plastic. The metal tips are sterilizable, while the plastic tips are discarded after one use. The surgical aspirating tips are long tubes that are very slender or tapered to small openings. The tips are used to aspirate blood and debris from the surgical site and tonsil suction for sedated patients (Figure 25-8). A stylet is used to clear blood and tissue from the surgical tips.

Surgical Curettes

Surgical curettes are used for curettage and debridement of the tooth socket or diseased tissue. They are double ended and have straight or curved shanks; the working end of the instrument is spoon shaped. Surgical curettes are available in various sizes (Figure 25-9).

(A)

(B)

FIGURE 25-6 (A) Hemostats. (B) Needle holder. (Courtesy of Miltex Instrument Co., Inc., Lake Success, NY.)

FIGURE 25-7 Surgical scissors.

FIGURE 25-8 Surgical aspirating tips.

FIGURE 25-9 Surgical curettes.

Surgical Chisels and Mallets

Surgical chisels are used to remove or shape bone. They can be used alone if the bone is soft, but if the bone is dense, a **surgical mallet** is used with the chisel. The chisel is positioned on the bone, and mallets are used to gently tap the end of the chisel. Chisels and mal-

lets also are used to split teeth into smaller portions for easier removal.

Chisels are available beveled on one surface or bi-beveled (beveled on both sides). The bi-beveled chisels are used to split a tooth, while the single-beveled chisel is used to remove and shape the bone (Figure 25-10).

Surgical Bone Files

Surgical bone files are usually double-ended instruments. They are supplied in various sizes and shapes. Bone files are used in a back-and-forth motion to smooth the edges of alveolar bone. They trim and smooth the bone after the teeth have been extracted and the rongeurs have contoured the bone (Figure 25-11).

FIGURE 25-10 Surgical chisel and mallet.

FIGURE 25-11 Surgical bone file.

Rongeurs

Rongeurs (**RON**-jeers) are hinged forceps with springs in the handle. They are used to trim and shape the alveolar bone after extractions. The beaks are sharp and have cutting edges, similar to fingernail trimmers. There are several sizes and shapes of rongeurs. When multiple teeth are removed and a denture is to be seated, rongeurs are necessary to contour the ridges of the alveolar bone and eliminate sharp edges (Figure 25-12).

Periosteal Elevator

The **periosteal elevator** is an instrument of many uses and is included on most surgical tray setups. It is often used to detach the periosteum (bone covering) and gingival tissues from around the tooth prior to the use of extraction forceps. The periosteal elevator is also used to reflect and lift the **mucoperiosteum** (mucosa and periosteum) from the bone.

Periosteal elevators are double-ended instruments with various working-end combinations. Often, one end is pointed and the other is rounded (Figure 25-13).

Elevators

Elevators are used by the surgeon to loosen and remove teeth, retained roots, and root fragments. Elevators are designed in different shapes and sizes to accommodate the variety of tasks, operating techniques, and tooth morphology. They are single-ended instruments with large, bulbous, or T-shaped handles to allow for a firm grip. Being able to firmly grip the elevator allows the surgeon to exert the necessary force. The working ends of

FIGURE 25-13 Periosteal elevators.

elevators may be straight or angular and are often paired left and right. Elevators are referred to by manufacturer's number or by designer names. Two common designer elevators are Potts and Cryers (Figure 25-14B and C).

Apical elevators are similar to the elevators with the large handle but have smaller working ends. They are straight or angular and have longer, narrower blades to loosen and remove roots or root or bone fragments (Figure 25-14A).

Root tip picks or elevators are even thinner and longer than apical elevators. They are paired left and right and are also straight or angled. The root tip picks are designed to tease the root tips or fragments out of the bone socket. They are delicate instruments that break if too much force is applied (Figure 25-15).

Forceps

Extraction forceps are used to remove teeth from the alveolar bone. They are hinged instruments with various handles and beak styles. Specific forceps are used on certain teeth or in certain areas of the mouth. Dental assistants should be able to identify which forceps their dentists routinely use. One way to learn forceps is by manufacturer's numbers. Each instrument has a number imprinted on the handle and is labeled with an "L" or "R" for left or right. For example, a #88R is used on the maxillary right first and second molars.

Another way to identify forceps is to learn how the design of the forceps applies to tooth morphology. Careful study of the various shapes of the beaks will allow determination of forceps for the:

- Maxillary or mandibular teeth
- Right or left quadrant
- Anterior or posterior teeth
- Accommodation of teeth anatomy

FIGURE 25-12 Surgical rongeurs.

FIGURE 25-14 (A) Apical elevators. (B) Potts or T-handled elevators. (C) Cryers elevators. *(Courtesy of Miltex Instrument Co., Inc., Lake Success, NY.)*

FIGURE 25-15 Root tip picks.

For example, on #53R for the maxillary molars, one beak is pointed for placement in the bifurcated buccal root. For the maxillary molars (#88L), there is a pointed single beak on the buccal to be placed between the two buccal roots and a split beak on the lingual to engage the single lingual root.

The curve of the shank of the forceps indicates whether the forceps should be used on the maxillary or the mandibular. Mandibular forceps are often at more of a right angle, and the maxillary are straight, slightly curved, or have two angles (like bayonets). For example, #17 forceps are used on the mandibular first and second molars; the beaks form an angle with the handle. The forceps for the maxillary first and second molars have two angles in the working end.

Some forceps are **universal forceps** and can be used on any of the four quadrants. Another example is, which #101 forceps can be used for bicuspids and deciduous teeth in either arch. Other forceps can be used on the left or right side in the same arch. Another example is #150 forceps, which can be used for maxillary incisors, bicuspids, and roots on the left or right quadrant.

Forceps used on the anterior or posterior teeth can be distinguished by beak width. For example, on mandibular forceps #151, the beaks are smaller to fit the incisors, bicuspids, and roots, while mandibular molar forceps #17 are wider to accommodate the width of the molars.

The shapes of forceps beaks are designed to accommodate the anatomy of specific teeth. For example, mandibular first and second molar forceps have narrow, pointed beaks to engage the bifurcated roots of these molars. These forceps are often called the "cow horns" because of their shape.

Extraction forceps are held in a palm grasp by the operator. Some handles are straight, while others have "finger rings" or hooks on the handles. The selection is the preference of the dentist.

To better visualize and learn forceps, divide them into the arches and teeth they are used on (Figures 25-16 and 25-17).

Asepsis in Oral Surgery

Like all dental offices, the oral and maxillofacial surgery office follows a plan for infection control. This plan is critical to prevent cross-contamination. The oral surgery office is a higher risk area because of the increased possibility of blood contact.

Extraordinary care of surgical equipment and supplies is necessary to prevent accidental exposure. In the sterilizing room, an area should be designated for "unclean" trays where the contaminated tray is taken apart and disposable sharps are placed in a marked sharps container. Expendable items, such as gauze, cotton rolls, and so on, are placed in marked hazardous waste containers. The instruments are cleaned, and then bagged or wrapped for sterilization. The bags are carefully marked with the procedure and date. The

(A) Upper incisor and root tip extraction forceps

(B) Upper incisor and cuspid extraction forceps

(C) Upper #150 extraction forceps used for incisors, cuspids, bicuspids, and roots

(D) Upper #88L extraction forcep–left first and second molars

(E) Upper #53R extraction forcep–right first and second molars

(E) Upper #53L extraction forcep–left first and second molars

(D) Upper #88R extraction forcep–right first and second molars

(F) Upper #210 extraction forcep–third molars–universal

FIGURE 25-16 Maxillary extraction forceps. *(Courtesy of Miltex Instrument Co., Inc., Lake Success, NY.)*

(A) Lower incisors, bicuspids, cuspids, and roots

(B) Lower #151 extraction forceps–incisors, cuspids, and roots–universal

(C) Lower #23 extraction forceps–first and second molars–universal "cow horns"

(D) Lower #15 extraction forceps–first and second molars–universal with ring on handle

(E) Lower #222 extraction forceps–third molars–universal

FIGURE 25-17 Mandibular extraction forceps. *(Courtesy of Miltex Instrument Co., Inc., Lake Success, NY.)*

instruments are sterilized according to various methods, such as steam autoclaving, dry heat, and chemical vapor. Current OSHA guidelines should be followed (see Chapter 11, Infection Control).

Storage of Contaminated Instruments

If contaminated instruments cannot be processed immediately, they should be presoaked to prevent blood and debris from drying on them.

The Dentist and the Dental Assistant

The dentist and the dental assistant must follow the routine requirements of personal protective equipment (PPE) for all surgical procedures. One change is in the handwashing procedure. For oral surgery, the surgical hand scrub is completed before donning sterile gloves. (See Procedure 25-1.)

Patient Considerations

During the first visit, a medical history is completed by the patient. If surgery is anticipated, the surgeon may consult with the patient's physician about the patient's medications and physical conditions that may affect the surgical procedure.

Radiographs are sent from the general dental office to the oral surgeon's office before the patient is scheduled. Periapical radiographs are commonly used for extractions, but occlusal and extraoral radiographs such as panoramic, lateral skull, cephalometric, and computerized tomography also may be required. (Specific extraoral exposures are explained in Chapter 22, Production and Evaluation of Dental Radiographs, and Chapter 23, Extraoral and Digital Radiography.)

 The oral surgeon completes a thorough examination. Once the diagnosis is made, the treatment options are explained to the patient. The patient

PROCEDURE 25-1

Surgical Scrub

This procedure is performed by the oral surgeon and the dental assistant before donning sterile gloves for a surgical procedure.

EQUIPMENT AND SUPPLIES

- Antimicrobial soap
- Sterile scrub brush or foam sponge
- Disposable sterile towels

PROCEDURE STEPS *(Follow aseptic procedures)*

1. Remove watch and rings before the scrub.
2. Use an antimicrobial soap, such as chlorhexidine gluconate.
3. Wet hands and forearms up to the elbows with warm water.
4. Dispense about 5 ml of soap into cupped hands and work into a lather.
5. Beginning with the fingernails, scrub the fingers, hands, and forearms with a surgical scrub brush.
6. Rinse thoroughly with warm water.
7. Repeat the procedure with soap but without the scrub brush.
8. Rinse with warm water, beginning at the fingertips and moving hands and forearms through the water and up so that the water drains off the forearms last (Figure 25-18A). This prevents the hands from being recontaminated.
9. Dry hands and arms thoroughly with disposable sterile towels.
10. Don sterile surgical gloves.

NOTE: The surgical scrub was commonly referred to as the "five-minute scrub," but studies have indicated that scrub times of three to four minutes are as effective as five-minute scrubs. The recommendation is to follow scrub product manufacturer's instructions and OSHA guidelines. Do not use a brush so stiff that it creates microscopic abrasions on the skin.

(A)

(B)

FIGURE 25-18 (A) Completion of surgical scrub. (B) Materials for surgical scrub.

must carefully read and sign an informed consent form prior to the procedure. The informed consent identifies and explains the surgery the patient is to receive and acknowledges any risks of the treatment.

Patient Preparation

Whether a general anesthetic is administered will determine the preoperative instructions given to the patient. It is important for the patient to follow the instructions carefully prior to his or her appointment.

Typical Preoperative Instructions for the Patient

1. Wear loose-fitting clothing and low-heeled shoes. Your shirt should be short sleeved or easy to roll up.
2. Remove contact lenses before surgery.
3. Notify the dentist if a cold, sore throat, fever, or other illness develops prior to surgery.
4. Do not consume alcoholic beverages twenty-four hours before surgery.
5. Arrange transportation to and from the office on the day of the surgery.
6. When a physical examination is requested by the oral surgeon, have the physician send written approval prior to surgery.
7. Some medical conditions, such as rheumatic heart disease or artificial heart valves, require prophylactic antibiotics to be taken prior to surgery.
8. If the surgery is in the morning, eat nothing after midnight. This includes medicines, food, and all fluids.*
9. If the surgery is in the afternoon, drink only water, juice, tea, or coffee prior to six A.M. After six A.M., take absolutely nothing by mouth.*

 *Food, liquids, or medications in the stomach when general anesthesia is administered may cause vomiting. The vomit may then be aspirated into the lungs.

Patient Preparation

1. The patient is escorted to the treatment room. The dental assistant checks any changes in the medical history, whether the patient followed the preoperative instructions, and whether prescribed medication was taken as directed.
2. The patient is given an antimicrobial rinse.
3. The patient is seated and a full-length drape is placed on him or her. The patient is then reclined to a routine position for the dentist.
4. A sterile towel is placed over the patient's chest.
5. Vital signs are taken and recorded. The patient is prepared for administration of the intravenous sedation.

Oral Surgery Procedures

 Common procedures performed in the oral surgeon's office are routine extractions, multiple extractions and alveoplasty, surgical removal of impacted third molars, biopsy procedures, and dental implant surgery.

Routine or Uncomplicated Extractions

Routine or uncomplicated extractions include the removal of permanent or primary teeth that are erupted into the oral cavity. These surgeries are usually less involved and performed more often than other surgeries. The dental assistant prepares the tray setup and selects forceps and elevators for the specific tooth to be extracted. (See Procedure 25-2.)

PROCEDURE 25-2

Routine or Uncomplicated Extraction

The dental assistant assists the oral surgeon throughout this procedure. The dental assistant must be prepared and thinking ahead to anticipate the surgeon's needs.

EQUIPMENT AND SUPPLIES (Figure 25-19)

- Mouth mirror
- Gauze sponges
- Surgical HVE tip
- University of Minnesota Retractor for the tongue and the cheek
- Local anesthetic setup
- Nitrous oxide setup (optional)
- Periosteal elevator

(continues)

PROCEDURE 25-2 *(CONTINUED)*

FIGURE 25-19 Tray setup for uncomplicated extraction.

- Straight elevator
- Extraction forceps
- Surgical rongeurs
- Hemostat/needle holder
- Surgical curette
- Surgical scissors
- Suture setup

PROCEDURE STEPS *(Follow aseptic procedures)*

1. The surgeon examines the site of extraction. The dental assistant transfers the mouth mirror and explorer to the surgeon. The patient's x-rays are mounted on the viewbox for the dentist to review.

2. Topical anesthetic is placed on the mucosa, and local anesthetic is administered. The dental assistant prepares the topical anesthetic and transfers it to the surgeon (if allowed by the state practice act, the dental assistant can place the topical anesthetic). The syringe is prepared and transferred to the surgeon. The dental assistant then observes the patient.

3. Either the periosteal or a straight elevator is used by the oral surgeon to determine whether the patient is adequately numb, to separate epithelial attachment from around the tooth, and to initiate alveolar bone expansion around the neck of the tooth (to accommodate forceps placement). The dental assistant transfers and receives elevators and has gauze ready to remove blood or debris from the instruments. The dental assistant maintains the operating field, adjusts the light, and retracts tissues as needed.

4. Once the tooth is loosened in the alveolus, forceps are placed securely on the tooth and, with a firm

grasp, the surgeon **luxates** (moves or dislocates) the tooth and then removes it from the socket. This may be easy, or the tooth may have to be subluxated (rocked back and forth), rotated, and lifted several times before the bone around the tooth is spread enough to lift the tooth out of the socket. During this time, the dental assistant transfers forceps and elevators as needed by the surgeon, keeps the instruments clean of debris, and retracts the cheek or tongue. The dental assistant should observe the patient for signs of anxiety or syncope. Once the tooth is extracted, the forceps beaks and tooth are received in the palm of the dental assistant's hand while transferring gauze to the surgeon (Figure 25-20). Once the forceps and tooth are placed on the tray, the tooth is examined for fractured roots.

5. The alveolus (socket) is examined for fractured root tips and debris. A surgical curette is used to remove bone chips, granulation tissue, and abscesses/cysts. The dental assistant evacuates the alveolus using the surgical HVE tip, and then transfers the surgical curette. A gauze is held close to the patient's chin to remove debris from the curette.

6. Once the tooth and any fragments are removed, the area is debrided and the wound is covered with a folded, moistened gauze as a pressure pack. The patient is instructed to bite down on the gauze to

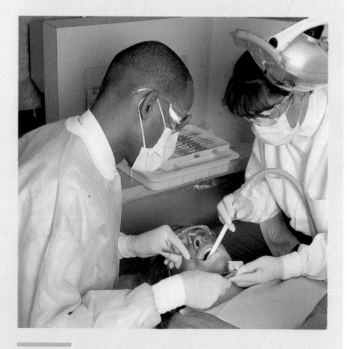

FIGURE 25-20 Dental assistant receiving extraction forceps with tooth in beaks.

(continues)

PROCEDURE 25-2 *(CONTINUED)*

apply pressure. This aids in controlling the bleeding and the formation of the blood clot.

7. The dentist may place sutures at this point in the procedure. The dental assistant prepares the sutures and assists during placement. The dental assistant debrides the area with the HVE and has a moistened

gauze folded and ready to place in the patient's mouth for biting on.

8. The dental assistant checks and cleans the patient's face, returns the patient to a sitting position, and allows a few minutes before giving postoperative instructions. The patient is then dismissed.

Multiple Extractions and Alveoplasty

Multiple extractions are needed when the patient is going to have a full or partial denture. The extraction process is similar for one tooth or for several teeth, but after several teeth have been removed, the bone and soft tissue must be contoured and smoothed. The contouring process is called an **alveoplasty**. The alveolar ridge must be free of

any sharp edges or points to achieve the most comfort and function for the patient. If both the maxillary and the mandibular teeth are to be extracted at one appointment, the maxillary teeth are extracted first. This prevents hemorrhage and debris from contaminating the mandibular extraction site during surgery. Routinely, the dentist starts at the most posterior tooth and moves anteriorly.

PROCEDURE 25-3

Multiple Extractions and Alveoplasty

The procedure is performed by the oral surgeon, who is assisted by the dental assistant. This sterile procedure involves the removal of several teeth and contouring the bone. Responsibilities of the dental assistant include evacuation and instrument transfer.

EQUIPMENT AND SUPPLIES (Figure 25-21)

- Mouth mirror
- Gauze sponges
- Surgical HVE tip
- Luer lok syringe and sterile saline solution
- Retractor for the tongue and cheeks
- Local anesthetic setup
- Nitrous oxide setup (optional)
- Scalpel and blades
- Surgical rongeurs
- Hemostat and tissue retractors
- Periosteal elevator
- Straight elevator

FIGURE 25-21 Tray setup for multiple extractions and alveoplasty.

- Extraction forceps (selected for the teeth being extracted)
- Surgical curette
- Root tip picks
- Bone file
- Low-speed handpiece and surgical burs

(continues)

PROCEDURE 25-3 (CONTINUED)

- Suture scissors

- Suture setup

PROCEDURE STEPS *(Follow aseptic procedures)*

1. The surgeon examines the teeth to be extracted.

2. When several teeth are going to be extracted, the patient may request general anesthesia. The patient will be prepared for intravenous sedation, which is followed by local anesthetic. The local anesthetic reduces bleeding at the extraction site and postoperative pain. The dental assistant prepares the materials necessary for the local and intravenous anesthetic, and then assists in the administration.

3. The teeth are removed by the same techniques described for the routine extraction.

4. After the teeth have been extracted and any root tips or debris removed, the alveoplasty procedure begins. The alveoplasty is usually accomplished one quadrant at a time. The surgeon makes an incision on the buccal and lingual surface to remove the interdental papillae and to expose the crest of the alveolar bone. The flap of tissue is reflected for clear vision. The dental assistant transfers the scalpel and evacuates the area as necessary, receives the scalpel, and transfers the periosteal elevator to reflect the soft tissue. The dental assistant uses tissue forceps to retract the tissue and maintain the operating area.

5. Rongeurs and/or surgical burs are used for the initial trimming and contouring of the alveolar bone. The dental assistant transfers the rongeurs and/or the low-speed handpiece with surgical burs and keeps them free of debris. The dental assistant intermittently uses the HVE and the irrigation syringe with sterile saline solution to maintain the operating field.

6. Final contouring and smoothing are done with the bone file. The area is rinsed with sterile saline solution. At this point, a **plastic stint** (clear denture base material, molded to the same shape and size as the denture) is placed in the patient's mouth. Areas impinging on the stint can be seen by the surgeon. The surgeon continues to contour the bone until all interferences are removed. The dental assistant transfers instruments and continues to maintain the surgical site. The stint must be kept clean, so the dental assistant removes blood and debris from the stint between placements.

7. The buccal and lingual flaps are repositioned and sutured into position. The dental assistant prepares the suture materials and, once the tissue is in position, transfers the suture for placement. The dental assistant assists during the suture procedure and holds the tissue as the surgeon places the sutures.

8. A folded moist gauze pack is placed over the surgical site or the immediate denture is seated. The dental assistant prepares the gauze pack and transfers it to the surgeon. If the patient receives an immediate denture, the dental assistant readies the denture and transfers it to the surgeon for placement.

9. The patient is allowed to recover, and then postoperative instructions are given verbally and in writing.

10. The patient is scheduled for a postoperative examination and suture removal.

Impacted Teeth Extractions

Often the jaw does not grow long enough to allow the third molars or wisdom teeth to erupt. These molars then stay trapped within the jaw. Many problems can arise when this situation occurs, such as infection, destruction of neighboring teeth, destruction of the bone, or movement of the permanent teeth out of proper alignment (Figure 25-22).

Extracting impacted teeth is one of the most common procedures the oral surgeon performs, especially third molar extractions. Many factors determine the difficulty of the impacted tooth extraction, including the depth, position, or angulation of the tooth in the bone. The teeth may be impacted in soft tissue or in the bone. If the teeth are impacted in bone, dental handpieces and surgical burs are required to gain access. Additional surgical instruments are used to facilitate the removal of the tooth from the bone. Often, all impacted third molars are removed at one appointment. (See Procedure 25-4.)

Biopsy Procedures

With every patient, the dentist and staff must be aware of any abnormal tissue. Through the clinical examination, x-rays, or patient complaints, pathology may be discovered. Early detection of premalignant and/or malignant conditions can save lives. Once the suspicious lesion or area is recognized, the dentist will want a **biopsy**. The biopsy procedure, performed by an oral surgeon, involves removal of tissue from a suspicious area, either totally or partially, for microscopic examination and diagnosis. There are three types of biopsy

1

Three roots

Wisdom teeth (No. 3 above) develop inside the bone. Crowns form first, then roots.

2

If the jaw grows long enough, the wisdom teeth can erupt and be used.

3

If the jaws are not long enough by age 16, wisdom teeth stay trapped (impacted) inside the bone.

4

Impacted wisdom teeth can cause:
(A) Infection of the gums over or around them.

5

(B) Infection in the bone around them

6

(C) destruction of the next tooth

7

I(D) Destruction of the bone by formation of a cyst.

8

Looking down on the biting surfaces of the lower teeth.

(E) Other teeth pushed out of line (arrows)

FIGURE 25-22 Problems caused by impacted wisdom teeth.

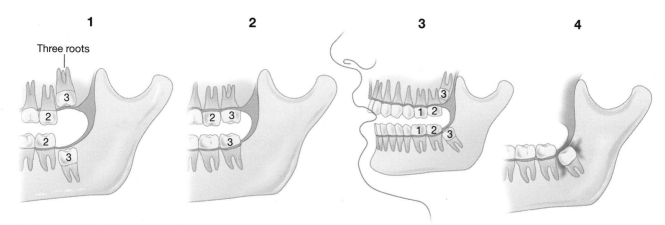

PROCEDURE 25-4

Removal of Impacted Third Molars

This procedure is performed by the oral surgeon, who is assisted by the dental assistant. This is a sterile procedure. Because the teeth are impacted, the surgeon will first have to expose the teeth by incising the tissue and removing the bone. The dental assistant transfers instruments and maintains the operating site.

EQUIPMENT AND SUPPLIES

- Basic setup: mouth mirror, explorer, and cotton pliers
- Gauze sponges
- Surgical HVE tip
- Irrigating syringe and sterile saline solution
- Retractor for the tongue and the cheek
- Local anesthetic setup
- Nitrous oxide setup (optional)
- Scalpel and blades
- Hemostat and tissue retractors

(continues)

PROCEDURE 25-4 *(CONTINUED)*

- Periosteal elevator
- Straight elevator
- Extraction forceps (if needed)
- Root tip picks
- Surgical curette
- Rongeurs
- Bone file
- Low-speed handpiece and surgical burs
- Surgical scissors
- Suture setup

PROCEDURE STEPS *(Follow aseptic procedures)*

1. The anesthetic is administered. Oral sedation may be used with local anesthetic, but the most common is intravenous (IV) anesthesia. The dental assistant prepares and transfers the anesthetic and/or assists with the IV.

2. When the patient is adequately anesthetized, an incision is made along the ridge, distal to the second molar. The scalpel incises the mucoperiosteum to the underlying bone. Depending on where the impacted tooth lies, a flap incision may be made to ensure adequate vision for the surgeon. The dental assistant transfers the scalpel and maintains the operating field with the surgical HVE (Figure 25-23A).

FIGURE 25-23 Steps to remove impacted third molars. (A) A flap incision is made; the assistant evacuates the area. (B) A periosteal elevator is used to retract the tissue. (C) A surgical bur is used to remove the bone over the tooth. The dental assistant evacuates and irrigates the area. (D) An elevator luxates and removes the tooth. (E) Sutures are placed. (F) The surgery is completed.

(continues)

PROCEDURE 2 5 - 4 *(CONTINUED)*

3. The periosteal elevator is used to retract the tissue from the alveolar bone. Once the tissue is incised, it must be reflected from the bone. The dental assistant transfers the periosteal elevator and evacuates. When the flap is completed, the dental assistant retracts the tissue (Figure 25-23B).

4. The surgeon uses a surgical bur and handpiece or a chisel and mallet to remove the bone over the tooth. The dental assistant receives the periosteal elevator and transfers the handpiece and bur or the chisel. The dental assistant continues to evacuate as needed (Figure 25-23C).

5. Once the tooth is exposed, it can often be luxated and lifted from the socket with elevators or forceps. If this is not possible, the tooth may be sectioned or divided for removal. This involves dividing the tooth into two or more parts. Burs and/or the chisel are used to separate the tooth in half to remove part or all of the crown of the tooth from the root portion. The dental assistant passes elevators and forceps. The dental assistant keeps the area clear with the HVE and periodically transfers the surgeon new gauze (Figure 25-23D).

6. When the tooth is removed, it is placed on a flat surface and examined to ensure that all of the tooth has been removed.

7. Curettes are used to remove the follicle (sac of thickened membrane) and debride the socket. The rongeurs, bone files, or burs may be used to contour the bone margins. The area is then irrigated with sterile water and evacuated. The dental assistant transfers instruments and removes debris from the working ends with gauze. The dental assistant prepares the irrigating syringe with sterile water and evacuates the area thoroughly.

8. The tissue flap is replaced to its normal position over the wound, and the operator sutures the area. The dental assistant prepares the suture and places it in the needle holder and transfers it to the oral surgeon. The cheeks are then retracted so that the surgeon can place the sutures (Figure 25-23E and F). The dental assistant has a folded moist gauze ready to place when suturing is completed.

9. The patient is allowed to recover and is given postoperative instructions, an ice pack, and a prescription for pain before being dismissed. The patient will need to schedule an appointment for suture removal in five to seven days. The dental assistant stays with the patient during recovery. When the patient is ready to leave, the dental assistant notifies the patient's escort and verifies that the patient has the necessary prescription(s) and postoperative instructions.

---

techniques: excisional, incisional, and exfoliative. (See Procedure 25-5.)

The Incisional Biopsy. The **incisional biopsy** involves removal of a small section of the lesion, which includes a small border of normal tissue (Figure 25-24A). This technique is often performed on lesions larger than 1 cm in all dimensions, where total removal is more difficult and patient appearance and function are impaired.

The Excisional Biopsy. The **excisional biopsy** involves removal of the lesion completely, including a border of the normal tissue surrounding it (Figure 25-24B). The excisional biopsy is performed for smaller lesions, such as fibromas. Total removal of the lesions does not interfere with the patient's appearance or functioning.

The Exfoliative Cytology. The **exfoliative cytology**, or "smear biopsy," involves removal of a layer of cells from the surface of the lesion. This is a nonsurgical procedure in which the gathered cells are spread on a glass slab. This technique is used as an adjunct to the surgical biopsy techniques and is also performed by an oral surgeon.

One way this procedure is done in many dental offices is by using the **oral brush biopsy**. This technique involves using a small sterile brush to "wipe" the sur-

face of the lesion firmly enough to remove the overlying keratin layer until pink tissue or pinpoint bleeding is evident. A kit available to dental offices contains everything needed to perform the biopsy and to prepare it for sending to the lab for computer-assisted analysis. These kits are used to test for dysplasia or cancer of oral lesions with abnormal epithelium (Figure 25-25).

Dental Implant Surgery

Dental implant technology has been around for more than 25 years and is becoming an increasingly popular choice for replacing missing teeth. Patients with one tooth, partial, or even all teeth missing may benefit from implants.

Dental implants have a great success rate, with the variance in success coming from where the implants are placed and what they do. For example, the anterior teeth success rate ranges from 90 to 100%, while the posterior teeth success rate ranges from 85 to 95%. Success also depends on the "load" that the implant carries; for example, with a denture the stress might be greater.

Implant failures are rare and usually can be corrected. The following are reasons implants may fail:

PROCEDURE 25-5

Biopsy

This procedure is performed by the oral surgeon, who is assisted by the dental assistant. The dental assistant readies all materials that are sent to the laboratory as well as the tray setup.

EQUIPMENT AND SUPPLIES

- Mouth mirror
- Local anesthetic setup
- Retractors (tongue, cheek, and tissue)
- Gauze sponges
- Surgical HVE tip
- Scalpel and blades
- Tissue scissors and hemostat
- Small container with a preservative solution, such as formalin
- Suture setup

PROCEDURE STEPS *(Follow aseptic procedures)*

1. The patient is anesthetized with local anesthetic.

2. A scalpel blade is used to incise or excise the lesion and a border of normal tissue. The dental assistant transfers the scalpel with the specific blade the surgeon prefers and has the HVE ready for use, if necessary. The dental assistant uses caution to remove only blood and saliva and not the tissue being removed for biopsy.

3. Tissue forceps are used to lift the biopsy specimen once freed from the underlying tissue and to place it in a small, covered container. The dental assistant retracts the cheeks and tongue, if needed, and uses gauze to control hemorrhage. The dental assistant has the specimen container ready for the surgeon. Care is taken not to touch the outside of the specimen container in order to prevent contamination. Once the tissue biopsy is placed in the container, the dental assistant replaces the cap tightly.

4. The biopsy site is closed with sutures. The surgeon then prepares the biopsy and the necessary information to be sent to the pathology laboratory. The dental assistant assists during the placement of sutures by transferring the suture needle and thread on needle forceps, retracting tissues, and transferring the suture scissors.

5. The patient is dismissed and scheduled for an appointment in one week for the results of the biopsy and suture removal. The dental assistant gives the patient postoperative instructions. The dental assistant gathers the pertinent information and prepares the biopsy container for pick-up by the pathology laboratory.

- Soft and/or hard tissues may have infections or inflammation that did not heal.
- Implant fails to integrate.
- Implant fractures or breaks.
- There is damage to the nerve in the mandible.
- There is damage to the maxillary sinus or nasal cavity.

The implant is a metal screw, cylinder, or metal framework that is surgically placed in the jawbone (Figure 25-26). Most often, the metal is titanium because it is compatible with human tissue. The implant fuses with the bone tissue through a biologic bonding process. This process is called **osseointegration**. Osseointegration usually takes three to six months following surgery.

Once the implant has begun to integrate and become stable in the bone, a fixed or removable prosthesis is fabricated. The prosthesis (artificial part) may be a single crown, a bridge, a partial, or a denture.

Considerations for Dental Implants. **Dental implants** give the option for a fixed restoration or removable appliance that provides function and esthetics. For patients with little bone to support a denture or a partial, many times the stability of the dental implants restores the patient's confidence and comfort and improves social interactions.

Patients considering dental implants should be in reasonably good overall health, have adequate jawbone that is healthy and strong, and have ample healing ability. Sometimes patients require bone grafting to build up the bone to ensure a successful dental implant. See Chapter 29, Periodontics, for information on bone grafting. The patient should also have a positive and cooperative attitude toward the implant treatment, be willing

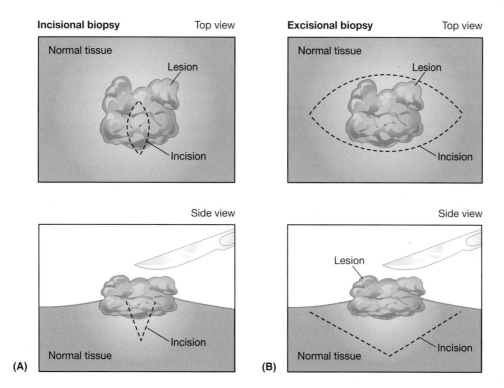

FIGURE 25-24 Biopsy techniques. (A) Incisional biopsy. (B) Excisional biopsy.

FIGURE 25-25 Oral CDX oral brush biopsy kit.

to follow all pre- and postoperative recommendations, and be dedicated to the care of the implants once they are in place.

Treatment Sequence. The success of dental implants depends on a coordinated team approach (surgical and restorative) and good patient cooperation. At present, it can take two to six months to complete all phases of the dental implant process. The process begins with the patient meeting with the restorative dentist. After a preliminary consultation, the restorative dentist refers the patient to the oral surgeon or periodontist. Some general dentists take additional specialized training to be able to do dental implants in their office. A diagnostic consultation is scheduled. Included in this appointment are panoramic and cephalometric radiographs,

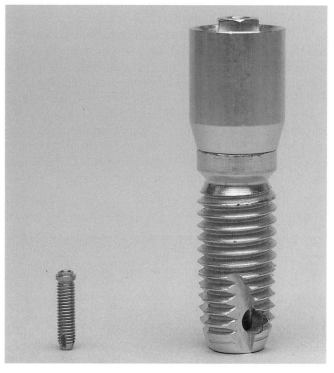

FIGURE 25-26 Dental implant system. (A) Actual implant size. (B) Model of the implant used to educate patients.

a medical and dental history review, an oral examination, and study casts. Study casts may also be used to fabricate a **surgical stint**. This stint is placed over the tissues during surgery to guide the dentist in placing the implant. The stint is made of clear acrylic and is sometimes called a template. At this time, the patient must also consider the time commitment, the expense of the procedures (implants are usually a little more expensive than traditional treatment), and the risks of a surgical procedure.

After the diagnosis is complete and the patient accepts the treatment plan, the patient completes the necessary consent forms, financial arrangements are completed, and treatment appointments are scheduled.

There are several techniques used today to place dental implants. Often one of the factors in selecting the technique is the amount of load the implant can tolerate and still be successful. The load is the amount of pressure or strain put on the implant once placed in the bone. Other factors include the dentist's preference and skill level.

There are usually two phases of treatment: surgical and restorative. The surgical phase includes:

In the **one-stage technique,** the implant is inserted into the bone but the extruding end is not covered with gingival tissue. The implant protrudes through the tissue and a healing cap is placed. There is no load on this implant during the healing time. The healing time is three to four months, during which the osseointegration process takes place.

In the **two-stage technique,** the implant is placed into the bone and gingival tissue is sutured into place to cover the implant. Sutures are removed in seven to ten days. If there is an old prosthesis (denture), it can be modified or relined by the restorative dentist so that the patient will not be without teeth during the three to four months of healing time. After the healing time, a second surgery is scheduled. During this surgery the implant is uncovered and checked for stability. If the implant is stable, a cap or abutment is placed. The cap protrudes out of the tissue. Once the soft tissues have healed, the crown, bridge, or other prosthesis can be fabricated and placed.

The restorative prosthetic phase includes the following:

1. Communication with the oral surgeon or the periodontist, if they placed the implant, and the patient before and during the surgical phase.

2. Taking impressions for the prosthesis to be placed over the implants.

3. Fabrication of the prosthesis (crown, bridge, partial, or denture).

4. Removal of the healing cap and placement of the prosthesis.

Types of Implants. The two most common types of dental implants include the subperiosteal and endosteal. A third type of implant called a mini (transitional) implant is also becoming very popular.

The **subperiosteal implant** is often used on patients whose dentures have failed because the alveolar bone has atrophied (wasted away). Subperiosteal implants are most commonly placed on the mandible. The titanium implant rests on top of the alveolar bone with abutment posts or bars above the mucoperiosteum in the cuspid and first molar area. The denture connects to this structure for support and retention (Figure 25-28).

The subperisoteal implant requires one or two surgeries, depending on the technique.

The single-surgery technique involves fabricating the impression for the implant on a model. The model is constructed by using computed tomography (CT) scans. After the implant is fabricated on the model, surgery is performed to incise the tissue and expose the alveolar bone. The implant is seated on the bone and the tissue is sutured back into place.

When using the *two-surgery technique,* during the first surgery the tissue is incised and the alveolar bone is exposed. Then an impression is taken. The impression is sent to the laboratory for the subperiosteal implant

FIGURE 25-27 Implants in place. *(Courtesy of Dr. Kenji W. Higuchi)*

FIGURE 25-28 Subperiosteal implant.

to be fabricated. Within a week, the patient returns to the office for the second surgery. The tissue is opened and the implant is seated. A transitional appliance is used while a final denture is made, which usually takes four to six weeks.

The **endosteal implants** (endosseous) are placed in the bone surgically. These implants are used to replace a single tooth and for patients who are partially or fully edentulous. The endosteal implants are placed when there is sufficient ridge width and at least 2 mm between the implant and the mandibular canal.

These implants are expensive, as is the equipment required to place them. There are two basic designs of the endosteal implants: the blade and the screw/cylinder. The screw implants come in a variety of shapes; they are straight or tapered as well as with or without threads (Figure 25-29).

The technique for endosteal implants is the one- or two-stage insertion (see Procedure 25-6). The endosteal implants are consistent and take into consideration the bone and the soft tissues.

The **mini (transitional) implants** were originally designed to be temporary implants to hold the restoration while the real implant heals. Today they are used on their own; these implants are easy to place and do not usually require an incision to be inserted. The best place for positioning these implants is the anterior of the mandible, but other areas work as long as there is sufficient bone height. The mini implants are smaller at around 2 mm in diameter, compared to regular implants, which are typically around 4 mm in diameter. They are used in many situations and work well to stabilize mandibular overdentures and for tooth replacement where the bone is narrow (Figure 25-30).

Postoperative Care and Home-Care Instructions. After implant surgery, the patient should follow these postoperative care instructions:

1. Only clear liquids should be taken during the first two days after surgery. Milk may be taken with medication. Blended/mashed food may be added after the second day. Smoking and alcoholic beverages should be avoided.

2. Softly biting for fifteen to thirty minutes on a gauze pad may control slight bleeding. If bleeding persists, contact the office.

3. Use extra pillows to elevate the head slightly during the first two nights after surgery.

4. Gently rinse the mouth with saline solution after each meal. Use no commercial mouth rinses.

5. Old dentures should not be worn until relining adjustments have been made.

(A)

(B)

(C)

FIGURE 25-29 Sample of endosteal implants. (A) The blade implant. (B, C) The screw/cylinder implant.

FIGURE 25-30 (A) and (B) The mini (transitional) implant placed during orthodontic treatment. (C) Panoramic radiograph showing the mini implants in place. *(Courtesy of Dr. Kenji W. Higuchi)*

PROCEDURE 25-6

Dental Implant Surgery

The following procedure is for the placement of an endosteal implant to replace a single tooth. This is the two-stage procedure in which appointments are scheduled three to four months apart. During the presurgery appointment, the treatment is explained in detail and the patient signs a written consent for the implant surgery. Radiographs are taken, impressions for diagnostic casts are made, surgical stent templates are fabricated, and financial arrangements are completed. The patient is given intravenous sedation for this procedure.

EQUIPMENT AND SUPPLIES (Figure 25-31)

For first surgical procedure:
- Intravenous sedation and local anesthetic setup
- Mouth mirror

- Surgical HVE tip
- Sterile gauze and cotton pellets
- Irrigation syringe and sterile saline solution
- Low-speed handpiece
- Sterile template
- Sterile surgical drilling unit
- Scalpel and blades
- Periosteal elevator
- Rongeurs
- Surgical currette
- Tissue forceps and scissors

(continues)

PROCEDURE 25-6 *(CONTINUED)*

(A)

(B)

FIGURE 25-31 (A) Tray setup for implant surgery. (B) Surgical barrier kit.

- Cheek and tongue retractors
- Hemostat
- Bite-block
- Oral rinse
- Betadine

- Implant instrument kit
- Implant kit
- Suture setup

For second surgical procedure:

- First seven items from first procedure
- Electrosurgical (cautery) unit and tips (Figure 25-32)
- Hydrogen peroxide

PROCEDURE STEPS

First Surgery for Endosteal Implants

1. The patient is prepared and IV sedation is administered. Local anesthetic is administered. The dental assistant prepares and assists during the administration of sedation and anesthetic.

2. The surgical template (stint) is seated in the patient's mouth. The target is marked through the template into the soft tissues.

3. The template is removed and the surgeon incises the tissue to expose the ridge of bone. The dental assistant prepares and transfers the scalpel and blade while maintaining the operating site.

4. A periosteal elevator is used to reflect the overlying tissues. Special spiral burs are used to prepare for the implant. The dental assistant changes burs as size increases and irrigates with the sterile saline solution.

FIGURE 25-32 Electrosurge cauterizing unit.

(continues)

PROCEDURE 25-6 *(CONTINUED)*

5. The implant is partially placed and then tapped or threaded into position. The dental assistant opens the sterile implant and transfers it to the surgeon. A special inserting mallet or ratchet wrench is transferred, and the dental assistant readies the healing cap and contra-angle screwdriver.

6. A healing cap is screwed into the implant. The dental assistant passes the healing cap and the contra-angle screwdriver (Figure 25-33). At this point in the one-stage implant technique, the healing cap is left exposed in the mouth. The patient does not see the dentist for three to four months while the osseointegration takes place. Then the patient sees the oral surgeon or periodontist for a final examination. If the

implant is stable, the patient returns to the dentist and final impressions are taken for the restoration to be fabricated.

7. Once the implant and healing cap are positioned, the flap is repositioned and sutured.

8. The patient is allowed to recover and given postoperative instructions.

Second Surgical Procedure

1. Local anesthetic is administered.

2. The template is positioned over the osseointegrated implant and a sharp-pointed instrument is used to mark the site. The dental assistant transfers the sterile template and a sharp-pointed instrument.

3. The template is removed and the soft tissue is excised with an electrosurgical loop. Once the healing screw is exposed, it is removed. The dental assistant receives the template and evacuates as the electrosurgical loop is used. Once the tissue is excised, the dental assistant receives the healing screw in a gauze sponge.

4. The inside of the implant is cleaned with hydrogen peroxide on a sterile cotton pellet. The dental assistant prepares the cotton pellet and transfers it to the surgeon.

5. The implant abutment is placed so that it extends slightly beyond the mucosa. The mucosa is then sutured around the abutment. The abutment is transferred to the surgeon and then the dental assistant prepares the suture material and assists during the suturing.

6. The patient is given postoperative instructions and is dismissed.

FIGURE 25-33 Implant placement procedures for (A) first-stage and (B) second-stage surgery for an endosteal implant.

6. Take daily requirements of vitamin C, D, B complex, and calcium.

7. If there are any questions or concerns about the healing process, contact the office.

Once the second surgery is completed, the exposed portion of the dental implant must be kept clean. The patient must perform daily hygiene maintenance on the implant and prosthesis. The instruments and techniques for implant hygiene are discussed in Chapter 30, Fixed Prosthodontics. The patient should also have routine dental examinations to evaluate the implants along with the rest of the mouth.

Postoperative Care of the Patient

Following oral surgery, the patient is given postoperative home-care instructions. The instructions are given routinely by a dental assistant at the direction of the surgeon. The dental assistant gives the instructions verbally to the patient and the patient's escort. In addition, a written copy of the instructions with the office phone number is given to the patient, along with necessary prescriptions.

Postoperative Home-Care Instructions

It is important to carefully read and follow postoperative home-care instructions to prevent needless worry. Have someone with you for twenty-four hours following the surgery. Treatment continues until the healing process is completed.

What to expect:

1. **Discomfort** reaches a peak when the anesthetic wears off and sensation returns.
2. **Swelling** is normal following a surgical procedure. The swelling will continue up to twenty-four hours after surgery and can persist for four to five days. Facial discoloration may appear but will disappear in a day or so.
3. **Bleeding** or oozing may occur for the first twelve to twenty-four hours after surgery. The surgeon will place a sterile gauze in your mouth to bite on immediately following surgery. Remove the gauze when the oozing has stopped.
4. **Difficulty opening mouth, a sore throat,** and **earaches** are not uncommon, especially if third molars were removed.

What to do:

1. Begin taking pain medication before the discomfort begins and the anesthetic wears off. Over-the-counter analgesics are suggested for minor discomfort, and the surgeon will prescribe a stronger medication for pain control, if necessary. Take medications as directed to avoid nausea and vomiting.
2. Use an ice pack to reduce the swelling as soon as possible. Apply the pack to the face over the extraction site for twenty minutes, and then remove for twenty minutes (twenty minutes on, twenty minutes off). Continue this cycle intermittently throughout the first twelve to twenty-four hours. After forty-eight hours if the swelling has not subsided, use moist heat.
3. The best means to control bleeding is pressure. To accomplish the pressure needed, place a folded gauze over the surgical site and bite down. Change the sterile gauze pads as needed. If the bleeding persists, insert a wet tea bag over the surgical site and bite down for about twenty minutes. Tea contains tannic acid, which assists in the clotting process.
4. A soft diet should be followed for twenty-four hours. Eat a well-balanced diet with soups, fruit juices, milk shakes, and other foods, as tolerated. Drink fluids to prevent dehydration and temperature elevation.
5. Take medications as directed to prevent infection.
6. Continue brushing and flossing areas not involved in surgery.
7. Sleep with your head elevated to reduce swelling.
8. Avoid vigorous physical exercise.
9. Rest as much as possible for the first couple of days following surgery to promote healing.

Things to avoid:

1. Avoid strenuous physical activity for forty-eight hours.
2. Do not suck through a straw and avoid spitting.
3. Do not smoke or chew gum.
4. Do not drive, drink alcohol, or operate machinery while taking pain medication.
5. If immediate dentures have been inserted, do not remove until your next appointment, usually within twenty-four hours of surgery.
6. Do not rinse vigorously for forty-eight hours after surgery. After this time, rinse gently with warm salt-water solution.

If you have any questions or problems, please call the office.

Dr. _____ Telephone # _____

Postsurgical Complications

Alveolitis (alveolar osteitis), or **dry socket**, is the most common complication following an extraction. The loss of blood clot leaves a dry socket, which is painful. Alveolitis usually develops between the third and the fifth day after surgery. In the normal process after an extraction, blood oozes into the socket and begins clotting. The clot is later replaced by connective tissue and eventually bone tissue. In some extractions, this process does not happen and the blood clot either does not form or forms and is lost. The exact etiology for this phenomenon is not clear, but insufficient blood supply to the area, infection, or trauma seem to play roles. The mandibular third molars seem to be the most frequent sites for dry socket.

The signs are extreme pain, foul breath and taste, exposed bone, and an empty socket. Procedure 25-7 describes the treatment for alveolitis.

Temporomandibular Joint Disease

The temporomandibular joint (TMJ) is made of muscles, bones, and joints of the jaw (refer to Chapter 7, Head and Neck Anatomy). These structures work closely together

PROCEDURE 25-7

Treatment for Alveolitis

This procedure is performed by the oral surgeon who is assisted by the dental assistant.

EQUIPMENT AND SUPPLIES (Figure 25-34)

- Mouth mirror
- Surgical HVE tip
- Local anesthetic setup (may be required)
- Surgical scissors
- Surgical curettes
- Irrigating syringe and warm sterile saline solution
- Iodoform gauze or sponge

PROCEDURE STEPS *(Follow aseptic procedures)*

1. Anesthetic may be administered. The sutures are removed.

2. The surgeon may gently curettage the area inside the socket to stimulate the formation of a new blood clot.

3. The alveolus (socket) is gently irrigated with the warm saline solution. The dental assistant prepares the syringe and maintains the area by retraction and evacuation.

4. The alveolus is gently packed with a medicated dressing. Narrow strips of iodoform gauze or iodoform sponge are used for packing the socket. The dental assistant prepares and transfers the materials to the surgeon for placement (Figure 25-35).

5. The surgeon prescribes medication for pain control, and the patient is scheduled to return in one to two days to repeat this process.

FIGURE 25-34 Tray setup for alveolitis treatment.

FIGURE 25-35 Examples of iodoform gauze and sponge packing materials. The dental assistant prepares to pass the gauze packing.

to make it possible to chew, speak, and swallow without discomfort. When these structures do not work together correctly, TMJ disease/dysfunction/disorder occurs. Other causes of TMJ problems include accidents, oral habits such as clenching or grinding the teeth (bruxism) (Figure 25-36), or disease such as arthritis.

Signs and Symptoms of TMJ Dysfunction

There are many signs and symptoms of TMJ disease/dysfunction/disorder. The most common are:

- Pain around the ear, which often radiates into the face
- Tenderness of the masticatory muscles

Compressed joint
Compressed, thinning disk
Tightened muscles
Clenched and worn teeth
Muscles of mastication tighten

FIGURE 25-36 Clenched teeth and tightened muscles cause TMJ disc to compress.

- Popping and clicking noise when opening or closing the mouth
- **Crepitus** (crackling sound) or **tinnitus** (ringing or tinkling sound)
- Limited mandibular movement when opening
- **Trismus** (limited opening of the mouth)
- Headaches or neckaches

Diagnosing TMJ Dysfunction

Diagnosis is an important step in TMJ treatment. A medical and dental evaluation should be completed to ensure the appropriate treatment. Diagnostic procedures may include:

- Complete dental and medical history to gather information about the patient's symptoms, overall health, and family history. The patient may be asked about stress, teeth grinding or clenching, diseases that may affect joint function, bite problems, or any injuries to the joint area.
- Physical examination of the joint, including palpating (touching) the muscles and jaw, listening for sounds as the jaw opens and closes, and measuring how wide the patient can open the mouth.
- Tomographic radiographs and magnetic resonance imaging (MRI) may be taken (see Chapter 22, Production and Evaluation of Dental Radiographs, and Chapter 23, Extraoral and Digital Radiography).
- Dental study casts (models) of the teeth, which help the dentist evaluate the patient's bite and occlusion. The study casts may be articulated so jaw movements can be simulated.

Treatment Options for TMJ Dysfunction

Once the evaluation process is complete, the dentist will decide which type of treatment the patient needs. Often, treatment involves several phases. Sometimes, only minor treatment may be needed, but if discomfort and other symptoms continue, a more involved treatment may be required. If the patient is unresponsive to treatment options, surgery may be advised.

Treatment options include:

- Alternately applying ice and heat to the TMJ area.
- Learning to rest the jaw.
- Medication, such as pain reliever, muscle relaxant, antibiotics, and/or nonsteroidal anti-inflammatory agent, or mood-elevator medications and/or anti-anxiety medication may be prescribed.
- Stress management, including relaxation techniques and biofeedback consultation.
- Physical therapy for jaw exercises, massage, good posture training, electrical stimulation, and ultrasound.
- Occlusal splint to relieve muscle spasms, balance the bite, relieve pressure on the joint, protect teeth from wear, and prevent grinding.
- Orthodontic treatment and restorative treatment may need to be completed.
- Intra-articular steroid injections.
- Arthrocentesis, which uses small needles to rinse the joint.
- Arthroscopic surgery, in which a tiny instrument (arthroscope) is inserted through a small incision to remove adhesions and place anti-inflammatory agents.
- Open joint surgery, which repairs severe soft tissue damage and restructures the joints.

Hospital Dentistry

Most procedures are performed in the oral maxillofacial surgeon's office, but some cases require a hospital setting. The surgeon follows the protocol of the hospital to meet scheduling, staffing, and credentialing standards.

Some hospitals allow dental assistants to assist oral surgeons, after the dental assistants meet hospital standards on asepsis and operating room protocol.

Patients who require hospitalization for dental treatment include:

- Trauma victims with facial and jaw fractures

- Patients with high-risk conditions or diseases (e.g., heart disease or diabetes)
- Patients with mental or physical disabilities who could not tolerate surgery in an office setting
- Patients who require extensive surgical procedures such as TMJ surgery or orthognathic surgery

ADVANCED CHAIRSIDE FUNCTIONS

Suture Removal

Sutures hold displaced or incised tissue in its original position; they close the wound to promote healing and limit contamination by bacteria and food debris. The dental assistant assists the dentist in the placement of sutures and observes the type and number of sutures, and then records this information on the patient's chart for later reference. In five to seven days, the patient returns to the office for the sutures to be removed. In some states, qualified dental assistants are allowed to remove the sutures under the supervision of the dentist. It is the responsibility of the dental assistant to gain the knowledge and the experience necessary to perform this task to the highest standard. The dentist must be aware of the patient's status and be notified immediately if diagnostic decisions are required.

Procedures Prior to Removal of Sutures

Prior to the suture removal, several steps and considerations are necessary to ensure patient comfort and safety. Included are preparing the equipment and supplies, reviewing the patient's chart, evaluating the suture site, and consulting with the dentist.

Prepare Suture Removal Equipment and Supplies. Before the patient's appointment, the tray is set up with the following items: mouth mirror, explorer, cotton pliers, suture scissors, gauze sponges, air-water syringe tip, and evacuator. This is a sterile procedure, so all aseptic guidelines are followed.

Review the Patient's Chart. After the patient has been seated and before the procedure has begun, check the patient's chart for information concerning the sutures. Ask the patient if any problems had occurred with the sutures since the last appointment.

Examine the Suture Site. Check the suture site for the following:

1. Location of the sutures
2. Number of sutures
3. Type or pattern of sutures
4. Healing of tissues in the wound area

Healing of the tissues depends on a number of factors, including the extent of the wound, the healing capabilities of the patient, whether a periodontal dressing was applied, and the amount of healing time. To evaluate the healing process, the dental assistant should debride (remove debris from) the suture site. Once the tissues have been cleaned, the suture site is evaluated for progress of healing and signs of infection. See Table 25-1 for descriptions of what to look for in the suture area.

TABLE 25-1   Suture Site Healing Signs

Size of Wound	Appearance
Large area for flap or multiple extractions without a periodontal dressing	Area is slightly red with granulation tissue present, but no infection.
Large area for flap or multiple extractions with a periodontal dressing	Area appears slightly red with granulation tissue present. A milky film is seen where the dressing was placed.
Small area for minor surgery without a periodontal dressing placed	Area appears almost healed, with dark pink granulation tissue and no inflammation.
Any size of wound that is red and inflamed, tender, and has some bleeding	This wound is infected or irritated or has not had enough time to heal.

ADVANCED CHAIRSIDE FUNCTIONS

Ways to Debride the Suture Site

1. Use light air and a warm water spray.
2. Use a cotton-tip applicator moistened with warm water or diluted hydrogen peroxide.
3. Use a moist cotton gauze to gently dab the suture site.

Consult with the Dentist. The dental assistant should always consult with the dentist when removing sutures. After the patient has been seated, the dental assistant should check the healing of the suture site and identify the correct number of sutures to be removed. Consult with the dentist prior to suture removal for instructions, especially if there is anything unusual in the healing process or sutures cannot be located.

Types of Suture Patterns

To remove sutures, it is necessary to understand how the sutures are placed. There are several basic patterns, although dentists may vary their suturing techniques depending on the procedure and the patient. Detailed charting when the sutures are placed will help the dental assistant during suture removal. Most sutures are tied with simple square knots, referred to as surgeon's knots. The dental assistant should ask the dentist to place a variety of sutures in a tissue simulation, such as cotton rolls rolled into 2 × 2 gauze or dental dam material, to practice suture removal.

Simple Suture. The simple suture is the most widely used suture stitch, is very versatile, and is used in many areas of the mouth (see Figure 25-37 for steps the dentist follows to place the simple suture). Once the suture is placed, it is tied with a surgeon's knot.

Continuous Simple Suture. The continuous simple suture is placed when there have been multiple extractions (Figure 25-38). This series of sutures looks like hem stitching, with a surgeon's knot at either end. The number of stitches depends on the wound site.

Sling Suture. The sling suture is used for interproximal suturing (Figure 25-39). When a flap has been necessary, the sling suture is especially useful. An example of when a sling suture would be used is on the facial surface of the tissue. The suture needle and thread are inserted through the tissue on the facial surface (distal-facial of the tooth), and then the thread is wrapped around the lingual of the tooth, where the needle and thread are placed through the facial tissue on the opposite side of the tooth (mesial-facial). The thread is then wrapped back around the lingual of the tooth and a surgeon's knot is used to secure the suture.

Continuous Sling Suture. The continuous sling suture is placed where a large flap involving several teeth has been used (Figure 25-40). This suture involves the same steps as with the single sling, except the suture thread is wrapped around to the next tooth instead of back to the beginning side. When the tissue has been secured interproximally of each tooth involved, the suture is tied off (see Figure 25-40 and 25-41 for a continuous sling suture securing the facial tissue of several teeth).

Mattress Sutures. Mattress sutures also are used when a flap is to be sutured. The difference between the simple and the mattress sutures is that the simple suture goes into the facial surface and then emerges from the lingual surface, while the mattress sutures go in and out of the tissue on the same surface. For example, on the facial surface, the suture goes into and comes back out of the tissue on the same surface. If the stitch, or bite, is taken horizontally, it is a horizontal mattress suture (Figure

Step 1   Step 2   Step 3   Step 4

FIGURE 25-37 Simple suture pattern.

ADVANCED CHAIRSIDE FUNCTIONS

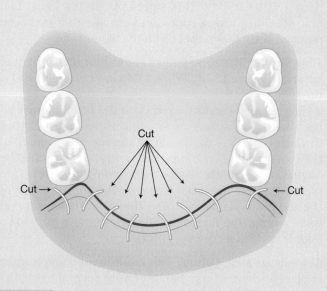

FIGURE 25-38 Continuous simple suture pattern with removable cuts.

25-42A). If the stitch is taken vertically, it is a **vertical mattress suture** (Figure 25-42B). With the mattress sutures, the same stitch is taken on the facial and lingual. The mattress sutures are tied with one surgeon's knot on the surface where the suture procedure began.

Suture Removal Criteria

The following are basic criteria to guide the dental assistant when removing sutures:

- Explain the procedure to the patient.
- The healing process should not be disturbed when removing the sutures.
- The suture is removed with the least amount of trauma to the tissues.
- All sutures are removed from the suture site.
- The knot is not cut.
- The suture is cut as closely to the tissue as possible.
- A suture that has been exposed in the mouth is not pulled through the tissue. (This suture is contaminated with saliva, food, and bacteria.)

FIGURE 25-39 Sling suture pattern.

ADVANCED CHAIRSIDE FUNCTIONS

FIGURE 25-40 Continuous sling suture pattern.

FIGURE 25-41 Patient with sutures in place. *(Courtesy of Dr. Kenji W. Higuchi)*

- ■ The knot is not pulled through the tissue.
- ■ The hemorrhage is controlled following established procedures.
- ■ The sutures are placed on a gauze so they can be counted.

Suture Removal

Each type of suture is placed in a specific pattern. To remove the sutures, identify the pattern and determine where the cuts are to be made. Then, follow the basic criteria and remove the sutures from the suture site. (See Procedures 25-8 through 25-10.)

Post-Suture Removal

If there was bleeding when the sutures were removed, apply pressure with gauze sponge for a few minutes until the bleeding stops. Check the patient's mouth for any debris, and wipe around the outside of the patient's mouth if necessary. After the sutures are removed, the dental assistant should instruct the patient to continue with a soft diet and rinse with warm saltwater for several days. Before the patient is dismissed, the dental assistant should document the procedure on the patient's chart. The chart entry should include any complications encountered and the degree of healing of the suture site. The dentist should examine the patient after the sutures are removed.

Summary of Suture Removal Steps

1. Review patient's chart and medical history.
2. Prepare armamentarium.
3. Seat the patient.
4. Explain the procedure and ask whether the patient has had any problems or has any questions.
5. Examine the suture site for healing.
6. Check the number and type of sutures.
7. Consult with the dentist.
8. Debride the suture site to prepare for suture removal.
9. Evaluate the sutures to determine where to make the cuts.
10. Gently secure and lift the sutures to position for cutting.
11. Using suture scissors or sharp, pointed surgical scissors, cut the sutures.

ADVANCED CHAIRSIDE FUNCTIONS

FIGURE 25-42 (A) Horizontal mattress suture pattern. (B) Vertical mattress suture pattern.

12. Remove the sutures and place on a gauze.
13. Blot the suture area if there is blood.
14. Count the sutures on the gauze.
15. Instruct the patient regarding care of the suture area.

16. Document the procedure on the patient's chart.
17. Call the dentist to check the patient.
18. Dismiss the patient.

PROCEDURE 25-8

Removal of Simple and Continuous Simple Sutures

This procedure is performed by the dentist or the expanded-function dental assistant. The patient returns to the office for suture removal. The dental assistant prepares the materials needed and the patient before beginning the procedure.

EQUIPMENT AND SUPPLIES

- Basic setup: mouth mirror, explorer, cotton pliers
- Suture scissors
- Hemostat
- Gauze sponges
- Air-water syringe tip, HVE tip

PROCEDURE STEPS *(Follow aseptic procedures)*

1. Using cotton pliers, gently lift the suture away from the tissues.

2. Take the suture scissors and cut the thread below the knot, close to the tissue.

3. Secure the knot with the cotton pliers and gently pull, lifting the suture out of the tissues.

4. Place the suture on a gauze sponge.

5. For continuous simple sutures, cut each suture and remove individually. Begin with one end and then proceed with each suture stitch.

(continues)

ADVANCED CHAIRSIDE FUNCTIONS

6. Loosen the suture with the cotton pliers and, while still holding the suture thread with the cotton pliers, cut the thread close to the tissue (Figure 25-43).

7. As each suture is removed, place it on a gauze sponge so it can be counted when finished with the procedure.

> Always carefully evaluate the sutures before cutting them to be sure sutures exposed in the oral cavity are not pulled through the tissue during removal.

FIGURE 25-43 Removal of simple and continuous simple sutures.

PROCEDURE 25-9

Removal of Sling and Continuous Sling Sutures

This procedure is performed by the dentist or the expanded-function dental assistant. The patient returns to the office for suture removal. The dental assistant prepares the materials needed and the patient before beginning the procedure.

PROCEDURE STEPS *(Follow aseptic procedures)*

1. The sling suture is cut in two places. With cotton pliers, lift the suture gently on each side of the tooth to loosen the suture from the tissue (Figure 25-44A and B).

2. Lift the knot gently and cut below the knot, near the tissue.

3. Lift the suture thread on the other side of the tooth, near the tissue, and cut it as close to the tissue as possible without cutting the tissue.

NOTE: When removing a continuous sling suture, this process is repeated, cutting on each side of the tooth until all sutures have been removed.

4. Using cotton pliers, remove each thread carefully, pulling toward the opposite surface, away from the flap. For example, if the suture is taken on the facial and wrapped around the lingual, pull toward the lingual to remove the sutures.

(continues)

ADVANCED CHAIRSIDE FUNCTIONS

5. Place each thread of the suture on a gauze sponge to be counted.

6. Examine the suture site.

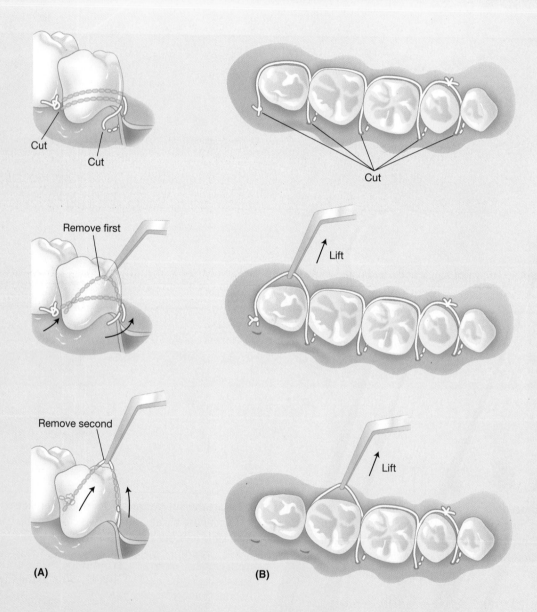

(A)   **(B)**

FIGURE 25-44 Removal of (A) sling and (B) continuous sling sutures.

ADVANCED CHAIRSIDE FUNCTIONS

PROCEDURE 25-10

Removal of Horizontal and Vertical Mattress Sutures

This procedure is performed by the dentist or the expanded-function dental assistant. The patient returns to the office for suture removal. The dental assistant prepares the materials needed and the patient before beginning the procedure.

PROCEDURE STEPS *(Follow aseptic procedures)*

Although the horizontal and vertical mattress sutures are placed differently, the basic placement steps are the same. This also holds true for their removal. Two cuts are made with each mattress suture, one on each side of the suture stitch (see Figure 25-45A for the horizontal mattress and Figure 25-45B for the vertical mattress).

1. Gently lift the knot with cotton pliers.

2. Cut the suture below the knot, close to the tissue.

3. Make the second cut on the opposite surface, close to the tissue.

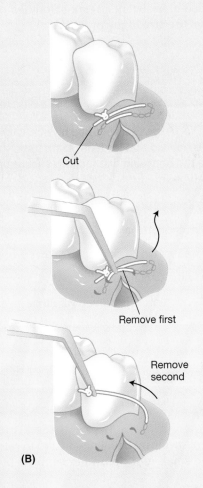

FIGURE 25-45 Removal of (A) horizontal mattress suture and (B) vertical mattress suture.

(continues)

ADVANCED CHAIRSIDE FUNCTIONS

PROCEDURE 25-10 *(CONTINUED)*

4. Remove one piece of the suture by holding the knot with the cotton pliers and lifting gently. Place it on a gauze sponge.

5. Remove the remaining suture thread.

6. Count pieces of the suture.

7. Examine the suture site.

CHAPTER SUMMARY

The dental surgery team may vary according to the surgeon's goals for the practice. In addition to the oral and maxillofacial surgeon, the team usually consists of the receptionist, the business office staff, the dental assistants, and, in some offices, a nurse or an anesthesiologist.

The surgical dental assistant's responsibilities often vary depending on the size of the practice.

Case Study

Josiah Scott, forty-five years old, had his maxillary first molar removed a few years ago. The patient is experiencing no pain but has noticed that his teeth seem to be shifting. The adjacent teeth are rotating into the space left by the first molar, and the opposing first molar is supererupting. Mr. Scott is scheduled for an examination by Dr. Manwell, who is an oral surgeon.

Case Study Review

1. Why would Mr. Scott make an appointment with an oral surgeon?

2. Which procedure would correct Mr. Scott's problem?

3. What would the dental assistant need to prepare for the examination appointment?

4. Which other dental professionals would be involved in Mr. Scott's treatment?

REVIEW QUESTIONS

Multiple Choice

1. Which of the following instruments is used to retract tissue, remove small root tips, and clamp off blood vessels?
   a. Needle holder
   b. Hemostat
   c. Tissue retractor
   d. Surgical curette

2. For which teeth are "cow-horn" forceps used to extract?
   a. Maxillary bicuspids
   b. Maxillary molars
   c. Mandibular bicuspids
   d. Mandibular molars

3. During surgical handwashing, the dental assistant scrubs with a scrub brush and then repeats the process with soap but without the scrub brush. How long does it take to complete this process?
   a. Fifteen seconds
   b. Thirty seconds
   c. One minute
   d. Five minutes

4. Before the surgery is scheduled but after the patient's records and examination are completed, the patient must
   a. sign an informed consent.
   b. sign a waiver from the patient's general dentist.
   c. register with the oral surgeon's office.
   d. bring proof of identification to the oral surgeon's office.

5. Which of the following biopsy techniques is non-surgical and is used as an adjunct to the other surgical techniques?
   a. Incisional biopsy
   b. Excisional biopsy
   c. Exfoliative cytology
   d. None of the above

6. Which of the following instruments comes in sizes #11, #12, and #15?
   a. Surgical curettes
   b. Needle holders
   c. Surgical bone files
   d. Surgical scalpel blades

7. This instrument is hinged and is used to trim and shape the alveolar bone after extractions.
   a. Periosteal elevator
   b. Rongeurs
   c. Apical elevators
   d. Extraction forceps

8. An alveoplasty is
   a. a surgical procedure to remove teeth from the alveolar bone.
   b. a surgical procedure to remove impacted teeth from the alveolar bone.
   c. a surgical procedure to contour and smooth the alveolar bone after several teeth have been extracted.
   d. a surgical procedure to remove tissue from a suspicious area, either totally or partially, for microscopic examination and diagnosis.

9. When a dental implant fuses with the bone tissue through a biologic bonding process, it is called an
   a. osseointegration
   b. alveoectomy
   c. alveolitis
   d. ostectomy

10. When removing sutures, follow all these statements except:
    a. Do not cut the suture knot.
    b. Do not pull the suture thread that was exposed in the oral cavity through the tissues.
    c. Cut the suture thread away from the tissues as far as possible.
    d. Place all sutures removed on a gauze following removal.

Critical Thinking

1. Why are the maxillary forceps designed for the left or the right quadrant and the mandibular forceps are not?

2. If a patient is having multiple extractions in preparation for a full denture, identify and explain the procedure that immediately follows the extractions.

3. List the dental assistant's responsibilities during surgical procedures.

4. When does the dental assistant have the dentist come in and check a patient having sutures removed?

5. List several questions the dental assistant may ask the patient who is experiencing pain or discomfort in the temporomandibular joint (TMJ) area?

6. Explain several considerations for dental implants as a treatment choice.

Web Activities

1. Visit http://www.enexus.com/dental-implant and learn more about dental implants by going to a dental office that offers this service through the patient's perspective as well as through the doctor/staff perspective.

2. Go to http://www.healthlinkusa.com and find links to Web sites that may include prevention, treatments, support groups, e-mail lists, message boards, personal stories, and more.

3. Find patient information pamphlets on various aspects of oral surgery treatments at http://aaoms.org. Click on Patient Information and then Public Information.

ORAL PATHOLOGY

SPECIFIC INSTRUCTIONAL OBJECTIVES

The student should strive to meet the following objectives and demonstrate an understanding of the facts and principles presented in this chapter:

1. Define oral pathology and identify the dental assistant's role in this specialty.

2. Characterize the process of inflammation.

3. Identify oral lesions according to placement.

4. Identify oral diseases and lesions related to biological agents.

5. Describe oral diseases and lesions related to physical agents.

6. Identify oral diseases and lesions related to chemical agents.

7. Identify oral conditions related to hormonal disturbances.

8. Identify oral conditions related to developmental disturbances.

9. Distinguish among oral conditions related to nutritional disturbances.

10. Identify the conditions and lesions of oral neoplasms.

11. Identify oral lesions related to HIV and AIDS.

12. Describe the conditions related to miscellaneous disorders affecting the oral cavity.

KEY TERMS

abscess *(569)*

actinomycosis *(569)*

amalgam tattoo *(572)*

amelogenesis imperfecta *(576)*

angular cheilitis *(579)*

ankyloglossia *(578)*

ankylosis *(576)*

anodontia *(576)*

antigenic *(567)*

aphthous ulcers *(570)*

basal cell carcinoma *(581)*

Bell's palsy *(584)*

bifid tongue *(578)*

biopsy *(567)*

blister *(568)*

bulla *(568)*

Candida albicans *(579)*

canker sores *(570)*

cleft lip *(576)*

cleft palate *(576)*

congenital *(576)*

cyst *(569)*

dentinogenesis imperfecta *(576)*

dysplasic cells *(580)*

ecchymosis *(569)*

etiology *(567)*

erosion *(569)*

erythroplakia *(580)*

exostosis *(577)*

fibroma *(581)*

fissured tongue *(578)*

Fordyce's spots *(577)*

fusion *(576)*

gemination *(576)*

gingival hyperplasia *(575)*

granuloma *(569)*

glossitis *(579)*

gumma *(571)*

(continues)

OUTLINE *(continued)*

KEY TERMS *(continued)*

INTRODUCTION

Oral pathology is defined as the study of oral diseases, their causes (if known), and their effects on the body. A dental assistant does not diagnose oral pathological diseases but may alert the dentist to abnormal conditions in the mouth. The dental assistant must recognize abnormal conditions and know how to prevent disease transmission, how the identified pathological condition may interfere with planned treatment, and what effect the condition will have on the overall health of the patient.

Oral pathology can originate from a number of different agents or disturbances. Biological, physical, and chemical agents may bring on a disease condition that exhibits signs in the oral cavity. Hormonal, developmental, and nutritional disturbances will also show disease signs in the mouth. Other disorders and reactions to stress and antigenic (capable of causing the production of an antibody) substances, as well as neoplasms and cysts, develop in the oral cavity. The dental assistant has a different viewpoint of the patient's oral cavity because she or he sits on the opposite side of the patient. Anything that appears to be atypical should be brought to the attention of the dentist for further investigation, without alarming the patient. Any unusual oral lesions, an all-encompassing term for abnormal structures in the oral cavity, must be closely observed by the dentist. The dentist may palpate (feel with fingers) or perform a procedure called a biopsy on the suspicious lesion. A biopsy (the removal of a small amount of the tissue surgically) is an accurate method of diagnosing many illnesses. After the diagnosis is made, further study is done to identify the etiology (cause of the disease). This biopsy is normally sent to a pathologist for examination under the microscope and further diagnosis. Dentists include any information they observe clinically or through palpation, such as size, location, color, and texture. Other information about the lesion may include how long it has been present, if it is painful to touch, whether the area seems hot, and what the patient believes caused the situation. All this information, as obtained from the patient, should be documented. Any additional information the doctor thinks is pertinent should be sent to the laboratory with the biopsy.

Inflammation

The body responds to disease and injury with a process known as **inflammation**. Specialized cells in the area release a number of chemicals, some of which are called **histamines**. Histamines are said to bring about inflammation by increasing blood flow to the involved area and causing redness and heat. They also make the blood capillaries more hyperemic (increased amount of blood), and fluid oozes from them into the tissues, causing swelling. When the nerve endings in the area are stimulated by these chemicals, pain occurs. Four conditions are an essential part of the body's response to injury or disease: redness (erythema), heat, swelling (edema), and pain. These symptoms were first defined as the clinical features of inflammation by Celsus Cornelius (c. 30 BC–45 AD), a Roman physician and medical writer. Often referred to as the *cardinal signs of inflammation*, they were known in Latin as rubor (redness), calor (warmth), tumor (swelling), and dolor (pain).

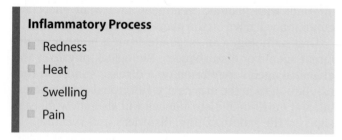

Inflammatory Process

- Redness
- Heat
- Swelling
- Pain

White blood cells, which are attracted to inflammation, help destroy the invading microorganisms and aid in healing. The area is encircled by a fibrous connective tissue to prevent the spread of the condition to any other area.

Diagnosing Oral Pathology

The dentist uses information from many sources to make a diagnosis for any oral pathology. She or he may use several diagnostic tools to identify the lesion or disease, or use a process of elimination to reach a conclusion. These diagnostic tools are radiographic, clinical, genetic history, surgical, microscopic biopsy, laboratory diagnosis, and therapeutic and differential diagnosis.

The dentist most often reads the radiographs and completes a clinical evaluation first. Radiographs provide views of the apical area, and the dentist can determine whether any areas of absorption have occurred. They

also indicate whether cysts or abscesses are present. The dentist performs a clinical diagnosis to assess the location, size, shape, color, and texture of the lesion. The patient's genetic and medical histories are often useful in making the diagnosis. There are a number of genetic disorders that may need to be illuminated. If these tools do not permit the dentist to reach a conclusion on which oral pathologic lesion is present, then further diagnostic information will be required. The dentist can then determine that a surgery is needed to help determine the diagnosis. If the diagnosis is still not clear (via visual examination during surgery), the dentist may decide to send a tissue sample to a laboratory for a biopsy, blood chemistry analysis, and/or other analysis.

The therapeutic/differential diagnosis is a commonly used tool. If prescribing a particular therapy (based on evaluation of clinical data, and thus, likely diagnosis) has no effect on the condition, the practitioner dentist moves on to the next likely diagnosis (and related therapy). In contrast, when the cause of a disease or disorder is unknown, it is said to be **idiopathic**.

Oral Lesions

 The abnormal tissues in the oral cavity, called lesions, are further classified according to their placement in the surface of the mucosa. They can be classified as above the surface, below the surface, or even or flat with the surface of the oral mucosa.

Above-Surface Lesions

- A **blister** is a raised area, usually oval or circular, filled with fluid, which protects the damaged tissue. This fluid leaks from the blood vessels to underlying layers of skin following some type of trauma, such as burn, friction, or disease.

- A **bulla** (**BULL**-ah) is a large (over one-half inch in diameter), fluid-filled blister.

- A **hematoma** is a lesion caused by bleeding from a ruptured blood vessel, which appears as a raised bruised area due to the collection of localized, clotted blood. Dental assistants should watch for a hematoma after oral anesthetic. Even the best clinicians may nick a blood vessel during an injection, resulting in a hematoma. The dental assistant alerts the dentist about the condition, and then applies pressure to the area to disperse the blood in the tissue, which alleviates pressure in the area.

- A **papule** is a small (less than one-half inch in diameter), solid, raised area of skin. The surface of the papule may be pigmented in color and smooth or bumpy.

- A **plaque** is any raised or flat patch in the oral mucosa. This term is not to be confused with dental plaque, which causes dental caries (see Chapter 4, Oral Health and Prevention Techniques).

■ A **pustule** is a small, pus-containing blister.

■ **Vesicles** are small, fluid-filled blisters.

Below-Surface Lesions

■ An **abscess** is a concentrated area of pus formed as a result of infection by microorganisms. Dental abscesses are periapical (at the apex of the tooth) or periodontal, caused by microorganisms invading the periodontal membrane of the tooth (see Chapter 29, Periodontics).

■ A **cyst** is a fluid or semi-solid, fluid-filled sac. The causes of cysts are numerous. In dentistry, cysts normally occur due to blockage of a duct leading from a fluid-forming gland. Cysts can develop around the crown of an undeveloped tooth before eruption.

■ **Erosion** is the defect left from a trauma or an injury. It may arise from biting the cheek. The margins of cheek erosion are red and painful.

■ An **ulcer** is due to destruction of the mucous membrane and appears as an open sore on the tissue. The ulcer may appear shallow or crated deeply and is normally inflamed and painful.

Even or Flat with Surface Lesions

■ **Ecchymosis** (eck-ih-**MOH**-sis) is a medical term for tissue bruising.

■ A **macule** (**MACK**-youl) is a spot of different texture or color on the skin.

■ A **patch** is an area of skin that is different in color and/or texture.

■ **Petechiae** (pee-**TEE**-kee-ee) are small spots, red or purple in color, that occur in the skin or mucosal tissue. They are caused by localized hemorrhage.

■ **Purpura** (**PUR**-pew-rah) is caused by bleeding within underlying tissues. These purplish or reddish brown areas or spots of discoloration can range in size from the diameter of a pin head up to one inch. Small purpura normally are called petechiae, and the larger are called ecchymoses or bruises.

Flat or Above-Surface Lesions

■ A **granuloma**, associated with chronic inflammation, appears as a neoplasm filled with granulation tissue. The suffix "oma" refers to a neoplasm.

■ **Neoplasm** is the medical term for tumor. This new, abnormal growth that serves no purpose can be either malignant (life threatening) or benign (not life threatening).

■ A **nodule** is a small lump of tissue, hard or soft, that is usually more than one-quarter inch in diameter. A nodule may protrude from the tissue or form beneath the surface of the tissue.

Biological Agents

A number of microorganisms cause oral diseases that are manifested through lesions in the head and neck.

Actinomycosis

Actinomycosis is an infection caused by bacteria. First, a painful swelling appears, and later pus and yellow granules discharge from the area. Poor oral hygiene or microorganisms obtaining access to the bone through the dental socket after tooth removal are thought to be contributing factors.

Herpes Simplex

Type I herpes simplex typically occurs above the waist (normally around the mouth), and Type II may appear in the oral cavity but normally appears below the waist, commonly called genital herpes. The Type I infection occurs in about three-fourths of middle-aged adults. Forms of the virus are responsible for cold sores (painful blisters around the mouth). These blisters, commonly called fever blisters, can appear solitary or in a cluster of small blisters on the lips, called **herpes labialis** (Figure 26-1). Normal inflammation encompasses the area.

The virus responsible for the disease is transmitted through physical contact and is seen normally in children around the age of six as **herpetic gingivostomatitis** (the initial infection). Adults often unknowingly pass the virus, which is infectious both during onset of the vesicular stage and throughout the crusted stage, to children during kissing. It exhibits symptoms much like the flu. Fever, along with body aches, is apparent, followed by

FIGURE 26-1 Herpes lesions on the lips, called herpes labialis. *(Courtesy of Joseph L. Konzelman, Jr., DDS.)*

scattered ulcers in the oral mucosa or on the lips. The lesions appear as nicks in the tissue and are extremely sore. These vesicle ulcerations vary in size from a pin head to one-quarter inch in size. The symptoms reappear throughout life and usually last from seven to fourteen days. If the condition is caught early, medication is available to alleviate discomfort (see Chapter 10, Microbiology).

Dental assistants must exert extreme care while working with patients who have herpes. Stretching and pulling of the lesion cause the patient significant discomfort. Dentists may choose to reschedule the patient until after recovery from the herpes outbreak. The dental assistant must pay special attention to eliminating cross-contamination by maintaining asepsis. The herpetic virus lasts on a countertop or work surface for up to four hours. Health care workers are known to develop the infection if barriers are not used. If exposure is significant, gloves are not worn, and a break in the skin is accessible to the virus, **herpetic whitlow** may occur. This is a crusting ulceration on the fingers or hands that is extremely painful.

Any patient with apparent ulcers from the herpes virus that last longer than a month should be tested for immunodeficient diseases, such as HIV.

Aphthous Ulcers

Common ulcerations that recur in the oral cavity are **aphthous** (**AF**-thus) **ulcers**. These painful ulcers appear circular with yellow centers and erythematous (red) halos surrounding the lesions (Figure 26-2). The yellow necrotic center is due to dead or dying epithelial cells. The cause of this ulcer is unknown, but streptococci bacteria have been identified in numerous cases. Recurrent aphthous ulcers (RAU) are referred to by patients as **canker sores**, and they are not contagious. A patient may have as few as one or as many as six sores at one time. Heredity, trauma, stress, food allergens, and hormonal changes are associated with the recurrence of this ulceration.

Recurrent aphthous ulcers start out as small bumps that begin with a sting. These ulcers develop on an area of unattached gingiva or mucosa inside the cheeks, and present as a whitish dished-out area that is surrounded with a red ring. Nerve endings are exposed. Bacteria can invade the area, resulting in inflammation, and the area becomes even more uncomfortable.

Aphthous ulcers last from ten to fourteen days, and topical anesthetics are used to treat the painful symptoms. Patients may have to be rescheduled for dental treatment, because these sores cause significant discomfort if they are touched or stretched.

Herpes Zoster

Herpes zoster (shingles) appears as unilateral, painful lesions that can last up to five weeks. This virus, which causes varicella in children, may be latent and then activate at a time when the person is immunodeficient. Patients with human immunodeficiency virus (HIV) or advanced cancers are predisposed to herpes zoster. Acyclovir™ has been used successfully to treat the symptoms of these painful ulcers in some cases.

Syphilis

Syphilis, the venereal disease caused by bacteria that may be treated with antibiotics, has three primary stages. The first stage presents with a primary lesion about one-half inch in diameter that is hard and raised (Figure 26-3). This lesion, called a chancre, appears nor-

FIGURE 26-2 Recurrent aphthous ulcer on buccal mucosa. *(Courtesy of Joseph L. Konzelman, Jr., DDS.)*

FIGURE 26-3 Lip chancre from primary syphilis.

FIGURE 26-4 Hutchinson's incisors from prenatal syphilis. *(Courtesy of Dale Ruemping, DDS, MSD.)*

FIGURE 26-5 Mulberry molars from prenatal syphilis. *(Courtesy of Dale Ruemping, DDS, MSD.)*

mally on the lip. The chancre first ulcerates and then becomes crusted over. It appears much like a herpetic lesion. The chancre disappears within five weeks, and no clinical manifestations of the disease appear in the oral cavity until two months to one year later.

The second stage begins with flu-like symptoms, followed by one of two types of lesions. These lesions, a mucous patch or a split papule, are both extremely infectious. In the tertiary or third and final stage of syphilis, a **gumma** or localized lesion appears. The final stage of syphilis may occur many years after nontreatment of secondary syphilis. This lesion destroys bone and cartilage.

Children born to mothers with syphilis may have teeth with enamel hypoplasia or teeth that have been altered, because of the infection, during the morphodifferentiation and dentinogenesis cycles of tooth development. The anterior dentition appears to be dented on the incisal edges, called **Hutchinson's incisors** (Figure 26-4). The permanent molars may appear more rounded with the occlusal surface, resembling a mulberry. Due to their appearance, they are called **mulberry molars** (Figure 26-5).

Thrush

Thrush is the common name for the fungal infection of candidiasis in children. It appears as a white, thick covering over the oral mucous membranes. The white covering can be removed by wiping it with a 2×2 gauze. This fungal infection often originates as the newborn travels through the birth canal. The fungal microorganism can grow in increasing numbers in this warm, moist environment and causes very little discomfort to the child. Treatment consists of wiping and then applying topical antifungal drugs to the area.

Physical Agents

Several physical agents can cause oral clinical manifestations. These trauma-induced ulcerations are most often self-induced. The patient may bite the inside of the cheek, fall on a blunt object, or wear an ill-fitting dental appliance, such as a denture. The dental team must use great care not to induce additional trauma during dental care. The HVE has a rough edge that can cut or lacerate the patient's tissue if not handled properly. Other physical agents, such as instruments, can cause trauma by tearing or bruising the tissue if not used carefully. The dental assistant must constantly watch as instruments and materials are transferred to and from the mouth.

Cotton rolls that are placed in an area that becomes overly dry and that are removed quickly can cause a gingival ulcer. The tissue adheres to the cotton roll so that when it is removed, the top layer of gingival tissue is also removed. To avoid this, the dental assistant can moisten the cotton roll prior to removing it.

Denture Irritation Causing Hyperplasia

An ill-fitting denture can cause small ulcers that, after continued irritation, become folds of excess tissue called **hyperplasia** (Figure 26-6). In the palatal area, the ruga(e) palatine become inflamed and swollen. Swelling is reduced and the redness disappears if the patient does not wear the denture for several days. Soft tissue lining material can be placed in the denture by the dentist to allow the palate to heal prior to relining or remaking the denture.

FIGURE 26-6 Hyperplasia from denture irritation. *(Courtesy of Joseph L. Konzelman, Jr., DDS.)*

Amalgam Tattoo

An amalgam tattoo can occur when amalgam particles become trapped in the tissue, either during oral surgery or during an amalgam or crown preparation procedure (Figure 26-7). The gingival tissue in the immediate area appears blue to gray. No treatment is necessary because the tattoo is asymptomatic and harmless. To prevent this condition from occurring, the dental assistant should flush the area with water to remove any amalgam particles after treatment, especially when the tissue is severely abraded. Use of a dental dam also aids in preventing amalgam tattoos.

Radiation Injury

Patients receiving excess radiation due to cancer treatment around the oral cavity may experience a number of side effects. Excess radiation may cause developing teeth to be malformed, dwarfed, or without roots. This deformity depends on the stage of tooth development. The soft tissue may show reddening, with apparent ulcers due to excess radiation. After the area has healed, the tissue within the area may appear pigmented. Spider-like vessels may appear in skin that appears to be atrophied.

Oral Piercing

Oral piercing (Figure 26-8) is a means of self-expression and body art, and the majority of them involve the tongue. A barbell-shaped piece of jewelry is placed in the midline of the tongue after a needle pierces the area. Often a temporary device is placed so that it can be adjusted if swelling occurs. When the barbell is placed through the tongue a ball is screwed on the lower side of the tongue to secure it. If a blood vessel is punctured during the piercing, severe bleeding may occur. In some instances, blood poisoning and/or blood clots will develop. Other sites include cheeks, lips, uvula, and the

FIGURE 26-7 Amalgam tattoo (A) in the oral cavity and (B) on a periapical x-ray. *(Courtesy of Joseph L. Konzelman, Jr., DDS.)*

FIGURE 26-8 Oral piercing. *(Courtesy of the University of Washington School of Dentistry.)*

FIGURE 26-9 Oral piercing shown to cause damage to teeth and tissues. *(Courtesy of the University of Washington School of Dentistry.)*

side of the tongue; sometimes multiple sites are pierced. Healing in any of these areas takes a month or more.

Before a person chooses oral piercing, possible outcomes and related symptoms should be investigated. Side effects are common. The most serious side effect is tongue swelling, which can actually close off the airway and thus hamper breathing. Other symptoms include pain, infection, and swelling, increased saliva flow, teeth and tissue damage (Figure 26-9), metal hypersensitivity, scar tissue development, and problems with mastication (chewing). Speech is often affected as well. Piercing has been identified by the National Institutes of Health as a possible factor in transmission of hepatitis B, C, D, and G.

Tongue Splitting

Another form of self-expression is tongue splitting, or separating the end of the tongue resulting in a reptilian

appearance. Reversing this procedure requires surgery. Compared to oral piercing, damage to teeth and tissue is less severe, speech problems are exaggerated, and the potential for infection is greater. Finally, swallowing may become more difficult.

Chemical Agents

A number of chemical agents can cause oral lesions. Some of the materials used in dentistry are caustic and may cause chemical burns. These agents include phenol, sodium hyperchlorate, zinc chloride, and aspirin. The chemicals in tobacco also cause oral lesions. Certain drugs will also induce oral lesions. The most common chemical agents seen in patients' oral cavities in the dental office are aspirin burns, nicotine stomatitis, and chewing-tobacco lesions.

Aspirin Burn

Some people place aspirin over the root area of the tooth to alleviate discomfort before seeking dental treatment. The placement of the aspirin causes a lesion that is white in color and rough in texture (Figure 26-10). Soreness is apparent after the aspirin is removed and before complete healing.

Nicotine Stomatitis

Nicotine stomatitis is another condition that the dental assistant is likely to see in the dental office (Figure 26-11). Pipe smokers are more likely to develop nicotine stomatitis than cigarette smokers. It is caused by the heat and the irritating effect of chemicals in tobacco.

FIGURE 26-10 Aspirin burn. *(Courtesy of Joseph L. Konzelman, Jr., DDS.)*

FIGURE 26-11 Nicotine stomatitis. *(Courtesy of Joseph L. Konzelman, Jr., DDS.)*

FIGURE 26-12 Chewing tobacco (snuff) lesion. *(Courtesy of Joseph L. Konzelman, Jr., DDS.)*

The reason for more frequent occurrence in pipe smokers is that they typically place the pipe in the same area. The pipestem then delivers a great deal of heat and tobacco to the same tissue every time the person smokes.

The affected area of tissue first turns red in response to the irritation. If the irritation continues, the tissue presents as whitened and red **hyperkeratinized** nodules. Hyperkeratinized tissue occurs where the epithelial tissue builds up a layer of keratin as a protective coating. The **orifices** (openings) of the salivary glands appear to be inflamed. The patient should be made aware of this condition and encouraged to stop smoking. Normally, the condition disappears if the patient ceases to smoke.

Chewing Tobacco (Snuff) Lesion

Snuff is a preparation of powdered tobacco (often mixed with other substances) for inhalation into the nose or formed into a wad for chewing. It contains nicotine and is addictive. In this chapter, snuff is referred to as chewing tobacco. Lesions caused by this form of tobacco appear in the oral vestibule, normally the lower anterior area between the lip and the teeth, as wrinkled, white, thickened tissue. Like nicotine stomatitis lesions, the severity of a snuff lesion depends on how often the smokeless tobacco is used and how sensitive the individual is to the product (Figure 26-12).

Individuals smoking other drugs, such as marijuana, may exhibit the clinical signs of tobacco irritation. Marijuana irritations normally are apparent in the middle anterior section of the lips, both maxillary and mandibular. This tissue appears red in the early stages and white with thick, wrinkled tissue in the later stages. This occurs primarily because a device such as a "roach clip" is used to hold the drug as it is smoked down to a very small piece; therefore, the heat and the drug are concentrated on the lips.

Hairy Tongue

A condition in which the filiform papillae of the tongue become elongated and appear like hairs is called **hairy tongue** (also called the black hairy tongue) (Figure 26-13). This "hair" normally becomes stained by tobacco, food, or other microorganisms, making it appear dark in color. Hairy tongue may appear without a known cause, but it is normally associated with chemotherapeutic agents such as drugs, hydrogen peroxide mouth rinses, and antibiotics. Treatment of this condition is to stop the known cause, if applicable, and use good oral hygiene, including brushing the tongue. In extreme cases, the filiform papillae grow so long that they cause the person to gag. If this happens, the papillae can be trimmed to alleviate gagging.

FIGURE 26-13 Hairy tongue.

FIGURE 26-15 Meth mouth. *(Courtesy of American Dental Association.)*

Gingival Hyperplasia

A condition known as **gingival hyperplasia** occurs when the connective tissue grows over the teeth (Figure 26-14). This fibrous mass is not uncomfortable to the patient but can inhibit eating and alter the patient's appearance. There are numerous causes of this condition: plaque, orthodontic braces, and various drugs. Phenytoin (Dilantin™) causes this symptom in about one-half of patients being treated with this medication. The condition is referred to as Dilantin hyperplasia.

The condition is normally reduced after the irritant is removed or the patient stops taking the drugs, but that solution is not always preferable. If ongoing drug therapy is necessary, the tissue can be removed surgically and recurrence is probable.

Meth Mouth

Methamphetamines have become a drug of choice in part because the drug is easily made with inexpensive ingredients, and the "high" from these drugs lasts up to 12 hours. Street names include ice, crank, crystal, meth, speed, fire, glass, and chalk, and the pills are called "yaba." Meth is consumed via injecting, smoking, snorting, or swallowing. Effects on the oral cavity may be devastating. The acid in the drug causes cravings for high-calorie carbonated drinks. Rampant decay is common in cases of "meth mouth" (Figure 26-15), and often teeth seem to have exploded. Dental treatment is typically complicated, long term, and expensive.

Hormonal Disturbances

Oral conditions can be caused by a change in hormonal balance. Puberty and pregnancy cause hormonal changes that affect the oral tissues. An individual who notices soreness in the gingival tissue must pay close attention to oral hygiene so that the condition does not progress.

Pregnancy Gingivitis

Pregnancy gingivitis occurs in about 5 percent of pregnant women. The gingival tissues appear enlarged and inflamed. A few pregnant women with this condition also develop tumors (see next section). Both of these

FIGURE 26-14 Gingival hyperplasia. *(Courtesy of Joseph L. Konzelman, Jr., DDS.)*

FIGURE 26-16 Pyogenic granuloma. *(Courtesy of Joseph L. Konzelman, Jr., DDS.)*

conditions clear up once the hormonal balance returns to normal, but good oral hygiene practices must be followed to control gingivitis and bleeding.

Pyogenic Granuloma

Often called pregnancy tumor, **pyogenic** (pie-oh-**JEN**-ick) **granuloma** is also found in males and nonpregnant females (Figure 26-16). This overgrowth of granulation tissue occurs as a result of local irritation. A red, vascular mass ranging in size from a few millimeters to several centimeters, the tumor grows rapidly. It normally is not painful and can be excised. The cause is hormonal disturbances, and the lesion may grow back if the situation continues. Therefore, it is not prudent to remove the lesion during the pregnancy unless the patient is uncomfortable. Other factors, such as calculus on the teeth, should be removed to eliminate irritation to the area.

Puberty Gingival Enlargement

Adolescents going through puberty can experience gingival enlargement due to hormonal changes. The condition appears much like pregnancy gingivitis as the gingival tissue is enlarged, bleeds easily, and appears soft and swollen. This condition is more common in girls than in boys. It corrects itself after hormonal balance is stabilized again and good oral hygiene practices are maintained.

Developmental Disturbances

A wide range of anomalies can take place if any stage of embryo development is disturbed. In the oral cavity, anomalies occur in about one in every 800 children born. These **congenital** (present at birth) conditions are genetic (inherited). Other anomalies are caused by outside agents, such as alcohol, drugs, or the mother's illness during pregnancy, such as syphilis (refer to biological agents).

One such developmental disturbance is clefting in the oral cavity, such as **cleft lip** and **cleft palate** (see Chapter 8, Embryology and Histology). The majority of these conditions is **innocuous** (harmless); however, some conditions cause eating, speaking, and esthetic difficulties. The construction of an obturator (an appliance to aid in swallowing) for the cleft palate may be necessary to treat the condition.

Disturbances in Tooth Development

As the teeth are developing, a number of disturbances can occur.

Amelogenesis Imperfecta. **Amelogenesis imperfecta** is a genetic (inherited) condition of the teeth in which the enamel is discolored, partially missing, or extremely thin. These teeth can be more susceptible to dental caries. Treatment may consist of composite restorations that cover the entire surface of the teeth.

Ankylosis. **Ankylosis** is a condition in which the tooth, cementum, or dentin fuses with the alveolar bone, restricting movement of the tooth as well as eruption. An ankylosed tooth appears below the normal occlusal plane of the adjacent teeth. If this condition affects a third molar, removing the tooth becomes quite difficult. The dentist may have to use a handpiece and a bur to separate the tooth from the bone to remove it from the socket.

Anodontia. **Anodontia** occurs when teeth are congenitally missing. This condition can affect primary or permanent teeth or both. It is most often seen in permanent third molars. Many individuals only develop one or two of their third molars, or "wisdom teeth." Some individuals develop no third molars.

Dentinogenesis Imperfecta. **Dentinogenesis imperfecta** is a condition in which the enamel appears to be opalescent and chips away from the dentin soon after eruption of the tooth. This hereditary condition normally appears in both deciduous and permanent teeth. The pulp chambers are missing, as are the root canals. Normally, these patients present with attrition (wearing away) due to lack of enamel.

Fusion. **Fusion** is a condition in which the enamel and dentin of two or more individual teeth join together. The incisal or occlusal surface may show an indentation between the two teeth, and they normally are much broader in appearance. This condition most often is seen in mandibular anterior deciduous teeth.

Gemination. **Gemination** may appear much like a fusion, but in this case one tooth bud attempts to divide. The indentation on the incisal or occlusal surface is apparent.

Macrodontia. Macrodontia teeth are abnormally large. The entire dentition may manifest itself in macrodontia teeth, or only two teeth may develop in this manner.

Microdontia. Microdontia teeth are the opposite of macrodontia: They are abnormally small. This condition is often seen in individuals with Down's syndrome and those born with congenital heart disease. Small teeth can be apparent in the entire dentition or only show up in one or two teeth. Commonly, the maxillary laterals show as microdontia teeth. In this area, the teeth are often peg shaped and small.

Neonatal Teeth. Neonatal teeth (natal teeth) are present at the time of birth or within the first month after birth. Normally, the baby sheds these teeth very quickly, because the roots are not formed yet.

Supernumerary Teeth. Supernumerary teeth are extra teeth. They appear dwarfed in size and shape but normal in all other aspects. Supernumerary teeth are seen most frequently in the maxillary anterior or third molar area, both maxillary and mandibular.

Twinning. Twinning is a condition in which the germination process has been successful and two separate teeth are made from a single tooth bud. The tooth appears as a clone of the original tooth in both shape and size.

Oral Tori

Bony outgrowths of tissue in the oral cavity that are benign (nonmalignant) in nature are called tori. In the maxillary hard palate, they are termed torus palatinus. In the mandibular canine or premolar region, they are called torus mandibularis.

Tori palatinus are normally seen close to the midline but can occur on the lateral borders (Figure 26-17). Approximately one in every five adults has a maxillary tori, and about one in every twenty has a mandibular tori. Tori mandibularis are more annoying, because food debris can collect under them (Figure 26-18). Both tori conditions present with surfaces of hard bone covered with thin coverings of tissue. The dental assistant must be careful while taking oral radiographs. He or she should examine the oral cavity carefully before placing the radiograph into position. The radiographs can abrade the tissue and cause the patient discomfort if placed directly on the tissue covering the bony growths.

These growths are not removed unless the patient needs a prosthetic appliance, such as a denture or a lower partial. The growths are then surgically removed to allow room for the dental appliance.

Exostoses

An enlargement or nodular outgrowth of dense lamella bone (thin structure extending from the facial surface) that appears on the facial surfaces of the mandibular

FIGURE 26-17 Torus palatinus. *(Courtesy of Joseph L. Konzelman, Jr., DDS.)*

FIGURE 26-18 Torus mandibularis. *(Courtesy of Joseph L. Konzelman, Jr., DDS.)*

and maxillary palates is called exostosis. These enlargements, which appear much like toris, may be variations of the same developmental disturbance. There is no treatment, unless a dental appliance is necessary or the enlargements hamper mastication (chewing) for the patient.

Fordyce's Spots (Granules)

In about 80 percent of the population, numerous light-yellow spots in the oral cavity are present. These round lesions, called Fordyce's spots, are sebaceous oil glands near the surface of the epithelium (Figure 26-19). They can be found anywhere in the oral cavity but most often

FIGURE 26-19 Fordyce's spots. *(Courtesy of Joseph L. Konzelman, Jr., DDS.)*

are on the buccal mucosa. No identified causes are known, and no treatment is necessary.

Fissured Tongue

A **fissured tongue** occurs in about 5 percent of the population (Figure 26-20). It appears as a wrinkled, deeply grooved surface on the tongue. Fissured tongue may be symmetrical or irregular in pattern. The patient may experience discomfort due to retention of debris in the

FIGURE 26-20 Fissured tongue. *(Courtesy of Joseph L. Konzelman, Jr., DDS.)*

FIGURE 26-21 Ankyloglossia. *(Courtesy of Joseph L. Konzelman, Jr., DDS.)*

deep fissures. No treatment is necessary, although the patient may use a home irrigating device to clean the fissures occasionally.

Bifid Tongue

If the two lateral halves of the anterior two-thirds of the tongue fail to fuse completely, a condition known as **bifid tongue** occurs. It appears as an extra tag of muscle at the end of the tongue. No treatment is necessary, unless the extra tag of tongue is annoying; then, it is surgically removed.

Ankyloglossia

The term commonly used for **ankyloglossia** is "tongue tied" (Figure 26-21). The lingual frenum is attached near the tip of the tongue, which limits movement of the tongue and may interfere with the enunciation of specific sounds. This condition can be corrected with a simple surgical procedure, which enables the individual to overcome related speech problems. A dental assistant should watch for this condition in children. Under direction of the dentist, while waiting for local anesthetic to take effect, ask the child to stick the tongue out and move across the upper lip from side to side. Note if a restriction is present, and bring this information to the attention of the dentist for further evaluation.

Nutritional Disturbances

The oral cavity can reveal a number of conditions resulting from inadequate diet. It is important to consult with all patients about eating a well-balanced diet (see Chapter 5, Nutrition).

Angular Cheilitis

Vitamin B complex deficiency results in a condition known as **angular cheilitis**. A lesion forms in the corner of the mouth, involving both the mucous membrane and the skin (Figure 26-22). This condition may also occur if the patient constantly licks the corners of the mouth (commissures) or if the patient loses vertical dimension of the face. A loss of vertical dimension occurs when a person overcloses the mouth because the occlusal plane is worn down or the bone structure beneath a denture is deteriorated. The end of the chin is closer to the tip of the nose and the corners of the mouth cave in, which allows saliva to pool in the corners. This condition permits the growth of microorganisms; as result, fungal **opportunistic infections** such as *Candida albicans* are often found in this area.

This condition is treated via correction of vitamin B deficiency or the use of antifungal drugs. Dentures can be remade or the teeth crowned and extended in length to correct the loss of vertical dimension.

Glossitis (Bald Tongue)

Another condition reportedly caused by the lack of the vitamin B complex is **glossitis**. Glossitis literally means "inflammation of the tongue." The filiform papillae on the tongue are absent, and the tongue appears to be smooth, hence the name "bald tongue." The tongue may be sore and the patient may experience difficulty in eating. A well-balanced diet aids in correction of this condition.

Neoplasms

As stated earlier, *neoplasm* is a medical term for tumor. This group of lesions has great potential for becoming **malignant** (cancerous). The dental assistant should be knowledgeable about the causes of these diseases and should perform careful clinical examinations for premalignant lesions. Even if it is known that a tumor is benign (harmless), it is important that all lesions are brought to the attention of the dentist, without alarming the patient. It could save the patient's life if the tumor is recognized early.

> ### Oral Cancer Warning Signs
>
> - Sore in the oral cavity that does not heal within a month
> - Lumps and swelling in the oral cavity, on the lips, or on the neck
> - White lesions or rough lesions in the mouth or on the lips
> - Dryness in the mouth over a period of time for no apparent reason
> - Numbness in or around the oral cavity
> - Soreness or burning sensation in or around the oral cavity
> - Difficulty speaking, chewing, or swallowing
> - Repeated bleeding in a specific area of the mouth for no apparent reason

Leukoplakia

A white, leathery patch that cannot be identified as any other type of lesion is termed **leukoplakia** (**loo**-koh-**PLAY**-kee-ah) (Figure 26-23). A biopsy is required to

FIGURE 26-22 Angular cheilitis. *(Courtesy of Joseph L. Konzelman, Jr., DDS.)*

FIGURE 26-23 Leukoplakia. *(Courtesy of Joseph L. Konzelman, Jr., DDS.)*

further identify the lesion. The dentist normally views these lesions with concern, because they may be precipitating factors to cancer. They are found throughout the oral mucosa and can be very dense or very diffuse. The operator is not able to wipe the lesion off with a 2 × 2 gauze as he or she could with thrush. Leukoplakia is often seen in the lower lip of a person who uses chewing tobacco. Excessive alcohol and tobacco usage, vitamin A deficiency, or trauma normally are associated with the lesion.

Biopsy results normally show **hyperkeratinization**, a thickening of the outer layer of the skin due to excess of keratin. This condition is similar to developing corns on the feet due to constant irritation. Biopsies also could reveal **dysplasic cells**, that is, abnormal cell features such as size, shape, and rate of multiplication. Dysplasic cells often become malignant.

Lichen Planus

The initial skin lesion of **lichen planus** usually appears on the lower leg or ankle. This lesion is a flat-topped papule, dark red or violet in color. The oral lesions (reticular lichen planus) begin as small, white papules that group and form interlacing white lines known as **Wickham's striae** (Figure 26-24). In most cases, they are on the buccal mucosa. An erosive form of the lesion (erosive lichen planus) causes the loss of oral epithelium in the infected area. Both types are fairly common, with reticular lichen planus being asymptomatic and erosive lichen planus usually being more tender and painful. A patient may exhibit pain while eating, and some foods may aggravate the condition. The treatment is topical steroid therapy.

Whether lichen planus is a premalignant condition is unknown. Patients should be examined periodically for any changes in this condition.

Erythroplakia

Any red patch of tissue in the oral cavity that cannot be associated with inflammation is termed **erythroplakia** (eh-rith-roh-**PLAY**-kee-ah). Most commonly, this condition appears in the soft palate, retromolar pad area, or the floor of the mouth. It is usually seen in patients over sixty who have used tobacco and alcoholic beverages on a regular basis.

This lesion is of great concern, because almost 100 percent of biopsies indicate premalignant or malignant tissue. Treatment depends on the extent of the lesion. In early stages, it can be removed surgically; however, in later stages, it is necessary to treat the lesion with radiation and chemotherapy.

Squamous Cell Carcinoma

A carcinoma is a malignant neoplasm (tumor) that can spread, or **metastasize**, into the surrounding tissue and lymph nodes. Typically, it first appears as an ulcerated area in the soft tissues of the mouth. **Squamous cell carcinoma** is cancer of the squamous epithelium (Figure 26-25). Nine out of ten oral cancers are of this type.

Factors associated with causing carcinomas are sunlight exposure and long-term use of tobacco and/or alcohol. Normally, squamous cell carcinomas are seen in adults over forty, but have also been found in younger patients. More cases have been documented in males than females. Squamous cell carcinoma is found primar-

FIGURE 26-24 Lichen planus. *(Courtesy of Joseph L. Konzelman, Jr., DDS.)*

FIGURE 26-25 Squamous cell carcinoma. *(Courtesy of Joseph L. Konzelman, Jr., DDS.)*

ily on the floor of the oral cavity under the tongue, on the sides or borders of the tongue, and on the soft palate tonsil area.

The lesion may first appear as a thickened, white plaque that develops into an ulcer. As it grows, this ulcer seems to encompass other tissues. Soon, a rolled border appears with the center tissue. The mass continues to grow, rising above the normal tissue level.

Treatment for squamous cell carcinoma depends on the size, site, and spread of the tumor. Early detection is essential, because if the carcinoma metastasizes into the lymph nodes, the survival rate is greatly diminished.

Basal Cell Carcinoma

The most common form of skin cancer is **basal cell carcinoma** (Figure 26-26). Lesions normally appear on the neck, ear, face, lip, and head. Because it is the area primarily exposed to the sun, the face is the principal site. Fair-skinned individuals are more susceptible to this carcinoma as are men over forty.

Unlike squamous cells, these cells typically do not metastasize. They invade the area around them as they grow. The lesion first appears as a nodule and then ulcerates, the borders rise, and the center develops into a crater.

Surgical removal of the lesion is the prinicipal treatment. Patients commonly develop more than one lesion. Careful clinical examinations of the head and neck can be performed during six-month recall appointments to identify other lesions at an early stage.

Papilloma

A lesion of squamous epithelial tissue that is benign is called a **papilloma**. A papilloma resembles a cauliflower

FIGURE 26-27 Papilloma. *(Courtesy of Joseph L. Konzelman, Jr., DDS.)*

in appearance because it seems to have a number of projections deriving from a single origin (Figure 26-27). It is not caused by continued irritation, as are many of the neoplasms, but rather occurs after the individual has been infected by a virus. A number of viruses have resulted in a similar type of lesion. This lesion ranges in color from white to red and is normally 1 to 3 cm in size.

Treatment of the papilloma is to surgically remove it and a small amount of normal epithelial cells at the base of the lesion.

Fibroma

A **fibroma** is a benign tumor of connective tissue cells (cells that surround and support structures) (Figure 26-28). A fibroma is a reactive hyperplasia rather than a

FIGURE 26-26 Basal cell carcinoma.

FIGURE 26-28 Fibroma. *(Courtesy of Joseph L. Konzelman, Jr., DDS.)*

true neoplasm. It presents in the oral cavity as a dome-shaped, pink-colored, smooth-surfaced lesion less than 2 cm in diameter. Normally, it is found on the buccal (cheek) surface, proximal to where the teeth occlude. The fibroma forms because of continued irritation of the teeth biting together. Continued trauma causes the connective tissue to grow. This benign tumor may be surgically excised or left without treatment. Recurrence of a fibroma is rare.

Oral Lesions Related to AIDS and HIV

AIDS is an immune system disorder that follows infection by the **human immunodeficiency virus (HIV)**. Healthy individuals can combat most microorganisms that cause disease, but individuals with suppressed immune systems do not fare as well. Opportunistic infections such as herpes virus, hepatitis, tuberculosis, candidosis, and pneumonia are common. There is no cure for AIDS, and treatment is focused on complications associated with it. Patients who are infected with HIV have specific oral manifestations related to the disease.

Patients with AIDS are much more susceptible to periodontal lesions than healthy individuals. The gingival tissue becomes inflamed, red, and bulbous, and bone loss occurs. Bacteria and yeast are found in the infected area. This condition is extremely painful and the tissue bleeds readily when touched. Normal oral hygiene techniques are not as effective as they are in a healthy individual.

Treatment consists of extremely good oral hygiene, root planing and curettage, rinses, and antibiotic therapy.

Hairy Leukoplakia

In the early 1980s, a raised, white-patch lesion called **hairy leukoplakia** was identified in patients known to be infected with HIV (Figure 26-29). It appears much like

the candidosis lesion but cannot be removed by wiping with gauze. Hairy leukoplakia is a white, patterned lesion normally found on the borders of the tongue. This lesion is not painful, and no treatment is available. If the patient has not been tested for HIV, the dentist may suggest testing.

Candida albicans

AIDS patients, and patients who have had cancer treatment such as chemotherapy and are immunodepressed, are likely to develop an infection called *Candida albicans*. Patients undergoing antibiotic therapy for a long time also may present with the lesions. This fungus infection is much like thrush or moniliasis, and is the first oral lesion manifesting from HIV infection. The membrane presents as a white, thick, plaque-like covering in linear patterns on top of a red, inflamed surface. It can be present on numerous oral membranes but normally appears on the tongue and buccal mucosa. Patients often report a burning sensation in the area of the infection. Treatment consists of antifungal medications such as Nystatin™ (see Chapter 15, Pharmacology).

Kaposi's Sarcoma

A number of AIDS patients present with an unusual malignant vascular tumor called **Kaposi's sarcoma** (Figure 26-30). AIDS patients are susceptible to other malignant tumors, such as squamous cell carcinoma and lymphoma, but, until the 1980s and the spread of AIDS, Kaposi's sarcoma was quite rare. In patients with AIDS, Kaposi's sarcoma is aggressive and spreads rapidly.

FIGURE 26-29 Hairy leukoplakia. *(Courtesy of Joseph L. Konzelman, Jr., DDS.)*

FIGURE 26-30 Kaposi's sarcoma. *(Courtesy of Joseph L. Konzelman, Jr., DDS.)*

The lesions, a diffuse blue-purple, appear all over the body, especially on the face, arms, and the palate. They are flat or nodular and, as the tumor enlarges, it becomes a hemorrhagic neoplasm. Bleeding and pain occur in the more advanced stages.

Treatment consists of low-dose radiation and/or chemotherapeutic drugs. The prognosis (outcome) is poor at this stage, and a number of people die from the lymphoreticular neoplasms related to this disease.

Miscellaneous Disorders

The dental assistant may see other disorders in the oral cavity. Any lesion appearing to be abnormal should be brought to the dentist's attention.

Acute Necrotizing Ulcerative Gingivitis

The tissues present with bleeding, infection, pain, and a foul odor in a condition known as acute necrotizing ulcerative gingivitis (ANUG) (Figure 26-31). This infectious disease is seen primarily in young adults and adolescents. Poor hygiene, lack of sleep, poor nutrition, and stress are precipitating factors. It was referred to as "trench mouth" years ago due to the fact that many soldiers who fought in "the trenches" developed ANUG. It is also seen on college campuses around final exam time.

ANUG is very painful and must be treated with thorough debridement and cleaning. Antibiotics may be prescribed along with oral rinses of hot water. Immaculate oral hygiene is also necessary to treat ANUG. After the

condition resolves, the tips of the papilla will, from that time forward, appear to be blunted or flat.

Mucocele

When trauma affects a minor salivary gland, a **mucocele** (**MYOO**-ko-seal) can result (Figure 26-32). This normally takes place on the mandibular anterior lip where a patient accidentally bites into the tissue. If this is at the place of a minor salivary gland, a duct may be closed off. The mucocele may appear like a bubble on the inside of the lip.

Occasionally, a stone-like particle may block the saliva duct opening. If this happens, the gland fills with fluid and enlarges. The gland may be opened and the fluid expressed from the area. Recurrence may necessitate total removal of the duct and gland.

Varix

Varix is a condition primarily seen in the elderly. The blood vessels become weakened and extended. Normally, this condition occurs in the oral cavity beneath the tongue or on the buccal mucosa. These dark-purple, extended vessels in the oral cavity are related to the varicose veins in other parts of the body. They should be noted on the patient's chart, but no treatment is necessary.

Geographic Tongue

Less than 2 percent of the population has an inflammatory condition that affects the tongue, called geographic tongue (Figure 26-33). It affects the dorsal and lateral sur-

FIGURE 26-31 Acute necrotizing ulcerative gingivitis. *(Courtesy of Joseph L. Konzelman, Jr., DDS.)*

FIGURE 26-32 Mucocele. *(Courtesy of Joseph L. Konzelman, Jr., DDS.)*

FIGURE 26-33 Geographic tongue. *(Courtesy of Joseph L. Konzelman, Jr., DDS.)*

faces of the tongue and presents as red, smooth patches absent of filiform papillae. Geographic tongue presents with patches that are normally surrounded by an elevated white or yellow border. The area of the patches make up an ever-changing pattern on the tongue that resembles a map of the world. The condition may have periods of remission. The condition is not painful, and treatment is unnecessary.

Anorexia Nervosa and Bulimia

The diseases anorexia nervosa (loss of 15 percent of body weight and an intense fear of gaining weight) and bulimia (episodes of out-of-control eating followed by purging) have several implications in oral pathology. Anorexia nervosa is a disease in which extreme aversion to food is present, and accompanying symptoms of induced vomiting (bulimia) have a direct impact on oral health.

Due to the constant vomiting, the lingual surfaces of the anterior teeth become decalcified and the enamel is eroded. The occlusal surfaces of the posterior teeth become eroded, causing existing restorations to deteriorate. Rampant caries and enlargement of the parotid glands are also problems, along with the other disease symptoms that are life threatening.

Treatment is for symptoms and maintaining comfort until the personality disorder can be reversed. The patient is encouraged to practice immaculate oral hygiene and to rinse the mouth after purging to decrease the number of microorganisms and acidity. The teeth may be sensitive where the enamel has eroded. Toothpaste for sensitive teeth is suggested as treatment.

Bell's Palsy

Bell's palsy (named for Scottish surgeon Sir Charles Bell) is a temporary paralysis of the muscles on one side of the face. The cause is unknown but thought to be related to herpes zoster (shingles). One side of the face droops down, and the patient cannot close the eye or smile. Some individuals have pain in the ear on the affected side. Taste is diminished, and sounds seem unnaturally loud. Most cases clear up without treatment, but analgesics can be given for symptoms of discomfort and corticosteroid drugs can be given to reduce inflammation in the nerves.

CHAPTER SUMMARY

The dental assistant, who sits opposite the dentist, has a different view of the patient's oral cavity. Anything that appears atypical should be brought to the dentist's attention, without alarming the patient.

The dental assistant does not diagnose oral pathological diseases but identifies abnormal conditions in the mouth. Further, the dental assistant must know how to prevent disease transmission, how the identified pathological condition may interfere with planned treatment, and what effect it will have on the overall health of the patient.

Case Study

Toby Edward, twenty years old, was just given an injection by Dr. Smile. The dental assistant notices that the area where the injection was given is swelling and appears to be a raised, bruised area. The patient feels no discomfort because the anesthetic has taken effect.

Case Study Review

1. What pathologic condition may be present in Toby Edward's mouth?

2. What should the dental assistant do to treat this condition?

3. What is the prognosis of this condition?

REVIEW QUESTIONS

Multiple Choice

1. The first stage of syphilis manifests in a lesion called a
   a. gumma.
   b. chancre.
   c. mucous patch.
   d. split papule.

2. An oral condition that is common in children and appears as a white, thick covering over the oral mucous membranes is called
   a. a papule.
   b. a bulla.
   c. a hematoma.
   d. thrush.

3. All of the following are caused by chemical agents except
   a. aspirin burn.
   b. hairy tongue.
   c. nicotine stomatitis.
   d. pustule.

4. A condition in which the tooth, cementum, or dentin fuses with the alveolar bone is called
   a. amelogenesis imperfecta.
   b. ankylosis.
   c. anodontia.
   d. fusion.

5. A vitamin B complex deficiency results in a condition known as
   a. *Candida albicans*.
   b. Fordyce's spots.
   c. glossitis.
   d. angular cheilitis.

6. All but one is involved in the inflammatory process. Identify the one that is not.
   a. redness
   b. swelling
   c. pain
   d. erosion

7. ____ or shingles appears as unilateral, painful lesions that can last up to five weeks.
   a. syphilis
   b. herpes zoster
   c. herpes simples
   d. actinomycosis

8. The common name for the fungal infection of candidiasis in children is _____.
   a. hyperplasia
   b. chickenpox
   c. measles
   d. thrush

9. A pregnancy tumor is called a _____.
   a. pregnancy gingivitis
   b. Dilantin hyperplasia
   c. pyogenic granuloma
   d. anodontia

10. Extra teeth are _____.
    a. germination
    b. supernumerary teeth
    c. neonatal teeth
    d. anodontia

Critical Thinking

1. If a dental assistant is taking radiographs on a patient who presents with tori mandibularis, what should be done?

2. A patient presents with a "bald tongue." What causes this condition? Is it uncomfortable for the patient? What will help correct the condition?

3. What are the warning signs of oral cancer?

Web Activities

1. Go to http://www.oralcancer.org and find the number of individuals who will develop oral cancer this year.

2. Go to http://www.hivatis.org and identify the number of people currently living with AIDS and the number of deaths in the most recent year data were collected.

3. Go to http://www.anad.org and identify the physical repercussions of anorexia nervosa and bulimia nervosa. Which of these physical repercussions are related specifically to dentistry?

ORTHODONTICS

SPECIFIC INSTRUCTIONAL OBJECTIVES

The student should strive to meet the following objectives and demonstrate an understanding of the facts and principles presented in this chapter:

1. Define orthodontics and describe the orthodontic setting.

2. Define the role of the dental assistant in an orthodontic setting.

3. Define and describe occlusion and malocclusion.

4. Identify the causes of malocclusion.

5. Describe preventive, interceptive, and corrective orthodontics.

6. Explain the process of tooth movement.

7. Describe the preorthodontic appointment for diagnostic records.

8. Describe the consultation appointment and the roles of the assistant, patient, and orthodontist.

9. Differentiate between fixed and removable appliances.

10. Identify and describe the function of basic orthodontic instruments.

11. Describe the stages of orthodontic treatment.

12. Explain the procedure for removing orthodontic appliances and how the teeth are kept in position after appliance removal.

KEY TERMS

activator *(599)*
Angle's classification *(589)*
arch wires *(595)*
brackets *(595)*
buccal tubes *(597)*
buccoversion *(589)*
corrective orthodontics *(592)*
deposition *(592)*
distoversion *(589)*
elastics *(597)*
fixed appliances *(592)*
headgear *(599)*

infraversion *(589)*
interceptive *(592)*
labioversion *(589)*
ligature wire *(596)*
linguoversion *(589)*
malocclusion *(589)*
mesioversion *(589)*
normal occlusion *(589)*
orthodontic bands *(595)*
osteoblasts *(592)*
osteoclasts *(592)*
overbite *(599)*

plastic rings *(596)*
preventive *(592)*
removable appliances *(592)*
resorption *(592)*
separators *(604)*
space maintainer *(598)*
springs *(597)*
supraversion *(589)*
tooth positioner *(600)*
torsoversion *(589)*
transposition *(589)*
transversion *(589)*

INTRODUCTION

Orthodontics is focused on the recognition, prevention, and treatment of malalignment and irregularities of the teeth, jaws, and face. Patients seek orthodontic treatment for esthetic and functional reasons.

> *Ortho* means straight; *odont* means tooth.

The Orthodontic Practice

The general dentist completes two additional years of study after finishing dental school to become an orthodontist. Although the general dentist may perform limited orthodontic treatment, most patients requiring tooth alignment are referred to an orthodontist. The general dentist and orthodontist work together to provide the best treatment for patients. Treatment may extend over several years as the child patient grows and develops.

Although the orthodontic practice treats mainly children and young adults, the number of adult patients who see an orthodontist is increasing. Adults seek orthodontic treatment for both cosmetic and functional reasons.

Office

The orthodontic office is designed to facilitate a number of patients at different stages of treatment. Specific rooms or areas are used for examination, diagnostic records, and treatment consultations before treatment begins. The treatment area contains several dental chairs and units. This area is an "open bay," meaning there are no walls separating the dental units (Figure 27-1). The laboratory in the orthodontic office is where appliances and models are fabricated. This area contains equipment and materials necessary to pour impressions, trim study models, and construct orthodontic appliances.

Team

The orthodontic team consists of the orthodontist, reception and business office staff, office coordinator, orthodontic/dental assistants, and laboratory technician(s).

Orthodontist. Orthodontists examine patients, make diagnoses for treatment, and perform orthodontic procedures. They check and evaluate the progress of patients throughout treatment.

Reception and Business Office Staff. The receptionist greets patients and schedules appointments. The business staff takes care of financial arrangements and manages the business administration of the office. They maintain communication with the patients, parents, and the general dentist during the course of treatment.

Office Coordinator. The office coordinator makes sure that the office is run smoothly and efficiently. The coordinator provides information to families considering orthodontic treatment and coordinates the orthodontic assistant's responsibilities during the various phases of patient treatment.

Laboratory Technician. The laboratory technician may pour and trim diagnostic models and working casts. The technician constructs orthodontic appliances and retainers to the specifications of the orthodontist.

Orthodontic Assistant. The orthodontic assistant has a variety of responsibilities depending on the size of the practice and the number of assistants. Functions also vary with each state's dental practice act. The orthodontic assistant works with the dentist but also functions independently to complete many orthodontic adjustments. Generally, the orthodontic assistant has the following responsibilities:

- Seat and dismiss the patient
- Take study model impressions
- Take and process intraoral radiographs (if not provided by the general dentist)
- Take and process extraoral radiographs (panoramic and cephalometric)
- Do the tracing on cephalometric radiographs
- Perform general chairside assisting responsibilities during treatment appointments
- Clean patients' teeth at various stages of treatment
- Maintain and sterilize instruments
- Maintain inventory and supplies
- Help dentist present the treatment plan during the consultation appointment
- Perform routine equipment maintenance

Figure 27-1 (A) Treatment area in orthodontic office. The chairs are arranged in an "open bay." *(continues next page)*

Figure 27-1 *(continued)* (B) Blueprint of an orthodontic office. *(Courtesy of Burkhard Dental Supply.)*

■ Give oral hygiene instructions

■ Give instructions on appliance wear and care

■ Prefit bands before cementation*

■ Remove excess cement from bands and brackets*

■ Apply sealants to teeth to be bonded*

■ Check for loose and broken appliances at each appointment*

■ Place and remove arch wires and ligatures*

■ Remove bands and brackets*

*If allowed by the state dental practice act.

Occlusion and Malocclusion

The dental assistant must understand the terminology related to occlusion to effectively assist the dentist during orthodontic treatment, as well as educate and motivate the patient during treatment.

Normal Occlusion

Normal (or ideal) occlusion describes the contact relationship of the mandibular arch with the maxillary arch. This usually focuses on occlusal contacts, alignment of teeth, and arrangement and relationship of the teeth within and between the arches.

Characteristics of normal occlusion follow:

- The mandibular teeth are in maximum contact with the maxillary teeth and the teeth are not rotated or spaced abnormally.
- The maxillary anterior teeth overlap the incisal edge of the mandibular anterior teeth by 2 mm.
- The maxillary posterior teeth are one cusp distal to the mandibular posterior teeth.
- The mesial buccal cusp of the maxillary first permanent molar occludes in the buccal groove of the mandibular first molar (Figure 27-2).

Figure 27-2 Example of normal occlusion.

Malocclusion

Malocclusion is any deviation from normal occlusion, including misalignment of a single tooth, a group of teeth, or an entire arch. There are many variations of malocclusion. Table 27-1 shows the most common method of classification, called Angle's classification. Also included in the table is the matching facial profile.

In 1899, Edward Angle established a system to classify malocclusion. It is still commonly used today.

Malpositions of Individual Teeth and Groups of Teeth

There are numerous variations in the position of individual teeth in the alveolar bone. The following terms describe these deviations:

- **Torsoversion**—Tooth is rotated or turned.
- **Mesioversion**—Tooth is mesial to normal position.
- **Distoversion**—Tooth is distal to normal position.
- **Linguoversion**—Tooth is lingual to normal position.
- **Labioversion** or **buccoversion**—Tooth is tipped toward the lip or cheek.
- **Supraversion**—Tooth extends above the normal line of occlusion.
- **Infraversion**—Tooth is positioned below the normal line of occlusion.
- **Transversion** or **transposition**—Tooth is in the wrong order in the arch.

Groups of teeth sometimes deviate from the normal tooth positions. Table 27-2 lists the term, provides a description of the variation, and shows an illustration.

Etiology of Malocclusion

The etiology or cause of malocclusion falls into one of three categories:

1. **Genetic or heredity** factors may be responsible for deviations such as supernumerary teeth, facial and palatal clefts, abnormal jaw relationships, abnormal teeth-to-jaw relationships, and congenitally missing teeth.

2. **Systemic** factors include systemic diseases and nutritional disturbances that upset the normal schedule of dentition development during infancy and early childhood.

3. **Local** factors include trauma and habits such as thumb sucking, tongue thrusting, tongue sucking, mouth breathing, bruxism (involuntary grinding or clenching of teeth), and nail biting.

TABLE 27-1 Angle's Classifications of Malocclusion and Facial Profiles

Class Name	Molar Relationship	Cuspid Relationship	Description	Illustration	Facial Profile
Neutrocclusion	Mesiobuccal cusp of maxillary first permanent molar occludes with the buccal groove of the mandibular first permanent molar.	Cusp of maxillary cuspid (canine) occludes between distal of mandibular cuspid and mesial of mandibular first bicuspid.	Similar to normal occlusion with individual teeth or groups of teeth out of position.	Class I	Mesognathic
Distocclusion	Buccal groove of the mandibular first permanent molar is distal to the mesiobuccal cusp of the maxillary first permanent molar.	Cusp of maxillary cuspid (canine) is moved forward and occludes between distal of mandibular lateral incisor and mesial of mandibular cuspid.	Division 1—Maxillary teeth in labioversion (teeth protrude outward, toward lips). Division 2—Linguoversion of mandibular teeth (teeth tilt backward toward the tongue).	Class II, Division 1 Class II, Division 2	Retrognathic Retrognathic
Mesioclusion	Buccal groove of the mandibular first permanent molar is mesial to the mesiobuccal cusp of the maxillary first permanent molar.	Cusp of maxillary cuspid (canine) is moved back and occludes behind mandibular cuspid and in the middle of mandibular first molar.	Mandibular teeth mesial to normal position.	Class III	Prognathic

TABLE 27-2 Malpositions of Groups of Teeth

Term	Description	Illustration
Anterior cross-bite	Abnormal relationship of a tooth or a group of teeth in one arch to the opposing teeth in the other arch. In anterior cross-bite, the maxillary incisors are lingual to the opposing mandibular incisors.	
Posterior cross-bite	Abnormal relationship of teeth in one arch to the opposing teeth in the other arch. In posterior cross-bite, the primary or permanent maxillary posterior teeth are lingual to the mandibular teeth.	Cross-bite Normal bite

(continues)

TABLE 27-2 Malpositions of Groups of Teeth *(continued)*

Edge-to-edge bite	Incisal surfaces of the maxillary anterior teeth meet the incisal surfaces of the mandibular anterior teeth.	
End-to-end bite	Maxillary posterior teeth meet the mandibular posterior teeth cusp-to-cusp instead of in normal fashion.	
Open bite	Failure of the maxillary and mandibular to occlude (meet).	
Overjet (horizontal overlap)	An abnormal horizontal distance between the labial surface of the mandibular anterior teeth and the lingual surface of the maxillary anterior teeth.	
Overbite (vertical overlap)	Normally, the maxillary teeth extend vertically over the incisal one-third of the mandibular anterior teeth. When the vertical overlap is greater than this, the person is said to have an overbite.	
Underjet	Maxillary anteriors positioned lingually to the mandibular anteriors with excessive space between the labial of the maxillary anteriors and the lingual of the mandibular anteriors.	

Types of Orthodontic Treatments

Orthodontic treatment involves much more than straightening teeth. The scope of treatments in orthodontics includes:

- Maintaining or establishing a normal or functional occlusion
- Improving the esthetic appearance of the face
- Eliminating problems that may disrupt normal development of the teeth and facial structures
- Correcting several facial and oral deformities through cooperative work with the oral and maxillofacial surgeon

Orthodontic treatments are divided into cases where malocclusion may be prevented or intercepted and cases where malocclusion already exists and correction is needed.

Preventive and Interceptive Orthodontics

Orthodontic treatment may be **preventive** and **interceptive**. Often, the general dentist and the pediatric dentist provide treatment. In complex cases, the general dentist works with the orthodontist on a treatment plan for the patient.

Common treatments that are considered preventive and interceptive include:

- Placing restorations to prevent premature loss of teeth
- Placing space maintainers to hold space for a missing tooth
- Recognizing any deviation from the normal
- Observing growth patterns and development of teeth and bones
- Correcting bad habits affecting the oral cavity as early as possible
- Extracting teeth to prevent overcrowding
- Removing deciduous teeth to provide space for permanent teeth

Corrective Orthodontics

Corrective orthodontics involves improving existing problems. This type of orthodontics is primarily accomplished on children in the last stage of mixed dentition entering full permanent dentition. Treatment of adults may also fall into corrective orthodontics.

Common treatments that are considered corrective orthodontics include:

- Placement of fixed or removable appliances. **Fixed appliances**, which are attached to the teeth and cannot be removed by the patient, include "braces," bands, brackets, arch wires, and ties. **Removable appliances**, which are inserted into the mouth and removed by the patient, include functional retainers.
- Orthognathic surgery for severe cases.

Process of Tooth Movement

Orthodontic appliances are devices that move teeth by applying force. They also hold teeth in position. The appliances are carefully designed to achieve the desired movement and position of the teeth. The teeth are allowed to be moved through the process of **resorption**, which eliminates tissues no longer needed by the body. The teeth are retained in position through the process of **deposition**, which creates and deposits new cells.

The force of the orthodontic appliance compresses the periodontal ligament and reduces the blood supply to one side of the tooth. Specialized bone cells called **osteoclasts** cause the bone to resorb, or break down. As the tooth moves into the new space, the periodontal ligaments on the other side of the tooth are stretched, causing tension. As the tension increases, bone cells called **osteoblasts** deposit new bone to hold the tooth in its new position.

The principles of tooth movement are the same for all patients regardless of age; however, the rate of movement may be slower in the adult patient. Redeposited bone tissue takes six to twelve months for osteogenesis to take place. Thus, appliances such as retainers are required to hold the teeth in position. Overall, tooth movement depends on the:

- Magnitude of force
- Duration of application of force
- Direction of force
- Distribution of force

Preorthodontic Treatment

Often, the purpose of a patient's first visit to the orthodontist is often preliminary examination. This enables the orthodontist to make an initial recommendation as to whether treatment is advisable at that time or should be delayed until there is further dental development. If treatment is delayed, follow-up appointments may be scheduled periodically to evaluate the patient's growth patterns. If treatment is advised, an appointment is scheduled for diagnostic records.

To ensure successful treatment, the orthodontist must have the cooperation of the patient and the support of the patient's family. This is an important aspect, because orthodontic treatment may take several years to complete. The patient must be willing to follow the directions of the orthodontist concerning appliances and also maintain good oral hygiene.

Diagnostic Records

Diagnostic records for orthodontic treatment include a medical and dental history, clinical examination, panoramic x-rays, cephalometric (**SEF**-ah-loh-meh-trick) x-rays, intraoral and facial photographs, and plaster study models of the teeth.

Medical–Dental History

Treatment begins with a complete medical history to evaluate the general health of the patient. Some conditions and medications have an effect on the patient's response to treatment or may require that the process proceed at a slower pace. Treatment may last for several years, so the medical history must be reviewed periodically.

The dental history provides information about the patient's past exposure to dental treatment. For example, caries incidence, missing teeth, and whether the patient has received routine dental care or only emergency dental care impact the outcome of orthodontic treatment. The dental history gives the orthodontist a guideline when designing the overall treatment plan to facilitate specific needs of the patient.

Clinical Examination

The dentist evaluates the results of an extensive examination of the face, jaws, and teeth, looking for symmetry between them. The teeth are evaluated for size, shape, color, and position. The jaws are examined for size, shape, and relationship to one another. The Angle classification of occlusion is often used to determine the classification on both sides of the mouth.

The oral cavity is also examined for abnormal functional and neuromuscular patterns, such as tongue sucking, tongue thrusting, mouth breathing, and bruxism.

Radiographs

The orthodontist takes radiographs as part of the diagnostic procedure. The most common types of radiographs for orthodontics are the panoramic and cephalometric. Some intraoral films are also taken for more detail of a particular area.

Panoramic x-rays are taken for an overall view of the dentition and surrounding area. Impacted teeth, abscesses, supernumerary teeth, or disorders of the temporomandibular joint can be determined from the panoramic film (Figure 27-3).

Cephalometric films are taken to evaluate the growth patterns and to determine the course of treatment. The cephalometric radiograph is a lateral view of the patient's head that shows the jaw and the teeth. Cephalometric radiograph tracings are performed to determine the relationship of certain landmarks.

Figure 27-3 Panoramic radiograph needed for diagnosis. *(Courtesy of Dr. Steven Gregg.)*

Once the measurements are obtained, they are used for diagnosis, treatment planning, and/or assessment of treatment effects. Cephalometric analyses help the orthodontist determine the shape of the face currently, how the face has grown, what the expected growth will be, and the changes that need to be made. These cephalometric tracings are either done manually using tracing paper and a special pen or by computer (Figure 27-4). Cephalometric radiographs are taken periodically during treatment to monitor the patient's oral facial growth.

Photographs

Intraoral and extraoral photographs are taken as part of the patient's records before and after treatment. Facial photographs include a full frontal view and a profile view (Figure 27-5A). These are used to evaluate the symmetry and balance of the face.

Cheek retractors and mirrors are used when exposing intraoral photographs (Figure 27-5B and C). Intraoral photos are a visual record of the teeth and are used for planning treatment.

Study Models

Study models or diagnostic casts are used as part of the patient's record. They show how the teeth, mouth, and arches relate to one another. The study casts allow the study of the sizes and positions of the teeth along with the widths and lengths of the arches.

The first step is to take an alginate impression of the patient's teeth. The impression is then poured in stone or orthodontic plaster, trimmed, and finished. Orthodontic models are very detailed and symmetrical (Figure 27-6). The finished study models are used in the case presentation as visual aids and are kept as a reference throughout the patient's treatment.

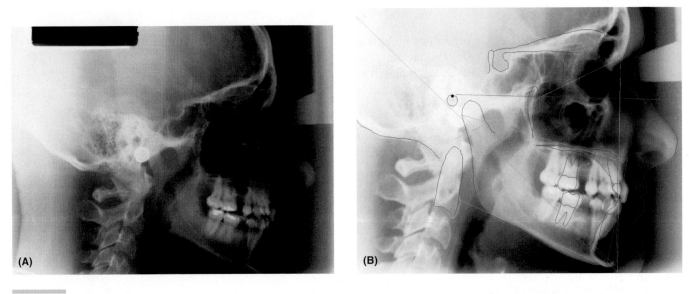

Figure 27-4 (A) Cephalometric radiograph. (B) Cephalometric tracing on a radiograph. *(Courtesy of Dr. Steven Gregg)*

Figure 27-5 Top row: patient profile view and frontal views. Middle row: Intraoral photographs of the maxillary and mandibular arches using mirrors. Bottom row: Dentition from various angles using mirrors and cheek retractors. *(Courtesy of Steven E. Gregg, DDS.)*

Figure 27-6 Orthodontic study model trimmed symmetrically.

Figure 27-7 Patient in full braces. The posterior teeth are banded; the anterior teeth have brackets only. *(Courtesy of Rita Johnson, RDH, and Dr. Vincent DeAngelis.)*

Consultation Appointment

After the diagnostic appointment, the patient (and a parent if the patient is under age eighteen) is scheduled for a consultation appointment. The orthodontist studies the information gathered, makes a diagnosis, and prepares a treatment plan before the patient's appointment. Sufficient time must be allowed to present all the information to the patient (and parents). Radiographs, photographs, study models, and other visual aids are used in the presentation. During the consultation, the treatment, duration of treatment, involvement, and costs are explained. The responsibility of the patient is reviewed at this time so that it is understood what he or she must do to facilitate treatment progress as planned. If the patient accepts the treatment plan, consent papers are signed and financial arrangements are made.

Sometimes, the age and development of the individual patient indicate that treatment be divided into several phases. The first phase may involve the patient wearing removable appliances and/or headgear. The patient often has mixed dentition, and treatment may last several months to two years. Next is the fixed appliance phase, which is started when the patient is in full permanent dentition.

Orthodontic Appliances

Orthodontic appliances are classified into two categories: fixed appliances and removable appliances.

Fixed Appliances

Fixed appliances are attached to the teeth and cannot be removed by the patient. The appliances are directly bonded onto the tooth or cemented into place with dental cement. The treatment is more controlled with fixed appliances, because the patient cannot remove them. Fixed appliances are commonly known as braces (Figure 27-7).

Orthodontic Bands. Orthodontic bands are thin bands of stainless steel that are carefully fitted around each tooth. Bands are supplied in a variety of sizes, and are presized on the patient's model before cementation. Glass ionomer, polycarboxylate, or zinc phosphate cement is commonly used for cementing orthodontic bands. Bands are used on the posterior teeth because they provide the means to hold and control tooth movement. Depending on the individual case, various attachments such as brackets or buccal tubes are placed on the bands (Figure 27-8A and B).

Brackets. Brackets are attachments that are either welded to the bands or bonded directly to the teeth. Brackets for the posterior teeth are made of stainless steel and are welded directly to the band. Brackets for the anterior teeth are made of stainless steel, ceramic, or acrylic, and are cemented or directly bonded to the teeth. Ceramic and acrylic brackets are popular because they are barely noticeable on the anterior teeth (Figure 27-8B). Tooth-colored brackets are also difficult to see on the teeth (Figure 27-8C).

The functions of the bracket are to hold the arch wire in place and to transmit the force of the arch wire to move the tooth.

Arch Wires. Arch wires fit into brackets and are secured by ligature ties or elastics. The arch wire is placed in the bracket and through a buccal tube on a posterior molar and then at each bracket; ligature wire or elastics are wrapped around the bracket. Arch wires are supplied in various shapes (square, round, and rectangular), diameters, and compositions, which alter the effect of the treatment (Figure 27-9A).

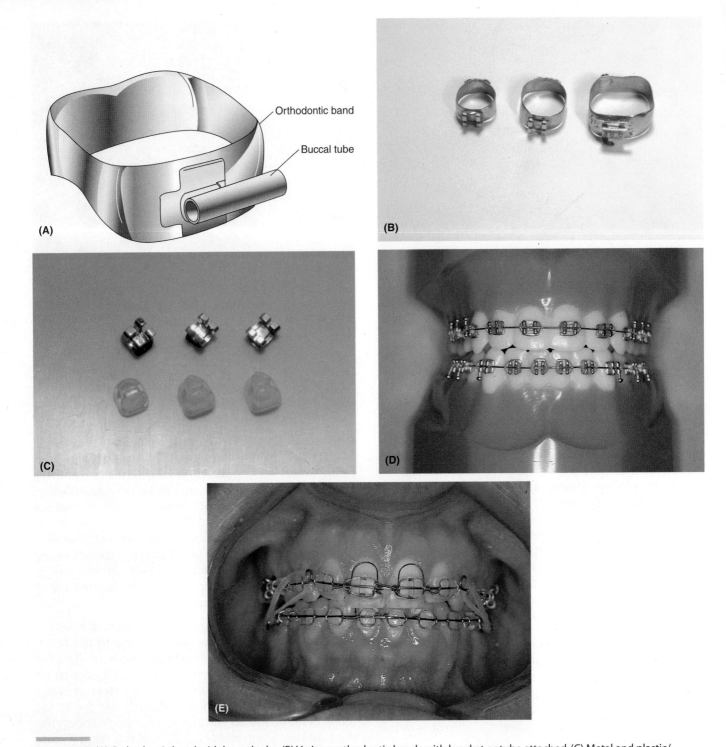

Figure 27-8 (A) Orthodontic band with buccal tube. (B) Various orthodontic bands with bracket or tube attached. (C) Metal and plastic/porcelain brackets. (D) Metal brackets on a model. (E) Tooth-colored brackets. *(D and E, Courtesy of Rita Johnson, RDH, and Dr. Vincent DeAngelis.)*

The function of the arch wire is to apply force to either move the teeth into or hold desired positions. The position of the arch wire is changed throughout treatment as the teeth move.

Ligature Wire and Plastic Rings. Ligature wire and plastic rings are used to hold the arch wire to the brackets. Ligature wire is a very thin, flexible wire that usually comes in precut lengths or on spools (Figure 27-9B). The wire wraps around the bracket and then is tightened by twisting the wire, which ties or "ligates" the arch wire to the bracket. Plastic rings, also called elastic ties, are small bands that are supplied in a variety of colors. The elastic bands slip over the bracket to secure the arch wire. Also commonly used are elastic chains. The chain is a continuous chain of "Os." The elastic chain attaches several adjacent teeth together. This continuous pressure brings the teeth together (Figure 27-9C).

Figure 27-10 Patient with full braces: bands with buccal tubes, brackets, arch wire, ligature wire, elastics, and finger springs. *(Courtesy of Rita Johnson, RDH, and Dr. Vincent DeAngelis.)*

Figure 27-9 (A) Various arch wires. (B) Ligature wire used to secure the arch wire to the brackets. (C) Elastic bands, "O's," and chain elastics are also used to secure the arch wire to the brackets.

Figure 27-11 (A) Finger spring on palate of retainer. (B) Coil spring.

Buccal Tubes. Buccal tubes are small cylinders of metal welded to the molar bands, usually on the buccal surface. Their function is to provide a means of attachment for the arch wire to the band in the posterior area (Figures 27-8 and 27-10).

Springs. Springs are specially bent or shaped wires that are attached to the main arch wire. There are two main kinds of springs: the finger spring and the coil spring. The finger spring provides gentle pressure on individual teeth (Figure 27-11A). The coil springs exert pressure to expand and compress spaces without losing the working force (Figure 27-11B).

Elastics. Elastics are rubber bands or elastic threads that are available in a variety of sizes. Elastics provide

Figure 27-12 Patient in full braces with rubber elastic from one arch to the other. The rubber bands provide the force for movement. *(Courtesy of Rita Johnson, RDH, and Dr. Vincent DeAngelis.)*

force for movement. They are often used between the upper and lower arches. Elastics are attached to hooks or buttons that are secured on the band or brackets.

 New developments in ligature ties include fluoride-releasing ties that aid in reducing decalcification of the tooth (Figure 27-12).

Special Fixed Appliances

There are several fixed orthodontic appliances that are not part of routine braces. These appliances are cemented in place and have a specific function for a specific treatment or phases of treatment. They include lingual braces, lingual arch wire, space maintainer, and the palatal expansion appliance.

Lingual Braces. Lingual braces, sometimes called invisible braces, are attached to the lingual surface of the teeth. These braces allow patients who are apprehensive about their appearance during treatment an option to conventional braces. When the braces are placed on the lingual surfaces they are much less noticeable. The disadvantages to lingual braces include placement and maintenance. It is difficult to keep the areas dry during cementation, and they are troublesome for the patient to maintain.

Lingual Arch Wire. The lingual arch wire is placed on the lingual surface instead of the facial. Orthodontic bands are placed on the first permanent molars, and the arch wire is closely adapted to the lingual surfaces of the teeth. The function of the lingual arch wire is to maintain the arch by holding the teeth in position until the permanent teeth erupt (Figure 27-13A and B).

Space Maintainer. The space maintainer is composed of a band and a wire loop soldered together (Figure 27-14). Its function is to maintain space for the permanent tooth

(A)

(B)

Figure 27-13 (A) Patient with a lingual arch wire. (B) Patient with a lingual arch bar from cuspid to cuspid.

Figure 27-14 Space maintainer to hold space when a tooth is lost prematurely.

to erupt after premature loss of the primary tooth. There are several varieties of space maintainers that can be adapted to the patient's teeth.

Maintaining this space until the permanent tooth begins to erupt is important. If the space is not held open, the adjacent teeth will drift in and begin to fill the space, which makes it more difficult for the permanent tooth to erupt as well as come in straight.

The space maintainer must be cemented in place to hold the teeth in position; if the maintainer loosens or comes out, it should be replaced as soon as possible to prevent the teeth from moving. If it is left out too long, a new impression must be taken and a new space maintainer must be fabricated.

Palatal Separating Appliance. The palatal separating appliance is composed of an acrylic palatal portion that is split along the midline. The acrylic palatal portion is attached to bands, and the bands are cemented to the posterior teeth for stability. In the middle of the acrylic is a screw-like device that can be adjusted to expand the arch. The function of the palatal separating appliance is to spread the mid-palatal suture. This process takes about two to three weeks. Bone tissue fills in the opening and closes the space (Figure 27-15).

The screw must be turned twice each day once the device is cemented in place. A "key" is inserted into one of the holes on the screw and pushed toward the throat. The next hole will then be exposed for the next turn. The key should always be secured by wrapping the string that is attached to the key around the wrist to prevent the possibility of swallowing the key. The tightening process may be a little uncomfortable until the palate separates to the desired space; subsequently, the patient may feel as if the roof of the mouth itches. The space between the maxillary central incisors may widen during the first two weeks as the appliance spreads the arch. The space will disappear soon when it is no longer necessary to turn the screw on the separator.

Removable Appliances

Removable appliances are designed to be inserted into the mouth and removed by the patient. There are numerous varieties of removable appliances and many ways to categorize them. The more commonly used removable appliances include headgear, functional appliances, retainers, and positioners. Also in this category of removable appliances is the invisible straightening of fully erupted permanent teeth with a series of removable custom plastic "aligners."

Headgear. Headgear consists of a strap that goes behind the patient's head or neck and a facebow that attaches to buccal tubes on molar bands. There are many designs to meet the individual patient's needs. Headgear is used to apply force to move teeth, to restrain or alter cranial-facial bone growth, and to reinforce stability of intraoral appliances. Usually, patients wear headgear for a specific number of hours per day (Figure 27-16).

Functional Appliances. Functional appliances are removable appliances that are routinely used before fixed appliances are placed. Functional appliances are used while the teeth and cranial-facial skeleton are still developing. There is a wide variety of functional appliances. Some guide newly erupting teeth into position, others change the direction of cranial-facial skeletal growth, and still others inhibit the growth rate of one arch. The activator is the original functional jaw orthopedic appliance, and it has been modified many times. The activator is used to expand the width of the maxillary arch, for minor tooth movement, to make changes in skeletal growth patterns, and to reduce overbite (projection of upper teeth over the lower). The most common activators are the Bionator, the Herbst, and the Frankel (Figure 27-17).

Retainers. Retainers are custom-made appliances fitted to the patient's arch. They are made of acrylic or metal wire and acrylic and are secured in the patient's mouth by wires braced against and/or around the teeth. They are used to retain the teeth in position after the fixed

Figure 27-15 Palatal separating appliance. *(Courtesy of Rita Johnson, RDH, and Dr. Vincent DeAngelis.)*

Figure 27-16 Headgear with adjustable straps used to apply force to move teeth.

appliances have been removed. The Hawley is an example of a retainer (Figure 27-18).

Tooth Positioner. The **tooth positioner** is a flexible rubber or soft-plastic appliance that surrounds the crowns of all teeth, in both arches, when positioned in the patient's mouth. Positioners are custom made for the patient after the removal of fixed appliances. Their function is to maintain the ideal position of the teeth upon completion of fixed treatment (Figure 27-19).

Esthetic Orthodontic Aligners. The aligner is an esthetic orthodontic appliance that, in conjunction with a dentist's diagnosis, treatment plan, and advances in medical imaging technology, corrects malocclusion using a series of custom-made, nearly invisible, removable aligners.

Patients wear each aligner for a minimum of two weeks, for about 22 hours per day. Aligners are only removed for eating, brushing, and flossing. Teeth are moved gradually as each aligner is replaced with the next, until the desired results are achieved (Figure 27-20).

The aligners are similar to whitening or fluoride trays in that they are custom made, but are thinner, even

Figure 27-17 (A) Patient with Bionator appliance. (B) Bionator appliance. (C) Herbst appliance. (D) Patient with Frankel appliance. (E) Frankel appliance. *(Courtesy of Dr. Steven Gregg.)*

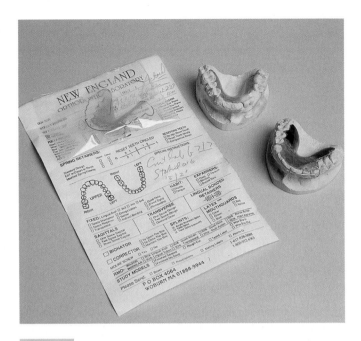

Figure 27-18 Various Hawley appliances with lab prescription.

Figure 27-20 Invisalign® esthetic orthodontic appliance. *(Courtesy of Invisalign-Align Technology, Inc.)*

Figure 27-19 Tooth positioner in storage container and in mouth.

practice building are presented. See Table 27-3 for an example of a sequence of treatment.

Orthodontic Instruments

Listed below are commonly used instruments and their functions.

- Coon ligature tying pliers—Manipulate ligature wire (Figure 27-21)
- Mathieu needle holder—Tie ligature wire and place elastic ligatures (Figure 27-22)
- Ligature director—Tucks twisted ligature wire ends into interproximal spaces (a small condenser may also be used) (Figure 27-23)
- Pin and ligature cutter or light wire cutter—Cut thin ligature wire (Figure 27-24)
- Howe pliers—Utility pliers to manipulate ligature wire (Figure 27-25)

more precise, and fabricated from a more rigid, proprietary material. The number of aligners and length of treatment depend on the complexity of the case. As with traditional braces, patients experience a brief period of adjustment as they transition to each new set of aligners. Since the aligners are removable, oral hygiene is easy to maintain, while patients eat, brush, and floss as they normally would.

Dentists must complete a program offered through the manufacturers in order to treat patients with their product. Dental auxiliaries attending the certification program will learn the submission process, which includes PVS impressions and bite, x-rays, intra- and extra-oral photographs, and the dentist's treatment plan. Additionally, modules on case management and

Figure 27-21 Coon ligature tying pliers.

TABLE 27-3   Sequence of Treatment for Invisalign® Aligners

Dental office evaluation	Complete examination and discussion of patient's chief complaint.
↓	Complete records • FMX or panorex (cephalometric optional) • PVS impressions (full maxillary and mandibular) • PVS bite • Series of intraoral and extraoral photographs • Prescription and diagnosis forms completed
Submit case to Align Technology ↓	Align receives records (x-rays, impressions, photos). Impressions are scanned to create a highly accurate 3D model of the patient's teeth. A computerized movie called ClinCheck® is then made depicting the movement of teeth from the beginning of treatment to the projected final result. This software allows the dentist to take an online virtual tour of the patient's teeth. You will see the patient's teeth the way they are at the beginning of treatment, the way they will look at the end, and each stage in between. Aligners are not manufactured until the treating dentist approves this ClinCheck file.
Dental office ↓	Dentist reviews ClinCheck file, makes any necessary modifications, and accepts the case to authorize fabrication of Aligners.
Manufacturing of aligners ↓	From the approved ClinCheck file, Align uses lasers to build a set of resin models for each stage/set of Aligners to be fabricated for the patient. From the resin models, Align Technology manufactures a series of clear Aligners with the specified movements built into the shape of each one sequentially. All aligners are shipped to the treating dentist.
Dental office	Dentist dispenses first set of Aligners to patient and schedules next appointment for two weeks to evaluate and deliver subsequent sets of Aligners. Normally after the second appointment, patients can be given two to three sets of Aligners at one time, with future visits scheduled 6 weeks apart.

Figure 27-22 Mathieu needle holder.

Figure 27-24 Pin and ligature cutter.

Figure 27-23 Ligature director.

- Band seater—Seats posterior metal bands (Figure 27-26)
- Bite stick band seater—Uses force of occlusion to seat the band (Figure 27-27)
- Band driver—Pushes the band into place (Figure 27-28)
- Posterior band removing pliers—Removes posterior bands (Figure 27-29)
- Band contouring pliers—Stretches and shapes the posterior bands to adapt to the tooth (Figure 27-30)
- Bracket forceps—Holds brackets for placement and positioning (Figure 27-31)
- "Bird-beak" pliers—Contours wire and forms springs (Figure 27-32)

Figure 27-25 Howe pliers.

Figure 27-26 Band seater.

Figure 27-27 Bite-block with band seater.

Figure 27-28 Band driver (pusher).

Figure 27-29 Posterior band–removing pliers.

Figure 27-30 Band-contouring pliers.

Figure 27-31 Bracket forceps.

Figure 27-32 Bird-beak pliers.

- Three-prong pliers—Adjusts and bends wire and clasps (Figure 27-33)
- Weingart utility pliers—Places the arch wire (Figure 27-34)
- Tweed loop pliers—Forms loops and springs in wire (Figure 27-35)
- Distal-end cutting pliers—Cuts the distal ends of the arch wire (Figure 27-36)

Figure 27-35 Tweed loop pliers.

Figure 27-33 Three-prong pliers.

Figure 27-34 Weingart utility pliers.

Figure 27-36 Distal end–cutting pliers.

Orthodontic Treatment

CDA Orthodontic treatment begins after the patient has finished the consultation appointment, the general dentist has restored all areas of decay, and the patient has been given a prophylaxis and fluoride treatment.

The orthodontic treatment sequence follows:

1. Application of separators
2. Placement of posterior bands
3. Placement of anterior brackets
4. Placement of arch wire
5. Interval checkups
6. Completion appointment

Separators

A few days before the bands are placed on the posterior teeth, the patient is scheduled for placement of **separators**. Separators are placed in the contact areas between the teeth, forcing the teeth to spread apart to accommodate the orthodontic bands. Types of separators include elastics, steel spring, and brass wire.

Elastic separators are used because they provide a constant force as the teeth move, are easy to apply, and are more comfortable for the patient. The elastic separators are small circles that are stretched for placement. They fit around the contact area and, when released, apply a constant pressure until the teeth move apart, usually within a couple of days. The dental assistant may be permitted, in some states, to place and remove these separators (Procedures 27-1, 27-2, and 27-3).

Selection of Orthodontic Bands

The patient returns to the office in a few days to have the separators removed and orthodontic bands placed. The bands may be selected and sized on the patient's study model before the appointment, or the selection may take place directly on the patient during the appointment. Bands are supplied in a wide variety of sizes for each tooth in the arch. They often have an identifying code printed on one surface. The code is helpful when selecting bands and replacing unused, sterilized bands.

PROCEDURE 27-1

Placement and Removal of Elastic Separators

After the diagnosis, the objective of the first treatment appointment is to place separators to prepare the teeth for the orthodontic bands. Following the dentist's directions, the dental assistant places the separators. The separators are removed and the bands placed several days following this procedure.

EQUIPMENT AND SUPPLIES (Figure 27-37)

- Basic setup: mouth mirror, explorer, and cotton pliers
- Separation pliers
- Separators (wire or elastic)
- Dental floss or tape (optional technique)
- Scaler

*Mathieu needle holder

PROCEDURE STEPS *(Follow aseptic procedures)*

Placement of Elastic Separators with Separating Pliers

1. Examine the patient's mouth using the mouth mirror.

2. Place elastic separator over the beaks of the separating pliers. Squeeze the pliers to secure the elastic on the pliers.

3. Further squeeze the pliers to stretch the elastic separator and place it between two teeth in a back-

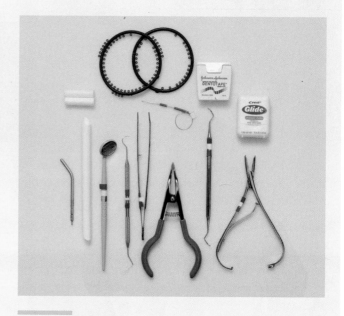

Figure 27-37 Tray setup for placement and removal of elastic separators.

(continues)

PROCEDURE 27-1 *(CONTINUED)*

and-forth motion similar to the motion used when flossing. Insert one side of the elastic band below the contact in the interproximal space.

4. Release the tension on the separating pliers and remove the pliers. Repeat this process on all interproximal spaces around the teeth that will receive metal bands.

Placement of Separators with Dental Floss (Figure 27-38)

1. Place two lengths of dental floss through an elastic separator.

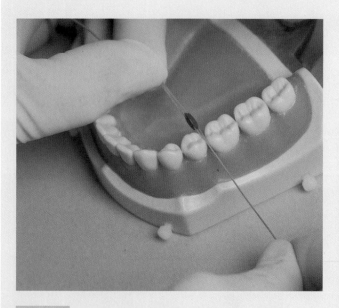

Figure 27-38 Placement of separators. Dental floss stretches elastic separator for placement. *(Courtesy of Rita Johnson, RDH, and Dr. Vincent DeAngelis.)*

2. Fold over each floss length until the ends meet. Pull each piece of floss by the ends to stretch the elastic.

3. Using a back-and-forth motion, insert the separator into place.

4. Once the separator is in place, release the floss and pull free.

Removal of Elastic Separators (Figure 27-39)

1. Using a scaler or an explorer, insert one end into the ring of the elastic separator.

2. Place a finger over the top of the separator to prevent the separator from snapping and injuring the patient.

3. Pull gently on the instrument toward the occlusal until the elastic is free of the contact.

Figure 27-39 Removal of elastic separators. *(Courtesy of Rita Johnson, RDH, and Dr. Vincent DeAngelis.)*

PROCEDURE 27-2

Placement and Removal of Steel Spring Separators

This technique involves placing and removing steel spring separators.

EQUIPMENT AND SUPPLIES

■ Basic setup: mouth mirror, explorer, and cotton pliers

■ Dental floss

■ Bird-beak or #139 pliers

■ Steel spring separators

(continues)

PROCEDURE 27-2 *(CONTINUED)*

PROCEDURE STEPS *(Follow aseptic procedures)*

Placing Steel Spring Separators (Figure 27-40)

1. Using the selected pliers, grasp the shortest side or leg of the spring separator.

2. Place the curve-hook of the spring separator under the contact from the lingual side.

3. Release the short side of the spring separator and slide it under the contact.

4. The coil is on the facial side; test the placement by gently pressing on the spring.

Removing Steel Spring Separators

1. Place the finger of one hand over the spring to prevent injury to the patient.

Long leg

Short leg

Figure 27-40 Steel spring separator.

2. Place one end of a scaler in the coil and lift upward.

3. Once the longest side of the spring is free of the lingual embrasure, pull the coil toward the facial aspect.

PROCEDURE 27-3

Placement and Removal of Brass Wire

This procedure involves placing and removing brass wire separators.

EQUIPMENT AND SUPPLIES

- Basic setup: mouth mirror, explorer, and cotton pliers
- Spool of brass wire (Figure 27-41)
- Hemostat
- Ligature wire cutter
- Condenser

Placing Brass Wire Separators

1. Bend brass wire into C-shape, leaving a "tail" portion.

2. Starting from the lingual surface, place one part of the wire under the contact using a hemostat.

3. Fold the other part of the wire over the contact and pull toward the facial. Bring the ends of the wire together and twist.

4. Cut the twisted ends with the ligature cutting pliers and tuck them into the gingival embrasure.

Figure 27-41 Spool of brass wire used to separate the teeth.

Removing Brass Wire Separators

1. Lift the brass wire carefully near the occlusal surface on the lingual side. Cut the wire using ligature cutting pliers.

2. Use the hemostat to remove both sections of the wire from under the contact on the facial side.

Once the bands have been selected, they are tied on the teeth in the following way:

1. Place the band over the occlusal and apply pressure with a finger. The band should move toward the cervical third of the tooth.

2. The band pusher is used to push the band onto the tooth so that the margins of the band are beyond the occlusion (Figure 27-42). The band is adjusted until it closely fits the tooth contours.

Figure 27-42 Band pusher is used to seat the band on the tooth. *(Courtesy of Rita Johnson, RDH, and Dr. Vincent DeAngelis.)*

3. After all bands have been sized, they are removed with band removal pliers and placed on a model or band block.

4. The orthodontist or lab technician then prepares the bands for final cementation by smoothing the margins of the bands with a handpiece and bur. If the bands have brackets or buccal tubes, the bands are fitted with pins or wax in the openings to prevent cement from filling the bracket holes and the buccal tubes.

Band Cementation

Orthodontic bands are cemented using a variety of cements, including glass ionomer, polycarboxylate, and zinc phosphate. Although zinc phosphate cement has been used for many years, glass ionomer cement is becoming the preferred cement because it releases fluoride, which helps prevent decay under the bands during treatment.

Generally, the cement is thick for orthodontic band cementation and has a long setting time to permit final seating and adaptation. Follow manufacturer's instructions and technique suggestions (Procedure 27-4).

Direct Bonding Brackets

The placement of brackets directly on the anterior teeth is a popular choice of treatment. Patients like the brackets because they are more esthetic than the full bands and it is easier to maintain good oral hygiene. The brack-

---

PROCEDURE 27-4

Cementation of Orthodontic Bands

Orthodontic bands are prepared for the individual patient. The orthodontist places the bands on the teeth to accomplish the task needed to correct the patient's malocclusion. The dental assistant mixes the cement and prepares the band for seating.

EQUIPMENT AND SUPPLIES (Figure 27-43)

- Basic setup: mouth mirror, explorer, and cotton pliers
- Cotton rolls and gauze
- Saliva ejector and HVE
- Slow-speed handpiece with rubber cup and prophy paste

- Selected and prepared bands
- Band pusher
- Bite stick
- Scaler
- Cement of choice
- Paper pad or glass slab
- Cement spatula
- Plastic filling instrument (PFI)

(continues)

P R O C E D U R E 2 7 - 4 *(C O N T I N U E D)*

Figure 27-43 (A) Selection of bands. (B) Tray setup for cementation of orthodontic bands.

Figure 27-44 (A) Assistant passes the band filled with cement to operator. (B) Excess cement is removed from the tooth around the band. *(Courtesy of Rita Johnson, RDH, and Dr. Vincent DeAngelis.)*

PROCEDURE STEPS *(Follow aseptic procedures)*

1. Once the separators are removed, the teeth are given a rubber cup polish.

2. The patient's mouth is rinsed thoroughly. The teeth are dried and cotton rolls are placed for isolation in the areas where the bands are to be placed.

3. Mix the cement according to manufacturer's directions and load the first band. Place cement from the gingival edge, covering the inside of the band. Once the band is ready, transfer it to the dentist. There are many methods to transfer the bands. Some orthodontists prefer placement on the mixing slab or pad in order. Others like the bands passed on the end of the spatula or on a piece of wax or masking tape. Transferring the band needs to be made as easy as possible. Position the bands so that the orthodontist can pick them up in order of placement sequence (Figure 27-44A).

4. The orthodontist seats the band on the tooth. Transfer the band driver and any other instrument the orthodontist requests until the band is properly seated.

5. The banding procedure is repeated. Continue to fill the bands and transfer them to the operator until all bands have been cemented or until the cement becomes too thick and a new mix is required. If a new mix is required, clean the instruments with a wet gauze or an alcohol wipe and mix additional cement.

6. Once all bands are in place, the cement is allowed to set. During this time, clean the cement off all used instruments.

7. After the cement is set, remove the excess cement with a scaler. When all the cement has been removed, the protective pins or wax is removed from the brackets and the patient's mouth is rinsed (Figure 27-44B).

ets are often purchased in kits or sets. The kit includes brackets from the left second bicuspid to right second bicuspid on both arches.

The brackets are bonded to the tooth surface with a similar material and technique used to restore anterior teeth composite resin (Procedure 27-5).

Placement of Arch Wire

The orthodontist selects and shapes the arch wire, so once the bands and brackets are placed, the arch wire can be positioned and secured in place (Procedure 27-6). The arch wire is commonly secured into the

---

PROCEDURE 27-5

Direct Bonding of Brackets

This procedure involves bonding the brackets to the teeth.

EQUIPMENT AND SUPPLIES (Figure 27-45)

- Basic setup: mouth mirror, explorer, and cotton pliers
- Cotton rolls and gauze
- Saliva ejector and HVE
- Slow-speed handpiece with rubber cup and pumice
- Bracket kit
- Retractors for cheeks and lips
- Bracket forceps
- Acid etchant
- Bonding agent
- Scaler

Figure 27-45 Tray setup for direct bonding of brackets.

PROCEDURE STEPS

(Follow aseptic procedures)

1. Polish the teeth that are to receive brackets with a rubber cup and pumice (Figure 27-46A). (Polishing paste with fluoride is not used because some of the ingredients will interfere with the bonding process.)

2. The patient's mouth is rinsed and dried. Cotton rolls are placed in the area where brackets are to be bonded and retractors are positioned.

3. The acid etchant is placed on the enamel surface. The etchant remains on the tooth for a specific amount of time, as per the manufacturer's directions. Prepare the etchant and transfer it to the operator. Maintain the operating field to be sure it stays dry.

4. Rinse the patient's mouth long enough to ensure that all the etchant is removed from the tooth surface (approximately thirty seconds) and then dry the tooth/teeth. The teeth will have a chalky appearance.

5. Prepare the bonding agent according to the manufacturer's directions and apply it to the back of the bracket (Figure 27-46B). Transfer the agent to the dentist for placement on the tooth. Then pass the bracket. The orthodontist positions it on the tooth. Any excess bonding agent is removed from around the bracket with a scaler or similar instrument.

6. The brackets are then held in position on the tooth until the bonding material is set chemically or with a curing light (Figure 27-46C).

7. Remove the cotton rolls and retractors from the patient's mouth.

(continues)

PROCEDURE 27-5 (CONTINUED)

Figure 27-46 Steps in placement of direct-bonded brackets. (A) Clean tooth surface. (B) Apply bonding agent to back of bracket (C) place bracket and light cure. *(Courtesy of Rita Johnson, RDH, and Dr. Vincent DeAngelis.)*

brackets with elastic or stainless steel ligatures (ties). There is also a bracket that does not require ligature ties; instead, the bracket has a slot that opens for placement and removal of the arch wire. It is called the "Damon SL" (Figure 27-47).

Oral Hygiene Instructions

Oral hygiene instructions are given to the patient once the braces are in place. With fixed braces, food and debris have many places to hide and attach to, making the patient more caries susceptible. Good oral hygiene is necessary to prevent plaque buildup in these areas. The dental assistant educates and motivates the patient. This process is continued throughout the treatment. Keeping some patients motivated can be a challenge, and numerous approaches must be used.

Instructions include the following:

■ Brushing—The patient is given an orthodontic toothbrush and shown how to brush around the fixed appliances in order to remove plaque. The toothbrush is contoured to fit around the brackets and into the space

Figure 27-47 Damon SL bracket. *(Courtesy of Dwight H. Damon, DDS, MSD.)*

PROCEDURE 27-6

Placement of Arch Wire and Ligature Ties

This procedure involves placing the arch wire and ligature ties.

EQUIPMENT AND SUPPLIES (Figure 27-48)

- Basic setup: mouth mirror, explorer, and cotton pliers
- Cotton rolls and gauze
- Saliva ejector and HVE
- Selected arch wire
- Weingart pliers
- Bird-beak pliers
- Elastics or ligature wire
- Ligature cutting pliers
- Ligature tying pliers
- Distal-end cutting pliers
- Condenser

PROCEDURE STEPS

1. Insert the arch wire into the buccal tubes on the molar bands using the Weingart pliers. If the wire is too long, cut off the ends with the distal-end cutting pliers.

2. The arch wire is placed in bracket horizontal slots along the arch (Figure 27-49A). This may be accom-

(A)

(B)

Figure 27-49 (A) Arch wire is cut to size with distal-end cutting pliers. (B) Place arch wire in buccal tubes. *(Courtesy of Rita Johnson, RDH, and Dr. Vincent DeAngelis.)*

Figure 27-48 Tray setup for placement of arch wire and ligature ties.

plished with plastic rings/elastic ties, ligature wire, or the Damon SL bracket.

Elastic Ties Placement

3. The elastic ties are slipped over the brackets using ligature tying pliers or a hemostat. The ring ties are spread and placed on the gingival extensions of the brackets, pulled over the arch wire, and then wrapped around the occlusal extensions of the brackets (Figure 27-50).

Ligature Wire Ties Placement

4. Hold the ligature wire between the thumb and the index finger. Wrap the wire around the occlusal and gingival wings of the bracket in a distal-mesial direction. Cross the ends of the wire together. Using a hemostat or ligature tying pliers, twist the ends of the wire together for several rotations. Repeat the process to secure the arch wire (Figure 27-51A).

(continues)

PROCEDURE 27-6 *(CONTINUED)*

Figure 27-50 Elastic rings being placed on anterior brackets. *(Courtesy of Rita Johnson, RDH, and Dr. Vincent DeAngelis.)*

5. The twisted ends of the ligature wire, called the "pigtail," are cut with ligature-wire cutting pliers to 3 to 4 mm (Figure 27-51B and C).

6. The pigtail is bent into the embrasure space with a condenser (Figure 27-51D).

7. After all the pigtail ends have been tucked into place, run a finger over the area to check for sharp ends.

8. Check the distal ends of the arch wire. Cut any excess with distal-end cutting pliers.

9. If the patient's treatment requires rubber elastic bands, they are placed at this appointment. The patient is shown how to place and remove them. The rubber bands stretch over time, so the orthodontist will give instructions on how often to change the rubber bands. The patient is given a sufficient number of elastics with instructions to call the office for more, if needed.

Figure 27-51 (A) Ligature wire being looped around brackets. (B) Ligature wire is twisted. (C) Ligature wire is cut with cutting pliers. (D) Ligature wire is tucked into embrasure space. *(Courtesy of Rita Johnson, RDH, and Dr. Vincent DeAngelis.)*

Figure 27-52 Toothbrushing with fixed orthodontic appliances. Toothbrush positioned properly on (A) maxillary teeth and (B) mandibular teeth.

Figure 27-53 Floss being threaded under arch wire.

- Fluoride rinses—These may be prescribed for the patient's home use during orthodontic treatment.

Periodic Office Visits for Adjustments

As time passes and the teeth begin to move, the patient will need to see the orthodontist for adjustments. These appointments are usually short, unless the arch wire needs to be changed. The orthodontist reviews the patient's progress, checks the appliances, and makes any adjustments. The dental assistant performs some of these tasks under direct supervision of the dentist.

These appointments are also used for oral hygiene checks. If the patient is not doing an adequate job, the dental assistant reviews brushing and flossing with the patient and talks with the patient to motivate and encourage.

Helping some patients stay motivated to maintain oral hygiene can be a challenge. Dental assistants are often responsible for this task. Educating the patient is the first step, followed by demonstrating various techniques for brushing and flossing with braces. Each orthodontic office has different ways to motivate and reward patients who maintain oral hygiene. Verbal and written encouragement, prizes, gift cards, passes to movies, and so on, and patient's name placed in drawing for a larger prize are just a few ways to encourage and motivate orthodontic patients.

Completion Appointment

Once the teeth have moved into position and the orthodontist is satisfied with the treatment, the braces are removed. The patient receives a coronal polish and an impression is taken for construction of a retainer (Procedure 27-7) or positioner to hold the teeth in position for the alveolar bone to stabilize the new positions of the teeth.

between the band and the gingival margin. The patient will need to spend more time after meals and at bedtime to keep the teeth clean (Figure 27-52A and B).

- Flossing—Supply the patient with a floss threader to thread the floss under the arch wire and through the interproximal area. Motivating the patient to take the time to floss routinely may be a challenge (Figure 27-53).

- Diet—The patient should avoid certain foods that may damage the bands, arch wire, or brackets. Foods that are sticky, crunchy, and hard should be avoided. Examples include caramels, chewing gum, popcorn, and raw vegetables (unless they are cut into small pieces).

PROCEDURE 27 - 7

Completion Appointment

When the orthodontist determines that the patient's teeth have moved to the desired positions, the appliances are removed.

EQUIPMENT AND SUPPLIES (Figure 27-54)

- Basic setup: mouth mirror, explorer, and cotton pliers
- Cotton rolls and gauze
- Scaler
- Ligature-wire cutting pliers
- Hemostat
- Bracket and adhesive removing pliers
- Posterior band remover
- Ultrasonic scaler (optional)
- Prophy angle, cups, and prophy paste
- Alginate impression material and selected tray

PROCEDURE STEPS *(Follow aseptic procedures)*

1. The ligature ties are removed first. They are loosened with a scaler or an explorer and then cut with the ligature-wire cutting pliers.

Elastic Bands

2. Elastic ties are removed with a scaler.

3. The tip of the scaler explorer is placed under the elastic and rolled over the bracket wings until the elastic is released (Figure 27-55).

Ligature Wire Ties

4. Place the beaks of ligature-wire cutting pliers where the wire is exposed and cut wire.

5. Carefully remove the wire from the wings of the bracket. Repeat on each tooth until all ligature wires are removed.

6. Using a hemostat, remove the arch wire from the brackets (Figure 27-56). Pull the arch wire from the buccal tube on one side. Then hold it securely to prevent injury to the patient while removing the opposite end.

7. To remove the anterior brackets, use a bracket and adhesive-removing pliers. The lower beak of the pliers, with a very sharp edge, is placed on the gingival edge of the bracket; the upper beak, with a nylon tip, is placed on the occlusal edge of the bracket. When the pliers are squeezed together, the sharp lower beak breaks the bond and removes some cement (Figure 27-57).

Figure 27-54 Completion appointment tray setup.

Figure 27-55 Removal of elastic rings. Insert end of scaler or explorer under elastic, and roll elastic rings over wings of bracket. *(Courtesy of Rita Johnson, RDH, and Dr. Vincent DeAngelis.)*

(continues)

PROCEDURE 27 - 7 *(CONTINUED)*

Figure 27-56 Removal of ligature wire. Pull twisted "pigtail" wire from embrasure. Cut wire. Unwind from wings of bracket in an occlusal direction. *(Courtesy of Rita Johnson, RDH, and Dr. Vincent DeAngelis.)*

8. To remove the posterior bands, band-removing pliers are placed with the cushioned end on the buccal cusp. The end with the blade is placed against the gingival edge of the band. The band is gently lifted toward the occlusal surface (Figure 27-58).

9. This process is repeated on the lingual surfaces until the band is free.

10. Cement and direct bonding materials are removed from the tooth surface with a hand scaler, an ultrasonic scaler, and/or a finishing bur.

11. A rubber cup polish is completed. Photographs may be taken.

12. An alginate impression is taken of both arches. The impressions are sent to the lab to be used in construction of the retainer.

13. The patient is reappointed for later that day or for the next day. The retainer or positioner is then placed.

14. The patient is given instructions on placement and removal of the retainer and the wearing schedule.

Figure 27-57 Bracket removal.

Figure 27-58 Band removal with band-removal pliers.

CHAPTER SUMMARY

The orthodontic team consists of the orthodontist, reception and business office staff, office coordinator, orthodontic assistants, and laboratory technicians. The orthodontic assistant has a variety of responsibilities, depending on the size of the practice and the number of auxiliaries. Assistants may work with the dentist or function independently under the direction of the dentist. The functions also vary with each state's dental practice act.

To become a certified orthodontic assistant, a specialty examination must be passed.

Case Study

Chaz Danton, twelve years old, had an appointment with the orthodontist, Dr. Snyder. Chaz has an overbite and a receded mandible. When eating crunchy foods, such as toast and pizza crust, his palate becomes inflamed and irritated. Chaz is missing his permanent bicuspids.

Case Study Review

1. What should the dental assistant prepare for Chaz's appointment?

2. Is Chaz's age a factor in the orthodontist's diagnosis?

3. What stage of tooth eruption should the dental assistant expect Chaz to be in? Which primary teeth are normally present?

4. Which of Dr. Angle's classes of malocclusion do you expect to see and record?

REVIEW QUESTIONS

Multiple Choice

1. When individual teeth are turned or rotated in the socket, they are said to be
   a. infraverted.
   b. linguoverted.
   c. transposed.
   d. torsoverted.

2. Which of the following types of orthodontic treatments involve fixing an existing problem?
   a. Preventive treatment
   b. Interceptive treatment
   c. Corrective treatment

3. Orthodontic tracings are made using which of the following types of radiographs?
   a. Bite-wing
   b. Periapical
   c. Cephalometric
   d. Panoramic

4. To secure the arch wire in position on the posterior bands, use
   a. buccal tubes.
   b. brackets.
   c. springs.
   d. plastic rings.

5. All of the following are true statements about orthodontic brackets except:
   a. Brackets are welded onto orthodontic bands or bonded directly to the teeth.
   b. Brackets are made of stainless steel, ceramic, or acrylic.
   c. Brackets hold the bands in place on the teeth.
   d. Brackets hold the arch wire in place.

6. An abnormal horizontal distance between the labial surface of the mandibular anterior teeth and the lingual surface of maxillary teeth is a(an)
   a. open bite.
   b. overjet.
   c. underbite.
   d. overbite.

7. Specialized bone cells that cause the bone to resorb or break down are
   a. osteoclasts.
   b. osteoblasts.
   c. odontoclasts.
   d. odontoblasts.

8. During the consultation appointment, which of the following is discussed?
   a. Cost of treatment
   b. Patient's responsibility
   c. Duration of treatment
   d. All of the above

9. Which of the following instruments is used to tie ligature wire and/or place elastic ligatures?
   a. Coons pliers
   b. Ligature director
   c. Mathieu pliers
   d. Ligature wire-cutting pliers

10. Elastic ties are removed with which of the following?
    a. Bird-beak pliers
    b. Weingart utility pliers
    c. Scaler
    d. Howe pliers

Critical Thinking

1. Do you have teeth that are out of alignment? Using orthodontic terms, describe the deviations and identify the malpositioned teeth.

2. Which foods should the orthodontic patient avoid? What are some alternatives?

3. Name the three categories of causes of malocclusion. Give three examples in each category. Have you or anyone in your family had an orthodontic condition? Trace the etiology to one of the categories.

4. Discuss the importance of using a space maintainer and why it should stay in the patient's mouth until the permanent tooth erupts.

5. List ways to motivate the orthodontic patient to brush and floss during orthodontic treatment.

Web Activities

1. Go to http://www.invisalign.com and find out if this treatment would work for you.

2. Go to http://www.ORMCO.com and watch the video on the Damon bracket system.

3. Go to http://www.braces.org and find out which month is orthodontic health month. Learn about the history of orthodontics.

CHAPTER 28

PEDIATRIC DENTISTRY AND ENAMEL SEALANTS

SPECIFIC INSTRUCTIONAL OBJECTIVES

The student should strive to meet the following objectives and demonstrate an understanding of the facts and principles presented in this chapter:

1. Define pediatric dentistry as a specialty.
2. Describe the pediatric office and team members.
3. Explain the common behavior characteristics of children of various ages.
4. Describe child behavior management techniques.
5. Explain the role of the parent or guardian in pediatric dentistry.
6. Identify common procedures in pediatric dentistry.
7. Identify the equipment unique to pediatric dentistry.
8. Explain common emergencies in pediatric dentistry and the treatment for these emergencies.
9. Identify the signs of child abuse and the procedure for reporting suspected child abuse cases.

ADVANCED CHAIRSIDE FUNCTIONS

10. Explain the purpose of using enamel sealants and where they are placed.
11. List the indications and contraindications of placing sealants.
12. Discuss the role of the dental assistant in the placement of enamel sealants.
13. Describe the types of sealant materials.
14. List and describe the steps of the application procedure.

KEY TERMS

apexogenesis *(629)*

avulsed tooth *(633)*

bonding *(636)*

behavior management *(622)*

cannula *(635)*

chemically cured *(637)*

coalesced *(635)*

color-changing sealants *(636)*

dental composite resin (BIS-GMA) *(635)*

direct pulp capping (DPC) *(627)*

etch *(636)*

fluoride applications *(624)*

glass ionomers *(636)*

hand-over-mouth (HOM) technique *(623)*

indirect pulp treatment (IPT) *(627)*

light cured *(637)*

maturation *(636)*

mechanical bond *(637)*

modeling technique *(622)*

mouth guards *(624)*

objective fears *(621)*

(continues)

KEY TERMS *(continued)*

INTRODUCTION

The pediatric dental practice provides dental care for children and is often referred to as pedodontics. The pediatric specialist treats children from birth through the eruption of their second permanent molars. The pediatric practice sometimes treats medically, mentally, or emotionally compromised adults. The scope of pediatric treatment for children includes restoring and maintaining the primary, mixed, and permanent dentition, and applying preventive measures for dental caries, periodontal disease, and malocclusion. Although there has been a decrease in the number of dental caries found in children, the restorative aspect is still a large part of the practice. The primary focus of the pediatric dental practice is preventive treatment and working with the compromised adult patient.

The pediatric specialist is concerned with the basic needs and special requirements for treatment of the young patient. The pediatric dentist has special training in child growth, development, and behavior management. This training enables the pediatric dentist to successfully treat the emotionally and physically developing child and the special needs patient.

The general dentist, other specialists, and physicians refer patients to the pediatric specialist for treatment. The general dentist, orthodontist, and pediatric dentist work closely together to ensure the best overall dental care and education for the child patient.

Pediatric dentists as a group have been very instrumental at all levels in improving dental care for children and to educate children and parents/guardians. Many programs are available, but the need to provide these services is still great. Some areas have federal, state, or local programs to provide dental care for children, while others have little, if any, assistance. So much can be done to prevent tooth decay and early loss of primary teeth. Dentists, dental hygienists, and dental assistants are working with communities to provide education and various services for children. The Surgeon General of the United States, along with the ADA and the American Pediatric Association, has expressed such concerns and seeks means and ways to meet this need.

The Pediatric Dental Office

The pediatric office is open and friendly to make the child patient feel comfortable and secure. Pediatric office settings are creative and imaginative. The decor is often bright and designed with things children are attracted to. The reception room usually has an area for coloring or reading, a cage for small animals or a fish tank, toys for various age groups, and a display area with pictures of patients (Figure 28-1).

In some pediatric offices, the treatment areas are designed with several dental chairs arranged in an open area. This open bay concept allows children to see each other. It is reassuring for the child patient to know that other children are there and receiving treatment. Many offices have headphones with a variety of programs or music available, or televisions with either movies or patient education programs running.

Often the pediatric office will include a "quiet room" for patients who are difficult to manage. This room is

FIGURE 28-1 Reception area in pediatric practice that includes various toys, activity area, books, television, and video games. *(Courtesy of Dr. Jay Enzler.)*

separate and closed off from the others so that if patient management problems occur, they will not upset the other children in the office.

Pediatric Dental Team

The composition of the pediatric dental team is the same as the general dental office team. The difference may be the personalities of team members and the desire to work with children. The entire staff needs to enjoy children and be sincere and honest in their actions and feelings. To be effective in managing children, the dental team must be upbeat, motivated, and aware.

The pediatric staff usually do not wear white uniforms but often wear bright colors and designs. Safety glasses, masks, and gloves are routinely worn. To make the mask look less threatening, some masks can be purchased that have designs printed on them, or the child or dental assistant can draw a happy face or a cartoon character on the mask.

Dental Assistant's Role in Pediatric Dentistry

The role of the dental assistant in the pediatric practice varies depending on areas of responsibility. One aspect is management of the child. Another is work at chairside. Skills that the assistant performs at chairside vary in every office and from state to state depending on the state dental practice act. When the assistant works independently, he or she assumes the authority role and must maintain control of the child.

In many offices, the assistant plays the dominant role in greeting the child, escorting him or her to the treatment area, and preparing him or her for treatment. When the dentist comes into the room, the assistant transfers attention and control to the dentist. The assistant's role during treatment is to support the dentist in a manner that the assistant and the dentist have discussed. Usually, this is office policy and a good topic for staff meeting discussions.

The dental assistant is also an educator, both for the child and the parents. The assistant answers questions or refers them to the pediatric dentist. Topics that might be discussed include oral hygiene techniques, dental nutrition, tooth eruption, and application of fluoride (Figure 28-2).

Behavior Characteristics of Children at Various Ages

Each child develops on his or her own special time schedule, but there are some common levels of psychological and physical growth. **Maturation** is growth to a certain level and then learning on that level. The child may be seven years old but not mature enough to learn on this level. Development takes longer for some than

FIGURE 28-2 Dental assistant showing children how to brush their teeth by demonstrating on a puppet.

for others, and environment, age, experiences, and other people all influence psychological growth. Table 28-1 provides general characteristics of behavior in children at various ages. These are generalizations and not meant to be comprehensive.

Understanding the behavior of children at various ages will give the dental assistant a better way to establish a relationship with children. Having some idea of their learning levels, communication abilities, and interests enables the assistant to understand the patient and effectively manage the child to make his or her experience with dentistry a positive one. Two to six years is the best age to introduce dental care in the dental office.

Patient Management

Patient management is a team effort. Successful treatment is the result of how well the patient is managed. The dental team must work together and know each other's responsibilities and roles. A positive, trusting relationship with some children takes time and effort. The dental team must have consistent management policies and procedure sequences, and consistently use the same terminology when speaking with patients.

Longevity of staff members provides the opportunity to better respond as a unit. Over time, the team will encounter various management problems; once the problems have occurred, discuss them and decide how they will be handled in the future.

Fear is a large factor in behavior problems with children. Some of the fears are based on feelings, attitudes, and concerns that have developed from suggestions of others, including parents, siblings, and friends. These are called **subjective fears**. Other fears, which are based on the child's own experiences, are known as **objective fears**.

TABLE 28-1 General Behavior Characteristics of Children at Various Ages

Age	Behavior
Two to six years overall	Likes to be with parents and siblings Likes to play (e.g., having a "ride" in the dental chair, seeing the "squirt gun") Can respond to dentist's instructions and understands simple explanations Transitional time from infantile behavior patterns to the more independent preschool child
Two to four years	Short attention span Wide variety of interests Parallel play without bothering other children Responds to fantasy
Four to six years	Shows feelings with facial expression Parents are very influential Greatest number of management problems Needs constant reassurance Moves to integrated play Shows some tolerance with dislikes
Six to twelve years overall	Period of socializing Asserts independence Differences in boys and girls more noticeable
Six to nine years	Learning to get along with people and regulations of society Friendships are important Usually prefers to come in for treatment without parent Likes to collect things Aware of place in society and likes to belong to a group Likes to be spoken to directly
Nine to twelve years	Usually not difficult to manage May respond passively Girls are more mature Will respond when things are explained Boys sometimes act like they know it all Likes to be treated as an adult

When a child has questions, the dental team should give honest, brief, and simple answers. Try to relate the answer to something the child already knows about or has experienced. For example, relate the pinch of an injection to the pinch of a mosquito.

Behavior Management Techniques

There are many **behavior management** techniques. A few are covered here to provide the dental assistant with some ideas. The following are taken from the American Academy of Pediatric Dentistry's published *Standards of Care for Behavior Management*.

Tell, Show, and Do. With the **tell, show, and do technique,** the assistant names a dental instrument and demonstrates its use, often using either his or her own hand or fingers or the child's hand. Once the child is comfortable, the instrument is used.

Voice Control. Speaking calmly but firmly lets the child know the dentist is in control and is serious about the treatment and the child's behavior.

Distraction. Distract the child's attention from perceived unpleasant procedures. Watching videos, listening to tapes, or getting the child to think of something pleasant are methods of distraction (Figure 28-3).

Nonverbal Communication. Nonverbal communication gains the attention of the child and guides his or her behavior. The dental team's facial expressions, postures, and contact with the child reinforce positive behavior.

Modeling. The **modeling technique** pairs a timid child in dental care with a cooperative child of a similar age. The open bay treatment areas provide the opportunity for the modeling process.

FIGURE 28-3 Child being distracted while receiving dental treatment with ceiling monitor showing a movie.

Positive Reinforcement. Give the patient positive reinforcement at the appropriate time. Every child does something right during the dental visit. Praise him or her in order to reinforce the positive behavior. Be sure the praise or positive reinforcement is honest, sincere, and for worthy behavior.

 Gentle Restraints. Sometimes a child's behavior during treatment requires management for his or her own protection from possible injury. Some children need gentle restraint of the arms and legs to reduce or eliminate movement. This is for the safety of the patient and the operator. A papoose board and pediwrap are used for this kind of restraint.

Hand over Mouth. The hand-over-mouth (HOM) technique works to gain the child's attention for establishing communication, eliminate inappropriate avoidance responses, enhance the child's self-confidence in coping during treatment, and ensure safety during delivery of care. The dentist places his or her hand over the patient's mouth and, in a very calm voice, explains behavior expec-

tations. The hand is removed when behavior is appropriate. The process is reapplied, if necessary. HOM requires informed consent and, although effective, this technique is not used often.

 Mild Sedation. An anxious child may benefit from sedation. Conscious sedation and nitrous oxide inhalation are two forms used in the pediatric office. Both require informed consent before being administered. Conscious sedation and nitrous oxide inhalation are preoperative or intraoperative. Both reduce anxiety and movement by the patient, increase tolerance for longer periods, and enhance communication. Sedation aids in the treatment of mentally, physically, or medically compromised patients.

 General Anesthesia. If a child is extremely fearful or uncooperative or if the patient has certain physical, mental, or medical conditions, general anesthesia is administered for treatment. This provides a safe, efficient, and effective means for dental care. General anesthesia requires informed consent from the child's parent or guardian and is usually administered in a hospital setting.

Role of Parent or Guardian

Parents or guardians often require assistance to best prepare the child for dental care. Sometimes, their past experiences influence how they feel about dental treatment, and this is transmitted to the child. Then the child becomes apprehensive and hesitant.

Many offices have suggestions for parents to help prepare the child for treatment. There are pamphlets, books, and videos to instruct the parents on how to explain what the child is going to experience in the dental office. It is important that the child's questions be answered truthfully but in terms they understand and with minimal explanation. If the parents are not sure of the treatment or how to answer the questions, they should tell the child to ask the dentist.

When the first appointment is made, the parent should be informed of what to expect. This usually means examining the child's teeth and taking x-rays. A treatment plan may include restorations and preventive treatment. The parents are encouraged to discuss concerns they might have with the dentist, away from the child.

Each office has a policy on parents coming into the treatment room with the child during the appointment. The dental assistants must know how the dentist feels about having the parents with the child during treatment. Some dentists feel that they can manage the child better if the parents are not in the treatment room. Others feel that as long as the parents do not interfere, they can remain. The parents usually are eager to cooperate with the office policies. If the child insists that the parent comes into the treatment area, offer him or her a chair near the foot of the patient's chair so he or she is not in the direct view of the child when the child is reclined and the dentist and dental assistant are seated. The dental team remains focused on establishing a relationship with the child. On occasion, the dentist may use the presence of the parents to control behavior. For example, the dentist might say that if the child cooperates, the parent can stay in the treatment area, but if the child does not cooperate, the parent will be asked to leave. Some dentists feel that if the child does not behave, it is the parent's responsibility to manage the child in order for dental care to be completed.

Parents generally are very supportive if they are informed, know what is happening, and know what is expected of them.

Procedures in Pediatric Dentistry

The first appointment with the pediatric dentist may be for a routine examination followed by treatment, or it may be an emergency appointment due to an injury. Dental care for children involves both the primary and permanent dentition. Sometimes the parents may question the need to restore primary teeth because they are not permanent and will be replaced. The primary dentition is restored for the following reasons:

- The primary teeth are needed to hold space for the permanent teeth.
- They maintain the functions of the teeth in chewing, speech, and esthetics.
- They act as guides for the permanent dentition during eruption.

Educating parents to understand the importance of the primary teeth is necessary with all types of pediatric dental treatments (see Appendix B, Development of Human Dentition).

The Examination

The examination of a child patient is similar to that of an adult. The gingiva, supporting tissues, and oral mucosa are checked. The surfaces of the teeth are examined with a mouth mirror and an explorer. Radiographs are exposed to show the conditions of the primary teeth and the positions and development of the permanent teeth (refer to Chapter 22, Production and Evaluation of Dental Radiographs, for suggestions and types of pediatric x-ray exposures).

The patient's medical/dental history is recorded by the parent or guardian. The medical history provides information about past dental experiences, any allergies, facial habits, illnesses, and general development of the child.

Preventive Procedures

Preventive procedures in pediatric dentistry include educating both the child and parent regarding diet suggestions, oral hygiene techniques, use of fluorides, pit and fissure sealants, use of mouth guards for sports activities, and preventive orthodontic treatment.

Oral Hygiene Techniques. Oral hygiene techniques are coordinated with the child's age and physical ability (see Chapter 4, Oral Health and Preventive Techniques, for oral hygiene techniques for children). The parent is given information on toothbrushing and flossing techniques in order to assist the child.

Coronal Polishes. Coronal polish is a rubber cup polish of the crowns of the teeth. Polishing paste is applied to the teeth with the rubber cup to remove plaque and some stains (see Chapter 29, Periodontics). This is routinely performed by the dental hygienist, but in many states dental assistants can also perform the coronal polish.

Pit and Fissure Sealants. Pit and fissure sealants are routinely placed to protect newly erupted teeth and teeth where sealants are indicated. The sealants protect the deep pits and fissure areas of the primary molars and the premolars and molars of the permanent teeth. Sealants have successfully reduced the number of cavities in children.

Fluoride Applications and Fluoride Varnishes. Fluoride applications and fluoride varnishes are routinely applied after the coronal polish and pit and fissure sealants have been placed. The dentist will determine a fluoride therapy plan with the parents periodically. How and when fluoride is given to a child often depends on if the water supply is fluoridated, oral hygiene techniques of the patient, and how often the patient visits the dentist. Fluoride is administered in the office as a gel, placed in the mouth in trays, or as a rinse (see Chapter 4, Oral Health and Preventive Techniques). Fluoride varnish is painted on the surfaces of the teeth after they are isolated and dried.

Mouth Guards. Children who are actively involved in contact sports should be fitted for mouth guards. The guards offer protection from premature loss of the teeth or from fractures. There are various types of mouth guards. Some are made in the dental office, such as the custom-fit mouth guard. This mouth guard is made in the office using a study model and vacuum-formed material (Figure 28-4A). There are also commercial "do-it-yourself kits" available, where the material comes in various sizes. It is heated under warm water and then molded to the individual arch (Figure 28-4B).

Preventive and Interceptive Orthodontic Treatment. Preventive and interceptive orthodontic treatment includes a variety of orthodontic treatments. Two common pro-

FIGURE 28-4 (A) Various mouth guards used in athletics. (B) Example of mouth guard material and formed mouth guard.

FIGURE 28-5 Space maintainer. *(Courtesy of Dr. Steven E. Gregg.)*

FIGURE 28-6 A crib appliance to stop a child from sucking his thumb. *(Courtesy of Dr. Steven E. Gregg.)*

cedures are placing space maintainers and correcting oral habits.

A space maintainer is designed to maintain a space until the permanent tooth erupts. The space is the result of the premature loss of a primary tooth. A space maintainer may be a fixed or removable appliance. The appliance is designed to meet the needs of the child patient. Fixed space maintainers are more commonly used because they are cemented permanently in place so that the patients cannot take them in and out (refer to Chapter 27, Orthodontics, for more information on space maintainers) (Figure 28-5).

Oral habits such as thumb sucking and tongue thrusting may need intervention because they can lead to abnormal muscle function, distorted growth of the jaw, malocclusion, changed facial contour, and problems with speech.

Thumb sucking is a controversial subject with many opinions on whether the habit should be "treated." Most orthodontists leave the thumb sucking of a child alone until the child's maxillary anterior teeth erupt; hopefully, by then, the habit will have disappeared. Most dentists begin some form of treatment if the child continues to suck his or her thumb at age five. Treatment includes counseling with the child and the parents, "gentle persuasion," and behavior modification tech-

niques. Fixed appliances, such as cribs and rakes, are also used if the habit continues (Figure 28-6).

Tongue thrusting is a habit in which the child's tongue pushes against the anterior teeth during swallowing, causing an anterior open bite. Treatment for this habit includes myofunctional exercises (therapy) or the use of appliances.

Restorative Procedures

Restorative procedures are similar to those performed on adult patients. The materials used in pediatric dentistry are the same as those used in the restoration of permanent teeth. Amalgam is used most frequently for posterior teeth, and it is approved by the ADA. Some dentists are placing more tooth-colored restorations because of their more natural appearance. These are placed in both the anterior and posterior regions of the child's mouth. Esthetic restorations include composites, glass ionomers, resin-modified glass ionomers, and compomers (combination of composite resins and glass ionomers) (see Chapter 34, Restorative Materials, Dental Dam, Matrix, and Wedge). Badly decayed teeth are protected with stainless steel crowns that are permanently cemented in place. In very rare cases, partials and dentures are made for pediatric patients.

The difference between pediatric and adult restorative procedures is the size of the instruments. Examples of instruments and materials that are reduced in size include the dental high-speed handpiece and burs, dental dam material, and dental dam clamps. The dental dam material is smaller in size and the width of the jaws of the clamps is smaller to accommodate the primary teeth. The high-speed handpiece has a compact head to allow for better access in the child's mouth, and the burs have shorter shanks.

Pedodontic Matrices. The dental matrices used in restorative procedures are adapted to the sizes and shapes of the teeth. The tofflemire matrix is used in pediatrics, but custom matrices are more common (see Chapter 34). Two custom matrices are the T-band matrix and spot-welded matrix band.

T-bands are designed for and used on primary teeth. Often made of brass strips that are "crossed" at one end, they are available in various designs and sizes. The T-bands do not require retainers, are adjustable, and can be secured on the tooth (Figure 28-7) (see Procedure 28-1).

Spot-welded matrix bands also are used for primary teeth (Procedure 28-2). The custom-made bands are used for Class II restorations. The matrix material comes in rolls of 0.25- to 0.18-widths and 0.002-gauge thickness. This custom matrix does not require a retainer to be secure on the tooth, but a spot-welding machine is required. The band is quickly made at chairside.

Dental Dam Procedure

Using a dental dam during pediatric procedures protects the patient's busy and curious tongue and prevents materials from being aspirated into the throat. It also provides a dry area while improving visibility, and often reduces procedure time by restricting the patient from talking and providing an isolated treatment area in the oral cavity.

Pediatric dental dams are smaller than dams for adults, typically comprised of 5-inch × 5-inch pieces of material. The dental dam punch is the same one used for adults, but holes are smaller and the distance between holes is shorter. To cover the area, usually three or four holes are punched in a quadrant. The dental dam clamps are smaller and sometimes have projections for better retention. (For more information and the procedure sequence, see Chapter 34, Restorative Materials, Dental Dam, Matrix, and Wedge).

(A)

(B)

FIGURE 28-7 (A) T-bands. (B) T-band correctly assembled on a tooth. (B. *Courtesy of Dale Ruemping, DDS, MSD.*)

Pulp Therapy in Primary and Young Permanent Teeth

Caries or traumatic injuries can damage both primary and permanent teeth. The teeth are assessed to determine the status of the pulp. The duration, frequency, and location of pain is recorded. The clinical assessment includes a visual examination and radiographs. The extent of the lesion is determined by the following: presence of fistula (pathway from abscess to mucosa), the tooth is mobile, presence of swelling, and/or sensitivity to heat or percussion.

PROCEDURE 28-1

T-Band Placement

For this procedure, the tooth has been prepared and a matrix is assembled and placed on the tooth. The dentist places the T-band unless the state dental practice act allows the dental assistant to perform this skill.

EQUIPMENT AND SUPPLIES (Figure 28-8)

- T-band assortment
- Burnisher
- Cotton pliers or hemostat
- Crown and collar scissors

PROCEDURE STEPS *(Follow aseptic procedures)*

1. Prepare the T-band ahead of time by selecting the appropriate band size.

2. Loop the band to shape the approximate diameter of the tooth.

3. Fold the "T" ends over the band loop, leaving a circle with long tail or end.

4. Place the band on the tooth in the interproximal space covering the margins of the preparation.

5. Place the portion of the band where the "T" is folded on the buccal surface, away from the margins of the preparation.

6. Tighten the band by pulling on the free end (tail) until the band is tight around the tooth.

7. Bend the free end back toward the "T" to secure the band. Remove excess band with scissors.

8. Burnish the band and place a wedge as needed.

9. To remove the T-band, fold back the overlapping section of band to loosen the band. Use cotton pliers to remove the band from the tooth.

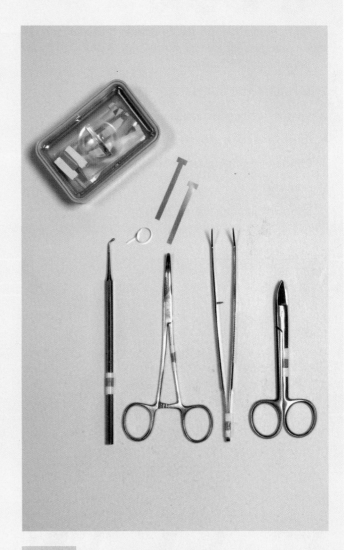

FIGURE 28-8 Tray setup for T-band placement.

Vital Pulp Therapy. Vital pulp therapy involves the removal of tissue that is potentially infected (this procedure will maintain the tooth in a healthy state so that the tooth is not lost) and focuses on the reparative ability of the pulp. There are three choices in treatment depending on the status of the pulp: **indirect pulp treatment (IPT)**, **direct pulp capping (DPC)**, or a **pulpotomy** (Procedure 28-3).

If the pulp is not yet exposed, indirect pulp treatment (IPT), also known as indirect pulp capping, is indicated

PROCEDURE 28-2

Spot-Welded Matrix Band Placement

For this procedure, the tooth has been prepared for restoration and the spot-welded matrix band is prepared by the dental assistant at chairside.

EQUIPMENT AND SUPPLIES

- Spot-welded matrix band material
- Crown and collar scissors
- Cotton pliers, hemostat, or Howe pliers
- Burnisher
- Spot-welding unit (Figure 28-9)

PROCEDURE STEPS *(Follow aseptic procedures)*

1. Cut an approximate length of matrix band material. Turn on the spot-welding unit to warm it up.

2. Loop the matrix material around the tooth, bringing the ends of the material together on the buccal surface.

3. Pinch the band tightly together with a hemostat, cotton pliers, or Howe pliers.

4. Bend the excess material to one side.

5. Take the band to the spot-welding unit and spot weld the band together to form a circle the diameter of the tooth (Figure 28-10).

6. Trim off the excess and sharp edges of the band.

7. Replace the band on the tooth with the welded area on the buccal surface. Place wedges in the interproximal and contour.

8. To remove the band after the amalgam has been placed, cut the lingual aspect of the band and pull it in an occlusal/buccal direction with cotton pliers.

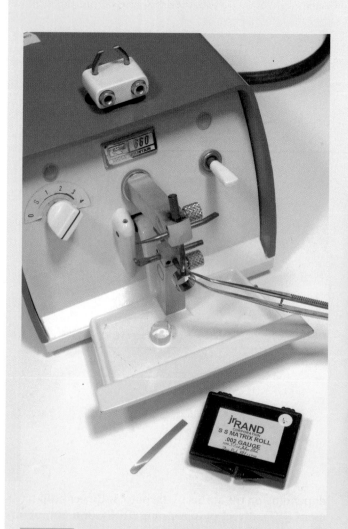

FIGURE 28-9 Spot-welding machine and matrix band material.

FIGURE 28-10 Spot-welding a matrix band.

(Figure 28-11A). In this case, the pulp has not yet been exposed, but there is a chance that the pulp will be exposed while removing the caries. The technique involves:

1. Leaving a thin layer of sound or carious dentin with no evidence of pulp exposure

2. Placing a medicament and a temporary restoration that seals completely

3. Leaving the medicament and restoration for six to eight weeks

4. Opening the tooth and removing the remaining caries

5. Placing restoration

If the pulp has been exposed through mechanical or traumatic means but there is a chance for a favorable response, a direct pulp capping (DPC) (Figure 28-11B) procedure is indicated. The patient should be informed of the possible outcomes with the direct pulp capping treatment. It may be successful and the pulp will heal, or the infection may continue and the tooth will abscess. In the case of an abscess, root canal treatment may be required. The DPC procedure involves placing a medicament, often calcium hydroxide, directly over the exposed pulp. The tooth is then restored or a temporary restoration is placed.

If the pulp of a primary or young permanent tooth has been exposed, a pulpotomy procedure may be indi-cated to remove a portion of the pulp. For primary teeth, a pulpotomy keeps the pulp vital, with no prolonged adverse signs, internal resorption, and harm to succe-daneous teeth. For the young permanent teeth, a pulp-otomy maintains pulp vitality and allows enough time for the root end to develop and close (in these cases, the treatment is referred to as **apexogenesis**).

Nonvital Pulp Therapy. Nonvital pulp therapy may be indicated for both primary and newly erupted per-manent teeth. The tooth is extracted or a **pulpectomy** is indicated. This procedure involves the complete removal of the dental pulp (see Chapter 24, Endo-dontics).

Stainless Steel Crowns

Stainless steel crowns are used on both primary and permanent teeth. On primary teeth, they are placed until permanent dentition erupts. On permanent teeth, these crowns are placed until the patient can have them replaced with cast gold or porcelain fused to metal crowns. Indications for use of a stainless steel crown include the following:

- Extensive carious lesions

- Hypoplastic or hypocalcified teeth

- Treatment following a pulpotomy or pulpectomy pro-cedure

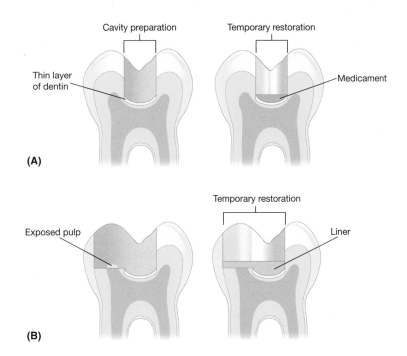

FIGURE 28-11 (A) Indirect pulp treatment/capping. (B) Direct pulp treatment/capping.

PROCEDURE 28-3

Pulpotomy

This procedure is performed by the dentist with the help of a dental assistant. The dental assistant prepares the treatment room, patient, equipment, and supplies. The tooth is opened and treated before a temporary restoration is placed.

EQUIPMENT AND SUPPLIES (Figure 28-12)

- Amalgam setup
- Formocresol
- Sterile round burs
- Zinc oxide-eugenol cement (ZOE or IRM)

PROCEDURE STEPS *(Follow aseptic procedures)*

1. Anesthetic is administered.
2. Place the dental dam.

3. Using the high-speed handpiece, a large opening is made in the occlusal surface of the tooth, exposing the coronal portion of the pulp (Figure 28-13A).

4. The coronal portion of the pulp is then removed with a spoon excavator or round bur (Figure 28-13B).

5. Prepare a sterile cotton pellet by wetting it in a Formocresol solution. The dentist places the pellet in the chamber for five minutes (Figure 28-13C). (Formocresol is bactericidal—it preserves a thin layer of the remaining pulp tissue to control hemorrhage.)

6. After the hemorrhage is controlled, the cotton pellet is removed and the pulp chamber is rinsed and dried.

7. Mix zinc oxide-eugenol to a base consistency and transfer it to the dentist. A layer of zinc oxide base is placed in the chamber over the remaining pulp (Figure 28-13D).

8. Place the restoration, such as amalgam, remove the dental dam, and check the occlusion. Stainless steel crowns are also used if little tooth structure remains. Sometimes, the dentist will choose to place a temporary restoration instead of a final restoration. This delays final treatment until the outcome of the injured pulp is known.

FIGURE 28-12 Pulpotomy tray setup.

FIGURE 28-13 Pulpotomy procedure showing direct pulp exposure.

- Primary tooth is used as an abutment tooth for space maintainer

- Temporary restoration of fractured teeth

Stainless steel crowns are available in various sizes, and can be purchased individually or in complete kits (Figure 28-14A and B). See Procedure 28-4 for an overview of the steps involved in placing a crown.

(A)

(B)

FIGURE 28-14 (A) Stainless steel crown kit. (B) Stainless steel crown placed on tooth. *(A. Courtesy of 3M Dental Products Division. B. Courtesy of Dale Ruemping, DDS, MSD.)*

PROCEDURE 28-4

Stainless Steel Crown Placement

This procedure is performed by the dentist with the help of the dental assistant. The assistant maintains the operating field, mixes materials, and assists in preparation of the stainless steel crown.

EQUIPMENT AND SUPPLIES (Figure 28-15)

- Basic setup: mouth mirror, explorer, and cotton pliers
- Cotton rolls and gauze
- HVE and saliva ejector
- High-speed handpiece with selected burs
- Low-speed handpiece with green stone and rubber abrasive wheel
- Spoon excavator
- Selection of stainless steel crowns
- Crown and collar scissors
- Contouring and crimping pliers
- Mixing spatula, paper pad, and permanent cement
- Articulating forceps and paper
- Dental floss

FIGURE 28-15 Stainless steel crown placement tray setup.

PROCEDURE STEPS *(Follow aseptic procedures)*

1. Local anesthetic is administered and the tooth is prepared, similar to preparation for a cast gold crown. The high-speed handpiece with tapered diamonds is commonly used. Transfer instruments and evacuate during the preparation of the tooth.

(continues)

PROCEDURE 28-4 *(CONTINUED)*

2. The circumference and height of the tooth are reduced.

3. Decay is removed using conventional methods and cavity medications are placed.

4. A stainless steel crown is selected from the kit, and it is tried on the tooth. The crown must fit around the circumference of the prepared tooth and contact the adjacent teeth, mesially and distally. Assist the dentist in the selection of the crown. (Some states do not allow dental assistants to perform the function of fitting the crown.)

5. Once the crown is selected, the crown and collar scissors are used to adjust the occlusal-gingival height (Figure 28-16A). The gingival margin of the crown should extend one millimeter beyond the margin of the tooth preparation.

6. A green stone is used to smooth the rough edges of the crown. This area is polished with a rubber abrasive wheel (Figure 28-16B).

7. Place the crown on the tooth and check the patient's occlusion with articulating paper. Make adjustments, if necessary. Use dental floss to check the contacts. Prepare the articulating paper, dry the tooth, and transfer the paper. Receive the articulating forceps and paper and prepare the handpiece, if necessary.

8. Using contouring and crimping pliers, contour the crown, and then crimp the cervical margins of the crown in toward the tooth (Figure 28-16C).

9. The crown is removed and the tooth is dried thoroughly.

10. The cement is mixed and placed in the crown and on the tooth (Figure 28-16D). Mix the cement and place it in the crown. Transfer the crown to the dentist for placement.

11. Remove the excess cement from around the crown.

12. Rinse the patient's mouth and then dismiss the patient.

(A) (B) (C) (D)

FIGURE 28-16 (A) Stainless steel crown selected and trimmed with crown and collar scissors. (B) Crown margins smoothed with green stone. (C) Crown contoured with contouring pliers; margins are then crimped with crimping pliers. (D) Crown placed on tooth.

Emergency Treatment for Traumatic Injuries

Children are prone to accidents as their bodies and coordination skills grow and develop. Traumatic injuries to children's teeth are not uncommon, resulting in fractured, displaced, or avulsed teeth. Another injury seen in the pediatric population is traumatic intrusion.

Fractured Teeth

Fractured teeth are a common emergency in the pediatric practice (Figure 28-17). The anterior teeth are most often involved. The child should be seen by the dentist as soon as possible after the accident. The dentist examines the teeth, documents the history of the accident, performs vitality tests, and takes radiographs. Treatment is determined by the extent of the injury and the vitality of the pulp (see Table 28-2 for classifications of fractures and suggested treatment).

At this initial appointment, the pulp is treated and a temporary restoration is placed if needed for protection. Generally, the dentist will wait three to six months for further treatment. This gives the pulp a chance to recover without additional injury. If the tooth recovers in six months, a permanent restoration is placed.

Traumatic Intrusion

Traumatic intrusion occurs when the teeth are forcibly driven into the alveolus so that only a portion of the crown is visible. The treatment for intrusion is to allow the teeth to re-erupt on their own, or the dentist will reposition the teeth and splint adjacent teeth to hold position. These teeth may become nonvital and later require endodontic treatment.

Traumatic intrusion of the primary teeth may cause damage to the underlying developing permanent teeth (Figure 28-18). The damage can result from the physical trauma or from infection of the traumatized teeth. The damage is determined when the permanent teeth erupt.

Displaced Teeth

Lateral or extrusive displacement of primary teeth should be repositioned by the dentist as soon as possible. The roots of primary teeth go through resorption faster after an injury and if the teeth are mobile. If infection occurs, the teeth are removed.

After the teeth are repositioned, they are held in place with a splint (Figure 28-19). The splint is left in place for two to four weeks in order to stabilize the teeth. Often with these injuries, the periodontal ligament is damaged extensively. The teeth are monitored for vitality and assessed for endodontic treatment.

Avulsed Teeth

An **avulsed tooth** has been completely removed from the mouth. Primary avulsed teeth are not replaced

FIGURE 28-17 Fractured anterior central incisors. *(Courtesy of Dale Ruemping, DDS, MSD.)*

TABLE 28-2 Classifications of Tooth Fractures and Treatment

Classification	Treatment
Enamel	Smooth the rough edges.
Enamel and dentin are involved in fracture	Exposed dentin is protected with glass ionomer, calcium hydroxide, and a bonding agent with composite restoration.
Enamel, dentin, and pulp are involved	Depending on the clinical examination, a direct pulp capping, pulpotomy, or pulpectomy may be indicated.
Crown is fractured with pulp exposure	Root canal treatment, if indicated. Post and cast crown are completed to stabilize and protect the tooth.

FIGURE 28-18 Traumatic intrusion. *(Courtesy of Dale Ruemping, DDS, MSD.)*

FIGURE 28-19 Child with teeth in splint. *(Courtesy of Dr. Steven Gregg, DDS.)*

because infection or ankylosis (**ANG**-kill-loh-sis) may occur. Ankylosis is the fusion of bone and cementum. Permanent teeth that have been avulsed should be replaced as soon as possible after the injury. Instruct the parents to replant the tooth immediately. The success rate is relatively high if this is done. If the tooth cannot be replanted, instruct the parent to place the tooth in milk, saliva, saline, or water and transport the patient and tooth to the dental office immediately. Caution should be taken with the avulsed tooth to place it carefully in liquid and not rinse it off.

Time is important if the tooth is to be saved. The patient should see the dentist as soon as possible and the dentist should be called immediately for instructions.

Replacing an Avulsed Tooth
1. The tooth is kept moist and the site in the mouth is examined.
2. Local anesthetic is administered.
3. X-rays are taken.
4. The blood clot is removed from the alveolus.
5. The avulsed tooth is cleaned off in a saline solution and then inserted into the alveolus.
6. A splint is placed to retain the tooth in position.
7. Antibiotics, analgesics, and chlorhexidine rinses are prescribed.
8. Endodontic treatment may be required later.

Child Abuse

Child abuse and neglect is a serious problem that all health professionals encounter. The dental office provides an opportunity for children who are abused to be observed and for the abuse to be reported. The entire dental team needs to be aware of types of child abuse and signs of abuse.

Types of child abuse include physical, sexual, neglect, and emotional. Injuries associated with child abuse that might be evident in the dental office include fractured teeth and jaw bones, lacerations around the labial frenum, missing teeth with no explanation, and bruises or scars on the lips. Marks on the child's arms, legs, and neck may also be noticed by the dental team. Lack of personal hygiene or appropriate clothing for the season, extensive caries, and lack of response to the need for the child to receive dental treatment are concerns of the dental team and should be noted and followed if the child's health and welfare are continually compromised.

The Law and Reporting Child Abuse

Laws regarding reporting child abuse may differ from state to state, but most require the dentist to report signs of abuse. The laws are designed to protect children and provide help for families.

Reports should include the following:

- The nature of the concern
- Description of the injury, including type, color, size, characteristics, and location
- X-rays and color photographs
- Child's name, age, address, sex, and date of birth
- Parent or caregiver names
- Physician's name
- Explanations by child and caregiver of the injury

Report the findings to a social service agency, the local police department, or a child protective service. The dentist may be asked to appear in court and/or file the report.

ADVANCED CHAIRSIDE FUNCTIONS

Enamel Sealants

Enamel sealants are hard resin materials that are applied to caries-free occlusal surfaces of premolars and molars. These pit and fissure teeth are particularly susceptible to caries because of the deep pits and fissures in the enamel on the occlusal surface. Toothbrushing is not always an adequate means of removing the bacteria and debris that are lodged in the pits and fissures. Fluoride is very effective in preventing decay on the smooth enamel surfaces but less effective in the pits and fissures. Sealants bond to the tooth to "seal" the pits and fissures, thereby preventing the decay process from starting. The barrier costs less than a restoration but does not last as long. On the average, sealants remain in place for five to ten years. The combined use of pit and fissure sealants and fluoride has proven to be an effective measure that greatly reduces dental caries in patients through age sixteen. Under the *Healthy People 2010* initiative, the U.S. government has set a goal that 50 percent of all children will have sealants by 2010. (*Healthy People* initiatives, which challenge private and public sectors at all levels, are managed by the U.S. Department of Health and Human Services.)

Indications and Contraindications for Sealants

Enamel sealants are indicated when the patient

- Has low to moderate caries activity.
- Practices good oral hygiene techniques.
- Teeth are erupted into mouth enough for occlusal surface to be accessible.
- Eats a balanced diet, preferably low in sugar.
- Has good quantity and quality of saliva.
- Has fluoride in water or takes fluoride supplement.

Sealants are most beneficial if applied:

- On occlusal pits and fissures of noncarious primary and permanent teeth
- On recently erupted teeth
- On patients with a high number of occlusal caries and deep fissures
- Along with preventive treatment

Contraindications to placing enamel sealants include:

- Teeth that have been caries free for four or more years (the chances are minimal that occlusal decay will occur)
- Teeth with shallow open grooves. Usually, these teeth are easy to keep clean, making them more resistant to decay. Also, sealants are not well retained in these areas
- Teeth with well-coalesced (blended) pits and fissures
- Patients with occlusal decay or who have occlusal restorations

Role of Dental Assistant

Applying enamel sealants is an expanded duty delegated to the dental hygienist or the dental assistant in some states. The laws governing the dental assistant's responsibilities vary greatly with each state, so become familiar with state practice acts. In some states, the dental assistant can assist the dentist in this procedure, in which help is always needed to isolate the teeth and keep them dry and free of debris until the sealant is placed. In other states, with education and training the dental assistant can place the sealants. The dental assistant can then follow through with the total preventive program and apply both the fluoride and the pit and fissure sealants.

It is important for the dental assistant to stay informed and current on enamel sealants. Research on sealant effectiveness, chemical properties, and potential is ongoing, so reading and attending seminars keeps the dental assistant well informed.

Enamel Sealant Materials

Several materials have been used as sealants for occlusal pits and fissures. The most commonly used are dental composite resins (BIS-GMA); composites have been diluted and are thus less viscous to enhance the flow typically required for sealants. Composites used as sealants are unfilled or contain a small amount of filler, and contain no inorganic fillers. Dental composites, which will last up to ten years, are inexpensive and come in kits with everything you need for application. They are quick and easy to use, which is important when working on active children. Composite sealants require no mixing because they usually come in syringes with disposable applicator tips, cartridges with a cannula (small hollow tube) for application, or single-use dispensing tips. Also available are dental-composite sealant materials containing fluoride for the added benefit of fluoride release under the sealant.

ADVANCED CHAIRSIDE FUNCTIONS

Composite materials come in clear, opaque, or lightly tinted colors. The advantage to the opaque and tinted composites is visibility, which makes placement less difficult and identification of the sealants at follow-up exams easier. Patients, however, prefer the clear or opaque options because of esthetic appeal. **Color-changing sealants**, a relatively new option, are popular. These sealants contain a photo-active color additive; they are tinted (usually pink or green) on the initial application, and then change to opaque white after being light cured. This is an improvement that allows for better visibility during sealant placement (Figure 28-20).

Glass ionomers, another common choice for pit and fissure sealant material, are popular because the office need not purchase a separate material for sealant procedures. In addition, they:

- Contain fluoride
- Require no etching or bonding agent

(A)

Before   After

(B)

FIGURE 28-20 (A) Color-changing composite resin sealant. (B) Sealant being placed on several etched teeth (Before); the teeth after the sealant has been light cured (After). (A. *Courtesy of 3M ESPE Dental.* B. *Courtesy of Dr. Chris Bryant.*)

- Can be used on smooth surfaces of the tooth because they are less fluid than composites
- Do not require that the area be completely dry for placement

The fluoride in the glass ionomer material is released continually for about two years, which is why glass ionomers are used if the patient has a high rate of caries or xerostomia (dryness of mouth caused by reduced saliva). Glass ionomers are available in powder/liquid form, and in capsules with cannula for dispensing the material and a syringe with disposable applicator tips.

Bonding, Etching, and Conditioning

Bonding or attachment to the tooth surface occurs differently for the composite sealants than the glass ionomer sealants.

Composite sealants bond to the tooth mechanically. The **mechanical bond** is accomplished by the sealant flowing into the irregularities of the treated enamel and locking into place. The enamel surface is **etched**, or conditioned, by phosphoric acid (or another type of acid) solution that is applied to a clean tooth with a brush, syringe, or small cotton-tipped applicator. The etchant comes in a gel or liquid, and is applied for a specified amount of time, usually fifteen to thirty seconds. During the application time, the etchant is "dabbed" or flowed over the area, but never rubbed. The phosphoric acid removes some of the matrix of the enamel, and leaves the enamel rods intact for the sealant material to bond to once it is light cured. If the etchant is rubbed during application, the enamel rods will be broken down and the sealant will not have an adequate surface to bond with. It is very important for the area to be dry and the phosphoric acid to be placed correctly for a good bond to occur and for the sealant to last. If the tooth is contaminated with saliva before the sealant is placed, the etching procedure must also be redone.

When the time for application has passed, the tooth is rinsed thoroughly for the specified amount of time, usually 30 to 60 seconds. After the tooth has been etched, the surface looks frosted or chalky and appears dull (Figure 28-21). If the enamel does not appear chalky and white, the procedure must be repeated. The etchant/conditioner is applied on the occlusal surface 2 to 3 mm beyond the area to be sealed. The tooth must be etched beyond the sealant to prevent fracture of the sealant and possible microleakage.

The glass ionomer sealant materials bond to the tooth chemically. An acid in the glass ionomer material breaks down the enamel and then fuses with it. This is a very strong bond with less chance of marginal chipping or poor bonding.

ADVANCED CHAIRSIDE FUNCTIONS

FIGURE 28-21 View of where acid etchant was placed.

- Air abrasion etchers and microetchers may also be used to prepare teeth for sealants. When using the air abrasion unit or microetchers, all debris from the tooth surface must be removed before placing the sealant.

- One-step etching and bonding materials are currently available. These materials are placed on the tooth and dried, but not rinsed; the tooth is then ready for sealant placement.

Curing Process

Another difference in the types of sealant materials is the curing or hardening process. The two methods of **polymerization** (hardening) follow:

1. **Chemically cured**, also known as self-curing or auto polymerization.

2. **Light cured**, in which a curing light is used to harden materials.

Chemically cured materials consist of a catalyst and a base. When the two are mixed together, they chemically react to polymerize in about one minute. Light-cured sealants are packaged as single-component systems that are activated by a curing light. The advantages of light-curing systems are that the operator has control of the setting time and no mixing is required.

Placement of Enamel Sealants

The dentist diagnoses which teeth need enamel sealants after a thorough examination that includes radio-graphs. Some dentists also use caries detection dye, magnified visual inspection, or the new nondestructive qualitative laser fluorescence. Children with newly erupted molars and premolars that are caries free benefit the most from sealants. Partially erupted teeth may be sealed provided there is not a flap over the occlusal surface that interferes with sealant application.

Isolation is a very important step during sealant placement, because the tooth must be kept dry and free from contamination after the etchant is placed. The dental dam is the best method of isolating the tooth/teeth. If placed correctly, the tooth is easier to see and the area is kept dry. The main disadvantage to using the dental dam is that placing it is time consuming.

Other means of isolating the tooth include cotton rolls or Garmer clamps with cotton rolls. Dri-Angles® or Dry-Tips® can also be used to block the Stenson's duct on the buccal mucosa and assist in keeping the mouth open.

It is the operator's preference when to isolate the teeth, before or after the polish. Usually, sealants are placed on one or two quadrants at a time to ensure adequate isolation of the teeth.

Typically, the tooth is cleaned before it is etched and sealed. The occlusal surface must be free of debris so the etchant can attach to the enamel surface. Prophy pastes, which are normally used for coronal polishing, should not be used because they contain flavoring oils and fluoride that may interfere with the mechanical bonding. Use flour of pumice with a rubber cup or bristle brush. Other means of cleaning the tooth include using an air port polisher or fissurotomy burs.

Always follow manufacturers' instructions for preparing the tooth and placing the sealant.

Helpful Hints

- The most likely cause of sealant failure is moisture control. Be sure to isolate the area well and maintain isolation throughout the procedure.

- Ask the patient to keep the tongue still to prevent contamination.

- Dri-Angles® can be placed to reduce saliva flow. Place on the buccal mucosa with the widest end toward the anterior of the mouth.

- Sealant patients can sometimes be a challenge, so be prepared and work quickly and efficiently in order to finish as soon as possible.

- Read manufacturer instructions to check for any changes in technique or product.

ADVANCED CHAIRSIDE FUNCTIONS

PROCEDURE 28-5

Procedure for Placing Enamel Sealants

This procedure is performed by the dental assistant, hygienist, or dentist depending on the state dental practice act. Before the sealant is placed, the teeth are evaluated for caries, then the tooth/teeth is/are polished with a rubber cup. Equipment for preparation of the tooth/teeth and the sealant procedure is listed below.

EQUIPMENT AND SUPPLIES (Figure 28-22)

- Basic setup: mouth mirror, explorer, cotton pliers

- Air-water syringe tip, HVE tips, and saliva ejector

- Rubber cup or brush

- Dri-Angles

- Low-speed handpiece with right angle (prophy angle) attachment

- Flour of pumice or prophy paste without fluoride, air polisher, dry toothbrush, or fissurotomy burs

- Dental dam setup, cotton rolls, or Garmer cotton roll holders and short and long cotton rolls

- Etchant/conditioner

- Sealant material: base material and catalyst (for self-cure) or syringe or capsule (for light cure)

- Applicators (microbrush, small cotton-tipped applicator, or syringe) for etchant

- Bonding agent

- Light-curing unit

- Articulating paper and forceps

- Assorted burs and/or stones for reducing high spots

PROCEDURE STEPS *(Follow aseptic procedures)*

1. Check tooth or teeth with explorer. Polish the occlusal surface of the teeth to receive sealants.

2. Use flour of pumice or a non-fluoride prophy paste with a rubber cup or bristle brush to clean the occlusal surfaces. An air polisher can also be used, a dry

FIGURE 28-22 Tray setup for placement of enamel sealants.

toothbrush, or fissurotomy burs. Once polished, rinse the teeth and dry thoroughly. If the pits and fissures are deep, check them with an explorer and then rinse and dry again.

3. Dental dam isolation is ideal because it keeps the teeth dry and protects the tissues from the etchant. Depending on the skill of the operator, the dental dam may be placed on more than one quadrant at a time. (Refer to information on dental dams in Chapter 34.) Cotton roll isolation is commonly used, but care must be given to ensure that the teeth are kept isolated. Garmer clamps used with long and short cotton rolls are very effective. Place cotton rolls on both buccal and lingual areas on the mandibular teeth and only on the buccal for the maxillary teeth. Place a Dri Angle on buccal mucosa.

4. After the tooth is isolated, completely dry the tooth. Following manufacturer directions, apply the etchant. Using an applicator, apply etchant to the occlusal surface, into the pits and fissures, and two-thirds up the cuspid incline. Use a gentle dabbing motion while

(continues)

ADVANCED CHAIRSIDE FUNCTIONS

applying the sealant for the designated amount of time (usually fifteen to thirty seconds).

5. Rinse the tooth with water, and use the evacuator tip to remove the remaining acid and water. Rinse for twenty to thirty seconds. Reisolate with dry cotton rolls if this method was used.

6. Dry the tooth with the air and examine the etched surface. It should appear dull and chalky white. If the tooth does not have this appearance, etch again for fifteen to thirty seconds (Figure 28-23).

7. Follow manufacturer directions to prepare and apply the sealant material. With the applicator selected, place the sealant so that it flows into the pits and fissures and reaches the desired thickness. Place the sealant on the mesial and allow it to flow toward the distal. The applicator tip or a microbrush can be used to carefully move the sealant and prevent air bubbles.

8. Allow the self-curing sealants to set (polymerize) for the time recommended by the manufacturer. For light-cured sealants, hold the curing light 2 mm directly above the occlusal surface and expose for the appropriate time (materials differ, so the curing time can range from twenty to sixty seconds).

NOTE: Use tinted protective eyewear during the curing process.

9. Evaluate the sealant (Figure 28-24). With an explorer, carefully check to see whether the sealant is hardened and smooth. If there are irregularities or voids, repeat the process to properly seal those areas. If the surface has been free of saliva, then additional sealant can be added without etching the tooth first. However, if saliva has contacted the tooth, then the process must be repeated.

10. After the sealant has set, rinse or wipe the surface with a moist cotton roll/pellet to remove the air-inhibited layer.

11. Remove cotton rolls or the dental dam. Check the contacts with dental floss, and look for any excess materials. Dry the teeth and, with articulating paper, evaluate for any high spots (Figure 28-25). If the markings are dark, use a bur or stone to reduce them. It does not take much to reduce the sealant, and areas just a little high will wear down in two to three days with very little patient awareness.

12. Apply fluoride to the sealed tooth to cover any areas that were etched but not sealed. Sealants are recorded on the patient's chart. Instruct the patient to have the sealants checked every six months to a year to ensure that they have been completely retained.

FIGURE 28-23 Isolated tooth with enamel etched. Appearance is white and chalky where etchant was placed.

FIGURE 28-24 Tooth with sealant in place.

(continues)

ADVANCED CHAIRSIDE FUNCTIONS

P R O C E D U R E 2 8 - 5 *(C O N T I N U E D)*

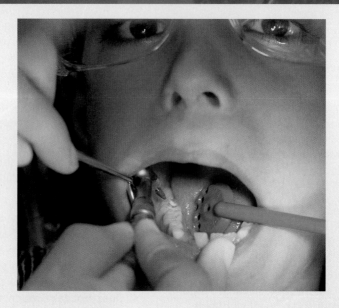

FIGURE 28-25 Articulating paper has marked high spots on the sealant. Before patient is dismissed, sealant is reduced with assorted burs and stones.

CHAPTER SUMMARY

The scope of pediatric treatment includes restoring and maintaining the primary, mixed, and permanent dentition, and applying preventive measures for dental caries, periodontal disease, and malocclusion. The primary focus of the pediatric dental practice is preventive treatment and dealing with the compromised child patient. The whole staff needs to enjoy working with children and be sincere and honest in their actions and feelings. To be effective in the management of children, the dental team must be upbeat, motivated, and aware.

The role of the dental assistant in the pediatric practice will vary according to areas of responsibility. One part that the assistant is involved in is managing the child. Another part is the tasks that the assistant performs at chairside. Depending on the state, when assistants work independently, they assume the authority role and must maintain control of the child. The dental assistant is also an educator of the child and parents.

Enamel sealants are an excellent means of preventing and reducing tooth decay. Depending on individual state dental practice acts, the dental assistant may or may not place sealants. If dental assistants are allowed to place sealants, they must obtain additional education and skills needed. Sealants are placed mainly on permanent teeth, preferably just after they erupt in the mouth. The technique for placing sealants requires practice to become proficient.

Case Study

On Friday afternoon, Mrs. Anderson brought her daughter, Noelle, age four years, to Dr. Bryan's office for emergency treatment. Noelle had fallen and hit her face. Her maxillary left central incisor was pushed into the alveolus so that only the incisal third of the tooth was exposed. Noelle had seen Dr. Bryan for an exam when she was three years old.

Case Study Review

1. What is the condition of Noelle's teeth called?

2. At what stage of tooth eruption is Noelle likely to be? What could happen to Noelle's teeth as a result of the physical trauma? Are the permanent teeth affected?

3. Because Noelle had only been in the office for one visit when she was three, would behavior management be a consideration?

REVIEW QUESTIONS

Multiple Choice

1. The best age range for introducing dental care in the dental office is
   a. two to six years old.
   b. four to eight years old.
   c. six to ten years old.
   d. ten to twelve years old.

2. Fear that is based on a person's own personal experiences is called
   a. objective.
   b. subjective.
   c. intraverted.
   d. extraverted.

3. If the pulp of a primary tooth has been exposed, which of the following procedures would be indicated?
   a. Pulpectomy
   b. Pulpotomy
   c. Apexification
   d. Root canal

4. Stainless steel crowns are indicated for all of the following *except*
   a. following a pulpotomy procedure.
   b. hypoplastic or hypocalcified teeth.
   c. incipient decay.
   d. extensive carious decay.

5. Tongue thrusting
   a. pushes the tongue against the posterior teeth.
   b. pushes the tongue against the anterior teeth when swallowing.
   c. pushes the tongue against the palate when swallowing.
   d. pushes the tongue against the floor of the mouth.

6. Enamel sealants are indicated for all of the following *except*
   a. recently erupted teeth.
   b. teeth that have been caries free for four or more years.
   c. on occlusal pits and fissures of noncarious primary teeth.
   d. on deep occlusal fissures.

7. Behavior management techniques used in the pediatric practice include
   a. voice control.
   b. positive reinforcement.
   c. distraction.
   d. all of the above.

8. A child with "mixed dentition" has
   a. deciduous and permanent teeth existing simultaneously in the mouth.
   b. deciduous teeth only.
   c. permanent teeth only.
   d. deciduous teeth with decay.

9. All of the following are true statements about enamel sealants except:
   a. Sealants bond mechanically to the tooth surface.
   b. The teeth are etched before sealants are placed.
   c. Sealants are light cured only.
   d. Sealants are placed on caries-free occlusal surfaces.

10. Where do you find out whether, in your state, dental assistants can legally place enamel sealants?
    a. American Dental Association
    b. American Academy of Pediatric Dentistry
    c. State dental practice act
    d. Dental assistants can place enamel in all states

Critical Thinking

1. Think of an office theme or design that would be attractive to children. Would the assistant be responsible for any maintenance?

2. List three behavior management techniques that would be effective with a young patient who is visiting the dental office for the first time.

3. A five-year-old child arrives at the dental office with bruising on the upper arms and cuts around and inside the mouth. List some steps that may be taken in the pediatric dental office with a suspected child abuse case.

4. On a six-month recall appointment for a child patient, you notice that a sealant is missing on tooth #30. Should the sealant be replaced? If so, can the sealant be replaced without etching the tooth first?

5. Discuss various methods for keeping the area dry when placing a sealant.

Web Activities

1. The American Academy of Pediatric Dentistry is a wonderful resource. Go to http://www.aapd.org and identify Children's Dental Health month. Also, examine the brochures available for parent and patient information.

2. Go to http://www.aapd.org to locate the questions parents most frequently ask about their children's teeth.

3. Sealants are a very important part of preventive treatment for children. To find out where to refer parents/guardians for more information on dental sealants, visit http://www.aadp.org.

PERIODONTICS AND CORONAL POLISH

SPECIFIC INSTRUCTIONAL OBJECTIVES

The student should strive to meet the following objectives and demonstrate an understanding of the facts and principles presented in this chapter:

1. Describe the scope of periodontics.

2. Identify members of the periodontal team and their roles.

3. Describe the stages of periodontal disease.

4. Explain the diagnostic procedures involved in the patient's first visit to the periodontal office.

5. Identify and describe periodontal instruments and their uses.

6. Describe nonsurgical procedures and the dental assistant's role in each procedure.

7. Explain surgical procedures and dental assisting responsibilities.

8. Identify the types of periodontal dressings and how they are prepared, placed, and removed.

9. Describe periodontal maintenance procedures and the patient's role relating to each.

ADVANCED CHAIRSIDE FUNCTIONS

10. Define coronal polish.

11. Explain the indications and contraindications for coronal polish.

12. Describe and identify dental deposits and stains.

13. List types of abrasives and explain characteristics of each type.

14. List and explain types of equipment and materials used to perform a coronal polish.

15. Explain how to maintain the oral cavity during coronal polish.

16. List auxiliary polishing aids and explain their functions.

17. Describe steps in the coronal polish procedure.

KEY TERMS

INTRODUCTION

The periodontist specializes in diseases of the tissue around the root of the tooth. This specialty deals with symptoms, probable causes, diagnosis, and treatment of periodontal disease.

Periodontal Team

The team in a periodontal office includes the periodontist, dental assistants, dental hygienists, and business office staff.

■ The periodontist coordinates treatment with the general dentist in the overall care of the patient. The periodontist screens the patient, performs the surgical care, and provides continual care according to the patient's needs.

■ The dental assistant performs chairside assisting duties and expanded functions allowed by state dental practice acts, including placing and removing periodontal dressing, removing sutures, and performing coronal polishes. The dental assistant takes radiographs, takes impressions for study models, places sealants, and administers fluoride treatments. The dental assistant also gives pre- and postoperative instructions and prepares the treatment room for surgery. These functions are in addition to treatment room preparation and maintenance and sterilization procedures. The dental assistant is involved in educating and motivating the patient throughout the treatment. In some offices, the dental assistant also may perform laboratory tasks, such as pouring study models or making periodontal splints.

■ The dental hygienist performs traditional hygiene procedures and, depending on the state dental practice act, may also administer local anesthetic. In a periodontal practice, the hygienist often sees patients who have more advanced periodontal disease; therefore, responsibilities include curettage, root planing, and clinical examination procedures.

Periodontal Disease

Ancient human skulls demonstrate evidence of bone destruction, and early civilizations had treatment methods such as using wire to tie loose teeth together. According to the American Academy of Periodontology, three out of four adults will experience, to some degree, periodontal problems at some time in their lives. Periodontal disease occurs in children and adolescents with marginal gingivitis and gingival recession, which are the most prevalent conditions (Figure 29-1).

FIGURE 29-1 View of patient with mild gingivitis.

Periodontal disease involves the **periodontium**, which represents the tissues that support the teeth and includes the following:

■ **Gingiva**—Tissues that surround the teeth.

■ **Epithelial attachment**—Area at the bottom of the sulcus where the gingiva attaches to the tooth.

■ **Sulcus**—Space between the tooth and the free gingiva. In healthy mouths, the sulcus is 1 to 3 mm deep.

■ **Periodontal ligaments or membranes**—Fibers of connective tissue that surround the root of the tooth and attach the cementum to the bone.

■ **Cementum**—Hard surface that covers the dentin on the root of the tooth.

■ **Alveolar bone**—Bone that forms the socket that encases the root of the tooth.

Symptoms of Periodontal Disease

The symptoms of periodontal disease include bleeding gums, loose teeth (mobility), inflamed gingiva, abnormal contour of the gingiva, periodontal pocket formation, malocclusion, halitosis, pain and tenderness, and recession and discoloration. All of these symptoms may be present or the symptoms may vary (Figure 29-2A).

Causes of Periodontal Disease

Local irritants are a significant cause of periodontal disease. One irritant, **bacterial plaque**, is a common cause of the inflammation of the gingival tissues. The bacterial plaque forms around the margin of the gingiva and, if left undisturbed, mineralizes and appears as a yellow or

FIGURE 29-2 (A) View of patient with unhealthy gingival tissues-advanced gingival inflammation. (B) Unhealthy gingival tissues and lingual calculus.

brown deposit on the teeth. This hard deposit is called calculus (tartar) (Figure 29-2B). If plaque and calculus are not removed, they continue to develop and grow on both supragingival and subgingival surfaces.

Poor oral hygiene results in the buildup of plaque and calculus. Lack of daily brushing and flossing leads to plaque and debris buildup on the teeth and appliances. (Proper brushing and flossing techniques are discussed in Chapter 4, Oral Health and Preventive Techniques.)

Improper nutrition leads to overall poor health, which often is evident in the gingival tissues. Eating a balanced diet, including foods that keep teeth strong and the tissues free of disease, can aid in maintaining a healthy mouth.

Malocclusion can be a factor in periodontal disease. Improper tooth alignment and occlusion can lead to plaque and calculus formation in areas where food and debris are not removed easily. Also, patients with sensitive teeth or who need dental restorations will favor these areas and alter chewing patterns, putting additional pressure on periodontal structures.

Stress can lead to bruxism (grinding of the teeth), which puts pressure on the teeth and surrounding tissues. Problems with the periodontium during times of stress may be evident because the patient may not eat healthy foods or maintain proper oral hygiene.

Systemic factors, including hormonal imbalances, hereditary predisposition, and certain diseases and medications, are often reflected in the gingival tissues. Examples include hormonal changes due to pregnancy, diabetes, cardiovascular disease such as hypertension, blood diseases such as leukemia, HIV infection, genetic conditions such as Down syndrome, emotional disorders, systemic drugs such as Dilantin or immunosuppressants, and thyroid deficiencies.

Classification of Periodontal Disease

There are two main classifications of periodontal disease: gingivitis and periodontitis. Through clinical research and improved technology, the understanding of periodontal disease has broadened in scope. Considering the course and characteristics of the disease, more classifications have been added. In 1999 at the International Workshop for a Classification of Periodontal Diseases and Conditions, the American Academy of Periodontology proposed a new classification system (Table 29-1). The revisions are inclusive and describe distinct types of periodontal diseases. The classifications are based on clinical (extent and severity of disease), radiographic, and historical data. Stages of periodontal disease have also been refined (Table 29-2).

Gingivitis. Gingivitis is inflammation of the gingival tissues. It is common in all ages. Causes may include buildup of plaque and calculus, poor-fitting appliances, and poor occlusion, and the condition may occur in association with certain systemic diseases (scurvy), hormonal changes (pregnancy), or prolonged drug therapy (phenytoin, which is an anticonvulsant drug). The tissues become reddish in color, interdental papilla may be swollen and bulbous, and tissues may bleed after brushing and flossing. Gingivitis precedes periodontitis but does not always progress to it. Proper brushing and flossing can reverse this condition in some cases by removing the plaque.

In the classification system, the section on gingival diseases is divided into plaque-induced gingivitis and non–plaque-induced diseases. Each section covers types of gingival conditions that are seen in periodontal and general dental practice. According to the section on plaque-induced diseases, gingivitis can be modified by systemic factors, medications, or malnutrition. The section on non–plaque-induced gingivitis includes a wide range of gingival diseases that are specific according to bacteria. This section also includes wide-ranging

TABLE 29-1 Classification of Periodontal Diseases and Conditions

I. Gingival diseases
  A. Dental plaque–induced gingival diseases*
    1. Gingivitis associated with dental plaque only
      a. Without other local contributing factors
      b. With local contributing factors (see VIIIA)
    2. Gingival diseases modified by systemic factors
      a. Associated with the endocrine system
        (1) Puberty-associated gingivitis
        (2) Menstrual cycle–associated gingivitis
        (3) Pregnancy-associated
          (a) Gingivitis
          (b) Pyogenic granuloma
        (4) Diabetes mellitus–associated gingivitis
      b. Associated with blood dyscrasias
        (1) Leukemia-associated gingivitis
        (2) Other
    3. Gingival diseases modified by medications
      a. Drug-influenced gingival diseases
        (1) Drug-influenced gingival enlargements
        (2) Drug-influenced gingivitis
          (a) Oral contraceptive–associated gingivitis
          (b) Other
    4. Gingival diseases modified by malnutrition
      a. Ascorbic acid–deficiency gingivitis
      b. Other
  B. Non–plaque-induced gingival lesions
    1. Gingival diseases of specific bacterial origin
      a. *Neisseria gonorrhoeae*–associated lesions
      b. *Treponema pallidum*–associated lesions
      c. Streptococcal species–associated lesions
      d. Other
    2. Gingival diseases of viral origin
      a. Herpes virus infections
        (1) Primary herpetic gingivostomatitis
        (2) Recurrent oral herpes
        (3) Varicella-zoster infections
      b. Other
    3. Gingival diseases of fungal origin
      a. *Candida* species infections
        (1) Generalized gingival candidiasis
      b. Linear gingival erythema
      c. Histoplasmosis
      d. Other
    4. Gingival lesions of genetic origin
      a. Hereditary gingival fibromatosis
      b. Other
    5. Gingival manifestations of systemic conditions
      a. Mucocutaneous disorders
        (1) Lichen planus
        (2) Pemphigoid
        (3) Pemphigus vulgaris
        (4) Erythema multiforme
        (5) Lupus erythematosus
        (6) Drug-induced
        (7) Other
      b. Allergic reactions
        (1) Dental restorative materials
          (a) Mercury
          (b) Nickel

(continues)

TABLE 29-1 Classification of Periodontal Diseases and Conditions *(continued)*

       (c) Acrylic
       (d) Other
     (2) Reactions attributable to
       (a) Toothpastes/dentifrices
       (b) Mouthrinses/mouthwashes
       (c) Chewing gum additives
       (d) Foods and additives
     (3) Other
   6. Traumatic lesions (factitious, iatrogenic, accidental)
    a. Chemical injury
    b. Physical injury
    c. Thermal injury
   7. Foreign-body reactions
   8. Not otherwise specified
II. Chronic periodontitis[†]
  A. Localized
  B. Generalized
III. Aggressive periodontitis[†]
  A. Localized
  B. Generalized
IV. Periodontitis as a manifestation of systemic diseases
  A. Associated with hematologic disorders
    1. Acquired neutropenia
    2. Leukemias
    3. Other
  B. Associated with genetic disorders
    1. Familial and cyclic neutropenia
    2. Down syndrome
    3. Leukocyte adhesion deficiency syndromes
    4. Papillon-Lefévre syndrome
    5. Chediak-Higashi syndromes
    6. Histiocytosis syndromes
    7. Glycogen storage disease
    8. Infantile genetic agranulocytosis
    9. Cohen syndrome
    10. Ehlers-Danlos syndrome (Types IV and VIIIAD)
    11. Hypophosphatasia
    12. Other
  C. Not otherwise specified (NOS)
V. Necrotizing periodontal diseases
  A. Necrotizing ulcerative gingivitis (NUG)
  B. Necrotizing ulcerative periodontitis (NUP)
VI. Abscesses of the periodontium
  A. Gingival abscess
  B. Periodontal abscess
  C. Pericoronal abscess
VII. Periodontitis associated with endodontic lesions
  A. Combined periodontal–endodontic lesions
VIII. Developmental or acquired deformities and conditions
  A. Localized tooth-related factors that modify or predispose to plaque-induced gingival diseases/periodontitis
    1. Tooth anatomic factors
    2. Dental restorations/appliances
    3. Root fractures
    4. Cervical root resorption and cemental tears
  B. Mucogingival deformities and conditions around teeth
    1. Gingival/soft tissue recession
     a. Facial or lingual surfaces
     b. Interproximal (papillary)
    2. Lack of keratinized gingiva

(continues)

TABLE 29-1 Classification of Periodontal Diseases and Conditions *(continued)*

      3. Decreased vestibular depth
      4. Aberrant frenum/muscle position
      5. Gingival excess
         a. Pseudopocket
         b. Inconsistent gingival margin
         c. Excessive gingival display
         d. Gingival enlargement (see IA3 and IB4)
      6. Abnormal color
    C. Mucogingival deformities and conditions on edentulous ridges
      1. Vertical and/or horizontal ridge deficiency
      2. Lack of gingiva/keratinized tissue
      3. Gingival/soft tissue enlargement
      4. Aberrant frenum/muscle position
      5. Decreased vestibular depth
      6. Abnormal color
    D. Occlusal trauma
      1. Primary occlusal trauma
      2. Secondary occlusal trauma

*Can occur on a periodontium with no attachment loss or on a periodontium with attachment loss that is not progressing.
†Can be further classified on the basis of extent and severity. As a general guide, extent can be characterized as localized ≤30% and generalized ≥30% of sites involved. Severity can be characterized on the basis of the amount of clinical attachment loss (CAL) as follows: slight, 1–2 mm CAL; moderate, 3–4 mm CAL; and severe, ≥5 mm CAL.
Source: Armitage, G.C. 1999. Development of a classification system for periodontal diseases and conditions. *Ann Periodontal* 4:1–6.

TABLE 29-2 Periodontal Disease Stages

Periodontal disease is caused by plaque, the colorless, sticky bacterial film that forms constantly on the teeth. The bacteria in plaque produce by-products that can irritate the gums and, over time, seriously damage the structures that support the teeth.

Healthy Tissues	Gingivitis	Early Periodontitis	Moderate Periodontitis	Advanced Periodontitis
Gum is firm, fits tightly to the teeth, and does not bleed.	Gum tissue may be inflamed, swollen, and bleeds easily during brushing, flossing, or examination by your dental professional.	Continued inflammation, loss of gum attachment and bone support.	Supporting gum and bone tissue have deteriorated, tooth loosens.	Severe destruction of tissue and bone, causing tooth loss.

manifestations of system conditions and allergic reactions.

Periodontitis. Periodontitis involves the formation of periodontal pockets. This occurs when margins of the gingiva and periodontal fibers recede and the supporting bone becomes inflamed and destroyed. There is an increase in tooth mobility as the pockets become deeper, and there may be **furcation** (area where the roots divide) involvement in multirooted teeth.

The classification system now refers to "chronic periodontitis" instead of "adult periodontitis" because adolescents as well as adults can develop periodontitis. Chronic periodontitis is a progressive disease process with the patient experiencing loss of tissue attachment and bone. Periodontitis can also be evaluated on the basis of extent and severity. Extent is characterized using

the following guideline: extent is localized if less than 30% of sites are involved, and generalized if more than 30% are involved. Severity is characterized by the amount of clinical attachment loss (CAL): slight = 1 or 2 mm CAL, moderate = 3 or 4 mm CAL, and severe = ≥5 mm CAL.

Aggressive periodontitis is a form of periodontitis that acts rapidly and aggressively destroys the tissue attachment and bone. Extent of the disease determines whether it falls under the localized or generalized classification.

Patients with periodontitis that is associated with complicated systemic involvement, such as diabetes, are addressed in the "Periodontitis as a Manifestation of Systemic Diseases" section (Table 29-1, section IV).

Necrotizing Ulcerative Gingivitis and Necrotizing Ulcerative Periodontitis. Necrotizing ulcerative gingivitis (NUG) occurs most frequently in young adults sixteen to thirty years old. Causes include stress, smoking, inadequate diet, and poor oral hygiene. Characteristics of this form of gingivitis are inflamed gingiva, metallic taste, bad breath, pain, and hemorrhage of the tissues. This condition is also known as Vincent's disease and trench mouth. It appears in individuals in the same unhealthy state and frequently occurs in college students around the time of final examinations (because of stress).

HIV periodontitis is now known as **necrotizing ulcerative periodontitis (NUP).** NUP is not limited to patients with HIV infections, but is also seen in patients who are severely malnourished and immunosuppressed. Patients with NUP are often in severe pain, the sites bleed easily, and tissue and bone destruction is extensive.

Periodontal Diagnostic Procedures

CDA The first appointment with the periodontist is often an information-gathering appointment. After completing the medical dental history, the patient is seated in the treatment room for an extraoral and intraoral examination. Radiographs and impressions are taken and a periodontal screening is completed. Developing rapport with the patient is essential for successful treatment. The patient must have confidence in the dentist and the staff. The patient has responsibility in the treatment of periodontal disease and should be educated and motivated. Information to share with each patient includes following oral hygiene instructions, diet suggestions and modifications, personal habit changes, and routine office visits.

Medical Dental History

The medical dental history gives the operator and the patient the opportunity to learn about each other. The operator gains information about why the patient is seeking treatment; if there is a systemic condition such as tuberculosis, HIV, AIDS, or diabetes; how the patient feels about his or her teeth; previous dental treatment; and if the patient has any oral habits that have contributed to the present condition. The patient has the opportunity to ask questions of the dentist and gain an understanding of what is involved with periodontal treatment. The patient's history must be accurate and complete. A history checklist should open the way for significant conversation between the patient, the dental assistant, and/or the dentist.

Sample Medical History Form. The following types of questions should be answered by the patient.

1. Chief complaints:
   - Why did you come to the periodontist?
   - Specifically, what area(s) of your mouth is (are) causing you concern?
   - Do you currently have pain in or near your ears?
   - Does any part of your mouth hurt when clenched?
   - Are there any areas in your mouth that have unhealed or inflamed sores?

2. Medical history:
   - Are you ill at this time? If so, what is (are) your ailment(s)?
   - Are you currently undergoing any medical treatment(s)? If so, what kind(s)?
   - Are you taking any medication(s)? If so, what kind(s)?
   - Have you ever had adverse responses to any type(s) of antibiotic? If so, what type(s)?
   - Have you ever had adverse responses to any type(s) of anesthetic? If so, what type(s)?
   - Are you pregnant?
   - Are you allergic to anything?
   - Do you have any of the following?
     Rheumatic fever
     Heart murmur
     Cardiovascular disease
     Hepatitis
     Kidney infection
     Tuberculosis
     Diabetes
     AIDS
     HIV
   - Do you have, or have you ever had, problems with any of the following?
     Prolonged bleeding
     Allergies
     Oral symptoms related to pregnancy, menstruation, or menopause
   - Do you have any oral conditions present? If so, how long have they been present and has there been any treatment for them?

3. Oral history:
   - Have you had any extractions? Have you had any restorations?
   - Do you have any problems after dental treatment, such as bleeding, pain, or swelling?
   - Do you have any problems with your teeth, such as bleeding gums, pain, mobility, or sensitivity?
   - Do you have difficulty with your joints when eating or opening and closing your mouth?

4. Oral habits:
   - Do you have any habits such as grinding, clenching, or mouth breathing?
   - Do you smoke?
   - Do you use alcohol or drugs?

5. Family history:

- Does anyone in your family have a history of periodontal disease?

6. Oral hygiene:

- Which brushing technique do you use?
- Do you floss? If so, how often?
- What type of toothbrush and toothpaste do you use?
- Do you use any other oral hygiene aids? If so, what kinds?

Clinical Examination

The clinical examination includes an extraoral examination of the face and neck; an intraoral examination of the tongue, palate, buccal mucosa, the teeth, the oropharynx area; and the periodontal examination.

Extraoral Examination. The extraoral examination includes observation of the skin and lips and palpation of the lymph nodes and the temporomandibular joint.

Intraoral Examination. The intraoral examination combines viewing and palpating the tissues in the oral cavity. The operator looks for abnormalities in color, size, texture, and consistency of all tissues. The intraoral examination includes an oral cancer screening. The condition of the teeth and any prosthetic appliances are examined, noting any areas that might cause or contribute to periodontal disease. Any necessary treatment is recorded on the patient's chart.

Periodontal Examination. The periodontal examination is a thorough examination of the periodontium using periodontal charts. The periodontal charts depict the condition of the patient's periodontal tissues. The charting is completed either manually or on a computer. The oral cavity is examined, and information is gathered by the operator while the dental assistant records the information on the periodontal chart (Figure 29-3).

- Patient oral hygiene is evaluated and the amount of plaque and calculus present is determined. This evaluation includes both supragingival and subgingival deposits.

- Periodontal probing measures the depth of the periodontal pocket with a periodontal probe (refer to Periodontal Instruments—Periodontal Probes section). A normal sulcus is 3 mm deep or less. When the depth is greater than 3 mm, it is termed a periodontal pocket. To determine the sulcus depth, six sites are probed and recorded on each tooth. There are three sites on the facial, including mesiofacial, midfacial, and distofacial, and three sites on the lingual, including mesiolingual, midlingual, and distolingual. The periodontal probe is inserted into the sulcus until the operator feels resistance. Tactile sensation indicates the level of the epithelium attachment. The calibrations on the probe measure the depth of the pocket. These are recorded on the chart.

- **Tooth mobility** measures movement of the tooth within the socket. The mobility test is accomplished by pushing the tooth in a buccolingual direction using the handle ends of two instruments or by using the automatic device for assessing mobility. Mobility is usually recorded using a scale of 0 to 3: 0 = normal, 1 = slight or 1 mm, 2 = moderate or 2 mm, and 3 = severe or 3 mm.

- Furcation involvement measures destruction of interradicular bone in the furcation area of multirooted teeth. A curved instrument is inserted in the furcation to determine the amount of involvement.

- Appearance of the gingiva is evaluated in terms of color, size, shape, texture, position, consistency, bleeding, and amount of exudate (pus).

- Bleeding/suppuration is the amount of blood/fluid present during probing. It is a major indicator of inflamed gingiva.

- **Recession** of the gingival margin is the loss of the gingival tissue exposing the underlying cementum/dentin, usually seen on the facial surface.

- Occlusion is evaluated and described. The occlusal bite relationship is checked with articulating paper or wax to identify areas that show excessive biting or chewing force.

> **Occlusal equilibration** is the process of removing areas showing excessive force. Once these "spots" have been determined, burs, discs, and stones are used to reduce and restore occlusion without interference.

Radiographic Interpretation

Radiographs are useful tools when evaluating the periodontium for periodontal disease. The radiographs show the teeth and the level and position of the alveolar bone. When periodontal disease is present, the alveolar bone recedes both vertically and/or horizontally. **Vertical bone resorption** is found on individual teeth on the interproximal surface (Figure 29-4A). **Horizontal bone resorption** occurs when there is equal crestal bone loss on the mesial and distal surfaces of the proximal teeth (Figure 29-4B).

Periapical x-rays supplemented with bite-wing radiographs are most commonly taken, and the x-rays must be as dimensionally accurate as possible. Usually, a full-mouth series is taken for comparisons throughout the mouth. Panoramic radiographs are also taken as an adjunct.

Examination of: John Snowton

Spokane, WA

Provider: Dr. G. Anthony

Age: 36 **Exam Done:** Chart

Sex: Male **Exam Type:** Initial

Exam Date:

Exam Time: 03:29PM

Spokane, WA

	1	2	3	4	5	6	7	8	9	10	11	12	13	14	15	16

Probing Depth

F: | | 646 | 725 | 626 | 625 | 636 | 767 | 735 | 537 | 736 | 636 | 635 | 636 | 636 | 655 | 676 |
L: | | 646 | 656 | 656 | 656 | 535 | 544 | 555 | 555 | 556 | 546 | 555 | 656 | 766 | 546 | 666 |

Bleeding / Suppuration

Furcation

Gingival Margin

F: | | 000 | 000 | 000 | 000 | 000 | 002 | 202 | 203 | 200 | 000 | 000 | 000 | 020 | 000 | 000 |
L: | | 000 | 000 | 000 | 000 | 000 | 000 | 000 | 430 | 320 | 000 | 000 | 000 | 020 | 000 | 000 |

Mobility

| | | | | | | | | | | | | | | 1 | | 1 |

Attachment Level

F: | | 646 | 725 | 626 | 625 | 636 | 769 | 937 | 731 | 936 | 636 | 635 | 636 | 656 | 655 | 676 |
L: | | 646 | 656 | 656 | 656 | 535 | 544 | 555 | 985 | 876 | 546 | 555 | 656 | 786 | 546 | 666 |

32	31	30	29	28	27	26	25	24	23	22	21	20	19	18	17

Probing Depth

F: | 635 | 536 | 636 | 637 | 644 | 435 | 545 | 535 | 535 | 655 | 566 | 535 | 636 | 737 |
L: | 546 | 646 | 646 | 636 | 636 | 444 | 444 | 444 | 434 | 444 | 435 | 656 | 656 | 645 |

Bleeding / Suppuration

Furcation

Gingival Margin

F: | 000 | 000 | 000 | 000 | 000 | 000 | 202 | 200 | 000 | 000 | 000 | 000 | 000 |
L: | 000 | 000 | 000 | 000 | 000 | 233 | 434 | 232 | 000 | 000 | 000 | 000 | 000 |

Mobility

Attachment Level

F: | 635 | 536 | 636 | 637 | 644 | 435 | 747 | 735 | 535 | 655 | 566 | 535 | 636 | 737 |
L: | 546 | 646 | 646 | 636 | 636 | 677 | 878 | 676 | 434 | 444 | 435 | 656 | 656 | 645 |

FIGURE 29-3 Periodontal chart.

FIGURE 29-4 (A) Vertical bone loss shown on x-ray, on the mesial of the maxillary left first bicuspid (#12). (B) Horizontal bone loss shown on x-ray between the maxillary right molar, bicuspids, and cuspid (#3, 4, 5, and 6).

Presentation of Treatment Plan

After gathering all the periodontal diagnostic information, the periodontist determines the appropriate treatment plan for the patient. The patient is scheduled for a consultation appointment. During this appointment, the prognosis (anticipated outcome) of the patient's condition and the treatment sequence are explained. Charts, radiographs, study models, and photographs are used to educate the patient. The patient's role in the treatment is discussed. The patient must be actively involved in the treatment and motivated to follow the home-care plan and keep treatment appointments. Once all questions are answered and the treatment plan is understood, appointments and financial arrangements are completed.

Periodontal Instruments

CDA Periodontal instruments are designed to probe, scrape, file, and cut the hard surfaces of the teeth, alveolar bone, and soft tissues of the gingiva. These instruments must be kept sharp. Usually, the hygienist or a specially trained assistant is responsible for maintaining periodontal hand instruments.

Instrument Sharpening

There are many benefits of using properly sharpened instruments. Sharp edges make the operator's work easier and faster, improve the quality of procedures, and enhance patient comfort. After repeated use, the cutting edges of instruments become dull and rounded, making the blades ineffective and more difficult to use. At this point, the operator applies more pressure and becomes fatigued more easily. The patient may feel the added pressure and discomfort.

There are manual and mechanical methods for sharpening periodontal instruments. Mechanical devices are more expensive, but they are effective and easy to use, and provide consistent, precision sharpening. These devices usually have sharpening guides that adjust for various instruments and mechanically rotating discs. Manually sharpening instruments involves using handheld sharpening stones. Sharpening stones are frequently used and are available in various shapes, sizes, and hardness (grits). Finer grits are often used to sharpen dental instruments because the finer grit (smaller particles) abrade metal slowly. There are several types of stones: Arkansas stone, India oilstone, and ceramic stones. Some of the stones are used with water to lubricate or, sometimes, honing oil. Oil is not used, because it may leave a residue that cannot be removed. The lubricant serves as a means for moving the metal particles of the instrument away from the blade and preventing them from becoming embedded in the stone. After use, the stones are thoroughly cleaned by scrubbing with a stiff brush, soap, and water or they are cleaned ultrasonically. The stones are then sterilized properly (Figure 29-5A).

There are many techniques for sharpening dental instruments; some use geometric concepts and terms

FIGURE 29-5 (A) Arkansas cylindrical dental instrument sharpening stone. (B) Arkansas thick wedge dental instrument sharpening stone. (C) Correct grasp and position when sharpening a dental instrument using the Arkansas stone.

while others use the "telling time" approach. The latter technique uses the face of a clock for orientation and positioning. With this method, the instrument is held stationary and the stone moves. The elbow is positioned on a stable surface with the hand upright. The end of the instrument to be sharpened is held downward, toward the wrist, in one hand; the other hand holds and moves the sharpening stone against the instrument (Figure 29-5B). The positioning and technique of sharpening dental instruments require additional information and training. It is a skill that takes time and practice but is extremely valuable to dentists and hygienists using these instruments.

Periodontal Probes

The **periodontal probe** is the primary instrument used in the periodontal examination (Figure 29-6). This is a calibrated instrument used to measure the depth of periodontal pockets. The probe is also used to measure areas of recession, bleeding, or exudate. The calibrations on the periodontal probe are in millimeters and vary depending on the manufacturer and the operator's preference. These markings may be indentations or color coded for easy reading. The probe may be flat, oval, or round in cross-section but must be thin enough to fit easily into the gingival sulcus.

A computerized probe system detects and stores information on pocket depth, recession, furcation involvement, and mobility. The information is shown on a computer screen and can be printed out.

Explorers

Explorers are used to detect and locate calculus, tooth irregularities, faulty margins on restorations, and furcation involvement. The explorer gives the operator the best tactile information for assessment.

The explorers used in periodontics are supplied in a variety of shapes, similar to those also used in general dental procedures. The working ends are thin and sharp. They may be curved or at near right angles to adapt to the curves of the tooth surfaces.

Curettes

The **curette** is a hand instrument used for removing subgingival calculus, smoothing the root surface, and removing the soft tissue lining of the periodontal pocket. The working end has a cutting edge on one or both sides of the blade and the end is rounded, not pointed like the scaler (Figure 29-7). The curette is a finer instrument that is designed to adapt to the curves of the root surfaces. There are two basic curettes: **universal curettes**, which are used throughout the mouth, and **Gracey curettes**, which are supplied in a set of several instruments that are designed and angled to be used in specific areas (Figure 29-8). The curette handles are similar to those on the scalers.

Scalers

Scalers are sharp hand instruments that are used to remove hard deposits such as **supragingival** (above the gingiva) and **subgingival** (below the gingiva) calculus from the teeth. Scalers are supplied in a variety of shapes and angulations to access all surfaces of the teeth. The working end of a scaler has two sharp edges that come to a point (Figure 29-7). The handles are often

FIGURE 29-6 (A) Varied periodontal probes. (B) Color-coded probe.

Working end of scaler ——— ——— Working end of curette

FIGURE 29-7 The working ends of a scaler and a curette showing how they are positioned on a tooth.

FIGURE 29-8 Types of periodontal curettes: Gracey curettes. (A) No. 5-6. (B) No. 7-8. (C) No. 9-10. (D) No. 13-14.

large and are ribbed, serrated, or knurled. Sometimes, the metal handles are covered with color-coded rubber grips to prevent muscle fatigue and for better control of the instrument.

Sickle Scalers. Sickle scalers are designed to remove supragingival calculus. The sickle scaler is also called the Shepherd's hook. These scalers have two cutting edges along the margins of the curved blade (Figure 29-9A and B).

Jacquette Scalers. Jacquette scalers, like sickle scalers, are designed to remove supragingival deposits. They

FIGURE 29-9 Types of periodontal scalers. (A) Combination instrument with a sickle scaler on one end and a Jacquette scaler on the other. (B) Sickle scaler. (C) Jacquette scaler.

have straight blades with cutting edges on both the sides. The Jacquette scaler has three angles in the shank of the instrument (Figure 29-9A and C).

Chisel Scalers. Chisel scalers are used most often in the anterior of the mouth. The blade of the chisel is slightly curved and the cutting edge is beveled (Figure 29-10A).

Hoe Scalers. The hoe scaler has a blade bent at a 90° angle at the end of the working end. This cutting edge is beveled and sharp. The hoe scaler is placed in the periodontal pocket to the base and then pulled toward the crown of the tooth with even pressure to plane and smooth the root surface (Figure 29-10B).

Files

Periodontal files are supplied in a variety of blade shapes and shank angulations (Figure 29-10C). They are used in a pulling motion interproximally to remove calculus and for root planing. Files are also used to remove overhanging margins of dental restorations.

FIGURE 29-10 Periodontal (A) chisel, (B) hoe, and (C) file. *(Courtesy of Miltex Instrument Co., Inc., Lake Success, NY.)*

Ultrasonic Instruments

Ultrasonic instruments are used to remove hard deposits, stains, and debris during scaling, curettage, and root planing procedures. Typically, they are used as an adjunct to manual scaling procedures. Ultrasonic units generate high-power vibrations to a handpiece with a variety of tips (Figure 29-11). These vibrations cause the calculus to fracture and be dislodged. Because ultrasonic vibrations cause heat, the units have cooling systems that circulate water through the handpieces and out openings near the tips. The water spray cools and also flushes the area. It is beneficial for a dental assistant to be present to evacuate the volume of water and debris. Although the ultrasonic units are effective and fast, care must be taken to prevent injury to the tissues and the teeth.

Periodontal Knives

Periodontal knives or gingivectomy knives are used to remove gingival tissue during periodontal surgery. The knives most commonly used are the broad-bladed Kirkland knives (Figure 29-12A). These knives are kidney-shaped and sharp around the entire periphery of the blade. They are supplied as either single- or double-ended instruments.

FIGURE 29-11 Ultrasonic scaling unit.

FIGURE 29-12 Gingivectomy knives. (A) Kirkland broad-blade knife. (B) Orban Interdental knife.

Interdental Knives

Periodontal knives that are used to remove soft tissue interproximally are called **interdental knives**. The Orban No. 1 and 2 are very popular interdental knives. These spear-shaped knives have long, narrow blades with cutting edges on both sides of the blade (Figure 29-12B).

Periotomes

Periotomes are fairly new instruments that are used to sever the periodontal ligament (PDL) prior to atraumatic extractions as well as to prepare the tissue for dental implants.

These instruments are available in a variety of shapes, including narrow, angled, and wide. Some are designed for use on anterior teeth and others for posterior teeth. Periotome blades are thin, flexible, and sharp to cause minimal damage to periodontal ligaments. Periotomes may be single- or double-ended, and are made of stainless steel (Figure 29-13).

Surgical Scalpel

Surgical scalpels are used for periodontal surgical procedures to remove gingival tissue. The surgical scalpel is also known as the Bard-Parker scalpel. The scalpel has two components: a sterilizible metal or plastic handle and a disposable blade. The blades come in different shapes and sizes. Disposable scalpels are also available (Figure 29-14).

Electrosurgery

The **electrosurgery** setup consists of a control box, foot-operated on-off controls, a terminal plate that is placed behind the patient's back or shoulders, and another terminal that is a probe with various cutting tips that the dentist uses for the surgery. The electrosurgery unit uses tiny electrical currents to incise the gingival tissue and also coagulate the blood during the procedure (Figure 29-15). The dental assistant must keep the oral evacuator near the surgical site to remove the debris and odors.

FIGURE 29-13 Periotomes. *(Courtesy of Hu-Friedy Mgf. Co., Inc.)*

(A)

Follow these easy steps.

1. Insert blade side up and align to guide.

(B)

2. Press downward.

3. Pull off handle.

(C)

(D)

FIGURE 29-14 (A) Surgical knife. Bard-Parker and blades. (B) Blade remover. (C) Disposable scalpels. (D) Various surgical blades. *(A to C, Courtesy of Miltex Instrument Co., Inc., Lake Success, NY.)*

FIGURE 29-15 Electrosurgical unit with various electrodes. *(Courtesy of Macon Engineering and Manufacturing Co.)*

(A)

(B)

FIGURE 29-16 (A) Pocket marking pliers. (B) Close-up of the working ends of the pocket marking pliers.

Pocket Marking Pliers

Pocket marking pliers are used to transfer the measurement of the pocket to the outside of the tissue so that the operator can see the depth level of the pocket. The pocket marking pliers have one straight, thin beak placed in the pocket, and another bent at a right angle at the tip. When the beaks are pinched together, the gingival tissue is perforated, leaving small, pinpoint markings (Figure 29-16).

Periosteal Elevators

A periosteal elevator is used to reflect soft tissue away from the bone. The elevators are usually double-ended, with a long, tapered end, and a round, bladed end (Figure 29-17).

FIGURE 29-17 Various periosteal elevators.

Periodontal Scissors, Rongeurs, and Forceps

Periodontal scissors are used during periodontal surgery, mainly to remove tags of tissue and to trim margins. There are other uses and many varieties, but most often the blades are long and very thin.

Soft tissue rongeurs or nippers are hinged pliers used to shape the soft tissue (Figure 29-18A).

Tissue forceps are used to retract tissue or to hold the tissue in place. They are designed similar to hemo-

(A)

(B)

FIGURE 29-18 (A) Soft tissue rongeurs. (B) Tissue forceps.

stats, except that the beaks are curved near the end at right angles to each other (Figure 29-18B).

Lasers

A dental laser is a medical device that generates a precise beam of concentrated light energy. The efficiency of the laser is based on the peak absorption rates of unique laser wavelengths by hard/soft tissues and other dental materials (e.g., composites or whitening solutions). There are many types of dental laser wavelengths to meet the needs of the dentist. Some standard dental laser wavelengths include the Erbium (Er: YAG), Nd: YAG, argon, diode laser. There is also a device that uses water, the YSGG hydrokinetic system, which has very similar uses and benefits (Figure 29-19).

The dentist must complete training to become qualified to use lasers. There are many courses available, and the companies that sell dental lasers offer comprehensive training and support packages. When the dental laser is used in the office, there is training for dental assistants and hygienists. The primary required safety measure is protective eyewear to be worn by the dentist, staff, and patient when the laser is being used. For more information, visit the Institute for Laser Dentistry (ILD) Web site at *www.laserdentistry.ca*.

Uses of the Dental Laser

Dental laser uses include procedures on hard and soft tissues. In periodontal practice, laser uses include the following:

- Sulcular debridement and laser curettage
- Gingivectomy, gingivoplasty, and frenectomy
- Fibroma and other tumor and lesion removal
- Excisional new attachment procedure (ENAP)
- Implant exposure
- Treatment for aphthous ulcers
- Tissue fusion, which eliminates the need for sutures
- Eliminates granulation tissue
- Biopsy
- Crown lengthening
- Control bleeding
- Osseous procedures

Other uses of the dental laser include tissue retraction for crown impressions, some cavity preparation and caries removal, diagnosis—transillumination for detection of caries microfracture, laser etching, composite curing, endodontic therapy, pulpotomy treatment, and in-office whitening (bleaching) (Figure 29-20).

Benefits of Lasers in Dentistry

Laser technology is rapidly advancing as applications expand and awareness of benefits increases. Following are some of the benefits of this technology:

- A near bloodless operating field so vision is improved
- Minimal or no anesthesia
- Minimizes postoperative swelling and discomfort
- Enhances coagulation (hemostasis)
- Minimizes healing time
- Reduces damage to surrounding healthy tissues
- Reduces chance of infection
- Accuracy of cutting
- Reduces chair time
- Less fear and anxiety for the patient

FIGURE 29-19 Dental laser.

FIGURE 29-20 Dental laser in use.

Nonsurgical Periodontal Procedures

Nonsurgical treatments for periodontal diseases include occlusal adjustment, scaling and polishing, root planning, and gingival curettage.

Principles of Periodontal Procedures

For periodontal treatment that is effective and efficient with minimal discomfort to the patient or stress to the operator, the following principles are followed:

- Comfortable position for the operator and the patient
- Effective pain control for the patient
- Use of a dental assistant to maintain the operating field for clear vision, good illumination, and retraction
- Maintain instruments properly (sharp and in order for use during the procedure)
- Correct instrument grasp, fulcrum, and instrument adaptation

Occlusal Adjustment

The occlusal adjustment or equilibration procedure involves adjustment of the occlusal surface to eliminate detrimental forces and to provide functional forces for stimulation of a healthy periodontium. The adjustment procedure is performed quadrant by quadrant and may require several appointments to fully equilibrate the patient's whole mouth (Procedure 29-1).

Scaling and Polishing

The purpose of **scaling** is to remove plaque, calculus, and stains from the surfaces of the teeth. The deposits above the gingival margin, supragingival deposits, and those just below the gingival margin are removed with scalers and curettes. After this, the coronal surfaces of the teeth are polished with rubber cups, brushes, an abrasive, porte polishers, and dental tape (Procedure 29-2). This procedure is called a **prophylaxis** and can be performed by the dentist or the dental hygienist. Depending on the state dental practice act, dental assistants can remove supragingival deposits and/or perform the **coronal polish** (discussed later in this chapter).

PROCEDURE 29-1

Occlusal Adjustment

The procedure is performed by the periodontist. It involves marking the patient's bite and adjusting the occlusal surfaces of the teeth. The dental assistant prepares the articulating paper or wax; maintains the operating field; and changes burs, discs, and stones in the handpiece.

EQUIPMENT (Figure 29-21)

- Basic setup: mouth mirror, explorer, cotton pliers
- Cotton rolls and 2 × 2 gauze sponges
- Saliva ejector, HVE tip, air-water syringe tip
- Articulation forceps and articulating paper and/or occlusal wax
- Low-speed handpiece
- Diamond burs, various discs, and stones
- Polishing wheels and discs

FIGURE 29-21 Occlusal equilibration armamentarium.

(continues)

PROCEDURE 29-1 *(CONTINUED)*

PROCEDURE STEPS *(Follow aseptic procedures)*

1. Seat and prepare the patient for the occlusal adjustment procedure.

2. Prepare the articulating forceps with paper, or prepare to transfer the wax. Dry the quadrant with the air syringe or a gauze sponge.

3. The periodontist places the articulating paper over the occlusal surfaces and instructs the patient to bite down and grind the teeth side to side.

4. The articulating paper is removed, and the colored marks left by the paper are evaluated. The markings indicate how teeth in the maxillary and mandibular arches occlude.

5. Change burs, discs, and stones as requested by the periodontist. Transfer the handpiece to the periodontist, and use the air-water syringe and the evacuator to keep the area clean and clear during the adjustment procedure.

6. This process is repeated until the teeth occlude evenly over the quadrant.

7. Each quadrant is evaluated and adjusted.

In a routine prophylaxis, deposits from above and just slightly below the gingival margins are removed. In a periodontal scaling, the subgingival deposits are more extensive and involve removal of irritants from deep pockets and smoothing of the root surface (Figure 29-22).

Root Planing

After the plaque and calculus are removed from the periodontal pocket and the root surface, the cementum is often rough and irregular. This provides a surface ideal for accumulation of plaque and calculus formation. The roughness is removed by **root planing**. This is a process of planing or shaving the root surface with curettes and other periodontal instruments to leave a smooth root surface. For the patient's comfort, anesthetic is sometimes given during this procedure.

Gingival Curettage

Gingival curettage, also known as soft tissue curettage, is a procedure that involves scraping the inner gingival walls of the periodontal pockets to remove inflamed tissue and debris. This is accomplished with curettes, and ideally performed after the scaling and root planing of the tooth. By removing diseased tissue and irritants, the edema is reduced and the gingival tissue may begin to heal itself (Figure 29-22).

Postoperative Treatment

- **Oral hygiene.** The patient is taught good brushing and flossing techniques. Periodontal aids such as interproximal brushes, soft wooden tips, and/or bridge threaders are selected to assist the patient in cleaning large interdental spaces or around fixed

(A)   (B)

FIGURE 29-22 Placement of instruments for scaling. (A) Supragingival scaling. (B) Subgingival scaling.

PROCEDURE 29-2

Scaling, Curettage, and Polishing

This procedure is done by the periodontist or the dental hygienist. A dental hygiene assistant assists during this procedure. Responsibilities include instrument transfer, rinsing the oral cavity, evacuation with the HVE, removing debris from instruments, retraction, and maintaining patient comfort.

EQUIPMENT (Figure 29-23)

- Basic setup: mouth mirror, explorer, and cotton pliers
- Saliva ejector, HVE tip, and air-water syringe tip
- Cotton rolls and gauze sponges
- Periodontal probe
- Scalers: Jacquette and Shepherd's hook
- Curettes: Universal and Gracey
- Dental floss and dental tape
- Prophy angle—rubber cups and brushes
- Prophy paste
- Optional—disclosing solution or tablets

PROCEDURE STEPS *(Follow aseptic procedures)*

1. The operator examines the oral cavity.

2. The operator uses scalers and curettes to remove calculus and debris from around the teeth. Often, the operator cleans all surfaces of the teeth in one quadrant before moving to the next quadrant.

FIGURE 29-23 Scale and polish (prophylaxis) tray setup.

3. After all the calculus has been removed, the operator polishes the teeth with prophy paste, rubber cup, and brush.

NOTE: Some practices use a prophy jet (spray saltwater) as an alternative to the rubber cup polish (discussed later in this chapter).

4. The operator uses dental tape and prophy paste to clean the interproximal areas. Then the entire mouth is flossed and rinsed.

---

appliances. Videos, pamphlets, and various other aids are used to motivate and educate the patient.

- **Antibacterial therapy.** Antimicrobial mouth rinses and antibiotic regimens are used in addition to routine treatments. Fluorides also are prescribed because they have bactericidal effects against the formation of plaque.

- **Diet and smoking.** Patients should be advised to avoid spicy foods, citrus fruits, and alcoholic beverages and to otherwise follow a normal diet. Smoking should be stopped, because the smoke irritates the tissues and delays the healing process.

Surgical Periodontal Procedures

The accepted rationale for periodontal surgery has been to arrest the disease process, reduce the periodontium to a level that is easier for the patient to keep clean, and perform effective scaling and root planing procedures.

Gingivectomy

A **gingivectomy** is the surgical removal of diseased gingival tissue that forms the periodontal pocket. The pocket must be eliminated to prevent the accumulation of debris and bacteria. This surgical procedure reduces the height of the gingival tissue, which provides visibility and access in order to remove irritants and smooth the root surface. This promotes the healing process and makes it easier for the patient to access the area during cleaning.

The gingivectomy procedure involves marking the pocket depths with pocket marking pliers and then excising the gingival tissue with periodontal knives, a scalpel, surgical scissors, or electrosurgery. After the tissue is excised, calculus and necrotic root tissue are removed and smoothed with scalers and curettes. The area is rinsed gently and covered with a gauze sponge until the hemorrhage is controlled. Once the blood clots have formed, a periodontal dressing is placed to promote healing, reduce the chance of infection, and prevent disturbance to the area (Procedure 29-3).

PROCEDURE 29-3

Gingivectomy

This procedure is performed by the periodontist in order to remove diseased gingiva and clean the periodontal pockets. The dental assistant prepares the instruments and materials, prepares the patient, and performs assisting responsibilities during the procedure. According to state dental practice act, the dental assistant may place and remove the periodontal dressing.

EQUIPMENT (Figure 29-24)

- Basic setup: mouth mirror, explorer, cotton pliers

- Periodontal probe

- Cotton rolls and gauze sponges

- Saliva ejector, HVE tip, air-water syringe tip, surgical aspirator tip

- Anesthetic setup

- Pocket marker

- Periodontal knives—broad bladed and interproximal

- Scalpel, blades, and diamond burs

- Scalers and curettes

- Soft tissue rongeurs and surgical scissors

- Hemostat

- Suture needle and thread

- Periodontal dressing materials

PROCEDURE STEPS (*Follow aseptic procedures*)

1. The anesthetic is administered to anesthetize the tissues and reduce blood flow to the area.

FIGURE 29-24 Gingivectomy tray setup.

2. The periodontist examines the patient's periodontal chart, and then the area is examined with a periodontal probe.

3. The depths of the pockets are marked with pocket markers (Figure 23-25A and B).

4. The broad-bladed knife or scalpel is used to incise the marked gingiva. Evacuate the area and transfer instruments (Figure 29-25C).

5. Interdental knives are used to remove interproximal tissue. Scissors, rongeurs, and burs are used to remove tissue tags. Have gauze ready to receive any tissue from instruments and to clean the area of debris.

(continues)

P R O C E D U R E 2 9 - 3 *(C O N T I N U E D)*

FIGURE 29-25 Gingivectomy procedure. (A,B) Marking pocket depth with pocket marker. (C) Incising marked tissue with periodontal knives.

6. After the tissue is removed, the periodontist scales and planes the root surfaces. Irritants are removed and the surfaces are smoothed to promote healing. Continue to pass instruments and evacuate the area. A sterile saline solution may be used to irrigate the area.

7. If sutures are needed, they are placed at this time. Prepare the suture needle and thread and have them positioned in a hemostat or needle holder, ready to pass to the dentist. Retract tissue as needed.

8. After the sutures are placed and the area is irrigated with the sterile saline solution, a periodontal dressing is prepared and placed. Assist the periodontist with the suture placement, evacuate the area, and prepare the periodontal dressing.

9. After the placement of the dressing is completed, the patient is given postoperative instructions and dismissed. Make sure the patient does not have any debris on his or her face, give postoperative instructions, and dismiss the patient.

Gingivoplasty

Gingivoplasty is reshaping the gingival tissue to remove deformities such as clefts, craters, and enlargements. A gingivoplasty does not involve the removal of periodontal pockets; it is completed to recontour the gingiva and often immediately follows a gingivectomy. A gingivoplasty is performed with periodontal knives, a scalpel, rongeurs, rotary diamonds, curettes, and surgical scissors. The gingival margin is tapered and thinned, creating a scalloped edge. Interdental grooves are contoured.

Postoperative Treatment Following Surgery

▪ **Oral hygiene**. Normal brushing and flossing should be completed in areas not involved in the surgery. Brush only the biting surfaces of the teeth involved in surgery. Gently rinse the mouth with warm salt-water after twenty-four hours.

▪ **Diet**. Avoid hot, spicy foods and citrus foods; eat soft foods; and chew on the healthy side of the mouth so that the periodontal dressing is not disturbed.

▪ **Pain**. The patient can expect mild to moderate discomfort, and medication should be prescribed.

▪ **Swelling and bleeding**. Some swelling may occur. Place an ice pack over the area for ten minutes and remove for ten minutes. Repeat as needed. Some seepage and bleeding may occur and is normal; however, if it persists, call the dentist.

Periodontal Flap Surgery

Periodontal flap surgery involves surgically separating the gingiva from the underlying tissue. The gingiva is incised with a scalpel and then separated with a periosteal elevator. Once the tissue is retracted, the periodontist has good visibility and access to bone, tooth, and the tooth roots (Figures 29-26 and 29-27).

The design of the flap depends on the objectives of the surgery and the periodontist. The amount of exposure necessary for the surgery and the repositioning of the flap are important considerations. The periodontist exposes an area large enough to remove the irritants completely with the periodontal instruments. The

FIGURE 29-26 Flap surgery to expose an impacted tooth. (A) Making incision. (B) Retracting tissue flap. *(Courtesy of Dr. Gary Shellerud.)*

FIGURE 29-27 Periodontal flap and osseous surgery. A flap is laid and alveolar bone exposed. *(Courtesy of Dr. Gary Shellerud.)*

appearance of the gingiva after the surgery depends on the proper repositioning of the flap. The tissue is positioned to heal in a manner that leaves as little evidence of the surgery as possible.

When the flap is retracted, the diseased tissue and debris are removed, the roots are planed, and the alveolar bone is trimmed and contoured. The area is rinsed with a saline solution and the flap is repositioned and sutured. A **periodontal dressing** may be applied to protect the surgical site.

Osseous Surgery

Osseous surgery removes defects/deformities in the bone caused by periodontal disease and other, related conditions (Procedure 29-4). Two types of bone surgeries that correct the deformities are **osteoplasty**, reshaping the bone, and **ostectomy**, removal of bone.

Osseous surgery can be either additive or subtractive. During additive osseous surgery (sometimes called augmentive surgery), bone or bone substitute is added to fill in areas. This is a **bone grafting** (moving tissue from one area to another) procedure.

Bone Grafting. Bone grafting offers some hope to restore lost bone and regeneration of a functional attachment of the periodontium. After careful patient evaluation, this procedure may be selected to improve the patient's condition. There are several types of bone replacement grafts: autogenous, allogeneic, xenogeneic, and alloplastic (see Table 29-3). Autogenous grafts have the best results, but because often only a limited amount of host bone is conveniently available in the oral cavity, other grafts may be indicated. Research reports all bone replacement grafts fill the original intrabony defects about 60 to 70 percent.

During subtractive osseous surgery, the bone is removed with chisels, rongeurs, files, diamond burs, and stones.

After the bone has been grafted or removed and contoured, the flap is repositioned and sutures are placed. The area is rinsed gently and blotted dry before a periodontal dressing is placed (Figure 29-27).

PROCEDURE 29-4

Osseous Surgery

This procedure is performed by the periodontist. It involves removing and recontouring diseased and defective bone tissue. The extent of the periodontal disease process determines the amount and type of surgery performed.

EQUIPMENT (Figure 29-28)

- Basic setup: mouth mirror, explorer, cotton pliers
- Periodontal probe
- Cotton rolls and gauze sponges
- Saliva ejector, HVE tip, air-water syringe tip, surgical aspirator tip
- Anesthetic setup
- Scalpel and blades
- Periodontal knives—broad bladed and interproximal
- Tissue retractor
- Periosteal elevator
- Diamond burs and stones
- Rongeurs, chisels, and files
- Scalers and curettes
- Hemostat and surgical scissors
- Suture setup
- Periodontal dressing materials

PROCEDURE STEPS *(Follow aseptic procedures)*

In osseous surgery, a flap of soft tissue is incised and reflected to expose the bone for reshaping and/or removal. This procedure is performed by the periodontist.

1. After the anesthetic is administered, the soft tissue is incised and loosened from the underlying bone. Transfer instruments and maintain good visibility for the operator.

2. The tissue flap is reflected and stabilized with tissue retractors. Retract and hold the tissue.

3. Once the bone is exposed, the diseased bone tissue is excised. Scalers and curettes are used to remove calculus and diseased tissue and the roots are planed. Transfer instruments, rinse the area with a sterile saline solution as needed, evacuate, and keep the instruments clean by removing debris from instruments with the gauze sponge.

4. The bone is shaped and contoured using diamond burs and stones, rongeurs, chisels, and files.

5. The tissue flap is replaced and positioned over the alveolar bone and then sutured in place. Prepare the suture and stabilize the tissue with tissue forceps during the suturing procedure.

6. Prepare the periodontal dressing materials and assist the operator in the placement. In some states, the dental assistant is allowed to place and remove the periodontal dressing.

7. Remove any debris from the patient's face, give postoperative instructions, and dismiss the patient

FIGURE 29-28 Osseous surgery tray setup.

TABLE 29-3 Descriptions of Bone Replacement Grafts

Autogenous (autografts)	Cortical and cancellous bone extracted from intraoral and extraoral sites. Examples are bone removed during an osteoplasty or an ostectomy, bone harvested from a healing socket after an extraction, donor bone from maxillary tuberosities, edentulous ridges, or retromolar areas.
Allogeneic (allografts)	An allograft is tissue transplanted between people of the same species. Bone tissue is carefully selected from donor cadavers; tested to ensure it is free of any transmissible pathologic condition; freeze dried; ground to average bone particle size; and placed in sterile, vacuum-sealed bottles with an indefinite shelf life.
Xenogeneic (xenografts)	Xenografts are tissues from different species. Cows and pigs are used most often for humans.
Allogeneic (alloplastic grafts)	Alloplastic grafts are various synthetic materials, including hydroxyapatite, calcium carbonate, polymers, bioactive glasses, and tricalcium phosphate.

Mucogingival Surgery

Mucogingival surgery is reconstructive surgery on the gingiva and/or mucosa tissues. The surgeries may involve covering exposed roots, increasing the width of the gingival tissue, and reducing frenum or muscle attachments. Periodontal disease can cause negative changes in the gingiva, and mucogingival surgery improves these areas. Two common examples of mucogingival surgery are gingival grafting and the frenectomy.

Gingival Grafting

During a **gingival grafting** procedure, tissue is taken from one site and placed on another. The procedure involves preparation of the site of the graft by eliminating any periodontal pockets and exposing a bed of connective tissue. Then, a graft (section of tissue) is obtained from the donor site, often the palate area. This graft is positioned carefully and sutured securely in place. The donor site is covered with a periodontal dressing or another protective material until it is healed, which usually takes one to two weeks (Figure 29-29).

Frenectomy

The **frenectomy** is a complete removal of the frenum, including the attachment to the underlying bone. The frenum may be removed if it is attached too close to the marginal gingiva. The procedure involves incising the frenum and removing a triangular section. The periodontal fibers are separated and cut to the bone. The labial mucosa is then sutured to the apical periosteum. The periodontal dressing is prepared and placed over the suture site.

FIGURE 29-29 Gingival graft. (A) Gingival recession shows need for graft. (B) Palatal tissue graft is positioned and sutured in place. (C) Graft after healing period. *(Courtesy of Dr. Gary Shellerud.)*

Guided Tissue Regeneration

Guided tissue regeneration, or selective cell reproduction, uses barrier membranes to maintain a space between the gingival flap and the root surface of the tooth in order for tissues to regenerate in a periodontal defect. Cells capable of forming new cementum, periodontal ligament, and supporting alveolar bone must move into the surgical site to produce these tissues, but they must not be interfered with. Therefore, apical epithelial migration must be delayed and gingival connective tissue from the flap must be kept away from the surgical area for regeneration to take place.

The membranes used as a barrier are classified as nonabsorbable or absorbable. Both have proven to be successful techniques. The technique involving nonabsorbable membranes has been on the market longer and requires a second appointment in about three to four weeks to remove the barrier. Selecting the type of membrane to be used is determined by the dentist's preference and the type of periodontal defect.

Periodontal Dressing

Periodontal dressings or packs are placed after periodontal surgical procedures. The dressings do not have any medicinal qualities; they are bandages used to protect the tissue during the healing process.

The following are objectives of the periodontal dressing:

- Minimizing postoperative infection and hemorrhage
- Protecting the tissues during mastication
- Covering the surgical site in order to reduce pain due to trauma or irritation
- Providing support for teeth that are mobile
- Helping to hold flaps in position

Types of Periodontal Dressings

The most common types of materials used as periodontal dressings are zinc oxide–eugenol materials, noneugenol materials, the light-cured dressings, and gelatin-based materials.

Zinc Oxide–Eugenol Materials. Zinc oxide–eugenol materials are supplied in a powder (zinc oxide) or liquid (eugenol) form that can be mixed before the procedure and stored for later use. In some offices the material is mixed, wrapped in wax paper, and then frozen until needed.

The presence of eugenol in this dressing can cause an allergic reaction. The area becomes red and a burning sensation is experienced by the patient.

Noneugenol Materials. The noneugenol materials come in a two-paste system: one tube of base material and one tube of accelerator. The two pastes are dispensed in equal portions on a paper pad and mixed together prior to placement (Procedures 29-5 and 29-6).

The noneugenol dressings do not cause sensitivity problems, and some noneugenol dressing materials have bacteriostatic agents added.

Light-Cured Periodontal Dressing. Light-cured periodontal dressing material comes in syringes. It can be placed directly on the surgical site or placed on a mixing pad. If it is placed directly on the tissues it can be

---

PROCEDURE 29-5

Preparation and Placement of Noneugenol Periodontal Dressing

The periodontist routinely places the dressing, but in some states the dental assistant is allowed to place and remove the periodontal dressing. The dressing is placed after the surgery to protect the tissues and promote the healing process.

EQUIPMENT

- Basic setup: mouth mirror, explorer, and cotton pliers
- Gauze sponges
- Noneugenol periodontal dressing material (base and accelerator)
- Paper pad and tongue depressor
- Lubricant
- Instrument to contour dressing (spoon excavator, sickle scaler)

(continues)

PROCEDURE 29-5 *(CONTINUED)*

PROCEDURE STEPS *(Follow aseptic procedures)*

1. After the hemorrhaging is controlled, the patient's lips are coated lightly with Vaseline.

2. The dressing materials are dispensed into equal lengths and mixed with a tongue blade until homogeneous. (Using a paper pad and tongue blade make cleanup easier.) The material is allowed to set for two to three minutes until the tackiness is gone (Figure 29-30A).

3. Lubricate gloved fingers with Vaseline so the putty-like material can be handled easily.

4. The dressing comes with a retardant to slow the setting time, if necessary; it can be molded easily for three to five minutes and worked for fifteen to twenty minutes.

5. The dressing is molded into a thin strip slightly longer than the length of the surgical site. Divide the strip into two equal lengths, one for the facial surface and one for the lingual surface (Figure 29-30B).

6. To begin the placement, form the end of one strip into a hook shape. Wrap this hook around the distal of the most posterior tooth (Figure 29-30C).

(A)

(B)

(C)

(D)

FIGURE 29-30 Preparation and placement of periodontal dressing. (A) Mixing the materials. (B) Preparing the materials for placement. (C) Placing dressing on tissue. (D) Contouring dressing.

(continues)

PROCEDURE 29-5 *(CONTINUED)*

7. Adapt the rest of the strip along the facial surface, gently pressing the pack into the interproximal areas (Figure 29-30D).

8. The second strip is applied to the lingual surface in the same manner. The pack is wrapped around the last posterior tooth and then adapted to the lingual surface, moving toward the midline.

9. The pack should cover the gingiva evenly without interfering with occlusion, tongue movements, or frenum attachments.

10. Check the dressing for overextensions. These areas are removed with a spoon excavator or scaler. Gently press the instrument into the dressing to detach the extra material. Smooth the pack and evaluate it for even thickness.

11. Ask the patient how the pack feels. Instruct the patient to move his or her tongue, cheeks, and lips to mold the pack. Make any adjustments to ensure that the dressing is securely in place, trimmed, and contoured.

12. Give the patient instructions about the periodontal dressing, including:

   - The pack is kept on for one week after surgery.

   - The pack will harden in a few hours and then withstand normal chewing stresses.

   - The pack may chip and break off during the week but should remain intact as long as possible. If there is pain when pieces of the pack come off or the pack becomes rough, the patient should call the office.

   - The patient should brush the occlusal surface of the teeth involved in the surgery and continue to brush and floss the rest of the teeth as normal.

PROCEDURE 29-6

Removal of Periodontal Dressing

This procedure is performed by the periodontist or the dental assistant depending on the expanded functions. The patient has worn the dressing for a week to ten days. The patient's mouth is examined before removing the dressing to check for areas where the dressing may have loosened or come off completely.

EQUIPMENT

- Basic setup: mouth mirror, explorer, and cotton pliers

- Saliva ejector, HVE tip, air-water syringe tip

- Gauze sponges and tissue

- Instruments to remove the dressing (spoon excavator, sickle explorer, surgical hoe)

PROCEDURE STEPS *(Follow aseptic procedures)*

1. After seating the patient, the surgical site is evaluated and the dressing is removed.

2. A surgical hoe or a spoon excavator is inserted along the margin. Lateral pressure is applied to pry the dressing away from the tissue (Figure 29-31).

3. The pack may come off in large pieces and then scalers and floss can be used to remove any particles

FIGURE 29-31 Removing periodontal dressing.

from the interproximal areas and tooth surfaces. Cotton pliers are used to remove particles of dressing embedded in the surgical site.

4. Gently rinse the entire area with warm water to remove any debris. The air-water syringe can be used carefully.

contoured into desired position, then light cured. The material may also be dispensed onto a paper pad, manipulated to the required shape and size, placed over the tissues, and then light cured.

Gelatin-Base Dressings. Gelatin-base dressings offer good stability and dissolve in 24 to 48 hours. They are excellent for use after soft-tissue augmentation.

Periodontal Maintenance Procedures

Periodontal surgery does not end the need for periodontal treatment. The patient determines the success of the treatment by being committed and following the designed therapy. Periodontal disease is an ongoing process, but continual care maintains the status of peri-

odontal health after surgery. Dedicated home oral-hygiene routines and periodic visits to the dentist are necessary for successful periodontal care.

Once the patient has accepted the treatment plan, plaque-control techniques are taught by the dental assistant and/or the hygienist. As the patient continues through treatment, the patient's hygiene skills and personalized intraoral aids are evaluated and adjusted according to the patient's individual needs. After surgery, the patient is instructed to keep the area as clean as possible to enhance the healing process. After the periodontal dressing is removed, interdental cleaners, floss, and water irrigators may be used to remove plaque and debris. When the tissues have healed sufficiently, the patient can begin the oral hygiene regimen prescribed.

ADVANCED CHAIRSIDE FUNCTIONS

Coronal Polish

The oral prophylaxis procedure is actually twofold. First, the hard deposits (scaling) are removed by the dentist or dental hygienist. Second, the teeth are polished with a rubber cup. In some states, a registered or an expanded-function dental assistant can perform this part of the prophylaxis, in addition to the dentist and the hygienist.

The coronal polish procedure involves removing soft deposits and extrinsic stains (stains removed by polishing) from the surfaces of the teeth and restorations. This is accomplished with an abrasive, dental hand-

piece, rubber cup (sometimes this procedure is called a "rubber cup" polish), brush, dental tape, and floss. The coronal polish is the polishing of the clinical crown, which may involve both enamel and exposed dentin that is visible in the mouth (Figure 29-32). Often, exposed dentin is not polished because of the possibility of increased sensitivity. Composite restorations, acrylic veneers, and porcelain-filled surfaces are also not polished or carefully polished because of the possibility of removing the finish and decreasing surface hardness. Different abrasives are used on each surface.

FIGURE 29-32 Varying length of clinical crown of tooth.

ADVANCED CHAIRSIDE FUNCTIONS

Rationale for Performing Coronal Polish

After the teeth have been scaled to remove the hard deposits, the polish is done to provide a smooth, polished surface. Additional benefits and indications include:

- A polish makes it easier for the patient to keep the teeth clean.
- The tooth surface absorbs fluoride better.
- The process of accumulation of new deposits is slowed.
- A clean tooth surface motivates the patient to maintain good oral hygiene habits.
- The teeth are prepared for placement of enamel sealant.
- The teeth are prepared for orthodontic bracket and band placement.

Contraindications and Modifications

Conditions that contraindicate a coronal polish involve the gingival tissues. The abrasive agents used in the coronal polish may cause problems, and the polish technique could traumatize the already irritated tissues. Whether the cause of the gingival irritation is systemic or local, whenever the gingival tissues are irritated, inflamed, sensitive, or hemorrhage easily, it is best to evaluate the necessity of the coronal polish. For some patients, the polish should be postponed until the condition of the tissue improves. For other patients, the polish removes the source of irritation. The dentist makes the decision on an individual patient basis.

The following conditions may require modification of coronal polish techniques:

- **Orthodontic appliances**—Use of a small rubber cup and a pointed or tapered brush, especially around the brackets.
- **Hypersensitive teeth**—Use a very wet abrasive agent with a light, intermittent stroke. Use a cotton roll or cotton swab to dry the area.
- **Green chromogenic bacterial stain**—Before beginning the coronal polish, use a solution of equal parts of 3-percent hydrogen peroxide and water. Apply to the stained areas with a cotton-tip applicator for a few seconds, and then rinse.
- **Minor oral irritations, such as cold sores**—Avoid the areas when polishing and retracting the tissues or establishing a fulcrum (position of stabilization). Apply a protective coating of lubricant.

 In states where the dental assistant can perform a coronal polish, legal and ethical issues must be considered. The following are guidelines when performing a coronal polish:

- Consistently meet the high standards of the profession in performing a coronal polish.
- Follow aseptic techniques and OSHA guidelines.
- Request assistance when needed to best serve the patient.
- Refer all diagnosing to the dentist.

Dental Deposits

Dental deposits is a collective term referring to various deposits and/or stains, intrinsic and extrinsic, that accumulate on the teeth and on appliances in the mouth. The dental assistant must be able to recognize these deposits and know how to remove them. Dental deposits are often classified as soft deposits, hard deposits, and stains (Table 29-4).

Soft Deposits

Soft deposits include the acquired dental pellicle, materia alba, food debris, and plaque. The dental assistant can remove these soft deposits while performing a coronal polish (Table 29-4) (Figure 29-33).

Calculus

Dental calculus is a hard, calcified deposit that forms on the teeth, restorations, and dental appliances. Another name for calculus is "tartar," which many people use. Calculus is mineralized plaque with few, if any, living organisms in its structure. It is often covered with a layer of plaque and is attached firmly to the tooth. The dental assistant should recognize both supragingival (above the gingiva) and subgingival (below the gingiva) calculus, even though the dental assistant is not legally allowed to remove it. Calculus may be present in a patient scheduled for a coronal polish (Table 29-5) (Figures 29-2 and 29-34).

Stains

Stains are discolorations of the teeth and are caused by foods, bacteria, tobacco, metals, drugs, imperfect tooth

ADVANCED CHAIRSIDE FUNCTIONS

TABLE 29-4 Soft Deposits

	Pellicle	Materia Alba	Food Debris	Plaque
Appearance	Thin, clear film, sometimes stained	Soft, bulky mass, cottage cheese-like, white to yellow	Small particles of food	Soft, dense, furry-like deposit
Composition	Acellular. Insoluble proteins, fats, and other materials	Unstructured, living and dead microorganism. Food debris, desquamated epithelial cells, disintegrating leukocytes, and proteins	Food particles	Organized mass of many types of microorganisms in a sticky matrix. Approximately 80 percent water and 20 percent organic and inorganic solids, with most of the solids being microorganisms
Source	Saliva and sulcular fluids	Accumulation of materials and bacterial growth	Diet	Microorganisms
Formation	Forms within minutes of removal	Time varies	Forms while eating	Forms within 12–24 hours of removal
Attachment	Tooth surface, restorations, and appliances	Loosely attached, collects in grooves and spaces on and between teeth, gingiva, and appliances	Loosely attached, collects in spaces and grooves in and around teeth and appliances	Gingival areas in difficult areas to clean and lingual and occlusal grooves
Classification	Unstained and stained surface	None	None	Location on tooth with pathogenic effect
Significance	May protect enamel or may provide attachment and breeding ground for plaque and calculus	Provides source for plaque development	Provides nutrients	Dental caries, gingivitis, and periodontal disease
Methods of removal	Polishing with an abrasive	Rinsing, toothbrushing, and flossing	Rinsing, toothbrushing, and flossing	Toothbrushing, flossing, and coronal polish

— Plaque

FIGURE 29-33 Soft deposits on teeth.

development, and excess fluoride among other things. Stains adhere to the tooth structure, plaque, and calculus or may be part of the internal structure of the tooth. They are classified according to location, either **intrinsic** or **extrinsic**, and by their origin, either **exogenous** or **endogenous**. Intrinsic stains are inside the tooth structure and are mostly permanent (in some cases, bleaching is successful). The origin of intrinsic stains can be both endogenous (originating from inside the tooth) and exogenous (originating from outside the tooth). Extrinsic stains are on the outside of the tooth structure and can be removed by scaling and polishing. Extrinsic stains are exogenous only.

Dental stains are significant because of their unattractive appearance. They also may provide rough surfaces for deposits to adhere to. Stains may indicate past or present physical habits or conditions, which aids the dental assistant in determining oral hygiene information and instructions to be given to the patient.

Intrinsic Stains. Categories of these stains are described below.

ADVANCED CHAIRSIDE FUNCTIONS

TABLE 29-5 Calculus

	Supragingival Calculus	Subgingival Calculus
Appearance	Chalky white, yellow, gray, or stained by food	Black, brown, or dark green
Formation	Surfaces above the gingival margin. Most common on lingual of mandibular incisors and buccal of maxillary molars	Surfaces below the gingival margin
Removal	Mechanical methods	Mechanical methods
Age of patient	Uncommon in children under age nine	Very rare in children under age nine

Calculus

FIGURE 29-34 Calculus on teeth.

(A)

(B)

FIGURE 29-35 (A) Severe dental fluorosis. (B) Mild dental fluorosis.

Dental Fluorosis. Dental fluorosis occurs as a result of high concentrations of fluoride received systemically during tooth development. The color of the stain varies from white to yellow-brown or gray-brown. The outer surface may be pitted and rough depending on severity. The stain is distributed relative to the stage of development of the teeth. Other names include brown stain and mottled enamel (Figure 29-35).

Pulp Damaged or Nonvital Tooth Stain. This type of intrinsic stain occurs when the pulp is damaged or removed. This stain can vary in color from light yellow to black to green to magenta and is caused by blood and pulp tissues seeping into the dentin tubules.

Tetracycline Stain. Tetracycline stain is the result of high concentrations of tetracycline antibiotics taken during the time the tooth was developing. The stain varies in color from light green or yellow to dark gray-brown.

Metallic Stain. Metallic stains can be intrinsic and/or extrinsic. Metals and metallic salts may be inhaled in industrial settings or taken orally in certain drugs, or comprise part of the materials used to restore teeth. The metals adhere to the pellicle and other soft deposits, or they penetrate the tooth surface to become part of the tooth structure. Several metals that can cause

permanent stains are copper dust, which causes green to greenish blue stain; amalgam; deposits that cause a gray to black or bluish black stain; iron dust that causes a brown stain; and iron drugs, which cause a black stain.

ADVANCED CHAIRSIDE FUNCTIONS

Extrinsic Stains. Extrinsic stains also have several classifications.

Yellow and Brown Stains. Yellow stains and brown stains are usually associated with poor oral hygiene and are dull yellow to a light brownish color. They are generally associated with plaque and most commonly found on the buccal surface of the maxillary molars and lingual surface of the mandibular incisors.

Tobacco Stain. Tobacco stains are the result of coal tar combustion in cigarettes and pigments from chewing tobacco penetrating the pits and fissures on the enamel and dentin surfaces. The stain is light brown to black in color, and the amount of stain depends on the individual's oral hygiene habits and how often the person smokes.

Green Stain. Green stain varies in color from light to dark green or a yellowish green and is found most frequently in children. It is found on the facial surface of the maxillary anterior teeth at the cervical third and contains chromogenic bacteria and fungi.

Black Line Stain. Black line stain forms a thin black to dark-brown line slightly above the gingiva and follows the contour of the gingival margin. It is found primarily in women and often where there is excellent oral hygiene. The black line stain forms on the facial and lingual surfaces of the teeth and tends to reform after removal.

Orange Stain. This extrinsic stain is believed to be caused by chromogenic bacteria often related to drug therapy, such as antibiotics. It is uncommon, but if it does occur, it can be found on the lingual and facial surfaces of the anterior teeth near the gingival margin.

Chlorhexidine Stain. This stain occurs with prolonged use of chlorhexidine, which is found in chewing gum and mouth rinse. It is yellowish to green to brown in color and appears on restorations, the tongue, in plaque, and in the cervical and interproximal surfaces of the teeth. This is not a permanent stain and can be removed with toothbrushing and/or a coronal polish.

Abrasives and Polishing Agents

Abrasives are materials that cut or grind the surface, leaving grooves and a rough surface, while polishing produces a smooth, glossy surface with fine abrasive materials. It is important to understand abrasives and their characteristics and their actions to select the best materials for the patient without damaging the tooth. Abrasives remove small amounts of enamel during the polishing procedure; therefore, it is best to follow the coronal polish procedure with a fluoride treatment and/ or to use a fluoride prophy agent.

Abrasives

Abrasives are materials composed of particles that come in powders or pastes. They are selected according to the amount of stain and soft deposits that are to be removed. Abrasives should always be as moist as possible yet easy to use without dripping or spattering. These particles have characteristics that affect their abrasiveness (Table 29-6).

TABLE 29-6 Characteristics of Abrasives

Characteristic	Effect on Abrasive
Particle shape	Sharp-edged particles are more abrasive than dull, rounded particles.
Particle hardness	Harder particles abrade faster. Particles must be harder than the surfaces they are used on.
Particle strength	Resistance of particles to break up during the polish; therefore, less material is used.
Particle size	The larger the particle, the more abrasive it is.
Grit or grade of abrasive particles	Materials are sifted through standardized sieves to grade fineness. Fine abrasives are called powders or flours and are graded F, FF, and FFF for increasing fineness.
Particle attrition resistance	Particles that do not dull or become embedded in the surface being polished are the most effective.

ADVANCED CHAIRSIDE FUNCTIONS

Rate of Abrasion. The rate of abrasion is the time it takes to remove stains and deposits from a surface. This depends on several factors:

- By *increasing the speed of the handpiece*, the rate of abrasion is increased accordingly. This also increases the heat production.

- The *pressure* can control the rate of abrasion. The firmer the pressure, the more abrasive. Also, frictional heat increases.

- The *amount of abrasive* material used affects the rate of abrasion. The more material that is used, the faster the abrasive works.

- The *type of abrasive* used determines the rate of abrasion. The larger and harder the particles, the faster the abrasion. Also, the rate of heat production increases.

- The *dryer the abrasive* materials, the more abrasive they are.

Select an abrasive material that is coarse enough to cut through the deposits and stains and polish until the surfaces are as smooth as possible. Then, select a finer material, if needed, to polish the surface until it is smooth and free of deposits and stains. Usually, one abrasive is enough to complete the task, but if the patient has a lot of stain, a more coarse abrasive should be used. In the case of gingival recession, a finer abrasive is used on these areas after finishing all other areas with a coarser abrasive. When using two types of abrasives, completely finish with one abrasive, and then rinse the patient's mouth thoroughly before beginning with another abrasive. Also, use separate dappen dishes, rubber cups, and brushes for each abrasive.

Types of Abrasives

The abrasives come in powders and pastes and in bulk form or individually packaged. Besides the abrasive, most commercial preparations contain water, a binder, humectant (retains moisture), color, and a flavoring.

- **Zirconium silicate**—Used for stain removal and polishing. This material may be used on gold restorations, exposed dentin, and tooth-colored restorations, as well as enamel.

- **Tin oxide**—A very fine polishing agent used on enamel and metallic restorations. Used in a paste form, it is mixed with water, alcohol, or glycerin.

- **Flour of pumice**—Used to remove stains from the enamel. It is relatively coarse and should be followed by a fine polishing agent. It is not used on exposed

FIGURE 29-36 Various types of abrasives.

dentin, tooth-colored restorations, or gold restorations because of its high abrasiveness.

- **Chalk** (also known as whiting)—A mild abrasive, it is used in some prophylactic pastes.

- **Fluoride prophylaxis pastes**—Available and very popular. Fluoride is added to commercially prepared prophylaxis pastes to replace the fluoride lost in the enamel surface during the polishing procedure due to abrasion. Fluoride prophylaxis pastes should not be used if the teeth are to receive enamel sealants after the coronal polish (Figure 29-36).

Equipment and Supplies

The tray setup for the coronal polish includes patient safety glasses, hand mirror, mouth mirror, explorer, cotton pliers, cotton swabs (Q-Tips), 2 × 2 gauze, cotton rolls, saliva ejector, evacuator, air-water syringe tip, low-speed handpiece, rubber cups, brushes, prophy paste, tongue depressor, dental floss, dental tape, disclosing solution, and dappen dish for disclosing solution (Figure 29-37). Barriers are placed on the dental unit, and the dental assistant follows OSHA guidelines and wears PPE.

Use of Dental Handpiece for Coronal Polish

For the coronal polish procedure, a low-speed dental handpiece is used with a prophy angle attachment (right angle). The handpiece is held in a modified pen grasp. The fingers should close up on the prophy angle attachment, and the body of the handpiece should rest in the "v" of the hand. This gives the operator control and prevents fatigue (Figure 29-38).

ADVANCED CHAIRSIDE FUNCTIONS

When the modified pen grasp is used, the ring finger is the fulcrum finger. The little finger is also used to supplement the ring finger as a fulcrum. During the procedure, tooth structure provides the most stable fulcrum. However, the soft tissue is used as a fulcrum. Cover the tissue with a 2 × 2 gauze first to prevent slipping. Using a fulcrum provides stability and control of the handpiece and patient comfort, and helps reduce fatigue of the dental assistant.

Points for Using Dental Handpiece

- Use a slow, even speed.
- Use light to moderate pressure.
- Always use a fulcrum.
- Start and stop handpiece inside patient's mouth.

FIGURE 29-37 Tray setup for coronal polish procedure.

Use of Rubber Prophy Cup

The rubber prophy cup is used with an abrasive agent to polish the teeth and dental appliances (Procedure 29-7). Rubber prophy cups are available in several designs to fit the prophy angles. On the back of the prophy cup there may be a small metal screw attachment that is screwed into the corresponding prophy angle or a small hole that slips over a knob on the prophy angle. Disposable prophy angles with attached prophy cups and brushes are also available (Figure 29-39).

Rubber prophy cups are made of either natural or synthetic rubber. Natural rubber cups are resilient and will not stain the teeth. Synthetic rubber cups are stiffer

FIGURE 29-38 Modified pen grasp and dental handpiece.

When the correct grasp is used, the procedure is performed efficiently and effectively. The speed of the handpiece is controlled by steady foot pressure on the rheostat. Keeping the speed even takes practice. An even, slow speed is desired, with just enough pressure to keep the cups and brushes rotating. Apply the handpiece to the tooth with light to moderate pressure. The handpiece should be started when it is in the mouth, near the tooth to be polished. This establishes the speed of the handpiece before placing the cup/brush on the tooth. When the handpiece is removed from the tooth for more than a moment, release the pressure on the rheostat so that the handpiece stops before being removed from the mouth. This prevents debris from splattering.

FIGURE 29-39 (A) Contra-angle with latch prophy cup. (B) Disposable prophy angle cup. (C) Right angle with snap-on prophy cup. (D) Right angle (prophy angle) for screw cup or brush. (E) Snap-on prophy brush. (F) Screw-on prophy cup. (G) Rubber point. (H) Screw-on prophy brush. (I) Latch brush. (J) Assortment of cups, brushes, and points.

ADVANCED CHAIRSIDE FUNCTIONS

PROCEDURE 29-7

Polishing with the Rubber Cup

This procedure is performed by the dental assistant, hygienist, or dentist. The following procedure for polishing with the rubber cup explains positioning techniques and action of the rubber cup. Examine rubber cup placement on both arches and each quadrant on the facial and lingual surfaces.

EQUIPMENT AND SUPPLIES

- Basic setup: mouth mirror, explorer/periodontal probe, cotton pliers
- Saliva ejector, HVE tip, air-water syringe tip
- 2 × 2 gauze sponges, cotton-tip applicator
- Dappen dish
- Lip lubricant
- Disclosing solution (optional)
- Low-speed handpiece
- Prophy angle attachment
- Assortment of rubber cups and brushes
- Prophy paste in different grits
- Finger rings to hold prophy paste cup
- Dental tape and dental floss (see Figure 29-37)

PROCEDURE STEPS *(Follow aseptic procedures)*

1. The patient is seated and prepared for the coronal polish procedure. Lip lubricant is sometimes offered for the patient's comfort. The dental assistant reviews the patient's medical history and inspects the oral cavity. The amount of extrinsic stain determines the grit of the abrasive to be used.

2. The dental assistant may dry the teeth and place disclosing solution on the teeth for easier detection of plaque.

3. After the teeth are dry, a cotton-tip applicator is used to place the solution on all surfaces of the teeth. This is accomplished one quadrant, one arch, or one side at a time.

4. After placing abrasive polishing agent in the cup, place the handpiece in the patient's mouth and start it. Then place the cup near the gingival sulcus and as far into the mesial or distal surface as possible. Establish a fulcrum as close to the tooth being polished as possible.

5. Apply light pressure to flex the cup and flare it into the sulcus 1 to 2 mm.

6. Sweep the rubber cup toward the incisal or occlusal edge. If the crown of the tooth is long, lift the cup halfway up the tooth and make a second stroke toward the occlusal.

7. At the incisal or occlusal edge, lift the cup slightly off the tooth and re-position it near the gingiva to repeat the stroke, moving toward the opposite side of the tooth.

8. Repeat the stroke, overlapping each time, until the entire tooth surface is polished.

9. When finished with one tooth, move to the adjacent tooth using the same steps until the surfaces of all teeth have been polished.

10. For the patient's comfort, rinse the mouth frequently, at least after polishing each quadrant.

11. When all teeth have been polished, rinse and evacuate the patient's mouth thoroughly, removing all debris (Figure 28-40A through F).

(continues)

ADVANCED CHAIRSIDE FUNCTIONS

P R O C E D U R E   2 9 - 7   *(C O N T I N U E D)*

FIGURE 29-40 Correct cup placement and fulcrum. A. Maxillary right posterior. Buccal surface and lingual surface. A1. Cheek is retracted to position cup on tooth. Fulcrum on same arch. A2. Use indirect vision and fulcrum on same arch. B. Maxillary anteriors. Facial surface and lingual surface. B1. Retract lip and fulcrum on incisal edge. B2. Use indirect vision. C. Maxillary left posterior. Buccal surface and lingual surface. C1. Retract cheek to position prophy angle and have patient close slightly. Fulcrum on same arch.

(continues)

(continues)

ADVANCED CHAIRSIDE FUNCTIONS

(C2)

(D1)

(D2)

(E1)

(E2)

FIGURE 29-40 *(continued)* C2. Adapt cup to lingual surface. D. Mandibular right posterior. Buccal surface and lingual surface. D1. Retract tissue to place prophy angle and have patient close slightly. D2. Retract tongue with mouth mirror. E. Mandibular anteriors. Facial surface and lingual surface. E1. Retract lip with a finger. E2. Use mouth mirror for indirect vision and retraction.

(continues)

(continues)

ADVANCED CHAIRSIDE FUNCTIONS

(F1)

(F2)

FIGURE 29-40 *(continued)* F. Mandibular left posterior. Buccal surface and lingual surface. F1. Retract cheek and position prophy cup. F2. Retract tongue with mouth mirror to position prophy cup.

than the natural rubber, and the black cups may stain the teeth during the polish.

The rubber cup should be soft and flexible to adapt to the contours of the teeth. Edges should not be rough or frayed, which could irritate the tissues. The number of cups needed for the polishing depends on the number of abrasives used. One cup is used for each polishing agent. The edge of the cup is the part that actually does the polishing. The center of the cup holds and transports the abrasive agent. The cup is flexed to adapt to the tooth surface by applying slight pressure to one edge (Figure 29-41). The cup is most efficient on the facial and lingual surfaces of the teeth and fixed appliances, along the gingival margin, and 1 to 2 mm into the sulcus.

The hand and wrist are used to move the handpiece to adapt the cup to the tooth surface. When working on the lingual or facial surfaces, move the edge of the rubber cup as far as possible into the proximal and manipulate the cup into the sulcus, *not* on the gingival margin. The next step in learning to use the prophy cup is to learn the stroke. A short, intermittent, overlapping stroke is used with a slow-revolving rubber cup. This stroke covers the tooth, leaves no unpolished surfaces, and minimizes the frictional heat produced (Figure 29-42).

Systematic Procedure

Follow a systematic procedure when polishing the entire mouth by developing a sequence that is always followed. For example, always start in the same quadrant or begin on the buccal surface of the most posterior tooth in the mandibular right quadrant and polish each tooth, moving around the entire arch; then make a loop around the most posterior tooth on the mandibular left quadrant and polish the lingual surface, ending on the right side.

Prophy Brush

The **prophy brushes** used for the coronal polish procedure come in several styles. Like the rubber cup, they are "snap on" or "screw on," depending on which prophy angle they are used (see Figure 29-39). Brushes are available with nylon or natural bristles. Some brushes are tapered, while others are flat on the end. For the coronal polishes, a soft and flexible brush is used. Softening can be accomplished by soaking the brush in hot water before using it.

Prophy brushes are used on the occlusal surfaces to effectively clean the deep pits and fissures and also on

ADVANCED CHAIRSIDE FUNCTIONS

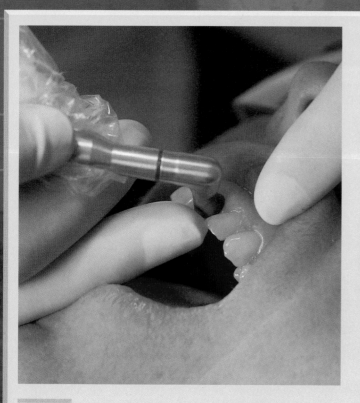

FIGURE 29-41 Adapting rubber cup to tooth surface.

FIGURE 29-42 Examples of polishing stroke.

the lingual of the anteriors, but the bristles should *never* contact the gingival tissues and should be positioned only above the gingival third of the tooth. This brush is used only on the enamel surface. Used in the same manner as the cup, the brush is flexed in the central fossa with a light, intermittent, and overlapping stroke. On lingual surfaces, the brush is placed in the lingual pit and moved toward the incisal edge. Procedure 29-8 outlines the use of the prophy brush for polishing.

Dental Tape and Dental Floss

Dental tape is used on the interproximal surfaces of the teeth with an abrasive agent. Care must be used not to damage the interdental papilla and free gingival margins when using the tape. After all the interproximal surfaces have been polished with dental tape and abrasive, the teeth must be flossed to remove any particles of abrasive that were left after rinsing. The **dental floss** is placed interproximally, wrapped around the tooth, and moved in an up-and-down motion (see Procedure 29-9).

Note: If fluoride is going to be applied as the next step of this procedure, unwaxed floss should be used instead of waxed floss. Waxed floss coats the teeth, preventing the fluoride from being absorbed by the teeth.

Maintaining the Operating Field

During the coronal polish, it is important to keep the mouth free of excess saliva and debris, direct the dental light for maximum light for the operator (dental assistant), keep the patient comfortable, and maintain correct positioning of the dental assistant and patient.

Dental Assistant Guidelines

The dental assistant should follow the guidelines for positioning discussed in previous chapters. When dental assistants become operators, they should sit on the side of the patient where they are most comfortable. For example, a right-handed dental assistant usually finds being on the right side of the patient more convenient. Dental assistants should adjust the operator's chair so that their feet are flat on the floor and movement around the patient's head is unrestricted. The dental assistant usually sits between the 8 and 9 o'clock positions when performing the polish if right-handed and between 3 and 4 o'clock if left-handed.

Patient Considerations

The patient is seated and reclined to the correct height for the dental assistant. During the coronal polish procedure, the patient's head may be positioned up and down and left and right depending on the arch and the quadrant that the dental assistant is working on.

Dental Light Use

The dental light needs to be adjusted for good direct and indirect vision. The dental assistant can maintain good

ADVANCED CHAIRSIDE FUNCTIONS

PROCEDURE 29-8

Using the Prophy Brush

This procedure is performed by the dental assistant, hygienist, or dentist. The prophy brush procedure follows the rubber cup polish, and includes the techniques used to manipulate and position the brush (Figure 29-43).

EQUIPMENT AND SUPPLIES

■ See Procedure 29-7, Polishing with Rubber Cup.

PROCEDURE STEPS *(Follow aseptic procedures)*

1. Place the softened brush on the prophy angle and apply prophy paste to the brush.

2. Establish a fulcrum close to the posterior tooth to be polished.

3. Move the brush bristles toward the mesial buccal cusp tip and continue until the brush comes off the occlusal surface.

4. Replace the brush bristles in the central fossa.

5. Apply slight pressure again, and move the brush up toward the distal buccal cusp until the brush comes off the occlusal surface.

6. Repeat this procedure on the occlusal surface of each posterior tooth until all of the occlusal surfaces are cleaned.

7. Repeat this process on the occlusal surfaces of all teeth.

FIGURE 29-43 Prophy brush on occlusal surface.

8. For the lingual surfaces of the anterior teeth, place the prophy brush in the lingual pit, above the cingulum.

9. Apply light pressure to flex and spread the brush bristles.

10. Move the brush toward the incisal edge to polish the lingual surface.

11. Repeat on all lingual surfaces that have deep pits and grooves.

12. When finished with the brush, rinse and evacuate the oral cavity thoroughly.

illumination of the mouth by remembering to adjust the light whenever the patient's head position is changed.

Oral Cavity Maintenance

The oral cavity should be rinsed frequently during the polish using the air-water syringe and evacuator. The saliva ejector helps to keep saliva to a minimum if placed in the patient's mouth during use of the prophy cup and brush. This also reduces splattering of the polishing agent. Another way to reduce splattering is to wipe the debris from the cup and the brush with a 2×2 gauze when removing the cup and brush from the mouth.

Auxiliary Polishing Aids

Several **auxiliary polishing aids** may be needed during a coronal polish. These aids include bridge threaders, abrasive polishing strips, soft wooden points, and small interproximal brushes (Figure 29-44).

Bridge Threaders

The **bridge threaders** are used to pull the dental tape and floss under fixed appliances, around orthodontic appliances, and around splints so that all proximal surfaces can be cleaned and polished. There are several

ADVANCED CHAIRSIDE FUNCTIONS

PROCEDURE 29-9

Polishing with Dental Tape and Dental Floss

This procedure is part of the coronal polish. After the rubber cup and brush have been used, the interproximal surfaces of the teeth are cleaned with dental tape and then dental floss is used.

EQUIPMENT AND SUPPLIES

- See Procedure 29-7, Polishing with the Rubber Cup.

PROCEDURE STEPS *(Follow aseptic procedures)*

1. Cut off a piece of dental tape twelve to eighteen inches long.

2. Wipe some abrasive agent into the interproximal contact areas of the teeth in a quadrant, with a cotton tip or finger.

3. Wrap the tape around the middle fingers of both hands, leaving a length of tape just long enough to wrap around the tooth while maintaining control.

4. Take the tape through the contact at an oblique angle (\) in a back-and-forth motion, using gentle pressure and holding the tape against the tooth. This assists in preventing the tape from snapping through the contact and damaging the gingiva.

5. Wrap the tape around the tooth to cover the line angles of the tooth on both the buccal and the lingual.

6. When the proximal surface of one tooth is complete, lift the tape up and over the interdental papilla without removing the tape through the contact and readapt the tape on the proximal surface of the adjacent tooth.

7. Polish this surface with the tape and abrasive and then remove the tape up through the contact. If the tape is pulled through the embrasure area, be careful not to injure the gingival tissues.

8. Continue around each tooth in both arches until all proximal surfaces have been polished, including the most distal surface of each quadrant. Use different areas of the tape as needed, and rinse areas thoroughly and evacuate all debris.

9. Follow the taping by using dental floss to remove any remaining debris. Floss all areas and rinse thoroughly.

---

types of bridge threaders. Usually, they are made of plastic with loops or eyes for the tape or floss to slide through and pointed ends (Figure 29-45). After the floss or tape is threaded through the eye of the threader on the facial side, slip the pointed end through the gingival embrasure. Once the bridge threader is through the embrasure, take hold of the floss or tape and proceed as described in the previous section on using the dental tape and floss.

Abrasive Polishing Strips

Abrasive polishing strips are used occasionally when a small stain is difficult to remove. Polishing strips or "finishing strips" are used only on enamel surfaces. They come in various grits and widths. The polishing strip is worked interproximally, pulled tight against the proximal surface of the tooth, and then moved in a back-and-forth motion until the stain is gone. Care must be taken not to cut surrounding soft tissues, because the edges of the strip are sharp.

Soft Wood Points

Soft wood points are sometimes used with polishing agents to polish occlusal grooves and pits, proximal surfaces of sensitive teeth, and areas other polishing instruments cannot reach. Soft wood points are made of balsa wood; orangewood sticks; round, wooden toothpicks; and several other types of soft wood. The soft wood points can be used alone or with handles. The points are narrow and come in either wedge shapes for the proximal surfaces or cone shapes for the pits and grooves.

ADVANCED CHAIRSIDE FUNCTIONS

FIGURE 29-44 Various auxiliary polishing aids. (A) Flossing aid. (B) Bridge threaders. (C) Abrasive polishing strip. (D) Disposable interproximal pick. (E) Various small interproximal brushes. (F) Soft wooden points.

FIGURE 29-45 Bridge threader going under fixed bridge near abutment tooth.

Interproximal Brushes

Interproximal brushes are small, soft-bristled brushes that come in a variety of shapes and sizes. The brushes come in packages of three or four and are used by attaching them to metal or plastic handles. After selecting the best shape of brush to clean a specific area, attach the brush to the handle and insert the brush with light pressure. Use a back-and-forth motion to work the brush.

Interproximal brushes are useful in the following conditions:

- Open contact areas
- Around orthodontic braces and wires
- Around exposed bifurcation or trifurcation of the roots
- On abutment teeth of a hygienic bridge

PROCEDURE 29-10

Coronal Polish

This procedure is performed routinely by the dental assistant and dental hygienist. The protocol for performing a coronal polish is described, including preparation of materials and the patient, positioning of the operator and the patient, sequence of procedure, and evaluating the procedure.

EQUIPMENT AND SUPPLIES (see Figure 29-37)

- Basic three setup: mouth mirror, explorer, cotton pliers
- Saliva ejector, HVE tip, air-water syringe tip

- 2 × 2 gauze sponges, cotton-tip applicators, tongue blade, and cotton rolls
- Lip lubricant and disclosing solution in dappen dish
- Low-speed handpiece with prophy angle attachment
- Prophy cups and brushes (dappen dish with warm water to soak brushes in)
- Prophy pastes, with a variety of grits and finger ring holder
- Dental tape and dental floss
- Auxiliary aids as needed

(continues)

ADVANCED CHAIRSIDE FUNCTIONS

The following items are needed off the tray:

- Patient's chart
- Red/blue pencil, lead pencil, and pen
- Barriers for the dental unit
- Patient napkin and napkin chain
- Patient safety glasses
- Patient hand mirror

PROCEDURE STEPS *(Follow aseptic procedures)*

1. After gathering the preceding equipment and materials, prepare the operatory for the patient.

2. Prepare the patient.

   - Following the established procedure, seat the patient and review and update the patient's records.
   - Explain the procedure to the patient.
   - Follow aseptic procedures to prepare the patient for the coronal polish.
   - Evaluate the patient's condition by performing an oral inspection.
   - Select abrasive agents to be used, based on the amount and type of stain.
   - Lubricate the patient's lips, dry the teeth, and apply the disclosing agent with the cotton-tip applicator.
   - Adjust the dental unit light for good vision.

3. Position the operator and the patient. When the operator is polishing the maxillary and mandibular right facial and the maxillary and mandibular left lingual, the patient's head is turned away from the operator (Figure 29-46). When the operator is polishing the maxillary and mandibular right lingual and the maxillary and mandibular left facial, the patient's head is turned toward the operator (Figure 29-47).

4. Initiate the procedure sequence.

   - Begin the polish on the quadrant or arch according to the predetermined, established routine.
   - Follow criteria previously discussed regarding the use of abrasives and the rubber cup, prophy brush, tape, and floss.

   - Rinse the patient's mouth after each quadrant is polished or as needed.

5. Evaluate coronal polish.

   - Once all steps of the coronal polish have been completed, rinse the patient's mouth thoroughly with spray from the air-water syringe and evacuator.
   - Apply disclosing solution to detect any areas of plaque or stain that were missed.
   - Using the mouth mirror and the air syringe, inspect each surface for any remaining soft deposits and/or stains. Note these areas on the patient's chart or paper for future reference.

FIGURE 29-46 Positioning patient's head away from dental assistant.

FIGURE 29-47 Positioning patient's head toward dental assistant.

(continues)

ADVANCED CHAIRSIDE FUNCTIONS

PROCEDURE 29-10 *(CONTINUED)*

- Polish the areas missed with a prophy cup and/or brush.

- Rinse the patient's mouth to remove all of the abrasive agent.

- Inspect the teeth for a lustrous shine showing no debris or extrinsic stains. The soft tissues should be free of abrasion or trauma. The patient is ready for a fluoride treatment. The dentist may want to see the patient before he or she is dismissed.

6. Chart the coronal polish. It is the dental assistant's responsibility to record the coronal polish completely and accurately on the patient's dental chart. The entry is recorded in ink, dated, and signed or entered into the computer system. Include any comments about the condition of the patient's mouth and type(s) of material(s) used.

CHAPTER SUMMARY

Periodontal disease is as old as the human race. According to the American Academy of Periodontology, three out of four adults will experience, to some degree, periodontal problems at some time in their lives. In children and adolescents, marginal gingivitis and gingival recession are the most prevalent conditions.

The dental assistant performs chairside assisting duties and the expanded functions allowed by the state dental practice act, including placing and removing periodontal dressing, removing sutures, and performing coronal polishes. The dental assistant takes radiographs, takes impressions for study models, and administers fluoride treatments. The assistant also gives pre- and postoperative instructions and prepares the treatment room for surgery. These functions are in addition to treatment room preparation and maintenance and sterilization procedures. The dental assistant is involved in educating and motivating the patient throughout the treatment. In some offices, the dental assistant may also perform laboratory tasks, such as pouring study models or making periodontal splints.

Performing a coronal polish, an expanded function, requires increased skill and responsibility. This task is delegated by the dentist according to the state dental practice act. Some states require additional education, certification, or registration to perform this function.

Case Study

Melissa Moore is forty-two years old. She has been Dr. Sanchez's patient for fourteen years. Melissa has her teeth examined and cleaned every six months. Over the years, she has developed several teeth with pocket readings of between six and eight. At Melissa's last cleaning appointment, the hygienist explained that she found over ten areas with periodontal probing readings of over six and areas where the tissues bleed easily. Melissa is in good general health but has been taking medication to reduce anxiety for the past six months.

Case Study Review

1. Are Melissa's periodontal readings within the normal range?

2. What questions should be asked in reference to the change in her condition over such a short period of time?

3. Explain how stress could affect Melissa's periodontal health.

REVIEW QUESTIONS

Multiple Choice

1. The periodontium includes
   a. gingiva, epithelial attachment, cementum, sulcus, enamel, and pulp chamber.
   b. gingiva, enamel, cementum, dentin, sulcus, and periodontal ligaments.
   c. gingiva, epithelial attachment, sulcus, periodontal ligaments, cementum, and alveolar bone.
   d. periodontal ligaments, sulcus, gingiva, salivary glands, and mucous membrane.

2. Periodontal disease is a virus that can be transmitted from one individual to another.
   a. True
   b. False

3. The working end of the periodontal instrument used to remove subgingival calculus and smooth the root surface is rounded and has cutting edges on both sides of the blade. This instrument is a
   a. hoe.
   b. file.
   c. scaler.
   d. curette.

4. The procedure to remove calculus and debris from the tooth and periodontal pocket is known as
   a. root planing.
   b. scaling and curettage.
   c. polishing procedure.
   d. occlusal adjustment.

5. Periodontal surgery that involves recontouring of the alveolar bone is called:
   a. mucogingival surgery.
   b. gingival grafting.
   c. osteoplasty.
   d. ostectomy.

6. When cleaning deep pits and fissures while polishing occlusal surfaces, which aid is most effective?
   a. Rubber cup
   b. Prophy brush
   c. Dental tape
   d. Dental floss

7. _____ are hinged instruments used to shape soft tissue.
   a. Pocket marking pliers
   b. Periosteal elevators
   c. Soft tissue rongeurs
   d. Tissue forceps

8. How many surfaces on a tooth are probed to determine the sulcus depth?
   a. Five sites
   b. Six sites
   c. Ten sites
   d. Twelve sites

9. The dental pellicle, materia alba, food debris, and plaque are all classified as
   a. dental stains.
   b. hard deposits.
   c. soft deposits.
   d. None of the above

10. When performing a rubber cup polish, all of the following statements are true *except*:
    a. Use a slow, even speed.
    b. Always use a fulcrum.
    c. Use the edge of the rubber prophy cup to polish.
    d. Start and stop the slow-speed handpiece outside the patient's mouth.

Critical Thinking

1. What are the signs and symptoms of periodontal disease?

2. Name the periodontal disease that occurs in young adults and results from stress, inadequate diet and sleep, and poor oral hygiene.

3. Patients must take an active part in the treatment of periodontal disease. List several means the dental assistant uses to aid the patient.

4. Review auxiliary polishing aids that are available, and then select the polishing aids that you would suggest to a patient who has a fixed bridge.

5. Discuss various ways to ensure that a fulcrum is always used when performing a coronal polish.

Web Activities

1. Go to http://www.perio.org for consumer information and the most frequently asked questions about periodontal disease and treatments.

2. To learn about periodontal disease and heart disease, visit http://www.perio.org.

3. Take the quiz at http://www.perio.org to see if you have periodontal disease.

FIXED PROSTHODONTICS AND GINGIVAL RETRACTION

SPECIFIC INSTRUCTIONAL OBJECTIVES

The student should strive to meet the following objectives and demonstrate an understanding of the facts and principles presented in this chapter:

1. Define the scope of fixed prosthodontics.

2. Explain dentist's considerations when recommending various prostheses to a patient.

3. Describe various types of fixed prostheses and their functions.

4. Describe dental materials used in fixed prostheses.

5. Identify and explain CAD/CAM restorative system.

6. Explain the involvement of the laboratory technician in the fabrication of fixed prostheses.

7. Describe the role of the dental assistant in all phases of fixed prosthodontic treatment.

8. Explain techniques for retaining the prosthesis when there is little or no crown on the tooth.

9. Describe implant retainer prosthesis.

10. Explain techniques for maintaining fixed prostheses.

ADVANCED CHAIRSIDE FUNCTIONS

11. Explain the function of gingival retraction.

12. Describe the different types of gingival retraction.

13. Explain the steps of placing and removing gingival retraction cord.

KEY TERMS

abutments *(692)*

bite registration *(703)*

CAD/CAM restorative systems *(698)*

CEREC *(698)*

chamfer *(702)*

dental casting alloy *(697)*

direct resin veneers *(693)*

direct restorations *(690)*

full-cast crown *(691)*

gingival retraction *(711)*

indirect resin veneers *(694)*

indirect restorations *(690)*

inlays *(691)*

ischemia *(712)*

Maryland bridge *(692)*

onlays *(691)*

partial crown *(691)*

pontic *(692)*

porcelain veneers *(694)*

porcelain-fused-to-metal crowns *(697)*

post-retained cores *(707)*

(continues)

INTRODUCTION

Fixed prosthodontics is the specialty that deals with replacement of missing teeth or parts of teeth with extensive restorations. The restorations or **prostheses** (artificial parts for missing tissues) are fabricated in a dental laboratory from detailed impressions taken in the dental office. When finished, the prostheses are cemented permanently in the patient's mouth.

Fixed prostheses replace missing teeth and tooth structures which:

- Restore masticatory function
- Improve esthetics and, often, self-esteem
- Improve speech
- Promote good oral hygiene
- Prevent further movement of the teeth because of support of the prostheses

The fixed prosthesis becomes part of the natural dentition and is maintained with routine brushing and flossing techniques. The main disadvantages are the expense of the prosthesis and the time involved in preparing the tooth, taking the impression, fabricating the restoration, and permanently cementing it in place. Restorations routinely take at least two appointments to complete. Dental insurance may cover some of the expense of prosthetic restorations.

There are several advantages of having a permanent restoration: The restoration is secure in the mouth, it is esthetic, and it restores function for many years. These advantages outweigh the initial monetary expense and time commitment.

The prosthodontist receives additional education and clinical practice to specialize in fixed and removable prosthodontic procedures. Patient cases may include fixed prosthetic procedures that are difficult, involved, and extensive. Such cases might include patients who have had extensive surgery due to cancer of the mouth, or patients who need full mouth reconstruction. The patients are referred by general dentists and other specialists to the prosthodontist.

There are many types of fixed prostheses and a variety of materials used for their preparation, fabrication, and cementation.

Patient Considerations

When a patient needs fixed prosthodontic treatment, the dentist performs an examination that includes:

- Medical and dental history
- Examination of the intra- and extra-oral tissues
- Radiographs
- Impressions for study models (diagnostic casts)
- Intraoral photographs taken with intraoral camera
- Extraoral photographs

Patients who are candidates for fixed prostheses should have healthy supportive tissues and be motivated to maintain the prostheses. Sometimes, patients need to have periodontal or orthodontic treatment prior to the fixed prosthodontic treatment.

Case Presentation

With less complicated cases, the dentist presents the treatment to the patient at the time of the examination. Other cases require time for the dentist to make the diagnosis and treatment plan before the patient is scheduled for the case presentation.

At the case presentation, the dentist recommends the type of prosthesis and explains what is involved in treatment, including the number of appointments and what the patient can expect. The dentist uses study models, radiographs, pictures of completed cases, samples of various dental prostheses on models, pamphlets, educational videos, and computer images in the presentation. The computer-imaging component shows the patient before and after images (Figure 30-1).

When presenting the treatment choices to the patient, the dentist or the office manager explains the cost of the prosthesis, whether insurance will cover any of the treatment, and the number of appointments required.

Types of Fixed Prostheses

Fixed prostheses are **indirect restorations**, meaning they cannot be placed directly in the mouth after the tooth is prepared like amalgam or composite restorations, which are **direct restorations**. Instead, impressions are taken and then the fixed prostheses are fabricated in a dental laboratory. The indirect restorations are designed to replace missing tooth structure in a variety of ways, including full crowns, partial crowns, inlays, onlays, bridges, and veneers.

Crowns

Crowns cover teeth with extensive decay or breakdown. The prepared tooth is covered with an anatomically shaped and fitted crown. Crowns are constructed of

FIGURE 30-1 Computerized imaging system shows patient before and after views of how prostheses will look.

various materials. The tooth may require a full crown, which is often referred to as a **full-cast crown** (Figure 30-2). A full crown covers the entire coronal surface of the tooth. Sometimes, the tooth is broken down so badly that means to retain the full crown on the tooth are required. (Retention is discussed later in this chapter.)

A **partial crown** is a cast restoration that covers three or more, but not all, surfaces of a tooth. A **three-quarter crown** normally is prepared so that the mesial, distal, and lingual surfaces are reduced but the facial surface is left intact (Figure 30-3). The incisal or occlusal surface of the tooth is also reduced.

Inlays and Onlays

Inlays and onlays are restorations that replace missing tooth structure within the tooth. **Inlays** cover the area between the cusps in the middle of the tooth and the proximal surfaces that are involved (Figure 30-4A). Inlays are MOD (mesio-occluso-distal), MO (mesio-occlusal), DO (disto-occlusal), or O (occlusal). **Onlays** are like inlays except they include the cusp ridges of the tooth (Figure 30-4B). Inlays and onlays are also cast restorations that are made of a variety of materials. The extent of lost tooth structure and the preparation determine which type of cast restoration is best suited to restore function and preserve the strength of the tooth.

Bridges

A bridge is a restoration that spans the space of a missing tooth or teeth. The bridge is divided into units, and

(A)

(B)

FIGURE 30-2 (A) Porcelain fused to metal crown. (B) Full porcelain crown.

FIGURE 30-3 Three-quarter gold crown.

FIGURE 30-4 (A) Gold inlay restorations. (B) Gold onlay restoration on a mandibular first molar.

Porcelain-fused-to-metal bridge

(A)

(B)

FIGURE 30-5 (A) Three-unit bridge abutments, pontics, and retainers. (B) Maryland bridge.

each unit of a bridge represents a tooth. A bridge may replace one or more adjacent teeth in the same arch. The missing tooth is replaced by a **pontic**, which can be designed in a variety of forms. Two common pontics are the hygienic (free cleansing/sanitary) and cosmetic (ovate). The hygienic pontics allow for space between the tissue and pontic, usually seen in the posterior area. The cosmetic pontics are tooth colored and fill in the entire space to the gingival tissue.

The teeth adjacent to the pontic are called **abutments**. Crowns, inlays, or onlays may be placed on the abutment teeth to support and stabilize the pontic (Figure 30-5A).

Bridges are made of a variety of materials to meet the patient's esthetic and functional needs. After the bridges have been fabricated, they are permanently cemented in the patient's mouth. Bridges also can be retained by one or two teeth on the same side. This type of bridge is known as a cantilever bridge.

The **Maryland bridge**, or resin-retained fixed bridge, is used to replace one tooth. Abutment teeth have very little tooth structure removed during preparation. The bridge consists of a pontic with extensions (retainers) of varying shapes. The extensions are designed to attach to the abutment teeth, on or toward the lingual surface. The retainers of the Maryland bridge are roughened by electrolytic etching to increase their bonding to the natural tooth structure (Figure 30-5B).

Preparation of the teeth for the Maryland bridge is usually minimal. The impressions are taken and temporaries may be placed. The laboratory procedures are the same for all cases except the electrolytic etching of the inside of the bridge retainers. Cementation steps are as follows:

1. The dental dam is placed to protect the tissues from the acid etching.

2. The abutment teeth are cleaned with pumice and water and then rinsed and dried thoroughly.

3. The prepared surfaces of the teeth are acid etched for thirty to sixty seconds, rinsed thoroughly, and dried.

4. A dual-cured composite cementing material is applied to the etched surfaces of the bridge retainers and the etched tooth surface.

5. The bridge is positioned on the abutment teeth.

6. Once the material has set, excess cement material is removed.

Veneers

Veneers are thin layers of tooth-colored material that cover much of the facial surface. They are used to cover badly stained teeth and to reshape the anatomy of teeth. Veneers improve appearance with very little removal of tooth structure. Examples include:

■ Full facial coverage on anterior maxillary teeth— Covered with veneers for a natural appearance (Figure 30-6).

■ Tetracycline stains on the maxillary anterior teeth— Veneers cover the stain for improved appearance (Figure 30-7).

■ Diastema (an abnormal space between two adjacent teeth in the same arch) on maxillary central incisors—Veneers close the space (Figure 30-8).

Veneer procedures are changing constantly as technology progresses. There are many types of veneers, materials used, and techniques. Direct resin veneers, indirect resin veneers, and porcelain veneers are three types.

Direct Resin Veneers. Direct resin veneers are made in the dental office directly on the patient's tooth. This procedure requires one appointment. In preparation for the veneer procedure, little, if any, tooth structure is removed. The tooth is etched, adhesive is applied, and opaquers and body shade are placed. The incisal shade follows. The shade can be varied between the incisal edge and body of the veneer. The veneers are contoured and finished. Generally these materials are light cured and require routine polishing and periodic maintenance.

(A)

(B)

FIGURE 30-6 Veneers on anterior teeth. (A) Before placement. (B) After placement. *(Courtesy of George J. Velis, DDS.)*

(A)

(B)

FIGURE 30-7 (A) Patient with tetracycline staining. (B) Patient with tetracycline staining after direct resin veneers have been placed. *(Courtesy of Kerr Corporation.)*

FIGURE 30-8 (A) Patient with diastema between two central incisors. (B) Same patient with diastema after indirect resin veneers have been placed. *(Courtesy of George J. Velis, DDS.)*

Indirect Resin Veneers. Indirect resin veneers require two appointments. At the first appointment, the tooth is prepared and an impression is taken. The impression is sent to the laboratory for fabrication of the veneer. During the second appointment, the veneer is bonded in place. These veneers do not bond well to resin cement. They lack strength and wear at a faster rate than porcelain veneers.

Porcelain Veneers. Porcelain veneers are similar to indirect resin veneers in that they require two appointments and are fabricated in the dental laboratory. Porcelain veneers are natural in appearance and are durable. The technique for the porcelain veneer is sensitive to shade selection and gingival margin adaptation if the veneer is to look natural and adapt well. Procedure 30-1 outlines the steps involved in placing porcelain veneers.

PROCEDURE 30-1

Porcelain Veneers

This procedure is performed by the prosthodontist and is completed in two appointments. During the first appointment, the tooth is prepared and impressions are taken; at the second appointment, the porcelain veneer is applied. Between appointments, the impressions are sent to a dental laboratory, where the porcelain veneer is fabricated.

EQUIPMENT *(For the preparation appointment)* (Figure 30-9)

- Basic setup: mouth mirror, explorer, and cotton pliers
- Cotton rolls, 2 × 2 gauze
- HVE tip, air-water syringe tip
- Anesthetic setup
- High-speed handpiece and assorted burs

- Shade guide
- Spoon excavator
- Low-speed handpiece with prophy angle, rubber cup, and pumice
- Retraction cord and placement instrument
- Bite registration materials
- Alginate impression materials for model of opposing arch
- Final impression materials (polysiloxane or polyether)
- Temporary veneer (optional)
- Laboratory prescription form

(continues)

PROCEDURE 30-1 (CONTINUED)

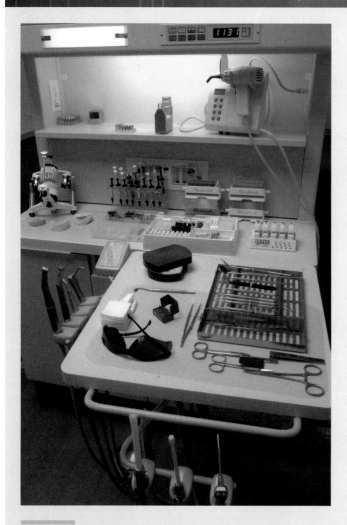

FIGURE 30-9 Porcelain veneers tray setup, preparation appointment, including the impressing materials, bite registration materials, curing light, shade guide, and provisional materials.

PROCEDURE STEPS *(Follow aseptic procedures)*

Preparation Appointment (First Appointment)

1. Bite registration and opposing arch impression are taken.

2. The teeth are cleaned with rubber cup and pumice to remove extrinsic stains. A shade is selected by the dentist to determine how light the patient wants the veneers and to estimate how light the finished shade will be.

3. The teeth are prepared according to the design of the veneer. The incisal edge and the cervical margin are prepared carefully so that the finished veneer is even with the gingival crest or just slightly subgingival.

4. The retraction cord is placed to achieve hemostasis and ensure visualization of the margins.

5. A final impression is taken with a dimensionally stable material such as polysiloxane or polyether.

6. Temporary veneers are placed if necessary, although most patients do not require temporary veneers.

7. The retraction cord is removed after the temporary veneers are placed.

8. The patient is informed that the gums will be tender for several days because of the retraction cord placement.

9. The patient is dismissed.

Laboratory Fabrication

1. The impressions are sent to the dental laboratory with a laboratory prescription.

2. The laboratory follows the dentist's prescription regarding length of veneer, shade, thickness, and texture. (Color photos of the patient are helpful in the designing and shading process.)

3. The laboratory fabricates the veneers and returns them to the office.

EQUIPMENT *(For the cementation appointment)*

- Basic setup: mouth mirror, explorer, and cotton pliers
- Cotton rolls, 2 × 2 gauze, cheek and lip retractors
- Saliva ejector, HVE tip, air-water syringe tip
- Porcelain veneers from the laboratory
- Low-speed handpiece with prophy angle, rubber cup, and pumice
- Silane coupling agent and small applicator (brush)
- Retraction cord and placement instrument
- Chlorhexidine soap
- Plastic or ultrathin metal strips
- Etchant and applicator
- Bonding agent and curing light (Figure 30-10)

Cementation Appointment (Second Appointment)

1. The second appointment should be scheduled as soon as possible after the first appointment because the patient is often without temporary coverage. The laboratory should be scheduled ahead of time so the turnaround time is minimal.

(continues)

PROCEDURE 30-1 *(CONTINUED)*

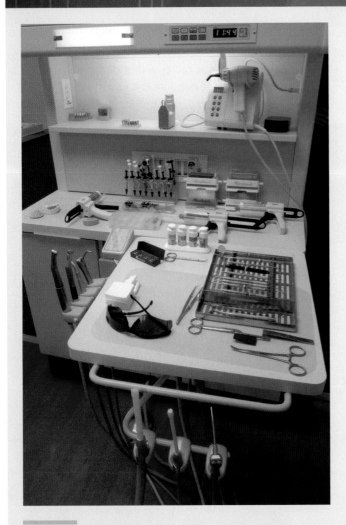

FIGURE 30-10 Porcelain veneers tray setup, cementation appointment, including veneers back from the lab, curing light, and permanent cement.

2. Complete a preliminary cleaning of the teeth with pumice to remove plaque and stains.

3. The veneers are tried on the tooth and adjustments are made with finishing diamonds. (The veneers are very fragile and require careful handling.)

4. Once all adjustments are complete, clean and dry the inside of the veneers thoroughly. Acid etchant is used to clean and decontaminate the inside surface of the veneer.

5. Apply a thin layer of silane coupling agent (this material allows bonding to porcelain).

6. Place the light-cured bonding agent in the veneers. Make sure there are no air bubbles. The material fills the veneer and is spread evenly. The veneers are then placed in a light-protected area or box until the teeth are prepared.

7. Prepare the teeth for bonding by placing a retraction cord on the facial surface. Clean the facial surface with chlorhexidine soap and a prophy cup or brush.

8. Isolate the teeth being bonded with cotton rolls, cheek and lip retractors, a saliva ejector, and plastic or ultrathin metal strips.

9. Etch the teeth to be bonded, following manufacturer directions of adhesive system.

10. Apply the adhesive to the teeth being bonded.

11. Seat each veneer in the correct position.

12. In some cases, the veneer is spot cured and excess cement is removed.

13. Light cure each veneer in place.

14. Remove excess cement with a scalpel.

15. Contour and refine the margins with finishing diamonds or burs (Figure 30-11).

16. Polish the veneers with rubber wheels, cups, and polishing paste.

FIGURE 30-11 Finishing porcelain veneer margins with diamond bur. *(Courtesy of Kerr Corporation.)*

Types of Materials Used for Fixed Prostheses

CDA The materials used for the construction of fixed crowns, bridges, inlays, onlays, and veneers depend, among other considerations, on their locations in the mouth, required strength, amount of tooth structure, and esthetics (natural-looking teeth are the current trend, while at one time having gold showing was desirable). Because patients want tooth-colored restorations, porcelain and composite materials are commonly used today.

Before discussing the types of materials used to construct fixed prostheses, many materials used during various procedures should also be mentioned. In the initial preparation appointment and final cementation appointment the following materials are used.

- Alginate impression material - Used to take an opposing arch impression and/or to make temporary restoration.

- Bite registration materials - Used to take an impression of how the patient bites. Materials used for bite registration include wax and polysiloxane.

- Retraction cord - Used to retract gingival tissue around prepped tooth.

- Final impression material - Used to take final impression of prepped tooth. Various types of final impression materials are used including silicone (modified polysiloxane and polyvinyl), polysulfide, polyether, and hydrocolloid.

- Temporary cement - Used to cement temporary restorations.

- Bonding agent - Used to assist in bonding of permanent restorations. The bonding agent is placed before permanent cement.

- Permanent cement - Used to cement permanent restorations. Permanent cements include polycarboxylate, glass ionomer, resins, and combinations of these materials.

To learn more about these materials and/or to review them, see Chapter 33, Dental Cements, Bases, Liners, and Bonding Agents, and Chapter 35, Laboratory Materials and Techniques.

Gold Casting Alloys

Gold used in crowns, inlays, and onlays is not pure gold but a combination of metals. When two or more metals are combined, they form an alloy. Pure gold is too soft for use in cast restorations, so other metals, such as platinum and palladium, are added, along with iron, tin, or zinc, to form a **dental casting alloy**.

Restorations made of gold alloy include full gold crowns, inlays, and onlays. These are fabricated mainly for the posterior teeth where they are less visible. Gold

FIGURE 30-12 Bridge with a full gold crown on the second molar and two metal crowns with porcelain facings on the first molar and the second bicuspid. *(Courtesy of Clifton O. Caldwell, Jr., DDS, FICD, FACD.)*

crowns are also fabricated with tooth-colored veneers. The veneers may cover the entire crown or just the facial surface. Crowns that have veneers are known as **porcelain-fused-to-metal crowns**, or ceramometal crowns (Figure 30-12).

Porcelain-fused-to-metal crowns are very popular and are commonly used where strength and esthetics are needed. These crowns resist fracture, abrasion, and discoloration, and are used in all areas of the mouth for single-tooth restorations or bridges. The disadvantages are that the tooth requires more reduction to allow for the thickness of the porcelain and the porcelain is abrasive and can wear down natural teeth or metal restorations.

Tooth-Colored Cast Restorations

Tooth-colored cast restorations are made either of porcelain or composite resin. Use of these materials is increasing for esthetic reasons. Porcelain is used for inlays, bonded veneers, porcelain-fused-to-metal crowns, and bridges. Porcelain cast restorations require at least two appointments, and are more expensive than gold cast restorations. Porcelain, a type of ceramic, resembles natural tooth structure but is not as strong when used alone. Porcelain is susceptible to fracture under occlusal stresses, but resin-bonding techniques have reduced this concern. Restorations that are solely porcelain are used mainly on single teeth and rarely for fixed bridges.

Composite-resin indirect technique restorations are fabricated in a dental laboratory. Inlays, onlays, and veneers are made from impressions taken at the first appointment; then the dental laboratory creates the restorations from composite resin material. This material is heated and placed under pressure. These restorations are stronger than direct composite resin restorations and are bonded in place during the second appointment (Figure 30-13).

FIGURE 30-13 Mirror view of composite resin inlays on patient's left mandibular. *(Courtesy of George J. Velis, DDS.)*

CAD/CAM Restorative Systems

In-office **CAD/CAM restorative systems** are becoming increasingly common. These systems allow metal-free, tooth-colored restorations to be fabricated in a single appointment. All types of restorations including inlays, onlays, posterior and anterior crowns, and veneers can be designed and milled at the chairside. With this type of system, there are no unpleasant impressions, no need for temporaries, and less reduction of healthy tooth structure.

The first CAD/CAM restorative system, called **CEREC** (Chairside Economical Restorations of Esthetic Ceramics), was developed in Switzerland in 1980. The CEREC 3 has the ADA Seal of Acceptance.

Several factors should be addressed before a dental team decides to add this technology to the practice. First, a time investment is required to integrate the system into office scheduling and routines. The dentist and staff must be trained and they need time to practice using both the hardware and software to become proficient. Training programs are available when the CAD/CAM system is purchased and as continued education. Second, a large financial investment is required for purchasing the system and for training. The learning curve may affect patient scheduling and production until the technique is mastered by dental team members. Third, the dentist and staff should be familiar with computers, be committed to learning the system, and be dedicated and enthusiastic about understanding and becoming skilled in this technology.

The first segment of the CEREC system is comprised of the machine that contains the intraoral camera to take the optical impression and the software that receives the impression data and then designs the restoration (Figure 30-14). The second part of the system is the milling chamber, which is usually located in the lab area of the office. The restoration that the dentist

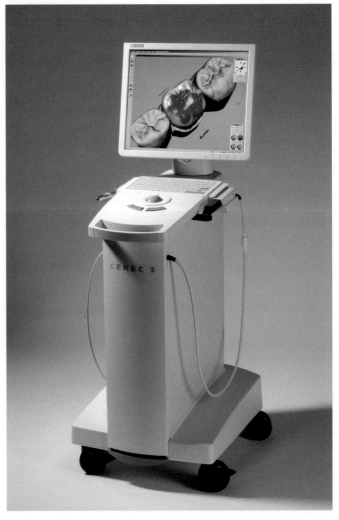

FIGURE 30-14 CEREC machine. *(Courtesy of Sirona Dental Systems.)*

designs with the CEREC software is transferred to the milling chamber (Figure 30-15). The milling chamber contains an attachment for the block of ceramic, two diamond burs, and water. A block of ceramic material that matches the patient's tooth color is selected and placed in the milling chamber; within minutes, the restoration is milled. Several ceramic materials available for the dentist to choose from include leucite-reinforced glass ceramic; fine-grained, feldspathic porcelain; and a polymer ceramic based on MZ100 composite restorative material (Figure 30-16).

Basic steps of the CEREC restoration system are summarized below.

1. Patient is seated and anesthetized.

2. Shade of ceramic material block is selected in the routine manner, and the block is placed in the milling machine.

3. The dentist prepares the tooth for a ceramic restoration.

4. The tooth preparation is coated with a reflective powder.

FIGURE 30-15 (A) CEREC system milling chamber. (B) Close-up of diamond burs inside milling chamber. *(Courtesy of Sirona Dental Systems.)*

FIGURE 30-16 A computerized image of the prepared tooth ready for the crown to be designed.

5. An instant optical impression is obtained by positioning the camera over the preparation.

6. The dentist designs the restoration using data from CEREC software and the optical image at chairside.

7. The information is transferred to the milling machine. Diamond burs will work simultaneously under the water coolant to mill the restoration.

8. The restoration is placed in patient's mouth and any adjustments are made if needed.

9. The restoration is bonded in place using standard bonding materials.

10. A polishing disc can now be used to bring out the natural "chameleon effect" of the all-ceramic material (Figure 30-17).

Since the introduction of the CEREC system, millions of restorations have been fabricated and placed. Patient satisfaction with this system has been very high, as the restoration is esthetically pleasing and comfortable, and obtaining the restoration takes a single appointment. Impressions and temporaries are nonexistent, and there are fewer injections. The CAD/CAM system provides the dentist with precision technology for creating dental restorations in the dental office.

Role of Laboratory Technician

The dental laboratory technician and dentist work closely together to give the patient quality restorations. The relationship between the laboratory and the dental office is critical. Good communication and clearly defined expectations are essential.

The laboratory technician performs the following procedures in fixed prosthesis construction: making custom trays, pouring impressions, articulating stone casts (models), preparing wax patterns, investing, and casting gold alloy restorations. The laboratory technician also constructs porcelain and porcelain-fused-to-metal restorations and fabricates the prosthesis according to the dentist's prescription and from the impressions sent from the dental office.

It is important that the impression materials be handled properly and that everything needed is sent to the laboratory. The dental assistant often is responsible for having everything ready for the laboratory pickup.

Role of Dental Assistant

The dental assistant is involved in all stages of fixed prosthodontic treatment. It is important to understand the sequence of the procedure and the various types of restorations when assisting the dentist. The dental assistant explains the steps of the procedure to the patient, answers questions, and gives postoperative and home-care instructions.

Responsibilities include preparation of equipment and supplies needed for both appointments. Each tray setup is arranged according to the sequence of the procedure, with auxiliary instruments and materials close at hand. The procedures require many different types of

FIGURE 30-17 (A) Teeth with amalgam restorations to be replaced. (B) Teeth are prepared. (C) Teeth restored with ceramic restoration designed and fabricated by the CEREC system.

dental materials, including alginate, bite registration materials, final impression materials, retraction cord, temporization materials, and final cements. The dental assistant prepares and/or utilizes these materials throughout the procedure.

The dental assistant assists the dentist in all aspects of the procedure, from selecting the shade of the tooth to general chairside assisting. In some states, the qualified dental assistant can perform procedures such as placing the retraction cord, placing and removing temporaries, taking preliminary impressions, and removing excess cement. The dental assistant also coordinates the patient's appointments and the laboratory schedule. In some offices, the dental assistant may perform selected laboratory functions, such as making custom trays and pouring study models.

Fabrication of Prosthesis in Dental Laboratory

Once the case is in the dental laboratory, several steps are involved in fabricating the prosthesis, depending on the number of units and types of materials used.

Laboratory steps include:

- Pouring alginate impression of opposing arch in plaster

- Pouring final impression to make master model and die (replica of prepared tooth)

- Creating a wax pattern on the die

- Investing and preparing wax pattern for casting

- Casting die once invested material and metal are heated to desired temperature

- Casting crown in gold alloy to prepare for making porcelain veneer

- Painting porcelain on crown in layers and then curing it in an oven at high temperatures

- Finishing and polishing porcelain-fused-to-metal crown

Retention Techniques

Often, the teeth being restored with a fixed prosthesis have substantial loss of tooth structure due to decay, fractures, or large deteriorated restorations. Also, root canal therapy may be required before crowns and bridges are made.

The dentist improves the retentive capability of the tooth if the tooth being restored will not retain the restoration alone. There are several options for building up the tooth including core build-ups, retention pins, and post-retained cores.

Core Buildups

A core buildup is treatment performed for vital teeth that have very little crown structure. For this procedure, the dentist removes any decay and defective restoration and then builds a core that supports and provides more retention for the cast restoration.

The core buildup or **retention core** is made of amalgam, composite, or a silver alloy/glass ionomer combination (Figure 30-18). These materials come in powder/liquid, syringe, or capsule form and are set chemically or light cured.

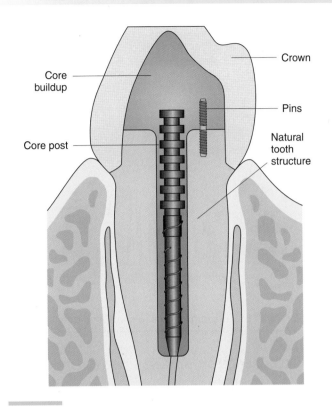

FIGURE 30-18 Tooth with core post, core buildup, and pins.

Preparation for Porcelain-Fused-to-Metal Crown

This procedure is performed by the prosthodontist and dental assistant. Like the porcelain veneer procedure, this process involves two appointments. The following procedure includes steps in the preparation appointment, including retention procedures, and steps in the cementation appointment.

EQUIPMENT (Figure 30-19)

- Basic setup: mouth mirror, explorer, and cotton pliers

- Cotton rolls, gauze, dental floss, articulating paper, and forceps

- HVE tip, saliva ejector, and three-way syringe tip

- Anesthetic setup

- Dental dam setup

- High-speed handpiece with a selection of diamonds, discs, and burs

- Irreversible hydrocolloid (alginate) impression materials

- Spoon excavator, scaler, plastic filling instrument, and cement spatula

- Tooth shade guide (optional)

- Retention materials depending on amount of tooth structure retained—core buildup materials and postretention pins (optional)

- Gingival retraction cord and placement instrument

- Final impression materials and tray (stock or custom tray)

- Bite registration materials

- Crown and collar scissors

- Provisional (temporary) coverage materials

- Low-speed handpiece with burs, discs, and stones

- Laboratory prescription and container for impressions (off-tray item)

(continues)

PROCEDURE 30-2 (CONTINUED)

FIGURE 30-19 Tray setup for preparation appointment.

PROCEDURE STEPS (Follow aseptic procedures)

1. The patient is given local anesthetic. Prepare the syringe, transfer the syringe to the prosthodontist, and, during the administration of the anesthetic, observe the patient.

2. Alginate impressions are taken for fabrication of certain types of temporaries and also for a model of the opposing arch. Select the trays, mix the irreversible hydrocolloid, and take the impressions. The impressions are stored properly until needed and/or poured in plaster or stone.

3. While waiting for the anesthetic to be effective before the tooth is prepared, the tooth shade is selected. A **shade guide** is used to match the natural teeth.

NOTE: This is a very important step for the esthetics of the crown and the appearance of the patient. The shade guide includes a variety of shades, and the shades can be variegated to match the varying shading of the patient's natural teeth (Figure 30-20A).

Moisten the shade guide and hold it close the natural teeth under natural light (Figure 30-20B). Record the information on the patient's chart and on the laboratory prescription.

4. Crowns are prepared with the high-speed handpiece and various diamonds and burs. (The tooth must be reduced to accommodate the thickness of metal and porcelain materials and to have enough strength.)

5. The margins of the preparation are either finished in a **chamfer** or **shoulder** preparation. The chamfer provides adequate bulk and extends easily into the

(A)

(B)

FIGURE 30-20 (A) Shade guide. (B) Matching shade guide to patient's natural teeth.

gingival sulcus. The shoulder provides a ledge that is sometimes beveled (Figure 30-21). Prepare and transfer the high-speed handpiece, and then evacuate and maintain the operating field with the air-water syringe. Retract and exchange instruments as needed.

The abutment teeth are prepared for full crowns by tapering margins of the preparation to the crown of the tooth. This preparation design allows for the placement and withdrawal of the finished restoration.

6. Once the tooth is prepared, the gingival tissue is retracted from the preparation so that a detailed

(continues)

PROCEDURE 3 0 - 2 *(CONTINUED)*

Preparations at the gingival margin

Crown

Prepared tooth

Preparation at gingival margin

Chamfer preparation

Shoulder preparation

Beveled shoulder preparation

FIGURE 30-21 Examples of cavity margins on preparation—chamfer, shoulder, and shoulder with beveled edge.

impression can be made of the margins. The margins of the preparation must be detailed in the impressions so that the finished crown fits snugly and securely on the tooth. The retraction cord is placed around the prepared tooth and pushed into the sulcus with a plastic filling instrument or a retraction cord-condensing instrument (Figure 30-22). (Gingival retraction techniques are discussed in detail later in this chapter.) In some states, the dental assistant is permitted to place the gingival retraction cord. Transfer a piece of retraction cord in cotton pliers to the prosthodontist. Then transfer the appropriate cord-condensing instrument. The retraction cord remains in place for five minutes.

7. The prosthodontist selects the tray and impression material to be used. There are a variety of materials that are suitable for final impressions (see Chapter 35, Laboratory Materials and Techniques). The tray and syringe are selected and prepared and the materials are mixed.

FIGURE 30-22 Placing retraction cord around prepared tooth.

8. Transfer cotton pliers to remove the retraction cord. Transfer the syringe material and receive the cotton pliers and cord. The prosthodontist removes the retraction cord, receives the syringe, and dispenses the material around the margins of the preparation (Figure 30-23A). During this time, mix and load the heavier material into the tray. The prosthodontist places and holds the tray with the impression material in the patient's mouth. Once the prosthodontist has seated the tray, move the light from the patient's face and clean up the impression materials. The final impression is rinsed, disinfected, and placed in a plastic laboratory container (Figure 30-23B).

9. The **bite registration**, also called the occlusal registration, is taken after the final impression is completed. The purpose of the bite registration is to record the way the patient occludes the maxillary and mandibular teeth. There are many types of materials that can be used to record the bite of the patient, including wax and vinyl polysiloxane materials (Figure 30-24). Prepare the materials and transfer them to the prosthodontist, who places the tray and takes the bite impression. In some states, the dental assistant can take the bite impression. After the bite registration is taken, rinse the patient's mouth. The materials are rinsed, disinfected, and placed in a plastic laboratory container.

The provisional (temporary) restoration is very important in crown and bridge construction. The temporary retains the teeth in the same position so that the adjacent and opposing teeth do not shift position. The temporary protects the prepared tooth so that the patient can function normally.

(continues)

PROCEDURE 30-2 *(CONTINUED)*

FIGURE 30-23 (A) Dental assistant receives syringe with light-bodies impression material, and transfers tray with medium- to heavy-bodied impression material to dentist. (B) Final impression. (C) Close-up of preparation margins in final impression. *(C. Courtesy of Kerr Corporation.)*

FIGURE 30-24 Materials for taking bite registration.

Between appointments, the temporary should look natural and be acceptable to the patient. Usually, the patient wears the temporary for seven to ten days, sometimes longer, depending on the extent of the prosthetics.

There are many types of temporary techniques and materials available (see Chapter 35, Laboratory Materials and Techniques). Some temporary crown forms are preformed, while others are custom made for each patient (Figure 30-25). The provisional must be fitted to the tooth in order to protect the margins, maintain the space, and be esthetically pleasing.

10. After trimming and contouring the temporary, it is polished and cemented with temporary cement. The dental assistant either assists the prosthodontist or makes the temporary restoration depending on the expanded functions laws. When assisting with the temporary, prepare the materials and trays as dictated by the technique. Some temporaries

FIGURE 30-25 Anterior and posterior preformed temporaries.

(continues)

PROCEDURE 30-2 *(CONTINUED)*

require crown and bridge scissors and crimping and contour pliers, while others need burs, discs, and stones to contour and finish. Transfer and receive the instruments and keep the area rinsed and dried. Once the temporary is completed, mix the temporary cement and place some in the crown. Transfer the bite stick for the patient to bite on, and then transfer a 2 × 2 gauze sponge to wipe off any excess.

11. Once the cement is dried, the bite stick is removed and a scaler is used to remove excess dry cement. Transfer dental floss to check the interproximal contacts.

12. Hold articulating paper in articulating forceps for the patient to bite on to test the bite. If adjustments are needed, transfer the low-speed handpiece with finishing burs. The patient's mouth is rinsed and evacuated before the patient is dismissed.

13. After the patient has been dismissed, the patient's impressions and models and the laboratory prescription are ready for the laboratory pickup (Figure 30-26). The following information is usually included on the laboratory prescription:

   ◾ Patient's name

   ◾ Description of the prosthesis

   ◾ Types of materials the prosthodontist wants the prosthesis to be constructed from

   ◾ Shade or shading desired

   ◾ Prosthodontist's name, license number, address, telephone number, fax number, and signature

   ◾ Date when the case will be back in the dental office

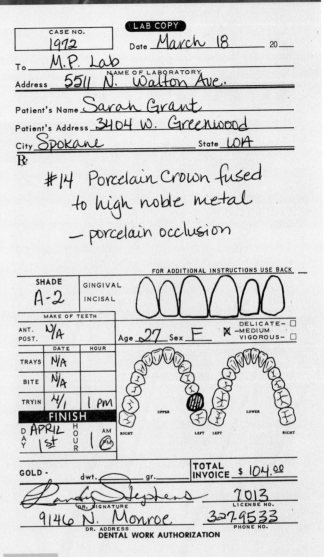

FIGURE 30-26 Laboratory prescription. *(Courtesy of Dr. Randall Stephens.)*

PROCEDURE 30-3

Cementation of Porcelain-Fused-to-Metal Crown

The following procedure is performed by the prosthodontist and the dental assistant. The temporary is removed, the permanent prosthesis is evaluated, and the final cementation is completed.

EQUIPMENT (Figure 30-27)

- Basic setup: mouth mirror, explorer, and cotton pliers
- Cotton rolls, gauze, dental floss, articulating paper, and forceps
- HVE tip, saliva ejector, and air-water syringe tip
- Low-speed handpiece with finishing burs, discs, and stones
- Anesthetic setup
- Spoon excavator and scaler
- Plastic filling instrument (PFI) and cement spatula
- Orangewood bite stick (crown remover, crown seater, and mallet are optional)
- Final cementation materials (glass ionomer cement, polycarboxylate cement, resin cements, or zinc phosphate cement)
- Porcelain-fused-to-metal crown from laboratory

FIGURE 30-27 Tray setup for cementation appointment.

PROCEDURE STEPS *(Follow aseptic procedures)*

1. The day before the patient's appointment, make sure the laboratory has completed the crown and that it is in the office.

2. Once the patient arrives for the appointment, prepare him or her and explain the treatment. Prepare the topical and local anesthetic, and then transfer the syringe and observe the patient. Once the anesthetic is placed, rinse and evacuate the mouth.

3. The provisional coverage is removed with a crown remover, scaler, and other instruments that fit under the margin of the temporary.

4. Remove the temporary, and then the excess cement. The dental assistant either assists during this stage of the procedure by transferring instruments and keeping the area clean and free of debris, or removes the temporary and excess cement as part of the expanded functions. Once the temporary is removed, rinse and dry the area and prepare the crown.

5. The cast crown is positioned on the preparation. If there is difficulty in seating the crown, a bite stick and/or mallet may be used. The occlusion, margins, and contacts are evaluated and adjustments made, if necessary. If the porcelain is adjusted, it is sent back to the laboratory to be refinished. Transfer instruments, dental floss, and articulating paper and forceps. Keep the area clean and dry and transfer the low-speed handpiece with finishing burs, discs, and stones. If the casting has to be returned to the laboratory, disinfect the crown and prepare it for return to the laboratory.

6. Before cementing the crown, the area is isolated with cotton rolls and protective liners and/or a cavity varnish is placed.

7. The permanent cement is mixed according to manufacturer's directions and placed in the crown and on the prepared tooth (Figure 30-28).

8. Prepare the permanent cement when the prosthodontist is ready and place some cement in the crown. Pass the plastic filling instrument, so the dentist can place cement on the preparation. Receive the PFI and transfer the crown and the bite stick for the patient to bite down on. Once the crown is seated on

(continues)

PROCEDURE 30-3 *(CONTINUED)*

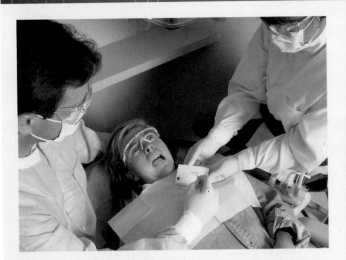

FIGURE 30-28 Dental assistant passes final cement and crown for cementation.

FIGURE 30-29 After crown is cemented permanently, excess cement is removed from margins of crown.

the tooth, the patient bites on a bite stick or crown seater until the cement hardens.

9. After the cement has hardened, remove it with a scaler, excavator, or explorer (Figure 30-29). The patient's mouth is rinsed and evacuated. Use dental floss to remove excess cement interproximally.

10. The patient is given instructions for brushing and flossing the area and told to call the office if questions or problems develop. Document the procedure and dismiss the patient.

Retention Pins

The dentist often places **retention pins** for additional retention of the core buildup. The pins are placed strategically depending on the amount of buildup needed and the type of restoration. They are placed before the core material; the core buildup material surrounds the pins (Figure 30-30).

Pins often come in kits with various sized pins, drills, and a hand driver or mechanical placement device (Figure 30-31). The drills are used in a low-speed handpiece to drill holes for the pins, which are retained in the holes.

Retention Pins in Amalgam

Retention pins also are used in an amalgam restoration for retention and support when a large surface of the tooth is being replaced. One example is replacing the distal-buccal cusp with amalgam.

Post-Retained Cores

Post-retained cores are often the treatment of choice when the tooth is nonvital and has root canal therapy (Figure 30-32). A portion of the root canal filling is

FIGURE 30-30 Pins placed in prepared tooth for support and retention.

removed and a post is fitted in the canal and cemented in place. The posts are made of materials such as titanium, titanium alloy, gold-plated metal, and stainless steel. They come in different sizes and are often purchased in a kit. The kits contain various sized posts,

FIGURE 30-31 (A) Retention pins kit. (B) Close-up of pins (maxillary restorative pins). *(Courtesy of Coltene/Whaledent, Inc.)*

drills, reamers used to prepare the tooth, and wrenches or keys for hand placement.

Once the post is fitted in the root canal, it is cemented in place. Core buildup materials are then placed around the post. The tooth is then ready for preparation of the prosthesis.

Implant Retainer Prostheses

 After six months, the dental implants have been in place long enough for substantial osseointegration. A fixed prosthesis stage can begin. Retainers that cover the implant may be a crown or part of a bridge. The abutments are fabricated in the dental laboratory and are either screw retained or cement retained (Figure 30-33).

The screw-retained prosthesis uses one screw to attach the abutment to the implant and a second screw to attach the abutment to the prosthesis. Sometimes, a composite restoration is placed over the screw for esthetic purposes.

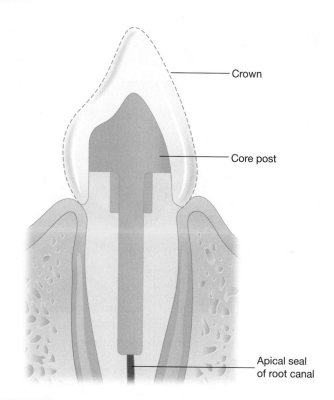

FIGURE 30-32 Core post in nonvital tooth.

The cement-retained prosthesis uses transitional cement to attach the prosthesis to the abutment. Transitional cement is used so that in case of problems with the implant, the entire system can be retrieved. The abutment is screwed into the implant like the screw-retained prosthesis.

Maintenance of Fixed Prosthodontics

The patient is given home-care instructions on how to properly maintain the new crown or bridge and is instructed to call the office if the restoration comes loose or falls out.

Fixed Prostheses Maintenance

Maintenance of the fixed prosthesis should become part of the patient's daily regimen. Brushing and flossing are continued. Depending on the patient's individual needs, various aids can assist in cleaning hard-to-reach areas. Toothbrushes should be soft and multitufted and have heads small enough to reach all areas in each quadrant. Dental floss works well under bridgework. A bridge threader can be used with the floss to clean under the pontic and along the abutment teeth. Interproximal brushes and tips are designed for removal of plaque around the fixed prosthesis.

Dental Implant Maintenance

Dental implants require maintenance just like fixed prostheses. Plaque builds up on the implant and needs to be

FIGURE 30-33 (A) Screw-retained implant prosthesis. (B) Cement-retained implant prosthesis. (C) Panoramic radiograph of dental implant on maxillary right lateral. (D) Patient's smile after the crown has been seated on the dental implant.

FIGURE 30-34 Dental floss used for dental implants.

FIGURE 30-35 Interproximal brush: one piece and handle with disposable brush.

removed routinely. The patient should be advised of the aids available, and a home-care regimen should be recommended. The toothbrush selected should be soft with multitufted nylon brush. There are numerous aids to choose from to use as adjuncts to the toothbrush, including threading systems, dental floss, interproximal brushes, water irrigators, and antimicrobial rinses.

Some dental flosses work well on dental implants or are designed specifically for implants. The floss is a wider band of ribbon to wrap around the implant and is moved in a back-and-forth motion (shoe-shine motion) (Figure 30-34).

Interproximal brushes and instruments provide easy access around the implant due to their small heads (Figures 30-35 and 30-36). The brushes and instruments must be plastic coated to prevent damaging the titanium surface of the implant. The brushes and instruments remove plaque and stimulate the gingival tissues to increase the blood flow in the surrounding areas. The interproximal brush and instrument are inserted interdentally and angled toward the occlusal or incisal surface. A gently rotating motion of the brush is suggested for around the implant, near the gingival margin.

Water irrigators are available to remove debris and plaque from around the dental implant. The patient should be advised, however, to use the irrigators at the lowest pressure setting in order to prevent damage to the tissues. The gentle spray should be directed interproximally and kept at a horizontal level along the gingival margin. The spray should not be directed into the gingival sulcus.

Antimicrobial rinses are recommended for many dental implant patients, such as chlorhexidine gluconate and phenolic compounds. The rinses are used once or twice daily depending on the type. The chlorhexidine gluconate rinses are safe and aid in the fibroblast attachment to the implant surface.

FIGURE 30-36 Plastic instruments used to clean and maintain dental implants.

ADVANCED CHAIRSIDE FUNCTIONS

Gingival Retraction

After a tooth is prepared for a crown, **gingival retraction** is done to ensure that an impression with clear margins can be obtained (Procedure 30-4). During this process, all hemorrhage must be arrested and all hard and soft tissue the operator wants to reproduce must be clean and dry. The margins ideally are supragingival, or above the gingiva, but many may be subgingival, or below the gingiva. The tissue must be retracted horizontally to allow room for sufficient impression material and displaced vertically to expose the margin completely.

Retraction cord is available in a variety of sizes, configurations, and chemical treatments (Figure 30-37). The

cord comes in a dispensing package for easy use, which may be twisted, braided, or woven to hold its shape.

Types of Gingival Retraction

Gingival retraction can be effectively accomplished by mechanical, chemical, or surgical methods. Recently, retraction systems have been used as an alternative to placing a retraction cord.

Mechanical Retraction

Mechanical retraction can be accomplished in a number of ways. Without the use of drugs, tissue shrinkage or hemostasis will not be accomplished; however, the tissue can be displaced to allow access to the margin. Retraction cord is placed in the sulcus of healthy and inflamed free gingiva. The cotton cord is left in place for ten to fifteen minutes (instead of the five minutes as it would be with the chemical retraction cord).

If any of the cords is placed too deep, the crevice opens at the bottom but is narrow at the top (Figure 30-38A). The operator may be able to get the impression material into the crevice after the cord is removed, but the material has a tendency to fracture near the edge of the preparation. If the cord is placed too shallow in the crevice, the space is inadequate to allow an accurate reproduction of the margin of the preparation (Figure 30-38B). The proper position of the tucked cord is 1 to 3 mm into the V-shaped crevice (Figure 30-38C). The dentist may want two cords placed to retract the gingival tissues. The crevice is V shaped, and this dictates the size of cords to use. The smaller cords are placed at the depth of the crevice, and the larger cord is placed on top (Figure 30-38D).

Another means of mechanical retraction is accomplished by lengthening a temporary crown form to cause tissue displacement and taking the impression at a later date. Another method uses a dental dam clamp and rubber dam to displace the tissue. The clamp and rubber dam are placed and then removed just before taking the final impression. Both of these techniques may cause the tissue to bleed and the impression to be distorted.

Retraction Systems

Gingival retraction systems are now available that offer alternatives to placing a retraction cord. These systems use a silicone material that is placed to retract the gingival tissues; aluminum chloride has been added to the material to prevent bleeding and

(A)

(B)

FIGURE 30-37 (A) Various types of retraction cords. (B) Tissue management gel kit. *(Courtesy of Pascal, Co., Inc.)*

ADVANCED CHAIRSIDE FUNCTIONS

Cord placed too deep in sulcus

(A)

Cord placed too shallow in sulcus

(B)

Proper cord position

(C)

Tucking additional cords, if necessary

(D)

FIGURE 30-38 (A) Retraction cord placed at root depth. (B) Retraction cord placed too shallow. (C) Retraction cord. (D) Double retraction cords placed properly.

crevicular seepage. The material is rigid enough to create a space between the tooth and tissue to expose subgingival margins and keep the area dry. The paste is dispensed into the sulcus with enough material to fill it. It is left in place for one to two minutes, and then rinsed before the final impression is taken (Figure 30-39A and B).

The material comes in a cartridge or capsule and is dispensed with a mixing/dispensing gun. Little pressure is needed to place the material, so the risk of trauma to the epithelial attachment is reduced. The dispensing cartridge makes placement easy and saves time compared to placing a retraction cord.

Chemical Retraction

Chemical retraction may be performed prior to placement of the cord, by impregnating the cord and then placing it, or both. One of the newer ways is to use a topical hemostatic solution, astringent with dento-infusion tubes, and a plastic Luer-Lok syringe. The solution is placed using a disposable metal tip bent to the desired area. As the solution is placed, the blood and the solution merge together and are washed away with the air-water syringe. What is left in the tissue is a temporary coagulum seal that does not allow any seepage. The tissue may appear slightly darkened, but this technique allows hemorrhage to be arrested. A retraction

FIGURE 30-39 (A) Expasyl material kit. (B–F) Steps for placing syringe-type gingival retraction cord. (*Courtesy of Kerr Corporation.*)

ADVANCED CHAIRSIDE FUNCTIONS

cord of interwoven cotton with or without solution is packed vertically to expose the prepared margin. This packing of the cord allows for horizontal retraction to allow for sufficient bulk of impression material to flow around the margin.

The retraction cord could also be impregnated with aluminum chloride or astringent of aluminum salts for chemical retraction. This technique causes a shrinking of the tissues, or *ischemia*, to obtain clear access to the margin of the preparation. A substance used to obtain this result is epinephrine, which is an astringent and a vasoconstrictor. It provides hemostasis and shrinks the tissues by constricting the blood vessels. Epinephrine brings on an increase in the heartbeat, or tachycardia, for the patient. The epinephrine definitely is contraindicated for a patient with heart disease, diabetes, or hyperthyroidism, or when taking certain drugs.

Note: The dental assistant should watch for patients who exhibit hypertension, knowing that most hyperthyroid and diabetic patients are usually hypertensive. Normally, the dentist prefers to use chemical retraction cord, so the patient's medical history should be reviewed carefully.

Surgical Retraction

Instead of retraction, the dentist may choose to remove the tissue around the preparation. This approach is accomplished by using a surgical knife or by performing electrosurgery. With the surgical knife, the dentist excises the tissue and exposes the margin of the preparation. The area where the tissue has been removed may bleed and cause additional treatment in order to get a good impression of the area.

The dentist may decide to use an electrosurgery unit, which cauterizes the tissues as it removes them. Therefore, the tissue is removed without bleeding. The unit passes high-frequency current to a small electrode passing through the tissue. The tip of the unit appears as a metal wire or loop. As the tip touches the tissue, the unit is activated to remove the tissue. It is especially important with this treatment that soft tissue anesthesia is maintained. Electrosurgery is not used with patients who are receiving radiation therapy, have cardiac pacemakers, or have any diseases that slow healing.

Constant use of a nonmetal HVE tip during the surgery is important due to the odor given off as the tissues are cauterized. The evacuator reduces the odor if it is placed near the surgical site. After the tissue is removed, the sulcus is cleaned with a hydrogen rinse. Immediately following the procedure, the final impression is taken.

PROCEDURE 30-4

Placing and Removing Retraction Cord

This procedure is performed by the dentist or the expanded-function dental assistant. After the tooth has been prepared, the retraction cord is placed. The equipment and supplies are included as part of the crown/bridge tray setup. Specific items needed to place and remove the retraction cord are listed.

EQUIPMENT (Figure 30-40)

- Basic setup: mouth mirror, explorer, cotton pliers
- HVE tip and air-water syringe tip
- Scissors
- Hemostat
- Retraction cord(s)

- Retraction cord placement instrument or plastic instrument
- Cotton rolls, 2 × 2 gauze sponges

PROCEDURE STEPS *(Follow aseptic procedures)*

1. The dentist prepares the tooth for the crown.

2. Rinse and dry the area in preparation for placement of the retraction cord.

3. Cotton rolls are placed on the facial and, if mandibular, on the lingual surface. The area is carefully dried.

(continues)

ADVANCED CHAIRSIDE FUNCTIONS

PROCEDURE 30-4 (CONTINUED)

FIGURE 30-40 Placing and removing retraction cord tray setup.

FIGURE 30-41 Retraction cord looped around prepared tooth for placement in gingival sulcus.

4. The dentist selects the retraction cord(s) to be placed around the tooth.

5. The length of the cord needed is determined by the circumference of the prepared tooth. *Note:* The desired length is determined by wrapping the cord around the small finger for an anterior tooth and around a larger finger for a molar.

6. The cord is cut to the appropriate length.

7. Twist the cord ends to compress the fibers together.

8. The cord is looped and placed in a hemostat or cotton pliers.

9. The cord is looped around the margin of the prepared tooth and tightened slightly (Figure 30-41). This aids in slipping the cord into the sulcus area. Normally, the ends of the cord are toward the buccal surface for easy access.

10. The hemostat or cotton pliers is/are released, leaving the cord in the sulcus.

11. The retraction cord is packed into position with a packing instrument or a plastic instrument.

12. The cord is gently packed around the cervical area, apical to the preparation.

13. The cord is packed around the tooth and overlaps, usually on the facial surface.

14. A tip of the cord is left showing out of the sulcus in order for easy removal just before taking the impression (Figure 30-42).

15. The retraction cord is left in place for five minutes when chemical retraction cord is used, and for ten to fifteen minutes for mechanical retraction.

16. The end of the retraction cord is grasped and removed in a circular motion just before the impression material being placed.

FIGURE 30-42 Retraction cord around prepared tooth with tag left out for easy removal.

CHAPTER SUMMARY

Fixed prosthodontics encompasses replacement of missing teeth or parts of teeth with extensive restorations. There are many types of fixed prostheses and a variety of materials used for preparation, fabrication, and cementation. The dental assistant is involved in all stages of fixed prosthodontic treatment. It is important to understand the sequence of the procedure and the various types of restorations when assisting the dentist.

The goal of this chapter is to assess the more common procedures to give the dental assistant the back-ground and sequence to assist the dentist. Restorations routinely take at least two appointments to complete. The assistant explains the steps of the procedure to the patient, answers questions, and provides postoperative and home care instructions.

Gingival retraction is an important step when preparing the tooth for the final impression. Margins of the preparations must be exposed so that the impression will reflect an accurate image of the tooth and preparation, and thus that the fixed prosthesis will fit perfectly. Learning about the various materials and techniques helps the dental assistant become more skilled when working with the dentist.

Case Study

Ann Arthur is unhappy with the appearance of her anterior teeth. The maxillary and mandibular incisors are a dull, medium-yellow shade. There is a slight diastema (space) between the maxillary central incisors. Ann has considered treatment for several years and has scheduled an appointment for next week. She has dental insurance through her husband's insurance plan.

Case Study Review

1. What are the two concerns Ann has about her anterior teeth?

2. What treatment options are available?

3. Once a treatment plan is in place, how might financial information, such as insurance, be considered by the business staff?

REVIEW QUESTIONS

Multiple Choice

1. Which of the following prosthetic restorations covers only the area between the cusps on the occlusal surface of the tooth?
   a. Three-quarter crown
   b. Inlay restoration
   c. Onlay restoration
   d. Veneer restoration

2. The dental bridge part that replaces the missing tooth is called the
   a. abutment.
   b. pontic.
   c. connector.
   d. retainer.

3. Materials used to fabricate crowns and bridges include all of the following *except*
   a. gold alloy.
   b. porcelain.
   c. composite resin.
   d. amalgam.

4. During the preparation appointment, the retraction cord is
   a. placed after the tooth is prepared but before the final impressions are taken.
   b. placed after the final impressions are taken.
   c. placed before the tooth is prepared.
   d. placed with the temporary restoration.

5. All of the following materials are needed during the preparation appointment *except*
   a. alginate.
   b. gingival retraction cord.
   c. bonding agent.
   d. temporary cement.

6. If a tooth is badly broken down, all of the following methods are used to add the needed support *except*
   a. glass ionomer cement base.
   b. core build-up.
   c. retention pins.
   d. post-retained cores.

7. All of the following are types of veneers *except*
   a. direct resin veneers.
   b. indirect resin veneers.
   c. direct glass ionomer veneers.
   d. porcelain veneers.

8. Which of the following materials is *not* used to take the final impression after the tooth is prepared?
   a. Polysiloxane
   b. Alginate
   c. Hydrocolloid
   d. Silicone impression materials

9. How many types of gingival retraction are used in fixed prosthodontic procedures?
   a. Two
   b. Three
   c. Five
   d. Six

10. Which type of gingival retraction is accomplished by placement of a retraction cord?
    a. Mechanical
    b. Chemical
    c. Surgical
    d. None of the above

Critical Thinking

1. Which expanded functions in your state relate to fixed prosthodontic procedures?

2. Name the restoration types that are fabricated of gold alloy, porcelain fused to metal, or porcelain.

3. Name possible techniques for building up a crown that is badly broken down.

4. Discuss what happens if the retraction cord is placed too deep in the sulcus.

5. Explain why the dentist may place additional retraction cord in the sulcus before the final impression is taken.

Web Activities

1. Go to http://www.aaid-implant.org to determine if you are a candidate for a dental implant.

2. For more information on cosmetic dentistry, go to http://www.ada.org.

3. Go to http://www.gingi-pak.com and continue in the area of technical help and techniques. Locate retraction techniques in this area. List three techniques for cord packing identified on this web page.

4. Find the lastest updates on the CEREC CAD/CAM system at http://www.cerec.net or http://www.sirona.com.

CHAPTER 31

COSMETIC DENTISTRY AND TEETH WHITENING

SPECIFIC INSTRUCTIONAL OBJECTIVES

The student should strive to meet the following objectives and demonstrate an understanding of the facts and principles presented in this chapter:

1. Define cosmetic dentistry and describe what is involved in cosmetic dentistry.

2. Describe who performs cosmetic dentistry and education requirements.

3. Explain the role of the dental assistant in cosmetic dentistry.

4. Explain the scope of cosmetic dentistry.

5. Describe fundamental principles that the cosmetic dentist must learn when creating the perfect smile.

6. Discuss the basic elements of psychology and sociology that are considered for cosmetic treatment.

7. Explain what the patient should consider when selecting a dentist for cosmetic treatment.

8. Identify and describe specific procedures performed in cosmetic dentistry, including diagnosis and treatment planning, legal forms, and documentation.

9. Describe the role that oral photography has in cosmetic dentistry, the equipment needed, and how the patient is set up for the photographs to be taken.

10. Describe why soft tissue surgery may be needed in cosmetic dentistry, how it is performed, and how lasers and electrosurgery are involved.

11. Explain why the dental team needs to know about occlusion in cosmetic dentistry.

12. Describe the types of restorations that are placed and materials used for cosmetic restorations.

13. Describe the marketing techniques for cosmetic dentistry.

ADVANCED CHAIRSIDE FUNCTIONS

14. Explain how teeth are whitened, and causes of intrinsic and extrinsic tooth staining.

15. Explain the benefits of whitening techniques used in dentistry.

16. Describe the role of the dental assistant in the whitening process.

17. List and describe types of whitening techniques.

18. Describe the procedures for dental office whitening for vital and nonvital teeth, and for home whitening and over-the-counter whitening materials.

19. Explain information given to the patient about outcomes, procedure, responsibilities, and precautions related to teeth whitening.

OUTLINE *(continued)*

KEY TERMS

INTRODUCTION

The search for means of enhancing the appearance of teeth dates at least to the Phoenicians in 800 BC. Carved animal tusks to resemble the shape, form, and hue of natural teeth were used as pontics to improve the appearance of their teeth. In the seventeenth century, gold shell crowns with enamel "veneers" were developed for improving esthetics. In the same century, a tooth powder was used to whiten teeth.

Porcelain teeth were first manufactured in the early part of the nineteenth century, while various techniques for esthetic crowns such as open-face crowns, porcelain jackets, and the three-quarter crowns were developed later. In 1904, the first truly cosmetic restorative material was developed, a combination of acid-soluble glass blended with a liquid containing phosphoric acid. Shortly thereafter, a chemically activated acrylic resin was developed and acrylic veneer facings were widely used. In the 1970s, composite resins almost completely replaced acrylic resins. Since that time, numerous refinements of the basic formula of resin matrix and glass filler have been introduced, and new and improved products are continually placed on the market. With the advancement of various materials and inventive techniques, cosmetic dentistry is increasingly popular.

Research continues, study groups are formed, continuing education courses/seminars are offered, and societies and journals are dedicated to cosmetic dentistry. Everyone wants a beautiful smile, and dentistry has changed from a need-based treatment to an elective-based treatment.

In this chapter, various aspects of **cosmetic dentistry** are discussed, but details and procedures on the various types of crowns and veneers are included in Chapter 30, Fixed Prosthodontics. Cosmetic dentistry also includes some orthodontic treatments (Chapter 27, Orthodontics) and oral surgery procedures (Chapter 25, Oral and Maxillofacial Surgery). If a patient requires either orthodontics or oral surgery, these become part of the treatment plan and are completed before cosmetic dentistry procedures are performed.

Cosmetic Dentist and Staff

The general dentist and prosthodontist perform many procedures that are part of cosmetic dentistry. Courses, seminars, and institutes on "smile designs or enhancements" provide extended training, both through lecture and clinical practice. Upon completing this training, dentists and staff members receive a certificate.

Established in 1984, the **American Academy of Cosmetic Dentistry (AACD)** is the largest international dental organization dedicated to the art and science of cosmetic dentistry. Members from all over the world include cosmetic and reconstructive dentists, dental laboratory technicians, educators, researchers, dental students, hygienists, corporations, and dental auxiliaries. To keep up-to-date with ongoing advancements in cosmetic dentistry, the AACD offers continued education through workshops, lectures, and publications. Dentists and their staff may also belong to local study clubs to provide support and updated information on products and techniques.

Two advanced credentialing programs are offered through the American Academy of Cosmetic Dentistry: Accreditation and Fellowship. To become an accredited member, the dentist must take continuing education courses and pass an examination process. This process includes a written exam and a clinical exam, in which the dentist submits clinical casework. Once the dentist successfully passes the written and clinical exams and becomes an accredited member of the AACD, she or he may choose to continue the pursuit of clinical education and fellowship. Fellowship is achieved when the dentist submits fifty clinical cases that exhibit competency in cosmetic dentistry.

Dental Staff

The staff of the dentist who performs cosmetic dentistry is similar to the staff of any dental office: front office personnel, business office staff, chairside assistants, and dental hygienists. Each member of the team plays an important part in the process of enhancing the appearance of a person's smile.

Office personnel ensure that the patient is scheduled in a convenient and timely manner. They also are the first to greet the patient and the last the patient sees before leaving the office. Their contact with the patient should be friendly and reassuring so that the patient is comfortable and confident in the treatment.

The business office staff will want to be familiar with the various dental insurance plans so that they can effectively communicate with the insurance companies. These staff members are also responsible for making financial arrangement with the patient that will work for both the dentist and the patient. Most dental offices cannot accept long-term payments for services rendered. Currently, dental offices are often affiliated with banks and savings and loan institutions and recommend that the patient make financial arrangements through them.

At chairside the assistant works with the dentist during cosmetic procedures that often include many expanded functions, such as placing and removing the rubber dam, taking detailed impressions, and creating esthetic temporaries for the patient to wear between treatments. The assistant is available to answer the patient's questions and provide reassurance and positive support throughout the procedure. The dental assistant may also accompany the dentist in additional training seminars, courses, and workshops, and therefore is knowledgeable about assisting with specific techniques and preparing various materials. Because they are close to both the dentist and patient, assistants may be involved in designing the right smile for a specific person (Figure 31-1).

FIGURE 31-1 Dental assistant talking to patient about cosmetic dentistry.

Dental hygienists often provide the patient with available options for improving the appearance of their teeth. They also speak with patients during hygiene treatment and learn about their desires regarding appearance. The hygienist can educate the patient about individual oral health needs and motivate them to talk to the dentist and other staff members. The hygienist may also be involved in providing oral hygiene care with detailed prophylaxis, fluoride treatments, and home-care instructions.

Scope of Cosmetic/Esthetic Dentistry

The scope of cosmetic/esthetic dentistry is very broad and diversified. General dentistry includes many aspects that we now consider to be part of "cosmetic dentistry," which sometimes makes the concept of this type of dental practice confusing. Most dentists do some cosmetic dentistry, but to be a "cosmetic dentist" the dentist needs continuing education at the postgraduate level and additional credentialing as mentioned previously.

Many procedures are included in cosmetic/esthetic dentistry. The cosmetic dentist performs some of these, and others are completed by various specialty dentists, including the orthodontist, periodontist, oral and maxillofacial surgeon, and prosthodontist. Selected cosmetic procedures are listed below:

- Bridges and crowns (Chapter 30, Fixed Prosthodontics).
- Veneers (Chapter 30, Fixed Prosthodontics).
- Tooth whitening (current chapter).
- Repositioning or straightening the teeth (orthodontics), including accelerated orthodontics (Chapter 27, Orthodontics).
- Lengthening the teeth (involves removal of gingival tissue with a laser and electrosurgery unit or scalpel). A periodontist often performs this stage of treatment (Chapter 29, Periodontics).
- Recontouring the gingival tissues (Chapter 29, Periodontics).
- Restoring length to crowns of the teeth. (Chapter 29, Periodontics).
- Changing bite relationships (Chapter 27, Orthodontics).
- Closing gaps (diastema) (Chapter 30, Fixed Prosthodontics).
- Repairing chips or fractures (Chapter 34, Restorative Materials, Dental Dam, Matrix, and Wedge).
- Changing shape and shade of the teeth (Chapter 30, Fixed Prosthodontics).
- Replacing old metal restorations with cosmetic restorations (Chapter 34, Restorative Materials, Dental Dam, Matrix, and Wedge).
- Replacing missing teeth with dental implants (Chapter 25, Oral and Maxillofacial Surgery).
- Dentures (Chapter 32, Removable Prosthodontics).
- Endodontic procedures (Chapter 24, Endodontics).

Cosmetic dentistry includes many procedures that improve patients' smile, appearance, and how they feel about their teeth. All of the listed treatments are covered in other chapters of this book (excepting whitening); this chapter focuses on cosmetic dentistry as compared to general dentistry. Figures 31-2 and 31-3 illustrate before and after results of cosmetic dentistry treatment designs.

Fundamentals of Cosmetic Dentistry

The cosmetic dentist looks at the entire picture of the patient's teeth and gingival tissues. Everything is taken into consideration, including the light, color, illusion, shape, and form to create a more esthetic whole than the original. In the following sections, aspects considered by the cosmetic dentist and staff are briefly described.

Light

Natural light must be used when selecting the shade of the teeth. Natural light is multidirectional, casting shadows and showing texture. Dental restoration can be manipulated to cast a shadow and provide a feeling of depth to match adjacent teeth.

Color

There is much to learn about principles of color and how color is interpreted. **Hue** is the color per se (e.g., bright white, beige, yellow). Younger permanent teeth appear to be similar in color throughout the mouth, but as the person ages and the teeth pick up intrinsic and extrinsic stains from smoking, foods, and restorative materials, hue will vary throughout the mouth. **Chroma** is the intensity or quality of the hue. Thus, to increase the chroma of a veneer, more color (hue) is added. The chroma of teeth responds to tooth whitening in both vital and nonvital teeth. **Value** corresponds to brightness, which is very important when matching shades.

FIGURE 31-2 (A) Patient with a large diastema between the central incisors. (B) Same patient after ceramic crowns have been placed to close the diastema. *(Courtesy of Chameleon Dental Products, Inc.)*

FIGURE 31-3 (A) Patient wanting to improve her smile. (B) The teeth are badly stained. (C) Patient after cosmetic dentistry with a beautiful smile. (D) Close-up of the cosmetic crowns. *(Courtesy of Dr. Steven Crump.)*

The dentist and lab technician strive to match primary, secondary, and complementary hues. Often a variety of lights are used in color selection for a patient. In the dental treatment room, three lights can be used: the overhead light, usually a white fluorescent light, natural light from a window, and the dental unit light.

The dentist also must consider the **opacity** and **translucency** of a material. Opaque materials reflect light, and thus do not permit light to pass through. For instance, an extra layer of opaque porcelain is applied in a porcelain-fused-to-metal crown to prevent metal from showing through the crown. Translucent materials are the opposite—they allow light to pass through. Translucency of crowns and veneers makes them appear more natural.

Illusion

Illusion is the art of making something appear to be different than it actually is. Teeth can be made to appear larger or smaller and of various shapes through illusion. An artistic principle is that light areas appear to be closer or highlighted, whereas dark areas appear to recede. Manipulating light in this fashion will give the tooth dimension (depth) along with length and width (Figure 31-4).

Another aspect of illusion concerns the horizontal and vertical dimensions. Horizontal lines make the tooth appear to be wider while vertical lines make the tooth appear longer (Figure 31-5). This phenomenon is analogous to a person wearing horizontal- versus vertical-striped clothing; horizontal stripes tend to make a person appear shorter and wider while vertical stripes make a person look taller and thinner.

Shape and Form

In cosmetic dentistry, a tooth is viewed in an environment of other teeth. We perceive certain qualities about a tooth based on individual and cultural assumptions. For instance, many people assume that stained, heavily worn, and dark teeth belong to an older person. We have cultural and artistic biases on how we perceive a person's teeth, which include gender-based features of the teeth and how the teeth are proportioned. For example, women's teeth are often perceived as more

FIGURE 31-4 Photograph showing the principle of illumination. The light side comes forward while the dark side recedes. *(Courtesy of Photo Disc.)*

FIGURE 31-5 Drawing of tooth with horizontal lines and tooth with vertical lines, which shows illusion of length and width, respectively.

rounded and translucent, while men's are more angled with a squared incisal edge (Figure 31-6). The cosmetic dentist can esthetically restore a person's teeth to persuade the eye of the observer that the latter conform to such biases.

FIGURE 31-6 (A) Feminine teeth: rounded. (B) Masculine teeth: square.

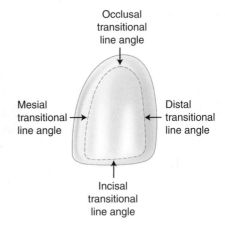

FIGURE 31-7 Face of tooth showing transitional lines.

The dentist can change the apparent size and shape of a tooth by shaping its face, the area on the facial surface that is flat and not running over onto the mesial or distal, incisal, or gingival surfaces. **Transitional line angles** surround the tooth and mark the boundaries of the face (Figure 31-7). Shaping the face of one tooth or several teeth to match each other will give the illusion that they are the same size and shape.

Cosmetic Dentistry and Psychology

Understanding a patient's feelings concerning their appearance and the appearance of their teeth is important. Knowledge of the patient's personality, motivations, desires, and expectations, and ability to accept change and cooperate will enhance and even determine the success of dental treatment. The dentist and dental team should be aware of Maslow's hierarchy of needs (see Chapter 2, Psychology, Communication, and Multicultural Interaction), as well as a general appreciation for the principles of psychology and sociology.

Psychological Influences

Psychological influences require learning about the patient's personality, and his or her motivations, desires, and expectations. Trust between dentist and patient, which requires that the dentist/dental team communicate empathetically and with a sincere desire to understand the patient and his or her dental cosmetic goals. Some dentists prefer the informal process of getting to know the patient's personality, which includes an interview and observation of the patient, while others prefer using questionnaires or personality tests.

Sometimes the dentist learns from the personality evaluation that the patient may need a family member to assist him or her in making decisions and to provide support during treatment. This person will be involved in all communications and may also come to appointments in which esthetic decisions are involved.

Psychological Environment. As it is true for all dental treatment, the need for a human touch is especially true for cosmetic treatment. Patients should feel that the entire office staff (or at least the individuals with whom he or she has contact) sincerely care about their welfare and are concerned with their dental treatment. The dentist and office staff should handle patients with respect and dignity throughout the treatment process. This is reflected in making patients comfortable, respecting their privacy, and being considerate of their time and schedules (Figure 31-8).

Sociological Influences

A number of social contemporary trends encourage individuals to seek esthetic dental treatment. The visual media (e.g., television, magazines, and advertising) exert a major influence on perceptions and attitudes about appearance. People are barraged with information on a daily basis about teeth whiting, veneers, orthodontic treatment, cosmetic surgery, and so on, and how much better they will feel and look once they partake in such services.

With escalating health care costs, many people are becoming more interested in disease prevention, and thus on maintaining health and fitness. The dental profession also endorses preventive care and clinical focus has shifted from caries to maintenance of oral health and esthetics. Meanwhile, people have become more involved in their medical/dental treatment, and they expect to participate and understand their options in order to make informed decisions.

How a Patient Selects a Cosmetic Dentist

If a patient is unhappy with the appearance or color of his teeth or avoids smiling because of embarrassment about his teeth, he may be a candidate for cosmetic dentistry. A smile makeover can change a person's whole outlook on life and with this enhance self-confidence and self-esteem.

Finding a cosmetic dentist who understands the type of results a patient wishes to achieve is important. Good communication between the dentist/dental team and the patient is key to successful cosmetic treatment. The American Academy of Cosmetic Dentistry suggests that the patient look for a dentist who is skilled in cosmetic dentistry procedures. Patients are encouraged to consult with the dentist to identify the right procedures to meet goals (Figure 31-9). Several areas that the patient should consider when selecting a cosmetic dentist are listed below.

- Get a referral—ask friends and family about the type and quality of care the dentist has provided.

- Ask the dentist for credentials on cosmetic dentistry. Has she or he completed continuing education courses to remain up-to-date on the latest techniques in clinical cosmetic dentistry?

- Examine before and after pictures—ask the dentist for such photographs of other patients who have completed cosmetic dental treatment in his or her office.

The patient might also consider the availability of appointments, that is, whether the office schedule is compatible with his or her timeframe. In addition, the patient should ask about how a patient is scheduled if a problem occurs or adjustment needs to be made.

Another consideration is available financial arrangements and options for payments. The patient should determine office policy, requirements, and communication responsibilities upon working with his or her insurance company.

FIGURE 31-8 Open, friendly, private, and caring office reception area. *(Courtesy of Dr. Charles Regaldo.)*

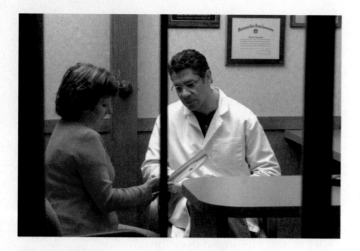

FIGURE 31-9 Patient interviewing cosmetic dentist. *(Courtesy of Dr. Charles Regaldo.)*

Procedures in Cosmetic Dentistry

Before any dental treatment begins, the dentist should thoroughly discuss with patients their expectations and esthetic desires. This discussion should include a history, as well as the patient's attitude towards previous treatments. These first steps can facilitate success of the cosmetic treatment by establishing clear and open communication between the patient and the dentist and dental staff. Patients need to explain their concerns with the appearance of their teeth in as much detail as possible. The dentist may inform the patient of ways that the appearance of their teeth can be enhanced, with the use of before and after pictures, models, videos, computer programs, and pamphlets (Figure 31-10).

Diagnosis and Treatment Planning

Listed below are items needed for the diagnostic records before a treatment plan can be designed for an individual patient.

- Medical and dental history
- Full-mouth x-rays
- Panoramic radiographs
- Periodontal charting
- Examination of existing restorations
- Occlusal analysis
- Study models
- Photographic series

Once all information is gathered, the dentist reviews it and designs a treatment plan. An appointment is set up with the patient for the case presentation. During the case presentation the dentist and staff members must educate the patient about oral health requirements for cosmetic dental treatment. With the use of visual aids, such as study models, photographs, and dental radiographs, the dentist can inform the patient about what needs to be done to attain his or her desired results. At this time the dentist explains to the patient everything involved in the treatment plan. Sometimes the patient needs to be referred to a specialist for treatment before cosmetic treatment actually begins. Once the patient understands what is involved in the treatment, the dentist and staff must motivate the patient to accept and make financial arrangements to pay for the treatment.

Legal Forms and Documentation

Because cosmetic dentistry involves increased risk, following a specific format with every patient is important. Legal forms should accurately describe the treatment and the expected outcome. The patient should sign a consent form that is specifically designed for the dentist and the expected treatment (Figure 31-11).

The dentist and staff must determine whether the patient fails to realize the limitations of dentistry. Special precautions must be taken by dentists who practice primarily cosmetic dentistry because subjective opinions about treatment results may determine whether a patient files a lawsuit. See Chapter 36, Dental Office Management for more information on consent and informed consent.

Careful and detailed documentation should be routine procedure for all treatments. Examples of information that should be documented are listed below.

- A detailed treatment plan was given to the patient, the patient signed a consent form before treatment began, and the patient was informed about all the risks and benefits of treatment.

- Comments made by the patient during the case presentation or course of treatment that indicate concerns or doubts.

- Adverse occurrences or problems that arose during the course of treatment.

- Request for consultation with other health care practitioners.

- Cancellations, late arrivals, and changes of appointments.

- Evidence that the patient did not follow the treatment plan involving dental specialists, such as orthodontic treatment or periodontal surgery required before cosmetic treatment can begin.

- Instances in which the patient did not follow home-care instructions.

Oral Photography

Oral photography is a new skill that many cosmetic dentists must acquire. The digital or 35-mm camera has become an indispensable piece of equipment in the cosmetic practice. Although the use of film as a storage medium has declined (due to use of computers, digital camers, and printers), at present conventional photography produces a clearer and higher-quality photograph.

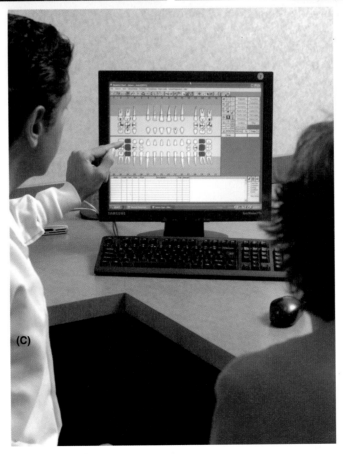

FIGURE 31-10 Everything needed for cosmetic case presentation: medical/dental history. (A) Photographs. (B) X-rays, panoramic x-ray. (C) Periodontal and restoration chart and occlusal evaluation. *(Courtesy of Dr. Charles Regaldo.)*

(A)

Consent to Dental Treatment

I, (print name) _____ have been

informed by Dr. (print name) _____ , of the need to

undergo dental treatment as presented to me on _____ .

I have been fully informed about the details of the recommended treatment and alternatives, and agree to accept the treatment as recommended by the doctor.

I understand that as the treatment proceeds there may be need to change the treatment plan. If this occurs I expect to be informed before any change is instituted.

I further understand that individual reactions to treatment cannot be predicted, and that if I experience any unanticipated reactions during or following any treatment, I agree to report them to the office as soon as possible.

I have been told that the success of the recommended treatment depends upon my cooperation in keeping scheduled appointments, following home care instruction, including oral hygiene and dietary instructions, and reporting to the office any change in my health status as soon as possible.

I have discussed all of the above with the doctor, and all my questions have been answered.

I acknowledge that no guarantees or assurances have been given by anyone as to the results that may be obtained.

Following the explanation, the discussion, and the answers to my questions, I authorize the doctor to complete the treatment as described.

_____   _____
Patient's Signature   If a Minor, Signature of Parent Or Guardian

_____   _____
Witness Signature   Doctor's Signature

_____
Date

FIGURE 31-11 (A) Consent to dental treatment form.   *(continues)*

(B)

Request for Release of Health Information

I, (print name) _____, hereby grant

permission to (print name of doctor or hospital) _____

to release information related to my health history, status, and treatment, and copies of my health

record, X-rays, and any test results to:

_____

At _____

_____

Signature _____ Date _____

(if a minor, parent or guardian must sign)

(C)

Permission to Take Photographs, Slides, & Videos

I, (print name) _____ , hereby

authorize Dr. (print name) _____ to take

photographs, slides, and/or videos of my face, jaws, and teeth.

I understand that the photographs, slides, and/or videos will be used as a record of my care, and may be used for educational purposes in lectures, demonstrations, and professional publications.

I further understand that if the photographs, slides, and/or videos are used in any publication, or as part of a demonstration, reasonable attempts will be made to conceal my identity.

_____   _____
Patient's Signature   If a Minor, Signature of Parent Or Guardian

_____   _____
Witness Signature   Doctor's Signature

_____
Date

FIGURE 31-11 *(continues)* (B) Request for release of health information form. (C) Permission form.

Uses of Oral Photography

- Case presentation—Close-up photographs should be taken before any dental treatment begins. These photos are used during the case presentation to explain the proposed treatment plan to the patient. These photos can also be used with a portfolio of before and after photographs of similar, successfully treated cases. Photographs are also taken once the treatment is complete.

- Patient records—Before and after photographs are kept as part of the patient's records. The dentist should have the patient sign a release form so the photographs can be used in office displays and in case presentations.

- Laboratory communication—Oral photographs give the dental laboratory technician another means of visualizing desired treatment outcomes for the patient.

- Insurance—Treatment plans may have a better chance of acceptance if photographs accompany insurance claims. Photographs will display certain things that are not evident on radiographs. Insurance programs may reimburse the patient for the cost of the photographs just as radiographs are covered.

- Quality control—A magnified image sometimes shows things that are not evident by viewing the patient. Photographs also are used by the dentist when she is studying a case in the patient's absence.

- Marketing and education—Before and after photographs are a wonderful marketing tool. The photographs can be displayed in the office or in pamphlets, newsletters, and so on that advertise a particular dentist's work. Photographs can also be used when the dentist is lecturing, sharing information at study clubs, or conferring with other dentists or dental specialists.

Basic Equipment for Dental Photography

The basic equipment necessary for taking quality photographs includes a 35-mm SLR camera, digital cameras, macro lens, flash unit to obtain proper lighting, film that is suitable for dental exposures, a variety of shapes and sizes of frontal surface glass mirrors to produce a clear view, and lip and cheek retractors (Figures 31-12 and 31-13). Some dental offices have a special area set up for photographs, while in others the photographs are taken when the patient is seated in the dental chair (Figure 31-14).

FIGURE 31-13 Various mirrors and cheek retractors used to take oral photographs of maxillary and mandibular arches.

FIGURE 31-14 Area in dental office where photographs are taken.

FIGURE 31-12 Camera used to take photographs in preparation for cosmetic dentistry.

FIGURE 31-15 Photograph of full-face view with (A) with the lips closed and (B) the patient smiling.

FIGURE 31-16 Photograph of side-face (profile) view.

FIGURE 31-17 Photograph of maxillary occlusal view.

Extraoral Techniques

Two views of the patient are necessary: full face view, in which the patient is seated with the head positioned looking straight ahead with the line from the ala of the nose to the tragus of the ear parallel to the floor (Figure 31-15); and a profile view, in which the patient's head is positioned showing one side of the face (the profile) with the ala of the nose to the tragus of the ear parallel to the floor (Figure 31-16).

Intraoral Techniques

Intraoral techniques involve using retraction means and mirrors. The anterior or frontal view, which can be taken with the use of cheek and lip retractors, shows the entire anterior dentition. Sometimes a more relaxed, casual view is also taken; in this photograph, a natural smile line with the teeth exposed (retractors are not used).

The maxillary occlusal and mandibular occlusal views are difficult to expose. The patient is positioned in a semi-upright position with his or her mouth open. Usually one assistant holds the lip and cheek retractors in the patient's mouth while another assistant positions the mirror so that it is resting on the maxillary tuberosity (Figure 31-17).

The mandibular occlusal view is the reverse of the maxillary occlusal view; the patient is positioned in the supine position parallel to the floor. The head is tilted back and the occlusal plane is parallel to the floor. One assistant places the retractors and another positions the mirror to rest on the retromolar pad (Figure 31-18).

The buccal views and lingual views are taken using mirrors and lip retractors. The buccal views are ideal for showing the patient's centric occlusion and bite relationship, while the lingual views show the lingual right or left side of the maxillary or mandibular arch (Figure 31-19).

FIGURE 31-18 Photograph of mandibular occlusal view.

FIGURE 31-19 (A) Buccal view. (B) Lingual view.

Contouring Soft Tissues in Cosmetic Dentistry

Cosmetic dental treatment may also include contouring of the soft tissues. As part of the evaluation, the dentist will examine and probe the gingival tissues and sulcus. The appearance of the gingival tissues is just as important as other elements in the mouth for achieving a pleasing smile.

Indications for Treatment

Indications for soft tissue contouring include incomplete passive eruption of one or more teeth. With this condition, the patient appears to have very short teeth with a lot of gum tissue showing, hypertrophied or malpositioned papilla, inflamed tissues as a result of orthodontic treatment, hypertrophied gingival tissue from drug therapy, such as Dilantin, and hypertrophied gingival tissue from poor oral hygiene or pathologic conditions (Figure 31-20).

Methods for Soft Tissue Contouring

Electrosurgery or lasers are used to remove and contour the gingival tissues. Both techniques require that the dentist become familiar with the equipment and skilled in the detailed application steps.

Electrosurgery equipment and techniques have been used for many years. The equipment has improved as have the precise techniques required for esthetic contouring. Electrosurgery equipment includes a unit that produces various current strengths, various styles of electrode tips, and a foot pedal control. See Chapter 29, Periodontics, for more information.

Dental lasers are becoming increasingly popular, and have proven to be an ideal technology for gum contouring and reshaping. Soft tissue lasers offer degrees of precision that surpass other techniques, while minimizing pain and other discomfort. The dentist will choose a dental laser among several types available based on primary intended use. Education and training for dentist and staff are provided by manufacturers when the dentist purchases a laser system.

FIGURE 31-20 Evaluation of gingival tissue symmetry.

Dental laser units include laser control system, handpiece with various tips, water reservoir, and a foot pedal. See Chapter 29, Periodontics, for more information.

Basic Clinical Technique for Soft Tissue Contouring

Ideally, the height of the gingival tissues of the central incisors is the same as the height of the cuspids (canines). The height of the gingival tissues of the laterals is just below the centrals or cuspids. If the first premolars (bicuspids) are included, the height of the gingival tissue should be 1 to 2 mm below that of the cuspids. The techniques involved to achieve these goals must be precise and accurate.

After the anesthetic is administered, the sulcular areas of the involved teeth are probed to determine the depth and orientation of the sulcus. A guide tooth is selected, usually an anterior tooth that is not involved in the surgical procedure. A straight-edge tangent is held to the gingival height and parallel to the pupils of the patient's eyes to determine the amount of gingival tissues to be removed for achieving symmetry. An explorer is used to penetrate the gingival tissue to mark the amount of tissue to be removed. The dentist evaluates whether sufficient gingiva exists to perform the contouring before proceeding (remember the adage "measure twice, cut once"). The tissues are then contoured and reshaped with a dental laser or electrosurgery. Typically, little bleeding occurs when either of these techniques is used. The gingival tissue height is evaluated throughout the procedure and then confirmed for accuracy using a straight line once all the tissue has been contoured.

Occlusion in Cosmetic Dentistry

Another area considered essential in successful esthetic treatment is occlusion. The cosmetic dentist will examine the patient's occlusion to determine whether any malocclusion exists. Malocclusions may result from skeletal, dental, or muscular problems. The mandible and maxilla are evaluated separately and in relationship to each other. A patient with occlusal problems involving orthodontic principles beyond the scope of the dentist should be referred to a specialist for a diagnosis. The orthodontist must consider whether restorative techniques may be a better means of treatment than extensive orthodontic therapy.

Traditionally, the dentist takes detailed, precise impressions of the patient's maxillary and mandibular arches. These impressions are poured up in stone and articulated. The dentist consults with a lab technician on the function of the patient's bite and how esthetic restorations will be affected.

Placing cosmetic restorations has a significant impact on occlusion, which is a topic in the neuromuscular dentistry subdiscipline. **Neuromuscular dentistry** is defined as "the science of occlusion that objectively measures the physiologic functions affected by occlusion to achieve an optimal relationship between the skull and the mandible."

Occlusion is evaluated and treated so that the muscles which control the jaw position are optimal for ideal function and the patient's comfort. Several devices are used to assist in evaluating occlusion before cosmetic treatment begins. One such analysis system uses a grid-based sensor to provide vivid graphics for the dentist to use in determining and adjusting a patient's bite to achieve the perfect bite (Figure 31-21).

(A)

(B)

(C)

FIGURE 31-21 (A) Patient having occlusion scanned/evaluated. (B) Arch marked with articulating paper and (C) graphic scan of occlusal analysis. *(Courtesy of Tekscan, inc.)*

Types of Restorations and Materials

While most types of restorations and materials used in cosmetic dentistry have been around for awhile, they are continually being improved and updated. Some materials are into respective fourth and fifth generations of development, such as dentin-bonding materials. The dentist and the dental staff must keep themselves up-to-date on new techniques and steps in a given procedure. This section provides a brief overview of selected types of restorations and materials used in cosmetic dentistry.

Composite resins are used in both direct and indirect techniques.

- The direct composite resin technique involves preparation of the tooth; placing liners and bonding agents; and insertion of the composite resin into the tooth, carving, and filling completion. Many types of composite resins are available, and resin selection depends on the design and location of the cavity. Most of these materials are light-cured and placed in increments or layers. Each layer is placed and then light cured before the next layer is placed. Direct composite resins are available in various shades to match the tooth and provide the patient with an esthetically pleasing restoration. More information on the various types of direct composite resins and their composition and characteristics is found in Chapter 34, Restorative Materials.

- The indirect composite resin technique involves preparation of the tooth, taking a final impression and sending it to a dental laboratory, fabrication of a restoration with a laboratory-processed composite resin. One advantage of this technique derives from rapid advances in composite resin technology. These materials have physical properties and appearance that are similar to porcelain, but without some of the problems associated with porcelain. For example, porcelain is harder than tooth enamel and can cause the opposing tooth structure to wear during normal function. In addition, if a porcelain restoration needs to be adjusted it cannot be polished as well as a composite resin restoration.

Composite resins used for direct and indirect restorations are improving rapidly, and systems for the office and laboratory use will be available soon. These systems are expected to meet both esthetic and functional expectations.

Ceramometal restorations are used in conditions of heavy occlusal stress and for multiple-unit fixed prostheses. These crowns offer both strength and acceptable appearance. A ceramometal restoration is comprised of metal alloy on the inside for strength, and porcelain on the outside for esthetics. The porcelain-to-metal bond is very strong and technique sensitive. In the dental laboratory, the first step is to make the metal crown, followed by fabrication of the porcelain cap, which is painted on and then fired. See Chapter 30, Fixed Prosthodontics, for further detail.

Porcelain restorations can be made as full crowns/coverage or as partial veneers/coverage. These ceramic restorations are esthetically advanced compared to metaloceramic restorations. Drawbacks of porcelain restorations are their relative lack of strength and the fact that usage is limited to single teeth.

All-ceramic (porcelain) materials are used in the following restorations: jacket crowns (Figure 31-22), Dicor crowns, Ips Empress crowns, and In-Ceram and Procera AllCeram crowns. Each of these systems has advantages and disadvantages, with the newer systems presenting improvements in the areas of strength, versatility, and natural appearance.

Veneers can be fabricated right in the office or at a dental laboratory. For more information, see Chapter 30, Fixed Prosthodontics.

Marketing Cosmetic Dentistry

Marketing cosmetic dentistry is similar to marketing for any other product or service. Various techniques are used to motivate a particular individual to become informed on available cosmetic services that would make possible that perfect smile they have always wanted. Marketing then motivates the person to take

FIGURE 31-22 Before and after of porcelain crowns.

action by finding a cosmetic dentist and going ahead with the treatment.

Marketing through advertising involves relaying a specific message by means of television, radio, magazines, and newspapers (Figure 31-23). Advertising also includes direct mailings, such as office newsletters or information on services and coupons for service. Marketing messages can be printed on pens, calendars, or cups, and then distributed to patients and prospective patients. All of these means should be considered as part of the dental practice's marketing plan.

Marketing Plan for Dental Office

Cosmetic dentistry is dental care above and beyond routine services, and patients typically use discretionary income to pay for these procedures. Basic market research is typically carried out to provide the dentist with a clear picture of how practice goals and objectives can be achieved. The dentist and dental staff work together as a team to formulate goals and objectives for the best working environment, utilizing the talents of each team member. Goals and objectives then are those of the dentist and staff.

A marketing plan may include the following:

- Goals and objectives of practice
- Assessment of target audience
- Specific marketing tools and activities
- Timeframes and budget
- Method to evaluate results

Goals and objectives may be specific, relating to cosmetic dentistry and marketing this aspect of the practice. Some dental practices are wholly dedicated to cosmetic dentistry, while others provide general dentistry and cosmetic dentistry services.

A profile of existing active patients and a profile of potential patients will assist the dentist and staff in determining the marketing plan direction. The practice should consider the age and income levels of their patients, and the most common types of treatments completed. Then the marketing plan can include ways to educate, motivate, and facilitate these individuals.

Specific marketing techniques should be discussed and then implemented for a predetermined time period. Marketing can be done in and out of the office. In-office marketing can be accomplished by dental team members answering patient questions, and using videos, pamphlets, and other means of suggesting cosmetic options during case presentations. Opening doors for questions about cosmetic treatment is a large part of motivating the patient to act (Figure 31-24).

Marketing outside the office may include mailing a newsletter to residents in the surrounding area, and ads in the Yellow Pages, on radio and television, billboards, on buses and subway cars, and in local magazines. Outside marketing must maintain professionalism to be effective and it can be very expensive.

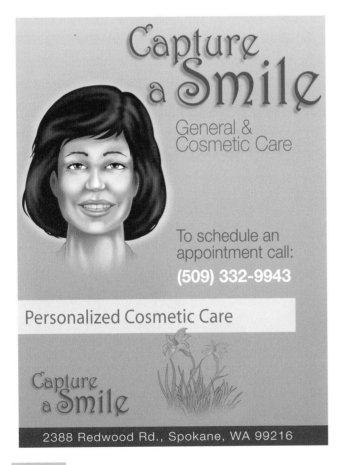

FIGURE 31-23 Cosmetic dentistry advertisement.

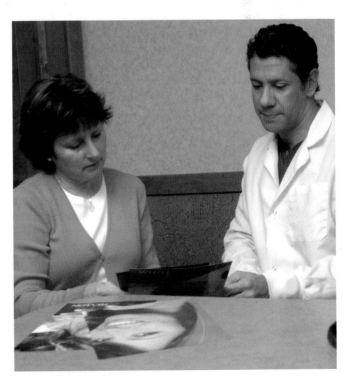

FIGURE 31-24 Cosmetic dentist showing before and after photos of patients who have completed treatment.

ADVANCED CHAIRSIDE FUNCTIONS

Introduction to Tooth Whitening

Many attempts have been made to esthetically improve the shade of one's teeth. Bleaching has become one of the most requested services provided by the dental profession, and is often delegated to a dental assistant. Specific training and clinical experience are required for the assistant to become confident and competent. Although the bleaching procedures have been proven safe and effective by the ADA and the Food and Drug Administration, research is continually being done and professionals must keep up-to-date on new information.

The procedure for lightening teeth is often referred to as tooth whitening or tooth bleaching. Causes of tooth stains or discoloration are varied, and lightening techniques are chosen based on these causes.

In this section, we discuss the causes of stains and discolorations, the types of materials used to whiten the teeth, procedures used to whiten the teeth, and certain precautions to be exercised during procedures.

How Teeth Are Whitened

The teeth turn a lighter shade when hydrogen peroxide or nonperoxide whitening material penetrates the enamel and into the dentin. The whitening process is accelerated mainly by the use of low-intensity heat or sometimes by a high-intensity curing light or a laser.

Today, the most commonly used materials are sodium perborate, hydrogen peroxide, and carbamide peroxide. Sodium perborate is a non-hydrogen peroxide system that contains sodium chloride, oxygen, and fluoride.

Hydrogen Peroxide

Hydrogen peroxide breaks down into water and oxygen. When this happens, free radicals of oxygen are released and they act with pigments in both intrinsic and extrinsic stains, producing a whitening effect. Available in liquid and gel forms, it varies in strength from a 5- to 35-percent solution.

Hydrogen peroxide may cause temporary sensitivity of the pulp when the solution penetrates the enamel and dentin. This is the most common side effect. Hydrogen peroxide will irritate the tissue and discolors clothing; therefore, precautions should be taken to protect the patient's eyes, face, lips, cheeks, tongue, and clothing when using hydrogen peroxide.

Carbamide Peroxide

Carbamide peroxide, a complex form of urea and hydrogen peroxide, is used in a 10- to 20-percent solution. It is weaker than hydrogen peroxide solution, but more stable. This solution is also available in liquid or gel form. A thickening agent is added to increase adhesion to the tooth and prolong exposure to the whitening agent (Figure 31-25).

Sodium Perborate

Sodium perborate, another weak oxidizing agent, is sometimes mixed with hydrogen peroxide and used to whiten nonvital teeth. This compound is the ingredient used in many household bleaching agents that are safe for colors.

FIGURE 31-25 (A) Nu Radiance whitening kit and (B) syringe. *(Courtesy of Nu Radiance.)*

ADVANCED CHAIRSIDE FUNCTIONS

Causes of Tooth Stains

Examples of extrinsic stains include stains from diets and habits, such as tobacco, tea, and coffee. These leave yellow to brown stains, and the success of the bleaching process depends on the amount of stain. Intrinsic stains include tetracycline stains, dental fluorosis, discoloration due to injury, and nonvital endodontically treated teeth. (See coronal polish section in Chapter 29, Periodontics, for more information on dental stains.) Sometimes, the shade of the teeth is naturally toward yellow or gray, and these patients can esthetically enhance the color of their teeth with bleaching.

Role of the Dental Assistant

The dental assistant and the hygienist may perform some or all aspects involving whitening, such as the following:

- Providing information and answering questions the patient may have about whitening
- Chairside assisting for whitening treatments
- Providers of home whitening information, including instructions for proper use of whitening and care of trays
- Fabricating custom whitening trays
- Obtaining informed consent form from the patient

Whitening Techniques

There are two methods of whitening: One method is performed in the dental office, and the other method at home. Patients can use one or the other or a combination to meet their needs. Both vital and nonvital teeth are bleached in the office. There are advantages and disadvantages to each method, and these should be presented to the patient. Considerations include the amount of stain and its origin, number of visits to the office versus the amount of time the bleaching trays are worn at home, expense of in-office bleaching (which is higher than in-home bleaching), and the amount of instruction and guidance the patient requires.

When patients inquire about teeth whitening, discussing available options and understanding their perceptions about their appearance are important. Factors to consider—and which determine the ultimate success of the whitening process—are summarized below.

- Degree of stains or discolorations
- Cause of stains or discolorations

- Whitening technique
- Whitening solution and strength of solution
- Vital versus nonvital teeth
- Presence or absence of restorations in teeth to be whitened

Nonvital Whitening

Endodontically treated teeth sometimes turn dark due to blood, pulpal debris, and restorative materials that are used to fill the canal. These teeth can be lightened by both internal and external bleaching. One of the most common bleaching techniques is the **walking whitening technique**. This technique calls for a thick paste of hydrogen peroxide, sodium perborate, or a combination of the two to be placed on the coronal portion of the nonvital tooth. With the bleach mixture temporarily sealed in place, the patient can leave the office and return for evaluation and another possible treatment as instructed by the dentist. Sometimes, heat is applied with a heated instrument/unit in order to achieve desired results.

An alternate method for whitening nonvital teeth consists of two major steps: (1) after the tooth has been treated endodontically, it is isolated with the rubber dam; (2) then a whitening agent is placed in the unfilled pulp chamber of the tooth. A 30- to 35-percent hydrogen peroxide solution (Superoxol) is applied with cotton tips or cotton pellets (Figure 31-26). A heated instrument is then placed in the pulp chamber to activate the peroxide. This procedure may be repeated several times to reach the desired whitening effect.

Vital Whitening in Dental Office

Bleaching vital teeth in the office involves the application of bleaching liquids or gels, often with the application of heat and a curing light. This is sometimes called **power whitening**. The patient's teeth are isolated tightly to prevent irritation to the gingiva by any chemicals, and then they are polished with a pumice or prophy paste. The actual bleaching steps depend on the types of materials used, but, for most, a fresh mix is applied every ten to fifteen minutes for three to four applications. The bleaching materials are evacuated between applications. Then when the procedure is finished, the teeth are rinsed thoroughly, the isolation removed, and the teeth polished with a fluoride prophy paste (Figure 31-27).

ADVANCED CHAIRSIDE FUNCTIONS

FIGURE 31-26 Superoxol 30–35% hydrogen peroxide. *(Courtesy of Sultan Healthcare.)*

Teeth dehydrate when they are isolated for a period of time and may appear whiter than they will be after they have dehydrated for several hours.

Dehydration may also cause the teeth to be more sensitive during the procedure.

Home Whitening Techniques

For home whitening, the patient applies a bleaching agent, usually carbamide peroxide or diluted hydrogen peroxide, in a custom-fit tray for specific amounts of time. There are multiple materials, and the techniques vary greatly. The dental staff must become familiar with materials being prescribed for their patients. The advantages of the home bleaching techniques include fewer visits to the dental office, less expense, and convenience. The disadvantages of these techniques are that the patients must be motivated to follow the routine, the time involved for the bleaching process can take several weeks, the bleaching materials can cause nausea and sensitivity to the gingiva, and there is lack of direct monitoring by the dentist. Home bleaching is very popular with patients because of the lower cost and the positive results when done properly. As an alternative, patients can come to the office for a startup, or assisted whitening, appointment and then complete the process with home bleaching. Usually, the two appointments are needed to set up the patient for home bleaching. At the first appointment, the impressions for the custom trays are made. The second appointment is for delivery of the bleaching trays; instructions are also given to the patient (Figure 31-28).

FIGURE 31-27 In-office whitening materials.

FIGURE 31-28 Home bleaching kit.

The patient is scheduled for his or her next appointment within one to two weeks. The patient should be told that the teeth may be sensitive. This process usually takes three appointments.

ADVANCED CHAIRSIDE FUNCTIONS

Over-the-Counter Whitening Materials

Many over-the-counter (OTC) whitening products are available, including whitening strips, gels, tray systems, toothpastes, mouth rinses, and even chewing gum. Although these methods do whiten the teeth to varying degrees, there is no professional guidance or evaluation. The ADA recommends that patients consult with their dentist to determine the most appropriate means of whitening their teeth. This is especially important if the patient has many restorations, crowns, and distinctive stains. If the patient chooses an OTC method, he or she must follow the manufacturer's directions carefully and proceed with caution. The most common side effects include temporary tooth and gingival sensitivity, and on rare occasions, irreversible tooth damage. These products generally contain a less-concentrated whitening agent (compared to agents used in dental practices), usually hydrogen peroxide gel or carbamide peroxide (Figure 31-29).

Whitening Strips

Whitening strips (e.g., Crest Whitestrips) are an alternative to tray-based whitening systems. Because the strips are very thin, they do not interfere with the user's normal routine. The number of strips in a kit depends on the concentration of the whitening agent. OTC products are available in a 6-percent hydrogen peroxide solution to be worn over a fourteen-day period, or a 10-percent solution that is worn for seven days. The user may achieve desired results before using all kit contents, and can stop at any time.

The strips are gently pressed on the facial surface of the anterior teeth to create maximum contact with the teeth. They are typically intended to be worn for thirty minutes two times a day.

Strip users should be aware that these products do not work on existing restorations and may cause temporary tooth and gingival tissue sensitivity. Patients are encouraged to consult with their dentist when using OTC teeth-whitening products.

Whitening Gel

OTC whitening gels are painted on the facial surface of the anterior teeth. Care should be taken to keep the gel on the tooth surface and away from the gingival tissues. Some gels contain 18% carbamide peroxide agent and can be used on a daily basis.

Home Tray Whitening Systems

Although many tray whitening systems are delivered through the dental office, OTC systems are available as well. The trays in these systems may be preformed stock trays or thermoplastic trays that can be heated and then molded to the teeth. The trays often do not properly adapt to the teeth and they are not trimmed or contoured to prevent excess whitening agent from contacting the gingival tissues. The manufacturer's instructions should be followed carefully, and a less-aggressive approach should be taken to prevent tooth and gingival sensitivity.

Whitening Toothpastes

Most toothpastes contain a "whitening agent," and some toothpastes are designed specifically as whitening agents. The whitening agents used in toothpaste include hydrogen peroxide, calcium peroxide, and sodium percarbonate. These agents contribute to the whitening effect, but the primary whitening is accomplished by the abrasive in the toothpaste. The abrasive agent (hydrated silica, dicalcium phosphate dehydrate, and calcium carbonate) rates very low on abrasive rankings. The ADA Seal on toothpaste packaging indicates that abrasive particles do not exceed the maximum acceptable abrasive ranking (Figure 31-30).

FIGURE 31-29 Over-the-counter whitening products.

ADVANCED CHAIRSIDE FUNCTIONS

FIGURE 31-30 Whitening toothpaste.

Mouth Rinses and Chewing Gum

Mouth rinses and even a few chewing gum products contain whitening agents. Like whitening toothpastes, the percentage of whitening agent in these products is very low. These products can be used daily. Discontinuation of use is advised if the teeth or gingival tissues become irritated or sensitive.

Patient Information

With all bleaching procedures, the patient needs to understand the procedure steps and the outcome possibilities. The bleaching process will "lighten" most teeth, but some teeth will never be the whitest or the brightest—but they will be improved. The patient's dedication to following procedures and limiting foods and habits that stain the teeth will enhance the process and bleach the teeth faster. The health of the gingiva and surrounding tissues must be protected by adhering to technique suggestions. Ingestion of the solutions should be kept to a minimum. The patient must realize that bleaching may be an ongoing treatment, with repeated bleaching necessary every few years.

Precautions with Tooth Whitening Techniques

Whitening materials may cause tooth sensitivity and/or irritation to gingival tissues in affected areas.

Sloughing of gingival, lip, and cheek tissues may occur.

Patients should contact their dentist if any of these side effects occur.

Tooth sensitivity is sometimes treated with sodium fluoride.

Patients should be instructed to discontinue whitening procedures until sensitivity has disappeared, and they have checked with their dentist.

ADVANCED CHAIRSIDE FUNCTIONS

PROCEDURE 31-1

Nonvital Whitening

This procedure is performed by the dentist. The patient has received information on the procedure and possible outcome before the procedure begins. More than one treatment may be necessary.

EQUIPMENT AND SUPPLIES

- Basic setup: mouth mirror, explorer, cotton pliers
- Cotton rolls, gauze sponges, cotton pellets
- HVE tip, air-water syringe tip, saliva ejector
- Dental dam setup
- Protective gel
- Waxed dental floss
- High-speed handpiece and assorted burs
- Low-speed handpiece
- Prophy brush
- Cement base materials
- Bleaching materials
- Heat source
- Temporary coverage and cement
- Finishing burs

PROCEDURE STEPS *(Follow aseptic procedures)*

1. The dentist examines and evaluates the root canal–treated tooth.

2. Place the dental dam and ligature of waxed dental floss on the designated tooth or teeth. Once the dam is in place, apply more protective gel to further seal the dam.

3. Remove the excess restoration and any debris in the crown. With the crown of the tooth open, some den-tists scrub the chamber with a soap solution and a prophy brush or cotton pellet.

4. The root canal is sealed with 2 to 3 mm of a thick base cement or with a light-cured resin ionomer or bonded composite. This is a critical step, because the tooth must be sealed in order to prevent the bleach from penetrating the root. This can be done using the gel bleach in the office, the walking technique, or a combination of both techniques. If bleaching results are not achieved, heat may be also used with the office-based bleaching gel technique. Stains caused by endodontic procedures and drugs often require application of heat with the bleaching agents.

   - Gel bleaching in the office involves the chamber being filled for thirty minutes. Change the bleaching gel every ten minutes. Then, place a cotton pellet and temporary in the crown. The patient should be reappointed in three to seven days for evaluation.

   - With walking bleaching, a thick mixture of bleach-ing agent is placed in the crown and covered with temporary cement. Reappoint the patient in two to five days to remove the cotton pellet.

5. Desired results should be achieved in three appoint-ments, but if the tooth remains darker than the patient prefers, a veneer should be considered. The shade can be altered slightly with the shade of the restorative materials. The temporary filling is removed, and the chamber is rinsed and evacuated. Etching is applied to the inside of the crown. Rinse. Apply the dental adhesive and then fill the chamber with restor-ative material and light cure.

6. Polish the restoration with finishing burs and polish.

7. Reappoint the patient in a few days to evaluate the color and whether there is the possible need of a veneer.

ADVANCED CHAIRSIDE FUNCTIONS

PROCEDURE 31-2

In-Office Whitening for Vital Teeth

This procedure is performed by the dentist in the dental office. The procedure is explained to the patient with the possible outcomes.

EQUIPMENT AND SUPPLIES

- Protective gel
- Rubber dam set-up
- Waxed dental floss
- High-speed handpiece and assorted burs
- Low-speed handpiece
- Prophy brush
- Cement base materials
- Bleaching materials
- Heat source
- Temporary coverage and cement
- Finishing burs

PROCEDURE STEPS *(Follow aseptic procedures)*

1. The procedure is explained and videos, photos, and pamphlets may be available for the patient. The teeth and surrounding tissues are examined. Before photos may be taken of the patient.

2. Cover all surrounding tissues with protective gel. Isolating with the dental dam is the safest method to protect the tissues. Place the dental dam, punching the holes as close as possible to match the tooth. With the dental dam on, place a ligature of waxed floss around each tooth, and pull the floss toward the cervix and secure.

3. Polish the crowns of the teeth to remove plaque and debris that may interfere with the bleaching process. Prophy paste or flour of pumice may be used.

4. Follow the manufacturer's instructions for the specific steps of the materials being used. Materials are mixed to a thick consistency and placed on the facial and lingual surfaces of the tooth or in a tray. Some materials require the use of a bleaching heat and/or light source and are used for approximately thirty minutes. The no-heat materials are applied every ten minutes, with fresh materials mixed each time for three to four applications. Rinse and evacuate between each application to remove the bulk of the bleaching gel.

5. After thoroughly rinsing the area, cut the ligatures and interseptal dental dam and remove these from the patient's mouth. Rinse again, and remove any protective gel with floss and wet gauze.

6. Polish the teeth with a composite resin polishing cup or a fluoride prophy paste. (This step may vary with different types of materials.)

7. Although the bleaching process may take some time before the shade can be evaluated, the patient's tissues are examined and the patient is instructed to avoid substances that may stain the teeth. The patient should also be warned that the teeth may be sensitive following the bleaching procedure. Usually, three appointments one to two weeks apart are required to reach the desired shade.

ADVANCED CHAIRSIDE FUNCTIONS

PROCEDURE 31-3

Home Whitening

This procedure is performed by the patient at home after an examination by the dentist. The patient is given a bleaching kit and step-by-step instructions from the dentist. This procedure is divided into appointments and steps that occur between appointments.

EQUIPMENT AND SUPPLIES

- Basic setup: mouth mirror, explorer, cotton pliers
- Alginate
- Rubber mixing bowl and spatula
- Impression trays
- Camera
- Custom-fit, vacuum-formed tray (see Chapter 35, Laboratory Materials and Techniques)
- Home bleaching kit
- Shade guide for before and after color comparisons.

PROCEDURE STEPS *(Follow aseptic procedures)*

First Appointment

1. The dentist examines the teeth, considering the shade of the teeth, sensitivity, restorations, and areas of abrasion and erosion. General procedures are completed before the bleaching process begins. The bleaching techniques are explained, and the procedure that best meets the patient's needs is selected.

2. Alginate impressions are taken of the arches being bleached. Before photographs are taken.

Between Appointments

1. The alginate impressions are poured in stone and prepared.

2. A custom-fit, vacuum-formed tray is made. This may be done in the office lab or at a commercial lab.

Second Appointment

1. With the home technique, the patient tries on the trays to ensure a good fit.

2. Instructions are given, including when and for how long to wear the trays, how to prepare the materials, how to place the custom-fit trays, what to do in case the gingiva becomes irritated, and how to handle other side effects.

3. In some cases, the patient receives one bleaching in the office, before beginning the home bleaching. The teeth are polished, and then the bleaching agent is prepared and placed in the trays. The trays are inserted into the patient's mouth for thirty to sixty minutes and then removed. The teeth are suctioned off and rinsed thoroughly.

4. Some offices schedule an appointment to follow-up with the patient's progress and to examine the tissues. This appointment is usually within two weeks of the second appointment.

CHAPTER SUMMARY

Cosmetic dentistry can be a life-changing experience for both the patient and the dental team. These procedures involve many and varied aspects of dentistry and provide esthetic services to patients. Cosmetic dentistry involves very detailed, comprehensive treatments that can involve orthodontics, oral maxillofacial surgery, occlusion adjustments, endodontic treatment, and periodontics. The fundamentals of cosmetic dentistry are discussed as well as the psychology of working with patients interested in improving their smile.

Tooth whitening also may be a part of esthetic treatments desired by patients to improve the appearance of their teeth. Various materials and techniques are discussed including nonvital and vital tooth whitening, in-office and home whitening techniques, and available OTC products.

The dental assistant plays an important role in all cosmetic and tooth-whitening procedures. The assistant must be educated and trained to assist the dentist and be actively involved in providing information to the patient.

Case Study

Chance Hall works with the public, and is very concerned about the color of his teeth. He scheduled several tooth-whitening treatments with Dr. Garrett. After several appointments, Chance's teeth became very sensitive and gingival tissues were irritated. Now he wonders if he will ever have the bright smile he wants without sensitivity.

Case Study Review

1. List tooth-whitening precautions.

2. What should the dental assistant have explained to Chance about the side effects of tooth whitening?

3. Discuss options available to Chance to achieve his goal of having whiter teeth.

REVIEW QUESTIONS

Multiple Choice

1. Porcelain teeth were first manufactured in the
   a. seventeenth century.
   b. eighteenth century.
   c. nineteenth century.
   d. twentieth century.

2. Soft tissue contouring is accomplished with a
   a. dental laser.
   b. electrosurgery unit.
   c. both a and b.
   d. None of the above

3. All of the following procedures are included in cosmetic dentistry, except
   a. amalgam restorations.
   b. veneers.
   c. tooth whitening.
   d. dentures.

4. _____ surround(s) the tooth and marks the boundaries of the face of the tooth.
   a. The dental hue
   b. The chroma
   c. Opacity
   d. Transitional line angles

5. _____ is the science of occlusion that objectively measures the physiologic functions affected by occlusion to achieve an optimal relationship between the skull and the mandible.
   a. Neurological dentistry
   b. Neuromuscular dentistry
   c. Skeletal dentistry
   d. Skeletal muscular dentistry

6. Bleaching can remove both intrinsic and extrinsic stains to varying degrees.
   a. This is a true statement.
   b. This is a false statement.

7. Which of the following agencies/organizations has proven the safety and effectiveness of whitening procedures?
   a. American Dental Association
   b. State drug administration
   c. Food and Drug Administration
   d. Both a and c

8. When a tooth is endodontically treated and turns dark due to blood, pulpal debris, and/or restorative materials, it can be lightened by
   a. vital whitening procedures.
   b. nonvital whitening procedures.
   c. home whitening procedures.
   d. None of the above, because it cannot be lightened with any whitening procedures.

9. All of the following are true statements about in-office whitening except:
   a. The teeth are polished before application of the whitening materials.
   b. The actual whitening steps depend on the type of materials applied.
   c. The patient is scheduled for another appointment in two to six months.
   d. The teeth are polished with a fluoride prophy paste after the whitening materials have been placed and then the mouth is rinsed thoroughly.

10. Which of the following whitening materials is typically used in home whitening techniques?
   a. Diluted hydrogen peroxide
   b. Sodium hypochloride
   c. Sodium fluoride
   d. Phosphoric acid

Critical Thinking

1. Discuss everything that would be needed to make a case presentation to a patient who wants to have a beautiful smile.

2. Explain why formal informed consents must be part of the patient's records.

3. When patients mention that they are interested in teeth whitening, what options could the dental assistant tell them about?

Web Activities

1. Go to http://www.lvilive.com (Las Vegas Institute for Advanced Dental Studies), and look up patient experiences and before and after pictures.

2. Go to http://www.cosmeticdentistry.com to view specific procedures included in cosmetic dentistry and locate a cosmetic dentist in your area.

3. To learn more about cosmetic dentistry certification, go to http://www.aacd.com.

4. To find out more about tooth whitening and recommendations by the American Dental Association go to http://www.ada.org, public information section.

PRACTICE   SKILLS

CHAPTER 32

REMOVABLE PROSTHODONTICS

SPECIFIC INSTRUCTIONAL OBJECTIVES

The student should strive to meet the following objectives and demonstrate an understanding of the facts and principles presented in this chapter:

1. Define removable prostheses and list the reasons for using them.

2. Describe considerations about the patient related to removable prosthetic treatment.

3. Explain dental assistant's role in removable prosthetic treatment.

4. Outline steps of the diagnostic appointment and list materials needed.

5. Describe the consultation appointment and materials required for case presentation.

6. Describe advantages and disadvantages of the partial denture, its components, and appointment schedule.

7. Describe the complete denture, considerations about the patient, and appointment schedule.

8. Explain types and steps of denture reline procedures.

9. Describe procedure for a denture repair.

10. List steps to polish a removable prosthetic appliance.

11. Explain the overdenture and the advantages and disadvantages related to it.

KEY TERMS

abutment *(746)*

anatomical *(753)*

artificial teeth *(749)*

bar-type clasp *(748)*

baseplate *(755)*

bite rim *(755)*

border molding *(757)*

centric occlusion *(758)*

circumferential-type clasp *(748)*

connectors *(747)*

denture base *(748)*

framework *(747)*

hinge *(747)*

immediate denture *(754)*

muscle trimming *(757)*

nonanatomical *(753)*

overdenture *(763)*

partial dentures *(745)*

prostheses *(745)*

relined *(760)*

rests *(747)*

retainer *(748)*

stress breakers *(747)*

vertical dimension *(755)*

INTRODUCTION

Removable prosthodontics, like fixed prosthodontics, refer to the replacement of missing teeth and tissues with artificial structures, or prostheses. The difference is that with removable prosthodontics, the prosthesis can be removed from the mouth by the patient for cleaning, examination, and repair. Removable prosthodontics involve two types of prostheses: partial dentures and complete (full) dentures.

The partial denture replaces one or more teeth in one arch and is retained and supported by the underlying tissues and remaining teeth.

The complete denture replaces all the teeth in one arch. A full denture is retained and supported by the underlying tissues of the gingiva and oral mucosa, the alveolar ridges, and the hard palate. In some cases, teeth are retained in the arch or implants are placed to support the denture.

The goals of removable prosthodontics are to restore lost functions, stabilize the arch, and improve esthetics. The lost functions include the ability to masticate food properly and to have clear speech. With removable prosthodontics, the patient regains these functions, improves appearance, and, within a short adjustment period, becomes very comfortable and confident with the prosthesis.

Most patients prefer to have fixed prostheses, but in some cases it may not be the treatment of choice due to existing conditions, such as unhealthy bone structure, not having the motivation to maintain good oral hygiene, or financial restrictions. Removable prosthodontics offers an alternative that restores function and esthetics for the patient.

Prosthodontics is a specialty that requires additional training upon completion of dental school. Routine prosthodontic procedures are performed by the general dentist as well as the prosthodontist. The prosthodontist may see patients who need surgery as a result of cancer, patients who have been in accidents involving severe facial/jaw trauma, and/or patients with anomalies such as cleft lip or cleft palate.

Patient Considerations

Good communication between the patient and the prosthodontic staff is required for successful removable prosthodontics. The patient should be in good health, have a positive attitude, and be cooperative. The patient's mental and physical capabilities must be such that he or she can adapt to wearing the prosthesis and be able to maintain good oral hygiene. Impaired health may contribute to a lack of muscle coordination that is needed to place and remove the partial prosthesis or to retain a denture in place. If the patient is in poor health, it is often reflected in the oral cavity. Also, the added stress of a new appliance may lower

FIGURE 32-1 Patient preparing to have full dentures placed compared to after placement and restoration of natural appearance.

the resistance of unhealthy tissue and complications may occur. Fluctuations in the patient's weight may alter the fit of the prosthesis, and it may need to be relined.

Some patients are very conscientious and require patience and understanding during the time of adjustment. There are also pamphlets and videos available to inform patients about their new prostheses (Figure 32-1).

Dental Assistant's Role

The dental assistant's main functions are to prepare materials, record measurements and details for the fabrication of the denture, provide patient education and support, and perform selective laboratory procedures. Procedures in removable prosthodontics do not require many instrument exchanges, and the dental assistant does not continually maintain the oral cavity throughout the appointment with the air-water syringe and the HVE. The steps in removable prosthodontics involve as many extraoral as intraoral procedures.

Diagnosis and Treatment Planning

The first appointment for a removable prosthesis is dedicated to examining the patient. A medical history is taken or reviewed to determine the patient's state of health. The dentist may also talk with the patient to determine how the patient feels about his or her existing oral condition and about the prospect of having a partial or full denture. The dentist examines the patient's remaining teeth and tissues.

After a prophylaxis, preliminary impressions for study models and working casts are taken. (Review Chapter 35, Laboratory Materials and Techniques, for more information on taking alginate impressions.) Radiographic films are exposed and processed by the dental assistant as part of the diagnostic aids. Photographs are made of the patient, including full face, frontal view, profile view, and a close-up. The patient is then scheduled for a consultation appointment a few days later.

Consultation Appointment

The patient is seated in an area designed for patient consultations. The following aids are present to help the patient better understand what is involved in the treatment:

- Study models of the patient's mouth
- Radiographs mounted on a viewbox
- Patient's photographs
- Visual aids to explain the types of removable prostheses (this may include pamphlets, models, pictures, or video programs)
- Proposed treatment plan

The dental assistant has all of the items prepared so that the dentist can explain the diagnosis, proposed treatment plan, and prognosis to the patient. The dentist answers any questions and concerns expressed by the patient. As with other dental procedures, a cost estimate is prepared and presented to the patient, along with the number of appointments the procedure will require. The treatment plan may involve restorative dentistry, periodontal treatment, endodontic treatment, and/or surgical procedures. These procedures must be completed and the patient must be completely healed before prosthodontic preparation can begin.

When the patient has accepted the treatment plan, a suitable financial plan is approved and insurance information collected. Often, the dental office takes insurance information at the first appointment and then contacts the insurance company for information on the patient's coverage. This information is presented at the consultation appointment. The necessary appointments are then made for treatment.

Removable Partial Denture

Partial dentures are designed to restore missing teeth and to preserve the remaining hard and soft tissues of the arches. The partial distributes the forces of mastication between the abutment teeth and the alveolar mucosa. The **abutment** is a natural tooth that becomes part of the support for the partial. The abutment teeth must be in good condition or be restored to withstand the stresses of chewing with a partial denture.

Advantages of a Removable Partial Denture

Listed below are reasons that a partial denture may be part of a patient's treatment plan when he or she has missing teeth.

- Partial dentures are repaired and adjusted easily. If teeth are lost in the dental arch, they can be added to the partial denture.
- When there are no teeth for a distal attachment, the removable partial denture is one treatment choice to restore function to that quadrant.
- Partial dentures require fewer intraoral procedures than fixed protheses. This means fewer appointments and less chair time for the patient.
- Maintaining good oral hygiene of the abutments and the appliance is easier for the patient because the prosthesis is removable.
- The partial restores the mesial-distal contacts between the teeth and the anterior-posterior continuity of the arch. This provides support that teeth standing alone do not have; therefore, the arch is stabilized.
- The partial maintains a proper occlusal plane by preventing supraeruption of the teeth on the opposing arch.
- The removable partial makes it unnecessary to reduce tooth structure. The partial appliance can be fitted to children and adolescents and is replaced easily to compensate for a child's growth.
- When several teeth are missing in both quadrants of an arch, a removable partial denture is designed to restore lost dentition in the long span.
- Removable prostheses may be designed to support periodontally involved teeth.
- Compared to a fixed prosthesis, the partial prosthesis is a less expensive treatment.

Considerations for a Partial Denture

Before choosing the partial denture as the treatment, the dentist must consider several factors. There must be a number of sufficiently positioned teeth in the arch to support and stabilize a removable prosthesis. To retain the appliance, there must be adequate root structure of the remaining teeth, and the alveolar bone and mucosa must be evaluated to determine whether they can support the partial denture. Another consideration is whether the patient exhibits interest in and is motivated to adjust to the partial denture. The patient must also maintain good oral hygiene, especially around the teeth to which the partial is attached.

Components of a Removable Partial Denture

CDA Components of the removable partial denture include the metal framework, rests, connectors, retainers, denture base, and artificial teeth (Figure 32-2). Partial dentures are designed for individual patients without set patterns.

Metal Framework. The metal framework is the skeleton of the removable partial (Figure 32-3A) to which the remaining units (such as the rests, connectors, and retainers) are attached. Part of the framework is a mesh or loop area designed to retain the acrylic base material. The acrylic portion of the partial denture surrounds the framework.

Rests. The rests are the part of the removable partial denture that contacts a tooth to provide vertical and horizontal support. The rests control the position of the partial in relationship to the supporting structures. To provide the best support, the rests are placed as close as possible to the center of the tooth so that they can direct functional forces to the long axis of the tooth. These rests are positioned on the occlusal, incisal, or cingulum (lingual) surfaces (Figure 32-3).

Connectors. The connectors unite the various parts of the partial into a single unit, hold the working parts in the proper position, and distribute the stresses. They are divided into major and minor connectors. The major connectors connect the left and right quadrants of the partial. On the mandibular, the major connector is often a lingual bar or plate. On the maxillary, the major connector is a palatal bar or strap or a complete palatal plate (Figure 32-4). A **stress-breaker**, or **hinge**, may be built into the partial. This is a metal device that relieves pressure on the abutment teeth. The stress-breaker is like a hinge that gives some release to the occlusal stresses during mastication.

(A)

(B)

(C)

FIGURE 32-3 (A) Partial denture with metal framework. (B) Placement of clasp with rest on tooth. (C) Partial in place.

FIGURE 32-4 Major connector for maxillary palatal strap.

FIGURE 32-2 Mandibular partial denture. (A) Denture base. (B) Denture teeth. (C) Connectors (lingual bar). (D) Occlusal rest.

The minor connectors connect the major connectors with the other units of the partial, such as the clasps and rests. They maintain the integrity of the arch by an anterior-posterior bracing action. The minor connectors protect against food impaction by filling the tooth-tissue junctions.

Retainer. Sometimes called a clasp, the retainer contacts the abutment teeth and prevents the partial from moving. The position of the prosthesis is controlled by the retainer and its relationship to the remaining teeth and support structures. Retainer designs are usually circumferential or bar type. The **circumferential-type clasp** (retainer) encircles and adapts to the contours of the abutment tooth (Figure 32-5). The **bar-type clasp** extends from a gingival direction toward the occlusal.

Partials can be designed with no facial clasp showing, and are made in several variations that will fit most patients. These partials are strong, have good retention, and reliably stay in place. The esthetic factor makes them appealing to most patients. The clasps are designed to fit on the lingual, wrapping interproximally without showing on the facial. In some designs the metal also extends onto the occlusal (Figure 32-6).

Denture Base. The **denture base** is most often made of acrylic resin with fibers to provide a natural appearance. It rests on the oral mucosa, providing coverage and stability. This portion of the partial is sometimes referred to as the saddle. The denture teeth are held in the denture base.

A flexible denture base resin is available that can be used for partial dentures. This material feels more natural and comfortable in the mouth because it is light-

FIGURE 32-6 Esthetic clasp on removable partial denture. *(Courtesy of Valplast International Corp.)*

weight and thin. The resin is available in basic shade categories of medium pink, light pink, and ethnic. This partial is an esthetic choice, and is suggested by some dentists for their patients.

The technique for the flexible resin base partial is very similar to the regular hard resin material, except that the flexible partial is immersed in very hot tap water before insertion in the patient's mouth. After about a minute, the partial is removed from the water and allowed to cool until it can be tolerated by the patient. The partial then adapts well with the natural tissues in the mouth. If adjustments need to be made, a green mounted stone is suggested followed by using a brown rubber wheel to smooth rough surfaces (Figure 32-7).

FIGURE 32-5 Circumferential clasp.

FIGURE 32-7 Flexible denture base resin for partial dentures. *(Courtesy of Valplast International Corp.)*

Artificial Teeth. The artificial teeth are made of acrylic resin or porcelain, and are available in a variety of shapes (molds), sizes, and shades. The artificial teeth are secured to the denture base by pins or holes on the undersides of the teeth (see Denture Teeth under Complete Dentures section in this chapter).

Partial Denture Procedure

The abutment teeth where the metal framework of the partial rests must be prepared before the final impressions are taken. The occlusal surfaces of the teeth are reduced to allow for clearance of the metal framework of the partial between the arches. This surface must be contoured so that the partial denture will be held firmly in place. The buccal and lingual surfaces are prepared to allow the partial to be inserted and removed without binding. If the teeth cannot be contoured adequately with burs, discs, and stones, they are prepared for fixed crowns before the partial denture is fabricated.

After the abutment teeth have been prepared, the dentist takes final impressions and a bite registration (Procedure 32-1). These are sent to the dental laboratory with a laboratory prescription form. The dental laboratory follows the dentist's instructions and constructs an appliance that consists of the cast framework and denture teeth set in the wax bite rim (Figure 32-8). The partial denture is articulated on the models to simulate how the appliance will occlude and mesh in various jaw positions. The laboratory then sends the partial to the dental office for the try-in and any adjustments (Procedure 32-2). The delivery appointment is outlined in Procedure 32-3. See Table 32-1 for the appointments for a partial denture.

(A)

(B)

(C)

FIGURE 32-8 (A) Wax up of a partial denture. (B) Metal framework made from wax up. (C) Metal framework with wax bite rims ready for placement of the denture teeth.

PROCEDURE 32-1

Final Impressions for Partial Denture

This procedure is performed by the dentist. After preparing materials needed for the final impressions, the dental assistant greets and seats the patient. A protective drape is placed on the patient and the procedure is explained to him or her.

EQUIPMENT (Figure 32-9)

- Basic setup: mouth mirror, explorer, and cotton pliers

- Mouthwash

- Custom tray (See Chapter 35, Laboratory Materials and Techniques) or stock tray

- Contouring wax for the impression trays

- Impression materials—spatula and mixing pad or dispensing gun and tips

- Wax or silicone bite registration materials

- Tooth shade and mold guides

- Laboratory prescription form

- Disinfectant and container for impressions and bite registration

FIGURE 32-9 Tray setup for final impression of partial denture.

PROCEDURE STEPS *(Follow aseptic procedures)*

1. The dentist examines the oral cavity and tries the custom or stock tray in the patient's mouth. Sometimes, wax is placed on the borders of the tray to secure a contoured fit. Once the tray is prepared, an adhesive is painted on the inside of the tray.

2. The final impression material is prepared and placed in the tray according to the manufacturer's directions.

3. Once the final impression is completed, receive the final impressions and either disinfect them immediately or set them aside to disinfect after the procedure is completed.

4. The occlusal or bite registration is taken. When completed, it is also disinfected in preparation for the laboratory. Prepare materials to be used for the bite registration. Soften the wax in warm water and then fold it several times before placing it in the patient's mouth. Mix other materials on a paper pad and place them on a quadrant tray. Then, place them in the patient's mouth or dispense them directly into the oral cavity with a dispensing gun and tip. After the bite materials set and are removed from the mouth, disinfect them and put them with the final impressions.

5. The shade of the artificial teeth is taken with a moistened shade guide under natural light. This can be completed at any point in the appointment sequence. Once the shade is determined, record it on the laboratory prescription and the patient's chart. Assist the dentist in shade determination and recording.

6. The dentist completes the laboratory prescription with details of the partial denture design. Make sure that the patient's face is clean of impression materials and debris and then dismiss him or her.

PROCEDURE 32-2

Try-In Appointment for Partial Denture

This procedure is performed by the dentist. The dental assistant prepares the materials and the patient.

EQUIPMENT (Figure 32-10)

- Basic setup: mouth mirror, explorer, and cotton pliers
- Hand mirror for patient viewing
- Articulating paper and forceps
- Adjusting instruments, including wax spatula, pliers, and a heat source
- Low-speed handpiece with burs, discs, and stones
- Contour pliers
- Partial denture from the laboratory

PROCEDURE STEPS *(Follow aseptic procedures)*

1. The appliance is placed in the patient's mouth and adjustments are made accordingly. If adjustments are made to the denture base and/or the position of the teeth, prepare the spatula by warming it in the heat source (alcohol torch or Bunsen burner) and transfer it to the dentist. Transfer the articulating paper and evaluate the occlusion. If adjust-

FIGURE 32-10 Tray setup for partial denture try-in appointment.

ments are needed, transfer the handpiece and burs.

2. The patient is given a hand mirror for viewing. Dismiss the patient and disinfect the partial to prepare it for the laboratory.

PROCEDURE 32-3

Delivery Appointment for Partial Denture

This procedure is performed by the dentist with assistance by the dental assistant. The partial denture is returned from the laboratory in a sealed container.

EQUIPMENT

- Basic setup: mouth mirror, explorer, and cotton pliers
- Partial denture
- Articulating paper and forceps

- Low-speed handpiece and acrylic burs and finishing burs

PROCEDURE STEPS *(Follow aseptic procedures)*

1. Preparations for the patient are completed.

2. The materials and equipment are similar to the try-in appointment with the exception of the wax adjustment instruments.

(continues)

PROCEDURE 32-3 *(CONTINUED)*

3. The patient is seated. If the patient has an old appliance, it is removed and placed in a cup with water.

4. The dentist seats the new partial denture (Figure 32-11) and makes any necessary adjustments. Rinse the partial denture and hand it to the dentist for insertion. Articulating paper is used to check the patient's occlusion. If adjustments are needed, transfer the low-speed handpiece with finishing or acrylic burs. Transfer contouring pliers for adjustments to the metal clasps.

5. The dentist instructs the patient on how to insert and remove the partial denture. Explain care of the partial and supporting teeth. Also explain that it may take several days to adjust to the partial and sore spots may appear. If the patient has any problems or questions, instruct him or her to call the office for an appointment right away.

FIGURE 32-11 Complete partial denture returned from dental laboratory.

TABLE 32-1   Appointments for Partial Denture

Appointment	Procedure
Examination	Prophylaxis is completed, preliminary impressions are taken, and radiographs and photographs are taken.
Consultation	Treatment is explained to the patient and treatment is chosen.
Final impressions	Abutment teeth are prepared, final impressions are taken, bite or occlusal registration is taken, and the shade and mold of artificial teeth are selected. *Note:* Sometimes restorative, periodontal, endodontic, or surgical procedures must be completed before the final impressions can be completed.
Try-in and adjustment	The framework is placed in the patient's mouth and adjustments are made accordingly.
Delivery	The partial is seated in the patient's mouth and instructions are given regarding how to place and remove the partial and about oral hygiene techniques.
Adjustment	As needed, adjustments are made at regular intervals to ensure proper fit

Complete Denture

The complete denture is also called the full denture. When all natural teeth are lost, a denture is fabricated to restore function and improve esthetics for the patient. (A person is said to be edentulous when he or she has no teeth remaining.) The denture is supported by the alveolar bone and oral mucosa. The shape and condition of the tissues determine how much support the denture will have.

Considerations for a Complete Denture

■ There is extensive bone loss and lack of support for remaining teeth in the arch.

■ The patient has exhibited lack of motivation and/or ability to maintain the remaining teeth.

■ The remaining teeth have gross decay, periodontal disease, or abscesses.

■ The patient is edentulous.

■ The patient lacks the financial means to have alternative treatments, including dental implants and fixed prostheses.

Necessities for Successful Denture Treatment

Dentures are not like natural teeth. They are prosthetic appliances that the patient must adjust to. For the patient to have success with dentures, he or she should have a positive attitude about the procedure and about wearing dentures. Dentures take time and patience to adjust to, and the patient who understands this will be more successful wearing them. Educate the patient so that he or she can prepare mentally. There are many pamphlets and videos available to explain to the patient what he or she can expect and how to function when wearing a denture.

The patient should be in good health. When a patient is in poor health, it is often reflected in the oral cavity. The added stress of a denture may lower the resistance of unhealthy tissues. Also, if there is weight loss or gain, the way the denture fits may change and a reline of the denture may be required. Impaired health may contribute to a lack of muscle coordination, which is needed to keep the denture in place.

The patient should have healthy alveolar ridges and oral mucosa. These tissues will be under stress from the denture and, if the denture does not fit properly, degeneration can occur at a much faster rate.

Components of a Complete Denture

The denture has two basic components: base and denture teeth (Figure 32-12). The external surface of the denture resembles natural tissues and extends over the retromolar pad on the mandible or the maxillary tuberosity area on the maxilla. The external sur-

FIGURE 32-12 Full maxillary and mandibular denture: denture base, artificial teeth, tissue side of denture on the left, and occlusal view on the right.

face is smooth and polished, while the internal surface matches the contours of the oral mucosa and the alveolar bone. The denture teeth are articulated to occlude with the natural or artificial teeth of the opposing arch.

Denture Base. The base is made of denture acrylic and may have a metal mesh embedded in the acrylic for additional strength. The acrylic is pigmented to resemble the normal gingiva; often, fibers are added to the acrylic to give the denture a natural appearance. The base covers the alveolar ridge and gingival tissues. The denture teeth are embedded in the denture base, just like the partial denture.

Denture Teeth. The denture teeth used in construction of the denture are made of porcelain or acrylic resin. The porcelain teeth are more resistant to stain and wear but are more brittle than the resins. They may wear away the opposing natural tooth structure, so they are used more often when the opposing teeth are also porcelain. Porcelain teeth sometimes cause a "clicking" sound when the patient is eating or talking.

Acrylic resin (plastic) teeth have the advantage of greater resistance to breakage. They are quieter and bond more efficiently to the denture base. The adjustments require less time, because the acrylic teeth can be polished in the office, whereas porcelain teeth must go to the laboratory to be refinished. The acrylic resin teeth are used when the patient has natural opposing teeth and in patients with poor ridges.

Porcelain teeth are secured in the denture base by mechanical means of pins on the anterior teeth and diatoric holes on the posterior (Figure 32-13A). The plastic teeth adequately bond to the denture base material and do not require mechanical retention.

Posterior denture teeth are either **anatomical** or **nonanatomical**. The anatomical teeth resemble natural teeth, with cusps and developmental grooves. The nonanatomical teeth do not have detailed anatomy on the occlusal surface but are concave and somewhat flat. Nonanatomical occlusals are designed for additional strength for patients with too little alveolar ridge to retain dentures.

FIGURE 32-13 (A) Porcelain teeth showing pins and diatoric holes. *Note:* These teeth are in a model in a flask preparatory to placing acrylic base material over them. (B) Sets of denture teeth showing shade and mold.

Denture teeth come in sets for the anterior and for the posterior. The anterior set includes six teeth: two cuspids, two laterals, and two central incisors. The posterior set includes eight teeth: four bicuspids and four molars. (Third molars are not placed in dentures.) These sets have matching shades and molds (shapes) (Figure 32-13B).

Immediate Dentures

The sequence of appointments for the complete denture depends on whether the patient is edentulous or has remaining teeth. When the patient is edentulous, he or she may already have a complete denture. This denture may have to be replaced with a new denture for better fit and retention, or the denture may have broken or been lost.

When the patient has remaining teeth, he or she will need to have the teeth extracted before receiving the denture. In this situation, there are two treatment sequences:

1. The patient can have all remaining teeth extracted and the alveolar bone shaped and contoured (alveoplasty). The patient waits for four to six months for the tissues and the alveolar bone to heal before the denture construction begins. The *advantage* of the sequence is that the tissues have healed and the alveolar ridge has resorbed to a stable position before impressions for the denture are started and the denture is fabricated. The *disadvantage* is that the patient is without teeth for the healing period. Esthetics and diet restrictions are concerns for the patient.

2. In the second treatment sequence, the patient has only the posterior teeth extracted—the anterior teeth remain. Construction of the denture begins as soon as the hard and soft tissues of the posterior areas have healed completely. When the dentures are completed, the anterior teeth are extracted, an alveolectomy is performed, and the denture is inserted. This is called an **immediate denture**. The advantages of the immediate denture are that the patient is never without teeth, the dentist and the laboratory have the patient's remaining teeth to reproduce the original appearance, there are no extreme diet restrictions, and the denture acts as a compress and bandage to protect the extraction sites. The disadvantages include no anterior try-in to evaluate the fit, the alveolar ridge changes after the extractions and alveoplasty, the denture needs to be relined in four to six months, and, because of the reline and the two appointments with the oral surgeon, this process is more costly to the patient.

The following sequence of appointments takes into consideration surgery appointments. Most patients elect to have the immediate denture sequence, and such additional appointments are noted in the procedure descriptions. For a brief overview of the appointments for a complete denture, see Table 32-2.

Examination and Diagnosis Appointments for Complete Denture

The examination appointment for complete dentures is similar to that of the examination for the partial den-

TABLE 32-2   Appointments for Complete Denture (Brief Overview)

Appointment	Procedure
Examination	An oral exam is completed. Preliminary impressions and radiographs are taken. The patient is asked to bring photos for the next appointment.
Consultation	Treatment is explained to the patient. Discussion of the treatment includes the dentist's and the patient's responsibilities.
Oral surgery	During the appointment, the posterior teeth are removed and the alveolar bone is contoured.
Final impressions	When the posterior extractions have healed completely, the patient returns to the dental office and final impressions are taken.
Jaw relationships	The jaw relationship is determined with baseplates and bite rims.
Denture delivery	The patient is scheduled for surgery to have the anterior teeth extracted and the immediate denture seated.
First follow-up (scheduled several days after the patient receives the denture)	With the immediate denture, the patient is seen the next day in the dental office.
Adjustments	As needed, adjustments are made

ture. The dentist completes a detailed examination of the condition of the tissues, the shapes and sizes of the ridges, the retromolar and tuberosity areas, the frenum attachments, and the undercut areas. Radiographs and preliminary impressions are taken. Current photographs are made and the patient is asked to bring in other photographs for reference to create a natural appearance for the patient.

Preparation of the diagnosis, treatment plans, and the financial estimate are similar to those of the partial denture prosthesis preparation.

Denture Construction between Appointments

Between the consultation and the final impressions appointment, the alginate impressions are poured in plaster or stone. On these models, custom acrylic trays are constructed. In the case of an immediate denture, the custom trays are fabricated to allow space for the anterior teeth present in the mouth and the posterior edentulous areas.

Between the final impression appointment and the measurements appointment at the dental laboratory, the master cast is poured in stone from the final impressions. The master cast is used to construct a **baseplate**. A baseplate is a preformed, semirigid, acrylic resin material that temporarily represents the denture base.

On the baseplate, several layers of baseplate wax are attached (Figure 32-14), called the **bite rim**. The bite

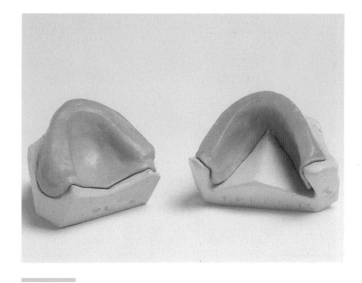

FIGURE 32-14 Baseplates and bite rims made in dental laboratory from final impressions.

rims represent the space provided by the teeth in normal occlusion. The bite rims, then, provide the **vertical dimension** for the denture and establish the position of the mandible to the maxilla. In the natural dentition, the length of the crowns of the teeth determines the distance between the upper and lower jaws. This distance is called the vertical dimension.

If the patient is receiving an immediate denture, the baseplate and bite rims are fabricated to fit over the posterior areas only. The patient's existing anterior teeth are used for jaw relationships and measurements.

Once the baseplate and bite rims are constructed, they are sent back to the dental office for the patient's next appointment.

Denture Construction between Appointments—Laboratory Procedures

Between appointments, the laboratory prepares a try-in denture. Denture teeth are mounted in the wax bite rim. They are positioned according to the dentist's directions, but the position can be altered at the try-in appointment (Figure 32-15).

FIGURE 32-15 Wax bite-rims with denture teeth on an articulator ready for try-in appointment. (A) Maxillary and mandibular dentures articulated in a closed position. (B) Maxillary and mandibular dentures articulated in an opened position.

PROCEDURE 32-4

Final Impression Appointment

This procedure is performed by the dentist. Materials are prepared and transferred to the dentist by the dental assistant.

EQUIPMENT (Figure 32-16)

- Basic setup: mouth mirror, explorer, cotton pliers

- HVE tip, air-water syringe tip

- Cotton rolls and gauze

- Mouthwash for patient to rinse with prior to impressions being taken

- Custom tray (see Chapter 35, Laboratory Materials and Techniques)

- Compound wax and Bunsen burner for border molding the rims of the trays

- Laboratory knife to trim border molding

- Impression materials—spatulas and mixing pads or dispensing gun and tips

- Laboratory prescription form

- Disinfectant and container for impressions and bite registration

PROCEDURE STEPS *(Follow aseptic procedures)*

1. The final impressions are taken after custom trays have been fabricated from the casts taken at the examination appointment. The custom trays are inserted into the patient's mouth and evaluated for fit.

2. The impression compound is heated and placed along the borders of the custom tray (Figure 32-17). The tray is cooled and then placed in the patient's mouth. With the tray in the patient's mouth, the lips, cheeks, and tongue are moved to establish accurate length for the periphery and adjacent tissues to be included in the final impression. This is called **border molding**, or **muscle trimming**.

3. Final impression materials are prepared and placed in the custom trays. The maxillary impression must include the tuberosities, frenum attachments, and other landmarks of the arch. The mandibular impression must include retromolar pads, oblique ridge, mylohyoid ridge, and frenum attachments.

4. Once the material has set, it is removed from the patient's mouth. The mouth is then rinsed thoroughly.

5. This procedure is repeated with the opposing arch if a full denture is being fabricated for both arches.

6. The impressions are disinfected and sent to the dental laboratory with the prescription form.

7. After the impressions have been taken, the patient is dismissed.

FIGURE 32-16 Tray setup for final impressions of complete denture with custom trays.

FIGURE 32-17 Custom tray that has been border molded to fit patient for the final impression.

PROCEDURE 32-5

Jaw Relationship Appointment

This procedure is performed by the dentist. During this appointment, the measurements, shape, and shade of the denture are determined. The dental assistant prepares equipment and materials and assists the dentist throughout the procedure.

EQUIPMENT (Figure 32-18)

- Basic setup: mouth mirror, explorer, and cotton pliers
- HVE tip and air-water syringe tip
- Hand mirror
- Laboratory knife, #7 wax spatula, Bunsen burner
- Shade guide
- Millimeter ruler and boley gauge
- Baseplates and bite rims
- Face bow
- Photographs of the patient, showing the shapes and shades of the teeth
- Laboratory prescription form
- Disinfectant

PROCEDURE STEPS *(Follow aseptic procedures)*

1. The baseplates and bite rims are inserted into the patient's mouth. The dentist determines and marks

FIGURE 32-18 Tray setup for jaw relationship appointment.

the midline of the maxillary and mandibular arches.

2. The bite rims represent the teeth and provide the vertical dimension. The dentist adjusts the wax bite rims with the laboratory knife and wax spatula until the patient has a natural lip drape and the correct amount of tooth and gingiva is visible when the patient is talking and smiling and the lips are in a resting position. The cuspid lines are determined to position cuspids at the corners of the mouth.

3. The **centric occlusion** is determined when the jaws are closed in a position that produces maximal contact between the occluding surfaces of the maxillary and mandibular arches. The jaw relationships are determined by evaluating how the mandible relates to the maxilla. The patient moves the mandible as far backward (retrusion) and forward (protrusion) as possible, and then as far to the right and then the left (lateral movement). Specially designed baseplates and materials assist in determining these measurements. Once determined, the information is used to articulate the casts to duplicate the normal motions of the patient. The laboratory technician constructs the complete denture in wax and with artificial teeth from these records.

4. After the jaw relationships are determined, the denture teeth are selected, and the appearance of the anterior teeth is discussed with the patient. The proper shade is determined using the shade guide and natural light. To achieve a natural look, the shade guide is compared with the patient's complexion and remaining natural teeth or photographs. Usually, the age of the patient indicates the shade range (the teeth stain and become darker with age). The shape (mold) of the teeth is determined by evaluating remaining natural teeth or from photographs. Sometimes, the shape of the patient's face also is used to guide the selection.

5. Because patients are concerned about the natural appearance of the teeth, some patients want to duplicate the arrangement of the teeth, including spaces, overlapping, and so on. Other patients want to correct the alignment of the natural teeth in the new denture. Spending a little more time at this point and having clear communication with the patient to determine what the expected outcome is often pays off when the patient receives the denture and is pleased with his or her appearance.

PROCEDURE 32-6

Try-In Appointment

This procedure is performed by the dentist. The dental assistant prepares the patient, instruments, and materials, and coordinates with the dental laboratory.

EQUIPMENT AND SUPPLIES

The equipment and supplies are the same for the try-in appointment as they are for the jaw relationship appointment.

PROCEDURE STEPS *(Follow aseptic procedures)*

1. The "try-in" denture is disinfected before being placed in the patient's mouth.

2. The patient is seated and the denture is inserted into the patient's mouth. The dentist and/or the dental assistant spends a few minutes talking with the patient. This allows the patient time to adjust to the denture.

3. The denture is evaluated for esthetics, retention, and comfort. The occlusion is checked with articulating paper.

4. The dentist makes adjustments to the position of the teeth. The shade can be changed by the dental laboratory technician in the dental laboratory, if necessary.

5. Once the dentist and the patient are satisfied with the denture, it is disinfected and placed back on the articulator to be returned to the laboratory.

Denture Construction between Appointments—Final Laboratory Procedures

The denture is returned to the laboratory for final processing. This is a multistep process that converts the wax try-in denture to a denture with an acrylic resin base and plastic or porcelain teeth. A dental flask is utilized for this process (Figure 32-19). The dental assistant should visit the dental laboratory and observe the steps involved in processing a denture to better understand and visualize the steps involved.

FIGURE 32-19 Dental flask and investment material used with denture teeth to fabricate the denture base.

Denture Adjustment Appointments

After receiving the immediate denture, the patient returns to the office the next day. The denture is removed and the tissues are examined. If any areas are uncomfortable to the patient at this time, the dentist performs minor adjustments. Because of the swelling and tenderness from the surgery, the dentist will not remove too much of the denture surface at this time. The patient is taught how to insert and remove the dentures and oral hygiene techniques. He or she is rescheduled in a couple of days for any adjustments.

The patient returns to the office after wearing the denture for several days. The dentist evaluates the tissues and may smooth rough areas, relieve pressure spots, and adjust the occlusion. The amount of adjustment varies with every patient, and this process may require several appointments over a period of time until the denture is comfortable.

The occlusion is adjusted with the burs, stones, and discs on the cusps of the denture teeth. Pressure spots are relieved on the tissue surface of the denture base. Pressure indicator paste is placed on the internal surface of the denture and then inserted into the patient's mouth. Pressure areas are marked and the dentist then uses acrylic burs and stones for adjustments.

PROCEDURE 32-7

Delivery Appointment for Complete Denture

This procedure is performed by the dentist. The dental assistant prepares the patient and coordinates with the dental laboratory. The dentures come back from the laboratory in a container that keeps them moist.

EQUIPMENT (Figure 32-20)

- Basic setup: mouth mirror, explorer, and cotton pliers

- HVE tip and air-water syringe tip

- Dentures from the laboratory

- Hand mirror

- Articulating forceps and paper

- High-speed handpiece and diamond and finishing burs

- Low-speed handpiece and assorted acrylic burs and discs

- Home-care instructions pamphlet, denture brush, and container to place dentures in when they are not in the patient's mouth

FIGURE 32-20 Tray setup for seating of complete denture.

PROCEDURE STEPS *(Follow aseptic procedures)*

1. The patient is seated and the appliances are removed and placed in a container to keep them moist.

2. If the patient is receiving an immediate denture, the denture is inserted after the extractions and alveoplasty. If there are more than simple extractions, the patient is scheduled with an oral maxillofacial surgeon. The dental laboratory sends the denture to the surgeon's office instead of to the dentist's office before the patient's surgery.

3. The new denture is inserted into the patient's mouth and the patient is given a few minutes to adjust. The dentist then begins the examination.

4. The patient's occlusion is evaluated and, if adjustment is needed, burs and discs are used. The denture is removed from the patient's mouth and the dentist uses a low-speed handpiece and acrylic burs to reduce any high spots on the inside of the base (the part of the denture that is against the tissues) of the denture. Sometimes after the adjustments, the denture needs to be polished in the laboratory. If this process is necessary, the denture must be disinfected before replacing it in the patient's mouth.

5. The dentist evaluates the retention of the denture and the jaw relationships by having the patient demonstrate various facial expressions, swallowing, chewing actions, and speaking.

6. The patient learns to insert and remove the denture and daily maintenance of the denture (see Table 32-3).

7. The patient is given instructions to call the office with any questions or problems and is scheduled for an adjustment appointment in a few days. The patient is then dismissed. As a courtesy, often the dentist or dental assistant calls the patient the following day to check on the patient's progress with the new denture.

Denture Reline

The tissue side of the denture bases may need to be **relined** to improve the fit of the denture and the comfort of the patient. After a period of time, the supporting tissues often shrink and change in size because of the pressure put on them by the complete or the partial denture. The denture relining adds a new layer of acrylic to the inside of the denture (Figure 32-21). This procedure can be done in the dental office (chairside) or sent to the dental laboratory (Procedure 32-8).

The chairside (soft) reline saves the patient time and makes it possible for the patient to never be without the denture. This reline process is a temporary solution,

TABLE 32-3   Home-Care Instructions

Keep the denture moist when not wearing it to prevent dimensional change.
Do not use abrasive dentifrice on the acrylic, because it abrades easily.
Do not clean acrylic dentures in hot water, because the acrylic can be deformed and distorted when exposed to high temperatures.
Dentures have low thermal conductivity, so the patient will notice a decrease in thermal changes to the tissues under the acrylic denture base.
Rinse thoroughly twice a day and after eating, if possible.
Use a soft denture brush and toothpaste designed for partials and dentures.
Remove the denture and rinse the oral cavity daily.
Denture adhesives are not needed with a well-fitting denture. As the tissues change and the denture does not adapt as well, adhesives will fill in the spaces so retention is increased.
Commercial cleaners are available for overnight soaking. Use warm water with these products.
The patient may wish to fill the sink with water or place a washcloth in the sink in case the denture or partial is dropped.

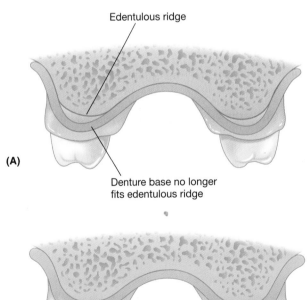

Edentulous ridge

(A)

Denture base no longer
fits edentulous ridge

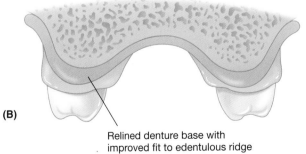

(B)

Relined denture base with
improved fit to edentulous ridge

FIGURE 32-21   (A) An ill-fitting denture. (B) Fit with denture reline.

Tissue Conditioning

Sometimes the tissues are irritated and inflamed due to an ill-fitting denture. These tissues must be healed before a denture reline is completed. This process is called tissue conditioning. A temporary soft lining material is placed in the denture to relieve the pressure and allow the tissues to heal. The healing usually takes several weeks and then the denture can be relined.

Denture Repair

The denture may need repair from time to time. Sometimes a denture tooth becomes loose or is lost or the denture is dropped and fractured. When the patient brings the denture or partial to the office for repair, the dental assistant should disinfect it before the repair process begins. Some of the repairs can be completed in the dental office, but other, more complex repairs must be sent to the dental laboratory. The patient may need to be seen by the dentist if an impression is needed or, in some cases, the dentures can be left at the office for repairs. The repairs often do not take long and the patient returns later in the same day or the next day to pick up the denture. Sometimes the patient is seen by the dentist for minor adjustments.

Polishing Removable Prostheses

After the dentist has adjusted the tissue surface of the removable prosthesis with acrylic burs, discs, and stones, it may need to be polished to smooth the sur-

because the soft reline is not as durable and will not last as long as the laboratory reline. The laboratory reline takes more time, and the patient may be without the dentures for a day. The laboratory reline replaces the tissue side of the denture.

PROCEDURE 32-8

Denture Relining

This procedure is performed by the dentist. The dental assistant prepares the patient and the materials. The reline materials are available in either hard or semi-soft materials. There is a variety to choose from, depending on the dentist's preference.

EQUIPMENT (Figure 32-22)

- Basic setup: mouth mirror, explorer, and cotton pliers
- Low-speed handpiece with acrylic burs
- Chairside reline materials
- Mouth rinse

Chairside Relining

PROCEDURE STEPS *(Follow aseptic procedures)*

1. Clean the denture by placing it in an ultrasonic unit for a few minutes.

2. The dentist uses acrylic burs to roughen the tissue side of the denture.

3. The material is mixed according to manufacturer's directions and then placed in the clean denture, covering the entire tissue surface. The materials have low thermal reaction and cure directly in the patient's mouth.

4. The patient rinses with mouthwash to clean saliva and debris from the tissues.

FIGURE 32-22 Tray setup for denture reline.

5. The denture is inserted into the patient's mouth and the patient is asked to bite until the material reaches the initial set stage. Explain to the patient that sometimes the tissue will have a slight burning sensation from the acrylic material during the setting time.

6. The denture is removed to complete the setting process.

7. Excess material is trimmed away and the denture is polished. Follow routine disinfecting before the denture is inserted into the patient's mouth.

Laboratory Relining

The patient's denture is prepared in the same manner as it is for the chairside relining procedure. The following are the impression and laboratory steps. The tray setup is the same as that in the chairside relining, except for the types of materials used. Often, the denture or partial is used as the tray for the impression materials. A variety of impression materials, including polysulfides, polyethers, and silicone, are used to take the impression.

PROCEDURE STEPS *(Follow aseptic procedures)*

1. The impression material is mixed and placed in the denture (tray) according to the manufacturer's directions. The material should cover the entire tissue surface of the denture evenly and without excess.

2. The denture is inserted into the patient's mouth and positioned firmly. The patient should occlude and hold until the material is set.

3. After the material sets, the denture is removed from the patient's mouth, disinfected, and prepared to be sent to the dental laboratory. The laboratory prescription is completed and the patient is dismissed.

4. The dental laboratory processes the impression materials into an acrylic resin base that is fused to the denture.

5. The patient returns to the dental office as soon as the laboratory can process the denture. The turnaround time varies from hours to several days. The procedure is scheduled with the laboratory to minimize the time the patient is without the denture.

6. When the patient returns to the office, the denture is seated and adjustments are made as needed.

FIGURE 32-23 Dental lathe with rag wheel and Tripoli to polish prosthesis.

FIGURE 32-24 Overdenture supported with abutments (roots are restored with cast-gold post and dome-shaped core combination). *(Courtesy of Clifton O. Caldwell, Jr., DDS, FICD, FACD.)*

face. The polishing can be accomplished on a dental lathe with rag wheels, pumice slurry, and various other polishing agents, such as Tripole or a paste of tin oxide and water (Figure 32-23). Care must be taken not to overheat the denture, because the denture base has a relatively low heat-transfer temperature. If the denture is overheated, it may be distorted, which affects the fit and the appearance of the denture. Also, the plastic teeth should be protected because they will abrade easily. Once the polish is complete, the prosthesis is washed in soap and water, disinfected, and stored in water until it is delivered to the patient. For each patient, separate burs, rag wheels, and pumice should be used to maintain infection control. Burs and rag wheels can be sterilized. The pumice is mixed with a disinfectant and green soap mixture and should be changed after each use.

Overdenture

Over time, the pressure applied during mastication on the mucosa and the supporting underlying alveolar bone causes the bone to shrink/absorb. The denture is not as stable, and retention becomes a problem for the patient. An **overdenture** can be fabricated to prevent or reduce this problem. The patient with overdentures has shown less alveolar bone loss.

To fabricate an overdenture, the dentist saves certain parts of the patient's remaining teeth or places dental implants in the dental arch on which the denture will attach. Instead of the denture base resting on the mucosa and the alveolar bone, the denture is supported by the retained prepared teeth (Figure 32-24) or the dental implants (Figures 32-25 and 32-26).

FIGURE 32-25 (A) Dental implants for a denture. (B) Denture to fit over dental implants. *(Courtesy of Paul A. Johnson, DDS.)*

Endosseous Implant and Overdenture for Implant

The retained teeth are endodontically treated and prepared with posts and cores or with special prefabricated attachments. The tissue side of the denture is constructed with part of the attachment aligned with the implant or retained tooth. There are various types of attachments, including magnets and a "snap" design.

FIGURE 32-26 (A) Panoramic radiograph showing dental implants to secure a denture. (B) Denture in place over the dental implants. *(Courtesy of Dr. Kenji Higuchi.)*

The advantages include retention and stability of the denture, especially if the patient does not have much alveolar ridge to retain a denture to begin with. The disadvantages include an increase in the cost and time involved because of the surgeries, endodontic treatment, and restorative procedures. Also, the patient must maintain the retained teeth and/or the dental implants. Plaque control is essential to prevent bone loss around the implants and the retained teeth and to inhibit root caries on the retained teeth. The patient must be diligent and motivated for the success of the overdenture.

CHAPTER SUMMARY

Removable prosthodontics, like fixed prosthodontics, refer to the replacement of missing teeth and tissues with artifical structures, or prostheses. With removable prosthodontics, however, the prosthesis can be removed from the mouth of the patient. Most patients prefer to have fixed prostheses, but in some cases it may not be the treatment of choice due to existing conditions.

The dental assistant's main functions are to prepare materials, record measurements and details for the fabrication of the denture, provide patient education and support, and perform some laboratory procedures. The procedures in removable prosthodontics do not require many instrument exchanges, and the assistant does not continually maintain the oral cavity throughout the appointment with the air-water syringe and the HVE. The steps in removable prosthodontics involve as many extraoral as intraoral procedures. The dental assistant has all the items prepared so that the dentist can explain to the patient the diagnosis, the proposed treatment plan, and the prognosis.

Case Study

Julie Davidson has been told by Dr. Jacobson that she needs a maxillary full denture. Mrs. Davidson has had problems with her teeth over the years because of advanced periodontal disease. She is an office manager for a group of physicians, and is very conscientious about her appearance and apprehensive about wearing dentures.

Case Study Review

1. What denture procedure would allow Julie to continue to function with her natural teeth while her maxillary denture is fabricated?

2. What types of patient information are available?

3. To prepare the patient for the denture procedure, what should the dental assistant consider?

REVIEW QUESTIONS

Multiple Choice

1. Removable prosthodontics include all of the following procedures except
   a. partial denture.
   b. full denture.
   c. crown and bridge.
   d. immediate denture.

2. Parts of the partial denture that contact the teeth to provide vertical and horizontal support are
   a. connectors.
   b. rests.
   c. retainers.
   d. denture bases.

3. Denture teeth are made of
   a. porcelain.
   b. plastic.
   c. both porcelain and plastic.
   d. amalgam.

4. When the jaws are closed to produce the maximum contact, _____ can be determined.
   a. vertical dimension
   b. centric occlusion
   c. vertical occlusion
   d. horizontal dimension

5. All of the following are correct home-care instructions for a patient just receiving a full denture *except*:
   a. Rinse the denture twice a day and after eating, if possible.
   b. Use a soft denture brush and toothpaste designated for dentures.
   c. Place water or a washcloth in the sink in case the denture is dropped while cleaning it.
   d. Use hot water when cleaning the denture to remove bacteria.

6. _____ abutment teeth may be prepared with rests to secure a removable partial denture.
   a. Incisor
   b. Cuspid
   c. Premolar
   d. Molars

7. The _____ retainer encircles and adapts to the contours of the abutment tooth.
   a. circumferential-type clasp
   b. bar-type clasp
   c. stress-breaker
   d. major connector

8. The part(s) of the partial denture that rest(s) upon the oral mucosa, providing coverage and stability, is(are) called the
   a. retainer.
   b. metallic framework.
   c. denture base.
   d. connectors.

9. All of the following statements are true about immediate dentures except:
   a. Patients are never without teeth with this technique.
   b. The patient has all teeth extracted, waits four to six months, and then the denture is fabricated.
   c. The patient's remaining teeth assist the laboratory to reproduce the original appearance of his or her teeth in the denture.
   d. This denture needs to be relined in four to six months.

10. The process of using impression compound to modify the custom tray is called
   a. centric rotation.
   b. vertical dimension.
   c. the smile line.
   d. border-molding/muscle trimming.

Critical Thinking

1. What types of materials can be used to take the final impression for a partial denture?

2. During which complete denture appointment must the baseplates and bite rims be ready for use?

3. When would a patient be a good candidate for an overdenture? What is an overdenture?

Web Activities

1. Find out how patients should care for their dentures. Go to questions patients frequently ask at http://www.ada.org, "dentures," and then "removable partial denture."

2. Go to http://www.nadl.org and find out if there is an accredited dental laboratory education program in your area.

3. Go to http://www.valplast.com to learn more about flexible partials.

4. Find out what metal partials are made of at http://www.austenal.com

SECTION

VIII

RESTORATIVE AND LABORATORY MATERIALS AND TECHNIQUES

DENTAL CEMENTS, BASES, LINERS, AND BONDING AGENTS

SPECIFIC INSTRUCTIONAL OBJECTIVES

The student should strive to meet the following objectives and demonstrate an understanding of the facts and principles presented in this chapter:

1. Explain the types of dental restorative materials.

2. List dental standards and organizations responsible for those standards.

3. Explain the role of the dental assistant.

4. List and explain the properties of dental materials.

5. Identify the types of dental cements. Explain their properties, composition, uses, and manipulation.

6. Describe bonding agents and their manipulation.

7. Describe the steps of cavity preparation.

8. Identify cavity preparation terminology.

ADVANCED CHAIRSIDE FUNCTIONS

9. Classify cavity preparations according to their relationships with the pulp.

10. Explain options for protecting the pulp with cavity liners, cavity varnish, and cement bases.

11. Describe the purpose of using cavity liners. List types of materials that can be used and explain the placement procedure.

12. Describe the purpose of using cavity varnish and explain the placement procedure.

13. Describe the purpose of using cement bases. List types of materials that can be used and explain the placement procedure.

KEY TERMS

adhesives *(786)*

axial wall *(791)*

base *(773)*

bonding *(771)*

bonding agents *(771)*

bonding resins *(786)*

bruxism *(770)*

calcium hydroxide *(773)*

cavity liners *(794)*

cavity preparation *(793)*

cavity varnish *(794)*

cavosurface margin *(791)*

cement bases *(794)*

chemical retention *(771)*

compomers *(773)*

copal varnish *(783)*

corrosion *(770)*

desensitizers *(790)*

dimensional change *(770)*

(continues)

INTRODUCTION

Although some materials used in dentistry have been around for a long time, there are constant changes and new products always being introduced. The dental team is updated by attending seminars and dental conferences, reading books and trade magazines, and through local sales representatives.

Generally, the materials are divided and categorized by function. Some materials have a broad spectrum of uses. After the tooth has been prepared and decay removed, certain materials are utilized to restore the tooth. Dental materials are regulated and tested for function and safety before they become available for use. The ADA and the Food and Drug Administration (FDA) regulate dental materials. The ADA Council on Dental Materials, Instruments, and Equipment is responsible for the testing of dental materials, and periodically publishes a listing of certified dental materials in the *Journal of the American Dental Association* and in *Clinical Products in Dentistry: A Desktop Reference.*

The ADA, in cooperation with the government, sponsored research on more than fifty types of dental materials. From this research, specifications and standards were established. These standards are updated continually and used to evaluate new materials. If a material meets specification requirements, the *ADA Seal of Certification* is awarded. This certifies that the material meets the criteria established by the ADA and the government, and that it is safe and effective.

For new types of dental materials, the ADA Council conducts the Acceptance Program for evaluation. The *Seal of Acceptance of the ADA* indicates that the material has proven to be safe and effective through biological, laboratory, and clinical evaluation, but that there are no physical standards or specifications by which the material can be measured for certification.

In addition, the following international organizations develop standards for materials, instruments, and equipment produced around the world: the Fédération Dentaire Internationale and International Standards Organization (ISO). (See Chapter 1, Introduction to the Dental Profession.)

Role of the Dental Assistant

The dental assistant's role when working with dental restorative materials depends on the expanded functions of individual state practice acts that regulate dentistry. The chairside dental assistant generally prepares and mixes the material while the dentist places the material in the oral cavity. Some states allow the dental assistant to perform these responsibilities in addition to placing the material in the oral cavity.

Knowledge of dental material properties is necessary for the dental assistant to properly prepare and manipulate the materials. The assistant's knowledge of dental materials is also beneficial for patient education and protection. Expanded-function dental assistants must understand and be competent in placing and finishing such materials.

Properties of Dental Materials

Replacing natural tooth structure has presented a number of challenges. The oral cavity environment and functions create complex situations. Properties that are considered for dental materials include:

Acidity

Acidity is viewed both in terms of its effect on a given material and on tissues in the mouth.

1. The normal pH of the oral cavity is about neutral (pH 7.0). Acidic foods, such as citrus fruits, and some bacteria found in the plaque are also acidic. Saliva aids in reducing the acidity of the mouth, but dental materials are subject to varying amounts of acid. How materials react to changing acidity levels in the mouth determines their use in the oral cavity.

2. The second consideration is that the acidity of the materials may cause irritation to the gingival tissues or damage to the pulp. These materials can be used successfully in the mouth, but care is taken to prepare them and/or place them following manufacturer's directions.

---

pH Scale

The pH scale, which ranges from 0 to 14, measures the level of acidity or alkalinity of a substance. A pH of 7 is neutral, a pH less than 7 is acidic, and a pH greater than 7 is basic.

Adhesion

Adhesion is the force or attraction that holds unlike substances together. Adhesion involves physical or chemical forces. Chemical adhesion is quite strong and preferable, but physical adhesion is more common. Adhesion is a way to attach solid structures to each other. An example of physical adhesion is dental plaque adhering to the tooth. Certain dental cements function on the basis of a chemical reaction, which results in (chemical) adhesion.

Biting Forces

Biting Force

The average biting force for a person with natural dentition varies from 130 to 170 pounds on the molars and progresses downward to about 40 pounds on the incisors. When force is applied on an individual tooth, this represents about 25,000 pounds per square inch (psi) on a single cusp or a molar.

Dental materials are subject to various types of biting forces. Natural dentition can withstand much more force than prostheses such as dentures and bridges. **Force** is defined as any push or pull on an object. The result of

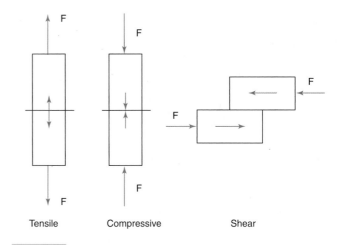

FIGURE 33-1 Tensile, compressive, and shearing stress and strain.

force on an object is resistance. The reaction of the object to resist the external force is called **stress**. Forces can cause stress over a large area, such as a quadrant, or over a small area, such as the occlusal surface of a tooth. Enough stress can be placed on an object to cause a change. This change or deformation is known as **strain**.

Types of stress and strain are described below (Figure 33-1):

1. *Tensile*—Pulls and stretches a material. Under tensile stress and strain, the structure tends to be elongated. An example of tensile stress and strain are wires that are pulled in opposite directions or elastic bands (rubber) used in orthodontics. The ability of a material to withstand forces of tensile stress without failing is known as **ductility**.

2. *Compressive*—Pushes or compresses a material. An example of compressive stress and strain is chewing or biting. The ability of a material to withstand compressive stresses without fracturing is known as **malleability**.

3. *Shearing*—Slides one part of a material parallel to another part in a back-and-forth motion. An example of shearing stress and strain is **bruxism**, or grinding of the teeth.

Corrosion

Corrosion is the result of chemical or electrochemical attacks of the oral environment on pure metal, such as gold, or an alloy, such as amalgam. Components of food and/or saliva react with the metals and cause deep pitting and roughness. Sometimes the metals become dull and discolored. This effect is referred to as **tarnish** (Figure 33-2).

Dimensional Change

Dimensional change in a material can occur from a variety of causes, such as the setting process of a material

FIGURE 33-2 Amalgam restoration showing corrosion and tarnish. *(Courtesy of Dr. Gary Shellerud.)*

or exposure to heat or cold. The change in a material usually is measured as a percentage of the original length or volume. If an impression material goes through dimensional change, the permanent restoration may not fit on the tooth because the impression material does not represent the exact dimensions of the prepared tooth.

Elasticity

Some materials have the property of **elasticity**, which is the ability to be distorted or deformed by an applied force and then return to its original shape once the force is removed. Rubber bands exhibit this property, but if they are stretched for too long or too far, they reach their *elastic limit* and will not return to their original shape.

The *elastic modulus,* or modulus of elasticity, is a measure of the stiffness of a material below the elastic limit. This is a measure of how a material can resist deformation or change.

Flow

Flow, or creep and slump, is a continuing deformation of a solid. Under a constant force, certain materials change and deform. Examples of materials where flow is a factor are dental waxes and certain impression materials. Amalgam is subject to flow under constant compressive forces.

Galvanism

When two different metals are present in the mouth there is potential for the creation of small electrical shocks. This is known as **galvanism**. The oral fluids act as a carrier between the two metals to cause an electrical shock. This can occur when a gold restoration in one arch contacts an amalgam restoration in the opposing tooth in the opposite arch. The same shock happens if an individual bites a piece of tin foil and it contacts a tooth with a restoration.

Hardness

The resistance of a material to scratch or indent is known as the material's hardness. There are various ways to measure the hardness of a material. Dental materials that can be dented or scratched will show wear.

Microleakage

When saliva and debris from the oral cavity seep between the tooth structure and the restorative materials, this is known as **microleakage**. The dentist prepares the cavity and places materials to prevent microleakage, but some microleakage still occurs. Recurrent decay and tooth sensitivity are some of the problems resulting from microleakage (Figure 33-3).

Retention

Retention in dentistry is one means by which materials are held in place. Different types of retention methods are used with the various types of restorative materials. Materials placed directly into the cavity preparation (direct restorative materials), such as amalgam and composites, are retained in place by mechanical means. **Mechanical retention** includes preparing the walls of the cavity preparation to be convergent (slanted in), by roughening the tooth surface with etchant, or by placing retentive grooves in the cavity walls.

Retention for indirect restorations such as gold inlays or crowns is accomplished with bonding agents and cements. Cements and bonding agents may be retained to the tooth surface by mechanical or chemical means. **Chemical retention** involves a chemical reaction between the tooth surface and the material.

Bonding

Bonding is the process by which materials adhere firmly or hold together. In dentistry, **bonding agents** are used

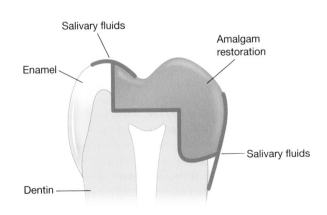

FIGURE 33-3 Microleakage can occur around the margins of an amalgam restoration.

to bond the dentin and enamel with restorative materials. These materials are discussed later in this chapter.

Solubility

When a material is soluble, it dissolves in fluid. The solubility of a dental material is one factor used to determine the success of the material in the oral cavity. A material that is soluble may be useful as a base or liner where it is not exposed to the oral fluids. If the material is exposed to the saliva, it dissolves and exposes the tooth structure.

Thermal Properties

Thermal conductivity is the ability of material to transmit heat. With some materials heat transmits rapidly, while with others the process is very slow. Thermal conductivity of a material is a consideration when it is placed near the dental pulp because a material that has a low rate of thermal conductivity offers more protection. Materials are placed in layers over the pulp to protect it from thermal changes. For example, the patient with a denture can drink hotter coffee because the denture base material has low thermal conductivity; thus, it protects the tissues under the denture.

Thermal expansion is another consideration for dental materials. With temperature changes, materials expand and contract. When materials are used in the oral cavity, they must expand and contract at a rate close to that of the tooth structure. Dimensional changes that occur from thermal expansion and contraction can lead to microleakage and sensitive teeth (Figure 33-3).

Viscosity

Viscosity of a material is the ability of liquid to flow. The thicker the material, the less it flows; therefore, it is said to be more viscous than a thin material that flows easily. Honey that is cool is thick and viscous, but when heated, it becomes thinner and less viscous. Materials that are more viscous do not spread easily over a surface. For example, if a cement is viscous, it will not flow over the tooth surface to produce adequate retention.

Wettability

The ability of a material to flow over a surface is wettability. This is an important property when applying certain dental materials. Wettability can be demonstrated by observing the shape of a drop on a solid material (Figure 33-4). If the drop spreads out (forming a low contact angle), the solid is readily wetted by the liquid. If the drop beads (forming a high contact angle), there is poor wetting of the solid. For instance, pit and fissure sealants should have good wettability to cover the grooves of the occlusal surface (Figure 33-4).

FIGURE 33-4 Example of material "wettability."

Types of Restorative Dental Materials

Dental materials used to restore teeth can be divided into two sections:

1. Liners, bases, cements, and bonding agents—Materials to prepare the teeth for restorative materials

2. Amalgam, composite, and glass ionomer restorative materials (see Chapter 34)

These materials are mixed at chairside by the dental assistant as indicated by the dentist, following manufacturer's instructions and the dentist's preferences. It is the dental assistant's responsibility to maintain the materials and the mixing equipment.

Dental Cements

Dental cements usually come in a powder/liquid form, two-paste system, capsule, or dispensing syringe. Most of these materials are mixed manually, but a few of the powder/liquid cements come in capsules that are mixed mechanically. Cements are mixed in a precise ratio to attain a specific consistency, ranging from a liquid solution to a putty consistency.

Dental cements set or cure by self-curing (chemical reaction between two materials), by means of a curing light (light cured) or by dual curing. Light-cured materials are becoming very popular because the operator has more time to place and manipulate the materials before curing them. These materials are sensitive to overhead lights, however, and must be protected from light if dispensed ahead of time. Dual-cured materials combine self-curing properties and light-curing techniques.

Several terms are used in conjunction with dental materials. Knowing these terms assists in understanding material uses and functions.

■ Luting—Bonding or cementing together. Dental cements may be used as luting agents to bond inlays, bridges, and so on to teeth.

■ Permanent luting cement—Long-term cementing agent.

- **Temporary luting cement**—Short-term cementing agent.
- **Intermediate luting cement**—Material that lasts six months to a year.
- **Liner**—Material placed in a thin layer on the walls and floor of the cavity preparation. The liner protects the pulp from bacteria and irritants.
- **Base**—Applied in a putty or thick layer between the tooth and restoration to protect the pulp from chemical irritation, temperature changes, electrical protection, and mechanical injury. Bases are strong enough to be placed under restorative materials and to support the materials from occlusal stresses.
- **Sedative** or **palliative effect**—Soothing effect that a material may have on a tooth. The sedative or palliative material may relieve pain but does not cure the problem.
- **Varnish**—Thin layer of material that is placed to seal the walls and floor of the cavity preparation.

Uses of Dental Cements

There are many types of dental cements, and each type of cement can have several uses (see Table 33-1 for the types of the cements and their uses). Some cements are combined with other materials to modify or expand their functions. Examples are reinforced zinc oxide eugenol cements and glass ionomers.

> Dental cements are usually mixed on a paper pad. Although the paper pads are easy to use and clean up, they present a disinfection problem. After mixing, the top sheet of the paper pad is discarded and rest of the pad is placed on the tray. Once in the sterilizing area, the paper pad is wiped with a disinfectant around the edges where the assistant may have held the pad. While this method works, after a while the edges of the paper pad begin to curl and the pad becomes difficult to use.
>
> An alternative to using paper pads is a Teflon slab, or for smaller mixes, the plastic that comes in x-ray packages. Be creative!

TABLE 33-1 Dental Cements and Functions

Type of Cement	Uses or Functions
Zinc phosphate	Permanent cementation of crowns, inlays, onlays, bridges, and orthodontic bands and brackets. An insulating base.
Zinc oxide eugenol	Temporary cementation of crowns, inlays, onlays, and bridges. A temporary restoration and a low-strength base (palliative base). Also a periodontal dressing after periodontal surgery. Root canal sealer.
Reinforced zinc oxide eugenol	Permanent cementation of crowns, bridges, inlays, and onlays. An insulating base and temporary restoration.
Polycarboxylate	Permanent cementation of crowns, bridges, inlays, onlays, and orthodontic bands and brackets. A high-strength base and a temporary restoration.
Glass ionomer	Permanent cementation of crowns, bridges, inlays, onlays, and orthodontic bands and brackets. A high-strength base and a low-strength liner. A permanent bonding liner for composites. Also a root canal sealer, restorative material, and core buildup material.
Calcium hydroxide	Low-strength liner.
Varnish	Thin liner.
Resin cement	Permanent cementation of cast crowns, bridges, inlays, onlays, and endodontic posts. Cementation of ceramic or composite inlays and onlays, cementation of resin-bonded bridges, and cementation of orthodontic bands.
Resin-reinforced glass ionomer	Used to cement metallic restorations or porcelain-fused-to-metal restorations to tooth structure. Core buildup material and high-strength liner.
Compomers	Referred to as polyacid-modified resins. They are used to cement all types of dental restorations.

Zinc Phosphate Cement

Zinc phosphate cement is one of the oldest, and while it does have some disadvantages, it is still a reliable choice for a luting and base cement. It comes in a powder/liquid form, and several brands are available.

Composition. The zinc phosphate powder is primarily zinc oxide with a small amount of magnesium oxide and pigments. The powder is available in shades of white, yellow, and gray. The liquid is a solution of phosphoric acid in water buffered by agents to slow down the setting reaction. Because the liquid is acidic and irritating to the pulp, the tooth must be protected with bases or liners before the cement is placed.

When the powder and liquid are mixed together, a chemical reaction occurs and heat is released. The reaction is called **exothermic**. As heat is produced, the reaction speeds up even more. There are specific guidelines to follow when mixing zinc phosphate cement to minimize the temperature rise and slow the reaction process. This provides reasonable working time and allows for maximum incorporation of powder.

Properties. When mixed, the zinc phosphate cement is high in strength and reaches two-thirds of this strength in less than an hour. Zinc phosphate sets (hardens) in five to nine minutes and has a long mixing time of up to two minutes. Viscosity is affected by mixing time and temperature. Zinc phosphate bonds to the tooth by means of mechanical interlocking.

Manipulation Considerations. When the zinc phosphate powder is mixed with the liquid, an exothermic reaction occurs. The cement is mixed on a cool glass slab to dissipate (spread) the heat of the mix. The slab is cooled in cold water and then dried completely. Any moisture left on the slab affects the properties of the cement. The glass slab should be clean and free of scratches and dried cement. A stainless steel cement spatula is used to mix the powder into the liquid. The spatula also should be cool.

The bottle of powder is fluffed, and the powder and liquid should be the same brand and type of cement. The powder and liquid may come in dispensing bottles, or a scoop for the powder and a dropper for the liquid may be required. The powder is placed on one side of the slab and then proportioned for mixing. Then the liquid is dispensed on the slab (Figure 33-5). The powder usually is divided into differently sized sections for easier mixing. Follow the manufacturer's instructions.

As mentioned, one objective in mixing the cement is to dissipate the heat from the exothermic reaction. If the heat is dissipated, the setting reaction is slowed and more powder can be incorporated to make the cement

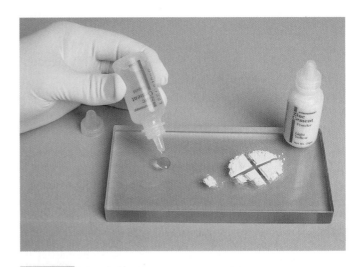

FIGURE 33-5 Zinc phosphate powder dispensed and divided into portions with liquid being dispensed.

stronger. To accomplish this, several mixing techniques are used:

- The glass slab is cooled.
- The first increment of powder is mixed into the liquid for ten to fifteen seconds before more powder is brought into the mix.
- Spatulate the mix slowly when incorporating the powder into the liquid.
- Mix slowly over a large area of the slab, wiping both sides of the spatula.

Of all the cements, mixing zinc phosphate is the most critical, and each procedural step must be followed (see Procedure 33-1). When zinc phosphate cement is mixed to a luting consistency, the cement is creamy and follows the spatula about one inch above the mixing slab. When zinc phosphate cement is mixed to a base consistency, the cement resembles thick putty.

Zinc Oxide Eugenol Cement

Zinc oxide eugenol cement, often referred to as ZOE, is another cement that has been used for many years. It is noted for its sedative or soothing effect on the dental pulp (refer to Table 33-1 for the various uses of zinc oxide eugenol). The functions of this cement are diverse because of additives that enhance its properties. There are two types: type I is not as strong and is used for temporary restorations and cementation; type II has been reinforced and is stronger and can be used for permanent cementation.

One type II zinc oxide eugenol cement is different from the rest in function. It is called an **intermediate restorative material (IRM)**. This material is placed in the patient's mouth and lasts up to one year. This mate-

PROCEDURE 33-1

Mixing Zinc Phosphate Cement

This procedure is completed by the dental assistant for the dentist. The equipment and materials are prepared and the material is mixed and passed to the dentist. Sometimes the dental assistant places the cement in the cast restoration while the dentist places material on the prepared tooth.

EQUIPMENT AND SUPPLIES (Figure 33-6)

- Zinc phosphate powder and liquid (dispensers, if needed)

- Cooled glass slab

- Flexible stainless steel cement spatula

- 2 × 2 gauze sponge

- Timer

- Plastic filling instrument

PROCEDURE STEPS *(Follow aseptic procedures)*

1. Shake the powder before removing the cap.

2. Place an appropriate amount of powder on one end of the slab. The amount of powder to be used is determined by the powder-liquid ratio and the amount of cement required for the procedure. For example, it would take less cement to cement a crown than a bridge.

3. Level the powder with the flat side of the spatula blade into a layer about 1 mm thick.

4. Divide the powder according to the manufacturer's instructions. One suggestion is to divide the powder into two equal portions with the edge of the spatula; divide each of these portions into quarters, and then two sections into eighths and one of the eighths into sixteenths.

5. Gently shake the liquid. Dispense the liquid from a dropper bottle onto the opposite side of the glass slab. Hold the liquid vertical while dispensing to produce uniform drops. Recap to avoid spilling and evaporation of the liquid.

6. Incorporate a small portion of powder into the liquid, following specific manufacturer's directions on mixing times. Use the flat side of the spatula blade to wet the powder particles (for about fifteen seconds).

7. Hold the spatula blade flat against the glass slab. Using a *wide sweeping motion,* spatulate the powder and liquid over a *large area of the glass slab* (Figure 33-7).

FIGURE 33-6 Zinc phosphate tray setup.

FIGURE 33-7 Mixing zinc phosphate powder and liquid. As powder is incorporated, a larger area of glass slab is used.

(continues)

PROCEDURE 33-1 *(CONTINUED)*

8. Adding small amounts of powder will help neutralize the acid, control the setting time, and achieve a smooth consistency of the mix. Incorporate each increment of powder thoroughly into the mix before adding more powder.

9. The mix will appear watery at first and then, as more powder is incorporated, the mix will become creamy. Gather all particles of powder and liquid from around the edges of the mix from time to time.

10. Turn the spatula blade on edge and gather the mass to check the consistency.

11. Continue to add additional increments to the mix until the desired consistency is reached and within the prescribed time.

12. Gather the entire mass into one unit on the glass slab.

13. The consistency for luting (cementing) will be creamy. It will follow the spatula for about 1 inch as it is lifted off the glass slab before breaking into a thin thread and flowing back into the mass (Figure 33-8A).

14. Consistency of the base should be putty-like, and you should be able to roll the base into a ball or cylinder with the flat side of the spatula (Figure 33-8B).

15. Once the cement has been mixed to the desired consistency, wipe off the spatula with a 2 × 2 gauze. Hold the glass slab under the patient's chin, and pass the plastic filling instrument.

16. Wipe the spatula and glass slab with a moistened 2 × 2 gauze.

17. To clean the glass slab and spatula, soak them in water or a solution of soda bicarbonate to loosen the hardened cement and then sterilize/disinfect.

(A)

(B)

FIGURE 33-8 (A) Demonstration of luting consistency. A spatula lifts cement one inch from the glass slab. (B) Base consistency—thick putty. *Note:* Most of the glass slab was used, and there is excess powder with which to pick up and manipulate the base.

rial comes in a powder/liquid form and in capsules (Figure 33-9). It is used when a tooth cannot be restored immediately, such as during illness, when the patient is moving, or because of economic reasons.

Composition. Zinc oxide eugenol is available in several forms, including powder/liquid, two-paste systems, capsules, and syringes. The powder for the conventional (type I) zinc oxide eugenol cement is zinc oxide, resin, zinc acetate, and an accelerator. The liquid, eugenol, is sometimes mixed with other oils, such as clove oil. The reinforced (type II) zinc oxide eugenol cement includes the addition of alumina and polymers (resins) to the powder, and ethoxybenzoic acid is added to the eugenol. Noneugenol zinc oxide cements are available for patients who are sensitive to eugenol. The noneugenol cements (type I) are formulated with other oils.

FIGURE 33-9 IRM-Type II (ZOE) comes in powder/liquid and premeasured capsule forms.

Although eugenol has long been known for its sedative effect on the pulp, it can also be irritating to the gingival tissues and the pulp when applied directly to these tissues. Sometimes when a product containing eugenol contacts the oral mucosa, the patient feels a burning sensation, and the tissues become red and irritated. The tissues will sometimes slough off and are tender to touch, thereby making eating and brushing uncomfortable. Several days may be necessary for the tissues to heal and become less sensitive.

Manufacturers of most products that previously contained eugenol, such as zinc oxide eugenol cements and periodontal dressings, now offer the same products containing a eugenol substitute. These materials are called noneugenol products.

Properties. Zinc oxide eugenol has several properties that affect the selection of this material. ZOE is very soluble in the mouth and dissolves quickly. The reinforced ZOE has the strength required for permanent cementation and retention, but it is not as strong as zinc phosphate. The pH of zinc oxide eugenol cements is neutral. With the sedative effect on the tooth, these materials do not require a protective base or liner.

Zinc oxide eugenol materials are not used under composites or acrylic restorations because the eugenol is not compatible with these materials. The eugenol retards the setting process.

Manipulation Considerations. Most zinc oxide eugenol materials are mixed on a paper pad with a stainless steel cement spatula (see Procedures 33-2 and 33-3). A glass slab may be used to control the setting time. Gently shake the powder before dispensing and swirl the liquid. Usually these materials have specific powder dispensers and liquid droppers. Care should be taken not to allow the eugenol into the rubber bulb of the dropper. The eugenol breaks down the rubber, thereby contaminating the liquid.

The type of material being mixed determines whether the powder is incorporated into the liquid in increments or brought in all at once. Usually, the mixing time is thirty to sixty seconds. All of the powder is mixed into the liquid to produce a uniform, smooth, creamy mix. Zinc oxide eugenol cements set quickly in the mouth because of the moisture and the warmth.

Some ZOE cements are two-paste systems comprised of an accelerator and a base. They are dispensed in equal lengths on a paper pad. The two pastes are different colors and are mixed until a uniform color is achieved, which takes about ten to fifteen seconds.

The setting time ranges from three to five minutes in the oral cavity for most zinc oxide eugenol materials. They are mixed to either a luting or base consistency depending on the use and the specific material.

Polycarboxylate Cement

Polycarboxylate cement, also known as zinc polycarboxylate, is used for permanent cementation and as an insulating base. This cement is said to be "kind" to the pulp and was the first cement that had the ability to chemically bond to the tooth structure. There are several brands of polycarboxylate cement, and the cement comes in a powder/liquid form and capsules.

PROCEDURE 33-2

Mixing Zinc Oxide Eugenol Cement— Powder/Liquid Form

This procedure is completed by the dental assistant when the dentist signals. The equipment and materials are prepared and the material is mixed and passed to the dentist. The dental assistant follows the manufacturer's directions for specific information on proportions, incorporation technique, and mixing and setting times.

EQUIPMENT AND SUPPLIES (Figure 33-10)

- Zinc oxide eugenol cement
- Dispensers for specific material
- Paper pad or glass slab
- Cement spatula
- Timer
- Plastic filling instrument
- 2 × 2 gauze sponges
- Alcohol or orange solvent

(continues)

PROCEDURE 33-2 (CONTINUED)

FIGURE 33-10 Tray setup for zinc oxide eugenol cement powder/liquid.

PROCEDURE STEPS (Follow aseptic procedures)

1. Fluff the powder before removing the cap.

2. Place the powder on the mixing pad according to manufacturer's directions. Replace the cap to avoid spilling and contamination.

3. After swirling, place the liquid on the paper pad. Hold the dispensing dropper perpendicular to the mixing pad and dispense the drops. Dispense near the powder but not touching it.

4. Incorporate the powder into the liquid in divided increments or all at once, according to the manufacturer's directions.

5. Spatulate with the flat part of the blade and with an even pressure to wet all particles of the powder. With some cements, a firm pressure is required to accomplish this.

6. Gather up the powder and liquid from the edges of the mix.

7. Gather up the entire mass into one unit on the slab to test consistency.

8. The consistency for temporary luting will be creamy, like frosting (Figure 33-11).

9. The consistency for an insulating base or IRM will be putty-like and can be rolled into a ball or cylinder.

10. Once the material has been mixed to the desired consistency, wipe the spatula with a 2 × 2 gauze. Hold the pad under the patient's chin and pass the cement on the plastic filling instrument.

11. Receive the plastic filling instrument and wipe it off. The top page of the paper pad is removed and folded to prevent accidental contact with the cement.

12. To clean material that has hardened on the spatula or glass slab, wipe it with alcohol or orange solvent as included in Figure 33-10, tray setup for zinc oxide eugenol cement.

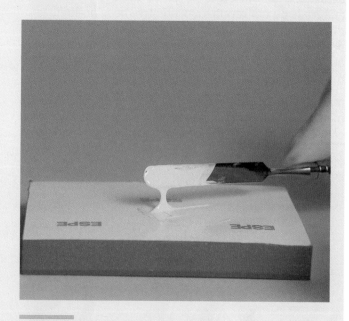

FIGURE 33-11 Consistency of ZOE temporary luting cement.

Composition. The powder of the polycarboxylate cement is similar to the zinc phosphate with zinc oxide as the main component and a small amount of magnesium oxide. Some stannous fluoride is added to most polycarboxylates to improve strength and reduce film thickness, not necessarily for anticarious effect. The liquid is what makes this cement different; it is a viscous solution of polyacrylic acid copolymer in water. The powder comes in a bottle with a specific dispenser, and the liquid comes in a squeeze bottle or a calibrated syringe (Figure 33-15). Polycarboxylate cement also comes in a capsule delivery system.

Properties. Polycarboxylate cement sets in three to five minutes and does not exhibit exothermic heat. This material bonds chemically to the tooth structure and

PROCEDURE 33-3

Mixing Zinc Oxide Eugenol Cement— Two-Paste System

This material is often used for temporary luting of provisional coverage. The dental assistant dispenses and mixes the material according to manufacturer's directions. The dental assistant assists the dentist during the placement of the temporary. Sometimes the dental assistant places the cement in the provisional coverage of the tooth, if this procedure is included in expanded function regulations.

EQUIPMENT AND SUPPLIES (Figure 33-12)

- Two-paste zinc oxide eugenol (accelerator and base)
- Paper pad
- Cement spatula
- 2 × 2 gauze sponge (moistened)
- Plastic filling instrument

FIGURE 33-12 Tray setup for zinc oxide eugenol cement two-paste system.

PROCEDURE STEPS *(Follow aseptic procedures)*

1. Dispense the amount of material required for the procedure. Equal lengths of the accelerator and the base are usually placed parallel to each other on the paper pad.

2. Gather the materials and mix into a homogeneous mass. Spread over a small area, and then gather. Repeat the process. The material should be a creamy mix that follows the spatula up for an inch (luting consistency).

3. Wipe both sides of the spatula and then gather all the material into one area.

4. Wipe off the cement spatula with the moist 2 × 2 gauze sponge.

---

mechanically to the restoration. The strength of polycarboxylate is similar to the reinforced ZOE and less than zinc phosphate cement. The material may appear quite viscous, but it flows readily when applied to a surface. Polycarboxylate cement is much less irritating to the pulp, with reactions similar to zinc oxide eugenol cement.

Polycarboxylate materials have a shelf life because of the water in the liquid. If the liquid discolors and becomes thick, it should be discarded.

Manipulation Properties. Polycarboxylate cements are mixed on a paper pad or a glass slab with a stainless steel cement spatula (Procedure 33-4). The powder is fluffed before the dispenser is used. The viscous liquid is dispensed from a squeeze bottle or a calibrated syringe. The liquid bottle is held perpendicular and squeezed until a drop begins to fall. The size of the drop varies because of this dispensing technique and the viscosity of the liquid. The syringe improves the accuracy of dispensing the liquid.

Polycarboxylate cements are mixed in thirty to sixty seconds and have a working time of about three minutes. The material loses its shine and becomes stringy or forms "cobwebs." At this point, the cement should not be used.

PROCEDURE 33-4

Mixing Polycarboxylate Cement

The dental assistant prepares and mixes the polycarboxylate materials to the desired consistency. The amount of materials dispensed depends on restoration size and number of units involved.

EQUIPMENT AND SUPPLIES (Figure 33-13)

- Polycarboxylate powder and liquid and dispenser for powder
- Paper pad or glass slab
- Flexible stainless steel spatula
- 2 × 2 gauze sponge (moistened)
- Timer
- Plastic filling instrument

PROCEDURE STEPS (*Follow aseptic procedures*)

1. The powder is fluffed before dispensing with the dispensing scoop.

2. The powder is measured and dispensed on one side of a paper pad or a glass slab.

3. Uniform drops of liquid are placed toward the opposite side of the powder. Follow the manufacturer's directions for the appropriate number of drops per scoop of powder.

4. Incorporate from three-fourths to all of the powder into the liquid and use a folding motion while applying some pressure to wet all the powder. Mix quickly until all the powder is incorporated. (Because the liquid is thick, it is harder to incorporate the powder.)

5. The mix will be slightly more viscous than zinc phosphate cement and is glossy. Gather all the cement, wiping both sides of the spatula.

6. For luting consistency, the mix should follow the spatula up 1 inch.

7. For a base consistency, the same amount of powder is used, but the liquid ratio is decreased. The mix for the base should be glossy, but the consistency is tacky and stiff.

8. The mix must be used immediately before it becomes dull and stringy and forms cobwebs (Figure 33-14).

9. The cleanup is done immediately by wiping the spatula with a wet 2 × 2 gauze or by soaking the spatula with the dried cement in a 10 percent sodium hydroxide solution. The paper pad sheet is removed, folded, and disposed of. (Fold the paper pad to prevent touching the cement and spreading it onto instruments and the patient's face.)

FIGURE 33-13 Mixing polycarboxylate cement tray setup.

FIGURE 33-14 When cement is mixed for too long, the mix become thick and "cobwebs" form.

FIGURE 33-15 Polycarboxylate powder and dispensing syringes of liquid. *(Courtesy of 3M-ESPE Dental Products Division.)*

FIGURE 33-16 Various brands of glass ionomer cements.

Glass Ionomer Cement

Glass ionomer cement is one of the newer systems. Its applications are diverse. Thus, there is more than one type of glass ionomer material. This cement has been modified for many uses, some of which are listed below.

- A fine-grain glass ionomer is used for cementation of crowns and bridges because it chemically bonds to the tooth structure. It is also used for orthodontic bonding.
- Pit and fissure sealant.
- A coarser-grain glass ionomer available in various shades for use in selected restorations, such as Class III and V and pediatric restorations (discussed in Chapter 34, Restorative Materials).
- Liner and dentin bonding agent.
- Silver or amalgam filings are combined with glass ionomer material used for crown and core buildups.

Glass ionomer cements are available in powder/liquid, paste systems, syringes, and capsule forms. The glass ionomers come in both self-curing and light-curing materials (Figure 33-16).

Composition. Glass ionomer powder is a silicate glass powder containing calcium, aluminum, and fluoride (calcium fluoroaluminosilicate glass). The liquid is an aqueous solution (the solution contains water) of polyacrylic acid.

Properties. Glass ionomer material is strong enough to act as a supportive base and is similar to zinc phosphate cement in strength. It mechanically and chemically bonds to the tooth structure and releases fluoride ions, which prevent secondary decay by strengthening the tooth structure. Glass ionomers have nonirritating qualities similar to polycarboxylate cements. The complete setting reaction of glass ionomers takes up to twenty-four hours.

Manipulation Considerations. Glass ionomer cements are mixed on a paper pad or a cool glass slab (Procedure 33-5). The paper pads are preferred for easy cleanup, but glass slabs may be used to retard the setting action. The materials should be mixed quickly, following manufacturer's directions, because of the water content. Water evaporation affects the properties of cement.

Although many properties are the same as those of the polycarboxylate cements, the liquid of the glass ionomers is not as viscous and is therefore easier to dispense and mix. The powder is dispensed first using the scoop and the amount indicated in the manufacturer's instructions, and liquid is dispensed just prior to manipulation. Mixing time is usually thirty to sixty seconds, and working time for the material is about two minutes.

The tooth must be completely isolated, cleaned, and dried before the cement is placed. The glass ionomer cement sets in the mouth in about five minutes.

Calcium Hydroxide Material

Calcium hydroxide cement is used as a low-strength base or liner under any restoration, such as indirect or direct pulp capping procedures (near or direct pulp exposures). This material has a therapeutic effect on the pulp; the area is sealed so that secondary dentin may form. Calcium hydroxide is not necessary to form secondary dentin, but its slightly irritating effect provides the mild irritant to encourage secondary dentin to form. Calcium hydroxide does also have antibacterial properties, which keep the bacteria from actively spreading.

PROCEDURE 33-5

Mixing Glass Ionomer Cement

This procedure is completed by the dental assistant. The equipment and materials are prepared and mixed when the dentist indicates. The material must be used immediately after it is mixed. This material requires that the tooth be clean of debris and dry, so the dental assistant should rinse and evacuate and then isolate the area before beginning to mix the cement.

EQUIPMENT AND SUPPLIES (Figure 33-17)

- Glass ionomer materials and appropriate dispensers
- Paper pad or cool glass slab
- Flexible stainless steel spatula
- 2 × 2 gauze sponges (moistened)
- Timer
- Plastic filling instrument

PROCEDURE STEPS *(Follow aseptic procedures)*

1. Fluff the powder and, using the recommended scoops, place the appropriate number of scoops on the paper pad or glass slab.

2. Swirl the liquid and then place the specified number of drops on the pad near the powder. Replace the cap on the liquid immediately to prevent evaporation (Figure 33-18).

FIGURE 33-18 Dispensed glass ionomer powder and liquid.

3. Divide the powder into halves or thirds and then draw the sections into the liquid one at a time.

4. Mix over a small area until all the powder is incorporated. The cement should be creamy and glossy for the luting consistency and tacky and stiff for the base consistency.

5. Once the cement has obtained the final consistency, wipe off the spatula with a 2 × 2 gauze. Hold the paper or glass slab under the patient's chin and pass the plastic filling instrument to the dentist.

6. To clean up, remove the top paper, fold it, and dispose of it. The instruments are wiped after use for easier cleanup.

7. Glass ionomer capsules are also available. They are activated by placement in an "activator" or dispenser to break the seal between the powder and liquid in the capsule.

8. The capsules are then placed in an amalgamator to be mixed (triturated) for a specific amount of time, usually ten seconds. Follow the manufacturer's directions.

9. Insert the capsule in the appropriate dispenser and pass it to the dentist for dispensing the material needed.

10. To clean up, the capsule is discarded and the activator and/or the dispenser are disinfected.

FIGURE 33-17 Tray setup for mixing glass ionomer cement.

FIGURE 33-19 Various forms of calcium hydroxide including the light cured material (in the dark tube) and the two paste materials.

Calcium hydroxide comes in powder/liquid, a two-paste system, or a one-paste system. The form many offices use is the two-paste system: catalyst and base. Calcium hydroxide comes in a self-curing and a light-curing formula (Figure 33-19).

Composition. Calcium hydroxide has complicated formulas with several ingredients in addition to calcium hydroxide. The light-cured calcium hydroxide formula also contains a polymer resin.

Properties. Calcium hydroxide is low in strength and is placed in a thin layer near or over the pulp. It is easy to mix and place. The cement has low thermal conductivity but is usually not used in a thick enough layer to provide thermal protection. An insulating base is often placed over the thin layer of calcium hydroxide.

Manipulation Considerations. The two-paste system is mixed on a small paper pad with a metal spatula, an explorer, or a small ball-ended instrument (Procedure 33-6). The base and the catalyst of the two-paste system come as a set and cannot be interchanged with those of other calcium hydroxide paste systems.

This material is dispensed in equal portions and mixed for about ten to fifteen seconds. Setting times vary from two to seven minutes.

Cavity Varnish

Cavity varnish is a material used to seal the dentin tubules that are exposed during an amalgam cavity preparation. This thin liquid is placed on the surface of the dentin only. There are various types of varnish, and some come with solvents.

Composition. Cavity varnishes are resin solutions of different compositions. The copal varnish contains organic solvents (ether, acetone, or chloroform) and is used only under metal restorations because the solvent material in the varnish may interfere with the setting action of composite and resins. The universal varnishes do not have the organic solvent and may be used under all restorations.

Properties. Varnishes are placed in a thin layer over the dentin tubules. The varnishes do not exhibit any strength and do not provide any thermal insulation. The cavity varnishes are insoluble in the oral fluids and reduce leakage around the margins of restorations, thereby preventing microleakage. Varnish also prevents penetration of the acids from some cements into the dentin. These materials are nonacidic and nonirritating.

Manipulation Properties. Cavity varnishes often are placed in two layers for greater protection and to prevent voids. Recap the varnish immediately to minimize evaporation of the varnish. The cavity varnish comes with a separate bottle of solvent. If the varnish becomes too thick, solvent can be added. The solvent also can be used to clean the applicator and to remove any varnish on the external tooth surfaces.

Cavity varnish is not mixed; it is placed directly on the tooth with one of various types of applicators, such as small cotton pellets or brushes (Procedure 33-7).

Resin Cement

Resin cements have multiple uses with a wide variety of procedures, including permanent cementation of cast metal restorations and porcelain/resin restorations and veneers, orthodontic brackets, and endodontic posts. Resin cements may be supplied in a two-paste system, powder/liquid set, or syringe. The manufacturer may supply etchant gel or liquid with the material. Some of these materials may be shaded to complement the translucency of the crown or inlay.

There are three types of resin cements: self-curing (chemical), light cured, and dual cured. Dual-cured materials contain chemicals for a self-curing as well as a light-curing reaction. The self-cured materials are used with metal or metal combination materials and endodontic posts; the light-curing materials are used with porcelain/resin restorations, veneers, and orthodontic brackets.

Composition. The resin cements are similar to composites in composition. Variation comes with individual products adjusted for different functions. The resin matrices are BIS-GMA (bisphenol A-glycidyl methaceylate) or dimethacrylate resin diluted with low-viscosity monomers. The resin cements are more fluid than direct filling composites because the amount of filler particles are reduced to create low viscosities for cementation purposes.

Properties. Most resin cements are radiopaque and exhibit adequate strength and wear resistance for luting. These materials are insoluble in oral fluids but are irritating to the pulp; thus, a protective cement is required. Some of the products contain fluoride.

PROCEDURE 33-6

Mixing Calcium Hydroxide Cement— Two-Paste System

This material is dispensed and mixed by the dental assistant. It is often the first step in restoring the cavity preparation.

EQUIPMENT AND SUPPLIES (Figure 33-20)

- Calcium hydroxide two-paste system
- Small paper pad
- Small ball-ended instrument or explorer
- 2 × 2 gauze sponge

PROCEDURE STEPS *(Follow aseptic procedures)*

1. Dispense small and equal amounts of both the catalyst and base onto the paper pad.

2. Wipe off ends of tubes and replace caps.

3. Mix the two materials together using a circular motion.

4. Mix until the materials are a uniform color within the ten- to fifteen-second mixing time.

5. Use a 2 × 2 gauze to remove excess material from the mixing instrument.

6. Pass the instrument to the dentist and hold the paper pad close to the patient's chin.

FIGURE 33-20 Two-paste calcium hydroxide tray setup.

7. Wipe off the instrument with a gauze for the dentist between applications.

8. Receive the instrument, wipe it off, tear and fold the top page of the paper pad, and dispose of it.

Manipulation Considerations. Resin cements do not adhere directly to metal or ceramic materials; these materials must be roughened with etchants to produce mechanical bonding or the tissue surfaces of ceramics are treated with a silane coupling agent to produce a chemical bond with the resin cements. Sometimes, a wire mesh or undercuts may be added to the tissue side of the prosthesis to aid in retention.

Self-cured materials come with an initiator and an activator. These are mixed on a paper pad for twenty to thirty seconds. Excess cement must be removed before the material is set completely to prevent any marginal leakage. Light-cured materials come in syringes and must be cured for at least forty seconds. Dual-cured materials come in two component systems that are mixed together for twenty to thirty seconds. Once mixed, these materials begin to set slowly, allowing for placement of the cement on the prosthesis and the prosthesis to be seated in the oral cavity. Once in position, the visible light unit is activated to harden the cement (Procedure 33-8).

Resin-Reinforced Glass Ionomer Cement

Resin-reinforced glass ionomer cement has been modified to include resin. This cement is stronger and more water insoluble and adheres to the tooth structure better than conventional glass ionomer cement. Like glass

PROCEDURE 33-7

Preparing Cavity Varnish

The materials needed for application of cavity varnish are prepared by the dental assistant. Depending on expanded function laws, the dental assistant applies the varnish or assists the dentist during placement.

EQUIPMENT AND SUPPLIES (Figure 33-21)

- Cavity varnish and solvent

- Two cotton pliers

- Cotton pellets or pieces of cotton rolled into small, football-shaped balls, or a small brush

- Cotton roll

PROCEDURE STEPS *(Follow aseptic procedures)*

1. Clean and dry the cavity preparation.

2. Prepare cotton pellets for application of two layers of varnish. The pellets must be small in order to apply the varnish on the dentin surface.

3. Remove the cap from the varnish bottle. Holding the two cotton pellets in the pliers, dip them into the varnish until they are moistened. Then replace the cap on the varnish.

4. Place the cotton pellets on a 2 × 2 gauze and dab off the excess varnish.

5. Using one pellet, apply the varnish to the cavity preparation. Coat the surface of the preparation.

FIGURE 33-21 (A) Varnish and (B) solvent with materials needed for placement. Micro-brushes are used for placement as well as cotton pellets and cotton pliers.

6. Allow the first coat to dry, and then apply a second coat in the same manner.

7. Dispose of the cotton pellets and clean the cotton pliers with solvent before sterilizing them.

8. To prepare the cotton pellets one at a time, two separate cotton pliers must be used to avoid contamination.

---

ionomer cement, it releases fluoride to protect the enamel against decalcification and demineralization.

Compomer Cement

Compomer cements are basically polyacid modified composites. They are like composites and do not contain water and have properties similar to resin cements. Compomers release fluoride, have self-adhesive properties, and come in light-cured and self-cured versions. They are used to cement all types of dental restorations.

Etchants

Etchants, which enhance retention/bonding between the tooth surface and dental materials, are used before the placement of bonding agents, restorative materials, dental cements, and pit and fissure sealants. Etching products are typically comprised of a thirty to forty percent phosphoric acid solution. The etchant comes in liquid or gel form and packaged in bottles or syringes. Liquids are placed with micro-brushes or small cotton pellets. Gel etchants placed with a syringe tip are the

PROCEDURE 33-8

Placing Resin Cement—Dual-Curing Technique

This procedure is performed by the dental assistant for the dentist. The equipment and materials are prepared, and the material is mixed and passed to the dentist. Because this material is dual curing, a curing light and eye protection are needed.

EQUIPMENT AND SUPPLIES (Figure 33-22)

- Resin cement system
- Paper pad
- Stainless steel spatula
- Plastic filling instrument
- Curing light and protective shield or glasses
- 2 × 2 gauze sponges

PROCEDURE STEPS *(Follow aseptic procedures)*

1. Clean and dry the tooth and isolate the area with cotton rolls.

2. Pass the etchant to the dentist.

3. Wait the required time for the etchant and rinse the tooth thoroughly.

4. Lightly air dry the tooth and apply the adhesive.

5. Dispense and mix the two components together to a homogeneous, creamy mixture.

6. Hold the pad close to the patient and pass the placement instrument. The dentist places the material on the tooth and restoration.

7. Hold a 2 × 2 gauze to remove any excess materials.

8. Receive the placement instrument and prepare the curing light.

9. Either the dental assistant or the dentist holds the curing light and uses the protective shield when the light is activated.

10. Clean up immediately. Wipe any excess cement off the instruments and discard disposable items.

(A)

(B)

FIGURE 33-22 (A) Resin cement tray setup. (B) Resin cement system. *(B. Courtesy of Kerr Corporation.)*

most common. Gels are packaged with a number of disposable tips (Figure 33-23).

Etchants are used both on enamel and dentin tooth surfaces and are tinted for more accurate placement. The etchant is usually left on for 30 to 60 seconds and rinsed thoroughly (Procedure 33-9).

Bonding Agents

Bonding agents are also known as **adhesives** and **bonding resins**. These materials are used to improve the retention between the tooth structure (enamel and dentin) and the restoration. These materials come in many forms and are

FIGURE 33-23 Various types of etchant materials.

often complete systems (Figure 33-25). These materials bond enamel and dentin to porcelain, resins, precious and nonprecious metals, composites, and amalgam.

The bonding materials are low-viscosity resins that may or may not contain fillers. Some of the bonding agents contain additives with adhesive enhancers, and some contain fluoride. These materials are mainly light cured or dual cured. Procedure 33-10 outlined the steps for placing a bonding agent.

Enamel Bonding

Adhesion of dental materials to enamel is accomplished by etching with phosphoric acid. This solution alters the surface of the enamel and creates microscopic undercuts between the enamel rod (Figure 33-26). Low-viscosity, unfilled resin bonding agents then penetrate

---

PROCEDURE 33-9

Placing Etchant

The dental assistant prepares the materials and isolates the area. The dentist places the etchant. When the allotted time has passed, the dental assistant thoroughly rinses the tooth.

EQUIPMENT (Figure 33-24)

- Acid etchant, usually a thirty to forty percent solution
- Isolation materials (rubber dam or cotton rolls)
- Applicator (syringe, cotton pellets, or small applicator tips)
- Dappen dish
- Air-water syringe
- Timer

PROCEDURE STEPS *(Follow aseptic procedures)*

1. Isolate the area.
2. Clean the surface thoroughly.
3. Prepare the etchant applicator or syringe.
4. Place the etchant on the surface for fifteen to thirty seconds depending on the manufacturer's directions.

FIGURE 33-24 Tray setup for placing etchant.

5. Rinse the tooth after the designated time for fifteen to twenty seconds with the air-water syringe and evacuate thoroughly for ten to twenty seconds.

NOTE: The etched surface will have a frosty appearance. This surface needs to be isolated until the cementation is complete. If saliva or other fluids contact the surface, the etching process must be repeated.

FIGURE 33-25 Bonding agents and systems.

FIGURE 33-26 Microscopic view of etched dentin. *(Courtesy of Kerr Corporation.)*

into these undercuts and mechanically lock into them. The restorative material then bonds to this layer and becomes a solid unit. Bonding to enamel is required before placement of composite restorations, pit and fissure sealants, veneers, resin-cemented crowns and bridges, and orthodontic brackets.

Dentin Bonding

Dentin bonding is more challenging than enamel bonding. Some of the obstacles are listed below:

- Dentin has a high water content, which can interfere with the bonding to the tooth.
- The composition of the dentin is more organic than inorganic and contains water. These factors make dentin difficult to bond to.

- Dentin is directly above the pulp, so the operator must take care not to injure the pulp.
- When the dentin is cut with a bur during the cavity preparation, it forms a **smear layer**. This layer of debris lies on the cavity floor and walls and prevents contact between the intact dentin and the bonding agent/adhesive.

Current dentin bonding materials use an etchant to remove the smear layer, because the smear layer is not attached firmly and is unreliable. When the smear layer is removed, the adhesives achieve a mechanical bond with the dentin. Many of the bonding agents are suitable for both enamel and dentin surfaces because of etchant application.

Restorative Dentistry

Restorative dentistry, also known as operative dentistry, involves various materials and techniques. There are many reasons a tooth needs to be restored, including decay, fracture, abrasion, esthetics, and attrition. Restorative materials such as amalgam and composites are used to restore the tooth. These materials are called direct restorative materials because they are mixed and placed directly in the cavity preparation in a single appointment.

Reasons for restoring teeth include:

- Arresting the loss of tooth structure. Stopping the decay process early allows the preparation to be conservative and small restorations to be stronger.
- Preventing the recurrence of decay by placing margins that can be reached easily for cleaning. This is known as *extension for prevention.*
- Restoring contour of the tooth (shape and design of crown). The proper contour prevents food impaction and gingival irritation.
- Restoring function of the tooth and establishing occlusion with opposing teeth for mastication of food.
- Restoring or improving appearance of the teeth.

Classification

Dental caries are classified to simplify the examination, charting, diagnosis, and patient communication. There are several ways to classify cavities and restorations (see Chapter 14, Dental Charting), including Black's, which identifies areas of decay according to the surfaces they are located on, such as Class I for occlusal caries on the posterior teeth and Class III for dental caries on the mesial or distal of anterior teeth where the incisal edge is not involved. Another classification is based on the number of surfaces involved, such as simple, compound, and complex. A third method of classi-

PROCEDURE 33-10

Placing Bonding Agent

Steps in the application of bonding agents vary by manufacturer, so follow the directions that come with the product. The dental assistant prepares the materials for each step and keeps the area dry and free of debris (sometimes cavity cleaners are used).

EQUIPMENT AND SUPPLIES (Figure 33-27)

- Bonding system that contains acid etchant, primer or conditioner, adhesive material

- Applicators (disposable tips or brushes)

- Dappen dish

- Isolation means

- Air-water syringe

- Curing light and shield

- Timer

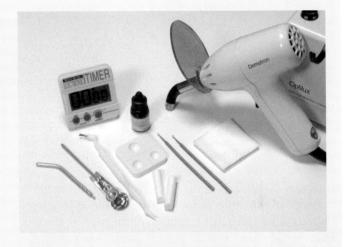

FIGURE 33-27 Tray setup and materials for placing bonding agents.

PROCEDURE STEPS *(Follow aseptic procedures)*

1. If the cavity preparation is near the pulp, place calcium hydroxide or glass ionomer lining cement over the area.

2. The etchant is placed on the enamel and the dentin for the specified amount of time, usually fifteen to twenty seconds. Usually, the etchant is placed on the enamel first and then the dentin, because the dentin is more sensitive to the etchant.

3. Rinse the tooth as soon as the time is up. Continue to rinse for at least five to ten seconds. Move quickly to prevent bacterial contamination of the dentin.

4. If the bonding involves both the enamel and dentin, a primer step is included. The primer or conditioner is placed with a brush or an applicator. This material wets the dentin and penetrates the dentin tubules.

5. The bonding resin is then applied, and the curing light is used to harden the material.

6. Cleanup involves disposing of applicator tips or brushes.

---

fying dental caries is based on whether the caries are pit and fissure areas or smooth surface areas.

Cavity Detection

Cavities can be detected with radiographs, probing with an explorer, or use of a special dye. This dye detects caries by distinguishing among good, sound, hard dentin and dentin that is infected with bacteria and softened. The dye is placed in the preparation early in the procedure to avoid removing too much tooth structure. The dye is applied for about ten seconds and then rinsed off. Burs and spoon excavators usually remove all the stained dentin. This process is repeated until no caries remain. This material also can be used to identify cracks and root canals.

Caries are also detected via manual probing with an explorer and through radiographs. Another noninvasive diagnostic tool, called the DIAGNOdent, is a Class II laser that measures fluorescence levels in the tooth structure to quantify caries progression. The DIAGNOdent comes in a battery-operated microprocessor-controlled display unit with handpiece and tips or a handheld pen unit for easier handling and greater mobility. Several tips are packaged with the units and the tips are sterilizible (Figure 33-28). Altered tooth

FIGURE 33-28 DIAGNOdent. *(Courtesy of KaVo Dental Corporation.)*

Therapy information according to KaVo DIAGNOdent pen	
Display value	**Therapy**
0–14	No special measures.
15–20	Usual prophylactic measures.
21–30	More intensive prophylaxis or restoration: indication is dependent on: ▪ Caries activity ▪ Caries risk ▪ Recall interval, etc.
≥30	Restoration and more intensive prophylaxis.

structure and bacteria fluoresce (give off light) when exposed to specific wavelengths of light. A clean, healthy tooth structure exhibits little or no fluorescence, while a tooth with decay fluoresces according to the extent of caries. Thus, healthy teeth register a low reading, while teeth with decay register higher readings. Laser units may also emit audio signals, which allow the dentist to hear changes as well as see display changes.

Benefits of using a laser caries detection unit include the following:

▪ Accurate diagnosis of tooth decay

▪ Simple, fast, and painless

▪ Quantification of caries over time

▪ Early detection of caries

▪ Can be used by hygienist to detect suspicious areas requiring further examination

▪ Provides accurate visual and sound representation of measured tooth structure

---

How to use KaVo DIAGNOdent pen

1. Clean tooth surfaces, preferably with an air polishing device (e.g., PROPHYflex) to remove plaque, stains, and calculus from fissure areas.
2. Dry the tooth.
3. Perform clinical examination (scanning of tooth surface).
4. Diagnose and evaluate quantitative measurement of DIAGNOdent pen (possible course of action):

   ▪ Chart readings and monitor over time.

   ▪ Initiate prophylactic treatment (fluoridation, etc.) and monitor success/result

   ▪ Restore and check for residual caries.

Cavity Cleaners/Disinfectants

Cavity cleaners/disinfectants can be used in the cavity preparation. Like any body wound, the cavity should be cleaned and disinfected to reduce bacterial growth under restorations that can lead to sensitivity. This step is completed before the tooth is etched.

Desensitizers

Desensitizers are used to treat or prevent hypersensitivity in the teeth. Hypersensitivity can be caused by cold, heat, or contact. In some procedures, etchants are used to increase bonding/retention of the tooth surface and restorative materials. The etchant opens and exposes dentin tubules, which sometimes cause hypersensitivity. In addition, patients who use certain whitening agents need to be treated with a desensitizer to reduce tooth sensitivity. Desensitizers can be used under all types of restorations, bonding agents, temporary fillings, and permanent cement. Some can also be used to desensitize exposed root surface.

Many types of desensitizers are available, some of which contain fluoride while others contain antimicrobial agent additives to remove residual bacteria from the tooth surface.

Desensitizers are available in liquid or gel form, and are placed with a brush or syringe. Some are single-dose or unidose cartridges. These materials may be self-curing or light-curing (Figure 33-29).

Cavity Preparation Identification

Once the tooth is prepared, there are terms used to describe the inside of the cavity preparation. Knowledge of these terms helps the dental assistant better communicate with the dentist and also understand the details of the cavity preparation.

FIGURE 33-29 Desensitizers.

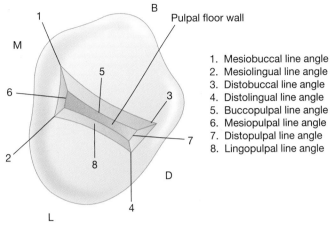

1. Mesiobuccal line angle
2. Mesiolingual line angle
3. Distobuccal line angle
4. Distolingual line angle
5. Buccopulpal line angle
6. Mesiopulpal line angle
7. Distopulpal line angle
8. Lingopulpal line angle

FIGURE 33-30 Cavity preparation line angles (looking down on occlusal view).

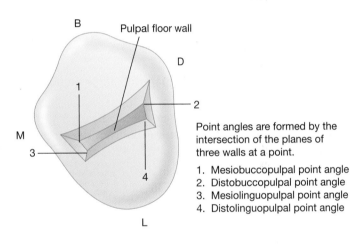

Point angles are formed by the intersection of the planes of three walls at a point.

1. Mesiobuccopulpal point angle
2. Distobuccopulpal point angle
3. Mesiolinguopulpal point angle
4. Distolinguopulpal point angle

FIGURE 33-31 Cavity preparation point angles.

The preparation of the tooth forms walls, lines, and angles. A wall is the side or floor of the cavity preparation. The wall is named according to the surface of the tooth it is nearest to, such as the buccal wall or distal wall. The internal wall that runs parallel to the long axis of the tooth is the **axial wall**. The wall that overlies the pulp is the **pulpal wall** or floor. The wall nearest the gingiva that is perpendicular to the long axis of the tooth is the **gingival wall**.

Lines are formed when two surfaces meet and form a **line angle**. The line angles are named according to the two surfaces, such as the distopulpal line angle or axiogingival (Figure 33-30). (Note that the names of the two surfaces are usually joined with an "o" between the words.) In the "corners" of the cavity preparation, three lines (surfaces) come together to form **point angles**. The point angles are named by joining the names of the walls, such as the mesiolinguopulpal line angle or the distobuccopulpal point angle (Figure 33-31).

The **cavosurface margin** is the angle that is formed by the junction of the wall of the preparation and the untouched surface of the tooth (Figure 33-32). The sealing of this margin is critical to prevent marginal leakage. Sometimes, this margin is beveled (slanted) during the preparation.

Elements of Cavity Preparations

The cavity preparation is a systematic cutting of the tooth structure that depends on location of decay, extent of decay, amount of lost tooth structure, and type of restorative material to be used. When the dentist prepares the cavity, some basic considerations are followed. Understanding these steps helps the dental assistant know what is coming next so that he or she can be prepared to change burs, rinse and evacuate the oral cavity, mix materials, and so on. It also keeps the focus on the preparation and the dental assistant more involved in the procedure.

Cavity Preparations. Cavity preparations include the following considerations (Figure 33-33):

■ **Outline form**—Designates overall shape of the cavity preparation. This form is determined by the extent of

1. Buccogingival line angle
2. Linguogingival line angle
3. Buccoaxial line angle
4. Linguoaxial line angle
5. Axiogingival line angle
6. Gingivobuccoaxial point angle
7. Gingivolinguoaxial point angle
8. Buccodistal line angle
9. Linguodistal line angle
10. Distopulpal line angle
11. Linguopulpal line angle
12. Buccopulpal line angle
13. Distobuccopulpal point angle
14. Distolinguopulpal point angle
15. Additional line angle, the pulpoaxial line angle is formed by the intersection of the pulpal and axial walls
16. Pulpolinguoaxial point angle
17. Pulpobuccoaxial point angle
18. Cavosurface margin

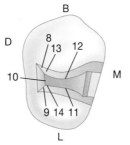

FIGURE 33-32 Cavity preparation line angles, point angles, and cavosurface margins. (The top figure is the view from the mesial, the bottom figure is the view from the occlusal.)

decay, type of restorative material, and retention of this material.

■ **Resistance form**—Internal shape of the cavity that protects the tooth and restoration from the stresses of mastication.

■ **Retention form**—Internal shape of the cavity walls that retains the restoration. In an amalgam preparation, the walls of the preparation are often slightly undercut to form mechanical locking of the amalgam and the cavity preparation.

■ **Convenience form**—Alteration to cavity preparation that is necessary for instrumentation during preparation and insertion of restorative materials. This is usually beyond the outline form and opens the tooth for the dentist to have enough space to prepare the cavity properly.

FIGURE 33-33 Steps of cavity preparation: opening cavity with a bur, outlining cavity, and refining and finishing cavity preparation.

■ **Finishing** or **refinement of the cavity preparation**—The final planing of the cavity walls before the placement of the restoration.

■ **Cleansing** or **debridement of the cavity preparation**—The spraying and rinsing of the cavity preparation to remove the debris. The dental assistant uses the spray from the air-water syringe and the HVE to cleanse the area.

ADVANCED CHAIRSIDE FUNCTIONS

Placing Cements, Bases, and Liners

The dental assistant should be familiar with and knowledgeable about the properties and preparation of cavity liners, varnishes, and cement bases. Cavity preparation and terminology also should be familiar so that the dental assistant can plan ahead and be ready to prepare and place the materials the dentist asks for. Some states allow dental assistants to place bases, liners, and cavity varnish; in others the dental assistant assists the dentist during this step of restorative procedures.

ADVANCED CHAIRSIDE FUNCTIONS

Cavity Preparation/ Pulpal Involvement

The cavity preparation for a restoration depends on the amount of decay, location of decay, and type of materials used to restore the tooth. If the dental assistant is placing the liners, base, or varnish, he or she should examine the cavity preparation to assess pulpal involvement (Table 33-2).

Treatment of Cavity Preparations

Treatment of cavity preparations varies with the amount of enamel and dentin removed and how near the prep is to the pulp. Using the categories from Table 33-2, possible treatments are summarized below:

1. Treatment of ideal cavity preparation:
   - A base is not required because only a minimal amount of enamel and dentin has been removed. Some dentists place only the restoration, while others prefer to place a fluoride-releasing liner. If an amalgam restoration is going to be placed, two thin layers of cavity varnish are often placed over the dentin.
   - If a composite restoration is going to be used, a glass ionomer liner or calcium hydroxide is placed over the exposed dentin.

TABLE 33-2 Depth of Cavity Preparations and Pulpal Relation

Pulpal Involvement	Illustration
1. Ideal level This preparation does not involve the pulp but is through the enamel and just in the dentin. It is large enough to retain a restoration.	
2. Beyond ideal More enamel and dentin are removed, but the preparation is not close to the pulp.	
3. Near exposure This cavity preparation involves a large amount of enamel and dentin being removed, but the pulp is not exposed. The floor of the preparation may be slightly pink due to proximity of the pulp.	
4. Pulp exposure Enough enamel and dentin have been removed to expose a portion of the pulp. There will be blood in the cavity preparation.	

ADVANCED CHAIRSIDE FUNCTIONS

2. Treatment of beyond-ideal cavity preparation:
   - With a beyond-ideal preparation, the level of the dentin is restored with a cement base.
   - With an amalgam restoration, there are several options. One option is to place two thin layers of varnish to seal the dentin tubules and then place a layer of a cement base, such as zinc phosphate.
   - Another option is a reinforced ZOE base, which has a soothing effect on the pulp. Varnish is not used with this material.
   - Other options include polycarboxylate or glass ionomer base, which also do not require varnish.
   - Under composite restorative materials, use a glass ionomer base or calcium hydroxide.

3. Treatment of near-exposure cavity preparation:
   - The closer the cavity preparation comes to the pulp, the more precautions that are needed. There are also several options of treatment of the near-exposure preparation.
   - With preparations that are going to be restored with amalgam, a liner of calcium hydroxide, glass ionomer, or ZOE is placed first over the deepest portion of the prep in the dentin. Once this layer is placed, two thin layers of varnish may be inserted over the exposed dentin. Then, a layer of cement base is applied. Zinc phosphate, polycarboxylate, or glass ionomer cements can be used for this layer.
   - Another option for amalgam restorations is to place a liner over the deepest portion of the preparation, then a layer of reinforced ZOE, polycarboxylate, or glass ionomer cement. This is then sealed with cavity varnish.
   - With some preparations, the dentist may choose not to place cavity varnish.
   - When composite materials are going to be used to restore the tooth, a liner is placed first, then a layer of either polycarboxylate or glass ionomer cement. Varnish is not placed and a ZOE base liner is not used because they inhibit the setting of the composite.
   - When a cavity liner is placed on a near exposure, the procedure is often referred to as an **indirect pulp capping**.

4. Treatment of exposed-pulp cavity preparation:
   - In an exposed pulp, the dentist must decide whether endodontic treatment is indicated or attempt to save the vitality of the tooth. If the treatment of choice is to save the pulp, a pro-

cedure called a **direct pulp capping (DPC)** is performed.
   - One treatment involves the placement of calcium hydroxide or glass ionomer liner and then reinforced ZOE as a temporary restoration. This gives the dentist time to see whether the pulp is going to heal.
   - Another treatment involves the placement of a liner, followed by a layer of ZOE cement, two thin layers of varnish, and a cement base.
   - Some dentists prefer to place a liner and then a layer of polycarboxylate or glass ionomer cement base.

Cavity Liners

Cavity liners are placed in the deepest portion of the cavity preparation on the axial walls or pulpal walls (Procedure 33-11). After the liners harden, they form a cement layer with minimum strength. They are placed on the dentin or on an exposed pulp, and protect the pulp from chemical irritations as well as provide a therapeutic effect to the tooth. Examples of cavity liners are calcium hydroxide, zinc oxide eugenol, and glass ionomer. Liners also are often called **low-strength bases**.

Cavity Varnish

Cavity varnish is used to seal the dentin tubules to prevent acids, saliva, and debris from reaching the pulp (Procedure 33-12). Cavity varnish is used under amalgam restorations to prevent microleakage and under zinc phosphate cements to prevent penetration of acids to the pulp. If cavity liners or medicated bases are used, varnish is placed after or on top of these materials.

Cement Bases

Cement bases are mixed to a thick putty consistency and placed in the cavity preparation to protect the pulp and provide mechanical support for the restoration. These cement bases are placed on the floor of the cavity preparation to raise the level of the floor of the preparation to the ideal height (Procedure 33-13). There are several different types of cements that can be used for bases. These include glass ionomers, hybrid ionomers, reinforced zinc oxide eugenol, zinc phosphate, and polycarboxylate. The preparation, sensitivity of the pulp, and type of restoration indicate which cement to use. These materials are often referred to as **high-strength bases**.

ADVANCED CHAIRSIDE FUNCTIONS

PROCEDURE 33-11

Placing Cavity Liners—Glass Ionomer

This procedure is performed by the dentist or expanded-function dental assistant. Preparation of the cavity has been completed, and this procedure begins the restorative process.

EQUIPMENT AND SUPPLIES (Figure 33-34)

- Cavity liner glass ionomer
- Application instrument—small, ball-shaped instrument or explorer
- Gauze sponges and cotton rolls
- Mixing pad and spatula, if material is mixed
- Curing light (if material is light cured)

PROCEDURE STEPS *(Follow aseptic procedures)*

1. Examine the cavity preparation. Determine the deepest portion of the cavity preparation and access to that area.

2. Clean and dry the cavity preparation. Remove any debris from the cavity preparation. Wash and dry the area with the air-water syringe.

3. Prepare the liner to be used. Dispense and mix according to directions. ***Note:*** Usually, light-cured materials do not have to be mixed but are placed directly in the preparation.

4. Place the liner in the cavity preparation. Using a small, ball-ended instrument, place the material in the deepest portion of the cavity preparation in a thin layer. Be careful not to touch the instrument to the sides of the preparation. The material will flow into the area and can be spread by pushing the liner in the direction desired with the small ball of the instrument.

5. Complete the placement. Remove the instrument, wipe it clean with a gauze, and repeat this procedure until the liner covers the deepest portion of the cavity preparation (Figure 33-35).

6. If the liner is self-curing, the mix must be allowed to harden. If the liner is light curing, the light is held over the tooth and activated to cure the material for the appropriate time (usually ten to twenty seconds).

7. Examine the cavity preparation. After the liner has cured, examine the preparation. If any material is on the enamel walls, remove it with an explorer.

FIGURE 33-34 Glass ionomer tray setup—placing cavity liners.

FIGURE 33-35 Placement of cavity liner in preparation.

ADVANCED CHAIRSIDE FUNCTIONS

PROCEDURE 33-12

Placing Cavity Varnish

This procedure is performed by the dentist or expanded-function dental assistant. Preparation of the cavity has been completed, and this procedure is part of preparing the tooth for the restoration.

EQUIPMENT AND SUPPLIES

- Cavity varnish (varnish and solvent)
- Cotton pliers
- Application instruments (cotton balls or cotton pellets, sponge applicators, brush applicators)
- Gauze sponges

PROCEDURE STEPS *(Follow aseptic procedures)*

1. Prepare two very small cotton balls or pellets about 2 mm in size to look like small footballs.

2. Evaluate the cavity preparation to determine access, visibility, and placement of liners or bases.

3. If the tooth has not been washed and dried, do so at this time with the air-water syringe.

4. To prevent contamination of the varnish, pick up both cotton pellets or balls with the sterile cotton pliers and place in the varnish. Then, place the cotton on gauze to remove excess varnish.

5. Using the cotton pliers, pick up one cotton ball or pellet and paint a thin layer of varnish on the dentin in the cavity preparation. A sterile disposable brush or sponge may also be used (Figure 33-36).

6. Allow the cavity to dry for thirty seconds. Place a second coat of varnish. Using the cotton pliers, pick up the second cotton pellet or ball from the gauze and apply a second layer of varnish (this prevents any voids). To prevent contamination, never place an applicator that has been used in the mouth back in the bottle of varnish.

7. Clean up after the procedure. If any excess varnish was placed on the enamel surface, remove it with varnish solvent and a small applicator.

Cavity varnish

FIGURE 33-36 Placement of cavity varnish in preparation.

ADVANCED CHAIRSIDE FUNCTIONS

PROCEDURE 33-13

Placement of Cement Bases

This procedure is performed by the dentist or expanded-function dental assistant. Preparation of the cavity has been completed, and this procedure is part of preparing the tooth for the restoration.

EQUIPMENT AND SUPPLIES (Figure 33-37)

- Cement base materials, usually powder/liquid
- Mixing pad
- Cement spatula
- Gauze sponges
- Plastic filling instrument
- Explorer or spoon excavator

PROCEDURE STEPS *(Follow aseptic procedures)*

1. Determine previous treatments and decide where to place the base and the size of the area. Evaluate access and visibility.

2. Prepare the preparation area. Remove any debris with the air-water syringe and HVE.

3. Prepare the cement base materials according to manufacturer's instructions. Mix the cement base to a thick putty consistency and gather into a small ball.

4. Collect the base on the blade of the plastic filling instrument. Place the base in the cavity preparation.

5. Using the small condensing end of the plastic filling instrument, condense the base into place on the floor of the cavity prep (Figure 33-38). If the material is sticky, place a small amount of powder on the mixing pad and dip the end of the condenser as needed. Continue until a sufficient base layer is placed.

6. Evaluate the placement. The base should cover the floor of the cavity preparation, leave enough room for the restorative materials, and should not be on pins or in retentive grooves.

7. Remove any excess materials with a spoon excavator or an explorer.

8. Clean up the mixing materials. Remove cement from the spatula as soon as possible and remove the paper from the pad.

FIGURE 33-37 Placement of cement base. (A) Cement base tray setup. (B) Base consistency.

FIGURE 33-38 Placement of cement base in cavity preparation.

CHAPTER SUMMARY

The general chairside assistant prepares and mixes the material, while the dentist places the material in the oral cavity. Some states allow the assistant to also place some of the materials in the oral cavity. Knowledge of dental material properties is necessary for the dental assistant to properly prepare and manipulate the materials. The assistant's knowledge of dental materials is beneficial for patient education and protection. Expanded-function dental assistants must understand and be competent in the placement and finishing of materials.

Case Study

Garrett Ruark is having a large filling placed in tooth #30. He has experienced sensitivity in the past after restorations, and is concerned he will have the same problem with this filling.

Case Study Review

1. Discuss steps that can be taken to reduce or eliminate sensitivity.

2. What information could the dental assistant give the patient about his concerns?

REVIEW QUESTIONS

Multiple Choice

1. Reaction of the object to resist external force is called
   a. strain.
   b. stress.
   c. shearing.
   d. elasticity.

2. All of the following are uses of dental cements *except*
   a. permanent luting.
   b. high-strength base.
   c. temporary filling.
   d. permanent restoration.

3. Which of the following cements, when mixed, exhibits an exothermic reaction?
   a. Calcium hydroxide
   b. Zinc oxide eugenol
   c. Zinc phosphate
   d. Glass ionomer

4. Luting cement that has reached the correct consistency
   a. is granular.
   b. is of a putty consistency.
   c. follows the spatula up an inch off the mixing pad.
   d. forms a ball.

5. The two types of retention are
   a. mechanical and chemical.
   b. mechanical and surgical.
   c. chemical and surgical.
   d. None of the above.

6. Dental cements are set or cured by
   a. self-curing.
   b. light-curing.
   c. dual-curing.
   d. All of the above.

7. Zinc oxide eugenol is used in all of the following *except*
   a. permanent cement.
   b. temporary cement.
   c. intermediate cement.
   d. temporary restoration.

8. _____ cement has many uses including as permanent cement, pit and fissure sealant, restorative material, and liner and bonding agent.
   a. Zinc phosphate
   b. Polycarboxylate
   c. Zinc oxide eugenol
   d. Glass ionomer

9. _____ is used as a low-strength base or liner, and is slightly irritating, which stimulates secondary dentin to form.
   a. Glass ionomer
   b. Zinc oxide eugenol
   c. Calcium hydroxide
   d. Cavity varnish

10. Which of the following materials is used to improve retention between the tooth structure and the restoration?
    a. Compomer cement
    b. Bonding agents
    c. Zinc phosphate cement
    d. Desensitizing materials

Critical Thinking

1. Give two examples of thermal conductivity relating to dentistry.

2. How is the amount of powder and liquid dispensed determined?

3. Would cavity varnish be placed under or over calcium hydroxide? Explain.

Web Activities

1. Go to http://www.kavo.com and donwload the video presentation on the DIAGNOdent pen.

2. To find out the latest information about cements and retraction materials, go to http://www.kerrdental.com.

RESTORATIVE MATERIALS, DENTAL DAM, MATRIX, AND WEDGE

SPECIFIC INSTRUCTIONAL OBJECTIVES

The student should strive to meet the following objectives and demonstrate an understanding of the facts and principles presented in this chapter:

1. Explain the properties, composition, and manipulation of dental amalgam.

2. Identify armamentarium and steps of an amalgam procedure.

3. Explain composition of composite resins.

4. Explain properties and manipulation of various composite restorations.

5. Identify armamentarium and steps of a composite restoration.

6. Explain the use of glass ionomer, resin, resin-reinforced glass ionomers, and compomer restorative materials.

ADVANCED CHAIRSIDE FUNCTIONS

7. Explain the purpose of the dental dam and identify who places it on a patient.

8. List and explain advantages and contraindications of the dental dam.

9. Identify armamentarium needed for the dental dam procedure and explain the function of each.

10. Explain how to prepare the patient for dental dam placement and how to determine the isolation area. Describe and demonstrate how dental dam material is prepared.

11. List and demonstrate steps of placing and removing the dental dam.

12. Explain and demonstrate the dental dam procedure for child patient.

13. Define matrix and wedge. List uses and types of matrices.

14. Describe functions, parts, placement, and removal of the Tofflemire matrix.

15. Explain and demonstrate placement and removal of the strip matrix.

KEY TERMS

automatrix *(830)*

alloy *(800)*

amalgam *(800)*

amalgamation *(803)*

amalgamator *(803)*

anchor tooth *(815)*

band *(830)*

burnish *(834)*

capsule *(802)*

cervical clamps *(817)*

circumference *(834)*

(continues)

OUTLINE (continued)

KEY TERMS (continued)

INTRODUCTION

This chapter discusses direct restorative materials, dental dam, and matrix and wedge. Direct restorative materials include dental amalgam and tooth-colored composite materials. Dental amalgam has been used successfully for filling posterior teeth for many years. Composition, types, and safety concerns are discussed as well as proper handling and mixing techniques. There are some concerns with the mercury in the dental amalgam and the dental assistant should keep up-to-date on current information to stay informed. Tooth-colored materials are the most popular and most widely used. Patients want the more natural look for the appearance of their teeth. There are several types and categories of materials used to fill both the anterior and posterior teeth. The various composites and combinations are discussed as well as their placement techniques.

Toward the end of the chapter, we discuss the dental dam and matrix and wedge materials and placement techniques. Placing the dental dam, matrix, and wedge are considered expanded/advanced functions. Each state has regulations delegating whether the dental assistant can actually place the dental dam and matrix and wedge or if the assistant can only assist during the placement and removal.

The dental assistant can stay current on restorative materials and dental dam, matrix, and wedge procedures by attending seminars and dental conferences, reading books and trade magazines, and through local sales representatives. The American Dental Association Council on Dental Materials, Instruments, and Equipment is responsible for information on and testing of dental materials and periodically publishes a listing in the *Journal of the American Dental Association and Clinical Products in Dentistry: A Desktop Reference.*

Amalgam Restorative Materials

After the cavity has been prepared and the liners and bases have been placed, the tooth is ready to be restored. One of the most common restorative materials is dental amalgam, which has been used for many years. Dental amalgam is an effective, long-lasting, and comparatively inexpensive restorative material. Amalgam is a combination of an alloy with mercury. An **alloy** is the combination of two or more metals.

Dental amalgam is pliable when first mixed, so it is easily placed in the cavity preparation. It is carved before hardening to resemble the tooth structure. This material is used on the posterior teeth only because of its strength and because it is not esthetically pleasing.

Composition

Dental amalgam is composed of silver, tin, copper, and zinc (optional) to form an alloy. This alloy is mixed with mercury to form the amalgam. The ADA has specifications that regulate the composition of dental amalgam (see Table 34-1 for the characteristics of each of the alloy components).

Types of Dental Amalgam

Dental amalgam consists of a low copper and high copper alloy. Metals for the alloys are prepared in several ways to produce the lathe cut (comminuted particles) and spherically shaped particles. The way these metals are prepared affects their properties. The low-copper alloys are available with comminuted and spherical particles. The high-copper alloys are supplied as comminuted, spherical, or combination particles (admix).

Spherical alloys have smoother surfaces that require less mercury when mixed. These alloys are also easier to condense and have improved carving and polishing properties. Combination alloys adapt better to the cavity preparation and produce better contacts with the adjacent teeth.

Mercury Used in Dental Amalgam

Dental mercury is a very toxic chemical and must meet specifications listed by the ADA. Dental professionals are aware of the hazards and safety measures when working with dental mercury to prevent problems from occurring.

Mercury is the only metal that is in a liquid state and vaporizes (particles of mercury scatter and float freely in the air) at a relatively low room temperature. Mercury

TABLE 34-1 Dental Alloy Composition

Silver	40 to 70 percent	High-copper amalgam
	68 to 72 percent	Low-copper mix
	• Used to form metallic compound with mercury (Hg) that determines dimensional changes that occur during hardening.	
	• Increases restoration strength.	
	• Increases expansion.	
	• Is slow to amalgamate.	
	• Hardens rapidly.	
	• Tarnishes easily.	
	• Decreases setting time.	
Tin	22 to 30 percent	High-copper amalgam
	26 to 37 percent	Low-copper amalgam
	• Aids in amalgamation (chemical combining) of alloy with Hg because of its strong Hg affinity.	
	• Reduces expansion during setting.	
	• Reduces strength.	
	• Setting time is slower.	
	• Is more susceptible to corrosion (conventional alloy).	
	• Tends to weaken amalgam.	
Copper	12 to 30 percent	High-copper amalgam
	4 to 5 percent	Low-copper amalgam
	• Increases strength and hardness.	
	• Increases expansion of amalgam during hardening.	
	• Reduces flow of finished restoration.	
	• Resists corrosion (high copper).	
	• Reduces marginal failure (high copper).	
Zinc	0 to 1 percent	For high- and low-copper amalgam
	• Minimizes oxidation of other metals in alloy during manufacturing. Zinc is a scavenger and reacts with oxygen, preventing it from combining with silver, tin, or copper. *Note:* Should moisture contamination occur during manipulation or condensation of the amalgam, delayed expansion may occur. Zinc-containing dental amalgams are particularly sensitive to moisture. Zinc reacts with water to form the zinc oxide and hydrogen gas that may cause the unwanted and excessive expansion of the set amalgam restoration.	

is absorbed through the pores of the skin and through inhalation. Some potential sources of mercury contamination in the dental office follow:

1. Mercury leaking out of a capsule during trituration

2. Mercury vapor that may occur during triturating and dispensing

3. Polishing an amalgam restoration

4. Removal of hardened amalgam restoration

5. Contacting amalgam during the procedure

6. Carpeting in the treatment rooms could retain amalgam particles and vacuuming these surfaces disperses the mercury through the air

7. Scraps of amalgam left in an open container

Studies have revealed that in most dental offices, the level of mercury vapor is well below the maximum safe environmental concentration levels. Another study testing the blood mercury level in dentists displayed a reading well below the level at which symptoms begin to show.

There has been some concern about the level of mercury in patients with numerous amalgam restorations. Recent studies have shown that these patients ingest a very low amount of mercury from the amalgam fillings, well below what they would ingest from food, water, and the atmosphere. A very small number of people are at possible risk of allergic reactions to mercury. The response manifests as a skin reaction that appears after the placement of an amalgam restoration. Including questions on the medical history is a step of prevention. Because of these concerns, the dentist and dental assistant should stay current with research and ADA recommendations.

The ADA recommends that a program of mercury hygiene be established at every dental practice. Potential office hazards involving mercury can be eliminated by practicing appropriate mercury hygiene. Guidelines should include the following:

1. Wear disposable gloves, face mask, and glasses when working with amalgam.

2. Educate all personnel regarding the potential hazards of mercury and good mercury hygiene practices.

3. A no-touch technique should be used when handling mercury. If the skin is exposed, wash with soap and water, and rinse under running water.

4. Use capsules containing a measured amount of mercury and alloy.

5. Use an amalgamator with a protective cover to reduce the chance of any mercury vapor being released and to confine mercury that might be sprayed from an ill-fitting capsule.

FIGURE 34-1 Mercury spill kit.

6. Store mercury and amalgam scraps in capped, unbreakable jars containing used x-ray fixer, finely divided sulfur, glycerin, or mineral oil.

7. Carpeting in dental treatment rooms is not recommended. Carpeting retains mercury, which is difficult to retrieve.

8. Use water spray and high-volume evacuation when cutting old amalgams or polishing new restorations. Wear a mask during these procedures.

9. Avoid working with mercury or amalgam near a heat source, such as the autoclave.

10. Handle mercury only over impervious surfaces. The area should have a continuous lip to retain any spillage.

11. The office should have proper ventilation to reduce the possibility of mercury vapor inhalation. Change the air filter frequently.

12. Office personnel should have periodic urinalyses to check for any mercury in the body.

13. Monitor the dental office to determine mercury levels.

14. Keep a mercury spill kit if the office uses large quantities of mercury. Clean up any mercury scraps or spills immediately, following OSHA recommendations (Figure 34-1).

Forms of Dental Alloy

Dental alloy is purchased in disposable **capsule** form. The capsule contains a premeasured amount of alloy and mercury and sometimes a **pestle**. The pestle, a small pellet, is made of metal or plastic and aids in the mixing of the alloy and mercury. In the capsule, a thin membrane separates the alloy and the mercury until they are mixed. Some capsules come with activators to break the membrane or the capsules are twisted or compressed before being mixed. The capsules are most often plastic and come with screw-type or friction-fit caps. Disposable capsules are color coded to distinguish single, double, and triple mixes (Figure 34-2).

Amalgam Properties

The strength of amalgam is not adequate to withstand occlusal forces alone. The preparation is designed so that the remaining tooth structure sustains the forces

FIGURE 34-2 Sample of amalgam capsules.

to the amalgam. Proper manipulation of amalgam is important in the overall strength and success of the restoration.

Amalgam is subject to dimensional change, such as expansion and contraction. The amount of expansion and contraction is controlled by the composition of the alloy and manipulation techniques.

Another property of amalgam is the ability of the material to creep. Creeping is a change in the material when under a constant load.

Amalgam restorations are subject to tarnish and corrosion in the oral cavity. Tarnish is the discoloration of the surface, and corrosion is the deterioration of the surface. The combination (admixed) and the spherical high copper amalgams are less susceptible to corrosion. Careful finishing and polishing of amalgams reduces tarnish and corrosion.

Amalgam Manipulation

Trituration is the mechanical means of combining (mixing) the dental alloy and mercury. Amalgamation is the actual chemical reaction that occurs between the alloy and the mercury to form the silver amalgam. Specially designed machines used to triturate (amalgamate) the alloy and mercury are called dental amalgamators or triturators. These machines have cradles to hold the capsules, cradle covers, timers, and variable speed controls (Figure 34-7). General steps for use of the amalgamator are outlined in Procedure 34-1. Each amalgamator must be set for the type of dental alloy used. Usually, trituration of the alloy and mercury is ten to fifteen seconds. This produces a homogeneous and uniform mix. Follow the manufacturer's directions and alloy specifications.

PROCEDURE 34-1
Using the Dental Amalgamator

This procedure is completed by the dental assistant. The materials and equipment are prepared before the procedure begins. The types of amalgamator and capsules vary.

EQUIPMENT (Figure 34-3)

- Amalgamator

- Premeasured capsule of dental alloy and mercury

- Amalgam well, dappen dish, or squeeze cloth

- Amalgam carrier/condenser

- Scrap container for excess amalgam

PROCEDURE STEPS *(Follow aseptic procedures)*

1. Assemble materials for the procedure. Select trituration time and speed for the type of alloy and amalgamator.

2. Prepare the capsule by twisting the cap, squeezing the capsule, or using an activator.

(continues)

PROCEDURE 34-1 *(CONTINUED)*

FIGURE 34-3 Tray setup for dental amalgamator.

FIGURE 34-4 (A) Placing capsule in amalgamator. (B) Activating amalgamator timer.

3. Insert the capsule into the cradle (prongs) of the amalgamator. Place one end first, then slide the other end down into place. Practice placing the capsules into the cradle with one hand (Figure 34-4A).

4. Close the cover of the amalgamator.

5. Activate the amalgamator for the prescribed time and speed (Figure 34-4B). (The timer will automatically switch off after prescribed trituration time.)

6. Lift cover and remove capsule.

7. Open capsule and empty amalgam into an amalgam well. Avoid touching the amalgam with gloved hands. Use cotton pliers, if necessary. A well-mixed amalgam will have a glossy appearance with a smooth, velvety consistency.

8. Reassemble the capsule and place it to the side.

9. Hold the carrier and load the amalgam (Figure 34-5).

10. Pack the carrier, applying pressure so that the cylinder is packed tightly. Wipe excess material from the end of the carrier on the sides of the amalgam well.

11. Pass the amalgam carrier to the dentist and prepare to exchange a condenser for the carrier. When practicing, dispense the amalgam from the carrier into a dappen dish and evaluate the mix. The cylinders of amalgam should be smooth and shiny.

12. Repeat the loading and dispensing of all the material. Toward the end of the manipulation, the amalgam becomes harder to load into the carrier because it begins to set. This is the stage that takes practice in order to become proficient.

FIGURE 34-5 Loading amalgam carrier.

(continues)

PROCEDURE 34-1 (CONTINUED)

13. To clean up, expel any excess amalgam into the appropriate container. The instruments are cleaned and sterilized (Figure 34-6).

FIGURE 34-6 Placing amalgam scraps in sealed container.

FIGURE 34-7 Kerr amalgamator. *(Courtesy of Kerr Corporation.)*

Trituration of the amalgam is an important step in restoration success. The quality of the mix is determined by the mixing time, speed of the amalgamator, and the force being applied during the trituration. Varying conditions in the trituration process can cause certain problems. If the amalgam is mixed too long (overtriturated), it will be soupy before hardening and difficult to remove from the capsule. If the amalgam is undermixed (undertriturated), it will be crumbly and dull in appearance and the strength of the amalgam will be reduced.

Amalgam Bonding

Amalgam bonding agents are available and used in many restorations to bond the amalgam to the tooth surface (Figure 34-8). The amalgam bonding increases the retention of the restoration and decreases marginal leakage. The bonding agent is a low viscosity resin, similar to those discussed in Chapter 33 Dental Cements, Bases, Liners, and Bonding Agents. The procedure describes the application of bonding agents. The placement of the amalgam follows immediately, before the bonding agent sets.

Note: Other retention methods, including the placement of retention pins and core buildups, are discussed in Chapter 30, Fixed Prosthodontics.

FIGURE 34-8 Amalgam bonding materials.

Complete Amalgam Procedure

The sequence of the procedure is for a complete amalgam restoration. The steps include administering anesthetic; placing the rubber dam; placing liners, bases, and bonding agents; assembling the matrix and wedge; and mixing, placing, condensing, and finishing the amalgam restoration. Procedure 34-2 gives the dental assistant an overall view of assisting during an amalgam procedure. Many of these steps, such as placing the rubber dam, are discussed in detail later in this chapter because they can be performed by an expanded function dental assistant.

PROCEDURE 34-2

Amalgam Restoration—Class II

This procedure is completed by the dentist and dental assistant. The tooth is prepared with the dental handpiece and assorted burs. Once the tooth is prepared, it is restored with dental amalgam.

EQUIPMENT AND SUPPLIES (Figure 34-9)

- Basic setup: mouth mirror, explorer, cotton pliers
- Air-water syringe tip, HVE tip, and saliva ejector
- Cotton rolls, gauze sponges, pellets, cotton tip applicators, and floss
- Topical and local anesthetic setup
- Rubber dam setup
- High- and low-speed handpieces
- Assortment of dental burs
- Spoon excavator
- Hand cutting instruments (hatchets, chisels, hoes, and gingival margin trimmers)
- Base, liner, varnish, and/or bonding agent
- Paper pad, cement spatula, and placement instrument
- Matrix retainer, matrix bands, and wedges
- Locking pliers or hemostat
- Amalgam capsules
- Amalgam well
- Amalgam carrier and condensers
- Amalgamator
- Carving instruments
- Articulating paper and forceps

FIGURE 34-9 Amalgam procedures tray setup.

PROCEDURE STEPS *(Follow aseptic procedures)*

1. Greet and prepare the patient for the procedure. Review the medical history.

2. Prepare for the administration of the topical and local anesthetic. Dry the injection site and apply topical anesthetic (Expanded Function—EF). Prepare the syringe and summon the dentist. Transfer the mirror and explorer to the dentist to examine the tooth before beginning the procedure. When the dentist is ready, transfer a 2 × 2 gauze in one hand and the syringe in the other. The dentist replaces the needle cap and places the syringe on the tray. After the injection, rinse and evacuate the patient's mouth.

3. Prepare the rubber dam materials and equipment to assist the dentist in the placement (EF).

(continues)

4. Transfer the mouth mirror and the high-speed handpiece with a bur. Position the HVE tip and maintain visibility throughout the procedure by retracting the cheek and tongue, keeping the mirror clear with the air-water syringe, and evacuating the site (Figure 34-10). Transfer and receive instruments at the dentist's signals. Instruments used at this point may include the explorer, the excavator, hatchets, hoes, angle formers, gingival margin trimmers, and chisels.

5. When the preparation is finished, transfer a cotton pellet with a cavity cleaning preparation to clean the inside of the tooth (EF). The area is then rinsed and dried. At the dentist's direction, mix the cavity liner (calcium hydroxide or glass ionomer), prepare the varnish if used, and the base (glass ionomer, polycarboxylate, zinc phosphate, or modified ZOE), and bonding agent if used, and transfer them to the dentist for placement. If the materials are light cured, hold the light tip near the material to be cured and, with the protective shield in place, activate the light to cure the material.

6. Assemble the matrix retainer and the band into the correct position according to the tooth being restored and transfer it to the dentist (EF). After the matrix is placed, transfer the wedge in cotton pliers (locking is best) or in a hemostat. The dentist places the wedge.

7. When the dentist is ready, prepare the amalgam capsule by twisting the cap, squeezing the capsule together, or placing it in an activator, and then placing the capsule in the amalgamator. The amalgamator is set for the specific type of amalgam material and size of the mix. When the amalgam material has been mixed, remove the capsule from the amalgamator and place it in the amalgam well or a dappen dish. The amalgam is loaded into the amalgam carrier. If the carrier is double ended, both ends are filled and the loaded carrier is passed to the dentist (Figure 34-11). The carrier and the condenser are used alternately until the restorative material fills the cavity. In some offices, the dental assistant loads the carrier and, at the dentist's direction, places the amalgam in the cavity preparation, eliminating the exchanging of instruments and allowing the dentist to focus on the condensing of the amalgam. After the last exchange, transfer the dentist an explorer to loosen amalgam from the matrix band. While the dentist is using the explorer, clean up any amalgam scraps from the carrier and the well and place them in a sealed container.

8. Receive the explorer and transfer carving and finishing instruments at the dentist's signals. Operate the HVE tip near the site to evacuate any amalgam particles. After the dentist completes the preliminary carving, pass the cotton pliers to remove the wedge and then receive the wedge, pliers, and matrix retainer. The cotton pliers may be used again to remove the matrix band. Receive the cotton pliers and band and then transfer the carver of the dentist's choice for finishing the carving of the anatomy in the restoration.

9. The rubber dam is carefully removed at this time (EF). Transfer the clamp forceps, receive the forceps with the clamp, and transfer scissors to cut the interseptal dam. Receive the scissors, frame, napkin, and dam material. Rinse and evacuate the patient's mouth.

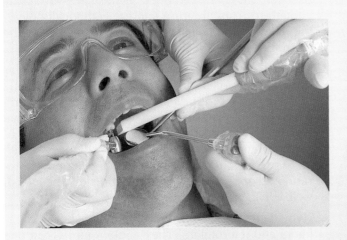

FIGURE 34-10 Cavity being prepared by dentist with dental assistant evacuating and keeping mirror dry and clean.

FIGURE 34-11 Loaded carrier, ready for use.

(continues)

PROCEDURE 34-2 *(CONTINUED)*

10. Dry the area and transfer the articulating paper, positioned on the forceps, to the dentist. The assistant may be instructed by the dentist to place the articulating paper over the restoration. The patient is instructed to gently tap the teeth together (Figure 34-12). Additional carving and checking of the occlusion are continued until the dentist is satisfied and the patient is comfortable.

11. The restoration is wiped off with a wet cotton roll to remove blue marks left by the articulating paper. Rinse and evacuate the patient's mouth thoroughly and clean any debris from the patient's face. The patient is cautioned not to chew on the side of the restoration for a few hours and is then dismissed.

FIGURE 34-12 Articulating paper for patient to gently close onto to check occlusion.

Composite Restorative Materials

Composite restorative materials dominate the field of esthetic restorations. These materials have natural appearances and were used primarily for anterior restorations but now have developed as esthetic restorations for the posterior teeth. Composite materials also are used for veneers of the anterior teeth that have been stained or that have some erosion. (These procedures are discussed in Chapter 30, Fixed Prosthodontics.)

Technology is expanding the types of materials available as alternatives to dental amalgam. With concerns over the mercury in amalgams and the desire for the natural appearance of teeth, there is ongoing research and development with composite restorative materials. Composites, glass ionomers, resins, and porcelain materials and combinations of these materials are used for esthetic restorations.

These direct restorative materials are inserted into the cavity preparation and then self-cured, light cured, or dual cured. They come in syringes or single-application cartridges (**compules**) and have a variety of shades or shade modifiers. The location and the size of the cavity determines which material the dentist chooses.

Composite Composition

Composite restorative material is composed of the following components:

- An **organic polymer matrix**, such as dimethacrylate, identified as BIS-GMA or urethane dimethacrylates.

- **Inorganic filler particles**, such as quartz, silica, and lithium aluminum silicate.

- **Organic silane coupling agents**. The inorganic filler particles are treated with an organic silane coupling agent to provide a bond between the inorganic fillers and the resin matrix.

Barium, strontium, zinc, or zirconium may be added to make the composite material more radiopaque.

The composites are classified according to the type, amount, and size of the filler particles, but all are referred to as composite resins. Composite particles are fine, microfill, and combinations of the fine and microfill filler particles, called *hybrids*. The filler particles can make up as much as 84 percent of the composite material by volume.

- **Macrofill composites** contain filler particles that range in size from 1 to 3 microns. These materials are used for Class IV restorations because they are strong enough to resist fracture and are esthetically pleasing. They do not polish to the same high finish as the microfill and the hybrids.

- **Microfill composites** contain fillers that range in size from 0.01 to 0.1 microns. They are used as a cosmetic filling material for Class III and V restorations. Microfills are also used for direct veneers and diastema closures. Some microfills are reinforced for Class IV restorations and the occlusal portion of Class I and II restorations. Microfill composites are esthetic restorations that resist wear due to abrasion and polish well, leaving a high-luster finish.

- **Hybrid composites** are a combination of both macrofillers and microfillers. They contain more than one type of filler particle, usually glass and silica. The glass particles are in the 1- to 3-micron range, and the silica is around 0.04 microns. These composites are stronger and less likely to fracture in high-stress areas than the microfill composites. The hybrids combine the strength and esthetics of the other com-

FIGURE 34-13 Flowable composite kit.

posites to make a restoration that is strong and polishable. They are used both in the anterior and posterior areas of the mouth.

Flowable Composites. Flowable composites are similar to microfilled and hybrid composites in filler content and particle size. They have a low viscosity that allows easy flow direct application into cavity preparations by small syringe tips. Flowable composites have many uses including adaptation to irregularities of cavity walls, flow into narrow preparations of conservative dentistry, pit and fissure sealant in some cases, large cavity preparation linings, additives to temporaries, and filling voids in noncarious areas, such as toothbrush abrasion areas or occlusal tooth loss due to bruxism. Advantages of flowable composites follow: they are easy to place, they can reach small areas, and they are esthetic, with many shades available. Disadvantages include lack of strength; they shrink more than the hybrid composites and cannot be used alone to fill large preparations (Figure 34-13).

Packable Composites. Packable composites are sometimes called condensable composites. They are more putty like and stiffer in consistency than other composites, and they are highly viscous and contain large amounts of fillers. They are used in posterior areas for core buildups, and places requiring a resistant, stronger restoration. Packable composites can be pressed into the restoration in layers. Sometimes various types of composite are layered for optimum results. Packable composites are not subject to as much shrinkage when polymerized as certain other composites because they contain less resin and more filler.

Composite Properties

Properties of composite resin materials vary depending on the type and size of the filler. These aspects of the composites are constantly being improved for a strong,

esthetic, long-lasting restoration. Overall, composites exhibit the following properties:

- Resistance to fracturing.
- Occlusal wear resistance is improving.
- Good esthetics for matching the tooth structure.
- Some composites are radiopaque, making them more visible on radiographic film.
- Composites bond efficiently to dentin and enamel.
- Composites are often placed in layers to reduce the effect of polymerization (setting) shrinkage.
- Composite resins have adequate strength for specific applications. The strength requirement varies for various classifications of cavities. For example, the anterior Class III and V cavities do not require great strength but do require color stability. The posterior Class I and II must exhibit enough strength to withstand occlusal stresses, but appearance is not as critical. All composite restorations require a smooth finish to reduce the potential for plaque and debris accumulation and for staining.
- Expansion and contraction rates of composite materials are similar to tooth structure.

Manipulation Considerations

To bond the composite material and tooth structure, the cavity preparation is acid etched for thirty to sixty seconds. The etchant is rinsed completely and the surface is dried. After etching, the tooth has a chalky, dull appearance. Adhesion of the composite to the etched surface is rated high, but it can be further improved by the use of a bonding agent. Bonding agents are applied as described previously to both the enamel and the dentin. The composite then adheres to the bonding agent.

Shrinkage of composites can be minimized by placing the composite in small layers in the cavity preparation. After each layer is placed, it is light cured to the hardened form. Layering of the composite is also a method to modify the restoration shade . The layers can be composed of various types of composites with diverse properties to enhance the qualities of the material.

Composites are mainly packaged as one-paste systems that are light-cured. The paste may come in a syringe for multiple applications or in single-dose cartridges that are used with a syringe (Figure 34-14). The pastes also come in a variety of shades. A specific shade guide comes with composite systems to assist in the selection of a shade that matches the patient's natural dentition.

The pulp can be protected with a cavity liner before the etching, bonding, and composite placement steps.

Often, a plastic or Teflon-tipped filling instrument is used to place and shape the composite. These instruments come in various sizes and shapes to aid in adapting the composite material to the cavity preparation.

FIGURE 34-14 Composite syringes and cartridges.

FIGURE 34-15 Celluloid matrix strip with metal clip.

Modifications

Procedure 34-3 is for a Class III restoration. Some modifications to the procedure may be required for Classes I, II, IV, and V. Most of the procedures are similar, but there are a few changes or considerations.

Classes I and II. Classes I and II are posterior restorations. Shade selection is not as critical with these restorations as it is with the anterior classes. The Class I restoration does not require a matrix, because only the occlusal surface is involved. For Class II restorations, some operators prefer the clear matrix band, which is used with a retainer, and wedges, which facilitate the light-curing process.

Some anatomy may be carved into the composite before the final curing. Discs may be difficult to use in some areas, but diamonds, finishing burs, and polishing points are used to smooth and finish the restoration.

Class IV. Class IV anterior restorations involve the proximal surface and incisal edge. In some cases, retention pins are required because of the amount of lost tooth structure. The pins are positioned once the tooth is prepared, before the placement of the composite material.

A matrix strip or preformed celluloid crown can be used to mold the composite (Figure 34-15). If the celluloid crown form is used, the dentist places the composite into the cavity preparation in layers, curing after each step. A crown form is partially filled and placed over the cured resin in the preparation to form the incisal angle of the restoration. The crown form is prepared with a small hole placed in the incisal edge to prevent air from being trapped. Excess material is removed, and the curing light is used to harden the composite.

After the material is cured, the crown form is removed and the final shaping and finishing are completed with finishing burs, polishing discs, and strips.

Class V. Class V gingival one-third restoration may not require a matrix strip. A precontoured matrix may be used, or a matrix may not be used at all. The restorative materials can be placed in the cavity preparation and shaped with a plastic or composite filling instrument, then light cured. Finishing should be minimal with these restorations.

Glass Ionomer Restorations

Type II glass ionomer materials are used as an esthetic restoration most often in non–stress-bearing restorations. Examples include restoring gingival one-third and root surface cavities. These materials are not suitable for areas that require strength or where esthetics are critical. They bond well to tooth structure and release fluoride to resist recurrent decay.

Hybrid (or Resin-Modified) Glass Ionomers

The combination of the composite resins and glass ionomers has improved the qualities of the glass ionomer restorations. They are used for Class III and V restora-

PROCEDURE 34-3

Composite Restoration—Class III

This procedure is completed by the dentist and dental assistant. The tooth is prepared with the dental handpiece and assorted burs. Once the tooth is prepared, it is restored with composite.

EQUIPMENT AND SUPPLIES (Figure 34-16)

- Basic setup: mouth mirror, explorer, cotton pliers
- Air-water syringe tip, HVE tip, and saliva ejector
- Cotton rolls, gauze sponges, cotton pellets, cotton-tip applicators, and dental floss
- Topical and local anesthetic setup
- Rubber dam setup
- High- and low-speed handpieces
- Assortment of dental burs (including diamond and cutting burs)
- Spoon excavator
- Hand cutting instruments (dentist's choice may include binangle chisel and Wedelstaedt chisel)
- Base and liner with mixing materials and placement instruments
- Bonding materials
- Etchant and applicator, if necessary (usually comes with composite system)
- Primer (usually comes with composite system)
- Composite materials, including a shade guide
- Composite placement instrument (plastic filling instrument)
- Curing light with protective shield
- Celluloid matrix strip and wedges
- Locking pliers or hemostat
- Finishing burs or diamonds
- #12 scalpel (optional)
- Abrasive strips
- Polishing discs
- Lubricant
- Articulating paper and forceps

PROCEDURE STEPS

(Follow aseptic procedures)

1. The patient is seated and prepared for the procedure. Confirm the procedure and review the medical history.

2. Rinse the patient's mouth, dry the injection site, and place the topical anesthetic (EF). Prepare the syringe. When the dentist comes in, remove the topical anesthetic applicator and transfer the mouth mirror and explorer to the dentist. After receiving the mirror and explorer, transfer 2 × 2 gauze to the dentist and then the anesthetic syringe is transferred. Following the administration of the local anesthetic, rinse the patient's mouth.

3. The shade is determined for the composite material before the placement of the rubber dam (Figure 34-17). Under natural light, the dentist compares a shade guide

FIGURE 34-16 Composite procedure tray setup.

(continues)

P R O C E D U R E   3 4 - 3 *(C O N T I N U E D)*

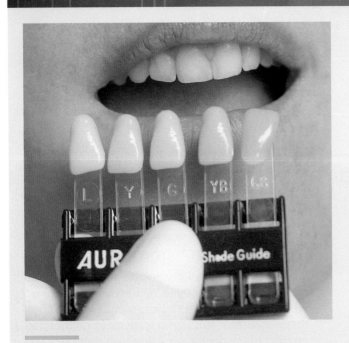

FIGURE 34-17 Determining shade before procedure begins.

to the patient's teeth. A shade or combination of shades is selected to match the patient's teeth as closely as possible. The shade is recorded on the patient's chart for future reference.

4. The dental dam is placed by the dental assistant or with the dental assistant helping the dentist.

5. Transfer a mirror, high-speed handpiece, and bur to the dentist. Maintain visibility throughout the procedure by cleaning the mirror, retracting the tissues, and evacuating the area. During the cavity preparation, transfer instruments and change burs as indicated by the dentist.

6. When the cavity preparation is complete, rinse and dry the preparation. Proximity of the pulp to the cavity preparation determines the type of base or liner needed for protection. Mix the appropriate materials, usually a calcium hydroxide or glass ionomer liner, and hold the mixing pad, applicator, and 2 × 2 gauze near the patient's chin. After each application, wipe the instrument. If the materials need the light for the curing process, the curing light is prepared and positioned.

7. Transfer a brush or applicator tip containing the acid etching materials to the dentist, who applies it to the cavity preparation. The etchant is rinsed thoroughly after the recommended time.

8. The celluloid matrix strip is placed by the dentist. If required, a plastic wedge is also placed (the plastic

wedges permit light curing of the bonding agent and the composite).

9. The bonding material is placed according to manufacturer's instructions. With some bonding resins, a **primer** or conditioner is placed before the bonding material.

10. Most composites are applied in a single-application syringe, which can be used to place the material directly into the cavity preparation. Sometimes, a composite placement instrument is used for placement. The matrix is held around the tooth to restore contour. If the material is light cured, it is placed in incremental layers and light cured after each layer is placed. The self-curing composites are mixed and placed in the cavity preparation. Within a few minutes, the material begins to chemically set.

11. Transfer cotton pliers to remove the wedge and the matrix strip. After receiving these items, an explorer is transferred to check the restoration.

12. Transfer the low-speed handpiece with finishing bur to the dentist. When the dentist is using the handpiece, use the air syringe. Finishing burs, diamonds, and abrasive discs may be used to finish the composite restoration. Abrasive strips may be used to smooth the interproximal areas. Composite polishing points, discs, and cups are then used to smooth the restoration (Figure 34-18).

13. The dental dam is carefully removed and the oral cavity is rinsed.

14. Transfer the mirror and explorer to the dentist for examination, dry the tooth, receive the mirror and explorer, and pass the articulating paper. The occlusion is checked and any high marks are removed. The patient's mouth is rinsed and the patient is given postoperative instructions.

FIGURE 34-18 Polishing burs and abrasive strip for composites.

tions. They come in various shades and are light-cured materials.

The technique for placement is similar to that for composites, with the following exceptions. The tooth is conservatively prepared with no need for mechanical retention or bevels. A retraction cord may be placed with the Class V preparations to expose the entire margin of the cavity preparation. The preparation is cleaned with a chlorhexidine soap solution. Follow the manufacturer's directions on the finishing and polishing of the restoration. Some need to be kept moist or have lubricants placed when polishing. A layer of light-cured enamel bonding agent is applied over the finished restoration.

Compomers

Compomers are a cross between composites and glass ionomers in characteristics and properties. They are single-paste, light-cured systems that release fluoride and are bonded to the walls of the cavity with dentin/enamel adhesives. Compomers are mostly used on Class III and Class V restorations on permanent teeth and on all types of restorations on primary teeth. They adhere to dentin without etching the tooth, but a primer/adhesive is used (Figure 34-19).

FIGURE 34-19 Compomer restorative material kit.

ADVANCED CHAIRSIDE FUNCTIONS

Dental Dam

Dental dam placement is one method of isolating teeth that are going to be restored. It can be used on almost any patient. The dental dam is a barrier that is applied by the dentist and, in some states, by the dental assistant and the dental hygienist. After the patient has received the anesthetic, the dental dam is prepared and placed. The dental assistant assists the dentist in the placement or places the dental dam before the dentist begins to prepare the tooth. The dam can be placed to isolate one tooth or one or more quadrants.

Advantages of Dental Dam Use

Advantages of using the dental dam follow:

- Greater visibility because of contrast between tooth and dental dam material

- Greater accessibility to operating field by retracting gingiva, tongue, cheeks, and lips

- Control of moisture to keep the area dry for better vision and to ensure a dry tooth when bonding agents, etchants, and restorative materials are used

- Protection for the patient from swallowing or aspirating debris during the procedure

- Protection of the gingiva during acid-etching procedures

- Improved patient management and decreased operating time because of limited patient conversation and because a clear, dry field is maintained

- Acts as a protective barrier for patient

- Decreased amount of contaminated aerosol exposure

Contraindications to Dental Dam Isolation

Conditions that contraindicate dental dam use include:

- Physical conditions of the patient, such as asthma, respiratory congestion, allergies to latex, herpetic lesions, or lesions of the commissures (corners of the mouth)

- Concerns the patient might have, such as if the patient is claustrophobic (cannot tolerate the dental dam) or the patient has had or has heard of a bad experience with the dental dam (hesitant to have the dam used for the dental procedure)

- Conditions in the oral cavity, such as partially erupted teeth or malaligned teeth

ADVANCED CHAIRSIDE FUNCTIONS

Materials and Equipment

The dental dam procedure requires a variety of instruments and materials. The materials and equipment may be on a separate tray stored at the dental unit, or in a tub for easy use. Materials include the dental dam material, dental dam napkin, dental floss, and tape. Dental dam clamps, forceps, frame, punching guides, and a punch are the specific equipment needed.

Dental Dam Materials

The dental dam is a latex or latex-free material that comes in various sizes, weights, and colors selected according to the office preference. The most common sizes of the dental dam are the 5×5 or the 6×6 precut squares. The 5×5 dental dam is used for endodontic procedures, anterior applications on adults, and for children. The 6×6 dental dam is used for adult procedures. These squares usually come in a box of fifty or more and are lightly powdered on one side to prevent sticking. The dental dam is also available in a continuous roll of five-inch and six-inch widths. This material is cut to the desired length by the operator.

The dental dam is available in different weights (thicknesses), including thin, medium, heavy, extra heavy, and special heavy. The thin or light dental dam materials are passed easily through contacts but tear easily and do not retract the tissues effectively. The medium and the heavy materials are often used because they do not tear as easily and provide greater tissue retraction. The heavier the material, the more difficult it is to place interproximally, but the retraction is excellent (Figure 34-20).

The dental dam is available in various colors (shades), from dark gray or green to pastels. The darker shades provide more contrast with the teeth and are easier for the operator. A scented dental dam is also available and is very pleasing to the patient (in comparison to the latex smell). It may be scented with mint or fruit.

The dental dam material has no definite shelf life but is sensitive to temperature changes and, like other latex rubber, to age. For a longer shelf life, store dental dam material in the refrigerator.

Dental Dam Napkin

Dental dam napkins are used for patient comfort and to absorb saliva, water, and perspiration. Disposable napkins are made of a soft, absorbent fabric and are precut. They are designed to prevent the dam material from

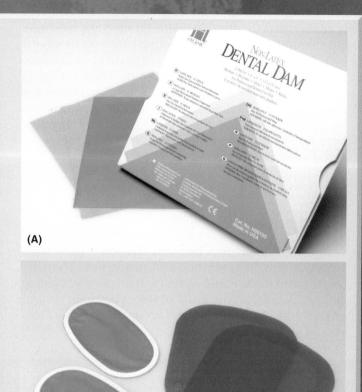

FIGURE 34-20 (A) Various colors and sizes of dental dam material. (B) Dental dam with frames.

touching the face by covering the area around the mouth and the cheeks (Figure 34-21).

Dental Dam Frame

The **dental dam frame**, or holder, is designed to stretch and secure the dam in place across the patient's face. The frame stabilizes the dental dam and keeps the operating area open. The frames are made of metal or plastic and have small projections around the borders to secure the dental dam.

Several styles of frames are available (Figure 34-22). The metal U-shaped frame is very common and is known as the **Young frame**. It is easy to apply and comfortable for the patient. The Young frame is made of stainless steel and can be autoclaved. The plastic U-shaped frame is also common and is known as the **U-frame**. It is also easy to apply and comfortable for the patient. This plastic frame is radiolucent and autoclavable. The **Ostby**

ADVANCED CHAIRSIDE FUNCTIONS

FIGURE 34-21 Dental napkins.

FIGURE 34-23 Dental dam punching guides. (A) Template. (B) Stamp with ink pad.

FIGURE 34-22 Dental dam frames.

frame is an oval-shaped plastic frame that was designed to follow the shape of the lower face. Projections on the outer borders secure the dental dam. The frame is radiotransparent and can be autoclaved.

Dental Dam Punching Guides

The dental dam may be marked by using a template or a stamp of the adult and pediatric arches. Both the template and stamp are marked to indicate where the holes for the teeth should be punched. The stamp is used with an ink pad and the dam may be stamped ahead of time. The template comes in both 5 × 5 and 6 × 6 sizes and also can be used to mark the dam ahead of time (Figure 34-23).

The dental dam guides are perfect dental arches, so they will not fit every patient. Instead, the markings act as guides. They are especially helpful when learning to punch the dental dam, but eventually they become

unnecessary and the operator uses the patient's teeth as the guide.

Dental Dam Punch

The action of the dental dam punch is similar to that of the paper punch, although the design is much different. The punch has a handle and a working end (Figure 34-24A). The working end of the punch has a stylus, which is a sharp projection to punch through the dental dam, and a punch table or plate. The table has four or five differently sized holes and rotates to facilitate punching holes for the various teeth (Figure 34-24B). The punch table should be adjusted so that the hole is centered under the stylus before the punch is made. This prevents damage to the holes of the punch table. When the punch table is rotated, it makes a clicking sound as it adjusts.

Dental Dam Clamps

Dental dam clamps come in numerous designs and sizes to fit around the teeth (Figure 34-25). Their purpose is to stabilize and secure the dental dam material in place. The tooth that the clamp is placed on is often called the anchor tooth. The anchor tooth is one or two teeth to the distal of the tooth or teeth being restored.

Dental dam clamps are made of high-quality stainless steel and are designed to be used on specific teeth. They are identified by numbers and letters, not by the teeth they are used on. The basic parts to a dental dam clamp include the following (Figure 34-26):

■ **Bow**—Arched metal joining the two jaws of the clamp

■ **Jaws**—Part of clamp that expands to fix over the tooth, and then releases to fit on the gingival one-third

ADVANCED CHAIRSIDE FUNCTIONS

(A)

(B)

Hole number 5–Molars and used for anchor tooth
Hole number 4–Molars
Hole number 3–Cuspids and premolars
Hole number 2–Upper incisors
Hole number 1–Lower incisors

FIGURE 34-24 (A) Dental dam punches. (B) Punch table with corresponding teeth.

(A)

(B)

(C)

FIGURE 34-25 Assorted clamps. (A) Cervical. (B) Winged. (C) Wingless.

of the tooth. Jaws secure the clamp to the tooth. The jaws are different sizes for different teeth in the arch.

■ **Forceps holes**—Located on the jaws of the clamp, the dental dam forceps attach to the clamp to place and remove the clamp from the tooth at these holes.

■ **Points**—Parts of jaws that actually contact the tooth. The points are located at different widths and angles to fit and secure the clamp on the tooth.

■ The jaws of the clamp are designed to be winged or wingless. **Winged clamps** have extra projections for better retraction, and they hold the dental dam in place because the wings are angled toward the gin-

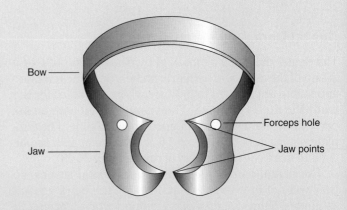

Bow

Forceps hole

Jaw

Jaw points

FIGURE 34-26 Parts of dental dam clamp.

ADVANCED CHAIRSIDE FUNCTIONS

giva. **Wingless clamps** have the letter *W* in front of the number of the clamp and have no projections.

- Some clamps are double bowed, and they are called **cervical clamps**. These clamps are used for Class V restorations on anterior teeth. These clamps assist in gingival retraction and often must be stabilized with stick impression compound after the teeth have been exposed. Examples are the SSW 212 or the Hygienic B6 and B5.

- Dental dam clamps that have the letter *A* following the number have jaws that bend sharply downward, toward the gingiva. Clamps without the letter *A* have jaws on a flat plane.

Selecting Clamp. The tooth to be clamped must be evaluated before the clamp selection is made. The mesiodistal width at the cementoenamel junction (CEJ) of the tooth must be evaluated to select a clamp. The width on the tooth must be about the same as the width between the points of the jaws of the clamp. The faciolingual width at the CEJ of the tooth must also be estimated to ensure that the clamp fits tightly. Once the tooth has been evaluated, a clamp can be selected. To place the clamp, the jaws are opened wide enough to clear the height of contour, which is the widest part of the tooth. Then, the jaws are closed slowly on the tooth to fit tightly at the CEJ. The points should rest securely all around the tooth.

Dental Dam Forceps

Dental dam forceps are used to place and remove the dental dam clamp. The forceps have two beaks that fit into the holes of the jaws of the clamp. Once the beaks are securely in the holes, pressure is applied to the handle of the forceps and the clamp jaws are opened slightly. There is a lock (sliding bar) on the handle that keeps the clamp in this position until it is placed on the anchor tooth. When the handle is squeezed again and the lock is released, the operator has control over the clamp and can make adjustments to the clamp position. As the clamp is placed properly, the tension that expands the clamp is eased and the clamp is secured on the tooth. Once the clamp is stable, the beaks of the forceps are removed from the clamp and the forceps are removed from the mouth (Figure 34-27).

Dental Floss

Dental floss is used for a variety of reasons with dental dam isolation.

1. A piece of dental floss, about eighteen inches long, is tied to the bow of the dental dam clamp before

FIGURE 34-27 Dental dam forceps.

the clamp is placed. If the clamp slips off the anchor tooth, the floss makes it easy to retrieve. The floss ends are always on the outside of the mouth for quick access. Sometimes the floss is called a ligature or safety line.

2. The floss is used to ease the dental dam material through tight contacts.

3. The dental floss assists in **inverting**, or tucking, the dental dam material around the teeth to prevent moisture leakage.

4. The clamp stabilizes the dental dam on one end of the arch and dental floss is sometimes used to secure the opposite end. On the distal of the last tooth on the opposite side from the clamped tooth, a piece of floss is placed interproximally and then looped over with a second piece of floss to secure the end of the punched dental dam (See Figure 34-32A).

Lubricant

A small amount of lubricant is placed on the back or underside of the dental dam. This facilitates slipping the dam material over the teeth. A water-based dental dam lubricant works better than a petroleum base, such as Vaseline, because it does not leave a film on the teeth, which makes the teeth slippery and makes it difficult to hold the dental dam material in place. For the patient's comfort, a light amount of petroleum jelly or another type of lip lubricant can be applied to the lips prior to placement of the dental dam.

Scissors

Scissors are used to cut the **interseptal** (between the teeth) dental dam during removal of the dam from the patient's mouth. **Dental dam scissors** or any small pair

ADVANCED CHAIRSIDE FUNCTIONS

of scissors the operator feels comfortable with can be used. When cutting the interseptal dam material, direct the scissors away from the tissues to prevent tearing of the dam material and to completely cut the interseptal dam.

Inverting or Tucking Instrument

The dental floss can be used to invert or tuck the dental dam, but sometimes an instrument is needed to accomplish this step. Some options include a periodontal probe, spoon excavator, or the flat side of the T-ball burnisher. These instruments are used to turn under the edge of the dental dam that is around the tooth. The instrument is started on one side of the tooth and run at an angle to the other side. The edge of the dam is tucked under to assist in keeping the area dry.

Ligatures

A **ligature** is a piece of floss or a cord that stabilizes the dental dam in different applications. Ligatures are used in fixed bridge isolation, in bleaching procedures, and on individual teeth isolation. Sometimes, the floss is tied into a slip knot and placed over the tooth, such as in isolation for bleaching a tooth. With some patients, the floss or cord is threaded between the teeth or under the pontics for placement and then tied into place to retain the dental dam material (see Figure 34-32A).

Stabilizing Cord

Stabilizing cord is an elastic cord that comes in different sizes and colors (see Figure 34-28). It is stretched and then placed interproximally to secure the dental dam material. The cord is used to stabilize the dental dam placement at the opposite end of the clamp or for individual teeth. For example, instead of using a dental dam clamp, use the stabilizing cord for an anterior dental dam placement (see Figure 34-32B).

Preparation Before Dental Dam Placement

Before the dental dam is placed, the procedure should be explained to the patient and the operator should examine the oral cavity to determine the area of isolation.

FIGURE 34-28 Stabilizing cord, various sizes.

Educating the Patient

Patients like to know what is going to happen during their appointments. The dental assistant should explain the purpose of the dental dam and then have the patient acknowledge acceptance of this part of the restorative procedure. If the patient has had the dental dam placed before, ask whether the patient has any questions before beginning the placement. If the patient has not had a dental dam application before, explain how the dam is placed and what to expect before beginning the placement. Some points that might be included are the pressure of the clamp on the tooth, to breathe through the nose, and that the patient can still swallow.

ADVANCED CHAIRSIDE FUNCTIONS

Determining Area to Isolate

Before the dental dam is punched, the area to be isolated needs to be determined and then examined. Follow these steps:

1. Determine the tooth to be restored and then determine the anchor tooth, which is usually one or two teeth distal to the tooth being restored. The number of teeth to be included in the punch is a personal preference. Some operators like only one or two teeth exposed, while others like eight or more teeth to be punched. When learning, a good rule of thumb is to punch to the canine of the opposite quadrant. This is good practice because one of the most difficult aspects of punching the dental dam is accurately punching the curvature of the arch. Once this skill is mastered, the dental dam should be punched precisely for any patient. For example, if tooth #14 was the tooth to be restored, the anchor tooth would be tooth #15 and holes would be punched around the arch to include tooth #6.

2. The size and the shape of the arch are examined so that they can be duplicated on the dental dam as closely as possible to the patient's arch.

3. The area is examined for missing teeth, teeth that are out of alignment, or fixed prosthetics. The dental dam can be punched and placed to accommodate most conditions in a patient's mouth.

4. The area is flossed to identify tight contacts and open spacing.

Dividing the Dental Dam

Select the size and weight dental dam that best suits the patient and the procedure. (Refer to the Materials and Equipment section of this chapter to review the information on the dental dam material.) When preparing the dental dam material for punching, it is first divided into sixths (Figure 34-29). One way to mark the divisions is to fold and then crease the dental dam. This leaves a faint mark on the dam for the operator to use when punching the dam.

To begin, fold the dam in half and then crease the fold. This horizontal line is the division between the maxillary and mandibular arches. With the dam folded in half, fold the dam vertically into equal thirds and crease along each fold. The center third is where the dam will be punched. This represents the width of the arches of most patients. Some operators prefer to divide the dam into thirds only, and some divide the dam into

FIGURE 34-29 Dental dam divided into sixths.

quarters and mark the center point as a reference point before punching.

Punching the Dental Dam

After the dental dam is divided, it is ready to be punched for the placement. There are many places to begin actually punching the dental dam, so it is important for the operator to visualize the patient's arch on the dental dam. Often, the key hole punch is punched first. The key hole punch is the largest hole punched in the dental dam. It is the hole that slides over the clamp and onto the anchor tooth. The next holes are punched moving forward, about 3 to 3.5 mm apart. This is the amount of dental dam that slides between the teeth. It is called the septum. The punch table is adjusted for the size of the teeth (see Figure 34-24).

Maxillary Arch. The maxillary arch is punched in the upper middle sixth portion of the dental dam (Figure 34-30).

- Holes punched for the anteriors should be one inch from the top edge of the dam. This assists in positioning the arch.

- Variations in this one-inch guide are for patients with full upper lips or mustaches or patients with thin upper lips. The distance is increased or decreased accordingly.

- Punch the pattern to follow the patient's arch, leaving 3 to 3.5 mm between each tooth.

- The punch includes from one to two teeth distal of the tooth to be restored and then all teeth to the opposite cuspid.

ADVANCED CHAIRSIDE FUNCTIONS

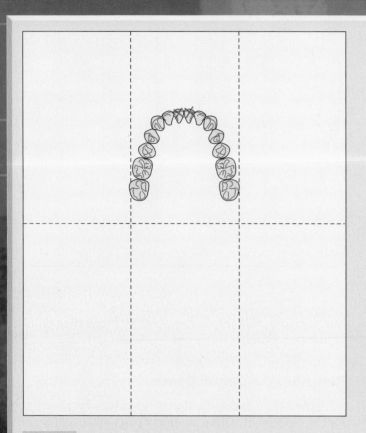

FIGURE 34-30 Maxillary arch punched for work to be done on the maxillary right first molar.

FIGURE 34-31 Mandibular arch punched for work on mandibular left first molar.

- Punch the two centrals first. Then continue to punch the remaining teeth. This centers the punch pattern on the dam.

Mandibular Arch. The mandibular arch is punched in the lower sixth portion of the dental dam (Figure 34-31).

- The first punch is the key hole punch. Teeth #17 and #32 are punched at the junction of the horizontal half and the vertical third. The more mesial the key hole punch is in the arch, the closer the punch is to the middle and bottom of the dam.

- The holes are not punched beginning with the central incisors, one inch from the lower edge of the dam. This would place the top part of the dam over the patient's nose. Instead, the central incisors are usually punched two inches from the lower edge of the dam.

- The rest of the punch follows the patient's arch, leaving 3 to 3.5 mm between each tooth.

- The punch includes one or two teeth distal of the tooth to be restored and all teeth to the opposite cuspid.

Maxillary and Mandibular Anterior Teeth. When placing the dental dam for the maxillary and mandibular anterior teeth, it is often unnecessary to use a clamp. Dental floss is doubled and a piece of dental dam or stabilizing cord is placed in the distal interproximals of each canine. This is usually enough to hold the dam in place without the placement of a clamp (Figure 34-32).

- There is no key punch.

- The punches for the two centrals are in the middle third of the dam, one inch from the top edge for the maxillary and two inches from the bottom edge for the mandibular.

Missing or Malpositioned Teeth. Punching for patients who have missing or malpositioned teeth is accomplished by the operator following the patterns of the teeth in the patients' mouths as the dental dams are punched.

- When teeth are malpositioned (out of normal alignment or position), they often are positioned either buccal or lingual of the normal curve of the arch, so the corresponding holes must be positioned either toward the buccal or the lingual to match the arch.

ADVANCED CHAIRSIDE FUNCTIONS

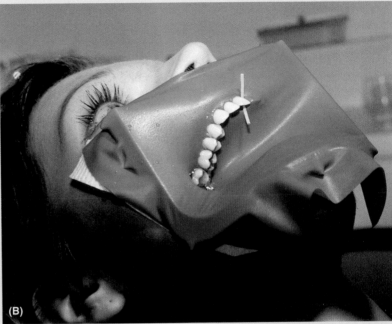

FIGURE 34-32 (A) Maxillary anterior placement with floss used as ligatures. (B) Patient with Wedjets stabilizing cord securing dental dam in place. *(Courtesy of Coltene/Whaledent, Inc.)*

■ Missing teeth or edentulous areas are accommodated by leaving a space on the dam between holes punched for teeth present in the mouth. So, if tooth #5 is missing, then tooth #4 would be punched, a space would be left, and teeth #6, #7, and so on would be punched.

Bridgework Placement. Patterns for patients with bridgework require punches similar to the punches with the missing teeth. It is impossible to punch holes for the pontics, so the punches are made for the abutment teeth and spaces are left for the number of pontics. Slits are cut between the holes with scissors to allow the bridges to be exposed.

Class V Restoration Placement. For a Class V restoration, the hole is punched facially to its normal position in the arch. A cervical clamp is often used with the Class V restorations, because they retract the gingiva and the dam beyond the borders of the cavity. The lower the cavity is on the facial surface of the tooth, the more the punch hole is moved toward the facial. The largest hole on the punch is used for this clamp, because the double wings allow an additional 1 to 3 mm between adjacent teeth.

Common Errors When Punching Dental Dam

The curve of the arch should match the arch curve of the patient. Punching the arch too flat or wide results in folds or bunching and stretching on the lingual. Punching the arch too curved or narrow results in folds and stretching on the facial. These errors make tucking the dental dam into the gingival sulcus difficult.

The punch table should be clean and free of previously punched dam material. Also, check for nicks in the holes of the punch table. If there are marks on the punch table or if the stylus does not line up directly, the punched holes may leave a tag of dam material or have a tear around the hole. The dam material will tear more easily when being stretched for placement with either of these errors, and the dam may leak once in place.

The hole spacing should match the space between the patient's teeth. If the holes are too close together, there will not be enough material to seal around each tooth, but the dam will be stretched and gingival tissue will be exposed. If the holes are too far apart, there will be excess material between the teeth. It may be difficult to get all the dam material interproximal when placing the dental dam, and the bunched dental dam material may get in the operator's way during the procedure.

ADVANCED CHAIRSIDE FUNCTIONS

Placement and Removal Procedures for Dental Dam

There are many techniques for placement of the dental dam, and the operator will find through practice which works best. Dental assistants help the dentist with the dental dam in states where it is not legal for them to place the dental dam, but in states where dental assistants can place the dental dam, the assistants punch the dam, select the clamp, and place and remove the dental dam without the chairside presence of the dentist (Procedure 34-4).

PROCEDURE 34 - 4

Placing and Removing Dental Dam

This procedure is performed by the dentist or dental assistant. The patient has been anesthetized before placement of the dental dam and before cavity preparation begins. The dental assistant has prepared all equipment and supplies needed for the entire procedure. Only the items needed for the dental dam are listed for this procedure.

EQUIPMENT AND SUPPLIES (Figure 34-33)

- Dental dam material (6 × 6 sheets)
- Dental dam napkin
- Dental dam punch
- Assortment of clamps
- Dental dam forceps
- Dental dam frame
- Dental floss
- Lubricant
- Cotton-tip applicator
- Tucking instrument (plastic instrument, T-ball burnisher, or spoon excavator)
- Scissors

PROCEDURE STEPS *(Follow aseptic procedures)*

Placement of Dental Dam

1. Inform the patient about the dental dam procedure.

2. Examine the patient's oral cavity to determine the anchor tooth, shape of the arch, tooth alignment,

FIGURE 34-33 Dental dam tray setup (labeled). (A) Dental dam punch. (B) Forceps. (C) Frame. (D) Dental dam napkin. (E) Tucking instrument. (F) Scissors. (G) Wedjets ligature. (H) clamp. (I) Dental dam material. (J) Floss.

missing teeth, and the presence of crowns and bridges. Also, examine the gingival tissues and check for tight contacts (Figure 34-34).

3. Prepare the dam material by dividing it into sixths and then punch the dam, aligning the stylus and the holes carefully.

4. Center the punch in the upper or lower middle third of the dental dam. Holes are punched according to size of tooth, with the key punch being the largest to accommodate the anchor tooth and the clamp.

(continues)

ADVANCED CHAIRSIDE FUNCTIONS

PROCEDURE 34-4 *(CONTINUED)*

FIGURE 34-34 Dental assistant checking patient's contacts with floss.

5. Holes are punched following the pattern of the patient's arch (Figure 34-35). Lubricate the dental dam on the tissue side of the dam with a water-soluble lubricant.

6. Select the clamp or several clamps to try on the tooth. Things to consider when selecting the clamp follow:

   ▪ Clamp design (if it is a winged or wingless clamp)

   ▪ Mesiodistal width at the CEJ of the anchor tooth

   ▪ Faciolingual width at the CEJ of the anchor tooth

   ▪ Height of the occlusal plane of the anchor tooth

7. Attach a safety line on all clamps that are to be tried on. When trying on the clamps, keep the end of the safety line in hand (Figure 34-36).

8. Secure the clamp on the clamp forceps and spread the jaws slightly to lock the forceps.

9. Place the clamp over the anchor tooth. To widen the jaws of the clamp, squeeze the forceps handle slightly to release the locking bar (Figure 34-37).

FIGURE 34-36 Clamp with floss safety ligature and dental dam clamp forceps.

FIGURE 34-35 Dental assistant punching dental dam material.

FIGURE 34-37 Dental dam clamp placed on anchor tooth.

(continues)

ADVANCED CHAIRSIDE FUNCTIONS

PROCEDURE 34-4 *(CONTINUED)*

10. Fit the lingual jaws of the clamp on the lingual side of the tooth first. Next, spread the clamp and slide the buccal jaws of the clamp over the height of contour of the buccal surface of the tooth. Release the pressure on the clamp forceps slightly against the tooth to evaluate the clamp, but do not release the clamp from the forceps.

11. The jaw points of the clamp should be at the CEJ, adapting to the gingival embrasures on the buccal and lingual. The clamp should be secure on the tooth, not pinching any gingival tissue. The clamp may be adjusted to the tooth by moving the wrist to the left and right and by putting more pressure on the distal or mesial of the clamp.

12. When the clamp is in place, confirm with the patient that the clamp position is comfortable (Figure 34-38).

13. Place the dental dam over the clamp bow by grasping the dam material and placing the index fingers on each side of the key hole punch. Spread the hole wide enough to slip over the clamp. Stretch the hole over the anchor tooth and one side of the clamp, then expose the other clamp jaw so that the entire clamp and anchor tooth are exposed. Pull the safety line through the dam and drape to the side of the patient's mouth.

14. Isolate the most forward tooth, usually the opposite canine. The dam material is secured on the distal of this tooth with a double loop of floss, a corner cut of the dental dam material, or stabilizing cord (Figure 34-39).

15. Place the dental napkin around the patient's mouth (Figure 34-40).

16. Place the frame or holder to stretch the dam to cover the oral cavity. The frame can be placed either under or over the dental dam material, depending on the type of frame and the preference of the operator (Figure 34-41).

17. Isolate the remaining teeth. The dental dam is worked gently between the contacts. Dental floss is used to assist in placing the dental dam and exposing the teeth. When using the floss, catch the edge of the hole with the floss and pull it over the tooth, into and through the contact (Figure 34-42). Using the air syringe to dry the teeth at this time facilitates the placement of the dam material.

FIGURE 34-38 Evaluate clamp placement and patient comfort.

FIGURE 34-39 Clamp with dental dam material on tooth and dam secured to opposite cuspid.

(continues)

ADVANCED CHAIRSIDE FUNCTIONS

FIGURE 34-40 Dental napkin being placed around patient's mouth.

FIGURE 34-41 Frame stretching dental dam material.

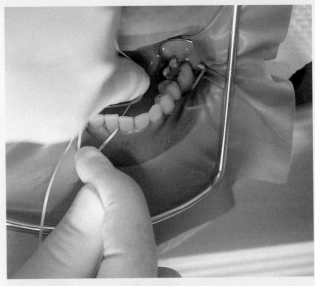

FIGURE 34-42 Dental assistant placing dam between contacts with floss.

FIGURE 34-43 Dental dam is in place and dental assistant is tucking dam with an instrument.

18. Invert or tuck the dam material. (The edge of the dam that surrounds the tooth must be inverted or tucked into the sulcus of the gingiva to seal the tooth and prevent leakage. There are several ways this is accomplished. Carefully pull the dental dam material slightly apically, and the dam will often invert when the dam is released. When using the floss to place the dam interproximally, the dam may be inverted. Or, use a T-ball burnisher, a plastic instrument, or a spoon excavator to tuck the buccal and lingual surfaces (Figure 34-43). Use the instrument with the air from the air-water syringe to dry the surface and then invert the edge of the dam. Continue until all edges of the dam are sealed.

19. Coat all tooth-colored restorations with lubricant.

20. Place and position a saliva ejector and/or a bite-block under the dam for patient comfort, if needed.

21. Double-check dam placement and patient comfort (Figure 34-44).

(continues)

ADVANCED CHAIRSIDE FUNCTIONS

PROCEDURE 34-4 (CONTINUED)

FIGURE 34-44 Patient with dental dam on and ready for dentist.

FIGURE 34-45 Dental dam clamp secured in forceps with dental dam material in position over bow of clamp for placement.

Alternate Technique for Placing Dental Dam

Some operators prefer to carry the clamp, dental dam material, and, in some placements, even the frame to the tooth when applying the clamp. This technique requires practice and confidence when placing the clamp but takes less time (Figure 34-45). The clamp is selected (usually a winged clamp) and the ligature is secured on the bow of the clamp. The bow of the clamp and the forcep holes on the jaws are exposed through the dental dam material. The clamp forceps are placed in the forcep holes and secured. The operator holds the rest of the dam material up and out of the way while placing the clamp and dam on the anchor tooth. After the clamp is secured on the tooth, the wings of the clamp are exposed and placement is completed following the procedure steps.

Removing the Dental Dam

When the operator is ready to remove the dental dam, the area is rinsed and dried using the evacuator and three-way syringe.

1. Explain to the patient the procedure to remove the dental dam and caution him or her not to bite down when the dam is removed.

2. Free the interseptal dam with scissors. To protect the patient, slip the index or middle finger underneath the dam material and stretch it facially, away from the tooth. Slant the scissors toward the occlusal surface, and clip each septum with the scissors (Figure 34-46). Pulling the dam material toward the facial, the operator cuts the interseptal dam.

3. Remove the dental dam clamp. Place the forceps in the clamp holes and squeeze the handles to open the clamp jaws. Usually, the clamp can be lifted straight off the tooth, but if this is not possible, rotate the clamp facially so the jaws clear the lingual and then rotate the clamp lingually to clear the buccal (Figure 34-47).

4. Remove the frame or holder and the dam material.

5. Remove the napkin, wiping the area around the mouth.

6. Examine the dam material by spreading the dental dam material out flat and examining to make certain that all the interseptal material is present (Figure 34-48). If there are any pieces missing, floss between the teeth. This should dislodge any small segment of remaining dam.

(continues)

ADVANCED CHAIRSIDE FUNCTIONS

PROCEDURE 34-4 *(CONTINUED)*

7. Massage the gingiva around the anchor tooth to increase circulation of the area.

8. Rinse and evacuate the patient's mouth thoroughly.

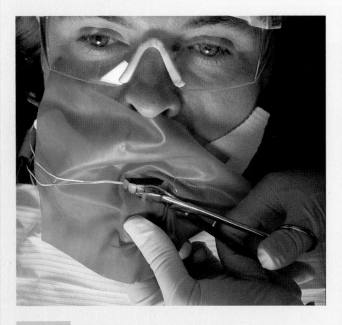

FIGURE 34-46 Pulling dental dam material toward facial, operator cuts the interseptal dam.

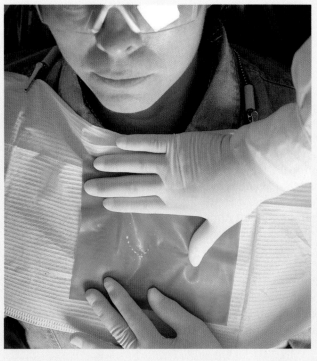

FIGURE 34-48 Dental dam material is placed on patient's bib or tray for operator to examine.

FIGURE 34-47 Clamp forceps remove clamp from anchor tooth.

(continues)

ADVANCED CHAIRSIDE FUNCTIONS

Dental Dam for Pediatric Patients

Dental dams are used on children as routinely as they are on adults. The key advantages become even more important when trying to control the busy tongue and lips of a child. The basic technique is the same for both adults and children. There are, however, several modifications.

It is important to explain to the child the parts of the dental dam and the procedure. Use terminology and explanations that are appropriate for the maturity of the child. Words that are commonly used to describe the dental dam include "raincoat" or "umbrella," the clamp might be the "button" or the "tooth raincoat holder," and the frame is the "coat hanger." Explain to the children how to swallow and breathe with the dental dam in place. Let them help by holding the saliva ejector during the procedure and establish a way for them to communicate, for example, raising a finger on the dental assistant's side. When people try to talk with the dental dam in place, it is amazing how well the dentist and the dental assistant understand "dental dam talk."

Look at the patient's dentition and determine whether all primary teeth are present, there are missing teeth, partially erupted teeth, and/or if the patient is in mixed dentition. The holes are punched according to these conditions. Generally, the holes are punched closer together and no holes are punched where teeth are missing or just barely erupted.

Placing Dental Dam for Pediatric Patients

When placing the dental dam for the pediatric patient (Figure 34-49), punch the holes in a 5 × 5 dental dam in the same manner as for adult patients, with the anchor hole the same but the holes for the individual teeth smaller (see Procedure 34-5). The arch is still punched fol-

FIGURE 34-49 Dental dam is placed on child patient.

PROCEDURE 34-5

Rubber Dam Application for Child Patient

The procedure is performed by the dentist or the dental assistant. The dental dam is quickly placed on the teeth. The patient's dentition must be evaluated to determine which teeth can be included in the isolation. Look for partially erupted teeth and teeth that are loose.

EQUIPMENT AND SUPPLIES

- Basic setup: mouth mirror, explorer, and cotton pliers
- Dental dam material (5 × 5)
- Dental dam napkin
- Dental dam punch

- Assortment of pedodontic clamps (bicuspid clamps)
- Dental dam clamp forceps
- Dental dam frame
- Dental floss
- Lubricant
- Cotton-tip applicator
- Tucking instrument (plastic instrument, T-ball burnisher, or spoon excavator)
- Scissors

(continues)

ADVANCED CHAIRSIDE FUNCTIONS

PROCEDURE 34-5 *(CONTINUED)*

PROCEDURE STEPS *(Follow aseptic procedures)*

1. Prepare the child for the dental dam placement by explaining the materials and the procedure at a level the child can understand.

2. Determine the number of teeth to be isolated and the size and shape of the arch.

3. Using the five-inch, square, heavyweight dental dam, punch the predetermined pattern. The holes are punched closer together than they would be for adults.

4. Select the clamp. Winged clamps are often selected because they retract the heavyweight rubber dam for better vision. The wings are also used to position the clamp below the height of contour of teeth that are partially erupted. Tie a piece of floss to the bow of the clamp for security.

5. The clamp is positioned on the tooth with the clamp forceps. Often, the clamp, dental dam, and frame are carried all in one to be applied to the tooth.

6. Check to see whether the clamp is securely positioned. Slide the dam over the wings of the clamp to expose the wings.

7. Place the dental dam over the remaining teeth.

8. A ligature of stabilizing cord or floss is placed to secure the dental dam.

---

lowing the pattern of the child's arch, going to the opposite cuspid. In some cases, the holes are punched only for the teeth that are directly involved. Dental dam clamps with projections are used on "short teeth" or teeth that are partially erupted. Bicuspid clamps are often used. Ligatures on the primary first molars or cuspids aid to retain the dam on the tooth. Wooden wedges are also used interproximally to depress the gingiva and the dental dam.

Alternatives to Full Dental Dam Placement

An alternative to the full dental dam placement is an oval piece of dental dam that has a border of flexible plastic. This dental dam comes with its own template to mark each tooth. The **quickdam** is punched using a regular punch and the same size holes (see Procedure 34-6).

PROCEDURE 34-6

Quickdam Placement

This procedure is performed by the dentist or dental assistant. The patient is anesthetized and quickdam is placed.

EQUIPMENT AND SUPPLIES

- Quickdam
- Quickdam template
- Dental dam punch
- Dental dam clamps
- Dental dam clamp forceps
- Dental floss
- Tucking instrument

PROCEDURE STEPS *(Follow aseptic procedures)*

1. Examine the patient's dentition to determine the punch pattern. Note any malpositioned teeth and the curve of the arch.

2. Use the quickdam template to mark each tooth to be punched and allow for any deviations. Mark with a felt-tip pen.

(continues)

ADVANCED CHAIRSIDE FUNCTIONS

PROCEDURE 34-6 *(CONTINUED)*

3. Punch the marked teeth according to the corresponding hole size for each tooth.

4. The quickdam can be used with or without a dental dam clamp. Without a clamp, fold the ends of the quickdam toward each other and press the sides together. Insert the quickdam into the patient's mouth and release the sides. The quickdam fits into the patient's vestibule. Slide the dam over the teeth to be isolated. Use dental floss to tuck the dental dam,

and secure the dam with floss ligatures on the distal of the last isolated teeth.

5. With a clamp, select a clamp and attach a ligature to the bow of the clamp. To place the clamp and dam in one step, secure the clamp in the hole punched for the tooth to be clamped. Apply the clamp forceps, and place the clamp over the tooth. Once the clamp is securely on the tooth, remove the clamp forceps. Place the dam over the teeth to be isolated and tuck the dam.

After the holes have been punched, the dam frame is folded and inserted into the patient's mouth, lying in the vestibular area. The dam must be fitted around the teeth to be isolated; sometimes, a ligature or dental dam clamp is used to secure the dam (Figure 34-50).

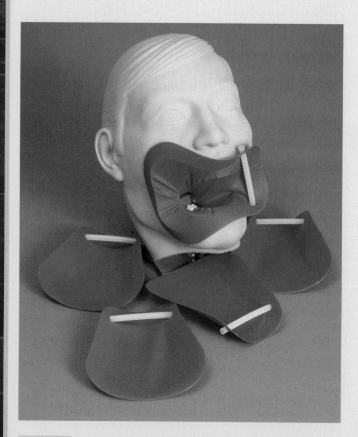

FIGURE 34-50 Alternative to full dental dam placement. *(Courtesy of Aseptico, Inc.)*

Matrix and Wedge

During the preparation of a tooth for an amalgam or a composite restoration, often one or more axial surfaces are removed. Once these surfaces are removed, the only way to restore the tooth is to have an artificial wall in place of the missing wall or surface. This wall holds the restorative materials in the preparation during the filling of the cavity. A matrix replaces the surface and acts as the artificial wall.

The **matrix** is a collective term used to refer to the matrix **band** and the **retainer**. The matrix band forms the missing surface or wall and reestablishes the normal contour of the prepared tooth while the tooth is being filled with the restorative material. The matrix band is inserted into the retainer and then placed on the tooth. The retainer is the device which holds the band. It is tightened on the tooth and secures the band in place.

In addition to replacing the missing tooth surface of the cavity preparation, the matrix restores the natural contours of the tooth and the proximal contact with the adjacent tooth. A matrix also contains the restorative material within the walls, thereby preventing any excess material from getting near the gingiva. In addition, the matrix must be stable enough to withstand the pressure of the restorative material being placed in the cavity preparation.

Matrices

Several different matrices are available, and the type of matrix selected depends on the type of restorative materials being used. For amalgam restorations, the **Tofflemire matrix** or the **Automatrix** is used. With the composite material, a **plastic strip matrix**, **shell matrix**, or a **sectional matrix system** is used.

ADVANCED CHAIRSIDE FUNCTIONS

Wedges

Once the matrix is in place, a wedge (small, triangular piece of wood or plastic) is inserted interproximally against the matrix band or strip near the gingival margin of the preparation. This wedge holds the band securely in place and also prevents excess filling material from escaping between the tooth and the matrix band. This excess is called an *overhang*. An overhang can be damaging to the gingival tissues if left in place, so the correct positioning of the wedge is important in order to prevent this from occurring. The wedge also separates the teeth slightly to compensate for the thickness of the band. This ensures good contact with the adjacent tooth after the band has been removed.

Wedge Types

Wedges come in different sizes that are either natural, clear, or colored. The clear or transparent wedges are used with light-curing restorative materials. These wedges deflect light into the restoration to ensure a thoroughly cured material without marginal gaps. They usually come in an assortment kit with various sizes, with the colors marking the different sizes (Figure 34-51).

Some wedges can be altered in shape with a knife, if needed. Once the procedure is complete, the wedges are discarded.

Wedge Placement

Wedges are only used when the preparation includes a proximal surface(s). For example, if the tooth had a mesiocclusal (MO) cavity preparation, only one wedge would be needed on the mesial. On the posterior teeth, either the wooden or plastic wedges can be used. On the anterior teeth, when light-cured materials are used, the plastic wedges are best.

The wedges are usually placed from the lingual on the posterior teeth. This makes placement easier and prevents interference with the retainer. Cotton pliers or a hemostat are used to place and remove the wedges. When placing the wedge, the smallest of the three sides is placed toward the gingiva. The wedge should fill the space and fit snugly (Figure 34-52A).

FIGURE 34-51 Assortment of wedges

FIGURE 34-52 (A) Occlusal aspect of Tofflemire matrix and wedge in place. (B) Parts of straight Tofflemire retainer: guide channels, vise, diagonal slot, spindle, inner knob, outer knob, and frame.

ADVANCED CHAIRSIDE FUNCTIONS

Tofflemire Matrix

The Tofflemire matrix is the most common matrix used for amalgam restorations. It has two parts: the retainer and the band (Figure 34-52B). The retainer can be sterilized and reused, but the bands are disposed of in the sharps container after the procedure.

Parts of Tofflemire Matrix Retainer

Table 34-2 identifies the parts and functions of the Tofflemire matrix retainer. This retainer has a top (occlusal) side and a bottom (gingival) side. The occlusal side is directed toward the occlusal surface and is the smooth side of the guide channels and the vise. The gingival side is directed toward the gingival tissues and has the diagonal slot on the vise and the open ends of the guide channels. Assembly of the matrix is outlined in Procedures 34-7 and 34-8.

Tofflemire Retainer Styles. The Tofflemire retainer is available in several styles so it can be positioned from either the lingual or the facial. The straight Tofflemire retainer is the most commonly used, and it is placed on the buccal or facial side, while the contra-angle Tofflemire retainer is placed on the lingual surface. It is angled slightly to accommodate clearance of the anterior teeth (Figure 34-53).

Matrix Bands

Matrix bands are made of stainless steel and are approximately all the same length. They differ in the shape of one edge and their widths (Figure 34-54). The size and

TABLE 34-2   Components of Tofflemire Matrix Retainer

Part	Function
Frame	Main body of retainer.
Guide channels	Slots in end of retainer that hold matrix band. The slots direct band to right or left of retainer.
Vise (locking)	Holds ends of matrix band in place in diagonal slot.
Spindle	Screw-like rod used to secure band in vise.
Inner knob (adjusting knob)	Adjusts size of matrix band loop by moving vise along retainer frame.
Outer knob (locking knob)	Tightens and loosens spindle against band in the vise.

FIGURE 34-53 Top: Contra-angle Tofflemire retainer (note angle of guide channel section). Bottom: Straight contra-angle Tofflemire retainer.

FIGURE 34-54 Examples of various matrix bands. The extension of cavity preparation determines the width of band selected. Gingival and occlusal edge of the matrix band is shown.

Occlusal edge

Gingival edge

ADVANCED CHAIRSIDE FUNCTIONS

PROCEDURE 3 4 - 7

Assembly of Tofflemire Matrix

This procedure is performed by the dentist or dental assistant. The assembly is completed before the procedure begins.

EQUIPMENT AND SUPPLIES

- Tofflemire retainer
- Assortment of matrix bands

PROCEDURE STEPS *(Follow aseptic procedures)*

1. Hold the retainer so that the guide channels and the diagonal slot on the vise are facing the operator.

2. Holding the frame of the retainer, rotate the inner knob (adjustment knob) until the vise is within one-quarter inch of the guide channels.

3. Turn the outer knob (locking knob) until the pointed end of the spindle is clear (below) of the slot in the vise.

4. Prepare the matrix band for placement in the retainer by holding the band to look like a smile, with the gingival edge on the top and the occlusal edge on the bottom.

5. Bring the ends together to form a teardrop-shaped loop (Figure 34-55). Be careful not to crease the band at any time. The larger circumference of the band, the

occlusal, will be on the bottom and the smaller, the gingival, will be on the top.

6. With the gingival edge still on the top, place the occlusal edge of the band in the diagonal slot of the vise. The loop is extended toward the guide channels.

7. Place the matrix band in the appropriate guide channels. The direction of the matrix band depends on the tooth being restored (Figure 34-56).

Hold matrix retainer with the guide channel up, facing the operator, and the matrix band looped. Then:

- If the matrix is to be applied to the maxillary right or mandibular left quadrant, place the matrix band in the guide channels toward the operator's right (Figure 34-57A).

- If the matrix is to be applied to the maxillary left or mandibular right quadrant, place the matrix band in the guide channels toward the operator's left (Figure 34-57B).

8. Once the band is placed in the vise slot with the guide channels, turn the outer knob until the tip of the spindle is tight against the band in the vise slot.

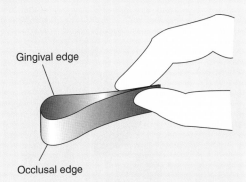

FIGURE 34-55 Hold matrix band in smile and loop ends of band together. Gingival edge will be on top and occlusal edge on the bottom.

FIGURE 34-56 Hold Tofflemire retainer with guide channels and slot facing up, and insert the matrix band into vise slot and guide channels.

(continues)

ADVANCED CHAIRSIDE FUNCTIONS

PROCEDURE 34-7 (CONTINUED)

(A)   (B)

FIGURE 34-57 Matrix band is positioned in guide channels for quadrants. (A) Maxillary right/mandibular left. (B) Maxillary left/mandibular right.

FIGURE 34-58 By turning inner knob of the Tofflemire retainer, the matrix band loop increases and decreases in size.

9. Move the inner knob to increase or decrease the size of the loop to match the diameter of the tooth (Figure 34-58).

10. If the band becomes creased or bent during the assembly, it can be smoothed out by inserting the handle of the mouth mirror into the loop and running it around the inside of the loop (similar to curling ribbon when wrapping a gift).

shape of the cavity prep indicate which band is used. The more the prep extends toward the gingiva, the wider the matrix band needs to be. The matrix band is slightly curved and when looped over so both ends meet, the small **circumference** edge faces toward the gingiva and the larger circumference edge faces toward the occlusal.

- Hold the retainer with the guide channels and diagonal slot on the vise facing the operator.
- Keep the guide channels and the vise within one-quarter inch of each other.
- The looped matrix band correlates to the shape of the tooth, with the smaller circumference at the gingiva and the larger circumference at the occlusal.

AutoMatrix

The AutoMatrix is a matrix without a retainer. The stainless steel bands are conical shaped and come in four sizes. The conical shape makes the band easy to **burnish** (smooth) for better contact in proximal areas. The bands are circles with autolock loops that lock the matrices on the teeth. The tightening coil on the outside of the band is where the matrix is adapted to the tooth.

There is no retainer to obstruct the operator's access or vision. The AutoMatrix comes in a kit that contains the clipping pliers, the tightening device, and bands in assorted sizes (Figure 34-59).

To place the AutoMatrix, position the matrix on the tooth following the same criteria as with the Tofflemire. Place the tightening device in the coil and rotate the handle to tighten the band around the

FIGURE 34-59 Automatrix kit: assortment of bands and tightening device. *(Courtesy of Dentsply)*

ADVANCED CHAIRSIDE FUNCTIONS

PROCEDURE 34-8

Placement of Tofflemire Matrix

This procedure is performed by the dentist or dental assistant. After the Tofflemire matrix is assembled, it is ready for positioning on the prepared tooth.

EQUIPMENT AND SUPPLIES (Figure 34-60)

- Assembled Tofflemire retainer and matrix band
- Cotton pliers or hemostat
- Ball burnisher
- 2 × 2 gauze sponges
- Assortment of wedges

PROCEDURE STEPS *(Follow aseptic procedures)*

1. Place the matrix band over the prepared tooth with the smaller edge of the band toward the gingiva. The slot on the vise is directed toward the gingiva. Keep the retainer parallel to the buccal surface as the loop is placed around the tooth.

2. Move the loop through the interproximal surface. Place one finger over the loop to stabilize the loop and the retainer.

3. Once the matrix band is around the tooth, adjust the guide channel to center the retainer on the buccal surface of the tooth (Figure 34-61).

FIGURE 34-60 Tray setup for placement of Tofflemire matrix.

FIGURE 34-61 Placing Tofflemire retainer with matrix band on tooth and centering retainer on buccal surface of tooth.

4. Turn the inner knob to tighten the band around the tooth. The band should be securely around the tooth and the retainer should be snug to the tooth. If the band is too tight or too loose, the contour of the restoration may change the contours of the tooth and the proximal contact.

5. Check the margins of the matrix band. The band should extend no more than 1 to 1.5 mm beyond the gingival margin of the cavity preparation on the gingival edge, and the occlusal edge should extend no more than 2 mm above the highest cusp (Figure 34-62).

6. To ensure contact with the adjacent teeth, the band needs to be contoured. To accomplish this, use a ball burnisher. Place the burnisher on the inner surface of the band and apply pressure until the band becomes slightly concave at the contact area.

7. Once the matrix band has been placed on the tooth, a wedge(s) is (are) placed to stabilize the band at the gingival margin of the preparation. (Refer to Wedges section for placement suggestions.)

8. Check the seal at the gingival margin of the preparation with an explorer. There should be no gap between the band and the preparation.

(continues)

ADVANCED CHAIRSIDE FUNCTIONS

PROCEDURE 34-8 (CONTINUED)

The band should be tight near the gingival margin.

The band should fit the circumference of the tooth near the occlusal surface.

1.0–1.5 mm

The band should extend 1.0 to 1.5 mm beyond the cavity preparation near the gingiva.

2.0 mm

The band should extend no more than 2 mm above the cusp of the tooth and occlusal ridge.

FIGURE 34-62 Criteria for correctly placing matrix band.

PROCEDURE 34-9

Removal of Wedge and Tofflemire Matrix

This procedure is performed by the dentist with assistance by the dental assistant. Once the tooth has been filled with restorative material, the matrix and wedge are removed to finish carving the anatomy of the tooth.

EQUIPMENT AND SUPPLIES

- Cotton pliers or hemostat
- 2 × 2 gauze

PROCEDURE STEPS *(Follow aseptic procedures)*

1. To remove the wedge, use cotton pliers or a hemostat. Grasp the wedge at the base and pull in the opposite direction of the insertion.

2. To remove the retainer, hold the matrix in place with a finger on the occlusal surface, then turn the outer knob of the retainer to loosen the spindle in the vise.

3. Separate the retainer from the band by lifting the retainer toward the occlusal surface.

4. Using cotton pliers, gently free the band from around the tooth, then lift one end of the band in a lingual occlusal direction.

5. Lift the band from the proximal surface and repeat with the other end of the band. The tooth is ready for the final carving.

ADVANCED CHAIRSIDE FUNCTIONS

PROCEDURE 34-10

Placement of Strip Matrix

This procedure is performed by the dentist or dental assistant. After the tooth has been prepared, the strip matrix is placed.

EQUIPMENT AND SUPPLIES

- Strip matrix
- Cotton pliers
- Mouth mirror
- Assortment of clear wedges

PROCEDURE STEPS *(Follow aseptic procedures)*

1. Contour the strip by drawing the strip over the rounded edge of the handle of the mouth mirror. The procedure is the same here as it is with the Tofflemire matrix band.

2. Place the strip matrix between the teeth. Hold the strip tightly and slide toward the gingiva.

3. Adjust the position of the strip so that the entire preparation is covered by the strip.

4. Seat the wedge to secure the strip in place.

5. Restorative materials are placed and the strip matrix is pulled tightly around the tooth to adapt the material to the convex surface of the tooth.

6. The strip matrix is held in place by hand or with a clip retainer until the material has been cured (Figure 34-63).

FIGURE 34-63 Strip matrix and wedges on tooth.

---

tooth. Once the matrix is securely on the tooth, place the wedges as needed. To remove the AutoMatrix, remove the wedges and then, using the removal pliers, clip the end of the auto-lock loop. The pliers clip the loop and then have a plastic cover to catch the ends of the loop as they fall after being cut. Open the matrix and slide toward the buccal or lingual while pulling it occlusally.

Plastic Strip Matrix

The thin, transparent, strip matrix is used with composite, glass ionomer, or compomer restorative materials on anterior teeth (see Procedures 34-10 and 34-11). The strip can be made of nylon, acetate, celluloid, or resin and is approximately three inches long and three-eighths inch wide. The functions of the strip matrix follow:

- Provide anatomical contour and proximal contact relation
- Prevent excess material at the gingival margin
- Confine the restorative material under pressure while the material is being cured
- Protect the restorative material from losing or gaining moisture during the setting time
- Allow the polymerizing light to reach the composite restorative material

Crown Matrix Form. The crown matrix form is a thin, plastic form that is shaped like the crown. On anterior teeth when the incisal edge is involved, Class IV, a crown

ADVANCED CHAIRSIDE FUNCTIONS

PROCEDURE 34-11

Removal of Strip Matrix

This procedure is performed by the dentist once the restorative material is placed and cured.

EQUIPMENT AND SUPPLIES

- Cotton pliers or hemostat
- 2 × 2 gauze sponges

PROCEDURE STEPS *(Follow aseptic procedures)*

1. Once the material has been cured and is completely hardened, remove the clip retainer if one was used. Then, remove the wedges with cotton pliers.

2. The strip matrix is gently pulled away from the restorative material.

3. Remove the strip by pulling the matrix strip in a lingual incisal or facial incisal direction.

form, is often used to restore the tooth. The crown forms come preformed in various designs and sizes. The restorative material is placed in the cavity preparation and in the crown form. The crown form is then placed on the tooth. These crown forms are clear and can be used with light-cured materials. Once the restorative material is set, the crown form is removed and the tooth is ready for final contouring and finishing.

Sectional Matrix Systems

A sectional matrix system is most often used on Class II restorations to restore anatomical contacts. The matrix is stable and produces a tight contact with no overhangs. The system consists of oval matrix bands, rings to hold the matrix bands, and forceps to place the rings. The oval-shaped matrix bands are contoured and come in different sizes. They are slightly thicker than the Tofflemire bands. The rings are used to hold the matrix bands in place and usually come in two different sizes. The forceps are designed to open the rings for placement and removal. They are like dental dam forceps except the ends are shorter, broader, and angled slightly for better retention (Figure 34-64).

FIGURE 34-64 Sectional matrix kit.

A separate matrix band/ring is used for each surface, so on an MOD two matrix bands/rings would be used. Placing the sectional matrix takes some practice, but once the procedure is learned it can be done quickly to produce a functional matrix. Wedges are used with this matrix system. They are usually placed after the band is

ADVANCED CHAIRSIDE FUNCTIONS

placed and before the ring is positioned. The main function of the wedge with this system is to prevent gingival overhangs (Figure 34-65).

FIGURE 34-65 Sectional matrix system in place for MOD restoration placement. *(Courtesy Garrison Dental Solution, Inc.)*

CHAPTER SUMMARY

The general chairside assistant prepares restorative materials for the dentist or hygienist (in states where hygienists can legally fill cavities) to place in the prepared cavity. Knowledge of the properties of the restorative materials is necessary for the dental assistant to properly prepare and manipulate the materials. Knowledge of the various types of restorative materials also allows the dental assistant to be prepared ahead of time. Some states allow dental assistants to place the dental dam and matrix before placement of restorative materials. Whether the assistant places the dental dam and the matrix or assists in the process, knowledge of sequence and techniques is necessary.

Case Study

Charlotte Larson needs to replace several restorations in her maxillary molars. Over the years, she has had numerous amalgam restorations placed throughout her mouth. Although Charlotte has never had any trouble, she is concerned after reading articles about restorations containing mercury. She also is interested in more natural-looking restorations.

Case Study Review

1. List some of the concerns Charlotte may have read regarding restorations containing mercury.

2. What information could the dental assistant give to Charlotte in response to her concerns? What resources are available for information?

3. Are there any alternative restorative materials available for Charlotte?

REVIEW QUESTIONS

Multiple Choice

1. If, after the amalgam has been triturated, it is crumbly and dull in appearance, it may have been:
   a. undermixed.
   b. overmixed.
   c. exposed to moisture before mixing.
   d. mixed at too high a speed.

2. The composite material that finishes to the highest luster and resists wear due to abrasion is the
   a. fine-fill composite.
   b. microfill composite.
   c. hybrid composite.
   d. extra-course composite.

3. Amalgam is a combination of
   a. alloy and copper.
   b. mercury and dental alloy.
   c. dental alloy and high copper alloy.
   d. mercury and copper.

4. _____ dominate the field of esthetic restorations.
   a. Composite restorations
   b. Dental amalgam restorations
   c. Glass ionomer restorations
   d. Resin-modified glass ionomer restorations

5. When is the shade taken when placing esthetic restorations?
   a. Before the procedure begins
   b. After the tooth has been prepared
   c. Before the bases and liners have been placed
   d. After the etchant and bonding agent have been placed

6. All of the following are true statements about the dental dam except:
   a. Dental dams are available in several sizes.
   b. Dental dams of various thicknesses are available.
   c. Medium and heavy dental dam materials do not tear as easily.
   d. Dental dam materials are available in one color only.

7. Which of the following stabilizes dental dam material and secures it in place?
   a. Dental dam frame
   b. Dental dam punch
   c. Dental dam clamp
   d. Dental dam material

8. Which of the following is used to place and remove the dental dam clamp?
   a. Dental dam frame
   b. Dental dam punch
   c. Dental dam clamp forceps
   d. None of the above

9. Once the matrix is placed, a(n) _____ is placed near the gingival margin of the preparation.
   a. overhang
   b. dental dam clamp
   c. automatrix
   d. wedge

10. All of the following are true about the Tofflemire matrix *except:*
    a. This matrix consists of two parts, the retainer and the band.
    b. Adjustment is not possible.
    c. Bands are made of stainless steel.
    d. The retainer has guide channels in which to place the band.

Critical Thinking

1. Discuss pros and cons of using amalgam as a restorative material.

2. How can pulp be protected when using a composite restorative material?

3. Discuss alternatives to composite restorations.

4. List advantages for dental assistant when dental dam is placed.

5. In your own words, describe how to assemble the band in the Tofflemire retainer.

Web Activities

1. To study the latest information about dental amalgam fillings, go to http://www.ada.org.

2. Go to http://www.kerrdental.com to compare types of composites.

LABORATORY MATERIALS AND TECHNIQUES

SPECIFIC INSTRUCTIONAL OBJECTIVES

The student should strive to meet the following objectives and demonstrate an understanding of the facts and principles presented in this chapter:

1. Identify materials used in the dental laboratory and perform associated procedures.

2. Demonstrate knowledge and skills needed to prepare, take, and remove alginate impressions and wax bites.

3. Demonstrate knowledge and skills necessary to prepare reversible hydrocolloid impression material for the dentist.

4. Demonstrate knowledge and skills necessary to prepare elastomeric impression materials such as polysulfide, silicone (polysiloxane and polyvinyl siloxanes), and polyether for the dentist.

5. Demonstrate knowledge and skills necessary to use gypsum products such as Type I, impression plaster; Type II, laboratory or model plaster; Type III, laboratory stone; Type IV, die stone; and Type V, high-strength die stone.

6. Demonstrate knowledge and skills necessary to pour and trim a patient's alginate impression (diagnostic cast).

7. Identify use of a dental articulator for dental casts or study models.

8. Identify various classifications and uses of waxes used in dentistry.

9. Demonstrate knowledge and skills necessary to fabricate acrylic tray resin self-curing and light-curing custom trays, vacuum-formed, and thermoplastic custom trays.

10. Demonstrate knowledge and skills necessary to contour prefabricated temporary crowns and to fabricate and fit custom temporary restorations.

KEY TERMS

accelerates *(852)*

articulator *(868)*

beading *(845)*

calcination *(858)*

catalyst *(852)*

distortion *(852)*

exothermic reaction *(858)*

gel *(842)*

gelatin time *(843)*

gypsum *(858)*

homogeneous *(874)*

imbibition *(843)*

irreversible hydrocolloid *(842)*

matrix *(881)*

monomer *(871)*

polymer *(871)*

polymerization *(853)*

polysulfide *(853)*

potassium alginate *(842)*

potassium titanium fluoride *(842)*

(continues)

INTRODUCTION

A number of materials that are used by dental assistants specifically in the dental laboratory are not used in the dental treatment room. Other materials are used initially in the treatment room and then taken by the dental assistant to the laboratory, where a second procedure is completed. Many models are taken to an in-office dental laboratory, where the laboratory technician completes the procedures, or the models are sent out to a commercial dental laboratory for additional procedures. It is always important to ensure that cross-contamination does not occur when working with laboratory materials. The dental assistant must pay special attention when taking materials from the treatment room to the dental laboratory.

Any dental assistant who has skills in performing laboratory duties is an asset to his or her employer. The better cross-trained the dental team members are, the better the dental office functions. A number of basic functions in the dental laboratory are routinely performed by the dental assistant, such as pouring and trimming study models, fabricating custom trays, and fabricating provisional temporaries. To accomplish these procedures, the dental assistant must understand the materials that are used, the properties of each material, and the steps in each procedure.

Hydrocolloid Impression Materials

Impressions are taken to reproduce an accurate three-dimensional duplicate of an individual's teeth and surrounding tissues. The impression makes a negative reproduction where gypsum material can be poured and therefore creates a completed positive model. Varying degrees of accuracy can be obtained depending on the type of impression material and gypsum used. The operator gives directions to the dental assistant on the type of model that is desired. Models can be used for many purposes. One of the most common models that the dental assistant will make is the study cast or primary model. Normally, the impression material used is irreversible hydrocolloid, which is commonly called alginate.

Alginate (Irreversible Hydrocolloid) Impression Material

Alginate is a generic name used for a group of **irreversible hydrocolloid** impression materials. Alginate is used when less accuracy is needed. One of the most common areas in which alginate is used is in making diagnostic casts or study models. Alginate impression material is used routinely in making opposing models for fixed and removable prosthetics, orthodontic appliances, mouth guards, bleach trays, provisional restorations, and custom trays.

Alginate material's primary ingredient is potassium alginate, therefore giving the generic name to the material. **Potassium alginate** is extracted from seaweed and kelp, which is a marine growth found primarily off the coastline of Japan. This material readily dissolves in water to form a viscous **sol** (liquid). Added to this potassium alginate is a calcium sulfate which, through a chemical reaction, forms a **gel** (solid). To control the setting time and allow for the material to be placed in a tray and into the patient's mouth, trisodium phosphate is added. Without this retarder, the material would be set before it could be inserted into the patient's mouth. A retarder slows the setting of the material. To increase the strength and stiffness and make up the bulk of the material, fillers are used. Some of the fillers that may be in alginate are diatomaceous earth, zinc oxide, color, and flavoring. The fillers constitute from one-half to three-quarters of the total composition of the material. A small amount of **potassium titanium fluoride** is added to the material to counteract a specific action of the alginate where it tends to soften the surface of the gypsum products, not allowing it to fully set on the surface.

Advantages and Disadvantages of Alginate. Alginate has a number of advantages that explain its extensive use in the dental office:

- Ease of manipulation

- Minimal equipment required

- Economical
- Meets the requirements for accuracy for a number of applications
- Rapid setting
- Comfort for the patient
- Can be used for both teeth and tissue impressions
- Withdraws over **undercuts** (recessed areas that are wider on the bottom than on the top) because of its elastic properties

The disadvantages of alginates primarily come from the loss of accuracy due to atmospheric conditions. If the impression is stored prior to pouring, it is susceptible to dimensional change due to loss or gain of water. If the impression loses water content due to heat, dryness, or exposure to air, it causes shrinkage. This condition is known as **syneresis** (sin-er-**EE**-sis). If the reverse happens and the impression takes on additional water and causes swelling, the impression will have a dimensional enlargement, known as **imbibition** (im-bah-**BIH**-shun). The material also can cause some tissue distortion due to its thickened consistency. Another disadvantage is that it is not as precise or accurate as some of the other materials on the market.

Setting Time for Alginate. The time from which the alginate powder material is mixed with water until it is completely set is called the **gelatin time**. The gelatin time is different depending on the type of material used. Most of the materials come in two types: Type I is a fast-set alginate and Type II is a regular-set alginate. The gelatin time for both is broken into two different increments. The first is the working time, where the dental assistant mixes the material to the desired consistency, loads it into the tray, and inserts and positions the tray into the patient's mouth. The working time for the regular set is approximately one minute and less than that for fast set. The second phase is the setting time, where the material remains in the patient's mouth and sets until the chemical reaction is completed, the gel is formed completely, and the tray is removed from the patient's mouth. Type I for both the working and setting times ranges from one to two minutes. Type II normally ranges from two to four and one-half minutes for both working and setting times. The setting times can be altered. The most convenient way to control the setting time is to adjust the temperature of the water. The suggested temperature of water to be used is room temperature (70°F or 21°C). If the temperature of the water is higher, working and setting times are shorter. If the water is cooled, the working and setting times are longer. Warm weather causes the alginate to set more rapidly as well. Some offices refrigerate the water during hot humid times.

The choice of whether to use Type I or Type II is made according to the preference of the operator and the conditions of the patient needing the impression. The outcome of both materials is the same. Cases in which the slower material, Type II, is beneficial would be where the operator is working alone or the tray is going to be difficult to insert into the oral cavity in the correct position in the patient's mouth. The faster set, Type I, is beneficial where the patient is a child or where the patient has a problem with gagging and the tray needs to be removed as rapidly as possible for patient comfort.

Alginate Packaging, Storage, and Shelf Life. Normally, alginate is purchased in air-tight plastic canisters the size of coffee cans (Figure 35-1). The powder may be inside, in a foil or plastic bag, to be placed in the container when ready for use. Along with the powder are the measuring devices for the powder and the water. Some of the canisters have built-in areas on the outside for the water-measuring devices. This makes it convenient for the dental assistant. Alginate can be bought in premeasured sealed bags, but it is much more costly and normally unnecessary because measuring the powder is not a difficult procedure.

Alginate is also available in a premixed package with a dispensing unit (Figure 35-2). This alginate unit is mounted on the wall or placed on the counter. The premixed alginate is placed in the dispensing unit, and the assistant places a dispensing tip on the unit. The material is then dispensed directly into the tray. This unit is similar to, or the same as, the unit for dispensing some polysiloxane or polyether materials (final impression materials). Most dental offices now use powder/water alginate.

It is important that alginate not be stored in an area that can have temperatures over 120°F because it causes loss of strength and lower resistance to deformation. If kept in an area where moisture can contaminate it, the material will demonstrate erratic setting times. Optimum storage is in a cool, dry place. Keeping the lid screwed tightly in place while not in use aids in preven-

FIGURE 35-1 Foil bags and plastic canister of alginate with measuring devices.

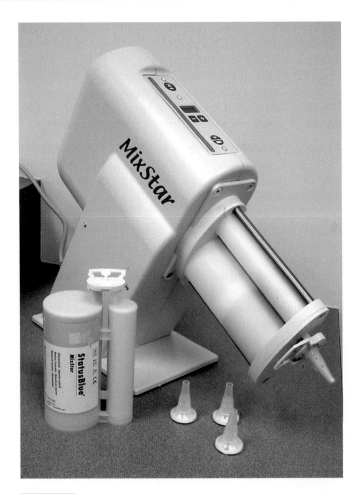

FIGURE 35-2 Unit for dispensing premixed alginate substitute.

tion of unintentional moisture contamination. The normal shelf life for alginate materials is not more than one year.

Alginate Powder/Water Ratio. All the alginate materials come with their own specific measuring devices for both the powder and the water. First, read the manufacturer's directions for dispensing the material. The dispensing of each material may be slightly different. For instance, some of the materials direct that the powder be fluffed with the lid on prior to putting it into the powder scoop, while others may indicate that the powder should be packed into the scoop. This makes a definite difference regarding the amount of powder that is used. The water measure is normally a plastic cylinder with lines on it to indicate the amount of water for each scoop of powder. Normally, it takes two scoops of powder to two increments of water for each mandibular impression. Three of each are normally needed for the maxillary impression. (These can change depending on the size of the patient's arches.)

It is important that the correct amounts of both powder and water are used. If a lower water-to-powder ratio transpires, a stiffer, thicker mix is produced. Along with being more difficult to use, the material has decreased

detail, decreased ability to pull from undercuts, decreased flexibility, increased tissue displacement, rapid setting time, increased strength, and a mix that is not as uniform in consistency. If a higher water-to-powder ratio is used, the impression has a decreased resistance to deformation, decreased strength, and increased setting time. Both increases and decreases in spatulation affect the setting time and decrease the strength of the material.

Bowls and Spatulas Used for Alginate Impressions. The operator can use a flexible rubber bowl and stiff spatula to mix alginate or a disposable bowl with built-in water measuring lines. The flexible rubber bowl allows easy mixing of the alginate but must be sterilized or disinfected after use. The disposable bowl comes with a disposable spatula that can be used for mixing alginate at one end and mixing plaster at the other end. The disposable bowl and spatula can be thrown away and they eliminate the aseptic procedures required after contamination of the rubber bowl and spatula (Figure 35-3).

Trays Used for Alginate Impressions. Several trays are available for alginate impressions (Figure 35-4). Most commonly used are the perforated trays that come in metal and plastic. The trays have holes in them for the material to ooze through and lock the impression material in the tray. If not using the perforated trays, the material may stay in the patient's mouth as the tray is removed.

(A)

Alginate   Plaster

(B)   Alginate bowl

FIGURE 35-3 (A) Bowl-Away and Spat-Away disposable bowl and spatula used for mixing alginate and plaster. (B) Bowl-Away and Spat-Away show water measuring lines in mixing bowl. The disposable spatula shows ends for alginate and one for plaster. *(Courtesy of Millennium Advantage Products, 1-888-798-5373.)*

FIGURE 35-4 Assortment of alginate trays.

FIGURE 35-5 Alginate tray with beading wax on the periphery. The wax aids in tray extension and patient comfort.

The impression then has to be retaken due to loss of accuracy from the flexible material coming loose from the rigid tray. Some operators use a rim lock tray in place of the perforated tray. The rim lock tray has a border around the top of it to aid in holding the material in place. This tray has no perforations in it. Both the perforated tray and the rim lock tray come in plastic and metal. The metal trays can be cleaned and reused after sterilization.

Whichever tray is used, the operator must make sure that the tray fits correctly in the patient's mouth. Selecting the correct tray is essential to obtaining an accurate impression. The trays come in several sizes. The operator first examines the patient's mouth and identifies a sterilized or disposable tray that he or she thinks will fit. The trays should be tried in the patient's mouth to ensure a correct fit and comfort for the patient. The tray should extend 2 or 3 mm beyond the last molar area and below both the lingual and facial tooth surfaces. Keep in mind that there should be enough room for 2 mm of the alginate material between the tray and all surfaces of the teeth and tissue. If the size of the tray seems appropriate but the tray does not extend over the last molar area, utility wax strips can be used. The wax is placed in layers until the desired length is achieved. The wax also can be placed around the border of the tray to lengthen it on the lingual and facial areas and to provide more comfort for the patient (Figure 35-5). The process of placing the wax around the border of the tray is called **beading**.

Taking Alginate Impressions for Diagnostic Casts (Study Models). In some states, dental assistants are allowed to take the alginate impressions, while in other states, the dental assistant can select the tray, mix the material, load the material into the tray, and pass the tray for the dentist to place in the patient's mouth.

The alginate material can be mixed using the Alginator II® method (Procedure 35-1) or the manual method (Procedure 35-2). The material can also be mixed in a plastic bag: place powder in the bag, add water, and knead. The "bag procedure" is very effective in ensuring aseptic technique because the bag can easily be disposed of, but mixing in this manner incorporates more air bubbles if not done properly.

The Alginator II device makes mixing easier, as well as increasing the likelihood of a bubble-free mixture. Rather than the operator rotating the bowl, the device spins the bowl about 300 times a minute.

Wax Bite Registration

A wax bite registration is taken to establish the relationship between the maxillary and mandibular teeth. It can be used to verify the occlusal relationship when trimming the diagnostic casts (**study models**). Normally, wax that is formed in a horseshoe shape is used, but the flat sheets of utility wax can be used as well.

Other materials are used in taking a bite. Polysiloxane impression material, specifically designed for occlusal registration, can be dispensed using a dispensing gun and cartridge tip. It is dispensed directly onto the occlusal surface, and the patient is asked to close in the normal biting position and remain closed until the material sets, normally within two minutes. The set material is removed, disinfected, stored, and used to establish the patient's occlusal relationship.

Accuracy of Alginate Impression

- Tray covers all necessary areas.
- Tray is centered on central incisors.
- Tray is not pushed down or up too far, allowing teeth to penetrate through material to tray.
- Impression is not torn.
- Impression is free of bubbles and voids.

PROCEDURE 35-1

Mixing Alginate with an Alginator II Mixing Device

This procedure is performed by the dental assistant in the states where allowed. The materials are prepared and the Alginator II mixing device is prepared and ready.

EQUIPMENT AND SUPPLIES

- Flexible spatula/broad blade or disposable spatula

- Flexible rubber bowl(s) or Alginator II flexible bowl only

- Alginate material with water and powder measuring devices

- Water

PROCEDURE STEPS *(Follow aseptic procedures)*

Material Preparation

1. Measure the impression water (room temperature) for the mandibular impression, normally two calibrations of the water measurement device supplied by the manufacturer. Place water in the rubber bowl attached to the Alginator II (Figure 35-6). Some operators use an additional bowl in the Alginator II so that it can be cleaned easily. Leaving the bowl attached allows for more control; attach it by rotating slightly to the side and fitting into the grooves on the bottom of the bowl.

2. Fluff the powder before opening the powder canister, if indicated by the manufacturer's directions.

3. Fill the measure with powder by overfilling and then leveling off with the spatula (use the flat blade, not the edge blade of the spatula). Dispense two corresponding scoops into the water in the rubber bowl.

4. Incorporate the mixture slightly.

FIGURE 35-6 Alginator II used for mixing alginate. *(Courtesy of DAX Dental Products.)*

5. Hold the spatula to the side of the bowl with the mixture and use slight pressure. Turn on the Alginator II; the material is mixed as the bowl rotates (300 times a minute). Use the side of the spatula blade during this process.

6. When the material is completely mixed, it can be easily collected by using the edge of the spatula starting from the deepest area in the bowl.

7. Upon completion, the material should be homogeneous and smooth without bubbles.

8. Remove excess material from bowls with paper towels, and then clean thoroughly and disinfect.

- Impression shows sharp anatomic detail of all teeth and tissues.

- Impression has a good "peripheral roll" and includes all vestibule areas.

- Mandibular impression shows good detail in retromolar area and shows lingual frenum and mylohyoid ridge area.

- Maxillary impression shows good detail in tuberosities and palate areas.

Reversible Hydrocolloid Impression Material (Agar-Agar)

One of the oldest impression materials that has good detail and is used for final impressions is **reversible hydrocolloid** impression material, sometimes referred to as agar-agar. The composition for this material is somewhat similar to alginate in that the main component is derived from seaweed and kelp. It also has fillers, additives, coloring, and flavoring. The unique difference between reversible and irreversible hydrocolloid mate-

PROCEDURE 35-2

Preparing for Alginate Impression

This procedure is performed by the dental assistant in states where allowed. The materials are prepared and the alginate impression is taken on the maxillary and mandibular arches.

EQUIPMENT AND SUPPLIES

- Flexible spatula/broad blade or disposable spatula
- Flexible rubber bowl(s) or disposable bowl
- Alginate material with water and powder measuring devices
- Water
- Impression tray(s)
- Beading wax (if necessary)

PROCEDURE STEPS *(Follow aseptic procedures)*

Patient Preparation

1. Health history is reviewed.
2. Patient is seated in an upright position with a patient napkin in place.
3. Patient's mouth is rinsed with water or mouth rinse to remove any food debris and to aid with removing thick saliva.
4. The procedure is explained to patient.
5. Impression trays are tried in the oral cavity to determine the correct size.

Material Preparation

1. Wax is placed around the borders of the impression trays, if necessary, to extend the borders of the trays or to provide additional patient comfort (Figure 35-5).

FIGURE 35-7 Mixing alginate material in a flexible rubber bowl, while pushing on sides of bowl to eliminate air bubbles.

2. The impression water (room temperature) is measured for the mandibular model, normally two calibrations of the water measurement device supplied by the manufacturer. The water is placed in the flexible mixing bowl. *Note:* Place the water in the bowl first to ensure that all the powder is incorporated into the mixture.

> Taking the mandibular model first allows the patient to build confidence and feel more secure before the maxillary impression, which often causes more gagging.

3. Fluff the powder prior to opening the powder canister, if indicated by manufacturer's directions.
4. Fill the measure of powder by overfilling and then leveling off with the spatula (use the flat blade, not the edge blade of the spatula) to get an accurate measure. Dispense two corresponding scoops into a second flexible rubber bowl.
5. When ready, place the powder in water.
6. Mix the water and powder first with a stirring motion. Then mix by holding the bowl in one hand, rotating the bowl occasionally, and using the flat side of the spatula to incorporate the material through pressure against the side of the bowl (Figure 35-7). The mixing time for Type I fast set is thirty to forty-five seconds, and for Type II regular set, one minute.
7. Upon completion, the mixture should be homogeneous and creamy. When the material is mixed correctly, load it into the impression tray. On the mandibular tray, the material should be loaded from both lingual sides (Figure 35-8). Use the flat side of the blade to condense the material firmly into the tray. If necessary to further smooth the surface, take a gloved hand, moisten, and smooth the top.

FIGURE 35-8 Loading mandibular alginate tray from lingual side to eliminate air spaces.

PROCEDURE 3 5 - 3

Taking an Alginate Impression

Refer to Procedure 35-2, Preparing for an Alginate Impression, to identify PPE, equipment, and supplies.

PROCEDURE STEPS *(Follow aseptic procedures)*

1. When taking the mandibular impression, face the patient, and retract the right cheek slightly.

2. Use the excess alginate material to rub onto the occlusal surfaces of the teeth in order to obtain more accurate anatomy.

3. Invert the impression tray so that the material is toward the teeth.

4. Turn the tray so that it passes through the lip opening with one side of the tray entering first, using the other hand to retract the opposite corner of the mouth.

5. When the tray is completely in the patient's mouth, center it above the teeth.

6. Lower the tray onto the teeth, placing the posterior area down first, leaving the impression tray slightly anterior.

7. Have the patient raise the tongue and move it side to side to ensure that the lingual aspect of the alveolar process is defined in the impression.

8. Pull out the lip from the center with other hand.

9. Finish placing the impression tray down and, as it is done, push slightly toward the posterior area with the tray. This pushes the impression material down into the patient's anterior vestibule area, therefore producing a good esthetic model. One area that often lacks detail in the impression is the anterior segment. By leaving the tray slightly anterior and pushing the tray toward the posterior while making sure the lip is out of the way, this problem can be overcome.

10. Allow the lip to cover the tray. It should be close to the handle portion of the tray.

11. Hold it in the patient's mouth with two fingers on the back of the tray, one on the right side, one on the left side, until set (Figure 35-9). Check the excess material around the edges of the impression tray, or in the bowl, to determine if the material is set. The material should feel firm and not change shape when pushed.

FIGURE 35-9 Holding mandibular alginate tray in patient's mouth, maintaining a stable force while material is setting.

12. The maxillary alginate impression is loaded from the posterior, making sure that the material completely fills the tray without voids (Figure 35-10A). Smooth the material (Figure 35-10B). Take a small amount of alginate out from the palate area to prevent the impression material from going down the patient's throat after insertion (Figure 35-10C). Place some alginate on the occlusal surfaces of the maxillary teeth.

13. Stand behind or to the side of the patient, place the maxillary tray in the patient's mouth by turning the tray so that it passes through the lip opening with one side of the tray entering first, using the other hand to retract the opposite corner of the mouth (Figure 35-10D). Raise the tray to the maxillary arch and hold out the lip before seating the tray in place. Hold it in position until the material is set in the bowl (Figure 35-10E).

(continues)

PROCEDURE 3 5 - 3 *(CONTINUED)*

FIGURE 35-10 (A) Load maxillary alginate tray from posterior area of tray. (B) Smooth the material. (C) Before seating tray in patient's mouth, remove a small amount of alginate from palate area. Doing so prevents material from descending into the patient's throat. (D) Insert tray into patient's mouth one side first, and then rotate the entire tray into patient's mouth. (E) Hold tray in place until material sets.

rial is the setting reaction. The setting of the irreversible hydrocolloid (alginate) is accomplished by a chemical reaction. Reversible hydrocolloid changes from a gel to a sol and back again due to thermal reaction. The material begins in a gel (solid) state and, after boiling in a hydrocolloid conditioner unit for ten minutes, it becomes liquid and remains in that state for hours if placed in a water storage bath of 150°F or 66°C until the operator is ready to use it. Five minutes before taking the impression, the tray material is moved into a water bath of 110°F or 45°C. It is further cooled in the mouth as cool water flows through the water trays, connected to hoses at the dental unit. Most units have two water connectors where the hoses can be attached.

Advantages and Disadvantages of Reversible Hydrocolloid. The primary advantage of using reversible hydrocolloid is accuracy of the impression. Accuracy is more precise and more detailed than that for alginate (irreversible hydrocolloid), and reversible hydrocolloid can be used for impressions for crown and bridge construction. This material can be used for impressions for both teeth and tissue. It is more economical than many materials on the market for final impressions, after the initial equipment has been purchased.

The disadvantage is the additional equipment needed to prepare the material. In addition, reversible hydrocolloid can lose accuracy due to atmospheric conditions. The preparation and setting time is increased to ten min-

PROCEDURE 3 5 - 4

Removing the Alginate Impression

Refer to Procedure 35-2, Preparing for an Alginate Impression, to identify PPE, equipment, and supplies.

PROCEDURE STEPS *(Follow aseptic procedures)*

1. When the material is completely set, remove it from the mouth by first loosening the tissue of the lips and cheek around the periphery with fingers to break the suction-like seal.

2. Place fingers of the opposing hand on the opposite arch to protect the adjacent arch as the tray is being removed.

3. Remove the tray in an upward or downward motion (depending on the arch) with a quick snap. Turn it to the side to allow it to be removed from the oral cavity.

4. Remove any excess alginate material from the patient's mouth with the evacuator and have the patient rinse. Check the patient's face for any excess alginate material. If present, give the patient a tissue and mirror to remove the material.

5. Check the impression for accuracy (Figure 35-11).

6. Rinse the impression gently with water to remove saliva or blood.

FIGURE 35-11 The alginate impression is checked for accuracy after removal from the patient's mouth.

7. Spray with approved surface disinfectant.

8. If there is a time lapse (maximum of twenty minutes) before pouring, wrap the alginate impression in an air-tight container or a moist towel and place it in a plastic bag labeled with the patient's name. If the impression is placed in a wet towel for an extended period of time, imbibition (taking up extra moisture) may occur.

PROCEDURE 3 5 - 5

Disinfecting Alginate Impressions

This procedure is performed by the dental assistant immediately after removing the alginate impressions from the patient's mouth and caring for the patient.

EQUIPMENT AND SUPPLIES

- Approved disinfectant
- Covered container

PROCEDURE STEPS *(Follow aseptic procedures)*

1. Rinse the impressions gently under tap water to remove any debris, blood, or saliva.

2. Spray the impressions with an approved disinfectant (see Chapter 11, Infection Control).

3. If not pouring immediately, place the impressions in a covered container.

4. Label the container with the patient's name.

PROCEDURE 35-6

Taking a Bite Registration

This procedure is performed by the dental assistant under direction of the dentist or by the dentist with the dental assistant assisting.

EQUIPMENT AND SUPPLIES

- Bite registration wax or wax horseshoe or polysiloxane and extruder gun and disposable tips
- Laboratory knife
- Warm water or torch

PROCEDURE STEPS *(Follow aseptic procedures)*

1. The patient remains seated in an upright position with a patient napkin in place after the impressions are taken.

2. Explain the procedure.

3. The bite registration wax is tried to determine correct length. If correction is needed, the laboratory knife is used to trim off the excess.

4. Instruct the patient to practice biting to establish occlusion. You may have to instruct patient in biting in occlusion.

5. Bite registration wax is heated in warm water or with a torch to soften.

6. Place wax on the mandibular occlusal surface of the patient. If using polysiloxane, the bite registration material is extruded from the disposable tip directly onto the occlusal surface of the mandibular teeth (Figure 35-12A).

7. Instruct the patient to bite together gently in the correct occlusion. You need to make sure the patient is in proper occlusion.

8. The wax will cool in one to two minutes while the patient keeps the teeth together in occlusion. If using polysiloxane, the patient gently occludes until the material sets (Figure 35-12B).

9. Gently remove wax or polysiloxane bite without distortion.

10. The wax or polysiloxane bite registration is disinfected, labeled, and stored for use during trimming of the diagnostic casts (Figure 35-12C).

(A)

(B)

(C)

FIGURE 35-12 (A) Bite registration material is extruded from the tip directly onto the occlusal surface of the mandibular teeth. (B) Patient occludes gently until the material sets. (C) Polysiloxane or wax bite taken on a patient for use in establishing patient's occlusion.

utes. This material was used widely in earlier years and now has declined some, due to the emergence of a number of elastomeric materials available with similar accuracy.

Reversible Hydrocolloid Packaging and Equipment. The tray material is supplied in collapsible plastic tubes (Figure 35-13). The syringe material is supplied in either cylinders in a jar or syringe carpules. Both materials come in several colors and strengths. Special water-cooled trays and attachment hoses to circulate the water must be used with this material.

A hydrocolloid conditioner unit is used to prepare the material for use. This electric unit has three compartments (Figure 35-14). As with all equipment and

FIGURE 35-13 Hydrocolloid. (A) Tubes. (B) Syringes and cartridges. (C) Trays used with hydrocolloid conditioning unit to obtain final impressions.

FIGURE 35-14 Hydrocolloid conditioning unit with boiling bath, storage bath, and conditioning bath. *(Courtesy of Van R)*

material, read the manufacturer's directions and specific time for the material to be placed in each compartment. Normally, a timer is built into the conditioner. Each compartment in the conditioning unit is filled with clean water. The first compartment on the left, facing the unit, is for boiling the material. The tubes are placed, with the lids tight and upside down, in the unit. The syringe material is placed in a holding case for the cartridges or inside the boiling syringes if cylinders are used. The material must stay in the syringes or tubes or it will disperse throughout the water and be unusable. There, the material is boiled for ten minutes. Digital machines can be set to start the timer for ten minutes as soon as the boiling temperature is reached. If not using a digital machine, the dental assistant has to monitor the boiling temperature and time carefully. After the boiling process is complete, the temperature drops to the preset storage temperature.

After the tubes and syringe material is boiled, it is moved to the middle compartment for storage. In this compartment, the temperature is set to maintain the material in a liquid state. The material can stay in this compartment for hours or days before use.

The third compartment on the right, facing the unit, is for tray material only. The material is placed in a water-cooled tray and then in the compartment to be tempered for five minutes. This cools the material so that it does not burn the patient's mouth upon insertion. The syringe material remains in the fluid state to get into the crevices around the prepared tooth and obtain the necessary anatomy on the adjacent teeth. Because of the small opening in the syringe, the amount coming from the syringe cools rapidly as it is used.

The hydrocolloid conditioner unit requires very little maintenance. The compartments should be emptied and rinsed out on a regular basis and then wiped with a soft cloth and refilled with clean water. A condition cleaner can be placed in the compartments and left for one hour to remove any buildup. The cleaner is then rinsed out prior to placing clean water in the compartments.

Elastomeric Impression Materials

Elastomeric impression materials have rubber-like qualities and are used for areas that require precise duplication. Materials in this classification are not as affected by atmospheric changes as hydrocolloids. They are more elastic and rubber-like when set, and thus allow removal from the mouth to take place without tearing and distortion. **Distortion** is a dimensional change in shape. There are three primary groups of materials in this classification: polysulfide, silicone (polysiloxane and polyvinyl siloxanes), and polyether. Each group has slightly different properties and characteristics, even though all have elastic qualities. All the materials have a catalyst and base that are mixed together to start the chemical self-curing process. The **catalyst** is the ingredient that **accelerates** or starts the process of setting the material. The process by which the catalyst and accelerator begin to cure and the material changes from a paste to an elastic, rubber-like material is called **polymerization**. The accelerator is dispensed as a paste from a small tube or in liquid form from a bottle with a dropper. The base that makes up the volume of the material is normally dispensed in a paste. Often, the tube openings of base and catalyst are different sizes, with the catalyst tube opening being smaller. Many of the materials are now dispensed in an "extruder gun" with a mixing tip. The mixing tip brings together the correct amount of each material and dispenses it, premixed (Figure 35-15). If this technique is used, there is no need for a mixing pad and spatula. A new tip is required for each application and the material must be purchased in special cartridges.

Polysulfide

Polysulfide impression materials have been around for a long time, and may be called mercaptan or rubber-base materials. They are supplied in two pastes: a base and a catalyst. The base is the larger tube and the white color of the two. It is made from liquid polysulfide polymer (thiodol polysulfide rubber) with filler added. The dark brown accelerator is made from lead peroxide. These pastes can be purchased as light (syringe material), regular, heavy, and extra heavy (tray material).

Advantages of the polysulfide material include relative stability after the final set has been achieved, good accuracy, sharpness of detail, and a relatively long shelf life (several years). Pouring the polysulfide impression within an hour is advisable, but impressions have been known to be left for days before pouring with no noticeable change in dimension. The disadvantages of polysulfide are the odor (it smells like sulfur because of the

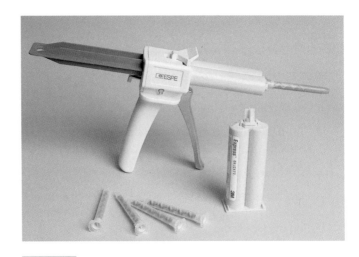

FIGURE 35-15 Extruder gun cartridge and tips used to mix and dispense material.

base), taste, staining (it permanently stains clothes because of the accelerator), and the relatively long setting time (ten minutes is required from the start of the mix to the setting of the material prior to removal from the patient's mouth). The setting time can be accelerated slightly by increasing temperature, moisture, and amount of accelerator. Procedure 35-7 outlines how to take an impression with polysulfide.

Silicone (Polysiloxane and Polyvinal Siloxanes)

A number of new silicone materials have been introduced in recent years. **Silicones** have the advantages of polysulfide without the disadvantages. They are more expensive than the polysulfide, however. Advantages of the material include high accuracy, no shrinkage, dimen-

---

PROCEDURE 35-7

Taking a Polysulfide Impression

This procedure is performed by the dentist with assistance by the dental assistant. This procedure can be four- or six-handed. Everyone should wear protective overclothing. Polysulfide is a material used in taking final impressions for which extreme accuracy is required.

EQUIPMENT AND SUPPLIES

- Two rigid laboratory spatulas
- Paper pad, provided by manufacturer

- Two pastes each (two syringes, two trays) from the same manufacturer (a base and an accelerator of the syringe material and a base and an accelerator of the tray material)
- Impression syringe with tip in place and plunger out of the cylinder
- Custom tray that has been painted with corresponding adhesive and permitted to dry

(continues)

PROCEDURE 3 5 - 7 *(CONTINUED)*

PROCEDURE STEPS *(Follow aseptic procedures)*

1. Health history is reviewed.

2. The patient is seated in an upright position with a patient napkin in place and a large drape over the clothes.

3. The procedure is explained to the patient.

4. The patient's mouth is rinsed with water or a mouth rinse to remove any food debris and aid with removing thick saliva.

5. The material is mixed concurrently by two individuals. The syringe material is mixed slightly ahead of the tray material.

6. Dispense the accelerator onto the pad in a long, even line about four inches long. If more material is needed, additional lines can be placed together on the paper pad. *Note:* Be sure to wipe the end of the tube before placing the lid back on to prevent mess and sticking of the top.

7. Dispense the base onto the pad in a long, even line the same length as the accelerator (Figure 35-16). Additional lines can be dispensed, but they should not touch the accelerator until the operator wants the process of polymerization to begin.

8. When ready, the individual with the syringe material begins mixing by first gathering up the accelerator with the spatula and placing it in the base material. Spatulate the pastes together with broad sweeps. After a minute has lapsed, the individual mixing the tray material begins the same process.

9. When the mix is homogeneous and lacks brown or white streaks, it is completely mixed. This process takes from forty-five seconds to one minute.

10. The syringe material is then loaded into an impression syringe using the back portion or the working end nozzle of the barrel and pushing the syringe over the material repeatedly to force the material into the chamber (Figure 35-17). When the material is in the syringe chamber, wipe the edges quickly and place the plunger in the syringe. Extrude the material slightly to make sure it is working and pass it to the dentist.

11. The tray material is mixed to the same consistency and within the same timeframe. The bulk of the tray material is picked up by the spatula and loaded into the impression tray and spread evenly. The tray is then transferred to the dentist after the syringe has been used. The mixing and loading (working time) must be completed within four minutes.

12. The impression must remain in the patient's mouth, held by the operator or the dental assistant, for six minutes in order to achieve a final set.

13. Cleanup is accomplished after the material has reached the rubber stage. The material peels off the spatula. The paper pad normally has a corner for the spatula to fit under to aid in removing the soiled top sheet (Figure 35-18). The disposable impression syringe and paper sheet can be disposed of and the spatula sterilized.

14. The removal of the tray is done in much the same manner as was the alginate. Remove the impression after releasing the seal, taking care to protect the opposing teeth from the quick snap.

FIGURE 35-16 Polysulfide material is dispensed and ready to mix. The lines are equally long, but amount of material differs.

FIGURE 35-17 Loading mixed polysulfide syringe material into syringe for placement directly around prepared tooth.

(continues)

PROCEDURE 35-7 *(CONTINUED)*

FIGURE 35-18 Polysulfide material cleans easily after it sets. The paper pad has a precut corner to allow the easy insertion of the spatula for cleanup and disposal.

sional stability, high tear resistance, no taste, and no odor.

The material comes in a number of forms, including putty for making a custom tray, in tubes of base and accelerator (catalyst) for injection, and regular and heavy type for impressions. It also is available in cartridge form to be used with the mixing tip and extruding gun (automix cartridge system).

The putty material comes in two colors. Each container of putty has a colored scoop that is used for either the base or the catalyst (Figure 35-19). Do not mix up the scoops because doing so will contaminate the material and cause the polymerization process to start, making the material hard and useless. The material is dispensed with an equal volume of base and catalyst putties. Knead and mix the putty quickly until a homogeneous color is achieved. This mixing takes about thirty seconds. Mixing putty with latex gloves will adversely affect the set of some materials—read the directions. The silicone is placed in the tray, covered with a thin plastic sheet, and placed in the patient's mouth or over the model. It takes about three minutes for the material to harden. Remove the plastic, and a custom tray is ready for the impression material. The putty material is not suitable for detailed impressions.

When ready for the impression, the tray is loaded by the operator squeezing the dispenser handle of the extruding gun and engaging the plunger. The plunger enters the cartridge and extrudes the material through the mixing tip and into the putty material in the impression tray. The syringe material can also be injected from the mixing tip into the impression syringe for use around the sulcus of the tooth. When ready, the tray is placed in

FIGURE 35-19 Two scoops of putty, or putty and a tube of accelerator, are dispensed for easy incorporation.

the patient's mouth and immobilized until set (three and one-half minutes for a fast set and five minutes for a regular set). The impression is removed after the seal is loosened and the opposing teeth are protected. The impression is run under cold water and sprayed with disinfectant. The impression is very stable and can be poured weeks later. The total time from mixing to the final set is from four to six minutes (see Procedure 35-8).

PROCEDURE 35-8

Taking a Silicone (Polysiloxane) Two-Step Impression

This procedure is performed by the dentist with assistance by the dental assistant. Silicone (polysiloxane) is a material used in taking final impressions for which extreme accuracy is required.

EQUIPMENT AND SUPPLIES

- Spatula
- Paper mixing pad
- Vinyl overgloves
- Two containers of putty (one base and one catalyst) with color-coordinated scoops or one putty base and liquid dropper of catalyst (Figure 35-20)
- Stock tray with adhesive painted on interior
- Plastic sheet for use as a spacer
- Extruder gun, mixing tip with intraoral delivery tip or injection syringe (Figure 35-20)
- Cartridges of impression material (light-body or wash material)

PROCEDURE STEPS *(Follow aseptic procedures)*

Patient Preparation

1. Health history is reviewed.

FIGURE 35-20 Extruder gun, mixing tips, and cartridges of impression material. *(Courtesy of Kerr Corporation.)*

2. The patient is seated in an upright position with a bib in place.
3. Retraction cord is placed around prepared tooth.
4. The procedure is explained.

Preliminary Putty Impression

1. Don vinyl gloves.
2. Equal scoops of the putty are mixed together, or the putty base and drops of catalyst are mixed together. The putty must be kneaded until a homogeneous mixture is obtained within the manufacturer's recommended timeframe (normally thirty seconds). The mixture must be a single color with no streaks.
3. After the material is mixed, pat it into a patty and load it into the prepared tray. With a finger, make a slight indentation where the teeth are located.
4. Place the plastic spacer sheet over the material and insert it into the patient's mouth. The objective is to create 2 mm of space for the final syringeable viscous impression material.
5. The setting of the putty takes about three minutes. The tray is then removed from the patient's mouth, the spacer is removed, and the putty is checked for accuracy and left to set further.

Final Impression

1. After the tooth has been prepared, the area cleaned and dried, the retraction cord placed, and the doctor indicates that he or she is ready for the final impression, prepare the material.
2. The tray with the preliminary impression is ready with the spacer removed. The extruder gun is prepared and loaded with the light-body or wash material.
3. The syringe (light-body) material is extruded through the mixing tip and placed in the preliminary impression (Figure 35-21).
4. The tip is wiped off and an intraoral delivery tip placed on for direct injection around the prepared tooth after the retraction cord has been removed. The extruder gun is transferred to the dentist. Instead of using the intraoral delivery tip, some dentists prefer to use an injection syringe, which can be loaded with the mixing tip.

(continues)

P R O C E D U R E 3 5 - 8 *(C O N T I N U E D)*

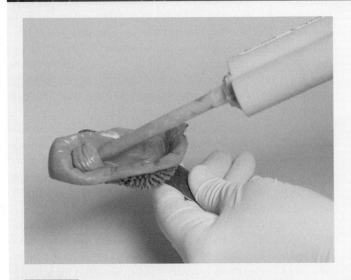

FIGURE 35-21 Syringe material extrudes from extruding gun into prepared tray.

5. The tray is seated by the dentist immediately into place and held steady for three to five minutes, depending on the material used.

6. After the material has set, the impression tray is removed after releasing the seal and taking care to protect the opposing teeth from the quick snap.

7. Immediately rinse the impression under water and lightly air blow dry. Disinfect according to manufacturer's directions.

8. Impressions should be poured immediately, but can be poured up to weeks later and still remain dimensionally stable.

Light-cured impression materials are also available. The advantage of this material is that the setting time is controlled by the operator. The disadvantage is that it is sometimes difficult to move the curing light over the complete surface of the material. A clear-plastic impression tray must be used. The light must hit all areas in order to bring about the curing. The light acts as a catalyst to set up the material.

Polyether

Polyether, impression material used for crowns and bridges, has excellent accuracy and dimensional stability. It is supplied in tubes as pastes, a larger one for the base and the smaller one for the catalyst. The material comes only in regular body and is stiffer than many other materials. It can be used for both the custom tray and the syringe. If used for a custom tray, a tray is chosen that is the correct size, painted with adhesive, and allowed to dry for one minute. The material is dispensed on a paper pad, supplied by the manufacturer, one inch per tooth involved in the impression. Equal lengths of material are placed on the pad, not equal amounts (Figure 35-22). This material is then mixed by placing the catalyst in the base in a figure-eight motion and obtaining a homogeneous mixture free of streaks. The mixing should not take longer than thirty seconds. When mixing is complete, the material is loaded onto the spatula and into the tray. The tray is seated by the dentist in the patient's mouth. After about two minutes of holding the impression in the patient's mouth, agitate the tray in all directions to make room for the final polyether impres-

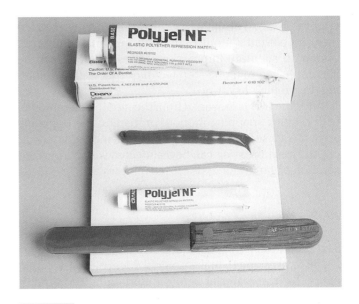

FIGURE 35-22 Polyether impression materials are dispensed on paper pad, ready to be mixed. Material swaths are equally long, but of unequal amounts.

sion material after the teeth are prepared. Remove the tray after three minutes.

To take the final impression after the teeth are prepared with polyether, dispense the material in a similar manner. Less material is needed because of the volume already in the preliminary tray. If a less viscous impression material is desired by the dentist, a thinner (or body modifier) can be added to the mixture. The catalyst and the modifier are mixed into the base material.

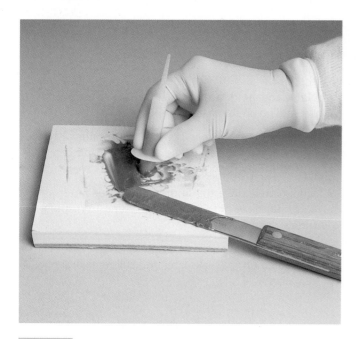

FIGURE 35-23 Mixed polyether is loaded into a syringe.

The material is loaded into an injection syringe, and the excess material is placed in the preliminary impression (Figure 35-23). The impression tray is then reinserted into the patient's mouth and held for four minutes to obtain an accurate impression. This technique can be accomplished in a one-step technique as well, eliminating the preliminary tray.

After the tray is loosened from the mouth and removed with a quick snapping motion, protecting the opposing arch, it is rinsed with cold water and then completely air dried. The impression can be disinfected with a 2 percent solution of glutaraldehyde for ten minutes.

Gypsum Materials

Several different **gypsum** materials are used when pouring an impression to make a model. Identifying the application for the material before determining the type of gypsum product to use is important. Gypsum materials vary in strength, dimensional accuracy, resistance, reproduction detail, water/powder ratio, and setting times.

Primary types of gypsum used in dentistry follow:

- Type I: Impression plaster
- Type II: Model or laboratory plaster
- Orthodontic stone/combination of Type II: Model or laboratory plaster and Type III: Laboratory stone
- Type III: Laboratory stone
- Type IV: Die stone
- Type V: High-strength, high-expansion die stone

During the process of manufacturing the various types of plasters and stones, the gypsum product (which is mined as a hard rock) is ground to a fine powder. It is then heated in large, cylindrical kettles equipped with agitators. The heating is controlled accurately and is continued until a specific amount of water is driven out of the gypsum. This process is known as **calcination**. Several methods of calcination are used to derive various stones and investment die stones. During this process, the gypsum, which is a calcium sulfate dihydrate (one molecule of calcium sulfate to two molecules of water), is changed to a hemihydrate powder (one water molecule to every two molecules of calcium sulfate). Because both plaster and stone are white in color, yellow, blue, and pink pigments are added to the stone to make it easier to distinguish which material is being used.

Strengths of the gypsum products are determined by the calcination process and the water/powder ratio needed to incorporate the mixture. Plaster (beta hemihydrate) comprises gypsum particles that are larger and more irregular than the particles of stone (alpha hemihydrate) that have undergone further processing and transformed into denser particles. It is important to follow the manufacturer's directions when mixing gypsum products. One of the chief obstacles to overcome when mixing these products is incorporating air and wetting each particle. Plaster particles are more irregular and require more water to wet each surface of each particle. The ratio of water to powder for plaster is 50 mL of water to 100 grams of powder; stone requires only 30 mL of water to 100 grams of powder. Die stones require even less water because the particles are smaller, less irregular, and more dense.

Incorporating the water is an important step in mixing gypsum products. Using a flexible rubber bowl and a stiff spatula allows the operator to stir the viscous material and press against the sides of the bowl to eliminate air bubbles. Avoid whipping the powder and the water together, because doing so adds air to the mixture. It should be mixed to a creamy, putty-like consistency. A grainy mixture will not pour into the impression. The incorporating and spatulating procedure should take about one minute. Overspatulating causes a breakdown of crystals and soft spots in the model.

Gypsum sets when the plaster or stone transforms back to the dihydrate through a chemical reaction. This process gives off heat, called an **exothermic reaction**. The temperature of the water increases or decreases the setting time. The hotter the water, the more rapidly the material sets. There are retarders such as borax and sodium citrate that can be added to the material to slow down the set. Potassium sulfate accelerates the setting time. The manufacturers add small concentrations of the retarders or accelerators to cause a decrease or an increase in the setting rate of the gypsum.

It is important to have the correct water-to-powder ratio. If less water is incorporated, the model can have greater setting expansion. It will have increased strength and hardness but may result in a thick mixture that becomes a dry, crumbly mass that cannot flow into the impression. At this stage, more water cannot be added to the mixture. It will need to be disposed of and a new mixture made. If too much water is incorporated into the mixture, the model will be weak, slow setting, and filled with air spaces. A plaster model will set in ten to twenty minutes and can be determined by feel. If the heat has dissipated, the model is set. It goes through a cycle and heats up and seems to perspire; then, the heat diminishes and the model is cool and dry. The final set occurs after twenty-four hours when the model reaches the optimum hardness. The gypsum powder is measured by weight and the water is calibrated by volume.

All gypsum products are packaged in some type of plastic bag or container to ensure that they do not become contaminated with moisture. If contaminated, the properties and the setting reaction may be altered. These plastic bags are normally further packaged in a cardboard box for easier handling.

Plaster

Plaster (plaster of paris) is a white gypsum referred to as beta-hemihydrate. It was one of the first gypsum products available to dentistry. It is the weakest and least expensive of gypsum products. It is calcinated in an open kettle method, and the result is particles that are rough, irregular, and porous. The final product is a powder that, when mixed with water, reverts to a gypsum product or dihydrate. Plaster takes more water to incorporate the powder. After the model dries and the water evaporates, the areas where the water was become air bubbles. This is the primary reason that plaster is weaker than stone. Stone is more compact and requires less water, therefore making a stronger model. Plaster is used in areas where detail and strength are not as important. Plaster is used to pour up study models, for opposing models, in mounting study models and casts, and for repairing casts.

Type I: Impression Plaster

Impression plaster (modified Type II: laboratory or model plaster) was used to take impressions before the newer, easy-to-manipulate impression materials now on the market. The plaster (Type I), mixed with a water-to-powder ratio of 60 mL of water to 100 grams of powder, is placed in the mouth carefully on the area to be duplicated, and then the operator must wait for the plaster to set. After the set (usually four to five minutes), the material is broken apart and reassembled in the laboratory. Because the material is so rigid, it fractures and breaks easily. Today, this material is rarely used for impressions; it is used primarily to mount casts on an articulator because of its quick setting time.

Type II: Laboratory or Model Plaster

Model plaster is used routinely in the dental office by the dental assistant to pour diagnostic casts or study models. It is normally white in color, and is slightly stronger than the Type I: impression plaster, because it requires a water-to-powder ratio of 50 mL of water to 100 grams of powder, making the material less porous.

Type III: Laboratory Stone

Type III: laboratory stone is stronger than plaster and is used where more strength is needed. It requires 30 mL of water to 100 grams of powder, making it denser, harder, and stronger. It is normally yellow in color due to the manufacturer's added pigments, more expensive than plaster, and referred to as alpha-hemihydrate. It is used for study models (diagnostic casts) that require greater strength, working casts, and models for partial and full dentures.

Orthodontic Stone

Orthodontic stone is a mixture of laboratory or model plaster and laboratory stone. This white stone allows for a stronger model to be used for the diagnosis and treatment of orthodontic cases.

Type IV: Die Stone

Type IV: die stone is calcinated by autoclaving in the presence of calcium chloride. This modified alpha-hemihydrate is referred to as die stone. A die is a positive replica of the prepared tooth made from stone. It requires much less water (less than 24 mL to 100 grams of powder) to incorporate its small, uniform particles. More stone with less water and air makes the model strong and resistant to abrasion. It is used most often for dies or where a very strong model or cast is needed.

Type V: High-Strength, High-Expansion Die Stone

Recently, the ADA added a new material to its list of gypsum products. Type V: die stone requires from 18 to 22 mL of water to 100 grams of powder, making it the strongest accepted gypsum product available for use in the dental office.

Trimming and Finishing Diagnostic Casts

Diagnostic casts (study models) are used to present the case to the patient. It is important that they have an attractive appearance. Not only are they part of the patient's permanent record, but they are also a direct reflection of the type of work the office performs for the patient. They can be trimmed in a geometric form that

Water-to-Powder Ratio Recommendations

Type I: Impression plaster	100 grams powder	to	60 mL water
Type II: Laboratory or model plaster	100 grams powder	to	50 mL water
Type III: Laboratory stone	100 grams powder	to	30 mL water
Type IV: Die stone	100 grams powder	to	24 mL water
Type V: Die stone	100 grams powder	to	18–22 mL water

PROCEDURE 35-9

Pouring an Alginate Impression with Plaster

This procedure is performed by the dental assistant in the dental laboratory.

EQUIPMENT AND SUPPLIES (Figure 35-24)

- Spatula, metal with rounded end and stiff, straight sides
- Two flexible rubber mixing bowls
- Scale
- Plaster (100 grams)
- Gram measuring device
- Water measuring device (calibrated syringe or vial)
- Vibrator with paper or plastic cover on platform
- Room-temperature water
- Alginate impression (disinfected)

PROCEDURE STEPS *(Follow aseptic procedures)*

Mixing the Plaster

1. Measure 50 mL of room-temperature water into one of the flexible mixing bowls (Figure 35-25).

2. Place the second flexible mixing bowl on the scale and set the dial to zero. This allows the plaster powder to be weighed (Figure 35-26).

3. Weigh out 100 grams of plaster in the second rubber bowl.

4. Add the powder from the second bowl to the water of the first bowl. Placing the water in first allows for all the powder to become incorporated into the mixture.

FIGURE 35-24 Equipment for pouring plaster.

Allow several seconds for the powder to dissolve into the water.

5. Use the spatula to slowly mix the particles together. The initial mixing should be completed in twenty seconds. The total mixing procedure should take about one minute.

6. Turn on the vibrator to medium or low speed.

7. Place the rubber bowl on the vibrator platform, pressing lightly.

8. Rotate the bowl on the vibrator to allow the air bubbles to rise to the top surface (Figure 35-27). The mixing and vibrating should be completed within a

(continues)

PROCEDURE 3 5 - 9 *(CONTINUED)*

FIGURE 35-25 Measure 50 mL of water into a flexible mixing bowl.

FIGURE 35-26 Measure 100 g of plaster powder into a bowl for pouring alginate impression.

FIGURE 35-27 Vibrator brings air bubbles to surface of plaster mixture.

FIGURE 35-28 Plaster's consistency should allow it to retain position as spatula slides through it.

couple of minutes. The mixture is ready if the spatula can cut through it and it stays to the sides without changing positions. It will appear like whipped cream with a smooth, creamy texture (Figure 35-28). Another way to check whether the powder/water is in correct ratio is to place a spoonful on the spatula and turn it upside down. If the material remains in place, the mixture is ready.

NOTE: When the spatula is held sideways, mixture will fall from it.

PROCEDURE 35-10

Pouring Alginate Impression for Study Model

This procedure is performed by the dental assistant in the dental laboratory immediately after mixing the plaster. The impression is ready to pour, the excess moisture is removed, and a laboratory knife has been used to eliminate any excess impression material that will hamper the pouring of the model.

EQUIPMENT AND SUPPLIES

- Metal spatula (stiff blade with rounded end) or disposable spatula

- Mixed plaster from Procedure 35-9, Pouring an Alginate Impression with Plaster

- Vibrator with paper towel or plastic cover on platform

PROCEDURE STEPS *(Follow aseptic procedures)*

1. Use the vibrator at low or medium speed.

2. Hold the impression by the handle with the tray portion on the platform of the vibrator. Allow a small amount of plaster to touch the most distal surface of one side of the arch in the impression (Figure 35-29).

3. When the plaster touches the impression that is on the vibrating platform, it flows down the back of the impression and into the anatomy of the teeth. Continue to add small increments of the plaster in the same area as the plaster flows around toward the anterior teeth and to the other side of the arch. (Using this technique allows the air to push ahead of the plaster material, and eliminates bubbles. This produces a model that has detailed anatomic qualities.)

4. Add the plaster in this manner until it flows out the other side of the impression and fills the anatomic portion of the model. Rotating the impression around on the platform of the vibrator aids in allowing the material to travel around the arch.

5. After the anatomy portion is filled with plaster, use larger increments to fill the entire impression, off the vibrator. When filled, place lightly on the vibrator to coalesce (combine). Overvibration can cause bubbles to form.

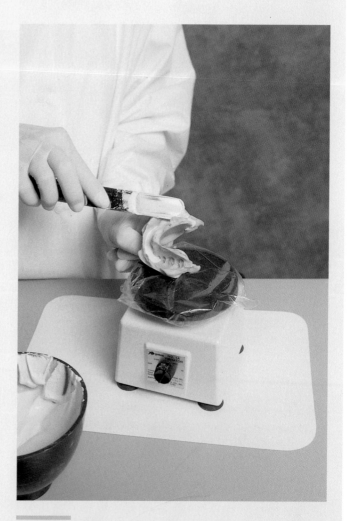

FIGURE 35-29 Mixed plaster is vibrated into alginate impression, starting at the posterior area of arch and continuing to fill from that area while material rotates around to opposite side of arch.

6. If a two-pour method is to be used, small blobs should be left on the top of the plaster so that it can attach to the art portion of the model. (A flat surface may break apart at a later date.)

PROCEDURE 35-11

Pouring Art Portion of Plaster Study Model Using Two-Pour Method

This procedure is performed by the dental assistant in the dental laboratory after the anatomic portion of the study model has set.

EQUIPMENT AND SUPPLIES

- Metal spatula (stiff blade with rounded end) or disposable spatula

- Flexible rubber bowl or disposable bowl

- Vibrator with a paper towel or plastic cover on platform

- Paper towels

- Plaster

- Calibration measurement device

- Room-temperature water

- Water measuring device

PROCEDURE STEPS *(Follow aseptic procedures)*

1. After pouring the anatomical portion of the impression, allow it to set for five to ten minutes.

2. Wipe the rubber bowl and spatula with paper towel and dispose of the material. Wash, clean, and ready the rubber bowl and spatula for a second pour of plaster.

3. The ratio of powder to water can be altered to create a thicker mix, which is desirable for bases. If pouring the bases or art portion of both the maxillary and the mandibular casts, use 100 grams of powder to 40 mL of water. If pouring only one model, mix half the amount of powder and water.

4. Mix the plaster in the same manner as before. It will appear much thicker. This part of the model is not as crucial as the anatomical portion. Areas that have bubbles can be repaired easily.

5. Gather the plaster on the spatula and place it on a glass slab or a paper towel (Figure 35-30). It is important to allow the material to mass upward and not to spread out like a pancake.

6. After all the material is on the paper towel, invert the poured anatomy portion onto the base material.

FIGURE 35-30 Plaster is gathered to make a base. The plaster must have enough body so that it does not flatten.

7. Hold the tray steady and situate the handle so that it is parallel to the paper surface or glass slab. It is important to get a base that is even and uniform in thickness. This makes it easier to trim the model later.

8. Carefully drag the excess plaster up over the edges of the cast, filling in any voided areas (Figure 35-31). Try not to cover any margins of the impression tray while doing this. This locks the plaster onto the tray and may cause the cast to fracture when removing the impression material and the tray.

NOTE: If using a one- or single-pour method, the base is poured immediately after the anatomical portion is poured. The two-pour method allows the material to initially set in the anatomical portion prior to inverting it and ensures that the plaster does not flow from any crucial areas.

FIGURE 35-31 Operator must smooth plaster sides of base after inversion of filled impression.

PROCEDURE 3 5 - 1 2

Removing Plaster Model from Alginate Impression

This procedure is performed by the dental assistant in the dental laboratory after the study model has set.

EQUIPMENT AND SUPPLIES

▪ Laboratory knife

▪ Maxillary and mandibular plaster models, set in alginate impressions

PROCEDURE STEPS *(Follow aseptic procedures)*

1. Allow the plaster to set for forty to sixty minutes before removing the impression material and the tray. The exothermic heat should be gone from the plaster material to indicate it is set.

2. Using a laboratory knife, gently remove any plaster on the margin of the tray (Figure 35-32).

3. Holding the handle of the impression tray, lift the tray straight upward.

4. If the tray does not come off, identify the area that is holding it back. Remove the necessary plaster in that area to release the tray and impression material. Be

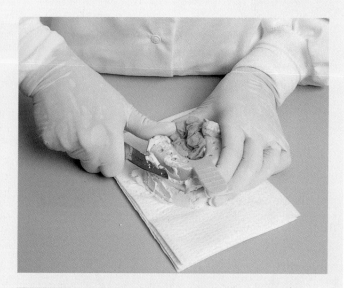

FIGURE 35-32 Before removing impression from the model, use knife to remove remaining plaster from impression.

sure to lift in an upward motion to remove the tray. Wiggling side to side or lifting sideways may fracture the teeth and anatomical portion of the cast.

is pleasing in appearance. Standard guidelines are used in trimming the casts.

Two-thirds of the trimmed model are made from the anatomical portion of the cast (Figure 35-33). The anatomical portion includes the teeth, the mucosa, and frenum attachments and is about one inch wide. This area was duplicated from the oral cavity. The remaining one-third is the base or art portion of the cast. This portion is trimmed in a geometric form with specific angles and is about one-half inch wide. When maxillary and mandibular models are trimmed and in occlusion, they should have an overall height of three inches.

Note: The grinding stone on the model trimmer can be cleaned with a brush and the water increased to run over the surface. Shut off the machine and clean the guide table and the reservoir beneath where the plaster accumulates. If this is allowed to build up, the

FIGURE 35-33 After trimming, the anatomical portion of the cast will make up two-thirds of the model.

PROCEDURE 35-13

Trimming Diagnostic Casts/Study Models

This procedure is performed by the dental assistant in the dental laboratory after the study model has set, been separated from the alginate impression, and prepared for trimming.

EQUIPMENT AND SUPPLIES

- Safety glasses
- Maxillary and mandibular models
- Two flexible rubber mixing bowls
- Laboratory knife
- Pencil
- Measuring straight edge

PROCEDURE STEPS *(Follow aseptic procedures)*

1. If the maxillary and mandibular plaster models are dry, soak the bases of the models in rubber mixing bowls for five minutes prior to trimming. The trimming wheel on the model trimmer is more effective if the models are wet prior to trimming.

2. Don safety glasses and adjust the model trimmer so that the water runs freely over the grinding wheel when the trimmer is on.

3. Invert the models so that the teeth are resting on the counter. Evaluate whether the base is parallel to the counter (Figure 35-34). Keep in mind that the art portion is one-half inch when completed.

4. Turn on the model trimmer and trim the base so that it is parallel to the occlusal plane. The model trimmer works best if light even pressure is used when applying the models to the grinding wheel. Hold the model as level as possible during this procedure (Figure 35-35).

5. Rest hands on the table of the model trimmer and keep fingers away from the grinding wheel.

6. The model may have to be returned to the counter for re-evaluation and then again to the model trimmer to achieve a parallel surface. Trim both models to this stage.

NOTE: Move the models back and forth once across the grinding surface as the model comes off the grinding wheel. This eliminates the circular grinding marks made as the wheel rotates.

7. Place the models together in occlusion (a wax bite may be necessary) and again evaluate whether the objective of obtaining parallel models has been achieved. If not, grind to get the models to this stage. All other cuts will be off if this stage is not achieved, because this flat surface is laid on the model trimming table guide to grind the other areas.

FIGURE 35-34 Before proceeding to trim study model, model base should be parallel to counter.

FIGURE 35-35 Study model base is trimmed as operator maintains even pressure on trimming wheel.

(continues)

PROCEDURE 35-13 *(CONTINUED)*

8. When the cut maxillary and mandibular models as a pair are parallel, keep them in occlusion and evaluate which posterior teeth are the most distal: maxillary or mandibular. When that has been determined, take that model and draw with pencil a line behind the retromolar area indicating where to trim (Figure 35-36).

9. Place the base surface of that model on the model trimmer table guide and cut the posterior area at a right angle with the base up to the indicated lines (Figure 35-37).

10. Put the two models back into occlusion and place the cut model on the top, whether maxillary or mandibular. Place the opposite base on the model trimmer table guide holding the models together and trim the posterior at a right angle to the base (Figure 35-38). The trimmed model acts as a guide to follow while trimming. When small particles of plaster are trimmed off the first base, it indicates that they are trimmed to the same plane. To evaluate this, the models are taken off the grinding wheel and placed on their backs (Figure 35-39). The occlusal plane is at a right angle to the counter. If the models stay in occlusion, the objective

FIGURE 35-36 Pencil line is drawn from 2 mm distal from the last molar to 2 mm distal from molar on opposite side of arch. This establishes a cutting line for back cut.

FIGURE 35-38 Models are placed together to trim back cut.

FIGURE 35-37 Posterior of model base is cut at right angle to base.

FIGURE 35-39 Models are placed on their backs on a hard, flat surface in occlusion to verify whether back cuts are correct.

(continues)

PROCEDURE 3 5 - 1 3 *(C O N T I N U E D)*

has been met. If they fall apart and out of occlusion, then place them back onto the grinding wheel until they stay in the correct position.

11. The top, bottom, and back now are trimmed. Left to trim are the heel, side, and anterior cuts. The first to be cut are the side angles. Take the pencil and mark the following areas: outward from the middle of the mandibular premolars to the edge of the model and the maxillary cuspids in the same manner. Draw a line running parallel to the teeth at the greatest depth of the buccal vestibule, from the molars to the premolars. This line will be about 5 mm from the buccal surface of the teeth. Mark both sides of the maxillary and the mandibular models in this manner.

12. Place the model base back on the model trimmer table guide and trim the model to the pencil lines on both sides (Figure 35-40). Repeat this procedure with both models.

13. Mark with pencil a dot at the midline of the maxillary model in the vestibule area. Using the straight edge of the measuring device, draw a line from the dot to the canine/cuspid line on each quadrant (Figure 35-41). Make both anterior cuts, forming a pointed area at the midline and center of both cuspids. If the teeth are highly irregular, adjustments may have to be done. After the lines are drawn, make sure that the cuts will not trim away the protruding teeth. If it appears that this may happen, move the lines out on each side to accommodate this. The model should appear symmetrical (Figure 35-42).

14. The mandibular model is marked in a rounded manner from the middle of the canine/cuspid on one side to the middle of the canine/cuspid on the other side.

FIGURE 35-41 Line is drawn from midline of central incisors to middle of cuspid to establish a cut line for anterior.

FIGURE 35-42 Maxillary anterior area is cut to a point, bringing both cuspid cuts to midline between maxillary central incisors.

A pencil line can be drawn at the depth of the anterior vestibule as a guide for trimming (Figure 35-43).

15. The heel cuts on both the maxillary and mandibular models are three-eighths to five-eighths inches wide and should appear symmetric in length. They can be drawn on the model by turning the base upward and placing an imaginary diagonal line from the cuspid (maxillary) premolar (mandibular) to where the side and back cuts meet. Draw a 90° angle across the base, opposite the anterior area. The heel cuts are small cuts on both the maxillary and the mandibular models that finish the trimming of the models (Figure 35-44).

16. After the models are trimmed symmetrically, a laboratory knife is used to trim the tongue area flat and smooth other areas on the art portion. Take care not

FIGURE 35-40 Vestibule or side area is cut at deepest area. A line can be drawn to establish a proper cut line.

(continues)

PROCEDURE 35-13 (CONTINUED)

FIGURE 35-43 A rounded line is drawn on mandibular from cuspid to cuspid to indicate where cut should be made.

FIGURE 35-44 Heel cuts are established on models and cut.

to destroy the anatomy of the diagnostic casts. Any air bubbles can be filled with plaster. Use dry plaster on the finger, and push it into the wet model to fill small air bubbles. To complete the smoothing of the flat surfaces, a fine wet/dry sandpaper can be used under water. Any small beads of plaster can be removed carefully from the surfaces of the teeth.

17. Place the models in a model gloss for ten minutes or spray with gloss to provide a professional appearance

and add strength. The models need to be polished with a dry cloth to buff the surface in order to achieve the desired high gloss.

18. Label both models with the patient's name and the date the models were taken. In an orthodontic office, the patient's age may also be identified on the models.

water will back up and cause water to splash out while trimming.

Trimmed Diagnostic Casts (Study Models) Evaluation

- Both maxillary and mandibular models are trimmed symmetrically following specific cut angles indicated.

- All anatomic portions of the model are accurate.

- Trimmed models sit on end and maintain occlusion.

- Models exhibit a one-half-inch base each and a one-inch anatomic portion each.

- Final finishing is accomplished and the models present a professional appearance (Figure 35-45).

FIGURE 35-45 Trimmed study models.

Articulating Casts or Study Models

An articulator is used to duplicate the patient's occlusion on models (Figure 35-46). An **articulator** is a frame that holds models of the patient's teeth in order to maintain the patient's occlusion and represent his or her jaws. Articulators can be simple, like hinges that only duplicate the up-and-down motions, or they can be complex, where they are adjustable and can duplicate the side-to-side motions as well as the up-and-down motions.

Articulators can be used to study malocclusion, to wax and carve teeth for crowns and bridges, and to demonstrate to the patient the action that is of concern.

FIGURE 35-46 Articulator.

FIGURE 35-47 Articulator that can duplicate an individual's bite and mastication.

They also have a number of other desired uses. The dental assistant may perform the task of mounting models or assist the dentist in this task.

Stephan Articulator

Offices may use a Stephan articulator (Figure 35-47), which allows both the up-and-down motion and has a spring that allows for some lateral movement as well. It has two support bows: one to stabilize the maxillary and one to stabilize the mandibular. The hinge represents the temporomandibular joints. The first step in using this articulator is to trim the models so that they fit within the two bows easily. The top portion of the bases can then be scored. To score a model is to make cut marks in the smooth surface so that the added gypsum can adhere. The models are placed within the bows in the correct bite. Normally, the wax bite is used to establish the correct occlusion. The models are then attached to the bows using impression plaster, which flows into the scored area and around the bow. After the plaster has set, the models remain fastened to the articulator and can be opened and the wax bite removed.

Dental Waxes

Waxes are among the oldest materials used in dentistry. Over two hundred years ago, impressions were taken of specific areas in the mouth with wax. The waxes are derived from a number of sources, including bees, plants, and minerals. Beeswax has to be refined and bleached to obtain uniformity of color and character. Differences in color and texture may take place if the bee has been feeding on something unusual, for example, plants all yellow in color. Plants in South America and Brazil bring to dentistry a hard wax that is gathered from the fronds of a tree. This wax also is used for polishing automobiles to a high gloss shine. From minerals come petroleum products, such as paraffin wax. In dentistry, only the highest grade of wax is used. It must be uniform and provide consistent results when used.

Wax Groups

Waxes are classified into three broad groups: pattern, processing, and impression. Pattern waxes are hard waxes used in crown and bridge casting (inlay wax) and the construction of the baseplate tray (baseplate wax). Processing and impression waxes have many uses in dentistry.

Pattern Wax

Pattern, or inlay, wax normally is supplied in dark-colored sticks (Figure 35-48A). It is used on a die, a positive replica of the prepared tooth made from stone. The wax is melted and applied to the die, making a wax pattern that is used to create the metal and/or porcelain restoration. The composition varies from manufacturer

FIGURE 35-48 Pattern waxes. (A) Inlay wax. (B) Baseplate wax.

FIGURE 35-49 Processing waxes. (A) Boxing wax. (B) Utility wax. (C) Sticky wax.

to manufacturer, but most have a certain degree of hardness, toughness, resistance to flaking, and ability to achieve a smooth surface. Desirable properties of inlay wax are that it flows at a temperature slightly above the mouth temperature, it achieves complete burnout at temperatures above 900°F, and it carves away easily without chipping or cracking. These properties are essential in using the lost wax technique of casting. The lost wax technique refers to the wax pattern after the wax is enclosed in investment stone and heated to high temperatures. The high temperatures cause the wax to vaporize, leaving behind a void or an empty space (lost wax) where the melted metal can be invested using centrifugal force.

The baseplate wax is a hard wax that can be heated to make the initial base on which to form a denture (Figure 35-48B). It comes in Types I, II, and III; Type III is the hardest. Type II is most often used in the fabrication of baseplates.

Processing Wax

Several waxes used in dentistry are in the processing wax classification (Figure 35-49). Boxing wax is a soft, pliable wax that is used to form a wax box around an impression prior to pouring it with gypsum. It comes in wax strips one and one-half inches wide and can be reused for the purpose of making a ring around the impression to hold the runny gypsum in place until it sets.

Sticky wax is another type of processing wax. It is very brittle at room temperature but when melted with a flame source becomes soft and sticky. It adheres to a number of surfaces, such as metal, gypsum, and porcelain. It is used to hold two fractured pieces together until they can be repaired.

Utility wax, also called periphery or bending wax, is a soft wax that is adhesive and pliable. It does not require additional heat and can be molded to most surfaces. This is the wax used to bead around trays to extend them and assist in patient comfort. This wax is also used for orthodontic patients to cover the brackets and uncomfortable areas until the cheeks and lips can adjust. It is supplied in long ropes or strips and in a number of colors.

Impression or Bite Registration Waxes

Normally containing copper or aluminum particles, impression waxes are used to take bite registrations. They are supplied in horseshoe shapes for obtaining the maxillary and mandibular biting surfaces.

Additional Waxes

Other waxes used in dentistry that are not in the three primary classifications are the study wax and the undercut wax. The study wax is hard wax supplied in blocks used for carving teeth and anatomy (Figure 35-50). Undercut wax is a putty-type wax used to fill in the undercuts prior to the impression being taken.

Custom Trays

The dentist may ask for a custom tray for the patient in order to obtain an accurate impression. This may be because a regular stock tray does not fit. The stock tray will not allow a minimum amount of space for the material to flow around the prepared area, or it may require that an overabundance of impression material be used to obtain the impression, therefore risking an inferior outcome. In any case, a custom tray can be fabricated to meet the need. Several materials are available to make a custom tray. It can be constructed from self- or light-curing acrylic resin, a vacuum resin, or a thermoplastic

FIGURE 35-50 Study wax blocks.

material. All materials must be rigid enough to provide subsistence for the material as it is inserted into and removed from the mouth. It is important that the material adapts well during the construction so that the final tray meets the required criteria.

Required Criteria for Custom Tray

- Stable enough to hold the material rigid during placement and removal
- Can be smoothed and contoured to the arch
- Can be adapted to an edentulous, a partially edentulous, and a full dentition
- Can be adapted to allow uniform thickness of impression material in all areas of the arch
- Can be altered and contoured to any irregular area
- Can be designed so that stops are in the spacer, therefore holding the material in a stable, specifically determined area, providing a more accurate impression

Acrylic Tray Resin Self-Curing Custom Trays

The most common material used to make custom trays is the self-curing acrylic tray resin (Procedure 35-14). It comes in a liquid catalyst (**monomer**) that mixes with a powder (**polymer**) to start the process of curing (polymerization). Polymerization occurs when material changes from a plastic pliable state to a rigid state. Once this process starts, it continues until the material is set completely. The material goes through several stages as it is cured. The first stage is after the liquid and the powder are mixed together. This initial set is when the material appears sticky and, if pulled apart, appears to have spider-web strands from particle to particle. The sec-

ond stage is where the material can be gathered into a ball, kneaded, and contoured to the model. The third stage is where the material goes through an exothermic reaction, giving off a great deal of heat while setting. When the heat has diminished and the material can no longer be shaped, the final set stage is completed. A custom tray should be allowed to set for twenty-four hours prior to use due to the fact that it is still dimensionally unstable.

Acrylic Tray Resin Light-Cured Custom Trays

Acrylic tray resin is supplied in light-cured custom trays. The primary difference between this material and the self-curing is that the setting time is operator controlled. The material stays pliable and workable until a light initiates polymerization. The polymerization process happens quickly. This technique requires special equipment: an oven-like appliance with a special curing light in it (Figure 35-51). The custom tray is designed and placed in the oven for a quick setting and then is ready for use.

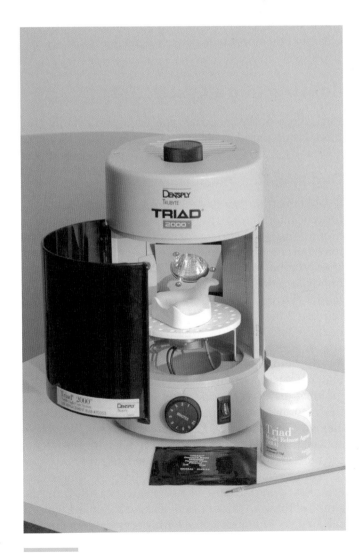

FIGURE 35-51 Triad® Visible Light Cure unit.

Vacuum-Formed Custom Trays

Like the acrylic tray resin that is light cured, the vacuum-formed custom trays require additional equipment (Procedure 35-15). This unit has a frame that holds the sheets directly under a heating element and, when they are softened, the frame drops the sheet onto the cast as vacuum pressure draws the material to the model. The vacuum-forming unit has other applications in dentistry. Acrylic resin sheets are supplied in several gauges for different applications. The custom tray requires the use of a rigid, heavy, plastic resin.

Thermoplastic Tray Material Custom Trays

Other materials used for making custom trays are the **thermoplastic** beads and buttons. When these small, round beads or buttons are placed in warm water, the thermoplastic reaction takes place. Thermoplastic means that the material becomes soft and pliable when exposed to heat. Once the material is soft, it can be conformed to the model in the desired shape. As the heat dissipates, the material hardens. It is easy to identify when the material is soft enough because it appears clear and then becomes dense when it hardens.

Constructing a Custom Tray

Regardless of the material type used, the custom tray model is prepared in the same manner.

Outlining Tray Margins

If a full custom tray is desired on an edentulous arch, draw a blue line at the bottom of the vestibule area around the facial surface, across the palate area on the maxillary model, around the posterior retromolar area, along the bottom of the vestibule area, and across the opposite posterior retromolar area on the mandibular model (Figure 35-52). From that first marking, make a red line 2 mm upward (toward the ridge). This gives a definite line to follow when adapting the spacer. A spacer is placed on the model to allow room in the tray for the impression material. This spacer normally is made of pink baseplate wax, but a commercial nonstick molding material may be used (especially when using the vacuum-formed custom tray because of the heating element) or a moist paper towel can be used. When the spacer is placed, the undercuts are filled in. Undercuts are recessed areas in the model that make it impossible to seat or remove the custom tray properly. Undercuts are caused by bubbles in the plaster, cavities, or the shape of the arch or dentition. If using baseplate wax for the spacer, it can be heated with warm water or butane torch (Figure 35-53) and conformed to the model. Cut it back to the red line in an angle-forming manner (see Procedure 35-14, Constructing Self-Cured Acrylic Resin

FIGURE 35-52 Tray margin is outlined on plaster or stone cast. The deepest area is marked in blue; 1 or 2 mm above this point, a red line indicating where wax spacer is to be located can be drawn.

FIGURE 35-53 Butane torch.

PROCEDURE 35-14

Constructing Self-Cured Acrylic Resin Custom Tray

This procedure is performed by the dental assistant in the dental laboratory on a working cast.

EQUIPMENT AND SUPPLIES

- Maxillary and/or mandibular casts
- Laboratory knife
- Pencil (plain or red and blue)
- Wax spatula
- Baseplate wax and heating source (warm water or laboratory torch)
- Tray resin with measuring devices
- Separating medium with brush
- Wooden tongue blade and wax-lined paper cup
- Petroleum jelly
- Tray adhesive

PROCEDURE STEPS *(Follow aseptic procedures)*

Preparing the Cast

1. Outline the area of the cast for the spacer to be placed (Figure 35-52). This is 2 to 3 mm below the margin of the prepared tooth or 2 to 3 mm above the lowest point in the vestibule if the arch is edentulous.

2. Fill any undercuts in the cast or cover with the spacer material. Heat the spacer material and contour to the pencil line.

3. Using a laboratory knife, trim the wax or spacer to the line using an angled cut instead of a blunt cut (Figure 35-54).

4. Cut the appropriate stops in the spacer (Figure 35-55).

5. Cover the spacer with aluminum foil or paint it with separating medium.

Mixing Custom Tray Acrylic Self-Curing Resin

1. Measure the powder and the liquid to the correct calibrations on the measuring devices according to the manufacturer's directions.

FIGURE 35-54 Wax spacer is trimmed to line on working cast.

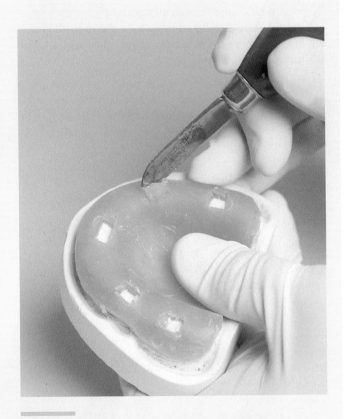

FIGURE 35-55 Stops cut into wax spacer allow room for impression material.

(continues)

PROCEDURE 35-14 *(CONTINUED)*

2. Mix the powder and liquid together in the wax-lined paper cup with the wooden tongue blade until **homogeneous** (uniformly mixed).

3. Allow the mixture to go through initial polymerization for two to three minutes. Some manufacturers indicate that a cover be placed over the material during the polymerization.

4. During this time, place petroleum jelly over the cast and on the palms of your hands.

Contouring Custom Tray Acrylic Self-Curing Resin

1. The material is ready to conform to the tray after the initial set when the material is no longer sticky and can be gathered into a ball. Knead the material to further mix the material and set a small amount aside for the handle (Figure 35-56). This doughy stage allows the material to be formed into a patty for the maxillary arch or a roll for the mandibular arch.

2. Place the dough-like patty for the maxillary cast, covering the wax spacer. Contour and adapt it to extend 1 to 2 mm over the wax spacer (Figure 35-57A). Try to complete the adaptation with a rolled edge at the designated area. If unable to accomplish this, a laboratory knife can be used to trim the material back. (Doing this causes rough edges that need to be smoothed back later.)

3. The material set aside for the handle is shaped and a drop of the monomer liquid placed on the tray where the handle is to be adapted and then on the handle

(A)

(B)

FIGURE 35-57 (A) Custom tray material is adapted to model over wax spacer. (B) Handle is attached to adapted custom tray.

where it will be placed on the custom tray. This allows the materials to join together for a better outcome.

4. Place the handle in the midline area of the arch (Figure 35-57B). If making an edentulous custom tray, the handle should come up from the ridge and then outward. A custom tray handle that is made for an area that has teeth can come directly outward.

5. Place the handle and hold it in the proper position until the material becomes firm.

Finishing Custom Tray Acrylic Self-Curing Resin

1. The setting takes about eight to ten minutes. Remove the custom tray from the cast and take out the spacer material.

2. If foil has been used, the cleaning will not take a great deal of time. If only wax was used, melt it. A wax spat-

FIGURE 35-56 Custom tray material is kneaded for use.

(continues)

PROCEDURE 35-14 *(CONTINUED)*

ula is used to remove it, along with hot water and an old toothbrush.

3. After the final set (thirty minutes minimum), use an acrylic bur (Figure 35-58) or an arbor band to trim the edges of the custom tray. Do not trim the inside of the tray.

FIGURE 35-58 Custom tray is trimmed with an acrylic bur.

4. Clean and disinfect the custom tray according to the manufacturer's directions. Write the patient's name on the tray.

5. Apply the adhesive provided by the manufacturer of the impression material to the inside of the custom tray and along the margins (Figure 35-59).

FIGURE 35-59 Adhesive is applied to custom tray in a thin coat and allowed to dry.

Custom Tray). This provides a smoother tissue side to the custom tray and is more comfortable to the patients than a blunt-edge cut. After the spacer is in place, take a warm plastic instrument to lute (secure) the edges of the wax to the cast. After the securing is accomplished, cut into the crest of the wax with a laboratory knife, making small rectangular or round holes. These stops (holes on the spacer that allow bumps to be formed on the tissue side of the tray) allow the tray to be seated 2 to 3 mm from the teeth or tissue and to prevent it from seating too deeply. This allows an adequate amount of impression material to flow around the prepared teeth or the tissue. There should be a minimum of four stops on an edentulous model, two on each first molar and cuspid area. When making a custom tray for crowns and bridges, the stops should be placed one tooth distal and mesial from the prepared tooth.

The self-curing material is exothermic. It heats up and causes the wax to melt slightly. It is advisable to place a layer of aluminum foil over the wax spacer and into the stops. The foil makes it easier to remove the wax from the tissue side of the tray after the custom tray is made. If foil is not used, a toothbrush and hot water will aid in getting the wax out of the inside (tissue side) of the custom tray.

After the cast is prepared, the custom tray material is mixed according to the manufacturer's directions and

formed to the cast. In the doughy stage, the maxillary material can be shaped into a patty and the mandibular can be rolled into a log shape prior to placing the materials on the cast. A handle can be made from the remaining material. It is placed on the anterior of the tray near the midline of the arch. It is secured by wiping the anterior area and the handle area that is to be attached with the resin liquid and then placing it on the custom tray. Because the handle is still soft when it is applied to the cast, it must be held in place until initially set up. Make sure the handle is large and strong enough to allow for leverage in placing and removing the custom tray from the mouth. Remember that the dentist will have his or her fingers and thumb on the handle while performing the procedure, so make sure it can be held easily. When working on edentulous custom trays, the handles should extend upward and outward from the model. If this is not done, the handle is placed so that it protrudes directly through the lip of the patient.

 When the exothermic reaction has completed and the model has cooled (about ten minutes), remove the spacer and evaluate the tray. The inside of the tray does not need to be smooth because the impression material covers this area. Any rough areas on the margins and on the outside of the tray can be smoothed for patient comfort. This can be accomplished by using an acrylic bur in a straight handpiece or with an arbor band on the laboratory lathe. Wear protective glasses when performing either of these trimming procedures. When completed, clean and disinfect the custom tray according to manufacturer's directions and place it in a barrier ready for patient use.

An adhesive is painted on the tissue side of the tray prior to taking the impression. It is normally applied in two coats. The first is allowed to dry and the second is placed ten minutes or so before the impression is taken. This secures the material to the custom tray. Some dentists may want holes placed in the custom tray to further lock the impression material into the tray. This can be accomplished by wearing protective glasses and using a straight handpiece with a round bur to penetrate the custom tray. Either or both techniques will secure the material into the custom tray.

Vacuum-Formed Tray

Trays that are vacuum formed can be used for a number of applications in the field of dentistry. Most often they are used for custom trays, bleaching trays, night guards, mouth guards, and matrices for provisionals. The material comes in several gauges and thicknesses for specific applications (Figure 35-60). Custom tray material is much more thick and rigid than the other applications. All use a vacuum former with a heating element, a cast, and material that can be heated and adapted through vacuum pressure.

FIGURE 35-60 Various vacuum-formed materials.

Temporary (Provisional) Restorations

After a tooth has been prepared for a crown and prior to the seating of the crown, a temporary restoration must be adapted and temporarily cemented on the tooth to protect it in the interim. These temporary

---

PROCEDURE 35-15

Constructing Vacuum-Formed Acrylic Resin Custom Tray

This procedure is performed by the dental assistant in the dental laboratory on a working cast.

EQUIPMENT AND SUPPLIES

- Maxillary and/or mandibular casts
- Laboratory knife
- Laboratory scissors
- Vacuum former with heating element
- Acrylic sheets

PROCEDURE STEPS *(Follow aseptic procedures)*

Preparing the Cast

1. The cast is soaked in warm water for up to thirty minutes prior to forming a custom tray on it. This eliminates small air bubbles. (These air bubbles coming to the surface [percolating] cause small spaces between the cast and the acrylic sheet. Then, the custom tray does not have the accuracy desired.)

2. Place the spacer, if indicated. (A wax spacer will melt under the heating element, if used.)

(continues)

PROCEDURE 35-15 (CONTINUED)

3. Mark the desired outer margin of the custom tray.

4. Place the cast on the platform of the vacuum-forming unit.

Contouring Acrylic Resin Sheets during Vacuum-Forming Process

1. Select the appropriate acrylic resin sheets to be used for the procedure.

2. Place the acrylic resin sheets between the heater frame and the gasket frame and tighten the anterior knob to secure the material in place. Place the cast on the platform (Figure 35-61).

3. Make sure the heating element is in the correct place above the acrylic resin sheet and turn it on.

4. Watch the resin as it heats. It will begin to sag downward (Figure 35-62). Allow this to continue until the resin droops downward about one inch. (Overheating causes air bubbles to form on the surface of the acrylic resin.)

5. After the material is heated properly, take both handles on the frame and pull the frame downward, over the cast. Only touch the handles because the entire area is extremely hot.

FIGURE 35-62 Resin sheet begins sagging as material is heated.

6. Turn on the vacuum immediately after the resin sheet is entirely over the cast (Figure 35-63).

7. Turn off the heating unit.

8. Allow the vacuum to continue for one to two minutes in order to cool the resin so it becomes firm again.

FIGURE 35-61 Resin sheets are secured in place, and cast is placed on platform of vacuum-forming unit.

FIGURE 35-63 When resin material has sagged 1 inch below holding ring, it is ready to be dropped into position over cast. The unit is held by handles to ensure that operator is not burned.

(continues)

PROCEDURE 35-15 (CONTINUED)

Finishing Vacuum-Formed Acrylic Resin Custom Tray

1. After the resin material is cooled, remove it from the vacuum form frame.

2. Separate the resin-formed custom tray from the cast and, using laboratory scissors, trim to the desired form (Figure 35-64).

3. Use a torch to heat and apply a cutout handle section to the custom tray.

4. Clean and disinfect the custom tray according to the manufacturer's directions and write the patient's name on it.

FIGURE 35-64 Vacuum form can be trimmed with scissors.

PROCEDURE 35-16

Sizing, Adapting, and Seating Aluminum Temporary Crown

This procedure is performed by the dentist or the dental assistant at the dental unit after tooth has been prepared for a crown.

EQUIPMENT AND SUPPLIES

- Maxillary and/or mandibular selection of aluminum temporary crowns (Figure 35-65)

- Millimeter ruler

- Basic setup: mouth mirror, cotton pliers, and explorer

- Crown and collar scissors

- Contouring pliers

- Acrylic or composite temporary material (optional)

- Sandpaper discs, rubber wheel, and mandrel

- Temporary cement, pad, and spatula

- Articulating paper

- Dental floss

FIGURE 35-65 Selection of Iso-Form temporary crowns. *(Courtesy of 3M Dental Products Division.)*

(continues)

PROCEDURE 35-16 *(CONTINUED)*

PROCEDURE STEPS *(Follow aseptic procedures)*

1. Measure the available space for the temporary crown from the mesial to distal with the millimeter ruler. This aids in the selection of a preformed crown having the appropriate mesial and distal contact.

2. Determine the correct crown to try in. The aluminum crown is for the correct tooth in the dentition and the size is chosen according to the measurement taken with the millimeter ruler. (Prevent cross-contamination while taking the crown from the container. Do not use contaminated instruments.) Any crown tried that does not fit must be sterilized before replacing it in the selection tray.

3. Try the selected crown on and check for mesial and distal width. The crown will be above the occlusal plane at this time.

4. The length of the crown is determined by placing the aluminum crown over the prepared tooth and using an explorer to mark the height (Figure 35-66). Another way to accomplish this is to scribe the tooth at the occlusal surface with an instrument where it aligns with the other teeth on the arch and then take that same amount off the gingival area. Either method shows that the margin of the gingival needs to be trimmed in order to fit.

5. Using a crown and collar scissors (with curved blades), trim the gingival margin. Crowns are never straight across the surface but are longer on the buccal and lingual margins. Use the rounded edges of the scissors to trim.

NOTE: Trimming a small amount at first allows refitting to further check the desired result (Figure 35-67). Taking too much off renders the crown useless. Making several trims to get the desired effect is a better method. Using the scissors in a continuous cutting action gives a much smoother surface. Avoid sharp, uneven edges that cause the patient discomfort around the gingival surface.

6. After the desired length is achieved, use the contouring pliers to invert the gingival edge in an inward manner. This crimping aids in the adaptation of the circumference edge of the aluminum crown to the finish line of the preparation.

7. Smoothing of the rough and jagged edges is accomplished through use of sandpaper discs and a rubber wheel. Check that all edges are smooth and polished (Figure 35-68).

8. Place the aluminum crown on the prepared tooth and check the occlusion with the articulating paper and the contacts with dental floss.

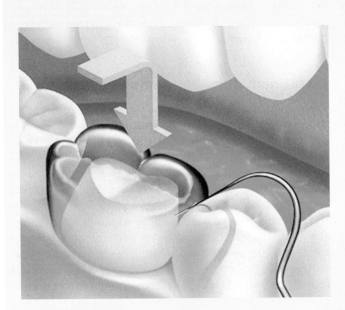

FIGURE 35-66 Explorer is used to establish height of temporary aluminum crown. *(Courtesy of 3M Dental Products Division.)*

FIGURE 35-67 Trimming aluminum crown with crown and collar scissors. *(Courtesy of 3M Dental Products Division.)*

PROCEDURE 35-16 (CONTINUED)

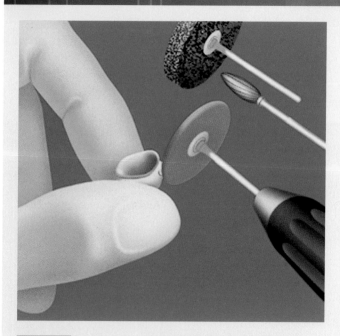

FIGURE 35-68 Smooth rough and jagged edges of temporary with rubber wheel. (Courtesy of 3M Dental Products Division.)

NOTE: If the contacts are weak, use a burnisher on the inside to extend the crown outward to get a better contact.

9. If an acrylic or a composite lining is used, the crown is filled with the material and placed on the prepared tooth. The patient is asked to bite into normal occlusion.

NOTE: The tooth may require light lubrication with petroleum jelly to avoid retention of the material.

The material sets according to manufacturer's directions and is then removed. Any excess material is polished away.

NOTE: Some operators prefer to do this step earlier in the procedure.

10. A final check for marginal fit, contour, and occlusion is done before cementation takes place.

---

restorations stabilize and protect the tooth for the two days to two weeks it takes to make the crown(s) or bridge(s).

Temporary Restoration Criteria

- Comfortable and esthetically acceptable to patient.
- Remains stable, with proper mesial and distal contacts and occlusal alignment, until permanent crown is cemented.
- Easily removed, without damaging tooth, when the permanent restoration is ready for placement.
- Fits snugly and accurately along prepared margin of the tooth. There is less than 0.05 mm of space between the temporary restoration and finish line of the margin.
- Contoured in a similar fashion to original tooth, therefore protecting gingiva from irritation and interproximal areas from food impaction.

Types of Temporary Restorations

Temporary restorations, also known as provisional restorations, can be made of a number of materials, both custom and preformed. In many states, the function of

fabricating and placing a temporary restoration is delegated to the dental assistant under the supervision of the dentist. Most offices use the preformed aluminum and acrylic crowns, along with the custom acrylic or composite crowns.

Preformed Aluminum Temporary Crowns

Preformed aluminum temporary crowns are supplied in different sizes and anatomic features. They are used on the posterior teeth because they lack esthetic value. Some are made without any anatomy and resemble thimbles with parallel straight sides and flat, occlusal surfaces. More contouring is necessary to adapt this model to the tooth. Others have anatomies similar to the natural teeth and are contoured much like stainless steel crowns. Both the crowns without anatomic features and the ones with anatomic features can be filled with acrylic or composite material to obtain a more custom fit prior to setting the temporary restorations in place over the prepared teeth.

Preformed Acrylic Temporary Crowns

Preformed acrylic or plastic temporary crowns are available in different sizes, shapes, and shades (Figure

PROCEDURE 35-17

Cementing the Aluminum Crown

This procedure is performed by the dentist or the dental assistant at the dental unit after the aluminum crown provisional has been prepared, sized, and contoured to prepared tooth.

EQUIPMENT AND SUPPLIES

- Fitted aluminum temporary
- Cotton rolls
- Temporary cementation material
- Mixing pad
- Plastic filling instrument
- Basic setup: mouth mirror, explorer, cotton pliers

PROCEDURE STEPS *(Follow aseptic procedures)*

1. The prepared tooth is rinsed and dried with cotton rolls in place.

2. The temporary cementation material, such as zinc oxide eugenol, is mixed with a spatula and placed in the aluminum crown.

3. The aluminum crown is placed in position over the prepared tooth and the patient is asked to bite in occlusion until the cement is set.

NOTE: Some operators like the patient to bite on a cotton roll over the aluminum crown while the cement sets.

4. After the cement is set, the excess is removed with an explorer.

5. The contacts are checked with floss and the margins are inspected to determine whether all excess cement has been removed and the crown fits correctly.

6. A final check for occlusion is done with articulating paper.

7. Instructions are given to the patient for care of the temporary aluminum crown.

35-69). The advantage of this type of crown is that it is more esthetically pleasing for anterior use. The plastic temporary crown is a form used to match the appropriate shape and contour of the tooth. It is filled with acrylic material and then removed. The preformed acrylic crowns have tabs on the incisal edge for easy placement. These tabs are removed prior to cementation. The preformed acrylic crowns are used more easily because they require little adjustment and can be seated immediately. One disadvantage is that they are shorter in length, or more closely trimmed to the optimum margin length of the prepared tooth. If a patient has had periodontal disease and the crown must be lengthened to cover any areas of recession, the clear-plastic crowns adapt better. They are supplied with longer "necks" on the crown for this purpose.

Custom Acrylic or Composite Temporary Restorations

When making custom acrylic or composite temporary restorations, a matrix is used. The matrix can be direct or indirect. A **matrix** is a form shaped in the pattern of

FIGURE 35-69 Preformed acrylic temporary crowns. *(Courtesy of Bosworth Co.)*

PROCEDURE 35-18

Sizing, Adapting, and Seating Preformed Acrylic Crown

This procedure is performed by the dentist or the dental assistant at the dental unit after the preformed acrylic provisional has been prepared, sized, and contoured to the prepared tooth.

EQUIPMENT AND SUPPLIES

- Maxillary and/or mandibular selection of acrylic temporary crowns

- Mirror, explorer, and cotton pliers

- Acrylic or composite temporary material (optional)

- Acrylic bur

- Temporary cement, pad, and spatula

- Articulating paper

- Dental floss

PROCEDURE STEPS *(Follow aseptic procedures)*

Preparing Preformed Acrylic Temporary Restoration

1. After the tooth has been prepared for a crown, a preformed acrylic temporary restoration is selected and adapted. Choose a crown that has enough width to contact on the adjacent teeth, is long enough to be in proper occlusion, and is the correct shade.

2. Retrieve this crown without cross-contaminating the other acrylic crowns. The tab at the incisal edge allows the operator to try the crown over the prepared tooth (Figure 35-70).

3. If necessary, adjustments are made with an acrylic bur. Polish with a rag wheel and pumice.

4. Take off the tag, place the crown, and check the occlusion with articulating paper.

5. Make adjustments, if necessary, and again polish the adjustment areas for a smooth surface for patient comfort.

Cementing Acrylic Provisional Crown

1. The prepared tooth is rinsed and dried with cotton rolls in place.

FIGURE 35-70 Acrylic crown is tried over prepared tooth, holding onto incisal tab. *(Courtesy of 3M Dental Products Division.)*

2. The temporary cementation material, such as zinc oxide eugenol, is mixed with a spatula and placed in the preformed acrylic crown.

3. The preformed acrylic crown is placed in position over the prepared tooth and the patient is asked to bite in occlusion or the operator holds the crown in place until the cement is set.

NOTE: Some operators like the patient to bite on a cotton roll over the preformed acrylic crown while the cement sets.

4. After the cement is set, the excess is removed with an explorer.

5. The contacts are checked with floss and the margins are inspected to determine whether all excess cement has been removed and whether the crown fits correctly.

6. A final check for occlusion is done with articulating paper.

7. Instructions are given to the patient for care of the temporary preformed acrylic crown.

the tooth prior to preparing the tooth (Figure 35-71). *Direct matrix techniques* (making the matrix directly from the tooth) uses alginate, impression material, freehand (block) technique, wax, thermo-forming beads, or a thermo-plastic button in the matrix. The *indirect matrix technique* (making the matrix on a model or cast) utilizes wax, a vacuum-formed shell, and thermo-forming bead and button matrices.

The alginate and impression materials render more anatomically accurate temporaries. The other materials meet the criteria for a temporary restoration form adequately and may prove to be less costly and more easily made. The utility wax is heated in warm water and then formed over the tooth or model to obtain the shape of the tooth and then cooled. Thermo-forming beads and buttons are heated in hot water and formed on the tooth prior to preparation or on a cast when using the indirect

matrix technique. The vacuum-formed shell is made on a vacuum unit using a cast covered with very thin sheets of acrylic resin. After it is heated, this sheet is cut to the desired size for use in making the temporary restoration.

Matrix Used for Direct Technique in Making Temporary Restorations

- Alginate impression
- Impression material
- Freehand (making a block of the material and covering the prepared tooth)
- Wax
- Thermo-forming beads or buttons

Matrix Used for Indirect Technique in Making Temporary Restorations

- Wax
- Thermo-forming beads or buttons
- Vacuum-formed shell

A custom acrylic or composite temporary restoration must have good proximal contacts, good occlusal contacts, good food deflection, and good marginal contours (Figures 35-72). Using the correct burs when making a temporary is essential. For making proper margins and contacts, use burs and discs (Figure 35-73) that have been developed specifically for this purpose, as the outcome of the temporary will be much more accurate.

Self-Cure Methyl Methacrylate. There are several categories of materials that achieve the desired outcome of a custom temporary restoration. Each material has advantages and disadvantages. One of the older materials that is routinely used is methyl methacrylate. The advantages of this material are that it has good physical properties, good esthetics, better color stability than the R′ methacrylates, and a lower cost. The disadvantages are the strong odor, high shrinkage, and high exothermic heat given off during the self-cure chemical setting.

Self-Cure R′ Methacrylate. The R′ (resin) methacrylates have one of the active ingredients, such as vinyl, ethyl, or isobutyl, in place of the methyl. In comparison to the methyl methacrylates, they have lower shrinkage and a lower level of exothermic heat given off during the self-cure chemical setting. They are similar in price per temporary, they are the weakest of the methacrylates, they have poor color stability, and they have the same strong odor that the methyl methacrylates have.

Both the methyl and the R′ methacrylates come in a powder and liquid form that is mixed together to form a creamy mix. After mixing, they are allowed to condition for approximately thirty seconds and then are placed in

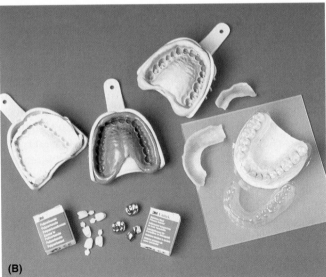

FIGURE 35-71 (A) and (B) Temporary matrices. *(Courtesy of 3M Dental Products Division.)*

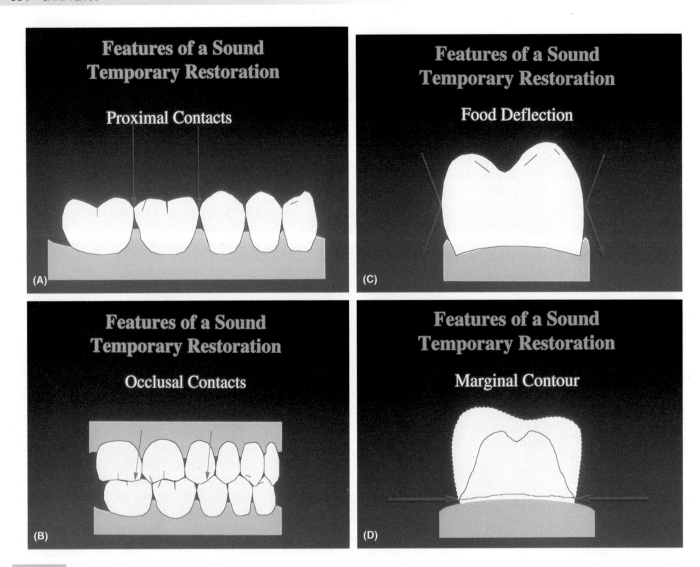

FIGURE 35-72 Criteria for custom acrylic or a composite temporary restoration. (A) Good proximal contacts. (B) Good occlusal contacts. (C) Good food deflection. (D) Good marginal contours. *(Courtesy of 3M Dental Products Division.)*

FIGURE 35-73 Provisional bur kit used when trimming temporary restorations.

the matrix. A dull surface appears on the top of the material, and it is placed in the mouth over the prepared tooth and held in place for the initial set. It has a rubber appearance at this time. Most manufacturers suggest that the material be taken off and on the prepared tooth during the time of four to six minutes. This is when the exothermic heat is the greatest. The excess can be trimmed off easily with scissors during this time. The final set is from six to eight minutes, and the material becomes hard plastic. The range of setting time from start to finish is from eight to ten minutes for the materials in these two groups. Many of the newer materials are completed in half the time. The temporary restorations are removed from the matrix and trimmed with an acrylic bur to the desired shape and size.

After the temporary has been trimmed, it is polished with pumice and a rag wheel. Some of the materials in this category come with glazes. This glaze is applied

PROCEDURE 35-19

Adapting, Trimming, and Seating Matrix and Custom Temporary Restoration

This procedure is performed by the dentist or the dental assistant at the dental unit after tooth has been prepared for a crown.

EQUIPMENT AND SUPPLIES

- Basic setup: mouth mirror, explorer, and cotton pliers
- Thermo-plastic buttons/hot water (one possible option for use in making a matrix)
- Composite temporary material
- Diamond bur
- Temporary cement, pad, and spatula
- Articulating paper
- Dental floss

PROCEDURE STEPS *(Follow aseptic procedures)*

Making Thermo-Forming Matrix before Tooth Preparation

1. Place the thermo-forming matrix buttons in hot water (one button per prepared tooth).

2. Allow the white color of the button to become clear. When that takes place, the material is pliable and able to be adapted.

3. Adapt the material over the tooth and tightly conform it to the tooth area and slightly below the gingival.

4. When the material cools (air can be used to make this more rapid), the matrix appears white and firm. Remove the matrix from the area and set it aside (Figure 35-74).

Preparing Custom Temporary Restoration

1. After the tooth has been prepared for a crown, coat the teeth with a light application of petroleum jelly.

2. If using the composite self-curing temporary material in two tubes, dispense on the paper pad by holding tubes at a 45° angle.

3. Rotate the end-dispensing handle of the base until a click is heard. (The base is the larger of the two tubes. The smaller of the two holds the catalyst and has two

FIGURE 35-74 Matrix is removed.

dispensing ends.) Rotate the end-dispensing handle of the catalyst. Two small amounts are expelled. Each click of the dispensing handle is enough material for one temporary.

4. If a shade is being used, mix it with the base. If a mottled effect is desired, mix the shade after the base and catalyst are mixed together.

5. Mix the material together to obtain a creamy substance (about thirty seconds).

6. Place the material in the matrix.

7. Place the matrix over the prepared tooth (manipulation time is about one and one-half minutes).

8. Hold it in place in the mouth for two minutes.

9. Remove it from the mouth and set it aside for two minutes.

10. Remove the crown or bridge from the matrix (Figure 35-75). The additional curing time takes one minute. There are seven minutes total time from start to finish of the set.

11. Remove the greasy layer with alcohol or any other organic solvent.

12. Trim with a diamond or an acrylic bur (Figure 35-76).

13. Check the contacts with dental floss.

(continues)

PROCEDURE 35-19 *(CONTINUED)*

14. Check occlusion by having patient bite on articulating paper.

FIGURE 35-75 Remove acrylic bridge from matrix. *(Courtesy of 3M Dental Products Division.)*

15. Check margins with explorer and mirror.

FIGURE 35-76 Trim temporary restoration.

PROCEDURE 35-20

Cementing Custom Self-Curing Composite Temporary Crown

This procedure is performed by the dentist or the dental assistant at the dental unit after the temporary restoration has been prepared and is ready to be cemented in place, over the prepared tooth.

EQUIPMENT AND SUPPLIES

- Basic setup: mouth mirror, explorer, and cotton pliers
- Cotton rolls
- Temporary luting cement
- Paper pad
- Mixing spatula
- Plastic filling instrument
- Dental floss

PROCEDURE STEPS *(Follow aseptic procedures)*

1. The prepared tooth is rinsed and dried with cotton rolls in place.

2. The temporary cement material is mixed with a spatula and placed in the custom composite temporary crown.

3. The temporary crown is placed in position over the prepared tooth and the patient is asked to bite in occlusion or the operator will hold the crown in place until the cement is set.

NOTE: Some operators like the patient to bite on a cotton roll over the preformed acrylic crown while the cement sets.

(continues)

PROCEDURE 35-20 *(CONTINUED)*

4. After the cement is set, the excess is removed with an explorer (Figure 35-77). Make sure that a fulcrum is used so that if the explorer slips, it does not go into the sulcus and cause tissue trauma. If feeling unsure with this skill, position the explorer so that the point is facing away from the tissue during removal of the cement.

5. The contacts are checked with floss and the margins are inspected to determine whether all excess cement has been removed and whether the crown fits correctly.

6. A final check for occlusion is performed with articulating paper.

7. Instructions are given to the patient for care of the temporary preformed acrylic crown.

FIGURE 35-77 Temporary is placed and excess cement is removed.

after the polishing and allowed to dry for five minutes before the temporary is cemented.

Self-Cure Composite Material. Materials in the category of self-cure composite are double the price of the methacrylates. They are much stronger materials because they are made as composites and not plastics. They do not have the odor, the shrinkage, or the exothermic reaction during setting, and they have excellent color stability.

Materials in this category come in two pastes. They are supplied in either two tubes or in a cartridge that fits into extruding guns with auto mixing tips. Both the tubes and the cartridge tips must remain clean and flowing to obtain the correct dispensed amount of the material. If they become clogged with old material, use an explorer to clear the old material out. Dispense a small, pea-shaped amount on the pad before beginning to ensure that everything is working properly.

The material is placed in the matrix and over the prepared tooth for up to two minutes. During the rubber stage (from four to six minutes), it is removed from the mouth to complete curing. The total time from start to finish for this material classification is up to seven minutes. After the material is set, the surface has a greasy layer due to the oxygen in the air, which can be removed with alcohol or any other organic solvent. The trimming is done with a diamond bur and no polish is necessary.

If additional material is required on the temporary, light-cured composite or flowable resin repair can be used and trimmed accordingly.

Multi-cured Temporary Materials. Several multi-cured temporary materials are on the market. They have extended working time in the rubbery stage and improved operator control because they can be light cured on demand. They have good strength and are higher in cost. Some of the materials in this group are methacrylates and some are composites having the characteristics of the self-curing materials. The biggest advantage of this group is light-curing control, which allows for a quicker set and unlimited setting time.

CHAPTER SUMMARY

A number of basic functions in the dental laboratory are routinely performed by the dental assistant, such as pouring and trimming study models, fabricating custom trays, and fabricating provisional temporaries. To accomplish these procedures, the dental assistant must understand the materials that are used, the properties of each material, and the steps in each procedure. Any dental assistant who has skills in performing laboratory duties will be an asset to his or her employer. The better crossed-trained the dental team members are, the better the dental office functions.

Case Study

Patrick Norman came into the dental office and wanted to talk to the doctor about a space in the anterior region of his maxillary teeth. After Dr. Smith completed a clinical examination, he asked the dental assistant to make diagnostic casts for further study. After talking to Patrick, the dental assistant found that Patrick has difficulty when anything is placed in his mouth and that gagging is a problem.

Case Study Review

1. What can the dental assistant do to help Patrick with the gagging problem while taking impressions for the diagnostic casts?

2. What material is used routinely for obtaining preliminary impressions?

3. Would the fast or regular set be more beneficial in this case?

4. Which arch would be taken first? Why?

REVIEW QUESTIONS

Multiple Choice

1. If an impression loses water content due to heat, dryness, or exposure to air, the condition is known as
   a. imbibition.
   b. syneresis.
   c. distortion.
   d. acceleration.

2. A final impression material that uses water-cooled trays is
   a. polysiloxane.
   b. polysulfide.
   c. reversible hydrocolloid.
   d. silicone.

3. The broad group title that encompasses the hard waxes used in crown and bridge casting (inlay wax) is
   a. pattern.
   b. processing.
   c. impression.
   d. study wax.

4. The liquid catalyst for the self-curing acrylic tray resin is a
   a. polymer.
   b. thermoplastic.
   c. monomer.
   d. spacer.

5. The strongest temporary (provisional) restoration is the
   a. aluminum shell temporary.
   b. self-cure methyl methacrylate temporary.
   c. self-cure R′ (resin) methacrylate temporary.
   d. self-cure composite temporary.

6. Storage bath temperature for the hydrocolloid unit is
   a. 110° F.
   b. 212° F.
   c. 150° F.
   d. 120° F.

7. Trays used for reversible hydrocolloid unit are
   a. disposable.
   b. water cooled.
   c. perforated.
   d. rim locked.

8. Trays used for irreversible hydrocolloid are
   a. water cooled.
   b. perforated.
   c. rim locked.
   d. b and c.

9. The final impression material that smells like sulfur is
   a. polysulfide.
   b. polyether.
   c. polysiloxane.
   d. silicone.

10. The highest-strength type of gypsum material is
    a. Type I.
    b. Type II.
    c. Type III.
    d. Type IV.

Critical Thinking

1. Name several types of final impression materials and identify factors that affect usage with each.

2. What are the effects of lower water-to-powder ratio in a mixture of irreversible hydrocolloid?

3. What are some of the advantages of polyether impression material?

Web Activities

1. Go to http://www.dentsply.com and review the product catalog for new products. Be prepared to discuss new products in class.

2. Go to http://www.bosworth.com, access techniques, and find the technique for Ultra Trim. Is this technique different from the one discussed in the book under temporary restorations? Compare and contrast information about each.

DENTAL PRACTICE MANAGEMENT

DENTAL OFFICE MANAGEMENT

SPECIFIC INSTRUCTIONAL OBJECTIVES

The student should strive to meet the following objectives and demonstrate an understanding of the facts and principles presented in this chapter:

1. Identify the dental office staff and their areas of responsibility.

2. Identify marketing ideas for dentistry.

3. Outline the proper procedure for answering an incoming call.

4. Describe the information every message should contain.

5. Describe telephone and business office technology and its uses.

6. Give examples of the ways in which computers are used in the dental office.

7. Explain how database management concepts can be used in the dental office.

8. Explain why ergonomics is important at a computer workstation.

9. Explain ways in which effective patient scheduling can be accomplished in the dental office.

10. Identify the equipment needed for record management.

11. Define key terms related to accounts receivable.

12. Identify computerized and manual systems for management of patient accounts.

13. Identify accounts payable expenses that the dental practice is responsible for.

KEY TERMS

OUTLINE *(continued)*

KEY TERMS *(continued)*

INTRODUCTION

The dental reception area needs to be an environment in which all patients feel welcome and comfortable. Dentists have worked long and hard to overcome the negative image of dentistry prevalent in the past. Today, dentistry can be a positive experience, and the dental treatment can be pain free. Many dentists have hired interior design consultants and space-planning advisors to aid the practice in developing an area that is inviting and pleasant for the patients. Some offices have themes while others are designed to be like warm, comfortable, home atmospheres. The creation of this area requires not only appealing colors, but a staff that greets patients with smiles and makes them feel welcome.

Reception Area

 The reception area is a place where patients are received (Figure 36-1). Calling it a waiting room gives it a negative connotation—patients are busy and their time is important and they do not want to wait. The colors, design, and artwork should be relaxing and adequate, and comfortable seating should be available so that each patient can have his or her own space. Keep in mind that individuals from different cultures have varying personal space requirements. The seating should be arranged in a way that allows people to cluster together or remain distant from others.

Have magazines containing short stories so that the patients can read while they are waiting. The magazines should be current. An office that has out-of-date magazines shows indifference to the patient, and it reflects negatively on overall care. Many dentists have brochures and pamphlets related to the procedures performed in the office. This is also an area in which to

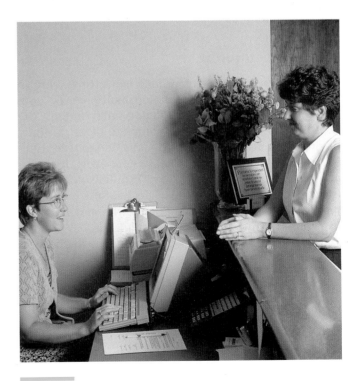

FIGURE 36-1 The reception area, where the patient first encounters the dental office, should be a welcoming environment.

display marketing materials. Some offices also have photo albums showing each staff member and his or her family. Patients like to feel that they can get to know staff members who are taking care of them. Some dental offices have areas where patients can relax with a beverage (coffee and juice).

Reception area requirements may change as the practice grows. In 1990, the **Americans with Disabilities Act** was passed by Congress. It mandated that individuals with disabilities have access to health care facilities having more than fifteen employees. Even though most dental offices have fewer than fifteen employees, access for all patients is still the goal. All doors and hallways should be wide enough for wheelchair access, and a ramp should be available in areas where stairs are present and no elevator is available.

The overall appearance and initial feeling obtained from the reception area should give the patients a feeling of well-being and confidence. The patients may not consciously realize the message that is being received, but the dental office should present an atmosphere that relieves feelings of anxiety.

Dental Receptionist and Business Office Staff

Front office staff has changed dramatically in recent years. One person used to greet patients and perform all the paperwork for the office. That no longer is the case due to the increased demand for skills that front office personnel are required to perform.

Dental Receptionist

The receptionist in a dental office needs to be able to organize time efficiently and handle multiple tasks concurrently. While constantly being interrupted, the receptionist must be able to complete tasks on time, paying close attention to details. The dental receptionist must be able to communicate effectively, listen to and observe patients, and serve as a liaison between the patient and office staff. This mature individual must be able to respond to patients who may be upset in a calm, tactful, and appropriate manner.

The receptionist is normally responsible for, but not limited to, the following tasks:

- Greeting patients
- Assisting patients in filling out initial paperwork required for treatment
- Answering the telephone and taking messages as necessary
- Scheduling appointments
- Maintaining patient chart system and records

Dental Office Bookkeeper

The dental office bookkeeper might be the same person as the dental office receptionist, or another individual, depending on the size of the office. This person must pay close attention to detail. All office finances are handled by this person, including **accounts receivable**, the money owed to the practice, and **accounts payable**, the money the office owes to others. These finances are normally handled in two separate bookkeeping systems. This individual may also handle patient dental insurance and make financial arrangements with the patients for payment of the dental service. The inventory and supply system may also be handled by this individual. This person must be organized, have a knowledge of dental treatments, and exhibit good communication and problem-solving skills. These tasks may be shared with other individuals, such as the dental receptionist, depending on the size of the practice. All individuals in the front office need to be knowledgeable using business machines, such as computers, faxes, and copy machines.

Dentistry Marketing

Even though the first priority of the office team is to care for patients' dental needs, this cannot be accomplished when patient numbers are inadequate. A dental office is a business as well as a health care facility. Marketing is a means of attracting and retaining patients who are satisfied with the practice. Dental assistants, along with all members of the dental team, need to be involved in marketing the practice. It can be rewarding for members of the dental team to use effective efforts in attracting patients to the practice, whether through external or internal methods.

Even in off hours, a dental assistant is still associated with the dentist with whom he or she is employed. When people ask what your occupation is, it provides an opportunity to do external marketing for the practice. Other planned external activities can be done, such as dental health education in the community, schools, and centers. Professionalism and enthusiasm enhance any marketing attempts.

Internal marketing can be accomplished in a number of ways. One person or the whole staff can participate. The ideas are limitless, but the following are suggestions:

- Monthly newsletters with tips for dental health
- Timed giveaways, such as teddy bears for children, and gift certificates for teens (CDs) and adults (dinners)
- Flowers distributed at every appointment or sent to patients for referral thank-yous
- Birthday greetings or cards for special occasions, such as new baby, anniversary, and graduation

- Bulletin board with patient pictures on it (for example, the good hygiene club)
- Map of the world with postcards from patients
- Special dental services coupons
- Bulletin board showing photos of patients flossing while on vacation and in various locations throughout the world
- Refrigerator magnets noting the dental office and phone number

Keep in mind that the goal of marketing is to attract new patients to the practice and retain current patients. Go that "extra mile" to make patients comfortable. Treat them with dignity every time they are in the office.

U.S. Postal Service

The U.S. Postal Service (USPS) has numerous ideas and plans for small businesses. Currently, the USPS has an online service that allows payment and receiving of bills at no cost for three months, and a small fee after that. This service can be used from any Web-enabled personal computer (PC). This service contains an online checkbook with an online payment history and e-mail bill reminder. The USPS can send certified mail through their online services. This allows the convenience of the Internet and the office is still able to have a hard copy of the mail. **Certified mail** gives the sender confirmation of delivery. Before the online services, the sender would send a copy and the mailperson would have the person receiving the mail sign for it. The copy was then given to the sender for the sender's records. Another service of the USPS is to send greeting cards and postcards, which are especially good for marketing. In addition, stamps can be purchased online. The dental office bookkeeper or office manager may want to check the services that the USPS offers to track mailing expenses and expand marketing. The Web site address for the USPS is http://www.usps.com.

USPS Services

As noted, there are many USPS services that a small business like a dental office can use, including:

- Certificate of mailing, which is a receipt showing that an item was mailed.
- Certified mail, which gives the sender a mailing receipt at the time of mailing and online access to the date and time of delivery. It also provides the recipient's signature at the delivery time.
- Collect on delivery (COD), which is when the mailer wants to collect payment when the merchandise is delivered.

- Delivery confirmation, which is an online service that verifies the delivery date, location, and time.
- Insured mail, which is like an insurance coverage that is purchased when the mailer sends the items.
- Registered mail, the most secure type of mail, which ensures the protection of important mail.
- Restricted delivery, which is when the mail is delivered only to the specified individual.
- Return receipt, which gives the sender proof of delivery.

Telephone Technique

The telephone may be the first contact the patient has with the office, and it sets the stage for the kind of care the person can expect to receive. The first impression tends to be a lasting one. Make sure that the tone of voice and message substance are informational and welcoming to the caller. Handle the call in the same manner as in meeting the patient face to face. Posture and the way the body is carried, along with attitude through facial expressions, are carried through the telephone line to the patient. If the telephone is answered by an individual who is slumped over, leaving the diaphragm constricted, it may be interpreted on the other end as being tired or frustrated. Correct posture allows an individual to sound alert and more professional. Attitude is "heard" by the patients over the phone. Never forget that the patients who are calling are not interrupting work but the reason that the job exists. Some reception areas have mirrors placed in front of the phone so that anyone answering can look at the expression on his or her face and be reminded of the importance of communicating a good attitude to the caller.

Answer the telephone in a manner that depicts pleasure that the individual called the office. Speak clearly and distinctly, identify the dental practice and yourself, and ask, "How can I help you?" Then, listen carefully. Personality and attitude sparkle through the telephone or come out flat and drab.

Basic Telephone Techniques

- No food or drink while on the telephone.
- Answer within two or three telephone rings.
- Smile because the patient can "hear your smile."
- Speak directly into the mouthpiece; keep it no more than one and one-half inches away.
- Use the same volume you would use if speaking to the person directly.
- Enunciate, speak clearly, and articulate carefully.
- Speak at a normal rate of speed.

- Pronounce the words correctly.
- Always use telephone **etiquette** (good manners).
- Get the caller's name and use it during the conversation.
- Listen carefully.
- Allow the caller to end the call.

Call Types

Several types of calls come into the dental office. They all should be handled in a professional manner. Some of the calls are more critical for patient care than others.

Answering Calls

A receptionist must be prepared to answer the incoming calls, at any time, while juggling the other responsibilities of the front desk. It is crucial that the caller feel that he or she has the total attention of the receptionist. Good listening and communication skills help portray an image of an organized, efficient, and courteous dental office. The receptionist must be able to listen carefully to the caller and make judgments after gathering information that will aid in the patient's care. It may be necessary to *screen* the calls to get the caller in touch with the right person to solve the problem. Patients may ask to speak to the dentist. The receptionist must first try to help, identify the patient's concern, and take a telephone number where the doctor can call back. Give the caller an idea of when to expect the call from the dentist. The dental receptionist must ensure that the dentist's time is managed efficiently. Most dentists prefer not to be interrupted at chairside while caring for another patient. With infection control concerns, the chance of being inconsiderate to the current patient, and the delay in patient treatment and a day's schedule, it is important not to disrupt the dentist with a telephone call. Some dentists will take calls from another dentist, the dental laboratory technician needing an answer to further a case, and/or family members. Know your doctor's policies in regard to taking incoming phone calls. Handle the calls with tact by saying something such as, "The doctor is with a patient. Can I help you?"

Placing Callers on Hold

If it becomes necessary to place the caller on hold and handle emergent situations or answer another phone line, ask the patient if he or she would mind holding for a minute and then listen to the answer. One of the rudest ways to handle patients on the telephone is by asking, "Can you hold?," then, without waiting, push the hold button and cut the patient off.

The caller should never have to wait any longer than one minute on hold. If necessary, check in and ask whether the caller would like to continue to hold or whether it would be more convenient to receive a call back. Handle on-hold calls in this manner and the patients will know that their time is being respected and their needs facilitated as soon as possible. Some offices have one-minute timers by the telephone to remind the receptionist of the person waiting and how long he or she has been on the other line. Do what is necessary to get back to the person on hold or that patient may be lost to the practice.

Taking Messages

When taking messages, be thorough. It is advisable to use standard telephone message pads with carbon so that the office can retain copies of all messages. Record and ask the caller the following information:

- Date and time the call was received
- Name and telephone number of the caller
- Who the message is for
- Message and urgency of the telephone call
- What action is required
- A good time to return the call
- The receptionist's initials or name in case the person receiving the messages has questions

After the message is written, repeat it to the caller to verify that it was written correctly. Give the caller an approximate time when to expect the return call to be placed.

Outgoing Calls

When telephone calls are made from the office, the same professional, positive approach should be followed. Be prepared and know the information that needs to be conveyed or sought. Most offices call the next day's patients to confirm their appointments. Performing this tedious task requires attention. More than one receptionist has called a patient to confirm the appointment and totally forgotten which individual was dialed. Use some type of indication system to keep track of which patients have been called. If calling an insurance company, have all the information, including the patient's chart and forms, handy so that any questions that come up can be answered readily.

If calling and leaving a message, take care with any information recorded on the answering machine. Remember that all health care issues are confidential and should be discussed only with the patient. Try not to leave the information with small children, because the information can become confusing and get passed on to the adult inaccurately.

It is best if no personal telephone calls are made at the office. If the need arises, make them during your lunch hour, if possible. The telephone is for dental office business, and personal matters belong outside the office.

Long-Distance Calls

Dental office assistants normally use direct-dial telephone calling for long-distance calls. This means that the number is dialed directly into the telephone and not placed through the operator. Most of the long-distance calls are made to insurance carriers to verify patient coverage or to follow up on payments. It is important to be aware of the location of the call and plan ahead according to the time zone (Pacific, Mountain, Central, and Eastern) (Figure 36-2). Keep in mind that there is a three-hour difference from one zone on the Pacific coast to the other time zone on the Atlantic coast.

English as a Second Language

 It is probable in the dental office to encounter many patients whose primary language is not English. The dentist is responsible for providing an interpreter, if necessary, for communication. Some patients bring family members who speak English to translate. It is important that communication on the telephone and in the office be handled in a manner that provides the patient with the pertinent information. Things to remember when speaking to patients whose first language is not English follow:

- Be patient.
- Speak at a normal volume. Raising the voice does not increase the other person's ability to understand the words.
- Speak more slowly, if necessary, and avoid complicated words.

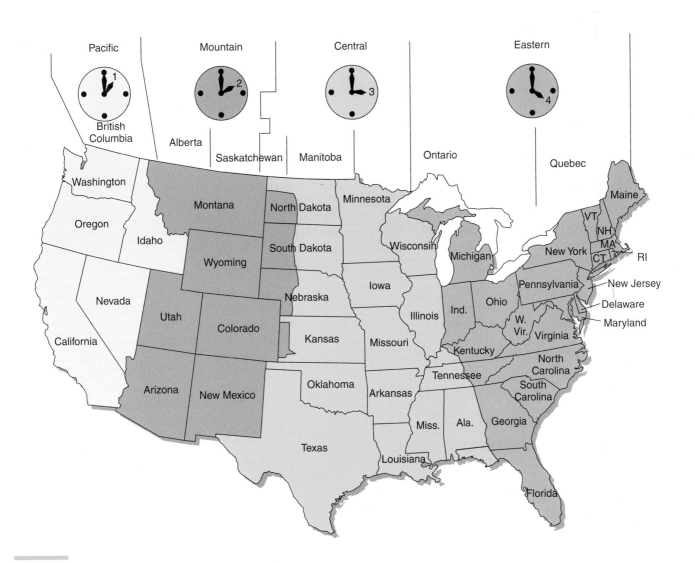

FIGURE 36-2 Pacific, Mountain, Central, and Eastern time zones.

- A patient who does not speak English may be able to understand English well. Do not assume that the patient does not comprehend what is being said.
- Ask the patient if clarification is needed.
- Repeat the information, if necessary, until understood.

Telephone and Business Office Technology

Most offices have multifunctional telephones. Normally, the telephones have a minimum of three lines and hold buttons. Spend time understanding functions so that if transfers are done, the patient is not lost. Spend time thoroughly learning the entire system. All telephone calls become a great expense to the dental office. Do research into the best service available at the most economical price. Check the statements and identify the highest-cost items, then contact the telephone services and tell them the office's needs. Service employees are happy to discuss current packages. Advances in telecommunications have a tremendous impact on dental office communication, so stay informed.

Answering Systems. Dental offices need to provide a way for patients to contact them in the event of an emergency. Answering machines are commonplace today, and patients have grown to accept them. They are not replacements for a live person answering but can be utilized to give patients emergency telephone numbers and information. Many offices use answering systems that are turned on each evening when the dentist and staff leave for the day and during lunch hour, staff meetings, and seminars. These systems are checked promptly each morning for messages and turned off during the day.

It is the responsibility of the receptionist to record the message on the answering machine and check frequently for messages. With heavy usage, the taped message may become difficult to understand. The receptionist should call the number occasionally to check that the message being received by the patients is acceptable. The phone message reflects the dental office and, like all other aspects, it is important that the recording is clear and of good quality.

Answering Services. Many offices have opted for answering services that are staffed by live operators. Having a person at the other end of the line is more reassuring to patients and other callers. These services also can provide flexibility in screening and routing calls. Most of the fees for the answering services are by the month or by the number of calls placed. This service is more expensive than that of an in-office answering machine.

Voice Mail. If working at a large group practice, a voice-mail or automated routing unit may be used. This system answers the call, and a recorded voice identifies choices for the caller to pick by pressing a specific number on a touch-tone telephone. Some of the automated routing systems have mailboxes for the caller to leave a message for the person being called. All the messages are done by a recorded voice. Some patients who are not familiar with a system like this can become frustrated by it, especially elderly patients who may have more difficulty hearing the directions. Some offices provide information sheets to patients to clarify the telephone options available with this type of system.

Fax Machines. Fax machines are common in the dental office. A fax is a facsimile transmission used to send and receive written messages through the telephone lines. It can contain typed or written data, pictures, and line art. It is important that it be sent to the correct address, taking care that confidential information be handled conscientiously. The fax is used to relay information to and from patients and insurance companies and to order dental supplies, among other things.

Electronic Mail (E-mail). Electronic mail (e-mail) is another form of communication done through the telephone lines via a computer. It is for sending, receiving, storing, and forwarding messages in digital form. It can be very convenient and saves time. A person can send a message to an electronic mailbox and the receiver reads it at a convenient time and responds, if necessary, by pushing the respond notation, typing the reply, and pushing send. Many of the new systems identify whether the person received and read the message that was sent. It is a great way to send inter-office memos to personnel in other areas. It also can be programmed to send the same message to a group of people.

It is possible to subscribe to on-line services that allow information to be transmitted around the world through the World Wide Web. These services also feature bulletin boards that are an electronic method of exchanging information publicly. Information regarding medical research and new treatment techniques can be found on the Internet.

Cellular Phones and Services. Patients, dentists, and staff members may use cellular phones routinely for communication. The person who owns the cellular phone pays for the time the call takes, even if that individual did not place the call. Cellular phone usage is more expensive than using traditional telephone lines. If a patient gives a cell phone number to the office, verify that he or she does not mind receiving a call on that phone and be mindful to keep the messages brief and to the point.

Paging Systems. Another telecommunication option available is a pager, or "beeper." Medical personnel have used the paging systems for years, and now they are available to individuals at a reasonable cost. The pagers are not as convenient as a cellular telephone, because they are one-way communication systems. The pager does have several options available:

- A beep or vibration to notify the person to call a designated phone number

- Voice alert in which the person hears the message from the caller along with a number

- Digital message display in which the receiver scrolls it out and reads it

Business Office Systems

 Historically, business office systems were manual, but today most offices have **computerized systems** (units of computer parts that function together to perform a particular task) of some sort. The office staff may choose to do only one or more aspects of the office business on a manual system. In today's fast-paced dental office, time and efficiency are important. Computers reduce the time involved in many routine office procedures. Once the dental assistant becomes familiar with the computer software and applications, he or she will find more and more uses for the computer. The responsibility of picking the correct **hardware** (computer physical equipment) and **software** (computer program or set of instructions that tells the hardware what to do) for the office may fall on the dental office manager or receptionist. Research the options available and know what is needed from the system. Talk to other office personnel about the systems they are using and the pros and cons of each system. Work with a trusted and knowledgeable vendor who understands the needs of the practice before purchasing a system.

After the research is completed, bring it to the staff members for their input. It is important that all the staff members be familiar with the system. It takes a great deal of time to convert all the information to the new system and staff training will be necessary, so it is best if everyone is involved in the process. Make sure the system that is purchased allows for expansion. Most dental offices purchase the microcomputers in the format of desktop PCs (Figure 36-3).

Common Dental Office Software

A variety of software applications are available for use in the dental office. Choose the software that meets the office's needs. It should have general-purpose software that includes word processing, graphics, spreadsheets, database, and on-line communication programs.

Word Processing. Word processing has largely replaced typing. It allows the user to type memos, letters and reports and to make corrections easily. Word processing software allows for spelling checks, deletions, cut and paste information, and much more. The documents can be stored for use at a later time and changed slightly for a different application. Typing a letter has been made much easier via the computer and word processing software.

Graphics. With the use of graphic software, numeric information can be transformed into graphs, pie charts, and bar graphs (Figure 36-4). This allows the informa-

FIGURE 36-3 The traditional desktop personal computer comes in various sizes and types.

tion to be summarized in a graphic format for easy visualization. Popular integrated packages of graphic software are Microsoft Works and Lotus Works. The dental software may allow usage with one of these possible systems.

Spreadsheets. Spreadsheets are the computerized format of the worksheets with calculations preprogrammed. Spreadsheets take numbers and electronically calculate the data to be analyzed. This calculation and recalculation that used to take hours is completed in seconds with spreadsheet software. Spreadsheets are used in the dental office to prepare monthly and yearly financial statements and accounts payable, along with other uses. The data from a spreadsheet can be converted to a graph or chart, therefore presenting information that can be interpreted at a glance.

Database Management

To organize large quantities of related data into useful forms, computer database management software is used. The office can design the basic database that would be beneficial to the practice. The general identifying information that is minimally required includes:

- Patient's name
- Spouse's name and/or other family members
- Patient's address

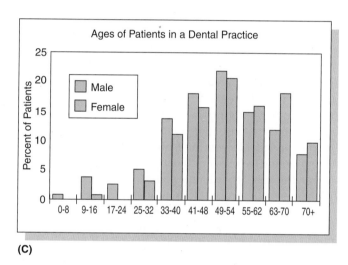

FIGURE 36-4 Graphs and charts make information easier to interpret. (A) Line graph. (B) Pie chart. (C) Bar graph.

- Patient's home phone number
- Patient's work phone number
- Patient's insurance

Most office database systems have information about the patient and spouse, the patient's insurer, Social Security number, patient's date of birth, primary care physician, phone number, type of insurance, identification of the insurance carrier or carriers, place of employment, and occupation. The patient's recall date can be placed in the computer with the other information.

Once the information is in the computer database, the information can be used with the word processor, graphs, or spreadsheets. This information can be grouped in a number of ways. For example, an office could identify all the patients who have birthdays in the current month and send birthday cards to them, or all the new patients could be identified so that welcome letters could go out to them. A large number of applica-

tions are beneficial to the dental practices both in marketing and collecting data.

Computer Safety

Use computer virus protection to protect the office system if there is any chance that the office downloads information from the Internet or accepts files from other computer systems. Everything could be lost if unprotected. Most offices download the files daily to make sure that a backup document is available if the system "crashes." Even if the possibility of losing the data is remote, it takes a great deal of time to reconstruct the system if this happens. Always have a back-up document or file or disk.

Computer Ergonomics and Eye Care. For those individuals who spend a great deal of time on the computer, it is important to practice recommended computer **ergonomics** (human factors that affect the design and operation of tools and the work environment). For instance, posture is critical in preventing injury. A recommended sitting posture for computer users was developed by Gary Karp, Ergonomics Consultant of Onsight Technology Education Services of San Francisco, California (Figure 36-5).

Other recommended aids include the ergonomic keyboard, which allows the wrists to remain in a flat position. A wrist rest for the mouse is used to keep the wrist in the level position. Screen glare protectors are utilized to deflect and reduce monitor glare. Eye care profes-

Sitting Diagram

This is the general diagram of the recommended sitting posture for computer users. Keep in mind that fixed postures contribute to the risk of cumulative trauma injury. Variety of posture is crucial, as is the habit of standing up often. The body needs movement. Nothing counts more than comfort, and this illustration is simply a tool to understand what is happening in your body at the computer. Keep these principles in mind as you develop a repertoire of comfortable postures to use throughout the workday, knowing that slumped and leaning postures demand more work from the body leading to early fatigue.

• Top of monitor just below eye level. This supports keeping the head over the shoulders. Comfortable viewing is generally 5 to 30 degrees below horizontal. Place in front of the body to prevent sitting in a twisted posture or turning the head.

• Head over the shoulders to allow the skeleton to carry the weight of the head, relieving overuse of neck, shoulder, and back muscles.

• Monitor distance so that chin doesn't jut forward while the trunk is against the chair back.

• Seat back should support curve in lower (lumbar) spine. Higher seat backs are recommended to relieve spinal pressures. A slight backward angle is preferred to allow the chair to take some load off the spine. Allow the chair to carry a share of the body weight.

• Keyboard height should allow for relaxed shoulders, flat wrists, and at least ninety degrees at the inside of elbow. Sit directly in front, close enough not to have to reach forward. Rest palms on rest only when fingers can remain relaxed.

• Armrests, if used, soft and wide. There should be no contact during keying. Close enough to not force extension of elbows, and low enough for shoulders to be relaxed without slumping or leaning.

• Thighs level with or just above knees to promote a neutral spine.

• Seat pan not so deep that comfortable contact with chair back is prevented. Contact behind the knees must be avoided. Optimal contact with thighs provides greatest degree of effortless support.

• Feet in firm contact with the floor to distribute load through the whole body. Use a footrest only if necessary. Leave space under desk free of any obstruction to legs.

FIGURE 36-5 Recommended computer operator position. *(Courtesy of Gary Karp, Ergonomics Consultant, Onsight Technology Education Services, San Francisco, CA.)*

FIGURE 36-6 Flat keyboard design and mouse allow for easy disinfection, with timed alert for users to become aware that disinfection has not occurred. *(Courtesy of Esterline Advanced Input Systems.)*

sionals advise that, for every hour of computer use, the user should relax the eyes by looking at a distance for ten minutes to reduce eye fatigue.

Infection Control for Keyboards. Infection control for keyboards in the dental office has long been a concern. Aerosol spray in the operatories from handpieces during treatment can land on computer keyboards, and using the keyboard with gloved hands causes cross-contamination. Keyboards are difficult or nearly impossible to clean and microorganisms multiply and are spread and transferred throughout the office. Many dental offices are covering keyboards and the mouse with a barrier during treatment. This barrier or keyboard overlay is acceptable, but it is still difficult to clean and keying in patient procedure data is cumbersome. Keyboards are available that act like a typical spring-key keyboard, but have a flat surface that can be disinfected. A timer on such keyboards can be set at intervals to alert the user to disinfect the keyboard (Figure 36-6).

Patient Scheduling

Effective patient scheduling is crucial to any dental office. Maintaining a smooth patient flow throughout the day determines the success and profitability of the dentist and the practice. Scheduling may seem to be a mundane task, but in reality it takes an organized person with good interpersonal and communication skills to schedule properly. If this task is done well, this job can be very challenging and satisfying. In this position, the receptionist acts as coordinator to help all team members work together, keep their timing perfect, and reach goals. One of the first steps in the process is to acquire the proper materials for scheduling effectively. Analyze the needs of the practice and plan accordingly. Understand that the needs may change and adjustments will have to be made.

Appointment Books

Appointment books are available in several forms. To choose the correct one for the office situation, evaluate the qualities of each. Manual appointment books come in ringed or bound copies. The ringed appointment book allows for the addition or deletion of additional pages. It lays open and flat on the counter during use. A bound appointment book needs to be replaced when the current one is filled. This leaves a timeframe in which two books are utilized, making it more difficult for the scheduling to be completed.

Another consideration is the number of appointment columns required. This is dependent on the unique needs of the physical facilities and staff. Solo practitioners have two or three columns for scheduling patients. Larger practices need six or more columns if multiple dentists practice together. Some practices have a separate column for each expanded-duty dental assistant or dental hygienist. Dental practices also may have separate appointment books for the dental hygienist's patient schedule.

Appointment book pages may have day headings printed in them. The blank headings can be filled in by the receptionist so only the days worked are used in the appointment book and a minimum number of pages are wasted. Some appointment books have the days of the week across the top of the schedule and the correct day can be circled or underlined. Identify the appointment book that works the best for the practice.

Many of the appointment books are set up so that the pages show a week at a glance. The days not worked can be crossed out, still allowing the user to see the entire week at one time.

The time intervals in an appointment book are normally ten- or fifteen-minute intervals and are described as units of time (Figure 36-7). There are six units in an

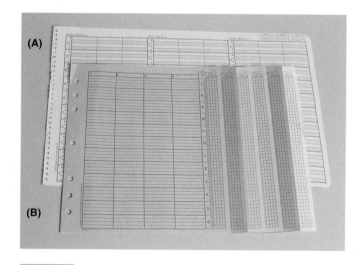

FIGURE 36-7 (A) Appointment book pages showing fifteen-minute units for patient scheduling. (B) Color-coded appointment book for efficient use of dentist's and dental assistant's time. Both allow for a week at a glance.

hour if using the ten-minute intervals and four units in an hour if using the fifteen-minute intervals. Most dental offices use the ten-minute unit because it allows for more effective patient scheduling. The fifteen-minute unit is routinely utilized in some offices. The treatment procedures are broken down into units, and the doctor may request five units for a crown preparation. This equals fifty minutes of time in the appointment book.

Receptionists who are advanced and production conscious can color code the scheduling of appointments. The appointment book indicates whether the dentist or expanded-duty dental assistant is performing treatment for the patient. For example, if using the crown preparation appointment, the schedule would reflect that the first five minutes of the fifty minute allotted time are for the dental assistant to set up and take the preliminary impressions; the next thirty minutes are for the dentist to anesthetize the patient, prepare the tooth for the crown preparation, and take the final impression; the final fifteen minutes are for the dental assistant to make the temporary (provisional) restoration and dismiss the patient. Therefore, the dentist's time can be scheduled for other patient care after the initial thirty-five minutes with the crown preparation patient. This method is utilized in a practice in which patients can be attended to by other staff members. This approach, called **double booking**, uses the dentist's time in the most productive manner. If patients are waiting for the staff or the dentist to attend to them, then the double-booking approach is not working effectively. Double booking can be done in a manual appointment book or on the computer.

Appointment Book Matrix. After the appointment book is selected with the appropriate days, columns, and units, the receptionist can begin establishing the appointment book matrix. This is where the whole year (if possible) can be mapped out to avoid scheduling patients when the dentist has other commitments or when the office is closed. It is advisable to use pencil, because even the best laid out plans may change. First, mark an X through the days when the office is closed. Identify all the continuing education seminars and meetings that the dentist and staff will be attending, along with the holidays when the office is closed.

In many offices, specific periods of time are set aside for emergencies. This time is referred to as buffer time. Each dental office identifies which time is best for buffer time. The most common buffer time is late morning, right before lunch, and late afternoon, right before closing. Buffer time is not previously scheduled but is reserved for emergency patients only.

Lunch time is marked out in the appointment book with an X or a diagonal line. The columns are identified for operatories or for specific dental team members, such as the dental hygienist. Color coding can be used in defining the appointment book matrix.

When scheduling the dental appointments or developing the treatment plan for patients, it is important to know the specific time intervals needed between appointments. For instance, after a crown is prepared and a provisional is placed, the dental laboratory needs time to process the case and return the finished product to the dental office before the next appointment. This interim time may be from two to seven days. Each dental laboratory varies in the amount of time needed to process the case. Whatever the time required by the laboratory, allow a couple of additional days to ensure that the case is complete prior to the patient's appointment. At times, multiple appointments are required in a series. The receptionist may have to consider healing time as well as laboratory production time when scheduling the advance appointments.

Special Patient Appointment Times. All practices have patients who require special scheduling of appointment times due to health concerns, age, or just nervousness. If young children are to be scheduled for dental appointments, it is best to care for them in the morning or after nap times. Treating a child prior to nap time when he or she is cranky and unhappy may make it difficult for everyone. Children of school age normally require appointments after school or during vacation days. Call the local schools to become aware of the academic calendar year so the appointment book can be scheduled according to the children's needs.

Elderly patients should be scheduled at a time when they are not fatigued or tired. They may have concerns about transportation, bus routes, and the weather. Arrange times for their appointments that are convenient for them. Morning appointments often work well.

It is well documented that patients who are extremely anxious about dentistry have a greater cancellation rate for their appointments. If a patient expresses fear, the assistant can reassure him or her and make a notation for the receptionist. This alerts the receptionist that a short, easy appointment should be scheduled the first time to build the patient's confidence and lessen the risk of cancellation. Calls may be made prior to the appointment to confirm the time, and follow-up calls may be made after the appointment to ensure that everything went well for the patient.

Health concerns impact patient appointment scheduling. If a patient has diabetes or hypoglycemia, schedule the patient after a mealtime. Confirm that the patient has eaten and verify that the diabetes patient has taken the needed medication. A patient with heart problems may require shorter appointments so that the patient does not become overfatigued.

Other Scheduling Concerns. Discuss the appointment book scheduling with the dentist and the staff. The dentist may have the highest energy level in the morning. Scheduling a difficult, tedious treatment at the end of the day may be overtaxing. Also, scheduling the same procedure repeatedly may make it difficult on the dental team members. Staggering the types of treatment allows the dental team to be prepared for the procedures and makes the day go smoother and faster. Also, scheduling the same procedure several times in a row may make it difficult to accomplish the sterilization procedures when only a limited number of specific instruments are available for the specific procedure. During staff meetings, talk over appointment scheduling that works well and define the best approach policy.

Computer Scheduling

Dental offices today most often use computer scheduling. Many software packages offering a variety of services are available. The office can determine the type of software needed for the practice. The same information is needed on a computer-scheduling package as was noted in the appointment books. Scheduling is, however, completed more rapidly and quickly for the patient and the receptionist.

When using computer scheduling, the program searches through the database for open appointment time frames. After finding a time and date that are convenient for the patient, the data is keyed into the computer schedule and the appointment is automatically scheduled. Software programs are available to develop any matrix that the practice desires for any specific database. The scheduling can be designed to highlight open appointment times with very few directions.

Appointment Book Entries

When making appointment book entries using the manual system, it is important to write in pencil. Of course, with a computer it is much easier. First, establish an appointment time with the patient, noting any special considerations, such as laboratory work that might affect the appointment. Record the entry in the schedule. The entry should include the patient's name, phone number, procedure to be completed (abbreviated), length of procedure identified by an arrow, and age, if the patient is a child. Write out the information on an appointment card for the patient, including the day, date, and time (Figure 36-8). Clearly repeat the information to the patient as the card is given to him or her, to verify it once again.

The receptionist must know the time units for each procedure in order to schedule patient treatment times. The more productive treatment procedures are called primary procedures. They tend to be the longer appointments dealing with crown and bridge preparations, amalgam and composite fillings, surgery, and endodontic treatment. With the increased time spent placing and removing barriers and sterilization, it is much more productive to take care of several teeth at the same appointment. Around the primary procedures, the dental receptionist can schedule a dovetail or conjunctive procedure that does not require the same concentrated attention by the dentist. These conjunctive procedures include routine examinations, consultations, or denture adjustments.

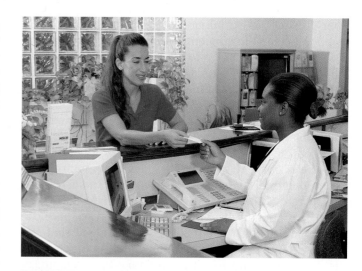

FIGURE 36-8 Patients are given appointment cards with next appointment and preoperative instructions printed neatly.

The receptionist's goal is to fill the appointment book with patient care so that the scheduling problems such as downtime, overtime, and overlap time are nonexistent for the dentist and dental assistants.

- **Downtime** is time in the appointment book that is not scheduled. If an appointment time using ten-minute units is open from 2:00 to 2:30, it is referred to as three units of downtime.

- **Overtime** is where the patient treatment time went beyond the estimated timeframe. This can affect the entire schedule. It can cause other patients to wait for their appointments, therefore making them unhappy.

- **Overlap of time** occurs when the dentist or dental assistant is required to be in two places at the same time or when two patients need to be seated in the same operatory at the same time.

All three scheduling problems occur, and care should be taken to eliminate them. Careful estimation of accurate time units reduces or eliminates some of these problems. If this is an ongoing concern, scheduling adjustments should be made accordingly. The office team should meet and discuss ideas to eliminate scheduling problems.

Office policies for handling patients with special needs, repeated appointment delays, and repeated missed appointments must be developed. The computer can note these and, after several missed appointments, it may be office policy to avoid rescheduling the patient. All these topics should be discussed so that the receptionist knows how to handle these situations.

Recall Patients

Established dental offices consider the recall system the backbone of the dental practice. A recall system ensures that patients return for continued care and maintenance of their dental needs. Bringing patients back into the office at regular intervals allows the dentist to assess their teeth and tissues and keep them in optimum condition. This preventive measure prevents serious discomfort for the patient. During the continued-care appointment (recall appointment), the dental team reinforces oral hygiene techniques and educates the patient concerning any new dentifrices or other dental aids on the market that will aid the patient in overall oral care. Questions may arise about whitening techniques, types of toothbrushes, and mouth rinses. It also allows the dentist to assess pathology concerns at an early stage.

Computer Recall. Recalling patients for their ongoing care can be accomplished with a number of methods. With increased computer use in the dental offices, most current recall is done from a computer-generated printout. Information is placed in the computer after the regular appointment is completed. The program allows a date for the recall or continued-care appointment to be indicated. At the end of the month, an alphabetical list of patients needing recall the following month, along with their addresses and phone numbers, can be generated. This list can be used to contact the patients by telephone or through the mail. The patients who schedule appointments can be removed from the list, while the others stay on the printout automatically.

Advance Appointment Scheduling. The appointment book allows for advance scheduling of continued-care appointments immediately after regular dental care is complete. This allows an appointment to be scheduled for the patient six months to a year in advance. The appointment book in this system is used as the primary listing. The patients need to reaffirm their appointments two weeks in advance as well as the day prior. The advantage to this system is that the task is completed immediately for the patient as well as the dental office. The disadvantage of this system is obvious: the patient does not always know what will be happening in his or her life that far in advance and may need to cancel or reschedule the appointment.

Chronological Card File. A minimum amount of time is invested in the chronological card file system. In this system, the patient fills out a postcard so that the next recall date will be mailed directly to him or her. The cards are filed according to the month the patient is to be recalled. The card is mailed to the patient two weeks before the given recall date. If this system is used alone, the card is sent to the patient and then all references for the patient recall are lost, unless someone goes through all the charts and makes a list of patients needing recall appointments. It is better to make a list and note the patients who do not schedule appointments and follow up with telephone calls to schedule the appointment.

Color-Tagged Card File. Another type of recall system is the color-tagged card file. In this system, every patient has an index card with name, address, telephone number, and any other special notations printed on it. The cards are filed alphabetically, and a colored tag is clipped to each card indicating in which month the patient requires a recall appointment. For example, a yellow tag is clipped to a card if the patient needs a recall appointment in January. The tagged file cards are reviewed each month, and calls are made to schedule the patients needing continued care. If they do not schedule, they can be moved up to the next month or later, if requested. After the patient is scheduled, the card is attached to the chart and updated at the time of the patient's appointment. A new color-coded tag is then attached to the card and filed in the index system. The advantage of this system is that the cards are available with information on them about prior appointments. Disadvantages are the time it takes to complete a card for each patient and the possibility of the tag falling off.

Regardless of which system is used, the goal is to make sure that every patient in the dental office is either under regular treatment or on a recall system.

Dental Records Management

Accurate dental records management is essential for quality patient care at any dental office. It is also necessary because of the legal issues that every dental office must face today. The records must be filled out completely, reflecting all pertinent information.

Equipment and Supplies for Record Management

The dentist decides on the type of file folder to use in the office, normally with the advisement of the receptionist and staff. File folders are designed in many different ways to meet office needs. They should provide easy accessibility and yet enclose the information and protect it during storing. A patient folder may be like an envelope or have a book-type opening. The envelope folder may have preprinted data on the outside and all the information sheets, x-rays, and so on placed inside. The book type normally keeps the patient information in constant order. The book type normally is more costly because it requires added pockets and fasteners to hold the information sheets secure.

File cabinets are also available in several primary types, such as vertical, open-shelf lateral, and movable. The vertical file cabinet is widely used in home filing (Figure 36-9A). The files are retrieved by lifting the appropriate file upward and outward. Open-shelf file cabinets seem to be the most widely used in the dental office, normally with a color-coding system that allows for easy chart identification (Figure 36-9B). The records from the open-shelf lateral files are retrieved by pulling them out laterally from the shelf. Some large offices

(A)

(B)

FIGURE 36-9 (A) Vertical file cabinet. *(Courtesy HON® Company.)* (B) Open-shelf lateral file cabinet.

FIGURE 36-10 Color-coded patient files. Yellow file selected for "Carl,""F" side tab selected for "Friend." *(Courtesy of KARDEX System, Inc., Marietta, OH.)*

may have the movable file units that are powered electrically or physically by easy handles. Patient names are typed on the labels and attached to the file for quick identification.

Patient Chart Filing

Make sure that the filing system used is organized alphabetically. Most systems index the individual names. The patient name is divided into three units: the last name, first name, and middle name or initial. File all the charts according to the last name; if two patients have the same last name, such as Smith, then use the first name. Therefore, if the office has a John Smith and a Jim Smith, Jim is filed before John in the file cabinet. Occasionally,

two patients with the same first and last names become patients. Use their middle names or initials to file properly. Alphabetical filing requires accuracy during the removal and replacement of the chart. These tasks must be done correctly or a lot of time can be wasted trying to find the chart.

Most dental offices use some form of color coding in regards to their patient filing (Figure 36-10). The file folder may be color coded so that all the patients with a last name beginning in A or S have yellow charts and all the patients with B or T have blue charts. Following this system reduces the lost charts because they will stand out if not in the proper color section. Other charts may have colored tabs that are placed on either plain or colored charts to make the filing and retrieval of files more efficient. The larger the practice, the more tabs required to break down the total charts into small groupings. However, this makes filing easier and reduces the number of errors that may occur, because any visible color differences are quickly identified. Color coding or adding date stickers helps dental assistants and receptionists track active and inactive accounts.

Tickler File. A well-organized office has a **tickler file** that serves as a reminder of any action that needs to be taken in the future. Most offices use sticky notes (reminder notes that have adhesive strips on one side) to remind office personnel of things that need to be taken care of immediately. A tickler file normally is index cards in an index box with approximate dates in which to complete the task (Figure 36-11). Many of the computer software programs have tickler files available so that the information can be stored and retrieved when necessary.

FIGURE 36-11 Tickler file for daily review and follow-up actions in patient management.

MONDAY, NOVEMBER 23			Dr. King	Dr. Lewis
7	00			
	15			
	30			
	45			
8	00			
	15			
	30			
	45			
9	00		Abigail Johnson-Black	Lenore McDonell
	15		466-2964 #140	535-4421 #29-DO
	30		Marge O'Keefe/296-7234	Consultation
	45			
10	00		#3 Full Gold Crown	Joseph Ortiz/New Pt
	15			462-3038 Exam
	30		Nora Fowler/466-2234	Maria Tover/296-2104
	45		#12-MO	
11	00		Jim Marshall/763-2067	Martin Gordon/763-6340
	15			Toothache
	30		Jeff Jones	Beverly Curtis
	45		296-7300	891-1970
12	00		#18-O #19-MO	#16 removal
	15			
	30			
	45			
			Lunch Meeting	Lunch Meeting
1	00		Matt Hanes/Consultation	Boris Bolski/New Pt
	15		763-3284	466-5529 Exam

FIGURE 36-12 Computer-generated daily patient schedule.

Record Confidentiality

The patient has the right to confidential treatment and records. (See Chapter 3, Ethics, Jurisprudence, and the Health Information Portability and Accountability Act, for more information and a list of the CTC codes.) The clinical record contains private information that must be kept confidential within the dental office. With the usage of computers and fax machines, great care must be used when placing anything on-line where others can access it. When sending a fax, attach a cover sheet that advises the receiver of the confidential nature of the material, and make sure that the fax machine that is receiving the material is located in an area where only the appropriate individuals can access it.

Archival Storage. Most dentists keep records for the entirety of their careers. This creates a storage concern for the practice. There is a process similar to microfiche and microfilm by which the records are copied with a laser beam and compressed onto an optical disc. These small discs can store a great deal of information, and this information can be easily retrieved and viewed, if needed.

Daily Schedule

The daily schedule is a form developed directly from the information in the appointment book for that day (Figure 36-12). It shows the time that each patient is scheduled and the treatment that is to be provided. Normally, several daily schedules are generated so that one can be placed in each operatory and one in the sterilization area. This schedule allows the clinical staff to plan ahead and set up for the upcoming patients. Any changes throughout the day are changed on each daily schedule. If a computer monitor is in each operatory, the daily schedule can be available through the network and changed more readily from the main computer at the front desk.

Accounts Receivable

The primary concern of the dental office is patient care, but without sound financial management, the office will not thrive and the patients will ultimately suffer. With the high cost of materials and equipment, profit management is critical. The accounts receivable of the dental office encompasses the money owed to the practice. The bookkeeping in this area must be accurate and carries with it a great responsibility. This position may be occupied by the receptionist or the business assistant. Like the information on the patient's records, the financial information must remain confidential. All transactions, payments, adjustments, and charges must be handled in a safe and professional manner. Any employee engaging in unlawful activities may be prosecuted under the law and required to repay the employer for any theft. Insurance fraud also brings with it prosecution and possible imprisonment.

Patient Fees

In the dental office, a fee schedule is used to define what patients are charged for each service. It is referred to as the usual, reasonable, and customary fee. The usual fee refers to the fee typically charged by the dentist for a specific procedure. The reasonable fee is the midrange of fees charged for this same procedure; therefore, if it is a difficult case, then the usual fee may be raised to reflect the difficulty of the case. The customary fee is the average up to the 90th percent that the dentists in the area charge for the same procedure. The impact that the fee schedule has on the dental practice is that if a dentist feels that he or she would like to charge a greater amount for one service, the insurance companies will not pay above the usual, reasonable, and customary fee schedule. The patient will be billed for the overage. Patients may question the additional charge and become upset with the practice if this has not been discussed previously in the treatment plan or at the consultation appointment. Most dentists stay within the fee range. This range can be adjusted yearly, rising by 5 percent, by area dentists, but seldom does it rise that much.

The dentists have the right to adjust the fees by means of a professional courtesy. This professional courtesy, a discounted amount, may be offered to other dentists for dental work or to employees, family, and friends. The dentist has the discretion to make any adjustments desired. Another area in which dentists may make adjustments is insurance. Dentists who accept assignments in specific programs agree to accept a payment in full by the provider. For instance, a patient is covered on a program and the dentist does a restoration on this patient for a fee of $75. The provider only pays $55 for this particular service. The dentist has to adjust, or "waive," the remaining $20 of the fee and the patient will not be responsible for it.

PROCEDURE 36-1

Preparing for the Day's Patients

This procedure is performed by the receptionist in preparation for the upcoming day.

EQUIPMENT

- File
- Patient charts
- Computer with word processor
- Telephone

Day Before

1. Dental receptionist pulls patient charts for the next day.
2. Laboratory work is checked to ensure that it is ready.
3. All patient appointments are confirmed via telephone calls.
4. Records are reviewed for any special concerns.

5. Patient account balances are reviewed and notations are made on chart.
6. Any premedications are identified and noted.
7. Daily schedule is typed and the appropriate number of copies are made.
8. Daily schedule is posted in the appropriate areas after the current schedule is completed for the day.

Day of the Appointment

1. Office staff meets in the morning to look over the daily schedule. This brief meeting (five minutes or fewer) allows the staff to dialogue any treatment or patient concerns that may transpire during the day.
2. Charts are ready for dental assistants as they seat the patients.
3. Patients are greeted and seated in dental treatment rooms by dental team.

Dental team members must be aware that the practice cannot survive if constant adjustments to the fees are made. Production must be balanced by other cases that meet the regular fee schedule to maintain a viable practice.

Patient Account Management

Patient accounts can be managed either through a computerized bookkeeping system or a manual system, such as the pegboard system. Many dental offices have converted the manual bookkeeping system to the computer system because it offers great versatility and reduces the need to record entries more than once. Changing from the manual system is, initially, time consuming until all the data is entered into the computer.

Pegboard System of Account Management

The pegboard system (Figure 36-13) is designed as a "write it once" system that uses no-carbon-required (NCR) paper, permitting the user to enter the data only once. The system consists of day sheets, charge slips, ledger cards, and receipt forms (Figure 36-14). The forms are designed to work together and are aligned on a pegboard with matching columns. The system is relatively inexpensive. Several companies have developed similar systems but their forms are incompatible. Therefore, it is important to use the forms from one company. The pegboard system is included in this chapter to show the components of the account management system. Most offices today have gone to computerized systems that use the same components but provide information much more easily.

Day Sheets. Day sheets record each charge, payment, and adjustment for the day. All transactions must be written legibly and accurately in order to maintain accurate records. The day sheets consist of five sections: the first three are for posting and the last two are for balancing (Figure 36-13).

- **Section 1** is where patient transactions are posted. All charges, credits, and previous and current account balances are noted.

- **Section 2** is where all deposits for the day are listed and transferred from section 1. This list includes the cash and check payments. Some companies have

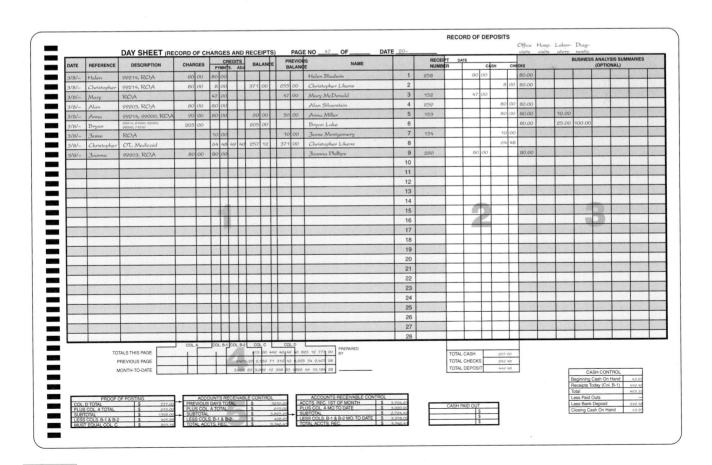

FIGURE 36-13 Pegboard system, shown with Section 1, record of charges and receipts; Section 2, record of deposits; Section 3, business analysis summaries; Section 4, daily and monthly totals; Section 5, proof of posting; and the accounts receivable control.

PROCEDURE 36-2

Day Sheet Preparation for Posting

The dental receptionist or office business assistant performs this task and prepares the day sheet before the first patient arrives.

EQUIPMENT

- Pegboard
- New day sheet
- Block of new charge slips and receipt forms
- Ledger cards for all patients scheduled that day (or ledger card file)

PROCEDURE STEPS

1. Place day sheet on pegboard.

2. Attach charge and receipt slips on first corresponding line (Figure 36-14).

3. At top of day sheet, fill in date and page number.

4. Transfer information from previous page and fill in previous day's totals from columns A through D and write in place at the bottom of the day sheet under "previous page."

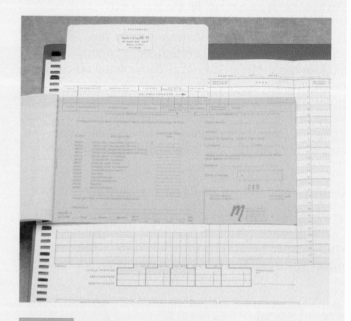

FIGURE 36-14 Pegboard accounting system with day sheet, ledger card, and charge slip in place.

5. Prepare ledger cards for patients scheduled that day by pulling or tabbing them or have storage file close by.

detachable portions or carbon overlays for use as deposit slips from this area.

- **Section 3** is where the business analysis summary can be recorded.

- **Section 4** is where all daily transactions are totaled and balanced. For example, the total of D is added to the total of A and the total of B1 and B2 are subtracted to equal the total of column C. What this means is that the previous balance is added to the charges and then the credits are subtracted to equal the new balance.

- **Section 5** is where the total cumulative accounts receivable is balanced. This is the amount that all patients owe the practice.

End-of-Month Balancing. When the last day sheet of the month is complete, there will be a total accounts receivable balance noted on it. The patient ledger cards (one ledger per family) need to be totaled (using the amount owed to the practice) to compare with the one on the last day sheet. These totals should be exactly equal; if they are not, the mistake must be tracked down before it

grows into a major problem. The most likely error is that a ledger card is misplaced. The patients are billed from the ledger cards, so this error needs to be rectified.

Computerized Account Management System

Most dental offices use computerized account management systems. They are much quicker and allow offices to gather information more rapidly. Patient ledgers that are computerized contain all the information about each patient, including name, address, telephone number, insurance coverage, and person responsible for the account. The ledger also has the office visits and the services provided and procedure codes. Each time the patient is in the office, the information about the service is entered from the charge slips. The computer automatically updates the ledger, posts the charges, and calculates the balance and the practice accounts receivable balance.

The patient account can be viewed on the computer monitor or printed out if the patient desires a copy (Figure 36-15). Specialized information such as missed

STATEMENT OF ACCOUNT

09/14/2003   Dentrix Dental Center   Page:1
                          5926 S. Dearborn Road
                          Spokane, WA 99223

Peter M. Barnes
4567 88th
Ronan, MT 59864   CHART#: BA0001

☐ Please check box if above address information is incorrect and indicate changes on reverse side.

DATE	DESCRIPTION	PATIENT	CHARGES	CREDITS
08/14/2003	Balance forward		1,708.40	
* 10/29/2002	Crown-porc fuse high noble mtl	John	613.00	
* 10/29/2002	Crown-porc fuse high noble mtl	John	613.00	
* 02/24/2002	Bitewings—two films	Peter	21.00	
* 02/24/2002	Emerg treatment, palliative	Peter	55.00	
* 02/24/2002	Intraoral—periapical—each add'l	Peter	10.00	
* 02/24/2002	Intraoral—periapical—1st film	Peter	13.00	
02/24/2002	Payment—Aetna Life and Casualty	Peter		–80.70

* Indicates that insurance has been billed for the procedure.

Charges on account over 90 days. PLEASE PAY IMMEDIATELY!

We have just converted to a new system. Your understanding is appreciated.

0-30	31-60	61-90	91=>
0.00	0.00	0.00	2952.70

                                            BALANCE: 2,952.70

Dentrix Dental Center 5926 S. Dearborn Road Spokane, WA 99223 (509) 448-3188

FIGURE 36-15 Computer-generated dental patient account showing services rendered and insurance and patient payments. *(Courtesy of Dentrix Dental Systems, Inc. © 1989-1999.)*

appointments or family discounts may be programmed into the computer.

Monthly Billing

Every patient owing the practice is billed monthly. If using the pegboard system, the ledger cards are copied and sent out for payment. The computer generates monthly bills from the ledgers on the database with an age analysis of the balance (Figure 36-16). Many offices include return envelopes to aid the patients in sending in payment. The patient statements are requests for payment and ask for the balance to be paid in full. Dental offices may charge a finance charge for balances that are not paid within the first thirty days after treatment.

Payment Options. At the time of treatment, the business assistant may set up financial arrangements. Often, an initial down payment is requested. The balance is then divided and this fixed amount is paid over

an arranged timeframe. For instance, a patient may have $1,000 worth of dentistry to complete. The office may request 20 percent as a down payment and that the other $800 dollars be paid in $200 increments over the next four months. The patient signs the payment plan along with office personnel or dentist. If payments extend over four months and finance charges are added to the unpaid balance, the patient must be notified in advance under the federal Truth in Lending Act (TILA). This law, which is designed to protect consumers in credit transactions, requires that clear disclosure of contract terms and any associated costs be given to the consumer. The dental office should use a truth-in-lending form that can be custom designed from a computer-generated template to notify the consumer of financial arrangements. Most dental practices add a finance charge of 1 percent to account balances that have not been paid within the first 30 days of the first statement. The patient is given one copy of the payment plan and the original is kept in the patient's record. This information may also be noted on the ledger to remind the patient of the arrangements when the statement is sent out.

Financial Information

When a patient calls for an appointment, it is beneficial to gather all the information in regard to dental insurance. When the patient comes in, be sure to get a copy of his or her insurance identification and have the patient complete and sign the patient portion of the insurance form. With this information, the business assistant can gather information concerning the patient's dental coverage. Insurance coverage can have yearly limits and may have restrictions for specific services. By having knowledge about the most commonly used insurance plans, the business assistant can help patients with making decisions concerning dental treatment.

Credit Reports. It may be necessary to obtain credit reports on patients who have large financial responsibilities for dental treatment. Essentially, the dental practice is loaning the patient the money to pay for this treatment. There are lab fees and overhead that must be paid, and the patient is requesting to be trusted to pay at a later date. Consumer credit reporting agencies provide financial profiles on individuals and verify whether they meet their obligations or are slow to meet their obligations through a rating system. The patient is to be informed prior to requesting a credit report. The patient's Social Security number and birth date may be necessary to obtain the pertinent information. Any bankruptcies and lawsuits are identified on the credit report. After the report is received, the dentist or business assistant can determine whether the patient can pay in installments for dental treatment.

FIGURE 36-16 Patient account showing age analysis.

Dental Insurance

Dental insurance represents a large portion of accounts receivable in most dental practices. By preparing the insurance forms accurately and submitting them in a timely fashion, payments are quickly submitted to the dental office. Dental insurance seldom covers the entire fee, and the patient is responsible for the balance.

Dental Insurance Terms

Assignment of benefits The patient assigns benefits to be paid directly to the dentist or the provider.

Beneficiary The patient who is entitled to dental insurance benefits.

Benefit-less-benefit refers to nonduplication of benefits pertinent to subscribers of more than one plan. Such plans allow reimbursement to be limited to the higher level allowed of two plans.

Birthday rule refers to cases when both parents have coverage for the child patient: the primary carrier is held by the parent whose birthday month and day (not year) comes earliest in the calendar year.

Carrier Usually the dental insurance company.

Coordination of benefits (COB) refers to provisions by two carriers to coordinate (share) benefits between them that are not to exceed 100 percent of dental charges for an eligible subscriber.

Coverage Benefits available to the person covered by dental insurance.

CDT codes Codes that are published in the *Current Dental Terminology* under ADA jurisdiction.

Deductible The amount paid before benefits take effect.

Dependents Children covered under dental insurance (normally up to age 18).

Dual coverage Two dental coverages; the primary is in first position and the balance is normally paid by secondary insurance.

Eligibility Determining if the patient is eligible for dental benefits.

Exclusions Items that dental insurance does not cover.

Fee for service Payment to providers on a service-by-service rather than a salaried or capitated basis.

Group plan Plan in which several individuals are covered.

Individual plan Plan in which an individual has a plan without a group of individuals.

Patient Person receiving treatment.

Predetermination of benefits Submitting the treatment plan to the carrier to determine what the insurance will pay on the dental services; this is often called the pretreatment estimate (estimate completed before treatment).

Premium Amount the carrier charges the subscriber.

Primary insurance Insurance of subscriber.

Provider Dentist who performs the dental service.

Reimbursement Payment made by the carrier to the patient or the dentist on behalf of the beneficiary toward the dental fee incurred.

Secondary insurance Insurance of the subscriber's spouse.

Subscriber Individual with dental insurance.

The individual who has dental insurance through employment or an individual plan is referred to as the subscriber. The patient who is entitled to benefits under any dental plan is referred to as the beneficiary. Some patients have dental insurance through their employment for themselves and have other coverage through their spouses. They would then be the subscribers for their primary insurance and the beneficiaries for the other dental insurance secondary insurance. This person is said to have dual coverage and may not have to pay for any additional expenses for dental treatment. If two coverages are used, the primary pays the normal fees and the secondary covers up to the amount owed. Together they pay the entire bill.

COB applies to patients eligible for benefits under two carriers, in which the primary carrier pays part of the allowed amount and the secondary carrier pays the balance. For instance, if allowed dental charges were $500 and the primary paid $350 of the fee, the secondary would only pay $150, regardless of allowed benefits for the services rendered under the secondary policy. Together the two carriers pay 100 percent of the dental fee.

Other plans may specify nonduplication of benefits, known as benefit-less-benefit. This provision applies to subscribers eligible for benefits under more than one plan. Reimbursement is limited to the highest level allowed by either plan, not a combined total or limit of 100% of the dental charge. For instance, assume that the dental fee is $500, the primary carrier allows $200, and the secondary carrier allows $300. In this instance, the secondary carrier would reimburse the dentist for $300, and the patient would be responsible for $200.

A person could also obtain insurance through an individual plan instead of a plan through an employer. A plan through an employer is normally a group plan, in which several individuals are covered. The larger the group in the plan, the better the benefit coverage and the more reasonable the premium or monthly costs. Individual plans are normally much more costly and often offer lesser benefits.

Children are normally covered under dental insurance until they are age eighteen or have completed their full-time education. They are referred to as dependents under the dental insurance carrier. The carrier is the dental insurance company that pays the agreed benefits for the patient treatment. Patients who have benefits are normally given benefit booklets that state the coverage that the patients are eligible for. Exclusions, items the dental coverage does not cover, are noted in this booklet. The coverage normally is negotiated with the employer for the employees. Limitations for benefits may be noted in the booklets along with the benefit plan. For children who are eligible under both parents' insurance, benefit payout may be determined by the birthday rule. Under this rule, the carrier for the parent subscriber whose birthday (day and month) comes first in the calendar year is the primary. This rule applies to parents who are not divorced, and is not applicable to stepparents.

Many of the insurance plans have an identified deductible amount. This means that a specified amount is deducted from the benefit amount before any benefits are paid. For example, if the policy has a $100 deductible each year, the individual must pay this amount before becoming eligible for payment of any benefits.

Some insurance plans have maximum amounts that can be paid out for the year. This means that no matter what the dental treatment is, the plan will not pay over a specified amount. So, if an insurance plan pays a maximum annual amount of $2,000 per year and a patient has ten crowns costing $400 each (total cost = $4,000), the insurance will only pay $2,000 of the bill. The patient would be responsible for the remaining $2,000 balance. So, for this patient, it would be beneficial to have five crowns completed each year for two years in order to utilize maximum benefits from the dental insurance.

If the dental coverage, or benefits available, is difficult to determine, send the planned treatment to the insurance company to get a predetermination of benefits. This predetermination is often referred to as a pretreatment estimate. The insurance carrier may request dental radiographs before the predetermination can be made. After receiving the predetermination, both the dentist and the patient will know the exact amount of benefits available toward the cost of the entire dental treatment.

Capitation Program

In a capitation program, the dentist or dentists contract with the program's administrator to provide subscribers all the services covered in the program for a payment on a per capita basis. The dentist receives a fixed fee for each patient in the program and is not paid for the services that are provided. The subscriber has a limited number of dentists from which to choose (only those contracted). This type of plan is used for health maintenance organizations (HMOs).

Contract Fee Schedule Plan

A contract fee schedule plan is a dental benefit plan in which participating dentists agree to accept the fees listed under the plan for the total fees. The government program Medicaid is a contract fee schedule plan. Dentists who accept Medicaid agree to accept the amounts paid by carriers and do not bill for the remaining amounts. Most contract fee schedule plans offer reduced payments.

Direct Reimbursement Plans

In the direct reimbursement plan, the patient pays the dental treatment fee and is reimbursed the agreed upon amount by the employer. An insurance carrier is uninvolved in this plan.

PROCEDURE 36-3

Posting Charges and Payments on Pegboard

The dental receptionist or office business assistant performs this task during or at the end of each day.

EQUIPMENT

- Pegboard
- New day sheet
- Block of new charge slips and receipt forms
- Ledger cards for all the patients scheduled that day (or ledger card file placed close by)

PROCEDURE STEPS

When Patient Enters Dental Office for Appointment

1. Place the patient's ledger under the next charge sheet and on the corresponding line on the pegboard.

2. Write in the date, responsible party's name, the patient's name, and the previous balance, if any, in the spaces provided for each on the charge and receipt sheet. The information will automatically copy onto the ledger card and the pegboard day sheet.

3. Remove the charge sheet from the pegboard and clip it to the outside of the patient's chart. The chart is then ready for the dental assistant and the dentist to use during treatment.

4. The dentist or dental assistant completes the chart and the charge sheet prior to dismissing the patient. The chart is given to the patient to take to the reception area or is brought to the reception area by the dental assistant while dismissing the patient.

After Patient Is Dismissed and Returned to Reception Area

1. Replace charge slip on pegboard, align it with patient's name, and insert patient's ledger card back into place under charge slip on the pegboard. Enter the charges and payments in the designated spaces in section 1 (Figure 36-13).

2. The final balance for the patient is totaled by adding the previous balance with the new charges and subtracting any payment the patient has made. Place the final charge in column C. Note that column D is the previous balance, column A is charges, column B1 is payments, and column B2 is adjustments. The proof of posting at the bottom on the day sheet indicates the procedure to be used for each entry as well as the entire day sheet.

Column D total + Column A total = Subtotal − (Column B1 + B2) = Column C

3. When posting is completed, the first copy of the charge slip is filed in the patient's chart and the second copy is given to the patient for the purpose of payment and the patient's records. The final copy is used for submission for insurance reimbursement.

Managed Care Plans

Managed care plans, or plans that provide minimum care to everyone, are becoming increasingly prevalent. These plans encourage preventive services and try to control costs. The idea is to provide high-level care for reduced fees. With more and more individuals losing dental insurance and requiring dental care, more plans will arise to try to control the rising cost of care.

Submitting Dental Insurance Claims

As a courtesy to patients, most dental offices submit insurance claims. The entire claim must be filled out. The patient fills in the patient and subscriber information and the dental office fills in the dentist's identification and the description of services. The American Dental Association developed a Code on Dental Procedures and Nomenclature to simplify the reporting of the confidential information regarding the patient's dental treatment.

The Current Dental Terminology (CDT) codes are published in the *Current Dental Terminology* under ADA jurisdiction. Until 2000, the codes were updated every five years. It is now anticipated that they will be updated every two or three years. The communities of interest and the ADA Council of Dental Benefit Programs update these codes, which follow a five-digit system for identifying dental procedures and services. The first digit of the code is the letter D for dental, which distinguishes the codes from medical ones. The second digit designates the category of service (e.g., preventative is 1). The third digit designates the class of service in the category, the fourth the subclass of service, and the fifth is open for expansion. An example of a CDT code is D1110 for adult prophylaxis. The CDT code for a child's prophylaxis is D1120. Most computer applications have the codes programmed. The dental assistant identifies the service and the code appears. As CDT codes change, applications must be updated. (See Chapter 3, Ethics, Jurisprudence, and the Health Information Portability and Accountability Act, for more information and a list of the CTC codes.)

It is advisable for the patient, the person receiving the treatment, to sign the area regarding **assignment of benefits**, as well as the area permitting payment from the insurance company directly to the provider dentist who provided the service. If this area is not signed, the dental office assumes that the patient is responsible for the entire fee. The business assistant must pay attention to and have the patients sign both areas in order to protect the practice.

The insurance can be completed on a paper claim form. These forms are available from the ADA. When the claim is completed manually, it is normally done in duplicate so one copy can go into the patient's chart and the other copy can be sent to the insurance company. The name and address of the carrier are noted on the form. The patient's name, address, date of birth, ID number (often the patient's Social Security number), sex, and phone numbers are also noted on the form. In addition, the employer, the relationship to the subscriber, the subscriber ID (again, usually the subscriber's Social Security number), and the group number are noted on the form. Other insurance is also written on the form when applicable. The claim form also has two boxes for patients to sign. One of the boxes is for *release of information*. The release of information allows the dentist to release the patient's dental treatment information to the carrier (insurance company). Without this box signed, the dentist cannot release this confidential information. The other box for the patient to sign is the *assignment of benefits*. Assignment of benefits authorizes the carrier to pay the dentist directly. If this box is unsigned, the check goes directly to the patient. When this box is unsigned, the office should arrange for payment of the entire dental treatment, because the office is not guaranteed to receive the insurance money. Another way to handle the assignment of benefits is to have a *signature on file*. This form is completed at patient registration and has boxes very like those on the dental claim form. The signature on file can be used instead of the assignment of benefits. It covers both the release of information and the assignment of benefits if the patient has signed both areas.

After the patient treatment is complete, the insurance is sent in for payment. The codes for service and their descriptions are completed, along with the fee and the date the service was performed. The form is submitted to the carrier through the mail or via electronic claims processing. Many software applications allow for the transmission of insurance claims through the modem. The claims are either transmitted to a national clearinghouse and then on to the carrier or directly to the carrier.

The business assistant is responsible for tracking the insurance claims and making certain that payment is received. A copy of each insurance claim submitted is essential for tracking. It is essential to follow up on claims that are not paid promptly in order to identify the problem so that it can be corrected.

The benefit checks received from the carrier are accompanied by an explanation of benefits. The benefit check is posted to the bookkeeping system on the patient ledger with information explaining the services covered. The check is then deposited along with other checks and cash in the daily deposit.

Insurance Schedule of Benefits. Insurance companies may list their schedules of benefits, also known as schedule or table of allowances. This is a list of specified amounts that the carrier will pay for the service. This schedule is not in any way related to the dentist's actual fees. The schedule of benefits also identifies the services that are covered under the plan. For instance, some carriers (insurance companies) will not pay for orthodontic benefits. They may provide **reimbursement** (the payment made by the carrier to the patient or the dentist on behalf of the patient toward the dental fee incurred). This amount might only cover two surface restorations at a $40 fee or a percentage of this established fee. The patient is responsible for the balance of uncovered fees. Medicaid, a government program, requires that the dentist accept the reduced amount as payment in full without being able to bill the patient for the balance.

Dental Service Payment

Ideally, every patient pays in full for the dental treatment he or she receives. Normally, however, the accounts receivable balance does not equal over three months of production. Offering several payment options helps the practice remain healthy and productive.

Cash Payments. Few patients pay for their dental treatment in cash. However, it is important to keep enough cash in the office to make change if the need arises. Some dental offices offer a discount to patients who pay cash in advance (checks included) for the entire treatment the patient is to receive. If a patient pays in cash, it is customary to give a written receipt showing payment on the account.

Check Payments. The majority of patients pay for their dental services with personal checks. Some offices require that the patient use a driver's license number on the check and/or another form of identification for the check. Some regular patients may take offense to this requirement, so be sure to identify how the dentist would like to handle this. Other checks that may be

PROCEDURE 36-4

Balancing Day Sheets and End-of-Month Figures

The dental receptionist or office business assistant balances the day sheets daily and totals the day sheets at the end of the month or prior to sending out patient statements.

EQUIPMENT

- Pegboard
- Day sheets totaled for month
- Ledger cards for all patients in storage file
- Calculator with tape that records entries

PROCEDURE STEPS

1. Total each column and place that total in the spaces provided at the bottom of the page in "Totals this page" (this section is identified as section 4 of Figure 36-13).

2. The column totals are added to the "Previous page" totals and these numbers are placed in the "Month to Date" total spaces.

3. The totals are verified in the "Proof of Posting" box in section 5 of Figure 36-13. This is where the total of column D is added to column A and subtotaled. The total of columns B1 and B2 are subtracted from the subtotaled amount of A + D. The final amount must equal column C. For example:

Column	D		A		Subtotal		B1–B2		C
	12	+	21	=	33	–	2	=	31
	10	+	14	=	24	–	9	=	15
	5	+	9	=	14	–	4	=	10
Column Totals	27	+	44	=	71	–	15	=	56

4. Once the proof of posting is complete, the accounts receivable control is totaled. This is accomplished by adding the total of column A to the previous day's total and subtracting the columns B1 and B2 from the subtotal. The amount owed to the practice is the accounts receivable total. By adding column A to this, the additional charges are added to the total (or additional money owed to the practice). The payments and adjustments (columns B1 and B2) are subtracted from the total, leaving a true balance of accounts receivable or a true amount that is owed to the practice.

5. The next step in balancing month-end figures is to total the amounts owed on the ledger cards. Use a tape to do this. The cards' totals can be verified on the tape to ensure that nothing was missed.

6. If the total of the ledger cards balances with the total on the day sheet, the accounts receivable is balanced. If it does not balance, recheck the figures and find the missing amount to balance the accounts receivable. Statements are sent out after the accounts receivable are balanced.

---

received in the dental office are cashier's checks. A **cashier's check** is guaranteed by the bank for the amount in which it is written. It is actually the bank's own check that the patient has paid for. Traveler's checks may be used by out-of-town patients. They are safer than cash for the user. They are written in specific denominations ($20, $50, and so on) and require a signature from the user that matches the one on the check, when used. A certified check could be used by a patient as well. A **certified check** is one that the bank has verified as "good" for the amount indicated.

Credit Cards. Patients may use credit cards to pay for services. The office takes the card and uses it with a credit card charge form. The totals are entered on the charge form and the patient signs it and is given a receipt. The dental office may call the credit card number in order to verify that the patient has not exceeded the limit available on the credit card. Credit card pay-

ments, accepted by the office, are assessed a service fee by the banks for handling the transaction. This service fee is actual funds collected. When credit card collections are used, they are documented on the ledger card as a payment. The bank charge is taken from the office checkbook as a fee and not added to the patient's account. The office may post the paid amount on the patient's account and post the bank charge as an adjustment. The patient is still given credit for the entire amount of the credit card transaction.

Loans. An additional payment option is a loan. Patients may have their own loan sources; many dental offices work with agencies or banks to provide their patients this service. To receive loans, patients must complete the appropriate paperwork. Some loan agencies can quickly verify that patients meet requirements; others need a day or two. In this system, the patient must pay additional loan fees, but payments can be established through loan agencies so those patients can pay on time.

Collection Management

Collection on some accounts is necessary no matter how effective the billing process. The best business assistant still has to collect from individuals who have past due accounts. There are individuals who have financial difficulties. Work with these patients so that they can continue paying small amounts on the accounts until they are in better financial states. There are also patients who are negligent in meeting their financial obligations. The longer the dental office puts off contacting these people, the less chance there is in receiving the delinquent amounts.

The dentist will give guidelines for patient collections. They must be handled carefully and tactfully. The best way to address this issue with a patient is in a manner of aiding the patient in finding a way to pay the account balance. The Fair Debt Collection Practice Act makes it illegal to telephone a debtor at inconvenient hours. It also prevents collection calls from being made to the debtor's employer, except to verify employment. It prevents anyone seeking collection from getting information through false pretense or by threatening violence.

The telephone is a more effective way to contact the debtor. First, identify that the person is the individual who is sought and then discuss methods for resolving the problem. Always set a date when the payment can be expected. If it does not arrive as promised, then contact the patient immediately to let the patient know that the dental office is not letting the debt slide.

Collection Letters. If unable to reach the debtor by telephone, a collection letter is necessary. The letters are sent to encourage patients to pay their overdue balances. Collection letters can be sent through certified mail (Figure 36-17). Any letters received via certified

---

Tamara Riegel, D.D.S.
909 Central
Rockford, LA 20011

December 1, 2003

Mr. John Cooper
41 Santiford Drive
Locust, LA 22011

Dear Mr. Cooper:

Your account with our office
is three months past due, and
you have not responded to our
previous requests for payment.
Please pay your balance of
$152 at this time, or contact
us with an explanation of why
you cannot pay.

Please call me at 555-7823 if
you have a question about your
account. Otherwise, we expect
your payment immediately.

Sincerely,

Natalie Short
Accounts Manager

Tamara Riegel, D.D.S.
909 Central
Rockford, LA 20011

December 29, 2003

Mr. John Cooper
41 Santiford Drive
Locust, LA 22011

Dear Mr. Cooper:

Your son, Royce, had a
seriously infected tooth in
March when he came to Dr.
Riegel for treatment. Dr.
Riegel was pleased to use her
experience and education to
treat Royce, and it was in
this same spirit of
cooperation that we expected
you to pay your account within
a reasonable amount of time.

Four months have passed and
you have still not remitted
the $152 outstanding balance
on your account. We cannot
continue to keep your unpaid
account on our books. If you
are experiencing financial
difficulties, please call the
office so we can arrange a
payment schedule that is
agreeable to both of us.

Sincerely,

Natalie Short
Accounts Manager

Tamara Riegel, D.D.S.
909 Central
Rockford, LA 20011

February 1, 2004

Mr. John Cooper
41 Santiford Drive
Locust, LA 22011

Dear Mr. Cooper:

You have not replied to our
previous notices regarding
your unpaid balance of $152.
Unless we hear from you
personally within 14 days,
your account will be given to
the Rockford Medical and
Dental Collection Service.

Do not wait any longer to
contact me at 555-7823 if you
wish to maintain your previous
good credit record with Dr.
Riegel. As previously
suggested, we will cooperate
in arranging a suitable
payment schedule, if needed.

Sincerely,

Natalie Short
Accounts Manager

FIGURE 36-17 Collection letters sent to patients with delinquent accounts, drafted to encourage patients to pay their bills.

PROCEDURE 36-5

Preparing a Deposit Slip

The dental receptionist or office business assistant creates the deposit slip and either takes it to the bank or the dentist takes it to the bank to be deposited. Deposits normally are made in person or placed in the night deposit box.

EQUIPMENT

- Deposit slip (Figure 36-18)
- Cash and checks received for that day
- Office stamp for endorsing the check
- Envelope in which to place the deposit slip, checks, and cash

PROCEDURE STEPS

1. Place the date on the deposit slip.

2. Separate the currency (coin and paper money) from the checks.

3. Tally the coins and place the total sum in the designated space on the deposit slip.

4. Tally the paper money and place the total sum in the designated space on the deposit slip.

5. On the back of the deposit slip, list each check separately, listing the patient's last name and the amount of the check in the space provided in the right-hand column.

6. Total the list amounts from the checks on the back of the deposit slip and place this sum in the area on the front of the check slip in the space identified as checks.

7. Total the currency (both coins and paper money) and the check amount and place this sum at the bottom of the deposit slip under total. This amount should total the total identified on the payments column on the day sheet. One way to further check that the total is accurate is to add up the coins, paper money, and each check. This verifies that the sum is correct.

8. Enter the date and the amount of the deposit into the checkbook stub.

FIGURE 36-18 Sample deposit slip.

mail are signed by the people receiving them. This receipt is sent back to the sender to verify that the letter was received. The receipt should be kept in the patient's chart, along with a copy of the letter.

Occasionally, dental offices have to turn highly delinquent accounts over to an outside collection agency. The agency will normally charge one-third of the balance collected as its fee. All accounts that reach collection are reported to the credit bureau. After the money is collected, the fees are subtracted and the balance is sent to the office.

Special Collection Situations

■ If the patient has declared bankruptcy, the dental office is notified. The dental office is no longer able to send statements or attempt to collect the amount owed. The patient's debt is written off as a loss for the dental office.

■ If the patient has died and his or her finances are tied up, a person is designated to execute the deceased individual's estate and oversee payment of outstanding bills. The statements should be addressed to the "Estate of" from that time forward until paid.

■ Some patients may "skip" town and leave no forwarding addresses. The statement will be returned with "no forwarding address" on the unopened envelope. Verify that the address was correct. If it is, the office needs to decide whether to pursue the unpaid debt or turn it over to a collection agency.

Recording Payments

All payments are written promptly onto the ledgers and into the bookkeeping system. The totals are deposited into the bank daily. The cash is noted separately and all the checks are endorsed with the office rubber endorsement stamp, which indicates the specific bank that is utilized. Most of the offices have restrictive endorsement stamps that state "for deposit only." This protects the office if the check is stolen or lost. A deposit slip with the date, practice name, account number, currency and checks listed, and total amount of the deposit identified on it is written for each deposit. Most offices keep carbon copies of these slips along with the bank's deposit receipt, as records of these transactions.

Accounts Payable

The accounts payable are the amounts that the practice owes others. Included are necessary expenses. The expenses that are required to run the dental practice are called **overhead**. The total accounts receivable is calculated as the **gross income**. Subtract the accounts payable from the gross income to identify the **net income**. The net income is the true profit the practice makes. The practice cannot remain vital if there is no

net income for the dentist. It is not advisable to operate a business in a non-profitable manner for long.

Some of the expenses are *fixed* (remain the same) each month. These include the mortgage, the full-time salaries, and some utilities. Other expenses are *variable*, meaning they fluctuate (do not remain constant), and are dependent on needs for the month. Variable overhead expenses include dental supplies, dental laboratory costs, and equipment repairs. The business assistant, along with the dentist, can document the monthly overhead and evaluate whether costs can be cut without decreasing patient service. One of the highest monthly variable overhead costs is in the area of dental supplies.

Inventory Supply Systems

There are different types of supplies utilized in the dental office. Some of these supplies are disposable and used up quickly. They are referred to as **expendable**. Examples of expendable supplies are cotton rolls and stationery. Other supplies are retained in the office for long periods of time and are referred to as **non-expendable** supplies. Examples of non-expendable supplies are an autoclave and a light-curing unit.

A number of things must be taken into account when developing an efficient inventory supply system. Products need to be looked at according to the following factors:

■ **Shelf life**—Length of time the product can be stored until it begins to deteriorate.

■ **Item price**—Cost of one item.

■ **Unit price**—Cost of a commonly grouped package of an item (for example, a dozen toothbrushes).

■ **Bulk price**—Reduced price for a minimum of units (for example, twelve dozen units of toothbrushes).

■ **Price break**—Minimum quantity of a supply at which the per unit or per item cost is reduced.

■ **Lead time**—Time between when an order is placed and the time it is received.

■ **Rate of use**—How much of a product is used in a specific period. For example, twenty toothbrushes per week are given out to patients.

■ **Reorder point**—Point ensuring that an adequate supply is available, taking into consideration the lead time and the rate of use for the product.

There are several inventory records systems that can be utilized in the dental office to keep track of the supplies. The goal of any system is that the supplies are available when they are needed. Maintenance of an adequate supply of materials and supplies is essential. Placing the supplies in a central location makes it easier to manage and restock. In most offices, one person is assigned to oversee the inventory system. The system should be simple, easy to use, and accurate. The computer has made an inventory list system easier to maintain. The system can be further designed to meet the needs of the practice. Another system that is routinely used in dental offices is the tag system. The tag system makes use of a reorder tag that is attached to the item in the inventory and represents the reorder point for that particular supply. Tags can be attached with rubber bands. The information on the tag may include only the name of the item. Some dental supply companies come into the dental offices and set up this system by placing the initial tags on the inventory.

When supplies get down to the tagged item, the tagged item is placed in an area to be ordered from the dental supply representative or mail-order supply company.

Mail-order supply companies require slight increases in lead time.

Another supply inventory system that has become more popular is the bar code system. This system allows dental assistants to use a bar code wand that reads the bar code information and electronically transmits this data to the dental supplier to be ordered (Figure 36-19). This system cuts down on the dental assistant's time spent ordering supplies.

Receiving Supplies. When the supplies are delivered, check them for damage. If there is damage, immediately notify the manufacturer or distributor. A **packing slip** listing everything that was shipped is enclosed with the supplies. Check the items received against the packing slip list; if there are any discrepancies, contact the manufacturer.

The packing slip does not have price information. That is sent separately on the *statement*, a monthly summary with charges of all supplies.

If any items are returned for any reason to a supplier, a *credit slip* is issued. The credit slip assures the office that they will not be charged for the returned item. If the supplier cannot supply an item on the order, a *back order slip* is issued. This slip lists the items the supplier could not ship immediately and gives an estimated date when the items will be available.

Storing Supplies. After supplies are received and checked, the dental assistant places them in the storage area. The supplies should be rotated so that the older supply items are used before the more recently purchased items. The older supplies are placed directly in the front, ready for use. Some of the supplies require special storage. For example, some of the dental medications and restorative materials require refrigeration, while others require dry, dark areas. Read the manufacturer's instructions for special storage concerns.

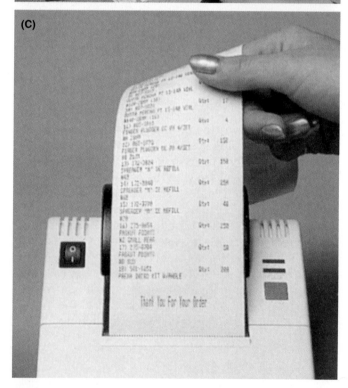

FIGURE 36-19 Electronic ordering system. (A) Scanner. (B) Assistant ordering supplies. (C) Receipt printout. *(Courtesy of Patterson Dental Supply, Inc.)*

PROCEDURE 36-6

Reordering Supplies

The dental assistant may be assigned specifically to order supplies or this task may be shared by several auxiliaries.

EQUIPMENT

Red Flag Reorder Tag System
- Red flag reorder tags that have surfaced for reordering
- Telephone
- Index card with order information

Electronic Bar Code System (Figure 36-20)
- Bar code wand
- Telephone

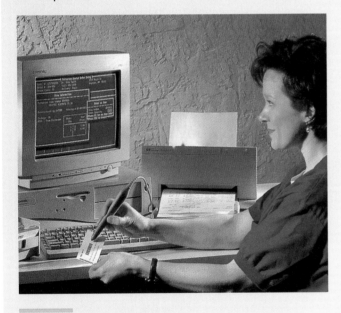

FIGURE 36-20 Electronic barcode ordering system. Assistant enters ID card using a portable barcode reader. *(Courtesy of Patterson Dental Supply, Inc.)*

PROCEDURE STEPS

Red Flag Reorder Tag System

1. Gather the red flags indicating the items that require reordering.

2. Check the index card to obtain the ordering information for each item.

3. Place an indicator in the upper-right corner to indicate that this item is to be ordered immediately.

4. After the item is ordered, place the indicator in the upper-left corner until the product arrives.

5. When the item arrives, remove the indicator from the tag, place the most recently received items to the back of the supply (using the older materials first), and place the red flag ordering tag on the minimum quantity needed in stock before reordering must be accomplished again.

Electronic Bar Code System

1. Identify the items that require reordering. (This system is used for the commonly ordered items.)

2. Obtain the book that has product information and bar codes identified.

3. Use the bar code wand to input the items needed. Run the wand over the bar codes of the items needing ordering. Indicate on the transmitter the number of items needed. The order is then transmitted directly to the dental supply company for ordering.

4. Place a date on the listed items and indicate the number that have been ordered.

Account Payment

The accounts payable for a dental office are paid monthly or bimonthly by the dentist. The dentist reviews the accounts payable and approves payment and then the business assistant prepares the checks for the dentist to sign. All statements are checked for accuracy prior to being paid.

The checks, which are orders for the identified banks to pay the specific amounts indicated to the payee, should be dated. The name of the **payee** must be clearly indicated following the preprinted "Pay to the Order of." The amount of the payment must be entered in both figures and in words. It is advisable to complete the check stub information needed for tax purposes. The **check register** is a record of all the deposits and checks made from the account. It provides a running balance of the funds within the account.

PROCEDURE 36-7

Reconciling a Bank Statement

Dental receptionist or business assistant reconciles the bank statement each month.

EQUIPMENT

- Bank statement (Figure 36-21)
- Checkbook
- Calculator

PROCEDURE STEPS

1. Make sure that all checks and deposits have been added to or subtracted from the checkbook.

2. Subtract any bank service charge from the last balance listed in the checkbook.

3. Check off each listed check in the bank statement against the checkbook and verify the amount listed.

4. Check off each deposit listed in the bank statement against the checkbook and verify the amount listed.

5. On the back of the bank statement, place the ending balance from the front of the statement in the ending balance space on the worksheet.

6. List all checks from the checkbook that have not cleared the bank in the section provided on the back worksheet.

7. List all deposits from the checkbook that have not been received by the bank on the space provided on the worksheet on the back of the statement.

8. Total the checks not cleared and the deposits not received. Subtract the checks not received from the ending balance on the bank statement and add the deposits not received to the ending balance on the bank statement. This balance should agree with the checkbook balance. (If there are any bank charges on the statement, make the corresponding adjustments to the checkbook balance.)

Summary of Account Balance   Closing Date 1/15/03

Account # 1257-164013   Ending Balance $8,347.62

Beginning Balance	$ 7,152.18	
Total Deposits and Additions	$ 8,643.86	
Total Withdrawals	$ 7,433.21	
Service Charge	$ 15.24	

Number	Date	Amount	Number	Date	Amount
201	12/18/02	173.82	234	1/4/03	96.31
223*	12/18/02	44.12	235	1/4/03	73.48
224	12/20/02	586.00	236	1/6/03	325.40
225	12/21/02	24.15	237	1/7/03	40.00
226	12/22/02	33.90	238	1/8/03	66.77
228*	12/23/02	1250.00	241*	1/9/03	15.55
229	12/24/02	11.75	242	1/10/03	12.45
230	12/24/02	19.02	243	1/10/03	4441.64
231	1/2/03	43.80	244	1/10/03	64.55
232	1/3/03	39.00			
233	1/4/03	71.50			

*Denotes gap in check sequence

Date	Deposit Amount	Date	Deposit Amount
18-Dec	361.75	4-Jan	825.00
19-Dec	586.00	5-Jan	1286.71
20-Dec	918.21	7-Jan	608.00
21-Dec	201.00	8-Jan	811.15
2-Jan	475.00	9-Jan	1092.68
3-Dec	1478.36		

Front

---

1. Enter ending balance from the front of this statement

$ _8,347.62_

2. Enter deposits not shown on this statement.

$ _3,162.50_

3. Subtotal (add 1 and 2)

$ _11,510.12_

4. List outstanding checks or other withdrawals here

Check #	Amount
222	37.89
227	161.15
239	11.50
240	92.12
245	835.17
246	21.75
247	586.00

5. Total outstanding checks.

$ _1,745.58_

Balance (subtract 5 from 3)

$ _9,764.54_

This should equal your checkbook balance

Back

FIGURE 36-21 Sample bank statement.

PROCEDURE 36-8

Writing a Business Check

The dental receptionist or business assistant writes out the office accounts payable for the dentist to review and sign.

EQUIPMENT

- Checkbook with check and stub (Figure 36-22)
- Calculator

PROCEDURE STEPS

1. Write or type in the date. Make sure the date is current.

2. Write or type in the name of the payee. Verify that this is the correct payee.

3. Write in the correct numbers for the correct amount and write out the amount in the designated area. Check that the numerical and written amounts agree and are correct.

4. Fill out the memo, indicating what the check is for.

5. Fill out the date, payee, memo information, and amount on the check stub.

6. Verify that everything is accurate, including spelling.

7. Have the dentist sign on the signature line after reviewing the account payable.

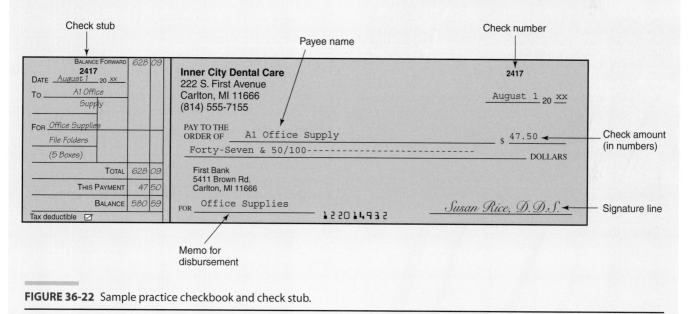

FIGURE 36-22 Sample practice checkbook and check stub.

Each month, the bank sends a statement showing any transactions that took place within the account during the month. It lists all checks that have cleared the bank, any deposits received by the bank, and any service charges that were deducted from the account. It should be reconciled against the entries made in the dental office check register.

Nonsufficient Funds. If any check is written in excess of the amount in the account, it is returned to the payee and marked NSF for nonsufficient funds. The bank charges the account for returned, or "bounced," checks. Most offices require the payer to pay an additional charge to the office for the returned check.

Stop Payment. If a check is written and has not cleared the bank, the payer can stop payment of the check. The bank may charge for stopping payment of a check. Normally, if the payee deposits the check in the bank immediately, it clears within a day of issue.

Petty Cash

The **petty cash** is the money kept in the office for minor expenses, such as for coffee supplies or postage-due letters. Most offices keep less than $100 in this account. The receptionist oversees this cash account. Each time it is used, a voucher or receipt is placed in the cash box until the money gets low. Then, the fund is replenished by writing another check to the cash fund, bringing it up to the original amount. The check is noted as petty cash and the receipts total the amount replenished to the account.

Payroll

The business assistant may complete the employee payroll. Each employee fills out a W-4 form, or the Employee's Withholding Allowance Certificate, when he or she begins employment, which includes his or her name, address, Social Security number, and the total number of allowances to be claimed. With this information, the payroll is calculated using charts provided by the Internal Revenue Service. Federal taxes are based on the amount earned, marital status, number and type of allowances (exemptions) claimed, and length of pay period. Most state and local taxes are calculated on the total gross earnings of the employee. A required deduction under the Federal Insurance Contributions Act (FICA), commonly called Social Security, is calculated on the basis of gross pay. The employer is required to match this deducted amount and send both contributions to the federal government quarterly. Other deductions that may be taken from the employee's paycheck are health and life insurance payments, along with retirement or savings that are put in another account.

At the end of the year, the employer is required to give each employee a W-2 wage and tax statement (Figure 36-23). This statement is used by the employee to submit his or her federal income tax. The statement includes total wages earned and tax deductions made for the year by that employee.

FIGURE 36-23 W-2 form, summarizing all earnings and deductions for the year. The employer prepares a W-2 form for each employee by January 31.

CHAPTER SUMMARY

The dental reception area must be an environment in which all patients feel welcome and comfortable. Today, dentistry can be a positive experience, and dental treatment can be pain free. That image is developed when the patient first steps into the reception area. Patients may not consciously realize the message that is being received, but the dental office should present an atmosphere that relieves anxiety.

Front office staff has changed dramatically in recent years. All individuals in the front office require knowl-edge of business machines such as computers, fax machines, and copy machines. These individuals must be organized, have a knowledge of dental treatments, and have good communication and problem-solving skills.

Marketing is also an important part of the dental practice. A dental office is a business as well as a health care facility. Dental assistants, along with all members of the dental team, need to be involved in marketing the practice.

Case Study

Melissa Jones is a new graduate of an accredited dental assisting program and has received her dental assisting national certification. She will be the dental receptionist in the office of Dr. Ward. Dr. Ward is using a computer-based patient management system and would like to expand on marketing ideas.

Case Study Review

1. Which types of effective marketing and practice management functions can be done from a computer-based practice management system?

2. What types of reports can be generated by a computer-based patient management system?

3. Identify the background knowledge Melissa received in her dental assisting program that will aid her in this task.

REVIEW QUESTIONS

Multiple Choice

1. When moving from a manual to a computerized bookkeeping system, office staff can expect
   a. a week or so turnaround time to input patient information.
   b. that the manual and computer systems may need to run concurrently for several weeks.
   c. the computer system to require a great deal of time until all patient information is entered into the system.
   d. all of the above.

2. A check guaranteed by the bank is called a
   a. certified check.
   b. cashier's check.
   c. voucher check.
   d. money order.

3. One of the primary reasons that dental patients do not pay their dental bills is that
   a. patients consider the cost of dental care to be too high.
   b. patients think that the insurance company should pay the entire dental bill.
   c. patients become unable to pay their dental bills because of financial hardship.
   d. the treatment plan was not discussed and sound financial arrangements were not made at the time of the dental services.

4. An example of a fixed cost is
   a. cost of supplies.
   b. cost of treating dental patients.
   c. salaries.
   d. cost of dental materials.

5. The Employee's Withholding Allowance Certificate, which is completed by all employees, is the
   a. W-2.
   b. W-4.
   c. accounts payable.
   d. accounts receivable.

6. In what year was the Americans with Disabilities Act passed by Congress?
   a. 1980
   b. 1990
   c. 2000
   d. 2005

7. Regarding ergonomics for computer workstations, comfortable monitor viewing level is generally ____ below horizontal.
   a. 1–5%
   b. 5–10%
   c. 5–30%
   d. 25–50%

8. Appointment books are normally set up in ____ minute units.
   a. 10
   b. 15
   c. 30
   d. a and b

9. The insurance birthday rule pertains to (the)
   a. primary carrier.
   b. dependent child of two parents who have dental coverage.
   c. stepchildren who have dental coverage.
   d. secondary carrier.

10. Assume that a patient had dental work totaling $600, and is eligible for benefits under two insurance carriers that have a benefit-less-benefit provision. One carrier allows $400 for this service and the other allows $450. The second carrier would pay $450 and the other would pay
    a. $0.
    b. $100.
    c. $450.
    d. $50.

Critical Thinking

1. Why is billing patients promptly and accurately critical to the success of the dental office?

2. List the five sections of the pegboard day sheet and describe the functions of each.

3. Explain why a color-coding system is used for filing charts.

Web Activities

1. Practice management is an important part of being successful in dentistry. Visit http://www.dentaleconomics.com and review articles in the current issue of the magazine. Review one of the articles.

2. Go to http://www.dental-resources.com and examine the many clinical software programs available to dental offices. Contrast one of these software programs with the one used in your school program.

3. Dr. Gordon J. Christensen, author of *Clinical Research*, a newsletter that evaluates many dental products, is also a well-known dentistry speaker. At http://www.dentaleconomics.com, visit the area where questions are asked and responded to by Dr. Christensen. Review the questions for the current month and be prepared to discuss them in class.

4. Go to www.advanced-input.com, click on medigenic, and find information about the alert system indicator that flashes at defined intervals to promote infection-control practices. Be prepared to discuss how this would help with infection control. In what other areas of the dental office would this be useful?

EMPLOYMENT STRATEGIES

SPECIFIC INSTRUCTIONAL OBJECTIVES

The student should strive to meet the following objectives and demonstrate an understanding of the facts and principles presented in this chapter:

1. Identify three pathways to obtain DANB certification.

2. Explain how to obtain employment and identify types of practices.

3. Set goals and identify sources to obtain employment in the dental field.

4. Identify steps of preparing a cover letter and a résumé.

5. Define how to prepare for the interview.

6. Explain the interview process and identify skills and preparation techniques that will aid in obtaining the job.

7. Identify the skills that a successful dental assistant possesses. Explain how to terminate employment.

KEY TERMS

American Dental Assistants Association (ADAA) *(928)*

American Dental Association (ADA) *(928)*

Dental Assisting National Board, Inc. (DANB) *(928)*

dental associate *(929)*

partnership *(929)*

INTRODUCTION

As the required formal training necessary to become a dental assistant nears completion, the student must switch his or her goals toward becoming an employed dental assistant. The first step in this process is obtaining national certification. Then, the employment search begins.

When conducting the search for suitable employment, it is necessary to be well prepared and goal oriented. Being knowledgeable about how to write a cover letter and prepare a résumé is very important. Effective cover letters and résumés lead to job interviews. Understanding the interview process and possessing the skills necessary to interview successfully lead to job offers.

Obtaining National Certification

National certification for dental assistants is not mandatory in every state. Once obtained, however, the patients and the dentist can be assured that the assistant has the basic knowledge and background necessary to perform as a professional on the dental team. The **Dental Assisting National Board, Inc. (DANB)**, assumes the responsibility for credentialing dental assistants. This board is independent of the **American Dental Association (ADA)** and the **American Dental Assistants Association (ADAA)**. Upon completing and passing the chairside dental assisting examination of DANB, the dental assistant can display the certificate that verifies successful completion of the DANB test (Figure 37-1). The assistant can also wear the official certified dental assistant (CDA) pin acknowledging that he or she is a certified dental assistant and can use that title (Figure 37-2). The DANB examination is divided into three major categories: radiology, infection control, and general chairside. An assistant must pass all three sections in order to become a certified dental assistant. Maintenance of the CDA credential is through yearly continuing education hours and a renewal fee.

A dental assistant is eligible to take the dental assisting examination and can obtain national certification by DANB through three pathways:

Pathway I

- Graduation from a dental assisting or dental hygiene program accredited by the ADA Commission on Dental Accreditation.

- Cardiopulmonary resuscitation (CPR) earned within two years prior to the examination date for which the application is being made.

Pathway II

- High school graduation or equivalent.

- Minimum of two (2) years full-time work experience (at least 3,500 hours accumulated over a 24-month period) as a dental assistant, verified by the dentist-employer;

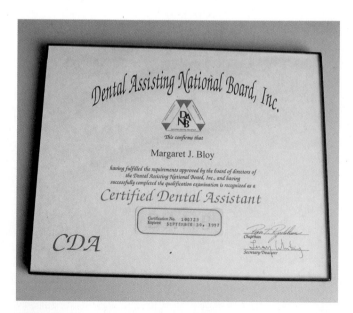

FIGURE 37-1 Dental Assisting National Board (DANB) certificate.

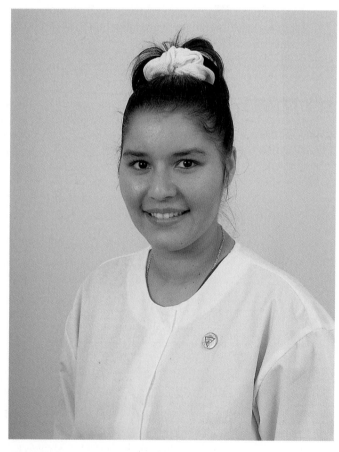

FIGURE 37-2 The official Certified Dental Assistant (CDA) pin of the Dental Assisting National Board worn by a certified dental assistant.

or at least 3,500 hours of combined full- and part-time or only part-time work experience earned over a minimum of 24 months and a maximum of 48 months as a dental assistant verified by dentist-employer.

- Cardiopulmonary resuscitation (CPR) earned within two years prior to the examination date for which the application is being made.

Pathway III

- Status as a current or previous DANB CDA or graduation from a DDS or DMD program accredited by the ADA or an equivalent foreign dental degree program.
- Cardiopulmonary resuscitation (CPR) earned within two years prior to the examination date for which the application is being made.

Reprinted with permission of the Dental Assisting National Board, Inc. (DANB)

Every dental assistant should obtain national certification to ensure that his or her patients receive the best care possible and to build self-esteem.

Employment

Whether graduating from an accredited program or just trying to obtain a position in the dental office, there are several important tasks that must be accomplished first. Planning future employment is important. It may be essential to obtain dental assisting national certification for the state in which employment is sought. If that is the case, reflect on the pathways available and seek the one that best suits your needs.

After obtaining the necessary credentials, the next goal is to prepare to obtain successful employment. Research should be done to identify the type of practice that will be the most interesting, stimulating, and enjoyable. When choosing an employer, find one who has a good reputation and whose philosophy is similar to your own. A dental assistant needs to feel that he or she is working together with the dentist and the other team members in order to care for the patients in the best manner possible. Do research and talk to employees who work for the dentist to make sure that a good match for employment will be accomplished prior to obtaining the position. The other aspect of the employment is working well with the other employees. Are they team players and is compatibility possible?

It is important to find employment that best suits the individual's needs and allows for the best possible situation for the dental assistant, the employer, and the patients. Before taking the first position offered, consider the following:

- What qualities are desired in an employer?
- What areas of growth are available in this situation?
- From an employee's position, what strengths can be brought to this position?

- What individual areas can be improved upon?
- Overall, what type of dentistry is interesting?

Solo or Partnership Practice

The majority of dentists practice in solo practices where there are single dentists. A dentist may hire another dentist under a contractual agreement; this hired dentist is a **dental associate**. An associate relationship may turn into a **partnership**, in which each dentist has equal rights and duties. A partnership is developed through a legal agreement and makes both dentists responsible for any accounts payable. A partner is not held responsible for malpractice suits against the other partner.

Partnerships in dental practices are increasing. This is due to the tremendous startup costs a dentist faces upon graduation from dental school. Therefore, a newly graduated dentist may work in an established practice as a dental associate for some time and then, after an allotted period of time, become a partner. Another way that dentists are dealing with the costs of a practice is to share a building and/or front office employees while still maintaining solo practices.

Group Practice

Another type of dental office is the group practice. In a group practice, any number of dentists (both general and specialty) can share a building and still remain independent. The positive aspects of this type of practice is the opportunity to talk over cases with each other, reduce overhead, and increase patient coverage on weekends and holidays. In addition, the total number of employees in the group practice may lend itself to offering more complete and extensive benefit packages. The more employees under the same insurance plan, the better the rates for the employer.

Dental Specialty Practice

If a dental assistant likes to assist primarily in oral surgery, endodontics, periodontics, orthodontics, prosthodontics, pathology, pediatric dentistry, or dental public health, specialty offices are available. Fewer employment opportunities are available in the areas of pathology and dental public health. The dental specialties work with the general dentists to care for specific cases. The general dentist refers the patient to a specialty office to obtain a special service and then the patient returns to the general dental office for routine care.

Other Employment Choices

Dental assistants can gain employment in government clinics that care for patients who are eligible to receive dental care at a reduced rate. Often, federal or state grants set up programs to meet the specific needs of people who cannot afford dental care. These programs may also collect data on specific diseases this group of people may have. Usually, the guidelines of the programs change or have to be renewed annually. A dental assistant is an employee hired by the overseer of the grant. This dental assistant may receive great satisfaction treating patients in this type of program.

School Clinics and Laboratories. Dental schools and dental assisting schools also employ dental assistants to either work in the clinic with students, teach, and/or be administrators for the program. In dental schools, the dental assistants work with student dentists to simulate four-handed dentistry or in dental laboratories to help the students perfect their skills.

Veterans Hospitals. Veterans hospitals hire dental assistants to assist the dentists on staff in the clinics. Employment in this area must be obtained through the civil service office. Points are given to individuals who have worked in the service or been employed in veterans programs before. A list of qualifications can be obtained from the civil service office that advertises the employment position.

Dental Supply Companies. Dental supply companies hire dental assistants as sales representatives for goods and supplies. Normally, a dental assistant in this position does not utilize his or her chairside skills, but becomes knowledgeable about the products and travels from dental office to dental office providing product information and ordering supplies.

Insurance Companies. Dental assistants are also hired by insurance companies to process dental insurance claims. Having knowledge and background in dental terminology and procedures is an asset in understanding situations and processing dental insurance claims.

Employment Search

After a decision is made about the desired type of dental practice, locating open positions is the next step. Many dentists advertise in daily newspaper classified sections. Other areas where employment opportunities are posted include the local dental and dental assistant societies. Most local societies have newsletters or other services that list the job openings. If graduating from a dental assisting program, career placement services may be available at the school. Some employment agencies have listings for dental assistant jobs, and most dental supply houses know of dentists who are hiring. Leaving a cover letter and résumé with some of these agencies may be a consideration.

An additional resource for an employment search is the Internet. On the Web, start with a search in employment in dental professions. This is especially helpful when planning to relocate.

Preparing a Cover Letter and Résumé

The next step in the employment search is to prepare a cover letter and a résumé. These documents introduce the prospective employee and present the individual's educational background, training, and previous employment experience. The cover letter states why the individual is right for the position and when he or she is available for employment.

The cover letter and the résumé should be printed on quality rag-bond paper (normally white, light gray, or off-white) and follow a professional format. It is crucial that the cover letter and résumé be prepared on a word processor, printed on a laser printer or high-quality dot matrix printer, and contain correct spelling, punctuation, and grammar. Every cover letter and résumé must be proofread several times before being submitted to a prospective employer.

Cover Letter

A cover letter is an introduction to a prospective employer (Figure 37-3). It communicates to the employer or hiring personnel the individual's potential value and any specific personal attributes that can be called attention to. A cover letter should accompany every résumé. A standard format can be used to develop a cover letter.

- **Return address**—Include a street address, city, state, and zip code.

- **Date**—Month, day, and year.

- **Inside address**—Addressee's name and title, company name, if different, street address, city, state, and zip code.

- **Salutation**—Make every effort to use the correct name. If unknown, and as a last resort, use "To Whom It May Concern:" At the end of every salutation, a colon (:) is used.

- **First paragraph**—Tell why the letter is being written and indicate where the information about the employment opportunity was obtained and which position is desired.

- **Second paragraph**—Identify the reasons for interest in the position (such as the dental office has a good reputation for providing quality dental care). List the qualifications that would be assets to the employer and dental team members (for example, a graduate of an accredited dental assisting program and an explanation of how the academic background makes for a qualified dental assistant). Mention any relevant work experience. Refer the employer to the résumé, which lists individual qualifications, education, training, and experience.

- **Third paragraph**—Ask for a personal interview, indicate flexible available times to be reached, and list a

625 "B" Street
Spokane, WA 99228

January 12, 2007

Dr. Conrad Jones
312 33rd
Spokane, WA 99205

Dear Dr. Jones:

I am writing in response to your advertisement in the April edition of the *Spokesman Review* for an expanded-function dental assistant.

I believe that I am the "gentle, caring, enthusiastic" dental assistant that you are looking for. You will find me to be flexible and capable of working individually or as a team member. A recent graduate of the Spokane Community College Dental Assisting program, I am currently awaiting the results of my Dental Assisting National Board examination. With the combination of my training, my desire to work, and my love of helping people, I will be a valuable asset to your office.

Looking at my enclosed résumé, you will see that I have worked in several offices during my training. I have also assisted several dentists in the volunteer clinic, provided dental education in the area schools, and worked with patients in my other health-related employment. Computer proficiency was obtained during my other employment opportunities.

Please contact me for a personal interview to further discuss the position and to answer any questions you may have. My schedule is flexible so feel free to call me at (509) 555-1857 as soon as is convenient so an appointment can be arranged.

Looking forward to meeting you and your staff and to getting the opportunity to demonstrate my abilities as a valuable member of your office team.

Sincerely yours,

Jean Lucas
Dental Assistant

Enclosure: résumé

FIGURE 37-3 Cover letter for employment as a dental assistant in a dental office.

phone number with area code, if applicable, and an e-mail address, if available. Close with a statement that encourages a speedy response: "I am available for an interview at your convenience and will be calling within the next five days to confirm an interview time with you," or "I am looking forward to meeting with you and your dental team in the near future."

- **Closing**—Close the letter with "Sincerely" and a comma. Then, type four returns and your name. The four spaces provide room for a signature, written in black ink. (Using other colors may detract from the professionalism that has been established in the cover letter.)

- **Enclosures**—After the typed name, type two returns and then type the words "Enclosure: Résumé" (any other enclosures can be listed beneath the word "Résumé," such as letters of recommendation).

Résumé

A résumé should fit on one page (Figure 37-4), and it should be attractive and professional. Present specific

625 "B" Street
Spokane, WA 99228

Phone: 509-555-1857
Fax: 599-555-3038
E-mail:
Jlucas@spokane.wa.us.com

Jean Lucas

Career Objective	To obtain a dental assisting position in which my education and skills can be utilized, in an office that uses the team approach to providing quality dental care.		
Education	1995–1997	Spokane Community College	Spokane, WA

AAS Degree, Dental Assisting
♣ Vice President's Honor Roll for academic achievement

Employment History	1997–Present	Community Clinic	Palouse, WA

Chairside Dental Assistant
♣ Assisted in a variety of dental procedures
♣ Developed and taught a program in oral hygiene to elementary children
♣ Provided patient care and service
♣ Maintained inventory and supplies
♣ Volunteered in community clinic care programs

	1994–1995	Ice Cream Delight	Seattle, WA

Senior Assistant Manager
♣ Supervised employees while providing customer service
♣ Created and decorated cakes
♣ Managed telephones
♣ Maintained accounts payable and receivable
♣ Organized employee work schedule

References: Available on request

FIGURE 37-4 Résumé for employment as a dental assistant in a dental office.

information and stress achievements and skills related to employment. Include personal data, career objective, education, employment history (including qualifications, skills, and abilities), and references.

- **Personal data**—Include the name, address, phone number, and e-mail address, if available, where the individual can be reached. Marital status and birth date are no longer appropriate for a résumé.
- **Career objective**—Identify the desired goal (for example, "To gain a position in a dental office as a dental assistant where I will utilize skills and abilities obtained in dental assisting school").
- **Education**—List certificates, registration, degrees, and continuing education courses that have been

completed. Do not include grade point average unless it is in some way pertinent to the position. Also, list any academic awards received, such as scholarships. List the most recent education first with corresponding dates. High school graduation information is not necessary.

- **Employment history**—Employment history should be listed with an idea of what was accomplished in each position. Use action words to explain what was done. For instance, instead of writing, "I worked as a cashier," it would be better to write, "I was responsible for maintaining cash payables while resolving daily problems, projecting a positive attitude, and developing good customer relations." Present the abilities in the best manner, but always be honest about the job description.

- **References**—It is appropriate to use the sentence "References are available upon request." In many areas of the country, it is beneficial to list three references using name, title, and phone number. It is likely that a dentist will call a fellow dentist to inquire about an individual's skills and abilities. Make sure that the references listed have been checked first to ensure that they will give positive references and that they are aware that they are listed as references. It is important to have references who relate specifically to the desired characteristics and who pertain to the employment that is sought.

Setting Up an Interview

Follow through on what was said in the cover letter. For example, if the letter mentions making a follow-up call in five days, be sure to call back on that fifth day. When making a follow-up call, make sure that background noises are not distracting. If you are nervous using the telephone to set up the interview, visit the dental office or practice in person or with a friend and identify a script that is comfortable to use while making the contacts. When setting up an interview, you should make sure that your schedule can accommodate the appointment time. It is also important to make sure that it is scheduled at a convenient time for the dentist and staff.

Interview Process

When preparing for the interview, there are several things to consider. It is important to be at least five minutes early for the interview, so allow additional time to get there. It is important that some research has been done regarding the dental office. The additional interest in the dental office will have a positive effect on the prospective employer. Know yourself and know your strengths and abilities in order to be prepared for the question that is most often asked: "Why should we hire you for this position?"

Develop questions that can be asked of the dentist and staff. Salary questions should not be the only thing that is brought up in the interview. Ask questions related to team work, prevention programs, or continuing education.

Prepare a portfolio with letters of recommendation, copies of certificates, radiographs you have taken, or any additional items that attest to your abilities and skills (Figure 37-5). Place them in a folder to present to the dentist and staff.

Practice the interview before actually going to one. Ask a friend or family member to do a mock interview and to give feedback on any areas that can be improved. A firm handshake, eye contact, and a smile are still

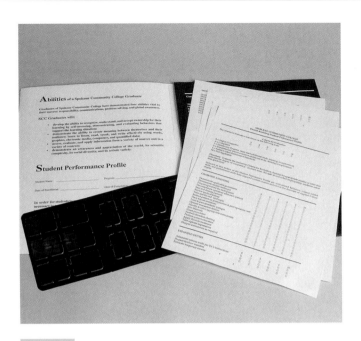

FIGURE 37-5 A personal portfolio is an effective way of sharing your certificates and letters of recommendation with the dental office.

important in the interview process. Sit up straight and speak distinctly. Try to relax and enjoy it. How is the situation going to be handled if the office staff ask you if you would like a cup of coffee? Identify the possible situations and plan ahead.

Appearance is crucial. Wear something that feels comfortable, but a rule of thumb is to dress like an individual who cares about being hired. Many individuals feel comfortable in jeans, but jeans are not appropriate attire for an interview. Dress appropriately and demonstrate good hygiene. Make sure that the clothes are clean and pressed. Do not wear clothes that appear to be flamboyant or dowdy; instead, err on the side of conservatism. Think about the small details, such as where your car keys or purse are going to be placed during the interview. Is a pen available if asked to fill out an application? If necessary, are references with addresses and phone numbers available? If asked to write a paragraph about yourself, can this be accomplished with the correct spellings of the words needed to express yourself properly? Would it be legible? Are the questions available to ask the dental team members? Many of these items may not be necessary, but it is important to be prepared.

Be yourself and, if nervous, say so, then continue on. Make sure that the dentist's name is pronounced correctly and always address the dentist as Dr. __ unless asked otherwise. The dentist may request a working interview. If that is the case, ask about time, uniform, and parking in order to be ready for the identified day. Stay calm and do the best work possible. The interviewer usually closes the session by asking if the interviewee has any further questions (Figure 37-6). This is

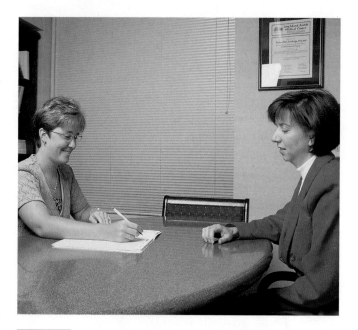

FIGURE 37-6 During the interview, be prepared and listen carefully to the interviewer before answering the question.

the time to ask prepared questions. If all areas have been covered, say, "The specific questions I had prepared to ask have been answered. Can I clarify anything in regard to my background and experience?"

Leaving Interview and Following Up

Be sure to thank the interviewers for their time and shake their hands. It is good to close by stating that you are interested in the position and look forward to hearing from them. If they have not stated it during the interview, ask when they anticipate making a decision on the open position. Dentists look for dental assistants who have positive attitudes, good interpersonal skills, good clinical skills, good dental educational foundations, flexibility, team player attitudes, and the willingness to learn.

If, after the interview, the interviewee confirms that he or she would like to obtain the position in that dental office, send a follow-up letter referring the office to the résumé and restate an interest in becoming part of the dental team (Figure 37-7).

Receiving an Employment Offer

Before accepting an employment offer, it is important to ask a few more questions. If it was not mentioned during the interview, now is an appropriate time to discuss salary. Also, ask about benefits and find out the office's policies on sick days, holidays, and vacation time. Know what the dental assistant's specific responsibilities are and what the office hours will be. Find out when performance evaluations are conducted and what performance objectives lead to a raise in pay.

Professional Conduct During Employment

Once the job is obtained, the dental assistant's goal becomes keeping the job. Basic requirements for keeping the job are to always be on time, be ready to accomplish the necessary skills, plan ahead, and prepare for success. Take care of all outside practical matters so that attention can be placed on fulfilling employment responsibilities. Make sure that child care is arranged (if applicable) and that backup care is available in case the primary caregiver has an emergency. Arrange for reliable transportation.

Maintain high standards of personal hygiene (Figure 37-8). As an employee in a health profession, it is important to present good health standards. Uniforms should be clean and well pressed; shoes should be clean and in good condition. Unfortunately, an employer's perception of an employee's abilities may be influenced by the employee's appearance. Therefore, dental assistants should always look and act like professionals and be well prepared for the job.

Make sure that expectations of the job are identified and then try to go above and beyond those expectations, especially if planning to advance. If expectations are unclear, talk with the office manager or employer to clarify areas of concern. A positive attitude is key to becoming an ideal employee. The dental office can be stressful, especially when a patient procedure changes and the schedule is off course, so tackling each challenge with a positive attitude and flexibility makes the office environment better for everyone. It is a well-known fact that the majority of patients who leave one dental office for another do so because of the poor attitude of one employee. Each dental assistant is responsible for maintaining a positive attitude at work.

Set goals to learn new skills, and stay current with the changes in technology and materials. One way to continue education is through the dental assistant association, other professional courses, and seminars. Other courses in the nearby community or four-year colleges may be of benefit to an individual's professional growth. Seek them out. Occasionally, perform a self-evaluation. Be honest and look at overall individual attitude, skill, and professionalism. Try not to look at others to correct these behaviors, because the only person an individual can change is himself or herself.

Terminating Employment

If you continue to dread going to work, determine where employment could be obtained that would correct the problem. Evaluate your career goals, the qualifications pertaining to these goals, and the new path that is desired. If it is determined that employment in a different office is the plan of action, submit a letter of termination or verbally notify the employer and allow him or

625 "B" Street
Spokane, WA 99228
Fax: 599-555-3038
E-mail: Jlucas@spokane.wa.us.com

Jean Lucas

April 24, 2006

312 33rd Street
Spokane, WA 99025

Dear Dr. Jones and Staff:

I wanted to thank you for your time and interest in interviewing me for the position of chairside dental assistant. I am extremely interested in working with you and your office in this position.

Your office reputation is one that above all provides quality dental care. My personal professional philosophy has always been that patient care is the number one priority and that teamwork is essential to the success of any dental office.

Dr. Jones, thank you again for taking time out of your schedule to interview me. Please review my résumé for my qualifications for the chairside position. I will look forward to hearing from you in the near future. I am available at (509) 555-1857.

Sincerely,

Jean Lucas

Certified Dental Assistant

FIGURE 37-7 Sending a follow-up letter is advisable after an interview.

her two weeks notice so that a replacement can be found. Do everything possible to leave a position on good terms with the employer. Then, if the new career does not proceed as planned, returning to the job when an opening is available is a possibility.

Continued Success

The career of dental assisting is a very rewarding one, both professionally and personally. The work environment is a pleasant one that usually does not require evenings or night shifts. The goal of dental offices is to provide the best care possible for the patients. The patients are appreciative of the dental assistants who care for their needs. The dental assistant who provides a pleasant smile while providing care makes everything go better for the patient. Most days, dental assistants go home feeling good about the skills and knowledge used to provide quality dental care to the patients. Continue to improve dental assisting skills and knowledge through continuing education, and stay challenged to stay knowledgeable about new techniques and materials. Be the best dental assistant possible. Good luck in your career!

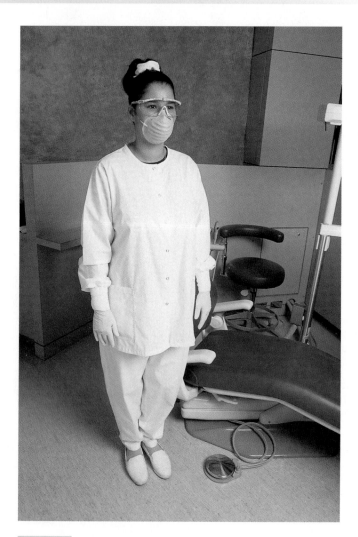

FIGURE 37-8 Maintaining a professional appearance on the job is important for the dental assistant.

CHAPTER SUMMARY

It is important to find employment that will best suit individual needs and that allows for the best possible situation for the dental assistant, employer, and patients. Before taking the first position available, plan ahead. It may be essential to obtain dental assisting national certification for the state in which employment is sought. National certification for dental assistants is not mandatory in every state, but it assures that the patients and the dentist that the assistant has the basic knowledge and background to perform as a professional on the dental team. Make sure that expectations of the job are identified and then try to meet and exceed those if planning to advance. Each dental assistant is responsible for maintaining a positive attitude at work. Set goals to learn new skills and stay abreast of changes in technology and materials. A dental assisting career is very rewarding, both professionally and personally. Be the best dental assistant possible.

Case Study

Drs. Bryan and Lucas are hiring a dental assistant to replace Phong Ho, a dental assistant who is leaving at the end of the month. Phong has been a chairside dental assistant for seven years for Drs. Bryan and Lucas. Svetlana Maklavic has applied for the position and will be the first dental assistant applicant to be interviewed.

Case Study Review

1. What paper work should Svetlana bring to the interview?

2. How should Svetlana prepare for the interview?

3. What clothes should Svetlana wear for an interview with Drs. Bryan and Lucas?

4. Why should Svetlana arrive for the interview five minutes early?

REVIEW QUESTIONS

Multiple Choice

1. A cover letter is a(n)
   a. listing of personal data for the employer.
   b. listing of education.
   c. introduction to your employer.
   d. career objective for the position that is being sought.

2. The interview
   a. does not require follow-up.
   b. is a time for questions and answers about salary and benefits.
   c. requires very little preparation.
   d. requires that you prepare, listen carefully, and think before answering questions asked.

3. If an individual is a graduate of an accredited dental assisting program, what would not be required in order to be eligible to take the Dental Assisting National Board?
   a. Current cardiopulmonary resuscitation care, health care provider level
   b. Verification of dentist employer of work experience
   c. Completed application
   d. Application fee

4. A _____ practice is one in which any number of dentists can share a building and still remain independent.
   a. group
   b. specialty
   c. general
   d. partnership

5. The key to becoming an ideal employee is
   a. a high standard of personal hygiene.
   b. skill.
   c. knowledge.
   d. a positive attitude.

6. The _____ provides national certification for dental assistants.
   a. American Dental Assisting Association
   b. Dental Assisting National Board, Inc.
   c. American Dental Association
   d. Commission on Dental Accreditation

7. To apply for the certification examination, Pathway I, the applicant must
   a. have graduated from a dental assisting or dental hygiene program accredited by the ADA Commission on Dental Accreditation.
   b. have earned a CPR card within two years prior to the examination date.
   c. pay a fee to take the examination.
   d. accomplish all of the above.

8. A dentist may hire another dentist under a contractual agreement; the hired dentist is a
   a. partner.
   b. dental associate.
   c. both a and b.
   d. neither a nor b.

9. The document that introduces the prospective employee and presents the individual's educational background, training, and previous employment experiences is a
   a. cover letter.
   b. resume.
   c. follow-up letter.
   d. interview.

10. Which of the following is one of the most frequently asked questions in the interview process?
    a. Do you have childcare for your child?
    b. Do you have transportation to and from home?
    c. Do you have a background in dentistry?
    d. Why should we hire you for this position?

Critical Thinking

1. Discuss methods of researching a prospective employer.

2. Identify the differences in a solo, partnership, group, or specialty dental practice.

3. Identify areas in which a dental assistant can obtain employment.

Web Activities

1. Identify possible employment opportunities by performing a Web search on dental assistant employment.

2. Find the site http://www.danb.org and download an application. At this site, also read the results of the salary survey "Show me the Money."

APPENDIX A

DENTAL AND DENTAL-RELATED ORGANIZATIONS AND PUBLICATIONS RESOURCE LIST

United States Organizations

American Dental Association (ADA)
211 E. Chicago Avenue
Chicago, IL 60611
(312) 440-2500
(800) 621-8091
online: *www.ada.org*

American Dental Assistants Association (ADAA)
35 East Wacker Drive Suite 1730
Chicago, IL 60601
(312) 541-1550
online: *www.dentalassistant.org*

Dental Assisting National Board, Inc. (DANB)
444 N. Michigan Ave. Suite 900
Chicago, IL 60611
(312) 642-3368
(800) FOR-DANB
online: *www.danb.org*

Centers for Disease Control and Prevention (CDC)
1600 Clifton Rd.
Atlanta, GA 30333
(404) 639-3534
(800) 311-3435
online: *www.cdc.gov.*

American Dental Education Association
1400 K St. NW
Suite 1100
Washington, DC 20005
202-289-7201
online: *www.adea.org*

American Dental Hygienists' Association
444 N. Michigan Ave. Suite 3400
Chicago, IL 60611
312-440-8900
online: *www.adha.org*

American National Standards Institute
25 West 43rd St. 4th Floor
New York, NY 10036
212-642-4900
online: *www.ansi.org*

ASTM International Standards Worldwide
100 Barr Harbor Drive
P.O. Box C700
West Conshohocken, PA 19428
(610) 832-9555
online: *www.astm.org*

Environmental Protection Agency (EPA)
Ariel Rios Building
1200 Pennsylvania Ave.
Washington, DC 20460
Waste Hotline: (800) 424-4372
(202) 260-2090
online: *www.epa.gov*

Food and Drug Administration (FDA)
5600 Fishers Lane
Rockville, MD 20857
Devices and Radiological Health (800) 638-2041
Drug Evaluation Research (301) 295-8000
online: *www.fda.gov*

United States Occupation Safety and Health Administration (OSHA)
Department of Labor
200 Constitution Avenue
Washington, DC 20210
(800) 321-6742
online: *www.osha.gov*

Latex Allergy Information Service
860-482-6869
online: *www.latexallergyhelp.com*

National Association of Dental Laboratories
325 John Knox Road # L103
Tallahassee, FL 32303
800-950-1150
online: *www.nadl.org*

Organization for Safety and Asepsis Procedures (OSAP)
P.O. Box 6297
Annapolis, MD 21401
800-298-6727
online: *www.osap.org*

Canadian Organizations

Canadian Dental Assistants' Association
1750 Courtwood Crescent, Suite 208
Ottawa, ON
K2C 2B5
Phone 1-613-521-5495
Fax: 1-613-521-5572
Toll-Free 1-800-345-5137
e-mail: info@cdaa.ca
online: *www.cdaa.ca*

Canadian Dental Association
1815 Alta Vista Drive
Ottawa, Ontario, Canada
K1G 3Y6
Phone 1 (613) 523 1770
Toll-Free 1-800-267-6354
e-mail: reception@ada-adc.ca
online: *www.cda-adc.ca*

College of Alberta Dental Assistants (CADA)
1102-10707 100 Ave. NW
Edmonton AB T5J 3M1
(780) 486-2526
online: *www.abrda.ca*

Certified Dental Assistants of British Columbia
103–3540 West 41st Ave.
Vancouver, BC V6N 3E6
Canada
(604) 714-1766
Email: info@cdabc.org
online: *www.cdabc.org*

Saskatchewan Dental Assistants Association
P.O. Box 294
Kenaston, SK S0G 2N0
Canada
online: *www.sdaa.sk.ca*

Ontario Dental Nurses & Assistants Association
869 Dundas Street
London, ON N5W 2Z8
Canada
(519) 679-2566
Email: odaainfo@ody.ca
online: *www.odnaa.org*

Nova Scotia Dental Assistants Association
Email: support@new-scotland.com
online: *www.nsdaa.ca*

Product Guides

CRA Newsletter
(Guide to dental products and techniques)
3707 North Canyon Road, Suite 6
Provo, UT 84604
(801) 226-2121
online: *www.cranews.com*

Reality
(Guide to dental products and techniques)
Reality Publishing Company
11757 Katy Freeway; Suite 210
Houston, TX 77079
(800) 544-4999
online: *www.realityesthetics.com*

The Dental Advisor
(Product and equipment guide and evaluation)
Dental Consultants, Inc.
3110 West Liberty
Ann Arbor, MI 48103
800-347-1330
online: *www.dentaladvisor.com*

Dental Products Report
(Product equipment guide and techniques)
2 Northfield Plaza, St. 300
Northfield, IL 60093
847-441-3700
online: *dpr@advanstar.com*

Dental Office
(Innovative ideas for dentists and assistants)
Penn Well Publications
online: *www.dentalofficemag.com*

APPENDIX B

STAGES OF TOOTH ERUPTION

Development of Human Dentition

Prenatal

4 months in utero

6 months in utero

Primary Dentition

Permanent Dentition

Infancy

Birth

4–8 months

8–12 months

9–15 months

15–21 months

Early Childhood

18–30 months

2–3 years

3–4 years

4–5 years

5–6 years

Late Childhood

6–7 years

7–8 years

8–9 years

9–10 years

Adolescence and Adulthood

10–11 years

11–12 years

14–15 years

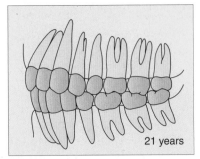

21 years

Copyright by the American Dental Association. Reprinted with permission, 1999.

GLOSSARY

abandonment desertion; refusal to treat a patient without notice (Ch. 31)

abdominal cavity includes most of the digestive tract and support organs necessary for the digestive process (Ch. 6)

Abraham Maslow (1908–1970) an American psychologist who founded the humanistic psychology movement (Ch. 2)

abrasive polishing strips used for small stains and only on enamel surfaces; also called "finishing strips" (Ch. 29)

abrasives materials that cut or grind a surface leaving grooves and a rough surface; in powder or paste form (Chs. 19 and 29)

abscess local area of pus and infection (Chs. 14, 24, and 26)

abscessed tooth an infected tooth that causes the patient pain (Ch. 16)

absorption process the process of transferring digested food to the bloodstream (Ch. 6)

abutment a tooth, a root, or an implant for retaining a fixed or removable prosthesis; the teeth adjacent to a pontic in a bridge (Chs. 14, 30 and 32)

accelerates speeds the process of (Ch. 35)

accessory organ aids in the digestive process, includes the teeth, tongue, salivary glands and ducts, liver, gallbladder, and pancreas (Ch. 6)

accounts payable amount a business or an office owes for goods or services (Ch. 36)

accounts receivable amount a business or an office is owed for goods or services (Ch. 36)

acetic acid chemical used in development of radiographs to stop the developing action and provide the required acidity for the sodium thiosulfate to work (Ch. 22)

acid etchant the process of applying phosphoric acid solution to a tooth (to alter the surface of the tooth enamel by creating microscopic undercuts between the enamel rod) to allow for adhesion of dental materials to the enamel by brush, syringe, or cotton pledget (Ch. 28)

acidulated phosphate fluoride APF solutions and gels are the preferred method of topical fluoride treatment because of patient acceptability and greater uptake of the fluoride by the surface enamel of the tooth (Ch. 4)

acquired immunity protection developed as a result of exposure to a pathogen (Ch. 10)

acquired immunodeficiency syndrome (AIDS) disorder of the immune system caused by the human immuno-deficiency virus (HIV) that ultimately destroys the body's ability to fight infection; not currently curable (Ch. 10)

actinomycosis an infection caused by bacteria, characterized by painful swelling followed by discharge of pus and yellow granules (Ch. 26)

activator orthopedic appliance that widens the maxillary arch (Ch. 27)

activity zones four zones of an area around the patient: operating, assisting, static, and transfer (Ch. 17)

acute fluoride poisoning this occurs when large amounts of fluoride are ingested, inhaled, or absorbed into the body at one time (Ch. 4)

addiction physical or psychological dependency (Ch. 15)

adhesives materials that improve retention between two objects; also known as bonding agents (Ch. 33)

adjacent next to, as in the teeth are adjacent to each other (Ch. 9)

aerobic bacteria require oxygen to grow and live (Ch. 10)

aerosol a spray of particle-containing air (Ch. 11)

agenesis occurs when the tooth buds do not form (Ch. 9)

agent 1. a person whose discussions and actions are a reflection and representation of the person he or she is working for (Ch. 3); 2. an entity that is capable of causing a disease (Ch. 11)

air abrasion a technique used for specific dental procedures to remove micro amounts of tooth structure in the cavity preparation (Ch. 19)

airborne transmission mode of disease transmission through contaminated droplets or dust particles that are suspended in the air (Ch. 11)

air compressor tool that provides compressed air for handpieces and air-water syringes (Ch. 17)

air-water syringe a device the dentist uses that provides air or water or a combination spray of air and water (Chs. 17 and 18)

ala of the nose the wing of the nose or outer edge of the nostril (Ch. 7)

ALARA the principle of keeping radiation exposure "as low as reasonably achievable"; it involves combining radiation protection procedures with commonsense practices (Ch. 21)

alimentary canal the tube of the digestive system from the mouth to the anus (Ch. 6)

alkalosis an increase in blood alkalinity (Ch. 16)

allergens substances that produce allergic reactions (Chs. 10 and 16)

allergic reactions the overreactions of the body to particular allergens; itching, redness of the skin, and hives are symptoms (Ch. 16)

allergy an overreaction of the body to an allergen (Chs. 6 and 16)

alloy combination of two or more metals (Ch. 34)

alveodental ligament five fiber groups (Ch. 8)

alveolar crest where two cortical bone plates come together between each tooth (Ch. 8)

alveolar crest fiber groups functions to resist rotational forces and tilting (Ch. 8)

alveolar mucosa thin, loosely attached mucosa covering the alveolar bone; alveolar process forms the bone that supports the maxillary and mandibular teeth (Chs. 7 and 8)

alveolar process the bone that supports the teeth in both arches (Chs. 7 and 8)

alveolar sac located at the end of the bronchioles, holds alveoli (Ch. 6)

alveoli part of the alveolar sacs in the lungs where gas exchange occurs (Ch. 6)

alveolitis complication following tooth extraction involving the loss of the blood clot, leaving a "dry socket" that can be very painful (Chs. 16 and 25)

alveologingival fiber groups aids in attaching the gingival to the alveolar bone; extends from the alveolar bone and diffuses into the overlying lamina propria of the marginal gingival (Ch. 8)

alveolus the bone that surrounds the root of the tooth, the socket (Ch. 8)

alveoplasty surgical contouring of the alvelar bone (Ch. 25)

amalgam an effective, long-lasting, and comparatively inexpensive material (an alloy with mercury) used for tooth restoration (Ch. 34)

amalgam tattoo blue to gray gingival tissue in an area where amalgam particles have become trapped in the tissue (Ch. 26)

amalgamation the actual chemical reaction that occurs between the alloy and the mercury to form the silver amalgam (Ch. 34)

amalgamator a small machine that mixes dental amalgam and other dental materials (Chs. 17 and 34)

ameloblasts enamel-forming cells (Ch. 8)

amelogenesis imperfecta genetic condition where tooth enamel is either discolored, partially missing, or extremely thin (Ch. 26)

amenorrhea absence of monthly menstrual periods (Ch. 5)

American Academy of Cosmetic Dentistry (AACD) largest international organization dedicated to the art and science of cosmetic dentistry (Ch. 31)

American Dental Assistants Association (ADAA) the national professional organization for dental assistants; local and state branches exist with a national office in Chicago (Chs. 1 and 37)

American Dental Association (ADA) the national professional organization for dentists (Chs. 1, 9, and 37)

American Dental Hygienists' Association (ADHA) the national professional organization for dental hygienists (Ch. 1)

American Dental Laboratory Technician Association (ADLTA) national organization that represents dental laboratory technicians (Ch. 1)

Americans with Disabilities Act legislation passed by Congress in 1990, to end discrimination against people with disabilities (Ch. 36)

analgesic a drug that relieves pain; (e.g., aspirin and morphine) (Ch. 15)

anaerobic bacteria can only survive without the presence of oxygen and are destroyed by oxygen (Ch. 10)

analog image an image depicted as a continuous spectrum of gray shades between black and white (Ch. 23)

anaphylactic shock an immediate, severe, sometimes fatal reaction to allergens (Chs. 10 and 16)

anatomical term for posterior denture teeth; resemble natural teeth with cusps and developmental grooves (Ch. 32)

anatomical crown portion of the tooth covered with enamel (Chs. 9 and 28)

anatomical root the portion of the tooth covered with cementum (Ch. 9)

anatomy the study of the body structure (Ch. 6)

anchor tooth tooth on which the dental dam clamp is placed; usually one or two teeth distal to the tooth or teeth being restored (Ch. 34)

anesthesia drugs that cause a loss of pain but not a loss of all sensation; usually used before surgeries (Ch. 15)

angina pectoris pain in the chest that may radiate into the jaw, neck, or arm (Ch. 16)

angioedema large urticaria (hives) brought on by an allergic reaction (Ch. 16)

angle of the mandible where the ramus meets the body of the mandible on the outside border (Ch. 7)

Angle's classification system used to classify malocclusion (Ch. 27)

angular cheilitis inflammation of the corners of the mouth (Ch. 26)

anklylosis a condition in which the tooth, cementum, or dentin fuses with the alveolar bone, restricting movement of the tooth (Ch. 26)

ankyloglossia a condition in which the lingual frenum is attached near the tip of the tongue thus limiting movement of the tongue (Ch. 26)

anode the positive terminal of an electrolytic cell (Ch. 21)

anodontia the congenital absence of teeth (Ch. 26)

anomaly extreme variation from the norm (Ch. 9)

anorexia nervosa an eating disorder characterized by severe weight loss, an extreme aversion to food, and a fear of being fat (Ch. 5)

antagonistic pair sets of muscles where one set contracts, the corresponding set relaxes; the body moves and functions through these coordinated efforts (Ch. 6)

antecubital space the indented area inside of the elbow as the arm is stretched straight (Ch. 13)

anterior alveolar nerve one of the two nerves that comes from the infraorbital nerve before it exits through the infraorbital foramen (Ch. 7)

anterior superior alveolar artery supplies blood to the anterior teeth (Ch. 7)

anterior tonsillar pillars folds of tissue that extend horizontally from the uvula to the base of the tongue (Ch. 7)

antibacterial effect the condition when the growth of acids is reduced (Ch. 4)

antibodies a disease-fighting protein developed by the body in response to the presence of an antigen (Chs. 10 and 16)

antigenic capable of causing the production of an antibody (Ch. 26)

antigens pathogens that stimulate the production of antibodies (Chs. 10 and 16)

antihistamines drugs that counteract the body's production of histamine (Ch. 16)

antimicrobial a microorganism growth inhibitor; (e.g., antimicrobial soap) (Ch. 11)

antipyretic an agent that reduces fever (Ch. 13)

antisepsis the inhibition of the growth of causative microorganisms (Ch. 11)

antitoxin an antibody produced in response to and capable of neutralizing a biologic toxin (Ch. 10)

aorta largest artery which receives blood directly from the heart (Ch. 6)

aorta valve path of blood into the aorta (Ch. 6)

apex at or near the end of the root (Ch. 9)

apex finder a unit which measures the distance to the apex of a tooth and displays the information on a digital readout (Ch. 24)

apexification the treatment of the apex of the root canal in a tooth that is necrotic (Ch. 24)

apexogenesis pulpotomy of permanent tooth whereby pulp vitality is maintained, allowing time for the root end to develop and close (Chs. 24 and 28)

aphthous ulcers painful ulcers that appear in the oral cavity; a circular lesion appears with a yellow center and red "halo" surrounding the lesion; sometimes called a canker sore (Chs. 10 and 26)

apical elevators similar to elevators but with a larger handle and smaller working ends; used to loosen and remove roots or bone fragments (Ch. 25)

apical fiber groups functions to resist forces that try to pull the tooth outward, as well as rotational forces; attaches at the apex of the tooth and radiates outward to attach in the surrounding alveolar bone (Ch. 8)

apical foramen an opening in the end of the tooth through which nerve and blood vessels enter (Ch. 9)

apical periodontitis pulpal inflammation that extends into the periapical tissues (Ch. 24)

apicoectomy removal of the apex of the root and infection surrounding the area (Ch. 24)

aponeurosis a specialized connective tissue extension, broad and flattened, attaches muscle to bone and binds muscle to muscle (Ch. 6)

appendicular skeleton one of the two main divisions of the skeleton, composed of the bones from the upper and lower extremities including arms, hands, legs, feet, shoulders, and hips (Ch. 6)

apposition in the life cycle of a tooth when the calcium salts and other minerals are deposited and when the tissues or enamel, dentin, and cementum are formed in layers (Ch. 8)

arch wires wires used to apply force to move or hold teeth in desired positions (Ch. 27)

argon laser a curing light technology, light amplification by stimulated emission of radiation, produces a relatively high intensity light that does not generate noticeable heat. Some disadvantages include lack of compatibility with some dental materials and the expense (Ch. 17)

arteriole smallest arteries (Ch. 6)

arteriosclerosis hardening of the arteries (Ch. 16)

artery carries oxygenated blood from the heart to the capillaries of the tissues (Ch. 6)

articular disc also known as meniscus, it is a dense, fibrous connective tissue that is thicker at the ends attached to the condyle (Ch. 7)

articulation joint where two or more bones meet or form a junction (Ch. 6)

articulator a frame representing the jaw that holds models of the patient's teeth to maintain the patient's occlusion; a mechanical device that represents the temporomandibular joints to which upper and lower casts of the dental arches may be attached to simulate mouth functions (Ch. 35)

artificial acquired immunity protection from a pathogen for an individual that has been vaccinated with a specific antigen (Ch. 10)

artificial teeth a component of the removable denture that is made of either acrylic resin or porcelain and secured to the denture base by pins or holes on the undersides of the teeth (Ch. 32)

asepsis the creation of an environment free of pathogens (Ch. 11)

aseptic technique steps necessary to ensure an environment free from pathogens; handwashing, for example (Ch. 11)

aspirating syringe most common type of syringe designed to allow the operator to check the position of the needle before depositing the anesthetic solution (Ch. 20)

assault threat of touching a person without consent (Ch. 3)

assignment of benefits area a patient must sign to authorize the insurance carrier to make payment directly to the dentist (Ch. 36)

assistant's cart a mobile cart that is usually set up with the air-water syringe, saliva ejector, and HVE (Ch. 17)

assisted bleaching initial in-office stages of home bleaching process; patient makes dental impressions, then returns to the office to obtain custom bleaching trays and instructions for home bleaching (Ch. 31)

assisted whitening combination of dental office and home bleaching process (Ch. 31)

assisting zone the area in which the dental assistant is positioned to easily assist the dentist and have access to instruments, the evacuator, and the dental unit or cart without interference (Ch. 17)

associate neuron also known as interneurons, transmits impulses from sensory neurons to motor neurons in the central nervous system (Ch. 6)

asthma muscular spasm of the walls of the bronchi occurs when air passages are constricted so the person cannot exhale easily (Ch. 6)

asymmetric unequal shapes, sizes, and relative positions of body parts on opposite sides (Ch. 13)

asymptomatic having no symptoms (Ch. 11)

atria upper chambers of the heart (Ch. 6)

atrophy muscle deterioration due to lack of use (Ch. 6)

attached gingiva extends from the mucogingival junction to the gingival groove; it is stippled and attached tightly to the alveolar bone (Ch. 8)

attrition the wearing away of the incisal or occlusal surfaces of the tooth during normal function; the final stage of the life cycle of the tooth (Ch. 8)

auricle upper chambers of the heart (Ch. 6)

autoclavable utility gloves gloves that can be sterilized in the autoclave after use (Ch. 11)

automatic processing processing of dental x-rays using automated equipment (Ch. 22)

automatrix a matrix without a retainer (Ch. 34)

autonomic nervous system (ANS) collection of nerves, ganglia, and plexuses through which visceral organs, heart, blood vessels, glands, and smooth muscles receive their innervation (Ch. 6)

auxillary polishing aids aids used during coronal polishing procedures, including bridge threaders, abrasive polishing strips, soft wooden points, and small interproximal brushes (Ch. 29)

avulsed tooth a tooth that has been removed from the mouth; avulsed teeth should be replanted immediately (if possible) or transported to the dentist in milk, saliva, saline, or water (Chs. 16 and 28)

axial plane plane around which computed tomography is achieved (Ch. 23)

axial skeleton one of the two main divisions of the skeleton includes bones of the cranium, face, spinal column, ribs, and sternum (Ch. 6)

axial walls walls parallel to the long axis of the tooth (Ch. 33)

axon nerve fibers that conduct impulses away from the cell body (Ch. 6)

bacteria tiny, simple, single-celled plants that contain no chlorophyll (Ch. 10)

bacterial endocarditis an inflammation of the heart lining (Ch. 6)

bacterial plaque a local irritant that is a common cause of the inflammation of the gingival tissues (Ch. 29)

band part of the matrix that forms the missing surface or wall of a tooth (Ch. 34)

barbed broaches endontic instruments used to remove soft tissue from the pulp canal (Ch. 24)

bar-type clasp a retainer design which extends from a gingival direction toward the occlusal (Ch. 32)

basal cells some of the deepest cells in the dermis (Ch. 21)

basal cell carcinoma most common form of skin cancer (Ch. 26)

basal metabolic rate (BMR) the energy that is used when a person is at rest (Ch. 5)

base material applied in a putty or thick layer between the tooth and restoration to protect the pulp from chemical, electrical, mechanical, or thermal irritation (Ch. 33)

baseline vital signs the initial reading of basic signs of life, including body temperature, pulse, blood pressure, and respiration rate (Ch. 13)

baseplate preformed, semirigid acrylic resin material that represents the denture base temporarily (Ch. 32)

battery according to the law, the actual touching of another individual without consent (Ch. 3)

beading process used with utility wax to curb impressions before boxing and pouring (Ch. 35)

behavior management plan to modify or maintain the desired behavior of a person or group of persons (Ch. 28)

Bell's palsy the temporary paralysis of the muscles on one side of the face (Chs. 6 and 26)

beneficiary the patient who is entitled to benefits under any dental insurance plan (Ch. 36)

benefit-less-benefit an insurance plan that allows reimbursement to be limited to the higher level allowed of the two plans so there is no duplication of benefits (Ch. 36)

bevel slanted edge or side on the working end of an instrument (Ch. 19)

bicuspid valve atrioventricular valve on the left side of the heart; mitral valve (Ch. 6)

bifid tongue the failure of the lateral halves of the anterior two thirds of the tongue to fuse completely (Ch. 26)

bifurcated one tooth with two roots (Ch. 9)

bilateral cleft lip when a cleft lip occurs on both sides of the upper lip (Ch. 8)

bile substance produced by the liver, emulsifies fat (Ch. 6)

binangle dental instrument on which the shank has two angles (Ch. 19)

binging over eating that is a response to stress or depression (Ch. 5)

biofilms microscopic communities that allow bacteria, fungi, and viruses to multiply (Chs. 10 and 11)

biopsy surgical removal of a small amount of tissue (Chs. 25 and 20)

biotin a vitamin found in both plant and animal foods; helps in energy metabolism (Ch. 5)

Birthday rule established for cases when both parents have coverage for a child; it establishes the parents' birthday month and day (not year) that comes earliest in the calendar year as the primary carrier (Ch. 36)

bisecting technique x-ray technique that applies the geometric principle in which the central ray bisects the angle formed by the dental film and the long axis of the tooth (Ch. 22)

bite registration an occlusal record of the relationship between the upper and lower teeth (Ch. 30)

bite rim several layers of baseplate wax that are attached to the baseplate to represent the space provided by teeth in normal occlusion, registering the vertical dimension for the denture and establishing the occlusal relationship of the mandibular and maxillary arches (Ch. 32)

bite-wing intraoral radiograph that shows the maxillary and mandibular crowns in occlusion (Ch. 22)

black line stain formation of a thin black to dark brown line slightly above the gingiva and following the contour of the gingival margin; found primarily in women and often in cases of excellent oral hygiene (Ch. 29)

Black's formula formula developed by G. V. Black to standardize the exact size and angulation of an instrument (Ch. 19)

blade flat working end on a dental instrument (Ch. 19)

blister a raised, fluid-filled area, usually oval or circular (Ch. 26)

blood main functions include transportation of nutrients, gases, waste products, and hormones; regulation of the amount of body fluids, pH balance, and body temperature; and protection against pathogens and blood loss after injury through clotting mechanism (Ch. 6)

Bloodborne Pathogens Standard effective in 1992, a federal standard instituted in the hope of reducing the occupational-related cases of HIV and hepatitis B infection among health-care workers (Ch. 11)

blurred images images on x-ray film that are out of focus (Ch. 22)

body substance isolation a system of techniques requiring personal protective equipment to be worn to protect against contact with all body fluids, whether or not blood is visible (Ch. 11)

bonding the process by which materials adhere firmly or hold together (Chs. 28 and 33)

bonding agents materials, usually low viscosity resins, used to improve retention between two objects (in dentistry, between the tooth structure [enamel and dentin] and the restoration); also known as adhesives, bonding resins; mainly light or dull cured (Ch. 33)

bonding resins materials used to improve the retention between the tooth structure (enamel and dentin) and the restoration; also called bonding agents and adhesives (Ch. 33)

bone grafting moving tissue from one area to another; adding bone or a bone substitute to fill areas (Ch. 29)

bone resorption bone loss caused during periodontal disease (may be horizontal or vertical) (Ch. 29)

border molding when receiving a final impression, the impression compound is heated and placed along the borders of the custom tray; the tray is cooled and placed in the patient's mouth and the lips, cheeks, and tongue are moved to establish accurate length for the periphery and adjacent tissues to be included in the final impression (Ch. 32)

brachial artery main artery of the arm (Ch. 13)

brackets devices attached to the teeth to hold the arch wire in place and transmit the force of the arch wire to move the tooth (Ch. 27)

bradycardia abnormally slow heart rate (Ch. 13)

bradypnea abnormally slow respiratory rate at rest (Ch. 13)

brand names drug names assigned by the manufacturer that are trademarked (e.g., Tylenol® is a brand name, aspirin is a generic name) (Ch. 15)

breach of contract   breaking of a contract (Ch. 3)

bridge   a fixed prosthetic device placed in the mouth to replace missing teeth (Ch. 14)

bridge threader   used to pull the dental tape and floss under fixed appliances, around orthodontic appliances, and around splints so that all proximal surfaces can be cleaned and polished (Ch. 29)

broad spectrum   refers to drugs, specifically antibiotics, that are effective against a wide range of bacteria, not just one specific bacteria (Ch. 15)

bronchi   two branches that form at the end of the trachea and enter the lungs (Ch. 6)

bronchioles   small branches of the bronchiole tubes that divide into alveolar sacs (Chs. 6 and 16)

bruxism   teeth grinding (Chs. 29 and 33)

buccal   the surface of the posterior tooth that is toward the cheeks (Ch. 9)

buccal branch   nerves that pass through the buccinator muscle to the cheek where it innervates the buccal mucosa, buccal gingiva, and the buccal of the mandibular molars (Ch. 7)

buccal groove   a linear depression forming a groove that extends from the middle of the buccal surface to the occlusal surface of the tooth (Ch. 9)

buccal mucosa   the inner surface of the cheeks (Ch. 7)

buccal tubes   small cylinders of metal welded to the molar bands providing a means of attachment for the arch wire to the band in the posterior area (Ch. 27)

buccinator   a muscle of facial expression (Ch. 7)

buccoversion   a tooth that is tipped toward the lip or cheek (Ch. 27)

bud stage   the first stage of odontogenesis, initiation of the tooth begins (Ch. 8)

bulimia   a psychological disorder that is characterized by secretive bouts of gross overeating followed by methods of weight control such as purging, laxative abuse, excessive exercise, and over usage of diuretics (Ch. 5)

bulla   a large, fluid-filled blister; greater than ½ inch in diameter (Ch. 26)

burnish   to smooth (Ch. 34)

burs   some of the dental rotary instruments; used to prepare the cavity, finish and polish restorations, aid in surgical procedures, and adjust dental appliances (Ch. 19)

business associates   indirect providers of health care services and supplies such as accounting firms, consultants, legal firms, management companies, data/record copying, storage and destruction companies, and suppliers (Ch. 3)

calcification   the process of depositing calcium salts and other materials in the formed tooth, it takes place in the apposition stage of tooth development (Ch. 3)

calcination   the process of driving a specific amount of water out of gypsum to create specific plasters, stones, or investment die stones (Ch. 35)

calcium   a major mineral found in bones and teeth and functions in muscle contraction, the nervous system, and the blood (Ch. 5)

calcium hydroxide   type of cementation used as a low-strength base under any restoration (Ch. 33)

calculus   hard, calcified deposit of mineralized plaque that forms on teeth, restorations, and dental appliances; also known as tartar (Ch. 29)

Calories   units of heat; the large Calorie (which is always capitalized) is the amount of heat needed to change the temperature of l gm of water from 14.5° C to 15.5° C.; one thousand kilo calories make up l calorie (Ch. 5)

cancellous bone   sponge-like tissue (Ch. 6)

candida albicans   yeast-like fungus (Ch. 26)

candidiasis   an infection, also called thrush, caused by the fungus Candida albicans, often on areas covered with mucous membrane like the mouth or vaginal area (Ch. 10)

canine   cuspid; third tooth from the midline; bulkier and aids in tearing food (Ch. 9)

canker sores   painful ulcers that appear in the oral cavity; circular lesions appear with yellow centers and red "halos" surrounding the lesion; sometimes called aphthous ulcers (Ch. 26)

cannula   small hollow tube (Ch. 28)

cantilever bridge   prosthetic device in mouth attached at only one side; useful in an area with little stress such as a missing lateral (Ch. 14)

capillary   the connection between the arteries and the veins where the exchange is made between the blood and body cells (Ch. 6)

cap stage   the bud of the tooth grows and changes shape (Ch. 8)

carbamide peroxide   a material used for teeth whitening and is used in a 10-20% solution; a thickening agent is added to increase adhesion (Ch. 31)

carbohydrates   one of the six broad categories of nutrients primarily found in fruits, grains, legumes, and some vegetable roots (Ch. 5)

cardiac muscle   found only in the heart, receives an impulse, responds and relaxes at a rapid pace which keeps the heart beating in an even rhythm (Ch. 6)

cardiopulmonary resuscitation (CPR)   rescue breathing and chest compressions performed on a patient experiencing cardiac arrest (Ch. 16)

caries   dental cavities; tooth decay (Ch. 4)

cariogenic foods   foods that break down into simple sugars in the mouth and can be used by the bacteria to cause dental caries (Ch. 5)

carotene   vitamin A that comes from plants (Ch. 5)

carpules   glass containers of anesthetic solution (Ch. 20)

carrier   dental insurance company that pays the agreed benefits for the patient treatment (Ch. 36)

cartilage   a tough nonvascular, resilient, specialized connective tissue (Ch. 6)

cartridges   glass containers of anesthetic solution (Ch. 20)

cashier's check   a check that is guaranteed by the bank for the amount the check is written for (Ch. 36)

cassette   a container for extra oral radiographic film containing intensifying screens; available in hard or soft light-proof containers (Ch. 23)

catalyst   an ingredient that starts or accelerates a process (Ch. 35)

cathode   the negative terminal of an x-ray tube (Ch. 21)

cavitation   a process where bubbles are formed (Ch. 11)

cavity liners   low-strength bases placed in the deepest portion of the cavity preparation, on the dentin or exposed pulp, which harden to form a cement layer to protect the pulp from chemical irritations and provide a therapeutic effect on the tooth (Ch. 33)

cavity preparation   preparation for a restoration; technique depends on the amount and location of decay, degree of pulpal involvement, and type of materials used to restore the tooth (Ch. 33)

cavity varnish   used to seal the dentin tubules to prevent acids, saliva, and debris from reaching the pulp; when used with cavity liner or medicated base, it is placed on top of these materials (Ch. 33)

cavosurface margin   angle that is formed by the junction of the wall of a cavity preparation and the untouched surface of the tooth; sealing of this margin is critical to prevent marginal leakage (Ch. 33)

CDT codes   Current Dental Terminology codes; five-digit codes used to submit insurance claims (Ch. 36)

cell   the smallest functioning unit of the body contains cell membrane, nucleus, cytoplasm, and chromosomes (Ch. 6)

cell membrane   the outer wall of the cell composed of proteins, lipids, and carbohydrates (Ch. 6)

cellulitis   swelling and discomfort of facial tissues caused by an abscess (Ch. 24)

Celsius   the centigrade measure of temperature; the freezing point is 0 degrees and the boiling point is 100 degrees (Ch. 13)

cement bases   high-strength bases of thick, putty-like consistency placed on the floor of a cavity preparation to protect the pulp and provide mechanical support for the restoration; preparation, pulp sensitivity, and type of restoration indicate which cement to use (Ch. 33)

cemental spurs   found near the cementoenamel junction (CEJ), it appears similar to calculus (Ch. 8)

cementoblasts   cementum-forming cells (Ch. 8)

cementum   the tooth structure that is located around the root covering the dentin on the root portion of the tooth (Ch. 8)

Centers for Disease Control and Prevention (CDC)   the organization that investigates, reports, and tracks specific diseases and public health concerns for the United States (Ch. 11)

central beam   the primary ray emitting from the x-ray tube head (Ch. 21)

central incisor   the first tooth starting from the midline; used to cut or bite the food that is ingested (Ch. 9)

central nervous system (CNS)   the brain and the spinal cord (Ch. 6)

central vacuum system   system that provides suction for saliva ejectors and oral evacuators (Ch. 17)

centric occlusion   closing of the jaws in a position that maximizes contact between the occluding surfaces of the maxillary and the mandibular arch (Ch. 32)

cephalometric radiographs   extraoral radiographs showing patient profiles, including bones and tissues (Ch. 23)

CERAC CAD/CAM retraction system   a restoration system that allows metal-free, tooth-colored restorations to be fabricated in one appointment (Ch. 30)

cerebral embolism   a blood clot that blocks the normal flow of blood to the brain (Ch. 16)

cerebral hemorrhage   rupture of a blood vessel in the brain (Ch. 16)

cerebral infarction   an interruption of the flow of blood to the brain (Ch. 16)

certified check   a check that the bank has certified is good for the amount it is written for (Ch. 36)

certified dental assistant (CDA)   a dental assistant who has obtained national certification through the Dental Assisting National Board (Ch. 1)

certified mail   mail sent that provides the sender confirmation of delivery (Ch. 36)

cervical clamps   double-bowed clamps used for Class V restorations on anterior teeth; help with gingival retraction; often must be stabilized with stick impression compound after the teeth have been exposed (Ch. 34)

cervical line   where the anatomical crown and root join (Ch. 9)

cervical third   the area on the crown of the tooth that is nearest the cervical (or nearest the gingival) (Ch. 9)

chain of asepsis   aseptic procedures ensuring that no cross-contamination occurs (Ch. 11)

chalk   a mild abrasive used in some prophylactic pastes; also known as whiting (Ch. 29)

Chapin A. Harris   (1769–1844) established the Baltimore College of Dental Surgery with Horace Hayden. This was the first dental college in the world (Ch. 1)

chamfer   a type of crown preparation that provides adequate bulk and extends easily into the gingival sulcus (Ch. 30)

charge-coupled device   an image receptor; converts x-rays to electrons (Ch. 23)

check register   record of all checking account transactions; includes deposits to and checks made from the account (Ch. 36)

cheilosis   a condition due to Vitamin B deficiency where lips become red and fissures develop in the corners of the mouth (Ch. 5)

chelating   a process by which an agent encloses or grasps a toxic substance and makes it nontoxic (Ch. 24)

chemical retention   a chemical reaction occurs between the tooth surface and a material which allows the material to be held in place (Ch. 33)

chemically cured   type of sealant material that is hardened by use of a catalyst and a base; also known as self-cure or autopolymerization (Ch. 28)

chicken pox   a childhood viral disease characterized by a rash and slight fever; virus remains dormant in nerve tissue and can result in shingles later in life (Ch. 10)

chisel scaler   a periodontal instrument used most often in the anterior of the mouth (Ch. 29)

chlorine   a mineral which maintains the correct pH balance in blood (Ch. 5)

chroma   the intensity or quality of the hue (Ch. 31)

chromium   a trace mineral involved in the process of metabolism (Ch. 5)

chromosome   located in the cell's nucleus and contains DNA which transmits genetic information (Ch. 6)

chronic fluoride poisoning   this occurs over a period of time with ingestion of high fluoride levels in the water or by a combination of several fluoride sources (Ch. 4)

chuck   a small metal cylinder in the head of the handpiece that holds rotary instruments (Ch. 19)

chyme   mixture of food and gastric juices (Ch. 6)

cingulum   a convex area on the lingual surface of the anterior teeth near the gingiva (Ch. 9)

circular ligament fiber groups   circles and tightens the gingival margin around the neck of the tooth; located in the lamina propria of the marginal gingival (Ch. 8)

circumference the distance around (Ch. 34)

circumferential-type clasp a retainer design which encircles and adapts to the contours of the abutment tooth (Ch. 32)

circumpulpal dentin the layer of dentin that surrounds the pulp (Ch. 8)

circumvallate papilla the largest papilla, mushroom shaped, are anterior to the sulcus terminalis in a row of eight to ten (Ch. 7)

cirrhosis liver deterioration (Ch. 15)

civil law law related to actions and circumstances between individuals; civil law can be broken into contract law and tort law (Ch. 3)

classifications of motion the five classifications that show the amount of motion with which the dental team is involved (Ch. 17)

cleaning the physical removal of organic matter, such as blood, tissue, and debris.

clear film a film that was not exposed to radiation (Ch. 22)

cleft lip cleft in or separation of the upper lip; also known as harelip; failure of the maxillary processes to fuse with the medial nasal process (Chs. 8 and 26)

cleft palate a fissure in the roof of the mouth that forms a passage between the nasal cavities and the mouth; failure of the palatal shelves to fuse with the primary palate or with each other (Chs. 6, 8 and 26)

cleft uvula the uvula is separated slightly (Ch. 8)

clinical crown exposed coronal portion of the crowns (Chs. 9 and 29)

clinical root the portion of the root seen in the oral cavity (Ch. 9)

closing prescription closing; area on the prescription where dentists sign their names and authorize whether prescriptions can be refilled and how many times; also notes whether a generic brand of the medication can be dispensed in place of that written (Ch. 15)

coalesced fused (Ch. 28)

cobalt a trace mineral that helps in the functioning of red blood cells (Ch. 5)

cold sore a blister (Ch. 10)

collimator a device used to eliminate peripheral radiation (Ch. 21)

color changing sealants sealants with a photo active color additive that change to opaque after being light cured (Ch. 28)

commissures corners of the mouth where the upper lip meets the lower lip (Ch. 13)

common carotid artery supplying blood to most of the head and the neck, divided into internal and external branches (Ch. 7)

common law standards and rules based upon previously determined cases in which everyone is now responsible to follow (Ch. 3)

communication exchange of information and ideas (Ch. 2)

compact bone the strong and hard section of a bone is dense and forms the main shaft of long bones and the outer layer of other bones (Ch. 6)

compomer polyacid-modified resin used to cement all types of dental restorations and to restore teeth in non-stress-bearing areas (Ch. 33)

composite direct, tooth-colored restorative material (Ch. 33)

Comprehensive Drug Abuse Prevention and Control Act of 1970 law that identifies drugs according to five schedules of potential abuse (Ch. 15)

compromised host an individual whose normal defense mechanisms are impaired (Ch. 11)

compules single-application cartridges (Ch. 33)

computed tomography (CT scanning) computer-produced image (Ch. 23)

computer-controlled local anesthesia used to administer all traditional infiltration and block injections; delivers a pressure and volume of anesthetic solution at a controlled rate (Ch. 20)

computerized systems units of computer parts that function together to perform tasks (Ch. 36)

concave recessed or indented (Ch. 9)

condensable composite also called packable composites, are putty-like and stiff in consistency; used in posterior areas (Ch. 34)

condyle the posterior projection at the top of the rami (Ch. 7)

condyloid process the posterior projection at the top of the rami; condyle (Ch. 7)

cone cutting partial image created when the central beam misses the x-ray film (Ch. 22)

congenital present at birth (Ch. 26)

congestive heart failure a condition that occurs as the heart weakens, rendering it unable to achieve the level of cardiac output that meets the body's needs (Ch. 16)

conjunctivitis also called pink eye, is an inflammation of the eye caused by infection or the herpes simplex virus type 1 (Ch. 10)

connectors elements that unite the parts of the partial into one unit; hold working parts in proper positions (Ch. 32)

conscious sedation a very safe means for patients to be free of pain and discomfort during dental procedures; patient can communicate during this process (Ch. 20)

contact area the proximal sides of where two teeth come together and touch; normally the medial of one tooth and the distal of another tooth (Ch. 9)

contact transmission the physical transfer of an agent from an infected person to an uninfected person through direct contact with the infected person (Ch. 11)

contamination the presence of an infectious agent (Ch. 11)

continuous simple suture series of stitches that look like hem stitching; placed in areas of multiple extractions and tied with a surgeon's knot at either end (Ch. 25)

continuous sling suture series of sling stitches placed in areas with a large flap involving several teeth (Ch. 25)

contour lines of Owen contour lines in dentin that demonstrate a disturbance in the body metabolism (Ch. 8)

contra-angle attachment head for the low-speed handpiece; contra-angles hold burs, discs, stones, rubber cups, and brushes for intraoral and extraoral procedures; type of Tofflemire retainer, placed on the lingual side, angled slightly to clear the anterior teeth (Chs. 19 and 34)

contract 1. exposure to infection (Ch. 6); 2. a binding agreement between two or more persons (Ch. 3)

contract law law that covers contracts that bind two or more parties (Ch. 3)

contrast difference between shades or colors (Ch. 21)

convex to bulge or curve outward (Ch. 9)

coordination of benefits (COB) when two insurance carriers coordinate the benefits not to exceed the total cost of the actual dental expense (Ch. 36)

copal varnish a cavity varnish containing organic solvents (ether, acetone, or chloroform) and is used only under metal restorations because the solvent material in the varnish may interfere with the setting action of composite and resins (Ch. 33)

copper a trace mineral involved in the process of metabolism (Ch. 5)

corneal ulcer an inflammatory condition of the cornea that results in the loss of the outer layer; can be caused by trauma, burns, infections, or the herpes simplex virus type 1 (Ch. 10)

coronal polish procedure whereby coronal surfaces of the teeth are polished with rubber cups, brushes, an abrasive, polishers, and dental tape (also known as prophylaxis) (Ch. 29)

coronid process the anterior projection at the top of the rami (Ch. 7)

corpuscle the cells or solid portion of the blood (Ch. 6)

corrective orthodontics the improvement of orthodontic problems (Ch. 27)

corrosion the result of chemical or electrochemical attacks (Ch. 33)

cortical bone compact bone plates on the facial and lingual surfaces (Ch. 8)

cosmetic dentistry dental specialty concerned with enhancing a person's smile and teeth appearance (Ch. 31)

Council on Dental Therapeutics part of the ADA, a body that gathers and releases to dentists information about drugs being used in dentistry (Ch. 15)

coverage benefits available through dental insurance (Ch. 36)

covered entity direct provider of health care services and supplies (Ch. 3)

cramp unpleasant sensations generally caused by a muscle contraction(Ch. 6)

cranial cavity large space inside the skull that contains the brain (Ch. 6)

creep a change in a material when under a constant load (Ch. 34)

crepitus crackling sound (Ch. 25)

criminal law law related to wrongs committed against the welfare and safety of society as a whole (Ch. 3)

cross-section technique technique used to expose occlusal radiographs (Ch. 22)

crown top or highest part of a tooth; often called a cap (Chs. 9 and 14)

crown matrix form a thin, plastic form that is shaped like a crown used on anterior teeth when the incisal edge is involved (Ch. 34)

culture the shared beliefs and values of a group (Ch. 2)

curette hand instruments for removing subgingival calculus, smoothing the root surface, and removing the soft tissue lining of the periodontal pocket (Ch. 29)

curing light a high-intensity light that hardens or sets many dental materials (Ch. 17)

curing light tester a device for testing the effectiveness of a curing unit (Ch. 17)

Current Dental Terminology (CDT) CDT represents the collaboration of dental vendors, payers, providers, clearinghouses, and the government for a standard code set. Initially developed in 1969, it is now revised every two years (Ch. 3)

Cusp of Carabelli a fifth cusp on the mesial lingual surface of most maxillary first molars (Ch. 9)

cusps pointed or rounded mounds on the crown of the tooth (Ch. 9)

cutting edge on a dental instrument, the sharpened edge used for refining the cavity preparation (Ch. 19)

cyst fluid-filled or semisolid fluid-filled sac (Ch. 20)

cytodifferentiation the development of different cells during the embryonic stage of pregnancy (Ch. 8)

cytoplasm everything within a cell except for the nucleus (Ch. 6)

dark room a small room near the treatment rooms where x-ray processing is done (Ch. 17)

day sheet sheets in a dental office which list the daily schedule with patient's names and their required services (Ch. 3)

debride to remove debris (dead tissue) (Chs. 25 and 26)

deciduous primary (Ch. 9)

deductible amount paid before benefits take effect (Ch. 36)

deep facial vein a tributary of the facial vein which connects the facial vein to the pterygoid plexus of veins (Ch. 7)

defamation of character causing injury to another's reputation, name, or character; can be verbal or written (Ch. 3)

defendant the individual a charge is brought against (Ch. 3)

deglutition also known as swallowing, provides the movement for the food to move from the mouth to the stomach (Ch. 6)

delivery systems types of dental units that are at various positions (e.g., front delivery, side delivery, and rear delivery) to accommodate dental team members (Ch. 17)

demineralization case in which calcium and phosphorus are lost from the enamel surface (Ch. 4)

dendrite nerve fibers that conduct impulses toward the cell body (Ch 6)

density degree of darkness on an x-ray (Ch. 21)

dental arteries supplies blood to the roots and periodontal ligaments of the molars and premolars (Ch. 7)

Dental Assisting National Board, Inc. (DANB) independent organization that administers the credentialing examinations for dental assistants (Chs. 1 and 37)

dental associate a dentist who works under contract, usually for a dentist with a solo practice (Ch. 37)

dental casting alloy combination of metals (gold, iron, tin, zinc) used in crowns (Ch. 30)

dental composites (BIS-GMA) material commonly used as a sealant for occlusal pits and fissures (Ch. 23)

dental dam latex material used to isolate teeth that are to be restored (Ch. 34)

dental dam clamps tools that stabilize and secure the dental dam material in place; come in numerous designs and sizes to fit around the teeth (Ch. 34)

dental dam forceps forceps with two beaks that fit in the holes of the jaws of the clamp; used to place and remove the dental dam clamp (Ch. 34)

dental dam frame holder designed to stretch and secure the dam in place across the patient's face; keeps the operating area open (Ch. 34)

dental dam napkins soft, precut, disposable, absorbent fabric pieces used for patient comfort and for absorbing saliva, water, and perspiration (Ch. 34)

dental dam punch a tool similar in action to a paper punch, although much differently designed, with a sharp projection to punch through the dental dam to create holes for the teeth (Ch. 34)

dental dam scissors any small pair of scissors the operator uses to cut the interseptal dental dam during removal of the dam from the patient's mouth (Ch. 34)

dental floss placed interproximally, wrapped around the tooth, and moved in an up-and-down motion (Ch. 29)

dental fluorosis a condition caused by an excess intake of flourides during tooth development; enamel surface appears mottled and stained but is caries free (Ch. 29)

dental implants fixed prostheses, attached to bone, used to replace missing teeth (Ch. 25)

dental jurisprudence the law(s) governing dentistry (Ch. 3)

dental lamina a growth from the oral epithelium that gives rise to the tooth buds (Ch. 8)

Dental Practice Act state regulations that describe legal restrictions and controls on the dentist, the hygienist, and other dental assistants (Ch. 3)

dental public health the specialty in dentistry that is concerned with dental disease; works with the community to promote dental health (Ch.1)

dental sac an enclosed area formed by the mesenchyme tissue that matures into the dentin, cementum, and the pulp of the tooth (Ch. 8)

dental tape used on the interproximal surfaces of the teeth with an abrasive agent (Ch. 29)

dental tubules tubules that pass through the entire surface of the dentin and contain dentinal fluid (Ch. 8)

dental unit positioned according to the dentist, unit that consists of handpieces, an air-water syringe, a saliva ejector, an oral evacuator (HVE), an ultrasonic scaling unit, and numerous other options (Ch. 17)

dentifrice toothpaste used with brushing and flossing for patient oral hygiene self-care (Ch. 4)

dentin makes up the bulk of the tooth structures located around the pulp cavity and under the enamel within the anatomical crown, and under the cementum within the root (Ch. 8)

dentinal fluid tissue fluid surrounding the cell membrane of the odontoblast (Ch. 8)

dentinal hypersensitivity pain which may occur if dentin is exposed (Ch. 8)

dentinal tubules tubules that pass through the entire surface of the dentin and contain dentinal fluid (Ch. 8)

dentinogenesis imperfecta a hereditary condition in which the enamel appears to be opalescent and chips away from the dentin soon after tooth eruption (Ch. 26)

dentition natural teeth in position (Ch. 9)

dentogingival fiber groups attached to the cementum and extends into the lamina propria of the marginal gingival; maintains the gingival integrity of the marginal gingival (Ch. 8)

dentoperiosteal fiber groups supportive fibers that anchor the tooth to the bone; originates from the cementum, near the CEJ, and extends across the alveolar crest (Ch. 8)

denture a prosthesis that replaces missing teeth in the same arch; a full denture is used when all the natural teeth are missing, a partial denture when some natural teeth are missing (Ch. 14)

denture base sometimes called the saddle, holds denture teeth (Ch. 32)

dependents children covered under dental insurance (normally up to age 18) (Ch. 36)

desensitizers materials that are used to treat or prevent hypersensitivity in the tooth (Ch. 33)

developer solution the first chemical solution used to process radiographs (Ch. 22)

developmental groove groove formed by the uniting of lobes during development of the tooth crown (Ch. 9)

diabetes mellitus insufficient insulin production in the pancreas leading to high levels of glucose in the blood (Chs. 6 and 16)

diabetic acidosis a serious consequence of hyperglycemia when the patient has too much sugar and not enough insulin. The body produces acids and the pH level is lowered often resulting in a coma and death if left untreated (Ch. 16)

diastema space between the maxillary central incisors in humans; can also be used to denote a space between two adjacent teeth in the same dental arch (Ch. 14)

diastolic blood pressure created as the arteries return to their original state when the heart relaxes between contractions (Ch. 13)

diet food an individual eats (Ch. 5)

digastric one of the muscles of the floor of the mouth that lifts the hyoid bone and assists in the opening of the mouth (Ch. 7)

digestion the process by which food is broken down into small nutrient molecules that the cells can use (Ch. 6)

digital image an image made up of many small pieces to make a whole picture (Ch. 23)

digital imaging technology imaging system that reduces x-rays received by the patient by over 90 percent (Ch. 23)

digital radiology a computerized system that allows the dentist to take an intraoral or extraoral radiograph and display the image on a computer screen without exposing and processing dental film (Ch. 23)

dimensional change change in length or volume of a material, usually from exposure to heat or cold (Ch. 33)

diphtheria a disease caused by the microorganism bacillus corynebacterium diphtheria appears as a severe throat infection and fever (Ch. 10)

diplocci pairs of bacteria (Ch. 10)

direct contact something an individual has with a lesion or microorganism while performing intraoral dental procedures; touching or first-hand contact (Ch. 11)

direct digital imaging the image is produced on a surface sensor, digitized, and then transmitted to a computer monitor (Ch. 23)

direct providers the HIPAA provisions apply to direct providers of health care services and supplies including hospitals, clinics, nursing homes, assisted living facilities, home health agencies, physicians, dentists, and alternative medicine (Ch. 3)

direct pulp capping (DPC) technique used to treat permanent tooth when pulp has been exposed due to mechanical or traumatic means but chance exists that the pulp will heal; involves placing of medicament directly over exposed pulp, followed by tooth restoration (Chs. 28 and 33)

direct resin veneers made in dental office directly on patient's tooth (Ch. 30)

direct restorations can be placed in the mouth after the tooth is prepared; examples include amalgam or composite restorations (Ch. 30)

disinfect to kill pathogens by physical or chemical means; does not destroy spores and resistant viruses (Ch. 11)

disinfection occurs when some microorganisms are destroyed; cleaning and sanitizing (Ch. 11)

distal the surface of the tooth that is away from the midline (Ch. 9)

distortion change in shape (Ch. 35)

distoversion a deviation in tooth positioning; the tooth is distal to normal position (Ch. 27)

diuretics substances that cause the body to lose water (Ch. 5)

Doctrine of Respondeat Superior simply put, the dentist is responsible for the actions of the dental assistant, as well as any assistant; when there is a complaint or an act of negligence on the assistant's part, the dentist is liable for the act (Ch. 3)

dorsal cavity posterior portion of the body that contains spinal canal and cranial cavity (Ch. 6)

double booking booking additional patients at down times with the initial patient's procedures (Ch. 36)

double exposure a technique error in which film was exposed twice (Ch. 22)

down time time in the appointment book that is not used for appointments (Ch. 36)

Dr. C. Edmund Kells (1856–1928) New Orleans dentist who took the first intraoral radiograph using his own equipment and techniques; hired a female to replace a male assistant in 1885 and started the popular "Ladies in Attendance" employment strategy (Ch. 1)

Dr. Greene Vardiman Black (1836–1915) known as G. V. Black and the "grand old man of dentistry"; taught in dental schools and as the dean increased the library holdings and authored more than 500 articles (Ch. 1)

drifting moving a tooth into the space created by a missing tooth (Ch. 14)

drug any substance that changes the body's life chemical processes (Ch. 15)

Drug Enforcement Agency (DEA) number number of the agency that regulates controlled substances; part of the U.S. Department of Justice (Ch. 15)

drug interaction the effect one drug can have on another when taken at the same time; intended results may be increased or decreased (Ch. 15)

dry angles triangular pads that absorb the flow of saliva and protect the cheek (Ch. 18)

dry socket common complication after an extraction where the blood clot has not formed or is lost; also called alveolitis (Ch. 25)

dual coverage two dental coverages; the primary is in first position and the balance is normally paid by secondary insurance (Ch. 36)

dual-cured materials materials containing chemicals for self-curing as well as materials set by light curing (Ch. 33)

ductility the ability of a material to withstand forces of tensile stress without failing (Ch. 33)

ducts of Bartholin route to the sublingual caruncles of saliva from the sublingual glands (Ch. 7)

ducts of Rivinus route to the mouth of saliva from the sublingual glands (Ch. 7)

due care the care that any reasonable and prudent dental care personnel would do in the same circumstances (Ch. 3)

duodenum first section of the small intestine where digestive juices enter and food breakdown process continues (Ch. 6)

duplication technique a technique whereby dental radiographs are reproduced on specialized film (Ch. 22)

dysplasic cells abnormal cell features such as size, shape, rate of multiplication (Ch. 26)

ecchymosis the bruising of tissue (Ch. 26)

ecotoderm one of the three embryonic layers formed in the early embryo stage that differentiates into skin, hair, nails, the brain, the nervous system, the lining of the oral cavity, and the enamel of the teeth (Ch. 8)

edema excessive amounts of fluid in body tissue; swelling (Ch. 16)

edentulous when all natural teeth have been lost (Ch. 32)

elasticity the ability to be distorted or deformed by an applied force and then return to its original shape once the force is removed (Ch. 33)

elastics rubber bands or elastic threads, often used between the upper and lower arches to provide force for movement (Ch. 27)

electrolytes minerals that have positive or negative charges (Ch. 5)

electromagnetic energy a form of energy that is the result of electric and magnetic disturbances in space (Ch. 21)

electronic anesthesia a method that has low to moderate levels of success but best used with nitrous oxide inhalation sedation or for a patient that can not tolerate local anesthetics (Ch. 20)

electronic pulp tester tool, usually battery operated, that creates an electrical stimulus to the tooth indicating whether pulp is vital or non-vital (Ch. 24)

electrosurgery procedure that uses tiny electrical currents to incise gingival tissue and coagulate blood; setup consists of control box, foot-operated on-off controls, a terminal plate that is placed behind patient's back or shoulders, and a terminal probe with various cutting tips (Ch. 29)

electrosurgery unit tool that cauterizes tissues as it removes them to prevent bleeding (Ch. 25)

elevators instruments that loosen and remove teeth, retained roots, and root fragments (Ch. 25)

eligibility determining if the patient is eligible for dental benefits (Ch. 36)

elimination a function of the digestive system that removes solid wastes from the body (Ch. 6)

elon a chemical reducer used in development of radiographs to blacken the exposed silver halide crystals (Ch. 22)

elongation a technique error that elongates the image of the teeth (Ch. 22)

emaciation extreme thinness (Ch. 5)

embrasure the triangular space in the gingival direction that is made when two adjoining teeth are contacting (Ch. 9)

embryology the study of prenatal growth and the developing process of an individual (Ch. 8)

enamel tooth structure that covers the outside of the crown of the tooth; the hardest living tissue in the body (Ch. 8)

enamel dysplasia a developmental disturbance during the apposition stage, perhaps from a nutritional loss, resulting in the surface of teeth becoming grooved and pitted (Ch. 8)

enamel hypocalcification   soft and undercalcified tooth enamel (Ch. 4)

enamel hypoplasia   incomplete development of tooth enamel (Ch. 4)

enamel lamellae   narrow and long enamel tufts that extend from the dentinoenamel junction to the enamel surface (Ch. 8)

enamel matrix   produced by the ameloblast cells (Ch. 8)

enamel spindles   short, dentinal tubules that seem to have crossed over into the enamel and were trapped there during the process of enamel mineralization.

enamel tufts   similar to enamel spindles but with bases near the dentinoenamel junction that appear as small, dark brushes (Ch. 8)

encoding   the use of specific signs, symbols, interpersonal communication or language used in communicating a message (Ch. 2)

endocardium   thin lining on the inside of the heart (Ch. 6)

endoderm   one of the three embryonic layers formed in the early embryo stage that gives rise to the epithelial linings of the respiratory system, some glandular organs, and the digestive tract (Ch. 8)

endodontic handpiece   an attachment to a low-speed handpiece that supplies quarter-turn motion consistently and evenly (Ch. 24)

endodontics   the branch of dentistry that deals with the diagnosis and treatment of diseases of the pulp and the periapical tissues (Chs. 1 and 24)

endogenous   originating from within the tooth (Ch. 29)

endospore   a dormant, non-reproductive structure produced by a small number of bacteria that's primary function is to ensure survival through periods of environmental stress (Ch. 10)

endosteal implants   implants placed into the bone surgically; used to replace single teeth and for patients who are partially edentulous (Ch. 25)

enteric-coated   a coating found on some medications that resists breakdown by gastric juices and dissolves in the intestines (Ch. 15)

Environmental Protection Agency (EPA)   a regulatory agency involved in the safety and effectiveness of disinfecting and sterilizing solutions (Ch. 11)

epiglottis   a leaf-shaped organ at the end of the larynx whose function is to close off the larynx during swallowing (Ch. 6)

epilepsy   a recurrent disorder of cerebral function, due to excessive neuronal discharge (Ch. 16)

epinephrine   the most common vasoconstrictor used in dentistry (Ch. 20)

epithelial attachment   the gingiva in the floor of the gingival sulcus that attaches to the enamel surface of the teeth just above the CEJ of the tooth (Ch. 8)

ergonomics   study of work and space, including factors that affect worker's health, productivity, and mental well-being (Chs. 17 and 36)

erosion   wearing away (Ch. 26)

eruption   when the tooth emerges from the gum tissue (Ch. 8)

erythema   redness or inflammation of the skin (Ch. 16)

erythrocyte   red blood cells (Ch. 6)

erythroplakia   any red patch of tissue in the oral cavity that cannot be associated with inflammation (Ch. 26)

esophagus   extends from the pharynx to the stomach; includes muscles that help food move toward the stomach (Ch. 6)

essential amino acids   (ten are needed) part of the protein molecule that the body cannot synthesize or produce; must be obtained through diet (Ch. 5)

etch   conditioned by a phosphoric or other type of acid solution that is applied to a clean tooth (Ch. 28)

ethics   although different from person to person, ethics are what is morally right or wrong (Ch. 3)

ethmoid bone   bone that forms part of the nose, orbits, and the floor of the cranium (Ch. 7)

ethmoid sinuses   contained within the thin, spongy ethmoid bone (Ch. 7)

ethnicity   a group that shares cultural characteristics (Ch. 2)

etiologic agent   causative agent of a disease (Ch. 10)

etiology   cause of a disease (Ch. 26)

etiquette   treating people/customers with respect; manners, politeness (Ch. 36)

eustachian tube   also known as auditory tubes, opens into the pharynx (Ch. 6)

evanesce   dissolve (Ch. 8)

excisional biopsy   complete removal of a lesion along with a small border of the normal tissue surrounding it (Ch. 25)

excitability   when muscle tissue responds to stimuli (Ch. 6)

exclusions   items dental coverage does not cover (Ch. 36)

exfoliated   shed from the oral cavity (Ch. 9)

exfoliative cytology   removal of a layer of cells from the surface of a lesion (Ch. 25)

exhalation   phase of respiration when muscles relax and the air is moved out of the lungs; breathing out (Chs. 6 and 13)

exogenous   originating from outside the tooth (Ch. 29)

exostosis   an enlargement of nodular outgrowth of dense lamella bone that appears on the facial surfaces of the mandibular and the maxillary palate (Ch. 26)

exothermic   a chemical reaction that releases heat (Chs. 33 and 35)

expanded functions   skills and functions beyond those normally associated with dental assisting that require increased skill and responsibility; delegated by dentists according to the Dental Practice Acts in their states (Ch. 3)

expendable   supplies that are used up or disposed of after use (e.g., cotton balls and envelopes) (Ch. 36)

expert witness   an individual specially qualified in a particular field or topic area who is called to testify to the standard of care expected within that field (Ch. 3)

expressed contract   a contract, written or verbal, that describes what each party in the contract will do (Ch. 3)

extensibility   the ability of the muscle to stretch or spread in order to perform tasks (Ch. 6)

external auditory meatus   opening for the ear (Ch. 7)

external carotid artery   supplies blood to the face and oral cavity and has many branches (Ch. 7)

external jugular vein   vein that drains the superficial veins of the face and neck into the subclavian vein (Ch. 7)

external oblique ridge   extending from the mental foramen, follows the length of the body of the mandible past the last tooth and up to the ramus (Ch. 7)

external pterygoid muscles   one of the muscles of mastication, opens jaw by depressing the mandible (Ch. 7)

extipate   to remove pulpal contents (Ch. 24)

extraction forceps instruments used to remove teeth from the alveolar bone (Ch. 25)

extraoral film film used outside the oral cavity (Ch. 23)

extrinsic muscles assist in the movement and functioning of the tongue; includes genioglossus, hyoglossus, styloglossus, and palatoglossus (Ch. 7)

extrinsic stains discolorations on the outside of the tooth structure that can be removed by scaling and polishing (Ch. 29)

exudate pus (Ch. 24)

facial either the labial surface of the anterior teeth or the buccal surface of the posterior teeth (Chs. 7 and 9)

facial artery contains six branches that supply blood to the pharynx muscles, soft palate, tonsils, the posterior of the tongue, submandibular gland, muscles of the face, nasal septum, the nose, and eyelids (Ch. 7)

facial vein drains the facial structures, beginning near the eye and descending toward the mandible (Ch. 7)

facsimile written message transmitted through the telephone line (Ch. 36)

facultative anaerobic bacteria grow with or without oxygen (Ch. 10)

Fair Debt Collection Practice Act legislation making it illegal to phone a debtor at inconvenient hours or to the debtors employers (Ch. 36)

Farenheit system used to measure temperature; the freezing point is 32 degrees and the boiling point is 212 degrees (Ch. 13)

fascia a fibrous sheet of connective tissue that covers, supports, and separates each group of muscle cells, or fibers (Ch. 6)

fats derived from solids, fat provides a source of energy in addition to carbohydrates. Fat insulates the body from heat loss, protects vital organs, and aids in the transportation of fat-soluble vitamins (Ch. 5)

fauces the space in the back of the oral cavity where food passes into the pharynx (Ch. 7)

Fédération Dentaire Internationale (FDI) system for numbering international system used for coding teeth and the oral cavity in charting (Ch. 14)

fee for service payment to providers on a service-by-service rather than a salaried or capitated basis (Ch. 36)

fever elevation of the body's temperature above the normal range (Ch. 13)

fiberoptic light sources available with high-speed handpieces, fiberoptic systems greatly improve visibility of the treatment area for the operator (Ch. 19)

fibroblasts cells that form connective tissue (Ch. 8)

fibroma a benign tumor of connective tissue cells; a reactive hyperplasia rather than a true neoplasm (Ch. 26)

fibromyalgia chronic pain in the muscles and soft tissues surrounding the joints (Ch. 6)

field block anesthesia injection method that places the anesthetic solution near larger terminal nerve branches (Ch. 20)

file folder an envelope or a book-type holder that stores patient information (Ch. 36)

files endontic instruments used to enlarge and smooth the canal (Ch. 24)

filiform papilla hair-like projections on the lateral border of the tongue near the base (Ch. 7)

fimbriated folds folds of tissue that are lateral to the lingual veins (Ch. 7)

fissure a developmental groove that has an imperfect union where the lobes join (Ch. 9)

fissured tongue a wrinkled, deeply grooved surface on the tongue (Ch. 26)

fistula a tube-like passage from an abcess to the external surface; used to drain the abscess (Chs. 16 and 24)

fixed appliances appliances attached to the teeth that cannot be removed by the patient (e.g., braces) (Ch. 27)

fixed prosthetic artificial part for missing tissue or tooth that becomes part of the natural dentition (Ch. 30)

fixer solution the second chemical solution used in processing radiographs (Ch. 22)

flagella long, threadlike appendage on protozoa that assist with movement (Ch. 10)

flex files endodontic files made of stainless steel or nickel-titanium and used for curved and narrow canals that require flexibility to negotiate (Ch. 24)

flowable composite similar to microfilled and hybrid composites in content and particle size; can be applied directly into cavity preparations by small syringe tips (Ch. 34)

floss holder a y-shaped device with a handle that makes flossing easier for individuals with arthritis, poor manual dexterity, or large hands (Ch. 4)

floss threader a device used to remove plaque and debris from under fixed bridges, orthodontic wires, and retainers (Ch. 4)

flour of pumice a relatively coarse (abrasive) material used to remove stains from enamel; should be followed by a fine polishing agent (Ch. 29)

flow continuing deformation of a solid; also called creep and slump (Ch. 33)

fluoridation the process of adding fluoride to the water supply (Ch. 4)

fluoride applications fluoride applied to the teeth in the dental office (Ch. 23)

fluoride prophylaxis pastes commercially prepared pastes with the addition of fluoride (Ch. 29)

fluorine a trace mineral that helps strengthen teeth and may help prevent osteoporosis (Ch. 5)

fluoroapatite crystal tooth structure formed when fluoride replaces the hydroxyl ion of the enamel (Ch. 4)

fluorosis mottled enamel; results from excessive fluoride during tooth development; tooth enamel appears pitted and multicolored (Ch. 4)

focal spot area on the anode that electrons hit during x-ray production (Ch. 21)

focal trough a three-dimensional curved zone in a panoramic radiographic machine in which the dental arches are positioned to achieve the sharpest image; also called the image layer or sharpness (Ch. 23)

focusing cup area on the anode that directs the electrons to the focal spot during x-ray production (Ch. 21)

foliate papillae slightly raised, vertical folds of tissue on the lateral border of the tongue near the base (Ch. 7)

folic acid also known as folacin, is a water-soluble vitamin found in plants such as spinach, asparagus, broccoli, and kidney beans; its primary function is the synthesis of red blood cells (Ch. 5)

fomite objects contaminated with infectious agents such as instruments or dressings (Ch. 11)

Food and Drug Administration (FDA) federal regulation agency (Chs. 11 and 15)

force the push or pull of an object (Ch. 33)

Fordyce's spots sebaceous oil glands near the surface of the epithelium that appear in the oral cavity as round, yellow spots (Chs. 7 and 26)

foreign body airway obstruction (FBAO) obstruction of normal breathing; dental instruments, crowns, amalgams, composite, cotton rolls, and gauze are items that may obstruct the airway (Ch. 16)

forensic dentistry area of dentistry that deals with identification of an individual through tooth restorations and morphology using dental records (Ch. 1)

foreshortening a technique error whereby the image of the teeth is shortened (Ch. 22)

fossa a shallow, rounded, or angular depression (Ch. 9)

four-handed dentistry system in which the dentist and dental assistant work together at the dental chair (Chs. 17 and 18)

fracture breaks of the bone or cartilage (Ch. 6)

framework the skeleton of the removable partial to which rests, connectors, and retainers are attached (Ch. 32)

Frankfort plane the imaginary horizontal plane from the bottom of the eye socket to the top of the ear canal (Ch. 23)

fraud a deliberate deception that is practiced to secure unfair or unlawful gain (Ch. 3)

free gingiva or marginal surrounds the teeth and is attached only at the gingival groove, appears lighter in color (if healthy) and is about 1 mm in width (Ch. 3)

frena raised lines of mucosal tissue found in the vestibule areas of the oral cavity (Ch. 7)

frenectomy complete surgical removal of the frenum, including the attachment to the underlying bone (Ch. 29)

frenum raised lines of mucosal tissue found in the vestibule areas of the oral cavity (Ch. 7)

frictional heat heat produced when a moving surface contacts another (Ch. 19)

front delivery system one of three types of dental unit with the equipment designed to be pulled over the patient's chest and located between the dentist and the assistant (Ch. 17)

frontal bone a bone in the human skull that resembles a cockle-shell in form and consists of vertical horizontal portions (Ch. 7)

frontal plane divides the body into front and back sections (Ch. 6)

fulcrum the support or point on which a level turns (e.g., position of fingerrest for support when working in a patient's mouth) (Chs. 13 and 29)

full-cast crown full covering over a tooth that has extensive decay or damage (Ch. 30)

furcation the dividing point of a multirooted tooth; division of the roots (Chs. 9 and 29)

fungiform papilla projections that give the tongue the "strawberry effect" (Ch. 7)

fusion a condition in which the enamel and dentin of two or more individual teeth join together (Ch. 26)

gallbladder muscular sac that stores bile from the liver (Ch. 6)

galvanism creation of electrical shock caused by two different metals coming together (Ch. 33)

gel a solid (Ch. 35)

gelatin time the time from which the alginate powder material is mixed with water until it is completely set and considered alginate (Ch. 35)

general anesthetic anesthesia that renders the patient unconscious (Ch. 20)

generic names drug names unprotected by trademark; are less expensive than brand names and may be used by any business (Ch. 15)

genial tubercles small, bony projections surrounding the lingual foramen (Ch. 7)

genioglossus extrinsic muscle of the tongue that does most of the work including protruding, retracting, and depressing the tongue (Ch. 7)

geniohyoid one of the muscles of the floor of the mouth that pulls the hyoid bone and the tongue anteriorly (Ch. 7)

germination a condition which is similar to fusion but in which one tooth bud attempts to divide (Ch. 26)

gestational period the period of carrying an offspring in the womb during pregnancy the fetus can grow from 19-21 inches (or 48-52 cm) (Ch. 8)

ghost image a radiopaque artifact seen on panoramic film caused by metal or dense objects being exposed twice by the x-ray beam (Ch. 23)

gingiva composed of a mucosa that surrounds the necks of the teeth, and covers the alveolar processes (Ch. 8)

gingival dense, fibrous tissue located between the alveolar mucosa and the teeth and covered with mucous membrane (Ch. 7)

gingival fiber groups found in the lamina propria, they support the marginal gingival tissues in relationship to the tooth, and lie above the alveolar bone crest and below the epithelium (Ch. 8)

gingival grafting procedure in which tissue is taken from one site and placed on another (Ch. 29)

gingival hyperplasia an overgrowth of gingival tissue (Chs. 16 and 26)

gingival retraction chemical, mechanical, surgical, or combination process used to ensure an impression with clear margins can be obtained when preparing a tooth for a crown (Ch. 35)

gingival sulcus the space between the attached gingiva and the tooth (Ch. 8)

gingival wall the side or floor of the cavity preparation nearest the gingival that is perpendicular to the long axis of the tooth (Ch. 33)

gingivectomy surgical removal of diseased gingival tissue (Ch. 29)

gingivitis inflammation of the ginigival tissues, marked by red, swollen, and/or bleeding gums; caused by buildup of plaque and calculus, poorly fitting appliances, or malocclusion; may occur with certain systemic diseases, hormonal changes, or prolonged drug therapy (Chs. 4 and 29)

gingivoplasty reshaping of the gingival tissue to remove such deformities as clefts, craters, and enlargements; performed only to recontour the gingiva (Ch. 29)

glass ionomer permanent cementation with diverse types and applications: Type I is a finer grain that bonds chemically to teeth; Type II is coarser grain and is used in selected restorations; Type III is used as a liner and dentin bonding agent; Type IV is admixtures of glass ionomers used for buildups (Chs. 28 and 33)

glenoid fossa a pit or depression found anterior to the mastoid process is where the mandible articulates with the skull (Ch. 7)

Glick #1 endontic instrument used to remove excess gutta percha (Ch. 24)

glossitis a condition due to Vitamin B deficiency causing inflammation of the tongue and Pellagra, where mucous membranes atrophy and ulcers develop (Chs. 5 and 26)

glossopharyngeal a cranial nerve that exits the brainstem out from the sides of the medulla (Ch. 7)

glutaraldehyde solution used for high-level disinfection and sterilization (Ch. 11)

glycogen stored glucose in a muscle (Ch. 6)

gold foil restoration created when several layers of pure gold are placed in the cavity preparation (Ch. 14)

Good Samaritan Law protection for people who provide medical assistance to those in emergency situations who are not seeking payment for it; those providing the assistance are given immunity (Ch. 3)

gram negative a cell wall's lack of dye color under a microscope (Ch. 10)

gram positive a cell wall's retention of dye color under a microscope (Ch. 10)

gram stain a procedure to differentiate cells into two specific groups using special dyes (Ch. 10)

grand mal seizure seizure marked by person becoming unconscious and the body jerking, twitching, and stiffening; usually lasts two to five minutes (Ch. 16)

granuloma a neoplasm or tumor filled with granulation tissue (Ch. 26)

Gray (GY) the Systeme Internationale unit of absorbed dose of ionizing radiation (Ch. 21)

gray scale the contrast found in an image related to the degrees of gray found in the image (Ch. 23)

greater palatine artery travels through the greater palatine foramen to supply the hard palate and the maxillary lingual gingival (Ch. 7)

greater palatine foramen the largest of three openings located in the posterior region of the hard palate (Ch. 7)

greater palatine nerve serves the soft palate, hard palate, medial gingival, and mucous membrane as far forward as the anterior teeth (Ch. 7)

green stain discoloration most often found in children; found on the facial surface of the maxillary anterior teeth at the cervical third, containing chromogenic bacteria and fungi; varies from light to dark green or yellowish-green (Ch. 29)

gross income total accounts receivable (Ch. 36)

group plan insurance plan that covers several individuals (Ch. 36)

guide channels slots in the end of a retainer that hold the matrix band and direct the band to the right or left of the retainer (Ch. 34)

guided tissue regeneration a technique that uses barrier membranes to maintain a space between the gingival flap and the root surface of the tooth in order for tissues to regenerate in a periodontal defect (Ch. 29)

gumma a localized lesion that occurs in the third stage of syphilis (Ch. 26)

gums the gingival that is composed of a mucosa that surrounds the necks of the teeth and covers the alveolar processes (Ch. 8)

gutta percha filling material; usually thermoplastic (Ch. 24)

Guy de Chaulic (1300–1368) a French surgeon who wrote hygienic rules for oral hygiene (Ch. 1)

gypsum calcium sulfate dihydrate; used when pouring an impression to make a model; water-powder ratio dictates strength, accuracy, resistance, reproduction detail, and setting times (Ch. 35)

habit forming leading to psychological or physical drug dependency (Ch. 15)

hairy leukoplakia a white, patterned lesion normally found on the borders of the tongue in patients infected with HIV (Ch. 26)

hairy tongue a condition in which the filiform papillae of the tongue become elongated and appear like hairs (Ch. 26)

halide crystals component of film's emulsion suspended in a gelatin; stores the energy from which they have been exposed and reacts with the chemicals in the processing tank to form a black region on the film (Ch. 21)

halitosis bad breath (Ch. 4)

hallucinate to cause the drug user to see images and hear sounds that do not exist (Ch. 15)

hand-over-mouth (HOM) technique act by which a medical or dental professional places the hand over the patient's mouth and calmly explains behavior expectations; requires informed consent (Ch. 28)

handpieces instruments used with rotary burs, discs, and stones; connected to power, air, and water sources (Ch. 17)

hard deposits hard, calcified deposits (mineralized plaque) firmly attached to teeth, restorations, and dental appliances; also called calculus or tartar (Ch. 29)

hard radiation short wavelengths with high frequency, high energy, and high penetrating power (Ch. 21)

hardware physical computer equipment that processes data (Ch. 36)

headgear orthodontic appliance composed of a strap that goes behind the patient's head or neck and a facebow that attaches to buccal tubes on molar bands; applies force to move teeth, restrain or alter facial bone growth, and reinforce the stability of intraoral appliances (Ch. 27)

heading portion of the prescription that includes the doctor's name and degrees, the DEA number, the office address, and the phone number (Ch. 15)

health information (HI) information provided to a health care institution related to a specific persons care and as well as personnel information (Ch. 3)

heart a pump that circulates blood throughout the body (Ch. 6)

heart valve maintains the unidirectional flow of blood by opening and closing depending on the difference in pressure on each side (Ch. 6)

heating unit recent technology that has many applications such as providing heat for vitality testing, warming the gutta percha for obturation, and providing heat for bleaching procedures (Ch. 24)

Hedström files endodontic files that are very sharp and cut aggressively; used in a push-and-pull motion (Ch. 24)

Heimlich maneuver the procedure performed when a person is in distress and unable to breathe due to a foreign body airway obstruction (Ch. 16)

hematoma appearing as a bruised area, a lesion caused by bleeding from a ruptured blood vessel (Ch. 26)

hemiplegia weakness, numbness, or paralysis on one side of the body (Ch. 16)

hemisection surgical removal of one root and the overlying crown (Ch. 24)

hemoglobin   a protein which gives the erythrocytes the ability to carry oxygen through the blood (Ch. 6)

hemophilia   a disorder causing failure of the blood to clot (Ch. 6)

hemostasis   to stop bleeding (Ch. 6)

hemostats   forceps instruments used during surgery to retract tissue, remove small root tips, clamp off blood vessels, and grasp objects (Ch. 25)

hepatitis   inflammation of the liver that is caused by several viruses (Ch. 6)

hepatitis A   also called infectious hepatitis, a bloodborne disease transmitted by person-to-person contact or by ingestion of contaminated water or food; symptoms are generally flu-like but could result in acute liver injury (Ch. 10)

hepatitis B   also called serum hepatitis, a bloodborne disease primarily transmitted through contaminated needles and syringes; symptoms include loss of appetite, digestive upset, upper abdominal pain, fever, weakness, muscle pain, and jaundice (Ch. 10)

hepatitis C   also called non-A and non-B, a bloodborne disease primarily transmitted through contaminated needles and syringes; symptoms are similar to Hepatitis B (Ch. 10)

hepatitis D   also called the Delta Agent, a bloodborne disease transmitted through contaminated needles and syringes; symptoms include loss of appetite, digestive upset, upper abdominal pain, fever, weakness, muscle pain, and jaundice (Ch. 10)

hepatitis E   a bloodborne disease transmitted through contaminated water and food with symptoms including loss of appetite, dark urine, fatigue, and nausea (Ch. 10)

herpes labialis   form of Herpes Simplex Type I; also known as fever blisters (Ch. 26)

herpes simplex   common and troublesome viral disease (Ch. 10)

herpes simplex virus type I   a viral disease usually associated with infections of the lips, mouth, and face is spread by contact with a fluid-filled lesion, or vesicle (Ch. 10)

herpes simplex virus type II   a sexually transmitted viral disease that displays fluid-filled lesions, or vesicles, on the sex organs or within the oral cavity (Ch. 10)

herpes zoster   unilateral, painful lesions that can last up to five weeks; also known as shingles (Ch. 26)

herpetic gingivostomatitis   inflammation of the gingiva caused by a virus (Ch. 26)

herpetic whitlow   exposure to the herpes virus that manifests itself as a crusting ulceration on the fingers or hands; may be very painful (Chs. 10 and 26)

herringbone pattern   a cross pattern that appears on film that has been placed backward in the mouth; caused by the pattern on the lead foil (Ch. 22)

high-speed handpieces   handpieces used to rapidly cut tooth structure and finish restorations; rotates between 10,000 and 800,000 rpm (Ch. 19)

high-strength bases   cement bases including glass ionomers, hybrid ionomers, reinforced zinc oxide eugenol, zinc phosphate, and polycarboxylate (Ch. 33)

high volume evacuation (HVE)   removing fluids from the patient's mouth; also called oral evacuation (Chs. 17 and 18)

hinge   a metal device—similar to a hinge—that may be built into the partial denture that relieves pressure on the abutment teeth; also called a stress-breaker (Ch. 32)

HIPAA   the Health Insurance Portability and Accountability Act of 1996 (HIPAA), also known as the Kennedy-Kassebaum Act, was enacted to establish safeguards for health care transactions transmitted electronically (Ch. 3)

Hippocrates   known as the father of medicine; the Oath of Hippocrates serves as the code of ethics for the medical and dental professions (Ch. 1)

histamine   chemicals released by specialized body cells as the body responds to disease and injury; brings about the inflammation process (Ch. 26)

histodifferentiation   the development of different tissues during the embryonic stage of pregnancy (Ch. 8)

histology   the study of the microscopic structure and function of tissues (Ch. 8)

Hodgkin's disease   a malignant disorder that causes enlargement of the lymph nodes (Ch. 6)

hoe scaler   instrument with sharp, beveled, 90-degree angled blade that, when placed in the periodontal pocket to the base and pulled toward the crown of the tooth with even pressure, planes and smooths the root surface (Ch. 29)

home whitening techniques   popular method used by patients that is less expensive, involves fewer visits to dental office, but requires high motivation by patient to follow routine (Ch. 31)

homeostasis   cells, tissues, organs, and systems all functioning together to maintain harmony in the body (Ch. 6)

homogenous   uniformly mixed (Ch. 35)

Horace H. Hayden   (1769–1844) established the Baltimore College of Dental Surgery with Chapin Harris. It was the first dental college in the world (Ch. 1)

Horace Wells   (1815–1848) Connecticut dentist who was the first to use nitrous oxide as an anesthetic during dental surgery (Ch. 20)

horizontal angulation   adjustment of angulation from left to right; improper angulation shows overlapping teeth (Ch. 22)

horizontal bone resorption   a result of periodontal disease when there is equal crestal bone loss on the mesial and distal surfaces of the proximal teeth (Ch. 29)

horizontal fiber groups   functions to resist rotational forces and tilting (Ch. 8)

horizontal mattress suture   used when suturing a flap, goes in and out of the tissue on the same surface; identified by a horizontal stitch or "bite"; tied with one surgeon's knot on the surface where suture procedure began (Ch. 25)

horizontal plane   also known as the transverse plane, divides the body into upper and lower regions (Ch. 6)

hormone   secretions released from the endocrine glands into the bloodstream (Ch. 6)

host   a simple or complex organism that can be affected by an agent (Ch. 11)

hue   color; the hue of mature teeth varies due to intrinsic and extrinsic stains from smoking, foods, and restorative materials (Ch. 31)

human immunodeficiency virus (HIV)   the AIDS virus; ultimately destroys immune system cells (Chs. 10 and 26)

humectant   material or substance that retains moisture (Ch. 29)

Hutchinson's incisors   the appearance of indentations on the incisal edges of the anterior dentition; this is characteristic of the teeth of children born to mothers with syphilis (Ch. 26)

hybrid composites includes more than one type of filler particle, usually glass and silica; stronger and less likely to fracture in high-stress areas (Ch. 34)

hydrogen peroxide material used for whitening teeth that causes temporary sensitivity of the pulp, irritates tissue, and discolors clothing (Ch. 31)

hydroquinone a chemical used in development of radiographs; a reducing agent used to blacken exposed silver hyalide crystals (Ch. 22)

hydroxyl ion located on the surface of the apatite crystal in the enamel (Ch. 4)

hyoglossus extrinsic tongue muscle that mainly depresses the tongue (Ch. 7)

hyoid bone a horseshoe-shaped bone lying at the base of the tongue; all the muscles of the tongue and the floor of the mouth attach to this bone for support (Ch. 7)

hypercementosis a thickening of cementum around the apex that is caused by trauma to the tooth (Ch. 8)

hyperglycemia too much glucose in the blood (Ch. 16)

hyperkeratinization a thickening of the outer layer of the skin due to an increased amount of keratin (Ch. 26)

hyperkeratinized epithelium tissue that has built a layer of keratin as a protective coating (Ch. 26)

hyperplasia excess tissue; in dentistry, resulting from ill-fitting dentures that initially cause small ulcers that, after continued irritation, become folds of excess tissue (Ch. 26)

hypersensitive repeated contact with an allergen which causes the body to overreact (Ch. 16)

hypersensitivity extreme sensitivity to certain allergens (Ch. 10)

hypertension higher-than-normal blood pressure (Ch. 13)

hyperthyroidism an overactive thyroid gland with excessive secretion of hormones (Ch. 6)

hyperventilation abnormally rapid and deep breathing resulting in decreased carbon dioxide levels (Ch. 16)

hypoglossal supplies motor fibers to all of the muscles of the tongue, except the palatoglossus muscle (Ch. 7)

hypoglycemia condition exhibited by too little glucose or sugar in one's blood (Ch. 16)

hypotension lower-than-normal blood pressure (Chs. 13 and 16)

hypothermic having a body temperature below normal (Ch. 13)

hypothyrodism an underactive thyroid gland (Ch. 6)

idiopathic a disease or disorder that has no known cause (Ch. 26)

illusion the art of making something appear different than it actually is (Ch. 31)

imbibition enlargement due to swelling or the absorption of fluid (Ch. 35)

imbrication lines small, curved lines running parallel to the CEJ near the gingival area of the labial of the crown of a tooth (Chs. 8 and 9)

imbrication lines of Von Ebner stained growth rings or incremental lines in dentin (Ch. 8)

implied consent consent for a procedure given by the patient's act (e.g., patients who roll up their sleeves for blood pressure readings or to receive injections (Ch. 3)

implied contract a contract implemented by actions, not words (Ch. 3)

immune deficiency disease a failure in some part of the immune system (Ch. 6)

immunization a process that increases an individual's resistance to a particular disease (Ch. 10)

immunotherapy injection of an allergen for treatment of an allergy (Ch. 16)

incipient beginning tooth decay that has not broken through the enamel into the dentin (Ch. 14)

incisal edge cutting or tearing edge of the anterior teeth (Ch. 9)

incisal-third the area on the crown of the tooth that is nearest the incisal edge on the anterior tooth (Ch. 9)

incisional biopsy removal of a small section of a lesion along with a small border of normal tissue (Ch. 25)

incisive arteries supplies blood to the roots and periodontal ligaments of the anterior teeth (Ch. 7)

incisive nerve branch innervating the anterior teeth and the labial gingiva; a branch of the inferior alveolar nerve (Ch. 7)

incisive papilla a raised area of tissue behind the maxillary central incisors (Ch. 7)

indirect contact contact with a microorganism through such means as contaminated instruments, supplies, and equipment (Ch. 11)

indirect digital imaging converts traditional x-rays to digital images (Ch. 23)

indirect providers the HIPAA provisions apply to indirect providers of health care services and supplies such as laboratories, pharmacies, surgical centers, and any others that would deal with any patient information (Ch. 3)

indirect pulp capping when there is a near pulp exposure a cavity liner is placed to protect the pulp before the restoration is placed (Ch. 28)

indirect pulp treatment (IPT) technique used when treating permanent teeth with potentially infectious tissue (due to caries or traumatic injury), when pulp is not exposed but when pulp may be exposed during tissue removal; also known as indirect pulp capping (Chs. 28 and 33)

indirect resin veneers requires two dental appointments; first an impression is made and then the fabricated veneer is bonded in place (Ch. 30)

indirect restorations impressions are taken and then these "fixed prostheses" are fabricated in a dental laboratory (Ch. 30)

individual plan insurance plan in which an individual has a plan without a group of individuals (Ch. 36)

infection control methods to eliminate or reduce the transmission of infectious microorganisms (Ch. 11)

inferior alveolar artery descends the ramus, enters the mandibular foramen, and bifurcates around the first premolar tooth to form the incisive and the mental arteries (Ch. 7)

inferior alveolar branch a main branch of the mandibular nerve (Ch. 7)

inferior nasal conchae scroll-like bones on the outside of the nasal cavities consisting of thin, cancellous bone (Ch. 7)

infiltration anesthesia an injection method that places anesthetic solution into the tissues near the small terminal nerve branches for absorption (Ch. 20)

inflamed the first response of the immune system to infection or irritation (Ch. 6)

inflammation body's defense against infection or trauma; redness, pain, and swelling may occur (Ch. 26)

informed consent agreement by the patient to the procedure that is about to be performed after being told of the procedure, risks involved, expected outcomes, and alternative treatments; patients acknowledge their understanding and acceptance by signing (Chs. 19 and 3)

infraorbital artery ascends from the maxillary artery and travels anteriorly to the infraorbital foramen, where it supplies the face with blood (Ch. 7)

infraorbital foramen located below the orbit on the maxillary bone and the maxillary sinus forming a large cavity above the roots of the maxillary molars (Ch. 7)

infraorbital nerve a branch of the maxillary nerve which branches into the middle superior alveolar nerve and the anterior alveolar nerve (Ch. 7)

infraversion tooth is positioned below the normal line of occlusion (Ch. 27)

inhalation breathing in; in the administration of drugs, the patient breathes in gas or aerosol; an individual contacts a microorganism by "breathing it in" (Chs. 6, 13, and 15)

inhalation sedation a general anesthesia used when IV sedation would be difficult to administer; the inhalation causes sleepiness and the patient doesn't remember much of the procedure (Ch. 20)

inhaler pressurized canister with a mouthpiece that administers antihistamines to a user (Ch. 16)

initiation when the tooth begins formation from the dental lamina (Ch. 8)

inlays restoration replacements for missing tooth structure in teeth; covers the area between the cusps in the middle of the tooth and the proximal surfaces (Ch. 30)

innocuous causing no harm (Ch. 26)

inscription name of the drug prescribed and the dosage; appears in the prescription (Ch. 15)

insertion point part of a muscle where the bone is moveable (Ch. 6)

insulin the hormone responsible for absorbing glucose into the cells for energy and into the liver and fat cells for storage (Ch. 16)

insulin shock caused by severe hypoglycemia and results in tremors, sweating, and nervousness. If not immediately treated, delirium, seizure-like jerkings, and collapse may follow (Ch. 16)

intensifying screens screens in cassettes used with extraoral films (Ch. 23)

intercellular substances substances between the cells (Ch. 8)

interceptive prevention and treatment of orthodontic problems (Ch. 27)

interdental knives periodontal knives used to remove soft tissue interproximally; spear shaped with long, narrow, double-edged blades (Ch. 29)

interdental ligament groups functions to resist rotational forces and hold teeth in interproximal contact (Ch. 8)

interdental septum a bony projection that separates each socket of the interradicular septum (Ch. 8)

intermediate restorative material a type II zinc oxide eugenol cement that is placed in the patient's mouth and lasts up to one year; used when a tooth cannot be restored immediately (Ch. 33)

internal carotid artery supplies blood to the brain and eyes (Ch. 7)

internal jugular vein vein that receives blood from the cranium, face, and neck and drains into the brachiocephalic vein, then into the superior vena cava, which drains into the heart (Ch. 7)

internal oblique ridge (mylohyoid ridge) follows the inside of the ramus and the body of the mandible (Ch. 7)

internal pterygoid muscles one of the muscles of mastication that elevates the mandible (Ch. 7)

interneuron also known as associate neurons, transmits impulses from sensory neurons to motor neurons in the central nervous system (Ch. 6)

interprismatic substance the weakest substance surrounding the inner portion, the red core, of each enamel rod (Ch. 8)

interproximal radiographs; also known as bite-wing radiographs (Ch. 22)

interproximal brush small, soft-bristled brush attached to a metal or plastic handle for cleaning open contact areas, around orthodontic braces and wires, around exposed bifurcation or trifurcation of the roots, or on abutment teeth of hygienic bridge (Chs. 4 and 29)

interradicular fiber groups found only in multi-rooted teeth; functions to resist rotational forces and to hold the teeth in interproximal contact (Ch. 8)

interradicular septum the bone that separates multiple roots in a tooth (Ch. 8)

interseptal dental dam material that goes between adjacent teeth (Ch. 34)

intertubular dentin dentin found between the tubules (Ch. 8)

intracanal instruments instruments used in endontics with precise diameters and lengths; made of stainless steel and nickel titanium alloy wire (Ch. 24)

intradermal administering drugs by injection under the epidermis (Ch. 15)

intramuscular administering drugs by injection into muscle tissue (Ch. 15)

intramuscular sedation an uncommon method when the sedative is injected into muscle in the upper arm or thigh; drug takes 20 to 30 minutes to take effect (Ch. 20)

intraoral film used inside the oral cavity (Ch. 21)

intraoral camera a small camera attached to the intraoral wand that transmits images to a television monitor (Ch. 17)

intraosseous anesthesia an injection of a local anesthetic directly into the cancellous bone (spongy bone) (Ch. 20)

intrapulpal injection a technique that deposits the anesthetic directly into the pulp chamber or root canal of the involved tooth (Ch. 20)

intravenous administering drugs by injecting directly into the vein (Ch. 15)

intravenous conscious sedation (IV) a very common way to keep patients relaxed, comfortable, and pain-free during dental procedures; sedative drugs are administered through an IV and directly into the patient's blood stream (Ch. 20)

intrinsic discolorations, usually permanent, inside the tooth structure (Ch. 29)

intrinsic muscles located within the tongue and are responsible for shaping the tongue during speech, mastication, and swallowing (Ch. 7)

inverting tucking of the dental dam material around the teeth to prevent moisture leakage (Ch. 34)

invisible aligners items that provide a method of tooth straightening without traditional braces; trays, similar to fluoride and bleaching trays, that are customized for each patient (Ch. 27)

iodine a trace mineral, found in the thyroid gland, regulates metabolism (Ch. 5)

iodophor solution used as an intermediate-level disinfection agent (Ch. 11)

ionization process by which atoms change into negatively or positively charged ions during radiation (Ch. 21)

iron a trace mineral whose primary function is to carry oxygen through the blood to the cells (Ch. 5)

irreversible hydrocolloid commonly called alginate, material used in the formation of dental impressions; setting of the material is accomplished by chemical reaction (Ch. 35)

irreversible pulpitis inflammation of the pulpal tissue to the point where it cannot recover; treatment includes root canal or extraction (Ch. 24)

irritability when muscle tissue responds to stimuli (Ch. 6)

ischemia shrinking of tissues

isometric contraction when there is no change in the length of a muscle but the muscle tension is increased (Ch. 6)

isotonic contraction when muscle tension remains the same but the muscles shorten (Ch. 6)

Jacksonian epilepsy condition characterized by a patient who remains conscious during seizure, recalling details of the events (Ch. 16)

James B. Morrison manufactured and patented the first dental engine with a functioning handpiece, motor, and foot-treadle (Ch. 1)

John Greenwood the favored dentist of George Washington; proponent for pediatric dentistry; constructed dentures (Ch. 1)

joint also known as articulations, areas where two or more bones meet or form a junction; composed of fibrous connective tissue and cartilage (Ch. 6)

Josiah Flagg (Late 1700s) notable dental surgeon; developed the first dental chair (Ch. 1)

Juliette Southard founded the American Dental Assistants' Association in 1924 (Ch. 1)

k-type files standard files used to scrape and widen the walls of the canal and to remove necrotic tissue (Ch. 24)

Kaposi's sarcoma malignant neoplasm, normally flat, reddish purple to dark blue; most commonly occurring in AIDS patients and men over 60 (Ch. 26)

key hole punch the largest hole punched in the dental dam; slides over the clamp and onto the anchor tooth; point from which next holes are punched (Ch. 34)

kilovoltage (kV) unit of electrical potential equal to 1,000 volts; dental kilovoltage is responsible for the quality of radiographs or penetrating power (Ch. 21)

labial the "inside" surface, which is toward the lips (Ch. 9)

labial commissures corners of the mouth where the upper and lower lips meet (Chs. 7 and 8)

labial mucosa the inner surface of the lips (Ch. 7)

labio-mental groove groove just below the lower lip that separates the lip from the chin (Ch. 7)

labioversion also called buccoversion, when a tooth is tipped toward the lip or cheek (Ch. 27)

laboratory area of the dental office where non-patient work is performed; may be used for finishing crowns, bridges, and so on (Ch. 17)

lacrimal bones small, delicate bones forming part of the corner of the eye; anterior to the ethmoid bone (Ch. 7)

lactic acid s waste product resulting from incomplete breakdown of glycogen in a muscle (Ch. 6)

lamina dura radioplaque line that represents the thin compact alveolus bone lining the socket (Ch. 8)

lamina propria the connective tissue of the marginal gingival and the location of the gingival fiber groups (Ch. 8)

lanugo baby-like hair on the body (Ch. 5)

large intestine extending from the small intestine to the rectum, stores and excretes the waste products of digestion (Ch. 6)

laryngopharynx the lower section of the pharynx (Ch. 6)

larynx also known as voice box, connects the pharynx and the trachea, is made up of cartilage and supported by muscles (Ch. 6)

laser a medical device that generates a precise beam of concentrated light energy (Ch. 29)

latent suppressed or dormant for a period of time (Ch. 10)

latent period time lapsed between exposure and response (e.g., time between exposure to the sun and sunburn) (Ch. 21)

lateral incisor the second tooth from the midline used for cutting (Ch. 9)

lateral jaw radiograph takes an image depicting a large area of the jaw and is used in dental offices lacking a panoramic x-ray machine (Ch. 23)

law the set of rules established and enforced by local, state, and federal governments (Ch. 3)

lead apron artifact a common panoramic radiography error resulting from a patient wearing a lead apron with a thyroid collar (Ch. 23)

leakage radiation the radiation comes out in all directions from the tube or tube head due to a malfunction or leakage (Ch. 21)

lesions tissue damage; in dentistry, all abnormal structures in the oral cavity (Ch. 26)

lesser palatine foramen two smaller openings located behind the greater palatine foramen in the posterior region of the hard palate (Ch. 7)

leukemia a malignant, progressive disease of the blood-forming organs that is marked by unrestrained growth of abnormal leukocytes (Ch. 6)

leukocyte white blood cells (Ch. 6)

leukoplakia a condition in the oral cavity with a white, leathery patch that cannot be identified as any other white lesion (Ch. 26)

libel false and malicious written comments (Ch. 3)

lichen planus a condition first appearing on the lower leg or ankle and then appearing in the oral cavity as small, white papules that group and form interlacing white lines (Ch. 26)

ligament composed of bands or sheets of fibrous tissue and act to connect or support two or more bones (Ch. 6)

ligature a piece of floss or a cord that stabilizes the dental dam in different applications; used in fixed bridge isolation, bleaching procedures, and tooth isolation (Ch. 34)

ligature wire a thin, flexible wire that holds the arch wire to the brackets (Ch. 27)

light cured type of sealant that is hardened by use of a single-component system activated by a curing light (Ch. 33)

light emitting diode (LED) A type of curing light that is durable, portable, produces minimal heat, does not require bulbs, and is quiet (Ch. 17)

line angle when two surfaces of a tooth meet (Ch. 33)

linea alba raised, white line on the buccal mucosa that runs parallel to where the teeth meet (Ch. 7)

liner material in a thin layer on the walls and floor of the cavity preparaton (Ch. 33)

lines of Retzius incremental lines or bands around the layers of the enamel matrix (Ch. 8)

lingual   surface of the tooth that is toward the tongue (Ch. 9)

lingual branch   nerve that innervates the floor of the mouth, ventral side of the tongue, tastebuds on the anterior two-thirds of the tongue, and the lingual gingiva (Ch. 7)

lingual foramen   the internal surface at the center of the mandible (Ch. 7)

lingual frenum   a line of tissue in the middle of the ventral side of the tongue that extends from the tongue to the floor of the mouth (Ch. 7)

lingual tonsil   located on the base of the tongue (Ch. 6)

lingual vein   located on either side of the lingual frenum and runs the length of the tongue (Ch. 7)

linguoversion   a deviation in tooth positioning; the tooth is lingual to normal position (Ch. 27)

lip retractors   used to hold the patient's cheeks away from the operating site (Ch. 25)

liver   largest of the glandular organs, main function is the production of bile as well as aiding in the digestive process (Ch. 6)

load   amount of pressure or strain put on a dental implant once place in the bone (Ch. 25)

lobes   divisions that join to form a tooth; often in molars, lobes become cusps (Ch. 9)

local anesthesia   anesthesia that produces a deadened or pain-free area (Ch. 20)

long wavelengths   in dental radiographs, wavelengths have low energy, low frequency, and are unsuitable for exposing dental radiographs (Ch. 21)

low-speed handpieces   handpieces used to polish teeth and restorations, remove soft carious material, and define cavity margins and walls; achieve between 6,000 and 25,000 rpm (Ch. 19)

low-strength bases   also called cavity liners, materials placed on dentin or on exposed pulp to protect the pulp from chemical irritation and provide therapeutic effect to the tooth; include calcium hydroxide, zinc oxide eugenol, and glass ionomer (Ch. 33)

lumbar   lower region of the back (Ch. 17)

lumen   the internal opening of the needle where the anesthetic solution flows through (Ch. 20)

lung   cone-shaped organ inside the rib cage (Ch. 6)

lung cancer   malignancy of the lung tissue often caused by cigarette smoking (Ch. 6)

luting   bonding or cementing together (Ch. 33)

luxates   moves or dislocates (e.g., the dentist uses forceps to luxate a loose tooth from the socket) (Ch. 25)

lymph   also called tissue fluid, is a clear liquid formed in tissue spaces. It enters the lymphatic capillary system and drains away excess fluid and carries proteins back to the blood stream (Ch. 6)

lymph node   found in groups along the lymphatic vessels, their purpose is to filter the lymph as it moves back to the blood stream and to manufacture antibodies and other active materials of the immunity process (Ch. 6)

lymphatic capillary   specialized network of vessels that transport lymph (Ch. 6)

macrodontia   abnormally large teeth (Ch. 26)

macrofilled composite   materials used for Class IV restorations because they are strong enough to resist fracture and are esthetically pleasing (Ch. 34)

macule   spot on the skin of abnormal texture or color (Ch. 26)

magnesium   a mineral involved in energy metabolism and stabilizing the components of the bones and teeth once they are formed (Ch. 5)

magnetic resonance imaging (MRI)   technique used mainly in the diagnosis of TMJ disease; allows the dentist to look at soft tissues of TMJ with little patient risk (Ch. 23)

malignant   cancerous (Ch. 26)

malleability   ability of a material to withstand compressive stresses without fracturing (Ch. 33)

malnutrition   disorder resulting from lack of correct nutrients for the body (Ch. 5)

malocclusion   any deviation from normal occlusion; may be a missing tooth, a group of teeth, or an entire arch (Ch. 27)

malpractice   incorrect or negligent treatment given to a patient by a doctor, dentist, or health-care provider (Ch. 3)

mamelons   three bulges on the incisal edge of a newly erupted central incisor (Ch. 9)

mandible   the only movable bone of the face (Ch. 7)

mandibular arch   lower arch in the dentition (Ch. 9)

mandibular artery   located behind the ramus of the mandible and branches into five arteries (Ch. 7)

mandibular foramen   located on the inside of the body of the ramus; the beginning of the internal oblique ridge (Ch. 7)

mandibular nerve branch   composed of both sensory and motor neurons and is the largest division of the trigeminal nerve (Ch. 7)

mandibular notch   a depression located between the condyle and the coronoid process; also known as the sigmoid or coronoid notch (Ch. 7)

mandibular occlusal view   patient is positioned in the supine position parallel to the floor with head tilted back. One assistant places the retractors and another positions the mirror (Ch. 31)

mandrels   rods of various lengths used in low-speed handpieces; mandrels are available in three shanks; latch, friction grip, or straight (Ch. 19)

manganese   a trace mineral involved in the process of metabolism (Ch 5)

mantle dentin   the first predentin that is formed and matures within the tooth (Ch. 8)

manual processing   processing dental x-rays using a manual tank with developer, running water, and fixer (Ch. 22)

manual toothbrush   a hand held toothbrush that only moves by the individual using it (Ch. 4)

manufacturer's number   number found on the handle of the instrument; used for ordering and identifying the instrument placement in a set (Ch. 19)

marginal ridges   elevated areas of enamel that form the mesial and distal borders of the lingual surface on the anterior teeth and the mesial and distal borders of the occlusal surface of the posterior teeth (Ch. 9)

Maryland bridge   a resin-retained, fixed bridge that replaces one tooth (Chs. 14 and 30)

Maslow's hierarchy of needs   ranking of human needs developed by Maslow in which physiological needs are on the lowest level and self-esteem and self-actualization are on the highest (Ch. 2)

masseter muscles   pairs of mastication muscles (Ch. 7)

master cone   the primary cone, normally gutta percha, used in a root canal (Ch. 24)

mastication   process of chewing (Ch. 7)

mastoid process   the bony projection found on the bottom border of the temporal bone (Ch. 7)

materia alba   soft, bulky, cottage-cheese-like mass of food debris and bacterial growth that collects in grooves and spaces on teeth, gingiva, and appliances; provides the source for plaque development (Ch. 29)

material safety data sheets (MSDSs)   health and safety information about chemicals; provided by the manufacturer (Ch. 11)

matrix   an essential artificial wall used to replace the missing or removed surfaces of a tooth during the filling of a cavity; composed of a band and a retainer (Chs. 34 and 35)

maturation   growth to and learning on a certain level (Ch. 23)

maxilla   the largest of the facial bones extending from the floor of each orbit and the floor and exterior walls of the nasal cavity to form the roof of the mouth (Ch. 7)

maxillary arch   upper arch in the dentition (Ch. 9)

maxillary artery   largest of the branches of the external carotid artery; moves anteriorly across the ramus of the mandible, near the condyle, and supplies facial structures (Ch. 7)

maxillary nerve branch   a sensory nerve that innervates the nose, cheeks, palate, gingival, maxillary teeth, maxillary sinus, tonsils, nasopharynx, and other facial features (Ch. 7)

maxillary occlusal view   patient is positioned in a semi-upright position with the mouth open. One assistant holds the lip and cheek retractors in the patient's mouth while another assistant positions the mirror (Ch. 31)

maxillary sinus   forms a large cavity above the roots of the maxillary molars (Ch. 7)

maxillary tuberosity   a rounded area beyond the last posterior maxillary tooth (Ch. 7)

maxillary vein   drains the pterygoid plexus of veins (Ch. 7)

maxillofacial   branch of dentistry focusing on the diagnosis and treatment of diseases, injuries, and malformations (Ch. 25)

maximum permissible dose (MPD)   the maximum dose of radiation that, in light of present knowledge, would not be expected to produce negative effects in a life (Ch. 21)

measles   a viral disease characterized by a rash and fever and spread by airborne droplets of nasal secretions (Ch. 10)

mechanical bond   bonding of sealant accomplished as sealant flows into the irregularities of the treated enamel and locks into place (Ch. 28)

mechanical retention   the attachment of materials to surfaces by means of grooves in the cavity preparation (Ch. 33)

mechanical toothbrush   a hand held toothbrush, powered by electricity or batteries, that moves the brush (Ch. 4)

medicines   drugs used to treat diseases (Ch. 15)

mental nerve branch   largest division of the trigeminal nerve (Ch. 7)

median sulcus   a groove that runs from the base to the tip of the tongue and divides the tongue in half (Ch. 7)

median suture   the juncture where the two sections of the maxilla bones come together (Ch. 7)

mental artery   branches off the inferior alveolar artery, then exits the mandibular canal at the mental foramen and supplies the chin and the lower lip (Ch. 7)

mental foramen   located on the body of the mandible near the apex of the premolars (Ch. 7)

mental protuberance   the tip of the chin (Ch. 7)

mentalis   one of the major muscles of facial expression (Ch. 7)

mercury   a toxic chemical element that is the main ingredient of dental amalgams (Ch. 34)

mesenchyme tissue   the primary embryonic mesoderm layer that develops during the morphodifferentiation period (Ch. 8)

mesial   surface of the tooth toward the midline (Ch. 9)

mesioversion   when a tooth is mesial to normal position (Ch. 27)

mesoderm   one of the three embryonic layers formed in the early embryo stage that differentiates into the lining of the abdominal cavity, the bones, the muscles, the circulatory system, the reproductive system, the internal organs, and the dentin, cementum, and pulp of the teeth (Ch. 8)

metabolism   sum of chemical and physical changes occurring in tissue (Ch. 5)

metabolism rate   the physical and chemical changes that take place in relationship to the usage of energy (Chs. 6 and 26)

metallic stains   discolorations of the teeth due to metals and metallic salts inhaled (in industrial settings), taken orally in certain drugs, or as part of the materials used in tooth restoration; copper dust, amalgam, iron dust, and iron drugs can cause permanent stains (Ch. 29)

metastasize   the spreading of a carcinoma (Ch. 26)

microbiology   the study of microorganisms (Ch. 10)

microdontia   abnormally small teeth; commonly seen in people with Down syndrome or people with congenital heart disease (Ch. 26)

microfilled composite   materials used as a cosmetic filling material for Class III and V restorations; used for direct veneers and diastema closures (Ch. 34)

microleakage   the seepage of saliva and debris from the oral cavity between the tooth structure and restorative materials (Ch. 33)

middle superior alveolar artery   branches to the maxillary premolar teeth (Ch. 7)

middle superior alveolar nerve   supplies the lateral wall of the maxillary sinus, gingival, mesial buccal root of the first molar, and all the roots of the bicuspids (premolars) (Ch. 7)

midline (median line)   imaginary line that divides the dental arches into two halves (Ch. 9)

midsagittal plane   equal left and right sides of the body (Ch. 6)

milliamperage (mA)   a measurement unit for electrical current (Ch. 21)

milliamperage seconds (mAs)   determines the amount of radiation exposure the patient receives (Ch. 21)

milliroentgen (mr)   one one thousandth (1/1,000) of a roentgen (Ch. 21)

mini (transitional) implant   used in many situations and work well to stabilize mandibular overdentures are for tooth replacement when the bone is narrow (Ch. 25)

mitosis   cell division in the sex cells in which the number of chromosomes in each is reduced by one-half (Ch. 21)

mitral valve   atrioventricular valve on the left side of the heart; bicuspid (Ch. 6)

mixed dentition   the period when primary teeth and permanent teeth are in the dentition lasting from approximately six to twelve years of age (Ch. 9)

mobile carts   movable cart that contains dental equipment (Ch. 17)

mobility   tooth movement in the socket; may be due to periodontal disease or trauma (Ch. 14)

mode of transmission   the process that bridges the gap between the portal of exit and the infectious agent from the reservoir and the portal of entry of the susceptible host (Ch. 11)

modeling technique   technique that aims to modify a patient's undesirable behavior by pairing the patient with another who demonstrates more desirable behavior (Ch. 23)

modified pen grasp   grasping an instrument as one would with a pen, except the pad of the middle finger is placed on the top of the instrument with the index finger (Ch. 18)

molar   teeth used to chew food (Ch. 9)

molybdenum   a trace mineral involved in the process of metabolism (Ch. 5)

monangle   a dental instrument with a shank that has one angle (Ch. 19)

monomer   self-curing acrylic tray resin (liquid catalyst) (Ch. 35)

morphodifferentiation   the development of different forms during the embryonic stage of pregnancy (Ch. 8)

motor neuron   carries a message away from the spinal cord and brain and directs the body to act (Ch. 6)

mottled enamel   fluorosis (Ch. 4)

mouth   part of the digestive system (Ch. 6)

mouth guards   protective devices that prevent premature loss or fracture of teeth (Ch. 28)

mouth props   devices used to prevent patients from closing the mouth (Chs. 18 and 25)

mucocele   trauma to a minor salivary gland resulting in a bubble on the inside of the lip (Ch. 26)

mucogingival junction   the line of demarcation between the attached gingiva and the alveolar mucosa (Ch. 8)

mucogingival surgery   reconstructive surgery on the gingiva and/or mucosa tissues; involves covering exposed roots, increasing the width of gingival tissue, and reducing frenum or muscle attachments (Ch. 29)

mucoperiosteum   mucosa and periosteum surfaces that combine to form a membrane (Ch. 25)

mucosa   the tissue that lines the inner surface of the lips and cheeks (Ch. 7)

mulberry molars   the appearance of a more rounded occlusal surface on the permanent molars; this is characteristic of the teeth of children born to mothers with syphilis (Ch. 26)

multiple sclerosis (MS)   a disease that destroys the myelin sheath of neurons in the central nervous system resulting in impulses that cannot transmit to their destinations (Ch. 6)

mumps   a viral disease with main symptom of swelling of the parotid (salivary) glands on one or both sides and spread by airborne droplets (Ch. 10)

muscle tone   the tension of the muscular system (Ch. 6)

muscle trimming   molding the borders of the custom tray to achieve margin adaption of the tray before final edentulous impression (Ch. 32)

muscular dystrophy (MD)   a congenital disorder characterized by progressive degeneration of the skeletal, and sometimes smooth, muscles (Ch. 6)

myasthenia gravis   an auto-immune disorder that leaves the muscles weak and fatigued; one of the first symptoms is weakness in the facial or swallowing muscles (Ch. 6)

myelin sheath   the protective and insulating covering of some nerves (Ch. 6)

mylohyoid   one of the muscles of the floor of the mouth that forms the floor of the mouth and assists in depressing the mandible and elevating the tongue (Ch. 7)

mylohyoid artery   branches off the inferior alveolar artery before entering the mandibular canal; supplies the mylohyoid muscle (Ch. 7)

mylohyoid nerve branch   supplies the mylohyoid muscle and the anterior belly of the digastric muscle (Ch. 7)

mylohyoid ridge   the internal oblique ridge (Ch. 7)

myocardial infarction   a condition in which the coronary arteries are blocked or severely narrowed; also known as a heart attack (Ch. 16)

myocardium   a tough, muscular wall (middle layer) of the heart (Ch. 6)

napkin   bib (Ch. 17)

nasal bones   form the bridge of the nose (Ch. 7)

nasal cavity   nostril (Ch. 6)

nasal mucosa   lines the inner surface of the nose; warms and humidifies the air as it passes through (Ch. 6)

nasal septum   divides the two nasal cavities (Ch. 6)

Nasmyth's membrane   a covering over the enamel of newly erupted primary teeth left over from the epithelium and the ameloblasts (Ch. 8)

naso-labial groove   also known as the sulcus, the groove from the ala of the nose to the corners of the mouth (Ch. 7)

nasolacrimal groove   extends from the medial corner of the eye to the nasal cavity along the maxillary process to the medial nasal process (Ch. 8)

nasopalatine nerve   innervates the anterior hard palate, gingival, mucous membrane, and the anterior teeth from the cuspids forward (Ch. 7)

nasopharynx   first section of the pharynx; located behind the nasal cavity (Ch. 6)

National Fire Protection Association's color and number method   labeling system for hazardous chemicals using data from MSDS (Ch. 12)

National Institute of Occupational Safety and Health (NIOSH)   the federal agency responsible for conducting research and making recommendations for work related sickness and health; it is part of the Centers for Disease Control (CDD) (Ch. 20)

natural acquired immunity   protection when an individual has had a disease and the body manufactured antibodies to the disease, and the individual recovers (Ch. 10)

natural immunity   the innate ability for our bodies to experience local inflammation and the existence of blood phagocytes to fight pathogens (Ch. 10)

natural light   multidirectional light that casts shadows and shows texture (Ch. 31)

necrotizing ulcerative gingivitis (NUG)   also called Vincent's disease or trench mouth, a common disease found in teenagers and young adults; causes include stress, smoking, poor diet, and poor oral hygiene (Ch. 29)

necrotizing ulcerative periodontitis (NUP)   disease found in patients with HIV infection and patients with severe malnutrition and suppressed immune systems; symptoms include pain, bleeding, and extensive tissue and bone destruction (Ch. 29)

needle holders   hemostat-like instruments with grooved beaks to hold the suture needles (Ch. 25)

Needlestick Safety and Prevention Act   passed by the U.S. Congress and became effective in April 2001, directs OSHA to revise the bloodborne pathogens standard (Ch. 12)

negligence   the failure to exercise the standard of care that a reasonable person would exercise in similar circumstances (Ch. 3)

neonatal line   an accentuated incremental line on the enamel matrix layer of a tooth that indicates the trauma of birth; found in all the primary teeth and several of the permanent teeth (Ch. 8)

neonatal teeth   teeth present at birth or within the first month after birth (Ch. 26)

neoplasm   an abnormal growth that can be malignant (cancerous) or benign (non-cancerous); a tumor (Ch. 26)

nerve block anesthesia   injection of anesthesia near a main nerve trunk (Ch. 20)

nerve cell   the basic structural unit of the nervous system (Ch. 6)

net income   the accounts payable subtracted from the gross income (Ch. 36)

neuritis   inflammation of nerves, or nerve tissue degeneration, that could be the result of a fall or blow (Ch. 6)

neuromuscular dentistry   the science of occlusion that objectively measures the physiologic functions affected by occlusion to achieve an optimal relationship between the skull and the mandible (Ch. 31)

neuron   basic structural unit of the nervous system comprised of a nucleus surrounded by a cell membrane with thread-like projections called nerve fibers (Ch. 6)

niacin   one of the B Complex vitamins found in animal products; helps prevent gastrointestinal and nervous system disturbances (Ch. 5)

nitrous oxide   odor-free gas derived from nitrogen and oxygen; used as a sedative before anesthesia; relieves anxiety and fear (Ch. 20)

nodule   small lump of tissue, hard or soft, usually more than ¼ inch in diameter (Ch. 26)

non-anatomical   term for describing posterior denture teeth; non-anatomical lack detailed anatomy on the occlusal, usually a concave and flat surface (anatomical teeth have cusps and developmental grooves) (Ch. 32)

non-compliant   unwilling to follow treatment plans or directions from the dentist or another party (Ch. 3)

non-cutting   not used for cutting tooth structure (e.g., mouth mirrors and cotton pliers) (Ch. 19)

non-expendable   supplies that are not used up or disposed of after use (e.g., the dental chair or an autoclave) (Ch. 36)

non-specific immunity   the body's defense against any harmful agents (Ch. 6)

non-verbal communication   communication that takes place without verbal communication (Ch. 2)

non-vital pulp   the pulp of the tooth that does not respond to sensory stimuli (Ch. 24)

non-vital whitening   lightening of endodontically treated teeth (Ch. 31)

normal flora   bacteria in the human body that perform tasks that are essential to human survival (Ch. 10)

normal occlusion   term that describes the contact relationship of the mandibular arch with the maxillary arch (Ch. 27)

nose   the passage for outside air to enter the body (Ch. 6)

nucleus   the controlling body of the cell containing the genetic codes (Ch. 6)

nursing bottle syndrome   tooth decay develops in infants who have erupted teeth and are given bottles of milk, fruit juice, or sweet substances over a long period of time (Ch. 5)

nutrients   chemical substances in food that provide the body tissues and structures with the elements needed for growth, maintenance, and repair (Ch. 5)

nutrition   the manner in which foods are used to meet the body's needs (Ch. 5)

objective fears   fears based on a person's experiences (Ch. 28)

oblique fiber groups   most abundant of groups, functions to resist intrusive forces that try to push the tooth inward (Ch. 8)

oblique ridge   elevated area of enamel that extends obliquely across the occlusal of the tooth (Ch. 9)

obturating   process of filling the root canal (Ch. 24)

occipital bone   forms the back and base of the skull containing a large opening, the foramen magnum, through which the spinal cord passes (Ch. 7)

occlusal   chewing surface of the molars and premolar teeth (Chs. 9 and 28)

occlusal equilibration   process of alleviating areas with an excessive force (Ch. 29)

occlusal radiographs   radiographs that expose the maxillary or mandibular occlusal surface of the dental arch (Ch. 22)

occlusal third   the area on the crown of the tooth that is nearest the occlusal surface of the posterior tooth (Ch. 9)

occupational exposure   any reasonably anticipated exposure to secretions of the eye, mucosa, skin, parenteral (cut, needlestick, puncture, abrasions, etc.), or any contact with blood or saliva that may be a result of employment tasks (Ch. 11)

Occupational Safety and Health Administration (OSHA)   regulating body that enforces the requirements established for employers to protect their employees (Chs. 11 and 10)

odontoblasts   dentin-forming cells (Ch. 8)

odontogenesis   origin of the tooth (Ch. 8)

olfactory receptor   facilitates the sense of smell (Ch. 6)

one stage technique   implant is inserted into the bone but extruding end is not covered with gingival tissue but with a healing cap; healing time is 3-4 months (Ch. 25)

onlays   replacements for missing tooth structure in the tooth (Ch. 30)

opacity   not allowing any light to pass through (Ch. 31)

open bay   treatment area with several dental chairs arranged in one open area; reassuring for patients to see others experiencing similar treatment (Ch. 28)

operating light   adjustable light used by the dentist during examinations and procedures (Ch. 17)

operating zone   the area where the operator (dentist) is positioned to access the oral cavity and have the best visibility (Ch. 17)

operator's cart   a mobile cart that is usually set up for two or three dental handpieces plus an air-water syringe (Ch. 17)

operatory   dental treatment room (Ch. 17)

opportunistic infections   infections resulting from a weakened immune system (Ch. 26)

oral   by mouth; with medications usually in tablet, capsule, pill, or liquid form (Ch. 15)

oral and maxillofacial pathology   dental specialty concerned with the diagnosis and nature of the diseases that affect the oral cavity (Chs. 1 and 26)

oral and maxillofacial radiology   dental specialty that covers radiology of the oral and maxillofacial area (Chs. 1 and 19)

oral and maxillofacial surgery   dental specialty concerned with the diagnosis and surgical treatment of the oral and maxillofacial region (Chs. 1 and 19)

oral brush biopsy   type of biopsy in which the surface of the lesion is wiped or scraped to remove a layer of the lesion (Ch. 25)

oral cavity   the mouth, a part of the digestive system (Ch. 6)

oral hypoglycemics   drugs taken orally to lower blood sugar levels (Ch. 15)

oral prophylaxis   two-fold procedure involving removal of hard deposits and polishing of the teeth with a rubber cup (Ch. 29)

oral sedation   a commonly prescribed drug is taken by the patient the night before their dental appointment (Ch. 20)

oral vestibule   pocket formed by the soft tissue of the cheeks and gingiva (Ch. 7)

orbicularis oris   arises from the nasal part of the frontal bone, from the frontal process of the maxilla in front of the lacrimal groove, and from the anterior surface and borders of a short fibrous band, the medial palpebral ligament (Ch. 7)

organ   group of tissues (Ch. 6)

organic   a product that is grown without the use of herbicides, chemical pesticides, or fertilizers. The seeds must not have been prepared with the use of hormones or any other enhancement (Ch. 5)

Organization for Safety and Asepsis Procedures (OSAP)   national organization that has members who are dental health-care workers, distributors of dental equipment and materials, health-care instructors, dentists, and others from the field of dentistry; has regional and annual meetings that cover topics of infection control and hazard communication for dental team members (Ch. 11)

orifices   openings of the salivary glands (Ch. 26)

origin   the part of a muscle that attaches to the more stationary bone (Ch. 6)

oropharynx   middle section of the pharynx behind the mouth (Ch. 6)

orthodontic bands   stainless steel bands fitted around teeth to hold and control tooth movement (Ch. 27)

orthodontics   dental specialty concerned with the diagnosis and supervision and guidance and correction of the malocclusion in the dental facial structures (Chs. 1 and 27)

orthodontics and dentofacial orthopedics   dental specialty concerned with the diagnosis, supervision, guidance, and correction of the malocclusion in the dental facial structures (Ch. 1)

orthognathic surgery   surgery involving the face, maxilla, and mandible (Ch. 25)

osseointegration   compatible interface between the bone and the dental implant (Ch. 25)

osseous surgery   restoration of bone by removal of defects and deformities caused by periodontal disease and related conditions; can be either additive (augmentive) or subtractive (Ch. 29)

osseous tissue   the connective tissue of bones is hard due to deposits of mineral salts (Ch. 6)

ostectomy   form of osseous surgery in which deformed bone is removed (Ch. 29)

osteoblasts   bone-forming cells (Chs. 6, 8 and 29)

osteoclast   dissolve and reabsorb the calcium salts of the bone matrix when bone is stressed or damaged (Chs. 6, 8 and 29)

osteomyelitis   an advanced stage of periapical infection that spreads into and through the bone (Chs. 6 and 24)

osteoplasty   form of osseous surgery in which deformed bone is reshaped (Ch. 29)

osteoporosis   the loss of bony material which leaves the bones brittle and soft (Ch. 6)

other potentially infectious materials (OPIMs)   any materials or bodily fluids other than blood; precautions should be taken to avoid contact (Chs. 11 and 10)

Otsby frame   a plastic dental dam frame that is oval-shaped and designed to follow the shape of the lower face; the frame is radiotransparent and autoclavable (Ch. 34)

over-the-counter (OTC) drugs   drugs that can be purchased without prescriptions (Ch. 15)

overbite   projection of the upper teeth over the lower (Ch. 27)

overdenture   retained roots providing support to a complete or partial denture (Ch. 32)

overglove   also known as food handler's gloves, are big, loose gloves that do not have the tactile touch that latex and vinyl gloves have, but quickly fit over the gloves to obtain something in a sterile area (Ch. 11)

overhang   excess restorative material projecting over the cavity margin (Ch. 14)

overhead   expenses required to run the practice (Ch. 36)

overlap of time   when a doctor/dentist is required to be in two different places at once, or when two patients are scheduled for treatment at once (Ch. 36)

overlapping   x-ray technique error resulting from improper horizontal angulation (Ch. 22)

overtime   treatment time beyond that scheduled (Ch. 36)

packable composite   more putty-like and stiff in consistency than other composites; used in posterior areas that need a stronger restoration (Ch. 34)

packing slip   list included with supply shipments stating everything that was included; contents of the package should be checked against the packing slip to make sure there are no discrepancies (Ch. 36)

palatine bones   joined at the midline are often referred to as the median palatine suture (Ch. 7)

palatine raphe   a slightly raised line extending from the back of the incisive papilla and down the middle of the hard palate (Ch. 7)

palatine rugae   the ridges that run horizontally across the hard palate behind the incisive papilla.

palatine suture   the median suture joining the bones of the palate (Ch. 7)

palatine tonsil   located on each side of the throat (Ch. 6)

palatine tonsils   a depressed area located between the anterior and posterior tonsillar pillars; appear red and inflamed when there is an infection.

palatoglossal arches   either of two ridges or folds of mucous membrane passing from the soft palate to the side of the tongue and enclosing the palatoglossus muscle (Ch. 7)

palatoglossus   a muscle of the soft palate that elevates the posterior portion of the tongue and narrows the fauces (Ch. 7)

palatopharygeal   one of the muscles of the soft palate that constricts the nasopharyngeal passage and elevates the larynx (Ch. 7)

palatopharyngeal arches   either of the two ridges or folds of mucous membrane passing from the soft palate to the wall of the pharynx and enclosing the palatopharyngeal muscle (Ch. 7)

palliative effect   soothing effect a material may have on a tooth; also called sedative effect (Ch. 33)

palm grasp   holding an instrument in the palm of the hand (Ch. 13)

Palmer System for numbering system of teeth identification that numbers permanent teeth 1 through 8, divided into quadrants; the deciduous teeth are labeled A through E, also by quadrant (Ch. 14)

palm-thumb grasp the grasping of an instrument that has the handle in the palm of the hand, four fingers wrapped around the handle, and the thumb extended upward from the palm (Ch. 18)

palpate to examine the body with the hands or fingers for detection of abnormalities, checking pulse rate, and so on (Chs. 13 and 20)

pancreas produces pancreatic juices that are emptied into the duodenum to aid digestion and produce insulin (Ch. 6)

panoramic technique rotation system used when taking radiographs that capture the entire dental arch on one film (Ch. 21)

panothenic acid a vitamin found in both animal and plant foods; helps in energy metabolism (Ch. 5)

papilla small, raised projection covering the dorsal side of the tongue (Ch. 7)

papilloma a benign lesion of squamous epithelium tissue resembling a cauliflower in appearance (Ch. 26)

papule a small, solid, raised area of skin less than 1/2 inch in diameter (Ch. 26)

paradigm how individual views life due to life patterns (Ch. 2)

paralleling technique x-ray technique, also known as the right-angle technique, whereby the film and tooth and PID are parallel (Ch. 22)

parenteral piercing of the mucous membranes of the skin through such events as needlesticks, cuts, and abrasions (Ch. 12)

paresthesia sensation of being numb (Ch. 20)

parietal bone forms most of the roof of the skull and the upper half of the sides (Ch. 7)

Parkinson's Disease a chronic nervous disease characterized by slowing spreading tremors, muscular weakness, and a peculiar gait (Ch. 6)

parotid duct also known as Stenson's duct, empties saliva from the parotid gland into the mouth (Ch. 7)

parotid glands largest of the salivary glands (Ch. 7)

parotid papilla a flap of tissue on the buccal mucosa opposite the maxillary second molar (Ch. 7)

partial crown covers only part of the tooth, not the entire crown of the tooth (Ch. 30)

partial dentures prosthetic devices containing artificial teeth supported on metal frameworks and attached by clasps to natural teeth (Chs. 14 and 32)

partial image an x-ray film processing error due to the film placement in the processing tank when the solution levels are low (Ch. 22)

partial seizures divided into two categories, can be simple (patient remains conscious and remembers all the event) or complex (patient is unconscious, remembers very little and experiences involuntary actions) (Ch. 16)

partnership legal agreement that makes doctors and dentists responsible for accounts payable; partners are not responsible for malpractice suits against the other (Ch. 37)

passive acquired immunity protection from a specific disease provided by an injection of antibodies from another animal or person (Ch. 10)

patch area of the skin that differs in color or texture (Ch. 26)

pathogenic disease causing (Ch. 9)

pathogens disease-producing microorganisms (Chs. 10 and 11)

patient the person receiving treatment

patient records patient histories; examined before procedures to see if there were any previous problems or concerns (Ch. 17)

Paul Revere (1735–1818) a silversmith who was known to practice dentistry; his greatest contribution was making artificial teeth and surgical instruments (Ch. 1)

payee the person to whom the check or cash is to be paid (Ch. 36)

pediatric dentistry dental specialty concerned with prevention of oral disease, diagnosis, and treatment of oral care in children from birth to adolescence (Chs. 1 and 22)

pediculosis infested with lice (Ch. 10)

pedodontics dental care for children (Ch. 28)

peg lateral a diminutive, peg-shaped crown with a smooth surface lacking contact on the mesial and distal surfaces.

pellicle thin, clear film of insoluble proteins, fats and other materials from saliva that forms within minutes of removal; may protect enamel or provide breeding ground for plaque and calculus (Ch. 29)

pelvic cavity the lower portion of the abdominal cavity contains the urinary bladder, rectum, and reproductive system (Ch. 6)

pen grasp the grasping of an instrument in the same manner as one would a pen or pencil (Ch. 18)

percussion examination of a tooth by tapping on the occlusal or incisal surface with fingers or instruments (Ch. 24)

periapical x-ray showing the tooth and surrounding tissues (Ch. 22)

periapical abscess localized destruction of tissue and accumulation of exudate in the periapical region (Ch. 24)

pericardial around the heart (Ch. 12)

pericardium double-wall sac that forms the outer layer of the heart (Ch. 6)

perikymata small grooves on some teeth (Ch. 8)

periodontal disease inflammation and deterioration of the periodontal tissues caused by protozoa with bacteria (Chs. 6 and 10)

periodontal dressing bandage-like material applied to protect a surgical site as it heals (Ch. 29)

periodontal fiber groups mostly principle fibers, organized into bundles or groups dependent on their functions, that allow for flexibility during mastication, speech, and other forces exerted on the teeth (Ch. 8)

periodontal flap surgery surgical separation of the gingiva from the underlying tissue (Ch. 29)

periodontal knives instruments used to remove gingival tissue during periodontal surgery; also known as gingivectomy knives (Ch. 29)

periodontal ligament connective tissue that is formed by the fibroblast cells and secures the tooth into the socket by a number of organized fiber groups; contains two types of nerves (Ch. 8)

periodontal ligament injection also known as an intraligamentary injection, has a variety of uses, and involves inserting the needle into the gingival sulcus along the long axis of the tooth to be treated (Ch. 20)

periodontal pocket space in the gingival sulcus (beyond the normal 1–3 mm) created by periodontal disease (Chs. 14 and 29)

periodontal probe calibrated instrument used to measure the depths of periodontal pockets, areas of recession, bleeding, or exudate; primary instrument in periodontal examinations (Chs. 19 and 29)

periodontal probing measuring of the depth of the periodontal pocket with a periodontal probe (Ch. 29)

periodontal scissors used during periodontal surgery mainly to remove tags of tissue and to trim margins. (Ch. 29)

periodontics dental specialty concerned with the diagnosis and treatment of the diseases of the supporting and surrounding tissues of the tooth (Chs. 1 and 23)

periodontitis the formation of periodontal pockets, occurring when margins of the gingiva and periodontal fibers recede and the supporting bone becomes inflamed and destroyed (Chs. 4 and 29)

periodontium a collective term for the periodontal tissues (Chs. 3 and 29)

periosteal elevator tool used to reflect soft tissue from the bone; usually double ended with one long, tapered end and one round, bladed end (Chs. 25 and 29)

periosteum tough, fibrous layer of tissue covering compact bone (Ch. 6)

peripheral nervous system (PNS) all of the nerves outside of the central nervous system (Ch. 6)

peristalsis the process of involuntary wave-like successive muscular contractions by which food is moved through the digestive tract (Ch. 6)

peritoneal abdominal (Ch. 12)

peritubular dentin the dentin that creates the wall of the dentinal tubule (Ch. 8)

permanent luting cement long-term cementing agent (Ch. 33)

personal computers (PCs) desktop computers; microcomputers (Ch. 36)

personal protective equipment (PPE) items that should be worn to protect against contact with all body fluids (e.g., protective eyewear) (Ch. 11)

pertussis also known as whooping cough, caused by the bacterium bordetella and mainly affects infants and young children (Ch. 10)

pestle a small pellet made of metal or plastic that aids in the mixing of the alloy and mercury (Ch. 34)

petechiae small red or purple spots that appear on the skin or mucosa tissue (Ch. 26)

petit mal seizure seizure marked by a momentary loss of consciousness; usually lasts 5 to 10 seconds (Ch. 16)

petri dish or plate a cylindrical shallow dish or plate with a cover used to grow bacteria under sterile conditions (Ch. 10)

petty cash small amount of money kept in the office for unexpected situations (Ch. 36)

pharmacology the study of all drugs (Ch. 15)

pharyngeal tonsil also known as adenoids, located on the posterior wall of the nasopharynx area (Ch. 6)

pharynx connects the oral cavity to the esophagus; where food is swallowed (Ch. 6)

philtrum vertical groove on the midline of the upper lip (Chs. 7 and 8)

phosphorus a mineral found in bones and teeth and involved in energy metabolism and maintenance of proper pH balance in the blood (Ch. 5)

Physician's Desk Reference (PDR) published annually, comprehensive listing of drugs and drug information; lists drugs by trade or product name, generic and chemical name, and category (Ch. 15)

physiology the study of how the body functions (Ch. 6)

Pierre Fauchard (1678–1761) founder of modern dentistry, organized all known information about dentistry and compiled it into a textbook (Ch. 1)

pit area on the occlusal surface of the teeth where the grooves come together or the fissures cross (Ch. 9)

pit and fissure sealants hard resin materials that are applied to the occlusal surface of caries-free posterior teeth to prevent decay; also known as enamel sealants (Ch. 28)

pixels picture element; a small dot in a digital image (Ch. 23)

plaintiff the individual who brings charges against another individual (Ch. 3)

plaque any raised or flat patch in the oral mucosa; common cause of inflammation of gingival tissues; a sticky mass that contains bacteria and grows in colonies on the teeth (Chs. 4, 26 and 29)

plasma liquid portion of blood is 91% water and carries nutrients, hormones, and wastes (Ch. 6)

plasma arc a type of light curing that is very fast and powerful. Disadvantages include the expense and some are not portable (Ch. 17)

plastic rings also called elastic ties, are small bands that are used to hold the arch wire to the brackets (Ch. 27)

plastic stint clear denture base material, molded to the same shape and size as the denture (Ch. 25)

plastic strip matrix a thin, transparent, strip matrix used with composite, glass ionomer, or compomer restorative materials on anterior teeth (Ch. 34)

platysma a sheet of muscle in the neck that draws down the mandible as well as the corners of the mouth and the lower lip (Ch. 7)

pleura a sac surrounding each lung (Ch. 6)

pleural pertaining to the pleura; the membrane surrounding the lungs (Ch. 12)

pluggers used in amalgam fillings and root canal filling to pack amalgam into the tooth; the working end is short and comes in a variety of shapes and sizes; endodontic versions have long working ends with blunt ends; also known as condensers (Ch. 24)

pocket marking pliers instruments with two beaks that, when pinched together, leave small pinpoint perforations on the gingival tissue; used to transfer measurement of a pocket to the outside of the tissue so the operator can see the depth of the pocket (Ch. 29)

point angle in the corners of a cavity preparation, the place where three lines (surfaces) come together (Ch. 33)

polishing process of using fine abrasives to produce a smooth, glossy surface (Ch. 29)

polycarboxylate type of permanent cementation for crowns, bridges, inlays, onlays, and orthodontic bands and brackets; sets in 3–5 minutes, does not exhibit exothermic heat (Ch. 33)

polymer self-curing acrylic tray resin (powder) (Ch. 35)

polymerization process by which a material changes from a plastic, pliable state to a rigid state (Ch. 35)

polynitrile autoclavable gloves sterilizable gloves used for disinfection and sterilization (Ch. 11)

polysulfide material used in taking final impressions; composed of a base and lead peroxide accelerator, resulting in good stability, accuracy, sharpness of detail, and a relatively long shelf-life (Ch. 35)

pontic portion of a bridge that replaces the missing tooth (Chs. 14 and 30)

porcelain-fused-to-metal crowns crowns with veneers (veneers are used to cover badly stained teeth and to reshape the anatomy of teeth) (Ch. 30)

porcelain veneers requires two dental appointments; natural in appearance and are durable (Ch. 30)

portal of entry the route by which an infectious agent enters the host (Ch. 11)

portal of exit the route by which an infectious agent leaves the reservoir to be transferred to a susceptible host (Ch. 11)

position indicator device (PID) the open-ended tube in a dental x-ray unit, commonly called the cone (Ch. 21)

posterior (teeth) molars in the primary dentition and the premolars and molars in the permanent dentition (Ch. 9)

posterior superior alveolar artery supplies the maxillary sinus, maxillary molar teeth, and surrounding gingival with blood (Ch. 7)

posterior superior alveolar nerve supplies the gingival, maxillary sinus, cheeks, and maxillary molars with the exception of the mesial buccal root of the first molar (Ch. 7)

posterior tonsillar pillars folds of tissue found farther back in the throat (Ch. 7)

posteruption stage immediately after the tooth has erupted into the oral cavity the absorption rate of fluoride is the highest (Ch. 4)

post-retained cores metal posts fitted into the pulp canal of endodontically treated teeth for crown retention (Ch. 30)

potassium a mineral that helps release energy and synthesize protein; works together with sodium to regulate the electrolyte balance (Ch. 5)

potassium alginate an ingredient extracted from seaweed and kelp used for alginate impression material (Ch. 35)

potassium alum a chemical used in development of radiographs that shrinks and hardens the emulsion gelatin (Ch. 22)

potassium bromide a chemical used in development of radiographs to slow the developing process to a practical speed and prevent film fog (Ch. 22)

potassium titanium fluoride an ingredient added to alginate impression material to counteract a specific action of the alginate where it tends to soften the surface of the gypsum products, not allowing it to fully set on the surface (Ch. 35)

power bleaching multistep application of bleaching liquids or gels, often with application of heat or curing light; patient's teeth are isolated to protect chemical irritation to the gingiva (Ch. 31)

power whitening process involving the reapplication of a bleach mix every 10-15 minutes (Ch. 31)

predetermine of benefits to submit a treatment plan to a carrier to find out what the insurance will pay on the dental services; often called the pretreatment estimate (Ch. 36)

preemption related to HIPAA, when state laws conflict with federal laws (Ch. 3)

preeruption stage before the tooth has erupted into the oral cavity (Ch. 4)

pregnancy depending on the stage of pregnancy, some dental treatments may need to be altered or delayed (Ch. 6)

premium amount the carrier charges the subscriber (Ch. 36)

premolar in permanent dentition, located after the canine are the first and second premolars; often called bicuspids because they usually have two cusps; used to pulverize food (Ch. 9)

prescription an authorization written by a doctor, dentist, or other that makes drugs available to patients (Ch. 15)

preservatives chemicals added to food to keep the contents fresh for a longer period (Ch. 5)

preventive orthodontic treatment to eliminate problems that may disrupt normal development of the teeth and facial structures (Ch. 27)

primary dentin formed before the completion of the apical foramen and represented the bulk of the tooth (Ch. 8)

primary insurance the subcriber's insurance (Ch. 36)

primary palate also known as primitive palate, appears as a triangular mass and contains the four maxillary incisor teeth; primary function is to separate the developing oral and nasal cavities (Ch. 8)

primary radiation central beam of the x-ray tube head (Ch. 21)

primer conditioner used before a bonding material is placed (Ch. 34)

privacy officer the person in the dental office responsible for keeping all office personnel updated on HIPAA (Ch. 3)

professional courtesy discount the provider gives the patient (Ch. 36)

proliferate rapid increase (Ch. 8)

proliferation the cap stage in the life cycle of a tooth where the primary embryonic ectoderm layer matures into the enamel of the developing tooth (Ch. 8)

prophy brush used for the coronal polish procedure; only used on the enamel surface and should never contact the gingival tissues (Ch. 29)

prophylaxis procedure whereby soft and hard deposits are removed from teeth; includes scaling and polishing (Ch. 29)

Protected Health Information (PHI) PHI, an integral part of HIPAA, covers any information that identifies the individual or reveals information identifying the individual. This includes information such as name, telephone number, email address, and birth date (Ch. 3)

prothrombin substance produced by Vitamin K which is responsible for blood clotting and coagulation (Ch. 5)

prostheses replacements for missing body parts; in dentistry, missing teeth and tissues are replaced with artificial structures (Chs. 30 and 32)

prosthodontics dental specialty concerned with the diagnosis and restoration and maintenance of oral function with replacement of missing teeth and supporting structures through artificial means (Chs. 1, 24, and 25)

provider dentist who performs the dental service (Ch. 36)

proximal nearest the point of attachment

psychologically dependent a person who develops an emotional need for taking a drug, even though there may no longer be a physical need to take it (Ch. 15)

psychology profession and science concerned with the behavior of humans and animals (Ch. 2)

pterygoid the wings of the sphenoid bone (Ch. 7)

pterygoid artery supplies blood to the temporal muscle, masseter muscle, pterygoid muscles, and buccinator muscles (Ch. 7)

pterygoid plexus of veins drains the region of the pterygoid muscles into the internal maxillary and anterior facial muscles (Ch. 7)

pterygopalatine nerve branch divides into the greater palatine nerve, the lesser palatine nerve, and the nasopalatine nerve (Ch. 7)

pulp vascular and nerve network of fleshy connective tissue that fills the center of the tooth in the cavity formed by the dentin (Ch. 8)

pulp canal is in the root of the tooth (Ch. 8)

pulp chamber a large portion of the pulp which is in the crown of the tooth (Ch. 8)

pulp horns pointed elongations of the pulp that extend toward the incisal or occlusal portion of the tooth (Ch. 8)

pulp stones calcified masses of dentin that can be attached or unattached to the pulpal wall (Ch. 8)

pulpal necrosis death of pulpal cells; often results from irreversible pulpitis (Ch. 24)

pulpal wall the side or floor of a cavity preparation that overlies the pulp (Ch. 33)

pulpectomy non-vital pulp therapy involving tooth extraction and complete removal of the pulp (Chs. 24 and 28)

pulpitis inflamed tissues due to injury (Ch. 8)

pulmonary circulation the pathway of blood circulation through the heart to the lungs and back to the heart (Ch. 6)

pulmonary valve blood is pumped through the tricuspid valve into the right ventricle and goes through the pulmonary valve into the pulmonary artery (Ch. 6)

pulpotomy removal of pulp exclusively in the coronal portion of the tooth (Chs. 24 and 28)

punch table/punch plate part of the working end of a dental dam punch that includes four or five differently sized holes and rotates to facilitate punching holes for the various teeth (Ch. 34)

Pure Food and Drug Act law passed in 1906 by the U.S. government; controlled and regulated the composition, sale, and distribution of drugs (Ch. 15)

Pure Food, Drug, and Cosmetic Act law passed in 1938 that made it mandatory for the FDA to have control of all food, cosmetics, and drugs sold, as well as their advertising (Ch. 15)

purging self-induced vomiting (Ch. 5)

purpura small purplish or reddish-brown areas or spots caused by bleeding in underlying tissues (Ch. 26)

purulence pus containing (Ch. 10)

pustule small, pus-containing blister (Ch. 26)

pyogenic granuloma an overgrowth of granulation tissue resulting from local irritation (Ch. 26)

pyogenic membrane the development of a wall to contain infection so that it does not spread to other parts of the body (Ch. 10)

quadrant two sections formed by the imaginary line dividing the dental arches in two halves; actually there are four quadrants each containing eight permanent teeth (Ch. 9)

quality radiograph a radiograph that shows all structures in a manner that makes assessment and diagnosis efficient and clear (Ch. 22)

quickdam an alternative to the full dental dam placement; an oval piece of dental dam with a border of flexible plastic that lies in the vestibular area of the patient's mouth (Ch. 34)

race grouping of people based upon biological resemblance (Ch. 2)

radiation absorbed dose (rad) amount of ionizing radiation absorbed in a substance (Ch. 21)

radiographs x-rays taken and processed to be used as a diagnostic tool (Ch. 21)

radiolucent black region on the x-ray indicating where radiation passed through the tissue (Ch. 23)

radiometer a meter that measures the intensity of a light bulb (Ch. 17)

radiopaque white or light region on the x-ray indicating where radiation was blocked by tissue or a substance (Chs. 22 and 23)

radiosensitive condition of being sensitized and affected by radiant energy (Ch. 21)

rami two vertical extensions of the mandible (Ch. 7)

"rare earth" phosphors substance used on the intensifying screens that are found in cassettes; rare-earth is green-light producing phosphors that are faster and reduce radiation exposure to the patient (Ch. 23)

reamers endodontic instrument with a tapered metal shaft used to clean and enlarge a root canal (Ch. 24)

rear delivery system one of three types of dental unit with the equipment located behind the patient's head (Ch. 17)

reception room area the patient initially enters in the dental office (Ch. 17)

recession movement of gingival tissue away from the tooth (Ch. 29)

reciprocity one who has passed the medical/dental requirements for one state that applies for the same "rights" in another state, without taking another written or clinical examination (Ch. 3)

recommendations guidelines and standards made by non-governing entities that have no power to enforce compliance (Ch. 11)

rectal administration of drugs through the anus; enemas and suppositories may be used (Ch. 15)

red bone marrow located inside the spaces of the cancellous bone and filled with blood vessels and small amounts of connective tissue. It manufactures red and white blood cells and platelets (Ch. 6)

reflex arc occurs when a stimuli is sent through the sensory neurons into the spinal cord and a response is automatically processed and sent back through motor neurons for an action (Ch. 6)

regulations guidelines and standards made by government agencies and licensing boards that have the authority to enforce compliance (Ch. 11)

regurgitation vomiting (Ch. 5)

reimbursement payment made by the carrier to the patient or the dentist on the behalf of the patient for the dental fee (Ch. 36)

relative biological effectiveness (RBE) measurement unit used to compare the biological effects of different tissues irradiated by different forms of radiation (Ch. 21)

relax muscles release and return to their normal form (Ch. 6)

relined resurfacing of the under surface or tissue surface of a full or partial denture to improve the fit (Ch. 32)

removable appliances devices inserted into the mouth and removed by the patient (e.g., retainers) (Ch. 27)

reservoir a place where the agent can survive (Ch. 11)

Res gestae meaning "part of the action"; any statements made during the time of an alleged act can be made admissible in a court of law (Ch. 3)

resin cement type of permanent cementation for cast crowns, bridges, inlays, onlays, and endodontic posts (Ch. 33)

resin-reinforced glass ionomer a dental material used to cement metallic restorations or porcelain-fused-to-metal restorations to tooth structure (Ch. 33)

resorption the body's process of removing bone (Ch. 27)

respiration   the process of breathing and exchanging oxygen and carbon dioxide between the body and its environment (Ch. 6)

restoration   process of replacing missing tooth structure; results in "fillings" (Ch. 14)

rests   the part of the removable partial denture that contacts a tooth to provide vertical and horizontal support (Ch. 32)

retainer   tool used to tighten and support the matrix band on the tooth while the tooth is being restored; part of a partial denture that contacts the abutment teeth and prevents the partial from moving (Chs. 32 and 34)

retention core   core buildup made of amalgam, composite, or a silver alloy/glass ionomer combination (Ch. 30)

retention pins   small metal pins placed for restoration retention (Ch. 30)

reticulation   processing error that shows on the dental film when the film emulsion is exposed to extreme temperature variations; normally shows as pitting or wrinkling of the emulsion (Ch. 22)

retinol   vitamin A that comes from an animal source (Ch. 5)

retractors   oral surgery instruments that clear tissue from the surgical site (Ch. 25)

retrograde filling   filling material placed in the apex of a tooth during an apicoectomy (Ch. 24)

retromandibular vein   drains the maxillary artery and the superficial temporal arteries (Ch. 7)

retromolar area   a triangular area located behind the last molar (Ch. 7)

reverse palm-thumb grasp   grasp with the evacuator tip held in the palm of the hand, thumb directed toward the assistant instead of toward the patient (Ch. 18)

reversible hydrocolloid   sometimes called agar-agar; used in the formation of dental impressions that can be converted from a gel to a sol back to a gel due to thermal reaction; produces accurate impressions (Ch. 35)

reversible pulpitis   inflammation of the pulp caused by an irritant; when irritant is removed, the pulp heals (Ch. 24)

revolutions per minute (rpm)   speeds of dental handpieces (Ch. 19)

Rh factor   blood variable that is either positive or negative and an important consideration for blood transfusions (Ch. 6)

rheostat   foot pedal on a dental handpiece that controls handpiece speed (Chs. 17 and 19)

riboflavin   also known as Vitamin B_2, found in milk, green vegetables, cereals, and enriched bread; it aids in growth, release of energy from food, and helps produce proteins (Ch. 5)

ridge   a linear elevation of enamel found on the tooth (Ch. 9)

Robert Woofendale   one of the first dentists from England to establish a practice in the United States (Ch. 1)

rod core   the inner portion of an enamel rod (Ch. 8)

roentgen equivalent man (rem)   radiation unit of measurement (Ch. 21)

roentgens   the amount of radiation that ionizes one cubic centimeter of air (Ch. 21)

rongeurs   forceps with sharp-cutting edges used to trim and shape the alveolar bone following tooth extraction (Ch. 25)

root   divided into anatomical and clinical portions; the anatomical root is covered with cementum and the clinical root is the root seen in the oral cavity (Ch. 9)

root amputation   surgical procedure to remove one or more roots of a multirooted tooth (Ch. 24)

root canal   where the pulp is removed and replaced with a filling material (Ch. 14)

root canal sealer   cement used with gutta percha to seal the pulp canal (Ch. 24)

root planing   process of smoothing the root surface with curettes and other periodontal instruments to leave a smooth root surface (Ch. 29)

root tip picks   delicate instrument used to tweeze the root tips or fragments from the bone socket (Ch. 25)

rotary instruments   instruments that are mechanically driven (Ch. 19)

rotational center   component of panoramic radiography machines that influence the shape and size of the focal trough (Ch. 23)

rubber dental stimulator   a device placed into the interproximal area that is angled toward the occlusal surface and rotated in a circular pattern (Ch. 4)

rubber stops   pieces of rubber placed on files and reamers to mark the length of the root canal (Ch. 24)

rubella   a viral disease, also known as German measles, with symptoms of a rash; can be serious when it affects pregnant women (Ch. 10)

sagittal plane   divides the body into left and right halves (Ch. 6)

saliva   clear fluid secreted from the salivary glands and mucous glands throughout the mouth (Ch. 7)

saliva ejector   a low-volume suction device that removes saliva and fluids from the patient's mouth (Chs. 17 and 18)

salivary gland   produces saliva to dissolve food, facilitates the process of chewing, and coats food for ease in swallowing; three types include parotid, submandibular, and sublingual (Chs. 6 and 7)

sanitized   similar to cleaning, an area has been decontaminated but does not mean that all microorganisms have been destroyed (Ch. 11)

scalers   sharp hand instruments used to remove hard deposits, such as supragingival and subgingival calculus, from the teeth (Ch. 29)

scaling   technique to remove plaque, calculus, and stains from the surfaces of the teeth (Ch. 29)

scatter radiation   radiation that is deflected from its path as it strikes matter (Ch. 21)

scored   when a drug capsule is cut superficially to allow it to separate or break apart more easily (Ch. 15)

sealant   enamel sealant is a resin material used to seal pits and fissures to prevent future decay (Ch. 14)

secondary dentin   forms after the completion of the apical foramen and slowly throughout the life of the tooth (Ch. 8)

secondary insurance   the subscriber's spouse's insurance (Ch. 36)

secondary palate   the separation between the oral and nasal cavities evolves to form the remaining two-thirds of the hard palate and contains remaining teeth (beyond the four maxillary incisor teeth), forming the soft palate and uvula (Ch. 8)

secondary radiation   formed when the primary X-rays strike the patient or come in contact with any matter or substance (Ch. 21)

sectional matrix system   system used to restore anatomical contacts during the filling process; consists of an oval matrix band, rings to hold the matrix band, and forceps to place the ring (Ch. 34)

Security Rule   the ability to control access and protect information from accidental or intentional disclosure to unauthorized persons and from alteration, destruction, or loss (Ch. 3)

sedative   a soothing effect a material may have (Ch. 33)

selective anesthesia   one area of a patient's mouth is selected for an injection to identify which tooth or arch is problematic (Ch. 24)

selenium   a trace mineral involved in the process of metabolism (Ch. 5)

self-curing   materials set by means of a chemical reaction (Ch. 33)

sensory neuron   carries messages from all over the body to the spinal cord and brain (Ch. 6)

separators   devices placed in the contact areas between teeth, forcing teeth to spread apart to accommodate the orthodontic bands; the separators are placed a few days before the patient is to have bands placed (Ch. 27)

septum   amount of dental dam that slides between the teeth (Ch. 34)

seroconversion   the process after exposure to a disease in which the blood changes from a negative to a positive serum marker for that disease (Ch. 10)

shade guide   samples of tooth shades used for tooth-colored restorations and denture teeth (Ch. 30)

shaft   the handle of an instrument (Ch. 19)

shank   the section of the instrument that connects the handle to the working end (Ch. 19)

Sharpey's fibers   collagen fibers from the periodontal ligament, found within the outer part of the cementum (Ch. 8)

shell matrix   a type of matrix used with composite material (Ch. 34)

short wavelengths   radiation wavelengths that have high frequency, high energy, and high penetrating power; also known as hard radiation (Ch. 21)

shoulder   a type of crown preparation that provides a ledge that is sometimes beveled (Ch. 30)

side delivery system   one of three types of dental unit with the equipment located on the dentist's side and mounted to a moveable arm or mobile cart (Ch. 17)

side effect   unintended result of drug use (Ch. 15)

sievert (Sv)   a radiation unit of measurement (Ch. 21)

silicones   materials available in various forms used in taking final impressions; benefits include high rate of accuracy, no shrinkage, dimensional stability, high tear resistance, no taste, and no odor (Ch. 35)

simple suture   most versatile, widely used stitch; suture goes into the facial surface and emerges from the lingual surface, and is tied with a surgeon's knot (Ch. 25)

six-handed dentistry   system in which the dentist and two dental assistants work together at the dental chair (Ch. 17)

slander   false and malicious spoken words (Ch. 3)

sling suture   used for interproximal suturing, stitch wraps around tooth to act like a sling; especially useful when a flap is necessary (Ch. 25)

small intestine   connects the stomach to the large intestine; includes the duodenum, where digestive breakdown continues, and villi where digested food is absorbed into the blood stream (Ch. 6)

smear layer   layer of debris (created when the dentin is cut with a bur during cavity preparation) that lays on the cavity floor and walls and prevents contact between the intact dentin and the bonding agent/adhesive (Ch. 33)

smile line   position of the lips when the patient smiles (Ch. 13)

smooth muscle   involuntary muscle that is under the autonomic nervous system's control. They are found in internal organs, blood vessels, skin, and ducts from glands (Ch. 6)

sodium   a mineral that maintains fluid balance in the blood; works with potassium to regulate the electrolyte balance (Ch. 5)

sodium carbonate   a chemical used in radiographs as an alkaline medium in developer (Ch. 22)

sodium fluoride   mouth rinses purchased at pharmacies generally contain .05% sodium fluoride and are fine for daily use. Prescribed mouth rinses generally contain 0.2% sodium fluoride. Sodium fluoride is used in the community water supply (Ch. 4)

sodium hypochlorite   the most common biomechanical cleaner; also known as household bleach (Ch. 24)

sodium perborate   a material used for teeth whitening that is a non-hydrogen peroxide system that contains sodium chloride, oxygen, and fluoride; used in household bleaching agents (Ch. 31)

sodium sulfite   a chemical used in radiographs to prevent oxidation and to increase the life span of the developer solution (Ch. 22)

sodium thiosulfate   a chemical used in development of radiographs for removal of unexposed and undeveloped crystals from the film (Ch. 22)

soft deposits   acquired dental pellicle, materia alba, food debris, and plaque, removed during coronal polish (Ch. 29)

soft radiation   long wavelengths with low energy, low frequency, and low penetrating power; also called Grenz rays (Ch. 21)

soft tissue rongeurs   also called nippers, hinged pliers used to shape the soft tissue (Ch. 29)

soft wood points   sometimes used with polishing agents to polish occlusal grooves and pits, proximal surfaces of sensitive teeth, and areas other polishing instruments can not reach (Ch. 29)

software   computer program (set of instructions) that tells the hardware what to do (Ch. 36)

sol   a liquid (Ch. 35)

soluble   ability of a material to dissolve in a fluid (Ch. 33)

space maintainer   device (fixed or removable) designed to hold a space (left from the premature loss of a primary tooth) until the permanent tooth erupts (Chs. 27 and 22)

spasm   when a muscle has a sudden, involuntary contraction (Ch. 6)

specific immunity   the body's defense against selected agents (Ch. 6)

sphenoid bone   one of the bones of the cranium; wedge-shaped bone that goes across the skull anterior to the temporal bones (Ch. 7)

sphenoid sinuses   contained within the anterior base of the skull behind the orbit of the sphenoid bone (Ch. 7)

sphygmomanometer   instrument used to measure blood pressure (Ch. 13)

spinal canal   also known as vertebral canal, is the space in vertebrae through which the spinal cord passes (Ch. 6)

spindle   screw-like rod used to secure the matrix band in the vise (Ch. 34)

spleen   largest lymphoid organ, functions include the removal of bacteria and other foreign materials, filtering out of old red blood cells, production of red blood cells before birth, and acts as a storage for blood in case of hemorrhage (Ch. 6)

spore   dormant stage of bacteria (Ch. 10)

sporulating   a means of survival for bacteria where spores become enclosed in several protein coats that resist drying, heat, and most chemicals (Ch. 10)

spot-welded matrix bands   custom-made bands constructed with the use of a spot-welding unit and used in class II restorations; does not require a retainer (Ch. 28)

sprain   an injury which occurs to the ligaments caused by sudden overstretching (Ch. 6)

spray-wipe-spray-wipe technique   a universally accepted technique for cleaning and disinfecting surfaces (Ch. 11)

spreaders   endontic instrument used when sealing the root canal (Ch. 24)

springs   specially bent or shaped wires attached to the main arch wire; used to exert pressure on the teeth (Ch. 27)

squamous cell carcinoma   a cancer of the squamous epithelium usually found in adults 40 years or older; lesions appear under the tongue, on the sides or borders of the tongue, and on the soft palate tonsil area (Ch. 26)

stainless steel crowns   used in the restoration of badly decayed teeth; usually used as a space maintainer in primary tooth replacement, or as temporary crown to be replaced by cast gold or porcelain (Ch. 28)

stamp   used with an ink pad to indicate where the holes for the teeth should be punched on a dental dam (Ch. 34)

standard precautions   precautions developed in 1996 by the Centers for Disease Control (CDC) that augment universal precautions and body substance isolation practices (Ch. 11)

stannous fluoride   a stannous fluoride mouth rinse prescribed by a dentist can be used for decreasing the sensitivity of the tooth to hot and/or cold dental hypersensitivity (Ch. 4)

staphylococcus infections   diseases such as staph infection, gangrene, toxic shock syndrome, venereal diseases, and some forms of pneumonia caused by bacteria groups that grow in clusters (Ch. 10)

static zone   the activity zone where rear delivery systems are located along with dental instruments and equipment used at the dental chair (Ch. 17)

status epilepticus   the experience of continually having one seizure after another (Ch. 16)

statutes   laws enacted by states (Ch. 3)

Stenson's duct   a duct that empties saliva from the parotid gland into the mouth; also known as the parotid duct (Ch. 7)

sterilization   process by which all forms of life are completely destroyed in a controlled area (Ch. 11)

sterilizing area   area of the dental office where all sterilization procedures are performed (Ch. 17)

sternocleidomastoid   a muscle located on each side of the neck that assists in elevating the chin (Ch. 7)

sternum   the breastbone (Ch. 16)

stethoscope   instrument used to listen to body sounds; for example, heartbeat and breathing (Ch. 13)

stimulant   a drug that speeds up the body's activities (Ch. 15)

stippled   healthy gingival tissue's appearance that is similar to the texture of an orange (Ch. 8)

stomach   an organ, extending from the esophagus to the small intestine, that acts as a storage area and a churn to mix food with gastric juices (Ch. 6)

stomedeum   primitive mouth (Ch. 8)

storage phosphor imaging   a type of indirect digital imaging; a wireless system that uses specially coated plates instead of sensors to record the image (Ch. 23)

strain   change or deformation of an object brought about by the object's resistance to a stress (Chs. 6 and 33)

strep throat   a common bacterial disease caused by the streptococcus microorganism with symptoms including sore throat, fever, and general malaise (Ch. 10)

streptococcus mutans   a species of streptococcus that has been implicated in dental caries and endocarditis; requires prompt use of antibiotics (Ch. 10)

stress   reaction of an object to resist an external force (Ch. 33)

stress breakers   a metal device that may be built into the partial denture that relieves pressure on the abutment teeth (Ch. 32)

striated muscle   also known as skeletal muscles, its function is to provide for external body movement. These are the only muscles under conscious control (Ch. 6)

stroke   a disruption of the blood flow to the brain because of a ruptured or blocked blood vessel (Ch. 13)

study models   diagnostic casts (Chs. 16 and 35)

styloglossus   one of the extrinsic muscles of the tongue that retracts the tongue and raises the tip of the tongue (Ch. 7)

stylohyoid   lies in front of and above the posterior belly of the digastric muscle (Ch. 7)

styloid process   a sharp projection on the under-surface of the temporal bone between the glenoid fossa and the mastoid process (Ch. 7)

subcutaneous   beneath the skin (Ch. 15)

subgingival   below the gingival margin (Ch. 29)

subjective fears   fears based on feelings, attitudes and concerns that have developed from suggestions by others (Ch. 28)

sublingual   in the administration of drugs, this method places the medication under the tongue and lets it dissolve (Ch. 15)

sublingual caruncles   two small, raised folds of tissue located where the lingual frenum attaches to the floor of the mouth (Ch. 7)

sublingual folds   begins at the caruncles on either side of the frenum and run backward to the base of the tongue (Ch. 7)

sublingual glands   smallest of glands located on the floor of the mouth; empties saliva either directly into the mouth through the ducts of Rivinus or through the sublingual caruncles by means of the ducts of Bartholin (Ch. 7)

sublingual sulcus   a horseshoe-shaped groove that follows the curve of the dental arch located to the lateral of the sublingual fold (Ch. 7)

sublingually   placed under the tongue (Ch. 16)

submandibular glands   the size of a walnut and lie on the inside of the mandible in the posterior area (Ch. 7)

subperiosteal implant   implanted beneath the periosteum, placed on top of the bone (Ch. 25)

subpoena   court order mandating an individual to appear at a particular time and date with a specific reason to testify (Ch. 3)

subscriber   individual with dental insurance (Ch. 36)

subscription   part of the prescription, it is the area where the doctor writes the name and strength of the drug being prescribed, the dosage, and the form in which the drug is to be dispensed (Ch. 15)

substance abuse   use of a drug for other than medicinal purposes (Ch. 15)

subsupine position   the patient is in a reclined position with the head lower than the feet (Ch. 17)

succedaneous (teeth) permanent teeth that replace primary teeth (Ch. 9)

sulfur a mineral found in protein and involved in energy metabolism (Ch. 5)

supernumerary teeth extra teeth, usually dwarfed in size or shape (Ch. 26)

superscription part of the prescription directly below the heading used for filling in patient information; includes blank lines where the dentist can fill in the name and address of the patient, space for when the prescription was written, patient's phone number, age, gender, etc. (Ch. 15)

supine position the patient is in a reclined position with the nose and knees on the same plane (Ch. 17)

supplemental groove shallow linear grooves that radiate from the developmental groove (Ch. 9)

supragingival above the gingival margin (Ch. 29)

supraversion when a tooth extends above the normal line of occlusion (Ch. 27)

surgical aspirating tips tools used to aspirate blood and debris from the surgical site (Ch. 25)

surgical bone files instruments used to trim and smooth the edges of the alveolar bone following tooth extraction (Ch. 25)

surgical chisels instruments used to remove or shape the bone (Ch. 25)

surgical curettes instruments used for debridement of the tooth socket or diseased tissue (Ch. 25)

surgical mallet instrument used to remove bone; shaped like a small hammer and used with a chisel (Ch. 25)

surgical scalpels surgical knives used to incise or excise soft tissue in a precise manner with the least amount of trauma (Chs. 25 and 29)

surgical scissors instruments made of stainless steel and available in various sizes; used to cut sutures and trim soft tissues (Ch. 25)

surgical stint made of clear acrylic and placed over the tissues during surgery to guide the dentist in the placement of the implant; sometimes called a template (Ch. 25)

susceptible host an individual who lacks resistance to an agent and is vulnerable to disease (Ch. 11)

symphysis a concave area where two bones of the mandible are fused in the center of the mandible on the external surface (Ch. 7)

symmetric shape, size, and relative position of body parts on opposite sides are equal (Ch. 13)

synapse the conduit through which nerve fibers move impulses from one to another (Ch. 6)

syncope fainting (Ch. 16)

syneresis shrinkage from a loss of water content due to heat, dryness, or exposure to air (Ch. 35)

synovial pertaining to the lubricating fluid of the joints (Ch. 12)

synovial fluid a thick, sticky fluid found in the joints of bones providing nourishment and lubrication that enables bones to glide over each other without friction (Ch. 7)

syphilis sexually-transmitted disease (Ch. 26)

system a grouping of tissues and organs (Ch. 6)

systemic circulation carries the blood from the aorta to the smallest blood vessels and back to the heart (Ch. 6)

systemic fluoride one of the two ways that fluoride is used for dental health care needs. The sources for systemic fluoride include fluoridated water, foods with fluoride, fluoride tablets and drops (Ch. 4)

systolic blood pressure created when the heart contracts and forces blood through the arteries (Ch. 13)

tactile the feeling sensed by touch (Ch. 18)

tachycardia abnormally rapid heart rate (Ch. 13)

tachypnea abnormally rapid respiratory rate at rest (Ch. 13)

tarnish dull and discoloration of metal resulting from chemical or electrochemical attacks of the oral cavity (Ch. 33)

taste buds oval structures located on the dorsal surface of the tongue that provide our sense of taste (Ch. 7)

T-band matrix restorative band made of brass strips that are crossed at one end; secured on primary teeth; adjustable, do not require a retainer (Ch. 28)

teeth begins the digestive process by biting, tearing, and grinding food (Ch. 6)

tell, show, and do technique technique for easing a patient's fears by introducing the patient to the instrument to be used, deomonstrating the instrument's use, then performing the technique (Ch. 28)

template guide showing the adult or pediatric arches indicating where the holes for the teeth should be punched (Ch. 34)

temporal bone located below each parietal bone forming the lower sides and the base of the skull (Ch. 7)

temporal muscles one of the four pairs of muscles of mastication (Ch. 7)

temporomandibular joint (TMJ) structure made of muscles, bones, and the joints of the jaw; work together closely to make it possible to chew, speak, and swallow without discomfort (Ch. 7)

temporomandibular joint disease (TMJ) degeneration or disease of the joint where the mandible articulates with the temporal bone (Ch. 6)

tendon skeletal muscle attached through specialized connective tissue extending beyond the muscle in the form of a cord (Ch. 6)

tertiary dentin forms quickly to localized injury and repairs and reacts to irritations (Ch. 8)

tetanus a disease caused by spores of bacterium clostridium tetani with stiffness of the jaw being the most common symptom (Ch. 10)

tetracycline stain discoloration of the teeth resulting from high concentrations of tetracycline antibiotics taken while the tooth was developing; vary in color from light green or yellow to dark gray-brown (Ch. 29)

thermal conductivity the ability for a material to transmit heat (Ch. 33)

thermal expansion the ability for a material to expand and contract with temperature changes (Ch. 33)

thermal property heat-related characteristic of a material (Ch. 33)

thermionic emission the process of heating the current to an extremely high temperature to allow electrons to be given off (during radiation production) (Ch. 21)

thermoplastic properties of becoming softer when heated and harder when cooled (Ch. 35)

thiamen a B-complex vitamin that provides energy as well as helps to prevent cardiovascular (Ch. 5)

thoracic cavity also known as the chest cavity, contains the lungs, heart, and all accessory parts needed for their functioning (Ch. 6)

three-quarter crown a fixed prosthesis that covers a tooth so that the mesial, distal, and lingual surfaces are reduced but the facial surface is left intact (Ch. 30)

thrombocyte   fragments or pieces of cells that are necessary for the blood to clot (Ch. 6)

thrush   fungal infection of candidiasis in children, appearing as a thick, white covering over the oral mucous membrane (Ch. 26)

thymus   located under the sternum, it is large and active before birth and through puberty but gradually shrinks; important to the development of the immune system (Ch. 6)

tickler file   system that serves as a reminder that events are to occur on specific dates (Ch. 36)

tin oxide   very fine polishing agent used on enamel and metallic restorations (Ch. 29)

tinnitus   ringing or tinkling sound (Ch. 25)

tissue   specialized group of cells (Ch. 6)

tissue fluid   clear liquid formed in tissue spaces (Ch. 6)

tissue forceps   instruments used to hold and retract tissue during dental procedures (Chs. 25 and 29)

tissue retractors   either a forceps (hinged) or cotton-plier style; the working end of both types has small teeth to assist in grasping the tissue securely (Ch. 25)

tobacco stains   light brown to black discolorations of the teeth caused by coal tar combustion in cigarettes and pigments from chewing tobacco penetrating the pits and fissures on the enamel and dentin surfaces (Ch. 29)

Tofflemire matrix   most common matrix used for amalgam restorations; the retainer can be sterilized and reused but the bands are disposable (Ch. 34)

tolerance   when a person requires larger amounts of a drug in order to produce the same effect (Ch. 15)

Tome's process   a secretory surface of the ameloblast that is responsible for laying down and guiding the enamel matrix into place (Ch. 8)

tomography   the fundamental principle governing panoramic radiography that shows the imaging of one layer or section of the body while blurring images from the other areas (Ch. 23)

tongue   moves food from the anterior teeth to the posterior teeth and gathers the food before it is swallowed (Ch. 6)

tongue retractors   spoon shaped or with long blades; used to retract the tongue or cheeks from the operating site (Ch. 25)

tongue thrusting   habit whereby a person's (usually a child's) tongue pushes against the anterior teeth during swallowing, causing an anterior open bite (Ch. 28)

tonsil   forms a protective circle around the inside of the oral cavity that guards against bacteria entering the body through the digestive and respiratory systems (Ch. 6)

tonsillitis   a chronic infection of the tonsil tissue (Ch. 6)

tooth decay   destruction of the tooth surface (Ch. 6)

tooth mobility   movement of the tooth within the socket (Ch. 29)

tooth positioner   a flexible or soft-plastic appliance that surrounds the crowns of all teeth, in both arches, when positioned in the patient's mouth (Ch. 27)

topical   administration of drugs to the skin's surface, usually in ointment, lotion, gel, or cream form; in dentistry, topical drugs are sometimes used as anesthesia prior to surgery (Ch. 15)

topical anesthetic   anesthesia that numbs the area about to be injected with local anesthesia; the patient will not feel the pain of the needle (Ch. 20)

topical fluoride   one of the two ways that fluoride is used for dental health care needs. The direct application of fluoride only penetrates the outer layer of the tooth enamel. It is available as a gel, rinse, foam, and liquid (Ch. 4)

topographic technique   technique used to expose occlusal radiographs (Ch. 22)

tori   boney outgrowths of tissue in the oral cavity that are benign (Ch. 26)

torsoversion   when a tooth is rotted or turned (Ch. 27)

tort   a wrongful act that results in injury to one person by another (Ch. 3)

torus   excess bone that is occasionally in the middle of the palate (Ch. 7)

torus mandibularis   excess bone formations that are sometimes under the tongue on the alveolar bone (Ch. 7)

toxic reaction   symptoms that appear due to overdose or excessive administration of the anesthetic solution (Ch. 20)

trabeculae   sponge-like appearance of the cancellous bone as seen on dental x-rays (Ch. 6)

trachea   also known as the windpipe, consists of C-shaped cartilage that allows for expansion of the esophagus during the process of swallowing (Ch. 6)

tragus of the ear   projection on the anterior portion of the ear that helps position the arches when exposing x-rays using the bisecting technique (Ch. 23)

transcranial temporomandibular joint radiograph   radiograph taken with the patient holding a cassette against the side of the head (Ch. 23)

transfer zone   the area below the patient's nose where instruments and materials are passed and received (Chs. 17 and 18)

transient ischemic attacks   a temporary interruption in the supply of blood to the brain; symptoms include weakness, dizziness, and loss of balance (Ch. 16)

transillumination test   reflection of fiberoptic light through the crown of a tooth to indicate vertical fractures (Ch. 24)

transitional line angles   surround the tooth and mark the boundaries of the face of the tooth (Ch. 31)

translucency   allows light to pass through (Ch. 31)

transposition   when a tooth is in the wrong order in the arch (Ch. 27)

transverse plane   divides the body into upper and lower sections (Ch. 6)

transverse ridge   the union of two triangular ridges produces a single ridge of elevation across the occlusal surface of a posterior tooth (Ch. 9)

transversion   when a tooth is in the wrong order in the arch (Ch. 27)

trapezius   a large neck muscle that moves the head backward and laterally (Ch. 7)

traumatic intrusion   occurs when the teeth are forcibly driven into the alveolus (Chs. 16 and 28)

treatment rooms   areas of the dental office where the patient is examined (Ch. 17)

Trendelenburg position   position in which the patient's head is low and the legs slightly elevated (Ch. 16)

triangular ridge   ridge or elevation that descends from the cusp and widens as it runs downward to the middle area of the occlusal surface (Ch. 9)

tricuspid valve   from the superior and inferior vena cava, blood enters the right atrium of the heart and is pumped into the tricuspid valve into the right ventricle (Ch. 6)

trifurcated   when there are three roots coming from the main trunk of the tooth (Ch. 9)

trigeminal the largest cranial nerve and most important to dental auxiliaries because it innervates the maxilla and the mandible dividing the semi-lunar ganglion into three branches (Ch. 7)

triglycerides neutral fats from plant and animal food found in a normal diet (Ch. 5)

trismus limited opening of the mouth (Chs. 23 and 25)

triturates mechanically combines dental materials (Ch. 17)

Triturator specially designed machine used to triturate the alloy and mercury; also called amalgamators (Ch. 34)

Truth in Lending Act (TILA) a United States federal law that is designed to protect consumers in any credit transactions (Ch. 36)

tubehead where the x-ray tube and step-up and step-down transformers are located (Ch. 21)

tubercle of the lip the small projection in the middle of the upper lip that sometimes enlarges or thickens (Ch. 7)

tuberculosis highly contagious disease of the respiratory system which can be spread to others by airborne particles released while coughing, from saliva contact, and, if cross-contamination occurs, by dental treatment (Chs. 6 and 10)

tungsten halogen the traditional curing light that is durable, less expensive, cures quickly, and is fairly effective. Disadvantages include emitted heat, requires a filter, and lack of portability (Ch. 17)

twinning a condition where two separate teeth are made from one tooth bud (Ch. 26)

two stage technique implant is placed into the bone and gingival tissue is sutured into place to cover implant; 3-4 months of healing time with second surgery to check for implant stability (Ch. 25)

U-frame a plastic dental dam frame that is easy to apply, comfortable for the patient, radiolucent, and autoclavable (Ch. 34)

ulcer an open sore, usually inflamed and painful, that forms on tissue (Chs. 15 and 26)

ultrasonic instruments instruments used to remove hard deposits, stains, and debris through the high-power vibrations of scaling, curettage, and root planing procedures (Ch. 29)

ultrasonic scaler through a vibrating action, removes hard deposits (e.g., calculus) from the teeth (Ch. 17)

unconscious a person who cannot respond to any sensory stimulation (Ch. 20)

undercuts recessed areas that are wider on the bottom than on the top (Ch. 35)

underexposed x-rays when the x-ray film appears light and has a thin image (Ch. 22)

undernourished lacking proper nutrients (Ch. 5)

unilateral cleft lip when a cleft lip occurs only on one side of the lip (Ch. 8)

universal distress signal clutching the throat with the hands (Ch. 16)

universal forceps forceps that can be used on any of the four quadrants (Ch. 25)

Universal/National System for numbering system adopted in 1968 by the ADA to identify the teeth; permanent teeth are numbered 1 to 32 (maxillary right to left; mandibular left to right); primary teeth are labeled A to T (Ch. 14)

universal precautions guidelines established by the CDC to help protect health-care workers and patients from the transmission of infectious diseases (Ch. 11)

universal varnish a cavity varnish that does not have the organic solvent and may be used under all restorations (Ch. 33)

urticaria eruption of wheals (welts) on the skin; also known as hives (Ch. 16)

usual, reasonable, and customary fee amount charged (fee) typically levied by the doctor/dentist for specific procedures; usual is the fee typically charged, reasonable is the midrange of fees charged for the specific procedure, and customary is the average charge physicians levy for the same procedure (Ch. 36)

utility glove thicker gloves used during disinfection and cleanup procedures (Ch. 11)

uvula small, soft structure that hangs from the soft palate above the rest of the tongue (Ch. 7)

varix weakening and extension of blood vessels in the oral cavity beneath the tongue primarily seen in the elderly (Ch. 26)

varnish thin layer of material that is placed to seal the walls and floor of a cavity preparation (Ch. 33)

vasoconstrictors drugs added to anesthetic solutions that constrict blood vessels around the injection site, reducing the blood flow in the area (Ch. 20)

vectorborne transmission mode of transmission of infectious agents through animate means such as mosquitos, ticks, lice, and other animals (Ch. 11)

vehicle transmission mode of transmission of infectious agents through contamination of inanimate objects such as water, food, meat, drugs, and blood (Ch. 11)

vein carries blood that has drained from the capillaries back to the heart (Ch. 6)

vena cava the large vessel where blood enters the heart (Ch. 6)

veneers items used to cover badly stained teeth and to reshape the anatomy of teeth; thin layers of tooth-colored material that cover much of the facial surface (Ch. 30)

ventral cavity anterior portion of the body (Ch. 6)

ventricles lower chambers of the heart (Ch. 6)

vermilion border line around the lips (Chs. 7 and 13)

vermillion zone the reddish portion of the lips (Ch. 7)

vertical angulation adjustment of angulation from top to bottom; improper vertical angulation shows teeth elongated or foreshortened (Ch. 22)

vertical bone resorption receding of the alveolar bone vertically on individual teeth and the interproximal surface (Ch. 29)

vertical dimension space provided by the teeth in normal occlusion, or, with the teeth in occlusion, a measurement of the face at the midline (Ch. 32)

vertical mattress suture used when suturing a flap, goes in and out of the tissue on the same surface; identified by vertical stitch or "bite"; tied with one surgeon's knot on surface where suture procedure began (Ch. 25)

vesicles small, fluid-filled blisters (Ch. 26)

vestibule fornix the deepest point of the vestibule that forms a U-shaped pocket that is continuous throughout the anterior and posterior areas (Ch. 7)

villi hair-like projections, as in intestinal mucous membrane (Ch. 6)

viral hepatitis disease that encompasses hepatitis A, hepatitis B, hepatitis C, hepatitis D, and hepatitis E; viral hepatitis can cause inflammation of the liver (Ch. 10)

virus smallest microorganisms known to date that reproduce inside host cells and are difficult to grow in a culture (Ch. 10)

viscosity the ability of liquid to flow (Ch. 33)

vise tool that holds the ends of the matrix band in place in the diagonal slot (Ch. 34)

vital pulp term used to describe healthy pulp (Ch. 24)

vital signs the basic signs of life; for example, body temperature, pulse, blood pressure, and respiration rate (Ch. 13)

vital whitening in office bleaching of vital teeth involves the application of bleaching liquids and gels with heat and a curing light (Ch. 31)

vitality scanner an electronic pulp testing unit that measures whether a tooth is vital or non-vital (Ch. 24)

vitamins a class of nutrients that do not provide the body with energy but perform other necessary functions (Ch. 5)

Vitamin B$_6$ essential in the synthesis and metabolism of protein, carbohydrates, and fat; if taken in large quantity, it could be toxic (Ch. 5)

Vitamin B$_{12}$ a water-soluble vitamin found in animal products; functions include the synthesis of red blood cells and maintenance of myelin sheaths (Ch. 5)

vocal cord mucous membrane stretched horizontally across the larynx (Ch. 6)

vomer a single bone on the inside of the nasal cavity (Ch. 7)

walking bleach technique technique using thick paste of hydrogen peroxide, sodium perborate, or a combination of the two, placed in the coronal portion of the nonvital tooth; heat application helps achieve desired results (Ch. 31)

walking whitening techniques teeth whitening techniques that are temporarily sealed in place and allows the patient to leave the office and return for evaluation at a later date (Ch. 31)

water irrigation device used to clean away debris from orthodontic brackets and other prosthetic devices (Ch. 4)

water reservoir bottle on the dental unit that supplies water to the water syringe and the dental handpieces (Ch.17)

wedge small, triangular piece of wood or plastic (Ch. 34)

Wells, Horace (1815–1848) Connecticut dentist who was the first to use nitrous oxide as an anesthetic during dental surgery (Ch. 20)

wettability ability of a material to flow over a surface (Ch. 33)

Wharton's duct duct that empties saliva into the mouth (Ch. 7)

Wickham's striae interlacing white lines formed by a grouping of white papules; usually on the buccal mucosa (Ch. 26)

Wilhelm Conrad Roentgen (1845-1923) discovered x-rays in 1895 (Chs. 1 and 17)

winged clamps clamps with extra projections (wings) that are angled toward the gingiva for better retraction and holding of the dental dam (Ch. 34)

wingless clamps clamps with no projections (wings) and with the letter *W* in front of the numbers of the clamps (Ch. 34)

withdrawal symptoms that occur when a person addicted to a drug stops taking that drug; nervousness, stomach cramps, diarrhea, shaking, and depression may be symptoms (Ch. 15)

wooden dental stimulator elongated, soft-wood wedges placed into the interproximal area, angling them toward the biting surface and rotating them in a circular pattern. The action stimulates the soft tissues and removes plaque in the area (Ch. 4)

working end part of the instrument that performs the instrument's function (Ch. 19)

xerostomia dryness of the mouth caused by saliva reduction (Ch. 4)

x-ray tube part of the dental x-ray unit that houses the coolidge, vacuum tube, filters, collimator, and cone (Ch. 21)

x-rays invisible, odorless electromagnetic radiation (Ch. 21)

yellow bone marrow contains mainly fat cells and is found in the center shafts of long bones; replaces red bone marrow as the body ages (Ch. 6)

yellow stains discolorations of the teeth usually associated with poor oral hygiene and plaque; dull yellow to light brownish (Ch. 29)

Young frame metal U-shaped dental dam frame that is made of stainless steel, easy to apply, and comfortable for the patient (Ch. 34)

zinc a trace mineral that aids in tissue growth and maintenance of the immune system (Ch. 5)

zinc oxide eugenol type of temporary cementation of crowns, inlays, onlays, and bridges (Ch. 33)

zinc phosphate permanent cement for crowns, inlays, onlays, bridges, and orthodontic bands and brackets (Ch. 33)

zirconium silicate material used for stain removal and polishing on gold restoration, exposed dentin, and tooth-colored restoration, and enamel (Ch. 29)

zygomatic one of the four branches of the maxillary nerve branch (Ch. 7)

zygomatic bones bones that form the cheeks (Ch. 7)

zygomatic major a muscle that controls facial expression drawing the angle of the mouth superiorly and posteriorly (Ch. 7)

zygote state during which cells proliferate (Ch. 8)

REFERENCES

American Dental Assistants Association. (1999). *Introduction to Basic Concepts in Dental Radiography.* Chicago, IL: ADAA.

American Dental Association. (1994). *ADA Principles of Ethics and Code of Professional Conduct.* Chicago, IL: The Association.

American Dental Association. (1994). *Dental Teamwork,* vol. 7(1). Chicago, IL: The Association.

American Dental Association. (2000). *OSHA: Refresher Course.* Chicago, IL: The Association.

American Dental Association, Council on Dental Education (1992, revised 1993). *Annual Surveys of Allied Dental Education Programs.* Washington, D.C.: U.S. Department of Health and Human Services, U.S. Department of Labor.

American Dental Association, Department of Education Surveys. (1992–92). *Allied Dental Education.* Chicago, IL: The Association.

American Dental Association, Department of Education Surveys. (1993). *Number of Accredited Dental Hygiene Programs* Chicago, IL: The Association.

American Dental Association, Department of Education Surveys. (1993). *Number of CDA Accredited Dental Assisting Programs.* Chicago, IL: The Association.

American Dental Association, Department of Legal Affairs. (1992). OSHA: *What You MUST Know.* Chicago, IL: The Association.

American Heart Association. (1991). *The American Heart Association Diet: An Eating Plan for Healthy Americans.* Dallas, TX: The Association.

American Heart Association. (1998). *Recipes for Low-Fat Low-Cholesterol Meals.* Dallas, TX: The Association.

American Heart Association. (1999). *Heartsaver AED.*

Anderson, K.N., Anderson L.E., Ganze W.D. (2002). *Mosby's Medical Nursing, & Allied Health Dictionary,* 6th ed. St. Louis, MO: Mosby.

Anderson, Pauline C., Pendleton, Alice E. (2001). *The Dental Assistant,* 7th ed. Clifton Park, NY: Delmar Learning.

Appleton & Lange's Health Professionals Drug Guide (2000). Stamford, CN: Appleton & Lange.

Aschheim, K.W., Dale, B.G. (2001) *Esthetic Dentistry: A Clinical approach to Techniques and Materials.* 2nd ed. St. Louis, Missouri, Mosby, Inc.

Ash, M., Nelson, S. (2003). *Wheeler's Dental Anatomy, Physiology, and Occlusion,* 8th ed. Philadelphia, PA: W.B. Saunders.

Ash, M.M. (1984). *Wheeler's Atlas of Tooth Form,* 5th ed. Philadelphia, PA: W.B. Saunders.

Babbush, C.A., Fehrenback, M. (1991). *Illustrated Dental Embryology, Histology, and Anatomy.* Philadelphia, PA: W.B. Saunders.

Bath-Balogh, M., Fehrenbach, M.J. (2005). *Illustrated Dental Embryology, Histology, and Anatomy,* 2nd ed. Philadelphia, PA: W.B. Saunders.

Beirle, J.W. (1993). "Dental Operatory Water Lines." *Canadian Dental Association Journal,* 211(2), 13–15.

Bergman, R., Adel, K., Heidger, P. (1996). *Histology.* Philadelphia, PA: W.B. Saunders.

Berkovitz, B.K.B., Holland, G.R., Moxham, B.J. (2002). *Oral Anatomy, Histology, and Embryology,* 3rd ed. St. Louis, MO: Mosby.

Bloodborne Diseases in the Workplace, Trainers Manual (1992). Spokane, WA: Scenic Bay Publications.

Bork, K. (1996). *Diseases of the Oral Mucosa and the Lips.* Philadelphia, PA: W.B. Saunders.

Bowen, R.F., Marjenhoff, W.A. (1993). "Adhesion of Composites to Dentin and Enamel", *Canadian Dental Association Journal,* 21(6) 19–22.

Brand, R.W., Isselhard, D.E. (2003). *Anatomy of Orofacial Structures,* 7th ed. St. Louis: Mosby.

Bressman, J.K. (1993). "Risk Management for the '90s." *Journal of the American Dental Association,* 124-63–67.

Burt, B.A., Eklund, S.A. (2005). *Dentistry, Dental Practice, and the Community,* 6th ed. Philadelphia, PA: W.B. Saunders.

Burton, G., Engelkirk, P. (2006). *Microbiology for the Health Sciences,* 8th ed. Philadelphia, PA: J.B. Lippincott Co.

Carranza, F., Newman, M. *Carranza's Clinical Periodontology,* 10th ed. Philadelphia, PA: W.B. Saunders.

Chapman, S. (1998). *Medical & Dental Associates, P.C. Insurance Forms Preparation,* 3rd ed. Clifton Park, NY: Delmar Learning.

Chasteen, J.E. (1997). *Chasteen's Essentials of Clinical Dental Assisting,* 5th ed. St. Louis, MO: Mosby.

Chernega, J.B. (2002). *Emergency Guide for Dental Auxiliaries,* 3rd ed. Clifton Park, NY: Delmar Learning.

Christensen, G.J. (1992). "Complex Fixed and Implant Prosthodontics: Making Nearly Foolproof Impressions." *Journal of the American Dental Association,* 123, 69–70.

Christensen, G.J. (2002). *A Consumer's Guide to Dentistry,* 2nd ed. St. Louis, MO: Mosby.

Christensen, G.J. (1993). "Removable Prosthodontic Impressions." *Journal of the American Dental Association,* 124, 112–113.

Cohen, B.J., Wood, D.L. (2005). *Memmler's The Human Body in Health and Disease* 10th ed. Philadelphia, PA: Lippincott-Raven.

Commission on Dental Accreditation, Council on Dental Education of the American Dental Association. (1993). *New Faces for Allied Dental Education.* Chicago, IL: The Association.

Corcoran, J.F. (1992). *Endodontics I,* 3rd ed. Ann Arbor, MI: University of Michigan. Dental Publications.

Cottone, J.A., Terezhalmy, G.T., Molinari, J.A. (1996). *Practical Infection Control in Dentistry,* 2nd ed. Philadelphia, PA: Lea & Febiger.

Council on Dental Materials, Instruments, and Equipment. (1994). "Choosing Intracoronal Restorative Materials." *Journal of the American Dental Association,* 125, 102–103.

Craig, R.G., O'Brien W.J., Powers, J.M. (2003). *Dental Materials: Properties and Manipulation,* 8th ed. St. Louis, MO: Mosby.

Craig, R.G., Powers, J. (2002). *Restorative Dentistry Materials,* 11th ed. St. Louis, MO: Mosby.

Crispin, G.J. (1993). "Expanding the Application of Facial Ceramic Veneers." *Canadian Dental Association Journal,* 21(6), 43–54.

Dale, B.G., Ascheim, K.W. (2000). *Esthetic Dentistry: A Clinical Approach to Techniques and Materials.* 2nd ed. Philadelphia, PA: Lea & Febiger.

977

Darby, M., Walsh, M. (2003). *Dental Hygiene Theory and Practice,* 2nd ed. Philadelphia, PA: W.B. Saunders.

Dental Dam Procedures, 9th ed. (1992). Akron, OH: Hygienic Corp.

Department of Veterans Affairs, American Dental Association, Department of Health and Human Services, Washington, DC: Learning Resources Services.

Dietz, E. *Dental Office Management* (2000) Delmar Thomson Learning. Clifton Park, New York.

Dietz, E., Badavinac, R. (2002). *Safety Standards and Infection Control for Dental Hygienists,* Clifton Park, NY: Delmar Learning.

Dionne, R.A. (1992). "Preventing and Treating Postoperative Pain." *Journal of the American Dental Association,* 123, 27–34.

Dofka, C. (1996). *Competency Skills for the Dental Assistant.* Clifton Park, NY: Delmar Learning.

Dorland's Pocket Medical Dictionary, 27th ed. (2004). Philadelphia, PA: W.B. Saunders.

Drafke, M.W. (2002). *Working in Health Care: What You Need to Know to Succeed.* 2nd ed. Philadelphia, PA: F.A. Davis.

Dunlap, C., Barker, B.F. (1991). *Oral Lesions,* 3rd ed. Kansas City, MO: Colgate-Hoyt.

Egelbery, J., Badersten, A. (1994). *Periodontal Examination.* Sweden: Munksgaard.

Ehrlich, A., Schraeder, C. (2004). *Medical Terminology for Health Professions,* 5th ed. Clifton Park, NY: Delmar Learning.

Ehrlich, A. (1994). *Nutrition and Dental Health,* 2nd ed. Clifton Park, NY: Delmar Learning.

Eversole, L. (1996). *Oral Medicine: A Pocket Guide.* Philadelphia, PA: W.B. Saunders.

Fanning, M. (1997). *HIV Infection: A Clinical Approach,* 2nd ed. Philadelphia, PA: W.B. Saunders.

Fedi, P.F. Jr., Bernino, A.R. (2002). *The Periodontic Syllabus,* 4th ed. Baltimore, MD: Williams and Wilkins.

Fehrenbach, M., Herring, S. (2006). *Illustrated Anatomy of the Head and Neck* 3rd ed. Philadelphia, PA: W.B. Saunders.

Ferracane, J.L. (2001). *Materials in Dentistry.* 2nd ed. Philadelphia, PA: J.B. Lippincott Co.

Finkbeiner B.L., Finkbeiner, C.A. (2001). *Practice Management for the Dental Team,* 5th ed. St. Louis, MO: Mosby.

Finkbeiner B.L., Patt J.C. (2001). *Practice Management for the Dental Team,* 5th ed. St. Louis, MO: Mosby.

Fordney, M.T. (2005). *Insurance Handbook for the Medical Office.* 9th ed. Philadelphia, PA: W.B. Saunders.

Frommer H.H. (2001). *Radiology for Dental Auxiliaries,* 7th ed. St. Louis, MO: Mosby.

Genco, R.J., Goldman, H.M., Cohen, D.W. (1990). *Contemporary Periodontics.* St. Louis, MO: Mosby.

Gershoff, S. (1995). *The Tufts University Guide to Total Nutrition.* 2nd Edition New York, NY: Harper & Row.

Gladwin, M., Bagby, M. (2004) *Clinical Aspects of Dental Materials Theory, Practice and Cases.* Lippincott Williams & Wilkins Baltimore, Maryland.

Glenner, R.A. (1984). *The Dental Office Pictorial History.* Montana: Pictorial Histories Publishing Company.

Gluck, G., Morganstein, W. (2003). *Jong's Community Dental Health,* 5th ed. St. Louis, MO: Mosby.

Gooch, B.F., Cardo, D.M. (1995). "Percutaneous Exposures to HIV Infected Blood." *Journal of the American Dental Association,* 126, 1237–42

Graber, T.M., Vanarsdall R.L. (2005). *Othodontics: Current Principles and Techniques,* 4th ed. St. Louis, MO: Mosby.

Grembowski, D. (1992). "How Fluoridation Affects Adult Dental Caries." *Journal of the American Dental Association,* 1123, 49–54.

Guerini, V. (1909). *A History of Dentistry from the Most Ancient Times Until the End of the 18th Century.* Philadelphia, PA: Lea & Febiger.

Hamilton, E.M.N., Whitney, E.N., Sizer, F.S. (1991). *Nutrition: Concepts and Controversies.* St. Paul, MN: West Publishing.

Haring, J.I., Lind, L.J. (1993). *Radiographic Interpretation for the Dental Hygienist.* Philadelphia, PA: W.B. Saunders.

Haring, J.I., Howerton, L.J., (2006) *Dental Radiography Principles and Techniques.* 3rd ed. Philadelphia, PA: W.B. Saunders.

Harris, N., (2003). *Primary Preventive Dentistry,* 6th ed. Stamford, CN: Prentice Hall.

Hatrick, C., Eakle, W., Bird, W., (2003). *Dental Materials: Clinical Applications for Dental Assistants and Dental Hygienists,* Missouri: Saunders.

Haveles, E. (2002). *Delmar's Dental Drug Reference,* Clifton Park, NY: Delmar Learning.

Haveles, E.B. (1997). *Pharmacology for Dental Hygiene Practice.* Clifton Park, NY: Delmar Learning.

Hazard Communication Program. (1992). Michigan: Health Career Learning Systems, Inc.

Helgeson, B. (1974). "American Dental Assistants Commemorate 50th Anniversary." *Journal of the American Dental Association,* 89, 539–544.

Herman, W. (1996). "Angina: An Update for Dentistry," *Journal of the American Dental Association,* 127, 98–102.

History of the American Dental Assistants Association. (1970). Chicago, IL: American Dental Assistants Association.

Hoag, P.M., Pawlak, E.A. (1990). *Essentials of Clinical Periodontology,* 6th ed. St. Louis, MO: Mosby.

Hodges, K. (1998). *Concepts in Nonsurgical Periodontal Therapy.* Clifton Park, NY: Delmar Learning.

Houston, W.J.B., Stephens, C.D. (1992). *A Textbook of Orthodontics* 2nd ed., Santa Rosa, CA: Redwood Press.

Hughes, T. (1992). "Electronic Claims Filing Shows Dramatic Growth." *Dental Economics,* 82(2), 80–83.

Ibsen, O.A., Phelan, J. (2003). *Oral Pathology for the Dental Hygienist* 4th ed. Philadelphia, PA: W.B. Saunders.

Incorporating New Technologies in Periodontal Diagnosis into Training Programs and Patient Care. (1992). "A Critical Assessment and a Plan for the Future." *New England Journal of Medicine* 63, (4) 383–393.

Infection Control in Modern Dental Practice. (1992). Rochester, NY: Eastman Kodak Co.

Ingle, John I., Bakland, L.K. (2002) *Endodontics.* 5th ed. BC Decker Inc. Hamilton, Ontario.

Ingersoll, B.D. (1986). *Patient Management Skills for Dental Assistants and Hygienists.* Connecticut: Appleton-Century-Crofts.

Intraoral Radiography with Rinn SCP/BAI Instruments. (1993). Elgin, IL: Rinn Corp.

Jacob, J.A. "New Technology Can Remineralize Teeth." *American Dental Association News,* 23(18) 27.

Jaroski-Graf, J. (2000). *Dental Charting: A Standard Approach,* Clifton Park, NY: Delmar Learning.

Jocobsen, P., Carpenter, W., Cunny, E. (1992). "Bloodborne Exposure Incidents: Complying with OSHA Regulations." *Canadian Dental Association Journal,* 20, 8.

Johnson, O.N. (2006). *Essentials of Dental Radiography for Dental Assistants and Hygienists,* 8th ed. Stamford, CN: Appleton & Lange.

Johnson, O., Thomsen E. (2007). *Essentials of Dental Radiography for Dental Assistants and Hygienists,* 8th ed. Upper Saddle River, NJ: Prentice Hall.

Karst, N.S., Smith, S.K. (1998). *Dental Anatomy, A Self Instructional Program* 10th ed. Stamford, CN: Appleton & Lange.

Kasle, M.J. (1994). *An Atlas of Dental Radiographic Anatomy,* 4th ed. Philadelphia, PA: W.B. Saunders.

Kimbrough, Vickie J., Lautar, C.J. (2006) *Ethics, Jurisprudence, & Practice Management in Dental Hygiene.* 2nd ed. Pearson – Prentice Hall, Upper Saddle River, New Jersey.

Kodak Recommended Dental Films & Intensifying Screens. (1993). Rochester, NY: Eastman Kodak Co.

Kratochvil, F.J. (1988). *Partial Removable Prosthodontics.* Philadelphia, PA: W.B. Saunders.

Kumar, V., Cotran, R.S., Robbins, S.F. (2003). *Basic Pathology,* 7th ed. Philadelphia, PA: W.B. Saunders.

Landgland, O., Langlais, R., Preece, J. (2002). *Principles of Dental Imaging,* 2nd ed. Maryland: Lippincott Williams & Wilkins.

Langlais, R., Miller, C.S. (2003). *Color Atlas of Common Oral Diseases.* 3rd ed. Philadelphia, PA: Lea & Febiger.

Langlais, R., Kasle, M. (1992). *Exercises in Oral Radiographic Interpretation,* 3rd ed. Philadelphia, PA: W.B. Saunders.

Leimone, C.A., Earl, E.M. (1988). *Dental Assisting Basic and Dental Sciences.* St. Louis, MO: Mosby.

Lindh,W.Q., Pooler, M.S., Tamparo, C.D., & Cerrato, J.U. (2005). *Delmar's Comprehensive Medical Assisting.* 3rd ed. Clifton Park, NY: Delmar Learning.

Little, J., Falace, D., Miller, C., Rhodus, N. (2002). *Dental Management of the Medically Compromised Patient,* 6th ed. St. Louis, MO: Mosby.

Mahan, L.K., Escott-Stump, S. (2003). *Krause's Food, Nutrition, and Diet Therapy,* 11th ed. Philadelphia, PA: W.B. Saunders.

Malamed, S.F. (2004). *Handbook of Local Anesthesia,* 5th ed. St. Louis, MO: Mosby.

Malamed, S.F. (1993). "Managing Medical Emergencies." *Journal of the American Dental Association,* 124, 40–52.

Malamed, S.F. (2007). *Medical Emergencies in the Dental Office.* 6th ed. St. Louis, MO: Mosby.

Malamed, S.F. (1993). "Pain and Anxiety Control in Dentistry." *Canadian Dental Association Journal,* 21, 10, 35–41.

Malamed, S.F., Sheppard G.A. (2000). *Handbook of Medical Emergencies in the Dental Office,* 5th ed. St. Louis, MO: Mosby.

Manson-Hing, L.R. (1991). *Fundamentals of Dental Radiography.* Philadelphia, PA: Lea & Febiger.

Matteson, S.R., Whaley C., Secrist, V.C. (1988). *Dental Radiology,* 4th ed. Chapel Hill, NC: University of North Carolina Press.

McMinn, R., Hutching, R., Logan, B. (2003). *Color Atlas of Head and Neck Anatomy,* 3rd ed. St. Louis, MO: Mosby-Wolfe.

Meltzer, M., Palau, S.M. (1997). *Acquiring Critical Thinking Skills.* Philadelphia, PA: W.B. Saunders.

Melfi, R.C. (1994). *PERMAR'S Oral Embryology and Microscopic Anatomy.* Pennsylvania: Lea & Febiger.

Miles, D.A., Van Dis, M.L ., Jensen, C.W., Ferretti, A. (1999). *Radiographic Imaging for Dental Auxiliaries,* 3rd ed. Philadelphia, PA: W.B. Saunders.

Miller, B., Keanne, B. (2003). *Encyclopedia and Dictionary of Medicine, Nursing, and Allied Health.* 7th ed. Philadelphia, PA: W.B. Saunders.

Miller, C.H., Palenik, C. (2004). *Infection Control and Management of Hazardous Material for the Dental Team.* 3rd ed. St. Louis, MO: Mosby.

Miller, M., Castellanos, R. *Reality Volume 20 2006.* Reality Publishing, Houston, Texas.

Mosby's 2007 Dental Drug Consult. Mosby Elsevier. St. Louis, Missouri, Mosby, Inc.

Mosby's Medical, Nursing, and Allied Health Dictionary, 6th ed. (2002). St. Louis, MO: Mosby.

Moyers, R.E. (1988). *Handbook of Orthodontics* 4th ed. Chicago, IL: Year Book Medical Publishers, Inc.

Muma, R.D., Lyons, B.A., Borucki, M.J., Pollard, R.B. (1997). *HIV Manual for Health Care Professional,* 2nd ed. Stamford, CN: Appleton & Lange.

Nathe, C. (2004). *Dental Public Health* 2nd ed. Upper Saddle River, NJ: Prentice Hall.

Neville, B.W., Damm, D.D., White, D.K., Waldron, C.A. (1999). *Color Atlas of Clinical Oral Pathology* 2nd ed. Philadelphia, PA: Lea & Febiger.

Newman, M.G., Nisengard, R. (1994). *Oral Microbiology and Immunology.* 2nd ed. Philadelphia, PA: W.B. Saunders.

Nield-Gehrig, J.S., Houseman, G.A. (2004). *Fundamentals of Periodontal Instrumentation,* 5th ed. Baltimore, MD: Williams & Wilkins.

Nisengard, R., Newman, M. (1994). *Oral Microbiology and Immunology,* 2nd ed. Philadelphia, PA: W.D. Sanders.

Nizel, A.E., Papas, E.S. (1989). *Nutrition in Clinical Dentistry,* 3rd ed. Philadelphia, PA: W.B. Saunders.

Olson, S. (1995). *Dental Radiography Laboratory Manual.* Philadelphia, PA: W.B. Saunders.

Periodontal Disease. (1990). *New England Journal of Medicine, 332(6),* 373.

Phillips, R.W., Moore, B.D. (1994). *Elements of Dental Materials for Dental Hygienists and Dental Assistants,* 5th ed. Philadelphia, PA: W.B. Saunders.

Pindborg, J.J. (1993). *Atlas of Diseases of the Oral Mucosa,* 5th ed. Philadelphia, PA: W.B. Saunders.

Poyton, H.G., Pharoah, M.J. (1989). *Oral Radiology.* Toronto, B.C.: Decker Inc.

Proffit, W.R. (2006). *Contemporary Orthodontics,* 4th ed. St. Louis, MO: Mosby.

Purtilo, R. (2005) *Ethical Dimensions in the Health Professions.* 4th ed. Elsevier Saunders, Philadelphia, Pennsylvania.

Reality Information Source for Esthetic Dentistry. (1996). Houston, TX: Reality Publishing Co.

Regezi, J., Sciubba, J.J. (2003). *Oral Pathology: Clinical-Pathologic Correlation's,* 4th ed. Philadelphia, PA: W.B. Saunders.

Reis, D., (1992). "Dental Professionals and the Disabled: A New Partnership. *Dental Products Report,* 26(9), 14–122.

Requa-Clark, B.S." (2000). *Applied Pharmacology for the Dental Hygienist.* 4th ed. St. Louis, MO: Mosby.

Ring, M.E. (1986). *Dentistry: An Illustrated History.* St. Louis, MO: Mosby-Year Book.

Rizzo, D. (2001). *Delmar's Fundamentals of Anatomy & Physiology,* Clifton Park, NY: Delmar Learning.

Robinson, D., Bird, D. (2001). *Torres and Ehrlich Essentials of Dental Assisting,* 3rd. ed. Philadelphia, PA: W. B. Saunders.

Robinson, H.B.G., Miller, A.S. (1990). *Color Atlas of Oral Pathology.* Philadelphia, PA: Lippincott.

Rosenstiel, S.T., Land, M.F., Fujimoto, J. (2006). *Contemporary Fixed Prosthodontics,* 4th ed. St. Louis, MO: Mosby.

Sarnat, B.G., Laskin, D.M. (1992). *The Tempororomandibular Joint: A Biological Basis for Clinical Practice,* 4th ed. Philadelphia, PA: W.B. Saunders.

Schluger, S., Yuodel, R., Page, R., Johnson, R.H. (1990). *Periodontal Diseases,* 2nd ed. Philadelphia, PA: Lea & Febiger.

Schoen, D., Dean, M. (1996). *Contemporary Periodontal Instrumentation.* Philadelphia, PA: W.B. Sanders.

Schuster, G.M., Wetterhus, G.J., Dryden, P. (1999). *Handbook of Clinical Dental Assisting.* Philadelphia, PA: W.B. Saunders.

Schwartz, M., Lamster, I., Fine, J. (1995). *Clinical Guide to Periodontics.* Philadelphia, PA: W.B. Saunders.

Short, M.J. (2000). *Head and Neck Dental Anatomy,* 3rd ed. Clifton Park, NY: Delmar Learning.

Snyder, H. (1994). "The Rise in Latex Allergy: Implications for the Dentist." *Journal of the American Dental Association* 125 1089–1097. J.A.D.A.

Soloman, E.P. (2003). *Introduction to Human Anatomy and Physiology.* 2nd ed. Philadelphia, PA: W.B. Saunders.

Stedman's Concise Medical Dictionary for the Health Professions, 4th ed. (2003) Baltimore, MD: Williams and Wilkins.

Roberson, T.M., Heymann, H., Swift, E. (2006). *Sturdevant's Art and Science of Operative Dentistry.* 5th ed. St. Louis, MO: Mosby.

Successful Intraoral Radiography. (1993). Rochester, NY: Eastman Kodak Co.

Taber's Cyclopedic Medical Dictionary. (2005). 20th Edition. Philadelphia, PA: F.A. Davis Company.

Tamparo, Carol D., Lewis, Marsha A. (2005). *Diseases of the Human Body* 4th ed. Philadelphia, PA: F.A. Davis.

TenCate, A.R. (2003). *Oral Histology: Development, Structure, and Function,* 6th ed. St. Louis, MO: C.V. Mosby Co.

Thibodeau, G.A., Patton, K.T. (2006). *Anatomy and Physiology,* 6th ed. St. Louis, MO: Mosby.

Thibodeau, G.A., Patton, K.T. (2005). *The Human Body in Health and Disease.* 4th ed. St. Louis, MO: Mosby.

Topazin, R.G. , Goldberg, M.H., Hupp, J. (2002). *Oral and Maxillofacial Infections,* 4th ed. Philadelphia, PA: W.B. Saunders.

U.S. Department of Health and Human Services, Centers for Disease Control and Prevention (1993). *Recommended Infection Control Practices for Dentistry.*

Walton, R.E., Torabinejad, M. (2002). *Principles and Practice of Endodontics.* 3rd ed. Philadelphia, PA: W.B. Saunders.

Watson, C.M. Whitehouse, R.L.S. (1993). "Possibility of Cross-Contamination between Dental Patients by Means of the Saliva Ejector." *Journal of the American Dental Association* 124-7-80.

Weisman, G. (1995). "Scope of Applications for Lasers in Dentistry Expanding." *Dental Products Report* 7, 26–29.

White, S.N. (1993). "Adhesive Restorative Dentistry: Introduction. Many New Adhesive Materials Can Offer Improved Clinical Results." *Canadian Dental Association Journal* 21(6), 17–18.

Williams, S.R. (2001). *Basic Nutrition and Diet Therapy,* 11th ed. St. Louis, MO: Mosby.

Woelfel, J.B. (2002). *Dental Anatomy: Its Relevance to Dentistry,* 6th ed. Connecticut: Lea & Faber.

Wood, J.T. (1996). *Everyday Encounters: An Introduction to Interpersonal Communication.* Belmont, CA: Wadsworth.

Woodall, I.R. (1993). *Comprehensive Dental Hygiene Care,* 4th ed. St. Louis, MO: C.V. Mosby, Co.

Your Teeth Can Be Saved by Endodontic Treatment. (1992). Chicago, IL: American Dental Association, Division of Communications.

Yu, X.Y., Joynt, R.B. (1993). "Adhesion to Dentin." *Canadian Dental Association Journal* 21(6), 23–28.

Zernik, J.H., Minken, C. (1992). "Genetic Control of Bone Remodeling." *Canadian Dental Association Journal* 20(12), 14–19.

Zwemer, T.J. (1998). *Mosby's Dental Dictionary,* St. Louis, MO: Mosby.

INDEX

Page numbers followed by "f" indicate figures; page numbers followed by "t" indicate tables; page numbers followed by "b" indicate boxes; page numbers followed by "n" indicate notes.

AACD. *See* American Academy of Cosmetic Dentistry
Abandonment, 30
ABCs of CPR, 301–303
Abdominal cavity, 87
Abrasion, x-ray artifact, 493, 493f
Abrasive polishing techniques, 684
Abrasives, 382–384, 382f, 383f
  air abrasion handpiece, 386, 387f
  sterilization and storage of, 383–384
Abscess
  gingival, 505–506, 506f
  periapical, 506
  periodontal, 648t
  tooth, 269
    charting symbol for, 271f
    definition of, 569
    emergency management, 316
    as x-ray artifact, 493
Absorption process, 100
Abutment, 269
Accelerates, 852
Accessory organ, 101
Acetic acid, 462
Acidosis, diabetic, 314
Acidulated phosphate fluoride (APF), 64, 66
Acquired immunity, 196–197. *See also* Acquired immunodeficiency syndrome;
      Immune system
  vaccinations, 187, 193, 194–195, 195t, 196–197, 207, 235f
Acquired immunodeficiency syndrome (AIDS), 194, 194b, 195–196. *See also*
      Human immunodeficiency virus
  asymptomatic, 207
  necrotizing ulcerative periodontitis with, 650
  transmission risk, 241
Acrylics. *See also* Restorations
  custom temporary restorations, 881, 883–884, 883f, 884f, 885–887, 885f,
    886f, 887f
  tray resin, 871, 871f
Acrylic bur, 381
Actinomycosis, 569
Activator, 599
Active acquired immunity, 197
Activity zones, 335, 337, 337f
Acute necrotizing ulcerative gingivitis (ANUG), 583, 583f, 649–650
ADA. *See* American Dental Association
ADAA. *See* American Dental Assistants Association
Adam's apple, 103
Addiction, drug, 282. *See also* Drugs
  Controlled Substances Act, 285–286, 286f, 286t
Adenoids, 105, 105f, 106f
ADHA. *See* American Dental Hygienists' Association
ADHD. *See* Attention deficit hyperactivity disorder
Adhesives, 786
Adjacent, 155
ADLTA. *See* American Dental Laboratory Technicians Association
Adrenal gland, 97f, 97t
AED unit. *See* Automated external defibrillation unit
Aerosol, 206
African Americans
  in dentistry history, 4t, 8b, 8f
  in U.S. population, 23f
Age characteristics, 621, 622t. *See also* Eruption
  developmental disturbances influencing, 576–578, 577f, 578f
  five through eight, 44, 622t
  gestational stage v. fetal size, 137f
  infants and preschool, 44, 44f, 622t
  nine through twelve, 44–45, 622t
  nineteen through sixty, 45
  sixteen through nineteen, 45
  sixty plus, 45–46
  susceptibility to infection v., 205
  thirteen through fifteen, 45
Agenesis, 167
Agent, 29, 204
AIDS. *See* Acquired immunodeficiency syndrome
Air compressor, 335
Airborne transmission, 204f, 205, 205t
Air-water syringe, 225, 226
  parts of, 360, 360f
  transfer of, 354, 355f
  usage guidelines, 360–361, 361f
Ala of the nose, 110
ALARA. *See* As low as reasonably achievable

Alaska Native Americans, 23f
Alcohol, 135, 216, 217f, 290
  isopropyl, 216, 228
  substance abuse, 288–289
Alginate impressions, 842–851, 843f, 844f, 845f, 850f, 860f, 861f
  application procedure, 848–849, 848f
  mixing procedures, 846–847, 846f, 847f
  packaging and equipment, 852, 852f
  plaster pouring procedure, 850–851, 850f, 851f
  removal procedure, 850, 850f
Alimentary canal, 101
Alkalosis, 312
Allergen, 197, 311
Allergic reaction, 312
Allergies, 106. *See also* Antigen
  antihistamines, 293t, 311, 311f
  emergency management, 309t, 311, 311f, 312
    anaphylactic shock/life-threatening, 197, 309t, 312
  gingival disease from, 647t
Alloy, 800
Aluminum temporary crown, 881, 881f
  preformed, 880
  sizing, adapting and seating procedure, 878–880, 878f, 879f, 880f
Alveoli, 103
  alveolitis, 316, 553
    treatment procedure, 554, 554f
      emergency, 316
  alveolodental ligament, 149, 148f
  alveologingival fiber groups, 149, 149f
  bone, 148, 148f
  crest, 490, 491f
    fiber groups, 149
  fetal development of, 139t
  mucosa, 150
  process, 147f
  sacs, 103
Alveolus, 148
Amalgam, 800–808, 801t, 802f, 803f, 804f, 805f, 806f, 807f, 808f
  bonding, 805, 805f
  carrier, 374, 375f
  composition of, 801, 801t
  condenser, 374, 375f
  disposable capsule, 802–803, 803f
  gun, 374
  mercury in, 801–802
  pediatric dentistry, 625
  properties of, 803
  restoration, 270t
    class II, 806–808, 806f, 807f, 808f
    symbol for, 273f
  shavings, as x-ray artifact, 493, 493f
  tattoo, 572, 572f
  trituration and amalgamation, 803, 805
    amalgamator usage, 803–805, 804f, 805f
    Kerr amalgamator, 805f
Amalgamation, 803
Amalgamator, 334, 334f, 803–805, 804f, 805f
Ambien, 286t
Ameloblasts, 144
Amelogenesis imperfecta, 576
Amenorrhea, 78
American Academy of Cosmetic Dentistry (AACD), 718–719
American Academy of Dental Radiology, 472
American Academy of Pediatric Dentistry, 622
American Academy of Periodontology, 646
American Board of Orthodontics, 4t
American Dental Assistants Association (ADAA), 4t, 11, 11f. *See also* Dental
      assistants
  code of professional conduct, 38, 38b
  liability insurance policy from, 28
  Southard as founder/president of, 11, 12f
American Dental Association (ADA)
  Council on Dental Therapeutics, 64, 283
  Health Insurance Portability and Accountability Act, 33–38, 34t, 35f, 36b, 36f
    privacy kit, 35, 36f
  history of, 3t, 8–9, 9f
  infection control recommendations, 201–203, 201b, 202b, 203b
  Journal of the American Dental Association (JADA), 9, 201
  mouth rinses, 48
  oral hygiene videos from, 44
  radiography recommendations, 426
  Seal of Acceptance for dentifrice, 46

IMPORTANT! READ CAREFULLY: This End User License Agreement ("Agreement") sets forth the conditions by which Delmar Cengage Learning will make electronic access to the Delmar Cengage Learning-owned licensed content and associated media, software, documentation, printed materials, and electronic documentation contained in this package and/or made available to you via this product (the "Licensed Content"), available to you (the "End User"). BY CLICKING THE "I ACCEPT" BUTTON AND/OR OPENING THIS PACKAGE, YOU ACKNOWLEDGE THAT YOU HAVE READ ALL OF THE TERMS AND CONDITIONS, AND THAT YOU AGREE TO BE BOUND BY ITS TERMS, CONDITIONS, AND ALL APPLICABLE LAWS AND REGULATIONS GOVERNING THE USE OF THE LICENSED CONTENT.

1.0 SCOPE OF LICENSE

1.1 <u>Licensed Content</u>. The Licensed Content may contain portions of modifiable content ("Modifiable Content") and content which may not be modified or otherwise altered by the End User ("Non-Modifiable Content"). For purposes of this Agreement, Modifiable Content and Non-Modifiable Content may be collectively referred to herein as the "Licensed Content." All Licensed Content shall be considered Non-Modifiable Content, unless such Licensed Content is presented to the End User in a modifiable format and it is clearly indicated that modification of the Licensed Content is permitted.

1.2 Subject to the End User's compliance with the terms and conditions of this Agreement, Delmar Cengage Learning hereby grants the End User, a nontransferable, nonexclusive, limited right to access and view a single copy of the Licensed Content on a single personal computer system for noncommercial, internal, personal use only. The End User shall not (i) reproduce, copy, modify (except in the case of Modifiable Content), distribute, display, transfer, sublicense, prepare derivative work(s) based on, sell, exchange, barter or transfer, rent, lease, loan, resell, or in any other manner exploit the Licensed Content; (ii) remove, obscure, or alter any notice of Delmar Cengage Learning's intellectual property rights present on or in the Licensed Content, including, but not limited to, copyright, trademark, and/or patent notices; or (iii) disassemble, decompile, translate, reverse engineer, or otherwise reduce the Licensed Content.

2.0 TERMINATION

2.1 Delmar Cengage Learning may at any time (without prejudice to its other rights or remedies) immediately terminate this Agreement and/or suspend access to some or all of the Licensed Content, in the event that the End User does not comply with any of the terms and conditions of this Agreement. In the event of such termination by Delmar Cengage Learning, the End User shall immediately return any and all copies of the Licensed Content to Delmar Cengage Learning.

3.0 PROPRIETARY RIGHTS

3.1 The End User acknowledges that Delmar Cengage Learning owns all rights, title and interest, including, but not limited to all copyright rights therein, in and to the Licensed Content, and that the End User shall not take any action inconsistent with such ownership. The Licensed Content is protected by U.S., Canadian and other applicable copyright laws and by international treaties, including the Berne Convention and the Universal Copyright Convention. Nothing contained in this Agreement shall be construed as granting the End User any ownership rights in or to the Licensed Content.

3.2 Delmar Cengage Learning reserves the right at any time to withdraw from the Licensed Content any item or part of an item for which it no longer retains the right to publish, or which it has reasonable grounds to believe infringes copyright or is defamatory, unlawful, or otherwise objectionable.

4.0 PROTECTION AND SECURITY

4.1 The End User shall use its best efforts and take all reasonable steps to safeguard its copy of the Licensed Content to ensure that no unauthorized reproduction, publication, disclosure, modification, or distribution of the Licensed Content, in whole or in part, is made. To the extent that the End User becomes aware of any such unauthorized use of the Licensed Content, the End User shall immediately notify Delmar Cengage Learning. Notification of such violations may be made by sending an e-mail to delmar.help@cengage.com.

5.0 MISUSE OF THE LICENSED PRODUCT

5.1 In the event that the End User uses the Licensed Content in violation of this Agreement, Delmar Cengage Learning shall have the option of electing liquidated damages, which shall include all profits generated by the End User's use of the Licensed Content plus interest computed at the maximum rate permitted by law and all legal fees and other expenses incurred by Delmar Cengage Learning in enforcing its rights, plus penalties.

6.0 FEDERAL GOVERNMENT CLIENTS

6.1 Except as expressly authorized by Delmar Cengage Learning, Federal Government clients obtain only the rights specified in this Agreement and no other rights. The Government acknowledges that (i) all software and related documentation incorporated in the Licensed Content is existing commercial computer software within the meaning of FAR 27.405(b)(2); and (2) all other data delivered in whatever form, is limited rights data within the meaning of FAR 27.401. The restrictions in this section are acceptable as consistent with the Government's need for software and other data under this Agreement.

7.0 DISCLAIMER OF WARRANTIES AND LIABILITIES

7.1 Although Delmar Cengage Learning believes the Licensed Content to be reliable, Delmar Cengage Learning does not guarantee or warrant (i) any information or materials contained in or produced by the Licensed Content, (ii) the accuracy, completeness or reliability of the Licensed Content, or (iii) that the Licensed Content is free from errors or other material defects. THE LICENSED PRODUCT IS PROVIDED "AS IS," WITHOUT ANY WARRANTY OF ANY KIND AND DELMAR CENGAGE LEARNING DISCLAIMS ANY AND ALL WARRANTIES, EXPRESSED OR IMPLIED, INCLUDING, WITHOUT LIMITATION, WARRANTIES OF MERCHANTABILITY OR FITNESS FOR A PARTICULAR PURPOSE. IN NO EVENT SHALL DELMAR CENGAGE LEARNING BE LIABLE FOR: INDIRECT, SPECIAL, PUNITIVE OR CONSEQUENTIAL DAMAGES INCLUDING FOR LOST PROFITS, LOST DATA, OR OTHERWISE. IN NO EVENT SHALL DELMAR CENGAGE LEARNING'S AGGREGATE LIABILITY HEREUNDER, WHETHER ARISING IN CONTRACT, TORT, STRICT LIABILITY OR OTHERWISE, EXCEED THE AMOUNT OF FEES PAID BY THE END USER HEREUNDER FOR THE LICENSE OF THE LICENSED CONTENT.

8.0 GENERAL

8.1 Entire Agreement. This Agreement shall constitute the entire Agreement between the Parties and supersedes all prior Agreements and understandings oral or written relating to the subject matter hereof.

8.2 Enhancements/Modifications of Licensed Content. From time to time, and in Delmar Cengage Learning's sole discretion, Delmar Cengage Learning may advise the End User of updates, upgrades, enhancements and/or improvements to the Licensed Content, and may permit the End User to access and use, subject to the terms and conditions of this Agreement, such modifications, upon payment of prices as may be established by Delmar Cengage Learning.

8.3 No Export. The End User shall use the Licensed Content solely in the United States and shall not transfer or export, directly or indirectly, the Licensed Content outside the United States.

8.4 Severability. If any provision of this Agreement is invalid, illegal, or unenforceable under any applicable statute or rule of law, the provision shall be deemed omitted to the extent that it is invalid, illegal, or unenforceable. In such a case, the remainder of the Agreement shall be construed in a manner as to give greatest effect to the original intention of the parties hereto.

8.5 Waiver. The waiver of any right or failure of either party to exercise in any respect any right provided in this Agreement in any instance shall not be deemed to be a waiver of such right in the future or a waiver of any other right under this Agreement.

8.6 Choice of Law/Venue. This Agreement shall be interpreted, construed, and governed by and in accordance with the laws of the State of New York, applicable to contracts executed and to be wholly preformed therein, without regard to its principles governing conflicts of law. Each party agrees that any proceeding arising out of or relating to this Agreement or the breach or threatened breach of this Agreement may be commenced and prosecuted in a court in the State and County of New York. Each party consents and submits to the nonexclusive personal jurisdiction of any court in the State and County of New York in respect of any such proceeding.

8.7 Acknowledgment. By opening this package and/or by accessing the Licensed Content on this Web site, THE END USER ACKNOWLEDGES THAT IT HAS READ THIS AGREEMENT, UNDERSTANDS IT, AND AGREES TO BE BOUND BY ITS TERMS AND CONDITIONS. IF YOU DO NOT ACCEPT THESE TERMS AND CONDITIONS, YOU MUST NOT ACCESS THE LICENSED CONTENT AND RETURN THE LICENSED PRODUCT TO DELMAR LEARNING (WITHIN 30 CALENDAR DAYS OF THE END USER'S PURCHASE) WITH PROOF OF PAYMENT ACCEPTABLE TO DELMAR CENGAGE LEARNING, FOR A CREDIT OR A REFUND. Should the End User have any questions/comments regarding this Agreement, please contact Delmar Cengage Learning at delmar.help@cengage.com.

STUDYWARE™ TO ACCOMPANY *DELMAR'S DENTAL ASSISTING: A COMPREHSENSIVE APPROACH*

Minimum System Requirements
- Operating System: Microsoft Windows 2000, Windows XP, Vista
- Processor: Pentium PC 500 MHz or higher (750 Mhz recommended)
- Memory: 64 MB of RAM (128 MB recommended)
- Screen Resolution: 800 x 600 pixels
- Color Depth: 16-bit color (thousands of colors)
- Macromedia Flash Player 9. The Macromedia Flash Player is free, and can be downloaded from http://www.adobe.com/products/flashplayer/

Installation Instructions
1. Insert disc into CD-ROM drive. The StudyWARE™ installation program should start automatically. If it does not, go to step 2.
2. From My Computer, double-click the icon for the CD drive.
3. Double click the *setup.exe* file to start the program.

Technical Support
Telephone: 1-800-648-7450, 8:30 A.M.-5:30 P.M. Eastern Time
Fax: 1-518-881-1247
E-mail: delmar.help@cengage.com

StudyWARE™ is a trademark used herein under license.
Microsoft® and Windows® are registered trademarks of the Microsoft Corporation.
Pentium® is a registered trademark of the Intel® Corporation.